OTOLARYNGOLOGY
HEAD & NECK SURGERY

OTOLARYNGOLOGY—HEAD & NECK SURGERY

VOLUME THREE

OTOLARYNGOLOGY
HEAD & NECK SURGERY

FOURTH EDITION

Charles W. Cummings, M.D.
Distingushed Service Professor
Department of Otolaryngology—Head and Neck Surgery
Johns Hopkins University School of Medicine
Baltimore, Maryland

Paul W. Flint, M.D.
Professor
Department of Otolaryngology—Head and Neck Surgery
Director, Center for Airway, Laryngeal, and Voice Disorders
Co-Director Minimally Invasive Surgical Training Center
Johns Hopkins University School of Medicine
Baltimore, Maryland

Bruce H. Haughey, MBChB, FACS, FRACS
Professor and Director
Head and Neck Surgical Oncology
Department of Otolaryngology—Head and Neck Surgery
Washington University School of Medicine
St. Louis, Missouri

K. Thomas Robbins, M.D.
Professor and Chair
Division of Otolaryngology, Department of Surgery
Southern Illinois University School of Medicine
Springfield, Illinois

J. Regan Thomas, M.D.
Francis L.Lederer Professor and Chairman
Department of Otolaryngology—Head and Neck Surgery
University of Illinois
Chicago, Illinois

Lee A. Harker, M.D.
Deputy Director
Boys Town National Research Hospital
Vice Chairman
Department of Otolaryngology and Human
Communication
Creighton University School of Medicine
Omaha, Nebraska

Mark A. Richardson, M.D.
Professor and Chairman
Department of Otolaryngology—Head and Neck Surgery
Oregon Health and Science University
Portland, Oregon

David E. Schuller, M.D.
Professor and Chairman
Department of Otolaryngology—Head
and Neck Surgery
Director, Arthur G. James Cancer Hospital
and Richard J. Solove Research Institute
Deputy Director, Comprehensive Cancer Center
The Ohio State University
Columbus, Ohio

Illustrator:
Tim Phelps, M.S., F.A.M.I.
Medical Illustrator and Associate Professor
Johns Hopkins University School of Medicine
Baltimore, Maryland

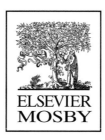

ELSEVIER
MOSBY

ELSEVIER
MOSBY

The Curtis Center
170 S Independence Mall W 300E
Philadelphia, Pennsylvania 19106

Cummings Otolaryngology—Head & Neck Surgery
Copyright © 2005, Mosby, Inc. All rights reserved.

NOTICE

Otolaryngology is an ever-changing field. Standard safety precautions must be followed, but as new research and clinical experience broaden our knowledge, changes in treatment and drug therapy may become necessary or appropriate. Readers are advised to check the most current product information provided by the manufacturer of each drug to be administered to verify the recommended dose, the method and duration of administration, and contraindications. It is the responsibility of the licensed prescriber, relying on experience and knowledge of the patient, to determine dosages and the best treatment for each individual patient. Neither the publisher nor the author assumes any liability for any injury and/or damage to persons or property arising from this publication.

Previous editions copyrighted 1998, 1993, 1986.

Library of Congress Cataloging-in-Publication Data
Cummings otolaryngology—head & neck surgery / [edited by] Charles W. Cummings . . . [et al.].—4th ed.
   p. ; cm
  Rev. ed. of: Otolaryngology—head & neck surgery. 3rd ed. c1998.
  Includes bibliographical references and index.
  ISBN 0-323-01985-4
    1. Otolaryngology, Operative. I. Title: Cummings otolaryngology—head and neck surgery.
  II. Title: Otolaryngology—head & neck surgery. III. Cummings, Charles W. (Charles William).
  [DNLM: 1. Otorhinolaryngologic Surgical Procedures. WV 168 C971 2005]
  RF51.O86 2005
  617.5′1059—dc22   2004055160

Acquisitions Editor: Rebecca Schmidt Gaertner
Developmental Editor: Mary Beth Murphy
Editorial Assistant: Suzanne Flint

Printed in the United States of America

Last digit is the print number: 9 8 7 6 5 4 3 2

Contributors

George L. Adams, M.D.
Professor and Head
Department of Otolaryngology—Head and Neck Surgery
University of Minnesota
Chair
Head and Neck Surgery
Lions 5M International Hearing Center
Minneapolis, Minnesota

Peter A. Adamson, M.D., F.R.C.S.C., F.A.C.S.
Professor
Department of Otolaryngology
University of Toronto
Adamson Associates Cosmetic Facial Surgery Clinic
Toronto, Ontario, Canada

Antoine Adenis, M.D., Ph.D.
Professor and Chairman
Department of Digestive Tract Cancer
Lille, France

Seth Akst, M.D.
Chief Resident
Department of Anesthesiology and Critical Care
The Johns Hopkins University
Baltimore, Maryland

David M. Albert, F.R.C.S.
Consultant
Paediatric Otolaryngology—Head and Neck Surgery
Great Ormond Street Hospital for Children
    NHS Trust
London, United Kingdom

William B. Armstrong, M.D.
Associate Professor
Department of Otolaryngology—Head and Neck Surgery
University of California, Irvine
Orange, California

Moisés A. Arriaga, M.D., F.A.C.S.
Director
Hearing and Balance Center
Allegheny General Hospital
Pittsburgh, Pennsylvania

Agustin J. Arrieta, M.D.
Resident
Department of Otolaryngology—Head and Neck Surgery
University of South Florida
Tampa, Florida

H. Alexander Arts, M.D., F.A.C.S.
Clinical Associate Professor
Department of Neurosurgery
Clinical Associate Professor
Department of Otorhinolaryngology
University of Michigan Medical Center
Ann Arbor, Michigan

Yasmine A. Ashram, M.D., D.A.B.N.M.
Surgical Neurophysiologist, Lecturer
Neurophysiology Division
Department of Physiology
Alexandria School of Medicine
University of Alexandria
Alexandria, Egypt

Nafi Aygun, M.D.
Assistant Professor
Department of Radiology
The Russell H. Morgan Department of Radiology and
    Radiological Sciences
The Johns Hopkins Medical Institution
Baltimore, Maryland

Douglas D. Backous, M.D.
Medical Director
The Listen for Life Center
Department of Otolaryngology—Head and Neck Surgery
Virginia Mason Medical Center
Seattle, Washington

Shan R. Baker, M.D.
Professor
Department of Otolaryngology
Professor
Center for Facial Plastic and Reconstructive Surgery
University of Michigan School of Medicine
Center for Facial Plastic Surgery
Livonia, Michigan

Thomas J. Balkany, M.D.
Chief
Division of Otology
Hotchkiss Professor
Chairman
Department of Otolaryngology—Head and
    Neck Surgery
University of Miami School of Medicine
Miami, Florida

Fuad M. Baroody, M.D.
Associate Professor
Division of Otolaryngology—Head and Neck Surgery
The University of Chicago Pritzker School of Medicine
Chicago, Illinois

Roberto L. Barretto, M.D.
Pediatric Otolaryngology—Head and Neck Surgery
St. Joseph Hospital Nasal and Sinus Center
Orange, California

Jonathan Z. Baskin, M.D.
Craniofacial Fellow
Department of Otolaryngology and Communication
    Sciences
Upstate Medical University, S.U.N.Y.
Syracuse, New York

Robert W. Bastian, M.D.
Bastian Voice Institute
Downers Grove, Illinois

Carol A. Bauer, M.D.
Associate Professor
Division of Otolaryngology—Head and Neck Surgery
Department of Surgery
Southern Illinois School of Medicine
Springfield, Illinois

Aaron Benson, M.D.
Resident
Department of Otolaryngology—Head and
    Neck Surgery
University of Illinois at Chicago
Chicago, Illinois

Nasir I. Bhatti, M.D.
Assistant Professor
Department of Otolaryngology—Head and
    Neck Surgery
The Johns Hopkins School of Medicine
Baltimore, Maryland

Carol M. Bier-Laning, M.D.
Clinical Assistant Professor
Department of Otolaryngology—Head and
    Neck Surgery
Loyola University Medical Center
Barrington, Illinois

James E. Blaugrund, M.D.
Department of Otolaryngology
Allegheny General Hospital
Allegheny Professional Building
Pittsburgh, Pennsylvania

Nikolas H. Blevins, M.D.
Assistant Professor
Department of Otolaryngology—Head and Neck
    Surgery
Tufts University New England Medical Center
Boston, Massachusetts

Andrew Blitzer, M.D., D.D.S., F.A.C.S.
Professor
Department of Clinical Otolaryngology
Columbia University
Medical Director
New York Center for Clinical Research
New York Center for Voice and Swallowing Disorders
New York, New York

Derald E. Brackmann, M.D.
House Ear Clinic
Los Angeles, California

Carol Bradford, M.D., F.A.C.S.
Director
Head and Surgery Division,
Director
Head and Neck Oncology Program
Associate Professor and Associate Chair
Department of Otolaryngology—Head and Neck Surgery
University of Michigan Health System
Ann Arbor, Michigan

Barton F. Branstetter IV, M.D.
Director
ENT Radiology
Associate Director
Radiology Informatics
Assistant Professor
Department of Radiology
University of Pittsburgh Medical Center
Pittsburgh, Pennsylvania

Hilary A. Brodie, M.D., Ph.D.
Professor and Chair
Department of Otolaryngology—Head and Neck Surgery
University of California
Davis School of Medicine
Otolaryngology Research Laboratories
Davis, California

Carolyn J. Brown, Ph.D.
Associate Professor
Department of Speech Pathology and Audiology
University of Iowa Hospitals and Clinics
Wendell Johnson Speech and Hearing Center
Iowa City, Iowa

Karla Brown, M.D.
Clinical Professor and Chief
Section of Pediatric Otolaryngology
Department of Pediatrics
Tulane Hospital for Children
Assistant Professor
Department of Otolaryngology—Head and Neck Surgery
Tulane University School of Medicine
New Orleans, Louisiana

Orval E. Brown, M.D.
Beth and Marvin C. (Cub) Culbertson Professorship in
    Pediatric Otolaryngology
Resident Selection Committee
Professor and Chairman
Department of Otolaryngology—Head and Neck Surgery
University of Texas Southwestern Medical Center
    at Dallas
Dallas, Texas

J. Dale Browne, M.D., F.A.C.S.
Professor
Department of Otolaryngology—Head and Neck Surgery
Wake Forest University School of Medicine
Winston-Salem, North Carolina

John Buatti, M.D.
Professor and Head
Department of Radiation Oncology
University of Iowa Hospitals and Clinics
Iowa City, Iowa

Daniel Buchbinder, D.M.D., M.D.
Associate Professor
Department of Otolaryngology—Head and Neck Surgery
Professor and Chair
Department of Dentistry
Professor and Chief
Division of Oral and Maxillofacial Surgery
Director of Residency Training
Division of Oral and Maxillofacial Surgery
Mount Sinai School of Medicine
New York, New York

Patrick J. Byrne, M.D.
Assistant Professor and Director
Division of Facial Plastic and Reconstructive Surgery
Department of Otolaryngology—Head and Neck Surgery
The Johns Hopkins University
Baltimore, Maryland

Joseph A. Califano III, M.D.
Associate Professor
Head and Neck Research Division
Department of Otolaryngology—Head and Neck Surgery
Associate Professor
Department of Otolaryngology
The Johns Hopkins University School of Medicine
Baltimore, Maryland

John P. Carey, M.D.
Assistant Professor
Department of Otolaryngology—Head and Neck Surgery
The Johns Hopkins University School of Medicine
Baltimore, Maryland

Eric Carlson, D.M.D., M.D.
Chief
Oral and Maxillofacial Surgery
University of Tennessee Memorial Hospital
University of Tennessee Cancer Institute
Director
Oral and Maxillofacial Surgery Residency Program
Professor and Chairman
Department of Oral and Maxillofacial Surgery
University of Tennessee Graduate School of Medicine
Knoxville, Tennessee

Ricardo L. Carrau, M.D.
Associate Professor
Department of Otolaryngology—Head and Neck Surgery
University of Pittsburgh School of Medicine
Eye and Ear Institute
Pittsburgh, Pennsylvania

Roy R. Casiano, M.D.
Director
Center for Sinus and Voice Disorders
Professor
Department of Otolaryngology—Head and Neck Surgery
University of Miami School of Medicine
Center for Sinus and Voice Disorders
Miami, Florida

Jon B. Chadwell, M.D.
Resident
Department of Otolaryngology—Head and Neck Surgery
University of Cincinnati Medical Center
Cincinnati, Ohio

Christopher Y. Chang, M.D.
Resident
Division of Otolaryngology—Head and Neck Surgery
Department of Surgery
Duke University Medical Center
Durham, North Carolina

Kristi E. Chang, M.D.
Assistant Professor
Department of Otolaryngology—Head and Neck Surgery
University of Iowa Hospitals and Clinics
Iowa City, Iowa

Burke E. Chegar, M.D.
Resident
Department of Otolaryngology and Communication
    Sciences
Upstate Medical University, S.U.N.Y.
Syracuse, New York

Sukgi S. Choi, M.D.
Associate Professor
Departments of Otolaryngology and Pediatrics
The George Washington University Medical Center
Associate Professor
Department of Otolaryngology—Head and Neck Surgery
Children's National Medical Center
Washington DC

Richard A. Chole, M.D., Ph.D.
Richard A. Lindburg Professor of Otolaryngology
Chairman
Department of Otolaryngology—Head and Neck Surgery
Washington University School of Medicine
St. Louis, Missouri

Martin J. Citardi, M.D.
Staff
Department of Otolaryngology and Communicative
    Disorders
The Cleveland Clinic Foundation
Cleveland, Ohio

Savita Collins, M.D.
Assistant Professor
Department of Otolaryngology—Head and Neck Surgery
University of Florida College of Medicine
Gainesville, Florida

Philippe Contencin, M.D.
Saint-Vincent De Paul-Hospital
Paris, France

Raymond D. Cook, M.D.
Assistant Professor
Department of Otolaryngology—Head and Neck Surgery
Wake Medical Center
Department of Otolaryngology—Head and Neck Surgery
University of North Carolina School of Medicine
Chapel Hill, North Carolina

Ted A. Cook, M.D., F.A.C.S.
Professor and Chief
Facial Plastic and Reconstructive Surgery
Department of Otolaryngology—Head and Neck Surgery
Oregon Health and Sciences University
Portland, Oregon

Robin T. Cotton, M.D.
Professor
Department of Otolaryngology—Head and Neck Surgery
University of Cincinnati Medical Center
Director
Department of Pediatric Otolaryngology—Head and Neck
    Surgery
Cincinnati Children's Hospital Medical Center
Cincinnati, Ohio

Marion Everett Couch, M.D., Ph.D.
Assistant Professor
Department of Otolaryngology—Head and
    Neck Surgery
University of North Carolina School of Medicine
Chapel Hill, North Carolina

Mark S. Courey, M.D.
Assistant Professor
Department of Otolaryngology—Head and
    Neck Surgery
Bill Wilkerson Center for Otolaryngology and
    Communication Sciences
Vanderbilt University
Nashville, Tennessee

Roger L. Crumley, M.D.
Professor and Chairman
Department of Otolaryngology—Head and Neck Surgery
University of California, Irvine Medical Center
Orange, California

Oswaldo Laércio M. Cruz, M.D.
Professor
Department of Otolaryngology
Federal University of Sao Paulo
Escola Paulista de Medicina
Sao Paulo, Brazil

**Bernard J. Cummings, M.B., Ch.B., F.R.A.N.Z.C.R.,
    F.R.C.R., F.R.C.P.C.**
Professor
Department of Otolaryngology
Professor
Department of Radiation Oncology
University of Toronto
Department of Radiation Oncology
Princess Margaret Hospital
Toronto, Ontario, Canada

Charles W. Cummings, M.D.
Distinguished Service Professor
Department of Otolaryngology—Head and Neck Surgery
Johns Hopkins University School of Medicine
Baltimore, Maryland

Calhoun D. Cunningham, III, M.D.
Costal Carolina OTO Associates
Charleston, South Carolina

Larry E. Davis, M.D.
Research Professor
Neuroscience, Microbiology, and Immunology,
Professor and Vice Chair
Department of Neurology
University of New Mexico Health Science Center
Albuquerque, New Mexico

Terry A. Day, M.D.
Associate Professor and Clinical Vice Chairman
Department of Otolaryngology—Head and Neck Surgery
Director
Division of Head and Neck Oncology Surgery
Hollings Cancer Center
Medical University of South Carolina
Charleston, South Carolina

Antonio De la Cruz, M.D.
Clinical Professor
Department of Otolaryngology—Head and Neck Surgery
University of Southern California Keck School of Medicine
Director of Education
House Ear Clinic
Los Angeles, California

Charles C. Della Santina, M.D., Ph.D.
Assistant Professor
Department of Otolaryngology—Head and Neck Surgery
Assistant Professor
Department of Biomedical Engineering
Division of Otology, Neurotology, and Skull Base Surgery
Johns Hopkins University School of Medicine
Baltimore, Maryland

Craig S. Derkay, M.D.
Professor
Departments of Otolaryngology and Pediatrics
Director
Pediatric Otolaryngology
Vice Chairman
Department of Otolaryngology—Head and Neck Surgery
Eastern Virginia Medical School
Norfolk, Virginia

Robert A. Dobie, M.D., F.A.C.S.
Clinical Professor
Department of Otolaryngology—Head and Neck Surgery
University of California, Davis
Sacramento, California

Newton O. Duncan, III, M.D.
Co-Director
Texas Pediatric Otolaryngology Center
Houston, Texas

Scott D. Z. Eggers, M.D.
Instructor of Neurology
Mayo Clinic College of Medicine
Senior Associate Consultant
Department of Neurology
Mayo Clinic
Rochester, Minnesota

David W. Eisele, M.D.
Professor and Chairman
Department of Otolaryngology—Head and Neck Surgery
University of California, San Francisco
San Francisco, California

Hussam K. El-Kashlan, M.D.
Medical Director
Vestibular Training Center
Associate Professor
Division of Otology and Neurotology
Department of Otolaryngology
University of Michigan Health System
Ann Arbor, Michigan

Ravindhra G. Elluru, M.D., Ph.D.
Assistant Professor
Department of Pediatric Otolaryngology
Cincinnati Children's Hospital Medical Center
Cincinnati, Ohio

Ramon M. Esclamado, M.D.
Vice Chairman
Department of Otolaryngology and Communicative
    Disorders
Cleveland Clinic Foundation
Cleveland, Ohio

Chun Y. Fan, M.D., Ph.D.
Assistant Professor
Department of Pathology and Otolaryngology
Department of Pathology
University of Arkansas for Medical Sciences and Central
    Arkansas Veterans Healthcare System
Little Rock, Arkansas

Edward H. Farrior, M.D., F.A.C.S.
Farrior Facial Plastic and Cosmetic Surgery
Tampa, Florida

Richard T. Farrior, M.D.
Boca Grande, Florida

Russell A. Faust, Ph.D., M.D.
Chief
Department of Otolaryngology—Head and Neck
    Surgery
Children's Hospital of Michigan
Detroit, Michigan

Willard E. Fee, Jr., M.D.
Edward C. and Amy H. Sewall Professor of
    Otolaryngology
Department of Otolaryngology—Head and Neck
    Surgery
Stanford University School of Medicine
Stanford, California

Berrylin J. Ferguson, M.D.
Associate Professor
Department of Otolaryngology—Head and Neck
    Surgery
University of Pittsburgh Medical Center
Eye and Ear Institute
Pittsburgh, Pennsylvania

Jill B. Firszt, Ph.D.
Director
Koss Cochlear Implant Program,
Director Department of Audiology
Assistant Professor
Department of Otolaryngology and Communication Sciences
Medical College of Wisconsin
Milwaukee, Wisconsin

Paul W. Flint, M.D.
Professor
Department of Otolaryngology—Head and Neck Surgery
Department of Anesthesiology and Critical Care Medicine
Director
Center for Airway, Laryngeal, and Voice Disorders
Co-Director
Minimally Invasive Surgical Training Center
Johns Hopkins University School of Medicine
Baltimore, Maryland

Robert L. Folmer, Ph.D.
Assistant Professor
Department of Otolaryngology—Head and Neck Surgery
Oregon Health and Science University Tinnitus Clinic
Portland, Oregon

Arlene A. Forastiere, M.D.
Professor
Departments of Oncology and Otolaryngology
The Johns Hopkins University School of Medicine
Baltimore, Maryland

L. Arick Forrest, M.D.
Associate Professor
Department of Otolaryngology—Head and Neck Surgery
The Ohio State University Medical Center
Columbus, Ohio

Oren Friedman, M.D.
Assistant Professor
Facial Plastic and Reconstructive Surgery
Department of Otolaryngology—Head and Neck Surgery
Mayo Clinic and Medical School
Rochester, Minnesota

John L. Frodel, Jr., M.D., F.A.C.S.
Director
Facial Plastic Surgery
Geisinger Medical Center
Danville, Pennsylvania

Gerry F. Funk, M.D.
Associate Professor
Department of Radiation Oncology
Associate Professor
Department of Otolaryngology—Head and Neck Surgery
University of Iowa Hospitals and Clinics
Iowa City, Iowa

Thomas J. Gal, M.D., M.P.H., Major, USAF-MC
Director
Head and Neck Oncology
Department of Otolaryngology—Head and Neck Surgery
Wilford Hall Medical Center
Lackland, Texas

Suzanne K. Doud Galli, M.D., Ph.D.
Adamson Associates Cosmetic Facial Surgery Clinic
Toronto, Ontario, Canada

Bruce J. Gantz, M.D.
Professor and Department Head
Department of Otolaryngology—Head and Neck Surgery
University of Iowa Hospitals and Clinics
Iowa City, Iowa

C. Gaelyn Garrett, M.D.
Associate Professor
Department of Otolaryngology
Vanderbilt Bill Wilkerson Center for Otolaryngology and Communication Sciences
Vanderbilt University Medical Center
Nashville, Tennessee

Holger G. Gassner, M.D.
Department of Otorhinolaryngology—Head and Neck Surgery
Mayo Clinic
Rochester, Minnesota

George A. Gates, M.D.
Adjunct Professor
Department of Epidemiology
Director
Virginia Merrill Bloedel Hearing Research Center
Chief Otology and Neurotology Service
Professor
Department of Otolaryngology—Head and Neck Surgery
University of Washington School of Medicine
Seattle, Washington

William Donald Gay, D.D.S., F.A.C.D.
Director
Division of Maxillofacial Prosthetics
Associate Professor
Department of Otolaryngology—Head and Neck Surgery
Washington University School of Medicine
St. Louis, Missouri

Norman Ge, M.D.
Surgery Fellow
Department of Otolaryngology—Head and Neck Surgery
University of California, Irvine Medical Center
Irvine, California

Eric M. Genden, M.D.
Associate Professor
Center for Immunobiology
Associate Professor
Department of Otolaryngology—Head and Neck
    Surgery
Mount Sinai School of Medicine
New York, New York

Elisa M. Ghezzi, D.D.S.
Adjunct Clinical Assistant Professor
Department of Dentistry
University of Michigan School of Dentistry
Ann Arbor, Michigan

Timothy G. Gillum, M.D.
Gillum Facial Plastic Surgery
Marion, Indiana

Marian Girardi, Ph.D.
Director
Clinical Research and Education
Vestibular Technologies, Inc.
Alexandria, Virginia

Douglas A. Girod, M.D.
Chairman and Professor
Department of Otolaryngology
Director
Division of Head and Neck Surgery
University of Kansas Medical Center
Kansas City, Kansas

George S. Goding, Jr., M.D.
Associate Professor
Department of Otolaryngology—Head and Neck
    Surgery
University of Minnesota, Twin Cities
Attending Staff
Department of Otolaryngology
VA Medical Center
Minneapolis, Minnesota

Andrew N. Goldberg, M.D., F.A.C.S.
Associate Professor
Department of Otolaryngology—Head and Neck
    Surgery
University of California, San Francisco
San Francisco, California

David Goldenberg, M.D.
Fellow
Department of Otolaryngology—Head and Neck
    Surgery
Johns Hopkins University School of Medicine
Baltimore, Maryland

W. Jarrard Goodwin, Jr., M.D.
Director
Sylvester Comprehensive Cancer Center
Professor
Department of Otolaryngology
University of Miami Hospital and Clinics
Sylvester Comprehensive Cancer Center
Miami, Florida

Daniel O. Graney, Ph.D.
Professor
Department of Biological Structure
University of Washington School of Medicine
Seattle, Washington

Patrick K. Ha, M.D.
Fellow
Department of Otolaryngology—Head and Neck
    Surgery
Johns Hopkins University School of
    Medicine
Baltimore, Maryland

Jeffrey R. Haller, M.D.
Rocky Mountain Ear, Nose, and Throat Center
Missoula, Montana

Jongwook Ham, M.D.
Associates in ENT Head & Neck Surgery
Elgin, Illinois

Ehab Y. Hanna, M.D., F.A.C.S.
Professor
Head and Neck Surgery
Director
Center for Skull Base Surgery
Chief
Section of Skull Base Surgery
Department of Head and Neck Surgery
MD Anderson Cancer Center
Houston, Texas

Marlan R. Hansen, M.D.
Assistant Professor
Department of Otolaryngology—Head and Neck Surgery
University of Iowa Hospital and Clinics
Iowa City, Iowa

Lee A. Harker, M.D.
Deputy Director
Boys Town National Research Hospital
Vice Chairman
Department of Otolaryngology and Human
    Communication
Creighton University School of Medicine
Omaha, Nebraska

Robert V. Harrison, Ph.D., D.Sc.
Professor
Department of Otolaryngology—Head and Neck Surgery
Professor
Department of Physiology
The Institute of Biomaterials and Biomedical Engineering
The Institute of Medical Science
The University of Toronto
Senior Scientist
Division of Brain and Behavior
Department of Otolaryngology
The Hospital for Sick Children
Toronto, Ontario, Canada

Bruce H. Haughey, MBChB, FACS, FRACS
Professor and Director
Division of Head and Neck Surgical Oncology
Department of Otolaryngology—Head and Neck Surgery
Washington University School of Medicine
St. Louis, Missouri

Gerald B. Healy, M.D., F.A.C.S.
Professor
Division of Otology and Laryngology
Department of Otolaryngology—Head and Neck Surgery
Harvard Medical School
Otolaryngologist-in-Chief
Department of Otolaryngology and Communication
  Disorders
Children's Hospital
Boston, Massachusetts

Michael L. Hinni, M.D.
Consultant
Department of Otorhinolaryngology
Head and Neck Surgeon
Mayo Clinic Scottsdale
Scottsdale, Arizona

Henry T. Hoffman, M.D.
Professor
Department of Otolaryngology—Head and Neck Surgery
Department of Radiation Oncology
Iowa City, Iowa

Eric H. Holbrook, M.D.
Instructor
Division of Otology and Laryngology
Department of Otolaryngology—Head and Neck
  Surgery
Massachusetts Eye and Ear Infirmary
Boston, Massachusetts

Lauren D. Holinger, M.D.
Professor
Department of Otolaryngology—Head and Neck Surgery
Northwestern University Feinberg School of Medicine
Professor and Chief
Division of Pediatric Otolaryngology
Children's Memorial Hospital
Chicago, Illinois

David B. Hom, M.D.
Associate Professor
Department of Otolaryngology—Head and Neck Surgery
University of Minnesota, Twin Cities
Associate Professor
Head and Neck Surgery Lions 5M International Hearing
  Center
Department of Otolaryngology
Minneapolis, Minnesota

John W. House, M.D.
Clinical Professor
Department of Otolaryngology—Head and Neck Surgery
University of Southern California Keck School of Medicine
President
House Ear Institute
House Ear Clinic
Los Angeles, California

J. W. Hudson, D.D.S.
Professor Department of Oral and Maxillofacial Surgery
University of Tennessee Graduate School of Medicine
Knoxville, Tennessee

Matthew C. Hull, M.D.
Radiation Oncologist
Mountain Radiation Oncology
Asheville, North Carolina

Timothy E. Hullar, M.D.
Assistant Professor
Department of Otolaryngology—Head and Neck Surgery
Washington University School of Medicine
St. Louis, Missouri

Kevin J. Hulett, M.D.
Clinical Assistant Professor
Department of Otolaryngology—Head and Neck Surgery
Loyola University Medical Center
Chicago, Illinois

Murad Husein, M.D., M.Sc., F.R.C.S.(C)
Assistant Professor
Department of Otolaryngology
University of Western Ontario
London, Ontario, Canada

Steven W. Ing, M.D.
Staff Attending
Department of Endocrinology
Geisinger Medical Group
Wilkes-Barre, Pennsylvania

Andrew F. Inglis, Jr., M.D.
Attending Surgeon
Division of Pediatric Otolaryngology
Children's Hospital and Medical Center
Associate Professor
Department of Otolaryngology—Head and Neck Surgery
University of Washington School of Medicine
Seattle, Washington

Robert K. Jackler, M.D.
Professor
Departments of Neurosurgery and Surgery
Edward C. and Amy H. Sewall Professor and Chair in
    Otolaryngology
Department of Otolaryngology—Head and Neck
    Surgery
Stanford University School of Medicine
Stanford, California

Herman A. Jenkins, M.D.
Professor and Chairman
Department of Otolaryngology—Head and Neck
    Surgery
University of Colorado Health Science Center
Denver, Colorado

John K. Joe, M.D.
Assistant Professor
Division of Otolaryngology—Head and Neck Surgery
Department of Surgery
Yale University School of Medicine
New Haven, Connecticut

Stephanie Joe, M.D.
Director
General Otolaryngology
Assistant Professor
Rhinology and Sinus Surgery
Department of Otolaryngology—Head and Neck
    Surgery
University of Illinois at Chicago
Chicago, Illinois

Jonas T. Johnson, M.D.
Professor
Department of Otolaryngology
University of Pittsburgh Medical Center
Eye and Ear Institute
Pittsburgh, Pennsylvania

Timothy Johnson, M.D.
William B. Taylor Professor of Dermatology
Departments of Otolaryngology, Dermatology, and Surgery
Director
Cutaneous Surgery and Oncology Unit Director
Multidisciplinary Melanoma Clinic
University of Michigan Health System
Department of Dermatology
Ann Arbor, Michigan

Kim Richard Jones, M.D., Ph.D.
Carolina ENT
Chapel Hill, North Carolina

Sheldon S. Kabaker, M.D.
Associate Clinical Professor
Division of Facial Plastic Surgery
Department of Otolaryngology—Head and Neck Surgery
San Francisco, California
Oakland, California

Lucy H. Karnell, M.D.
Associate Research Scientist
Department of Otolaryngology—Head and Neck Surgery
University of Iowa Hospitals and Clinics
Iowa City, Iowa

Matthew L. Kashima, M.D.
Assistant Professor
Department of Otolaryngology—Head and Neck
    Surgery
The Johns Hopkins University School of Medicine
Baltimore, Maryland

Robert M. Kellman, M.D.
Professor and Chairman
Department of Otolaryngology and Communication
    Sciences
Upstate Medical University, S.U.N.Y.
Syracuse, New York

Paul E. Kelly, M.D., F.A.C.S.
Private Practice
Riverhead, New York

David W. Kennedy, M.D.
Professor
Department of Otorhinolaryngology: Head and Neck
    Surgery
Vice Dean for Professional Services
Senior Vice President, University of Pennsylvania Health
    System
University of Pennsylvania School of Medicine
Philadelphia, Pennsylvania

Merrill S. Kies, M.D.
Professor of Medicine
Department of Thoracic/Head and Neck Medical Oncology
MD Anderson Cancer Center
Houston, Texas

Paul R. Kileny, Ph.D., F.A.S.H.A.
Director
Audiology and Electrophysiology
Director
Hearing Rehabilitation Program
Geriatric Center Member
Professor
Department of Pediatrics and Communicable Diseases
Professor
Department of Otolaryngology—Head and Neck Surgery
University of Michigan Medical Center
A. Alfred Taubman Health Care Center
Ann Arbor, Michigan

David W. Kim, M.D.
Assistant Professor
Department of Otolaryngology—Head and Neck Surgery
Director
Division of Facial Plastic and Reconstructive Surgery
University of California, San Francisco
San Francisco, California

John Kim, M.D., FRCPC
Assistant Professor
Department of Radiation Oncology
University of Toronto
Department of Radiation Oncology
Princess Margaret Hospital
Toronto, Ontario, Canada

William J. Kimberling, Ph.D.
Professor
Biomedical Sciences
Director
Center for the Study and Treatment of Usher Syndrome
Boys Town National Research Hospital
Omaha, Nebraska

Jeffrey L. Koh, M.D.
Director
Pediatric Pain Management Center
Associate Professor
Department of Anesthesiology and Pediatrics
Oregon Health and Sciences University
Portland, Oregon

Peter J. Koltai, M.D., F.A.C.S., F.A.A.P.
Chief of Otolaryngology
Lucile Packard Children's Hospital
Stanford University
Stanford, California

Horst R. Konrad, M.D.
Professor
Division of Otolaryngology—Head and Neck Surgery
Southern Illinois University School of Medicine
Springfield, Illinois

Frederick K. Kozak, M.D.
Clinical Instructor
Division of Otolaryngology—Head and Neck Surgery
Director
Continuing Medical Education
University of British Columbia
Staff
Division of Pediatric Otolaryngology
British Columbia's Children's Hospital
Vancouver, British Columbia, Canada

Paul R. Krakovitz, M.D.
Associate Staff
Section of Pediatric Otolaryngology
The Children's Hospital
Cleveland Clinic Foundation
Cleveland, Ohio

Russell W. H. Kridel, M.D., F.A.C.S.
Clinical Associate Professor and Fellowship Director
Division of Facial Plastics and Reconstructive
    Surgery
Department of Otolaryngology—Head and Neck Surgery
University of Texas Health Center at Houston
Facial Plastic Surgery Associates
Houston, Texas

Manoj Kumar, M.S., F.R.C.S.
Specialist
Registrar in Otolaryngology
Singleton Hospital
Swansea, Wales, United Kingdom

Parvesh Kumar, M.D.
Professor and Chair
Department of Radiation Oncology
University of Southern California Keck School of Medicine
Los Angeles, California

Dario Kunar, M.D.
Greater Baltimore Medical Center
Ear, Nose, and Throat Associates
Towson, Maryland

Ollivier Laccourreye, M.D.
Professor
Department of Otorhinolaryngology—Head and Neck Surgery
Hôpital Européen Georges Pompidou
University of Paris
Paris, France

Stephen Y. Lai, M.D., Ph.D.
Fellow
Head and Neck Surgical Oncology
Department of Otolaryngology—Head and Neck Surgery
University of Pittsburgh Medical Center
The Eye and Ear Institute
Pittsburgh, Pennsylvania

Anil K. Lalwani, M.D.
Mendik Foundation Professor of Otolaryngology
Chairman and Professor of Physiology and Neuroscience
Department of Otolaryngology—Head and Neck Surgery
New York University School of Medicine
New York, New York

Paul R. Lambert, M.D.
Professor and Chairman
Department of Otolaryngology—Head and Neck Surgery
Medical University of South Carolina
Charleston, South Carolina

George E. Laramore, M.D., Ph.D.
Chairman and Director
University Cancer Center
Professor and Chairman
Department of Radiation Oncology
University of Washington Medical Center Cancer Center
Seattle, Washington

Peter E. Larsen, D.D.S.
Professor and Chair
Department of Oral and Maxillofacial Surgery
The Ohio State University College of Dentistry
Powell, Ohio

Daniel M. Laskin, D.D.S., M.S., D.Sc.
Professor and Chairman Emeritus
Division of Oral and Maxillofacial Surgery
Professor of Psychology (Affiliate Appointment)
Virginia Commonwealth University
Richmond, Virginia

Richard E. Latchaw, M.D.
Chief
Section of Neuroradiology
Professor
Department of Radiology
University of California, Davis School of Medicine
Sacramento, California

Christine L. Lau, M.D.
Fellow
Division of Cardiothoracic Surgery
Washington University School of Medicine
St. Louis, Missouri

Ken K. Lee, M.D.
Assistant Professor
Department of Dermatology
Oregon Health and Science University
Portland, Oregon

Nancy Y. Lee, M.D.
Assistant Attending
Department of Radiation Oncology
Memorial Sloan-Kettering Cancer Center
New York, New York

Stephen Lee, M.D.
Resident
Department of Otolaryngology—Head and Neck Surgery
University of Arkansas for Medical Sciences
Fayetteville, Arkansas

Jean-Louis Lefebvre, M.D.
Professor and Chairman
Department of Head and Neck Cancer
Lille, France

Susanna Leighton, F.R.C.S.
Consultant
Paediatric Otolaryngology
Great Ormond Street Hospital for Children NHS Trust
London, United Kingdom

Donald A. Leopold, M.D.
Professor and Chair
Department of Otolaryngology—Head and Neck Surgery
University of Nebraska Medical Center
Omaha, Nebraska

Daqing Li, M.D.
Director of Gene and Molecular Therapy
Division of Otolaryngology—Head and Neck Surgery
University of Maryland School of Medicine
Baltimore, Maryland

Timothy S. Lian, M.D.
Assistant Professor
Residency Program Director
Division of Facial and Reconstructive Surgery
Department of Otolaryngology—Head and Neck Surgery
Louisiana State University Medical Center
Shreveport, Louisiana

Greg R. Licameli, M.D.
Assistant Professor
Division of Otology and Laryngology
Department of Otolaryngology—Head and Neck
    Surgery
Harvard Medical School
Children's Hospital
Boston, Massachusetts

Charles J. Limb, M.D.
Assistant Professor
Department of Otolaryngology—Head and Neck
    Surgery
Johns Hopkins University School of Medicine
Baltimore, Maryland

Jerilyn A. Logemann, Ph.D.
Director
Voice, Speech, Language, and Swallowing Center
Northwestern Memorial Hospital
Professor
Department of Otolaryngology—Head and Neck Surgery
Department of Neurology
Ralph and Jean Sundin Professor
Department of Communication Sciences and Disorders
Northwestern University Feinberg School of Medicine
Evanston, Illinois

Brenda L. Lonsbury-Martin, Ph.D.
Professor and Vice Chair of Research
Department of Otolaryngology—Head and Neck Surgery
University of Colorado Health Sciences Center
Denver, Colorado

Benjamin M. Loos, M.D.
Clinical Instructor and Fellow
Division of Facial Plastic Surgery
Department of Otolaryngology—Head and Neck
    Surgery
University of California, San Francisco
San Francisco, California

Manuel A. Lopez, M.D.
Fellow
Department of Otolaryngology—Head and Neck Surgery
University of Illinois at Chicago Medical Center
Chicago, Illinois

Rodney P. Lusk, M.D., F.A.C.S., F.A.A.P.
Alpine Ear, Nose, and Throat
Fort Collins, Colorado

Lawrence R. Lustig, M.D.
Associate Professor
Otology, Neurotology, Skull Base Surgery
Department of Otolaryngology—Head and Neck Surgery
Johns Hopkins University School of Medicine
Baltimore, Maryland

Anna Lysakowski, Ph.D.
Associate Professor
Department of Anatomy and Cell Biology
University of Illinois at Chicago College of Medicine
Chicago, Illinois

Richard L. Mabry, M.D.
Clinical Professor
Department of Otolaryngology—Head and Neck
  Surgery
University of Texas Southwestern Medical Center
Dallas, Texas
University of Texas Medical Branch
Galveston, Texas
University of Texas Health Science Center
San Antonio, Texas

Carol J. MacArthur, M.D.
Assistant Professor
Department of Otolaryngology—Head and Neck
  Surgery
Oregon Health and Sciences University
Portland, Oregon

Allison R. MacGregor, M.D.
Fellow
Facial Plastic and Reconstructive Surgery
Edgewood, Kentucky

Robert H. Maisel, M.D., F.A.C.S.
Professor
Department of Otolaryngology—Head and Neck
  Surgery
University of Minnesota, Twin Cities
Hennepin County Medical Center
Minneapolis, Minnesota

Patrizia Mancini, M.D.
Ear, Nose, and Throat Department
Università Degli Studi di Roma La Sapienza
Rome, Italy

Susan J. Mandel, M.D., M.P.H.
Associate Professor of Medicine and Radiology
Associate Chief for Clinical Affairs
Director Endocrinology Fellowship Training Program
University of Pennsylvania Medical Center
Division of Endocrinology, Diabetes, and Metabolism
Philadelphia, Pennsylvania

Scott C. Manning, M.D.
Associate Professor
Department of Otolaryngology—Head and Neck Surgery
University of Washington Medical Center
Chief Division of Pediatric Otolaryngology
Children's Hospital and Medical Center
Seattle, Washington

Lynette J. Mark, M.D.
Associate Professor
Department of Anesthesia and Critical Care Medicine
Associate Professor
Department of Otolaryngology—Head and Neck Surgery
Johns Hopkins University School of Medicine
Department of Anesthesiology and Critical Care Medicine
Johns Hopkins Hospital
Baltimore, Maryland

Jeffery C. Markt, D.D.S.
Assistant Professor
Department of Hospital Dentistry
University of Iowa Hospitals and Clinics
Iowa City, Iowa

Bradley F. Marple, M.D.
Associate Professor and Vice Chairman
Department of Otolaryngology—Head and Neck Surgery
University of Texas Southwestern Medical Center
Dallas, Texas

Michael A. Marsh, M.D.
Arkansas Center for Ear Nose Throat and Allergy
Sparks Medical Plaza
Fort Smith, Arkansas

Glen K. Martin, Ph.D.
Professor and Director of Research
Department of Otolaryngology—Head and Neck Surgery
University of Colorado Health Sciences Center
Denver, Colorado

Douglas D. Massick, M.D.
Assistant Professor
Department of Otolaryngology
The Ohio State University
Columbus, Ohio

Douglas E. Mattox, M.D.
Professor and Chair
Department of Otolaryngology—Head and Neck Surgery
Emory University School of Medicine
Atlanta, Georgia

Thomas V. McCaffrey, M.D., Ph.D.
Professor and Chair
Department of Otolaryngology
Program Leader
Head and Neck Cancer
University of South Florida
H. Lee Moffitt Cancer Center and Research Institute
Tampa, Florida

Timothy M. McCulloch, M.D.
Professor
Department of Otolaryngology—Head and Neck Surgery
University of Washington Medical Center
Chief
Department of Otolaryngology—Head and Neck Surgery
Harborview Medical Center
Seattle, Washington

Thomas J. McDonald, M.D.
Professor and Chairman
Department of Otolaryngology—Head and Neck Surgery
Mayo Clinic
Rochester, Minnesota

JoAnn McGee, Ph.D.
Staff Scientist
Developmental Auditory Physiology Laboratory
Boys Town National Research Hospital
Omaha, Nebraska

Trevor J. McGill, M.D., F.A.C.S.
Professor
Department of Otology and Laryngology
Harvard Medical School
Senior Associate
Department of Otolaryngology and Communication
   Disorders
Children's Hospital
Boston, Massachusetts

John F. McGuire, M.D., M.B.A.
Resident Physician
Department of Otolaryngology—Head and Neck Surgery
University of California, Irvine
Irvine, California

W. Frederick McGuirt, Sr., M.D., F.A.C.S.
James A. Harrill Professor and Chairman
Department of Otolaryngology—Head and Neck
   Surgery
Wake Forest University Baptist Medical Center
Winston-Salem, North Carolina

Sean O. McMenomey, M.D., F.A.C.S.
Associate Professor
Cochlear Implant/Implantable Hearing Aid Program
Chief
Division of Otology, Neurotology, Skull Base Surgery
Associate Professor
Department of Otolaryngology—Head and Neck
   Surgery
Oregon Health and Science University
Portland, Oregon

J. Scott McMurray, M.D., F.A.A.P., F.A.C.S.
Assistant Professor
Division of Otolaryngology—Head and Neck Surgery
Departments of Surgery and Pediatrics
University of Wisconsin School of Medicine
Madison, Wisconsin

Khosrow (Mark) Mehrany, M.D.
Fellow
Department of Dermatology
Oregon Health and Science University
Portland, Oregon

Nancy Price Mendenhall, M.D.
Rodney R. Million, M.D., Professorship for the Chairman of
   Radiation Oncology
Department of Radiation Oncology
University of Florida Health Science Center
Gainesville, Florida

Saumil N. Merchant, M.D.
Associate Professor
Department of Otology and Laryngology
Harvard Medical School
Department of Otolaryngology—Head and Neck
   Surgery
Massachusetts Eye and Ear Infirmary
Boston, Massachusetts

Jennifer L. Mertes, Au.D.
Assistant
Department of Otolaryngology—Head and Neck
   Surgery; and The Listening Center
Johns Hopkins University School of Medicine
Baltimore, Maryland

Anna H. Messner, M.D.
Service Chief and Assistant Professor
Department of Otolaryngology—Head and Neck
   Surgery
Department of Pediatrics
Lucile Packard Children's Hospital at Stanford
Pediatric Otolaryngology
Palo Alto, California

Ted A. Meyer, M.D., Ph.D.
Fellow
Department of Otolaryngology—Head and Neck
   Surgery
University of Iowa Hospitals and Clinics
Iowa City, Iowa

James Michelson, M.D.
Professor
Department of Orthopaedic Surgery
Director of Clinical Informatics
The George Washington University School of Medicine and
   Health Sciences
Washington DC

Henry A. Milczuk, M.D.
Assistant Professor
Division of Pediatric Otolaryngology
Department of Otolaryngology—Head and Neck Surgery
Oregon Health and Sciences University
Portland, Oregon

Lloyd B. Minor, M.D.
Andelot Professor and Director
Department of Otolaryngology—Head and Neck
  Surgery
Johns Hopkins University School of Medicine
Baltimore, Maryland

Steven Ross Mobley, M.D.
Assistant Professor
Facial Plastic and Reconstructive Surgery
Department of Otolaryngology
University of Utah School of Medicine
Salt Lake City, Utah

Jeffrey Morray, M.D.
Medical Director
Surgery Pain Management
PACU and Pre-Procedure Unit
Department of Anesthesiology
Phoenix Children's Hospital
Phoenix, Arizona

John B. Mulliken, M.D.
Professor
Department of Surgery
Harvard Medical School
Director of Craniofacial Center Division of
  Plastic Surgery
Children's Hospital
Boston, Massachusetts

Harlan R. Muntz, M.D., F.A.A.P., F.A.C.S.
Professor
Department of Otolaryngology—Head and Neck
  Surgery
University of Utah School of Medicine
Salt Lake City, Utah

Craig S. Murakami, M.D., F.A.C.S.
Department of Otolaryngology—Head and Neck
  Surgery
Virginia Mason Medical Center
Seattle, Washington

Charles M. Myer, III, M.D.
Professor
Department of Otolaryngology—Head and
  Neck Surgery
University of Cincinnati Medical Center
Director
Hearing Impaired Clinic
Children's Hospital Medical Center of Cincinnati
Cincinnati, Ohio

Robert M. Naclerio, M.D.
Professor and Chief
Section of Otolaryngology
The University of Chicago Pritzker School
  of Medicine
Chicago, Illinois

Joseph B. Nadol, Jr., M.D.
Walter Augustus Lecompte Professor and Chairman
Department of Otology and Laryngology
Harvard Medical School
Director Otology Service
Chief Department of Otolaryngology
Massachusetts Eye and Ear Infirmary
Boston, Massachusetts

Philippe Narcy, M.D.
Professor
Department of Otorhinolaryngology
Paris University
Hôpital Robert Debré
Paris, France

Paul S. Nassif, M.D., F.A.C.S.
Assistant Clinical Professor
Department of Otolaryngology
University of Southern California School of Medicine
Los Angeles, California
Assistant Clinical Professor
Department of Otolaryngology
University of California, Los Angeles
Attending Clinical Assistant Professor
Department of Otolaryngology
West Los Angeles VA Medical Center West
Los Angeles, California
Attending
Department of Otolaryngology
Century City Hospital
Century City, California
Spaulding Drive Cosmetic Surgery and Dermatology
Beverly Hills, California

Julian M. Nedzelski, M.D., F.R.C.S..C.
Professor and Chair
Department of Otolaryngology—Head and Neck
  Surgery
University of Toronto
Otolaryngologist-in-Chief
Sunnybrook Health Science Centre
Toronto, Ontario, Canada

John K. Niparko, M.D.
Division Director
Otology, Audiology, Neurotology, and Skull Base
  Surgery
Director
The Listening Center
Professor
Department of Otology
Johns Hopkins School of Medicine
Baltimore, Maryland

George T. Nager
Professor
Department of Otolaryngology—Head and Neck Surgery
The Johns Hopkins University School of Medicine
Baltimore, Maryland

Susan J. Norton, Ph.D., CCC-A
Professor
Department of Otolaryngology—Head and Neck
	Surgery
University of Washington School of Medicine
Director
Research and Clinical Audiology
Division of Otolaryngology
Children's Hospital and Regional Medical Center
Seattle, Washington

Daniel W. Nuss, M.D., F.A.C.S.
Professor and Chairman
Department of Otolaryngology—Head and Neck Surgery
Louisiana State University Health Sciences Center
New Orleans, Louisiana

Brian Nussenbaum, M.D.
Assistant Professor
Department of Otolaryngology—Head and Neck Surgery
Washington University School of Medicine
St. Louis, Missouri

Bert W. O'Malley, Jr., M.D.
Chair
Department of Otorhinolaryngology—Head and Neck
	Surgery
University of Pennsylvania Medical Center
Philadelphia, Pennsylvania

Patrick J. Oliverio, M.D.
Neuroradiologist
Fairfax Radiological Consultants, P.C.
Fairfax, Virginia

Kerry D. Olsen, M.D.
Professor
Department of Otorhinolaryngology—Head and Neck
	Surgery
Mayo Medical School
Mayo Clinic
Rochester, Minnesota

Juan Camilo Ospina, M.D.
Pediatric Otolaryngology Fellow
Division of Pediatric Otolaryngology
British Columbia's Children's Hospital
Vancouver, British Columbia, Canada

Robert H. Ossoff, D.M.D., M.D.
Associate Vice Chancellor for Health Affairs
Director
Vanderbilt Bill Wilkerson Center for Otolaryngology and
	Communication Sciences
Guy M. Maness Professor and Chairman
Department of Otolaryngology—Head and Neck
	Surgery
Vanderbilt University School of Medicine
Nashville, Tennessee

Brian O'Sullivan, M.B., F.R.C.P.C.
Associate Professor
Department of Radiation Oncology
University of Toronto
Associate Director
Radiation Medicine Program
Princess Margaret Hospital
Department of Radiation Oncology
Princess Margaret Hospital
Toronto, Ontario, Canada

John F. Pallanch, M.D.
Ear, Nose, and Throat Consultant
Department of Surgery St. Lukes Medical Center
Merly Medical Center
Sioux City, Iowa

James N. Palmer, M.D.
Assistant Professor
Department of Otorhinolaryngology—Head and Neck Surgery
Hospital of the University of Pennsylvania
Philadelphia, Pennsylvania

Stephen S. Park, M.D., F.A.C.S.
Director
Division of Facial Plastic and Reconstructive Surgery
Associate Professor and Vice Chair
Department of Otolaryngology—Head and Neck Surgery
University of Virginia Health System
Charlottesville, Virginia

Nilesh Patel
Associate Adjunct Surgeon
Department of Otolaryngology—Head and Neck Surgery
New York University School of Medicine
New York, New York

G. Alexander Patterson, M.D.
Joseph C. Bancroft Professor of Surgery
Chief Section of General Thoracic Surgery Division of
	Cardiothoracic Surgery
Washington University School of Medicine
St. Louis, Missouri

Bruce W. Pearson, M.D., F.R.C.S., F.A.C.S.
Serene M. and Francis C. Durling Professor of
	Otolaryngology
Department of Otorhinolaryngology—Head and Neck Surgery
Mayo Clinic
Jacksonville, Florida

Phillip K. Pellitteri, D.O., F.A.C.S.
Associate Professor of Clinical Surgery
Penn State College of Medicine
Staff Attending
Section of Head and Neck Surgery
Department of Otolaryngology—Head and Neck Surgery
Geisinger Health System
Danville, Pennsylvania

Jonathan A. Perkins, D.O.
Assistant Professor
Department of Otolaryngology—Head and Neck Surgery
University of Washington School of Medicine
Attending Otolaryngologist
Department of Otolaryngology
Children's Hospital and Regional Medical Center
Seattle, Washington

Stephen W. Perkins, M.D., F.A.C.S.
Private Practice
Meridian Plastic Surgery Center
Department of Otolaryngology—Head and Neck Surgery
Indiana University School of Medicine
Indianapolis, Indiana
Perkins Van Natta Center for Cosmetic Surgery and
    Medical Skincare
Indianapolis, Indiana

Shirley Pignatari, M.D., Ph.D.
Associate Professor and Head
Division of Pediatric Otolaryngology
Department of Otolaryngology—Head and Neck Surgery
Federal University of Saõ Paulo
Sao Paul, Brazil

Randall L. Plant, M.D., M.S., F.A.C.S.
Department of Otolaryngology—Head and Neck
    Surgery
Alaska Native Medical Center
Anchorage, Alaska

Steven D. Pletcher, M.D.
Resident
Department of Otolaryngology—Head and Neck
    Surgery
University of California, San Francisco
San Francisco, California

Gregory N. Postma, M.D.
Associate Professor
Department of Otolaryngology—Head and Neck
    Surgery
Wake Forest University School of Medicine
Winston-Salem, North Carolina

William P. Potsic, M.D., MM
E. Mortimer Newlin Professor
Department of Otorhinolaryngology—Head and
    Neck Surgery
University of Pennsylvania Medical Center
Medical Director
Pediatric Cochlear Implant Program
Medical Director
The Center for Pediatric Childhood
    Communication
Director
Department of Otolaryngology
The Children's Hospital of Philadelphia
Philadelphia, Pennsylvania

Vito C. Quatela, M.D.
The Lindsay House Center for Cosmetic and
    Reconstructive Surgery
Rochester, New York

C. Rose Rabinov, M.D.
Bakersfield, California

Reza Rahbar, M.D., D.M.D.
Associate in Otolaryngology
Department of Otolaryngology and Communication
    Disorders
Children's Hospital
Assistant Professor
Department of Otology and Laryngology
Harvard Medical School
Boston, Massachusetts

Gregory W. Randolph, M.D., F.A.C.S.
Assistant Professor
Department of Otolaryngology—Head and Neck
    Surgery
Harvard Medical School
Director
Endocrine Surgery
Director
General Otolaryngology
Director
General and Thyroid Services
Department of Otolaryngology—Head and Neck
    Surgery
Massachusetts Eye and Ear Infirmary
Boston, Massachusetts

Christopher H. Rassekh, M.D.
Director
Head and Neck Oncology and Reconstructive Surgery
Co-Director
Center for Cranial Base Surgery
Associate Professor
Department of Otolaryngology—Head and Neck
    Surgery
West Virginia University
Morgantown, West Virginia

Steven D. Rauch, M.D.
Associate Professor
Department of Otology and Laryngology
Harvard Medical School
Coordinator
Medical Student Education
Department of Otolaryngology—Head and Neck Surgery
Massachusetts Eye and Ear Infirmary
Boston, Massachusetts

Lou Reinisch, Ph.D.
Associate Professor
Department of Physics and Astronomy
University of Canterbury
Christchurch, New Zealand

Dale H. Rice, M.D.
Professor and Chair
Department of Otolaryngology—Head and Neck
    Surgery
University of Southern California Keck School of Medicine
Los Angeles, California

Mark A. Richardson, M.D.
Professor and Chairman
Department of Otolaryngology—Head and Neck
    Surgery
Oregon Health and Sciences University
Portland, Oregon

K. Thomas Robbins, M.D.
Professor and Chair
Division of Otolaryngology
Department of Surgery
Southern Illinois University School of Medicine
Springfield, Illinois

Kimsey Rodriguez
Resident
Department of Otolaryngology
Tulane University
New Orleans, Louisiana

Richard M. Rosenfeld, M.D., M.P.H.
Director
Department of Pediatric Otolaryngology
Long Island College Hospital
Professor
Department of Otolaryngology—Head and Neck
    Surgery
Downstate Medical Center, S.U.N.Y.
Brooklyn, New York

Jason K. Rockhill, M.D., Ph.D.
Assistant Professor
Department of Radiation Oncology
University of Washington School of Medicine
Seattle, Washington

Jay T. Rubinstein, M.D., Ph.D.
Associate Professor
Department of Otolaryngology
Associate Professor
Department of Physiology and Biophysics
Associate Professor
Department of Otolaryngology—Head and Neck
    Surgery
Iowa City, Iowa

**Michael J. Ruckenstein, M.D., M.Sc., F.A.C.S.,
    F.R.C.S.C**
Associate Professor
Department of Otorhinolaryngology—Head and Neck
    Surgery
University of Pennsylvania Medical Center
Philadelphia, Pennsylvania

Christina L. Runge-Samuelson, Ph.D.
Assistant Professor
Department of Otolaryngology and Communication
    Sciences
Koss Cochlear Implant Program
Medical College of Wisconsin
Milwaukee, Wisconsin

Cynda Hylton Rushton, D.N.Sc., R.N.
Assistant Professor
Undergraduate Instruction
Johns Hopkins School of Nursing
Baltimore, Maryland

Leonard P. Rybak, M.D., Ph.D.
Professor
Division of Otolaryngology—Head and Neck
    Surgery
Department of Surgery
Southern Illinois School of Medicine
Springfield, Illinois

Alain N. Sabri, M.D.
Assistant Professor and Consultant
Department of Otorhinolaryngology—Head and Neck
    Surgery
Mayo Clinic and Mayo Graduate School of Medicine
Rochester, Minnesota

John R. Salassa, M.D.
Assistant Professor
Department of Otorhinolaryngology—Head and Neck
    Surgery
Mayo Clinic
Jacksonville, Florida

Thomas J. Salinas, D.D.S., M.S.
Assistant Professor
Section of Maxillofacial Prosthodontics
Department of Otolaryngology—Head and Neck Surgery
University of Nebraska Medical Center
Omaha, Nebraska

Sandeep Samant, M.D., F.R.C.S.
Assistant Professor
Department of Otolaryngology—Head and Neck Surgery
University of Tennessee Health Science Center
Memphis, Tennessee

Robin A. Samlan, M.S., CCC-SLP
Department of Otolaryngology—Head and Neck Surgery
Center for Laryngeal and Voice Disorders
The Johns Hopkins University
Baltimore, Maryland

Ravi N. Samy, M.D.
Assistant Professor
Department of Otolaryngology—Head and Neck Surgery
University of Texas Southwestern Medical Center at Dallas
Dallas, Texas

Peter A. Santi, Ph.D.
Director
Cochlear Anatomy Laboratory
Professor
Department of Otolaryngology
University of Minnesota, Twin Cities
Minneapolis, Minnesota

Steven D. Schaefer, M.D.
Professor and Chairman
Department of Otolaryngology—Head and Neck Surgery
New York Eye and Ear Infirmary
New York, New York

Richard L. Scher, M.D.
Assistant Clinical
Professor Division of Otolaryngology—Head and Neck
    Surgery
Department of Surgery
Duke University Medical Center
Durham, North Carolina

David A. Schessel, Ph.D., M.D.
Associate Professor
Departments of Otolaryngology and Neurosurgery
George Washington University School of Medicine
    and Health Sciences
Washington DC

Joshua S. Schindler, M.D.
Clinical Instructor
Department of Otolaryngology
Vanderbilt University Medical Center
Nashville, Tennessee

Cecelia E. Schmalbach, M.D.
Chief Resident and House Officer
Core Otolaryngology
Department of Otolaryngology—Head and Neck
    Surgery
University of Michigan Health System
Ann Arbor, Michigan

Ilona M. Schmalfuss, M.D.
Assistant Professor
Department of Radiology
University of Florida
Gainesville, Florida

David E. Schuller, M.D.
Professor and Chairman
Department of Otolaryngology
Director
Arthur G. James Cancer Hospital and Richard J. Solove
    Research Institute
Deputy Director
Comprehensive Cancer Center
The Ohio State University
Columbus, Ohio

James J. Sciubba, D.M.D., Ph.D.
Professor
Department of Otolaryngology—Head and Neck
    Surgery
Dental and Oral Medicine
The Johns Hopkins School of Medicine
Baltimore, Maryland

Jon K. Shallop, Ph.D.
Consultant and Associate Professor
Department of Otorhinolaryngology
Mayo Clinic and College of Medicine
Rochester, Minnesota

Clough Shelton, M.D., F.A.C.S.
Medical Director
Otolaryngology Clinic
Neurotology Fellowship Program
Director
Residency Program
Professor and Assistant Chief
Division of Otolaryngology—Head and Neck
    Surgery
University of Utah Medical School
Salt Lake City, Utah

Neil T. Shepard, Ph.D.
Director
The Balance Center
University of Pennsylvania Medical Center
Professor
Department of Otorhinolaryngology—Head and Neck
    Surgery
University of Pennsylvania School of Medicine
Philadelphia, Pennsylvania

Samuel G. Shiley, M.D.
Resident
Department of Otolaryngology—Head and Neck Surgery
Oregon Health and Science University
Portland, Oregon

Edward J. Shin, M.D.
Assistant Professor
Department of Otolaryngology—Head and Neck Surgery
Mt. Sinai Medical Center
Regional Director
Department of Otolaryngology—Head and Neck
    Surgery
Elmhurst Medical Center
Elmhurst, New York

Jonathan A. Ship, D.M.D.
Professor
Departments of Oral Medicine and Medicine
Director
New York University Bluestone Center for Clinical Research
New York University College of Dentistry
New York, New York

Kevin A. Shumrick, M.D.
Professor
Department of Otolaryngology—Head and Neck Surgery
University of Cincinnati Medical Center
Cincinnati, Ohio

Kathleen C.Y. Sie, M.D.
Assistant Professor
Department of Otolarygnology—Head and Neck Surgery
University of Washington Medical Center
Assistant Professor
Division of Pediatric Otolaryngology—Head and Neck
    Surgery
Children's Hospital and Medical Center
Seattle, Washington

Patricia Silva, M.D.
Sacramento Radiology Medical Group, Inc.
Sacramento, California

Alfred Simental, M.D.
Chief
Department of Otolaryngology—Head and Neck
    Surgery
Loma Linda University School of Medicine
Loma Linda, California

Ranjiv Sivanandan, M.D.
Clinical Instructor
Department of Otolaryngology—Head and Neck
    Surgery
Stanford University School of Medicine
Stanford, California

Marshall E. Smith, M.D., F.A.A.P., F.A.C.S.
Associate Professor
Department of Otolaryngology—Head and Neck Surgery
University of Utah School of Medicine
Salt Lake City, Utah

Richard J.H. Smith, M.D.
Professor
Interdepartmental Genetics Ph.D. Program
Professor and Vice Chairman
Department of Otolaryngology—Head and Neck
    Surgery
University of Iowa Hospitals and Clinics
Iowa City, Iowa

Russell Smith, M.D.
Assistant Professor
Department of Otolaryngology—Head and Neck Surgery
University of Iowa Hospitals and Clinics
Iowa City, Iowa

Robert A. Sofferman, M.D.
Professor and Chief
Division of Otolaryngology—Head and Neck Surgery
University of Vermont School of Medicine
Burlington, Vermont

Peter S. Staats, M.D.
Associate Professor
Department of Oncology
Associate Professor
Department of Anesthesia and Critical Care Medicine
Johns Hopkins University School of Medicine
Anesthesiology and Critical Care Medicine
Division of Pain Medicine
Baltimore, Maryland

Hinrich Staecker, M.D.
Assistant Professor
Division of Otolaryngology—Head and Neck Surgery
University of Maryland Hospital-North
Baltimore, Maryland

Aldo Cassol Stamm, M.D., Ph.D.
Professor
Department of Otolaryngology—Head and Neck
    Surgery
Federal University Sao Paulo
Director ENT Sao Paulo Center
Professor
Edmundo Vasconcelos Hospital
Sao Paulo, Brazil

James A. Stankiewicz, M.D.
Professor, Vice Chairman, and Residency Program
    Director
Department of Otolaryngology—Head and Neck Surgery
Loyola University Medical Center
Maywood, Illinois

Laura M. Sterni, M.D.
Assistant Professor
Division of Pediatric Pulmonary Medicine
Department of Pediatrics
The Johns Hopkins Children's Center
Baltimore, Maryland

Holger Sudhoff, M.D.
Associate Professor and Vice Chairman
Department of Otolaryngology—Head and Neck
    Surgery
University of Bochum
St. Elisabeth Hospital
Bochum, Germany

James Y. Suen, M.D., F.A.C.S.
Professor and Chairman
Department of Otolaryngology—Head and Neck
    Surgery
University of Arkansas for Medical Sciences
Little Rock, Irkansas

John B. Sunwoo, M.D.
Assistant Professor
Department of Otolaryngology—Head and Neck Surgery
Washington University School of Medicine
St. Louis, Missouri

Neil A. Swanson, M.D.
Professor and Chairman
Department of Dermatology
Oregon Health and Science University
Portland, Oregon

Veronica C. Swanson, M.D.
Director
Pediatric Cardiac Anesthesiology
Assistant Professor
Department of Anesthesiology and Peri-Operative Medicine
Oregon Health and Science University
Portland, Oregon

Jonathan M. Sykes, M.D., F.A.C.S.
Professor
Facial Plastic and Reconstructive Surgery
Department of Otolaryngology—Head and Neck Surgery
University of California, Davis Medical Center
Sacramento, California

M. Eugene Tardy, Jr., M.D., F.A.C.S.
Professor of Clinical Otolaryngology
Division of Facial Plastic and Reconstructive Surgery
Department of Otolaryngology—Head and Neck Surgery
University of Illinois at Chicago
Chicago, Illinois

Sherard A. Tatum III, M.D.
Director
Division of Facial Plastic Surgery
Director
Center for Cleft and Craniofacial Disorders
Associate Professor
Department of Otolaryngology and Communication Sciences
Upstate Medical University, S.U.N.Y.
Syracuse, New York

Helene M. Taylor, M.S., CCC-SLP
Speech and Language Therapy
Primary Children's Medical Center
Salt Lake City, Utah

S. Mark Taylor, M.D., F.R.C.S.C.
Assistant Professor
Division of Otolaryngology
Department of Surgery
Dalhousie University
Halifax, Nova Scotia, Canada

Steven A. Telian, M.D.
John L. Kemink Professor of Otorhinolaryngology
Director
Division of Otology, Neurotology, and Skull Base Surgery
Medical Director
Cochlear Implant Program
Department of Otolaryngology—Head and Neck Surgery
University of Michigan Medical Center
Alfred Taubman Health Care Center
Ann Arbor, Michigan

David J. Terris, M.D., F.A.C.S.
Porubsky Distinguished Professor and Chairman
Department of Otolaryngology—Head and Neck Surgery
Medical College of Georgia
Augusta, Georgia

J. Regan Thomas, M.D., F.A.C.S.
Francis L. Lederer Professor and Chairman
Department of Otolaryngology—Head and Neck Surgery
University of Illinois at Chicago
Chicago, Illinois

James N. Thompson, M.D., F.A.C.S.
President and CEO
Federation of State Medical Boards of the United States
Clinical Professor
Department of Otolaryngology
University of Texas Southwestern Medical Center at Dallas
Dallas, Texas

Robert J. Tibesar, M.D.
Resident
Department of Otorhinolaryngology
Mayo Clinic
Rochester, Minnesota

Evan J. Tobin, M.D.
Clinical Assistant Professor
Department of Otolaryngology
The Ohio State University School of Medicine
Columbus, Ohio

Travis T. Tollefson, M.D.
Fellow
Facial Plastic and Reconstructive Surgery
Department of Otolaryngology—Head and Neck Surgery
University of California, Davis Medical Center
Sacramento, California

Dean M. Toriumi, M.D.
Department of Otolaryngology—Head and Neck Surgery
University of Illinois at Chicago Medical Center
Chicago, Illinois

Joseph B. Travers, Ph.D.
Associate Professor
Department of Psychology
College of Social and Behavioral Sciences
Professor
Section of Oral Biology
Department of Dentistry
The Ohio State University
Columbus, Ohio

Susan P. Travers, Ph.D.
Associate Professor
Department of Psychology
College of Social and Behavioral Sciences
Professor
Section of Oral Biology
Department of Dentistry
The Ohio State University
Columbus, Ohio

Robert J. Troell, M.D., F.A.C.S.
Director
The Center for Facial Plastic and Reconstructive
    Surgery
Las Vegas, Nevada

Terrance T. Tsue, M.D., F.A.C.S.
Associate Professor, Co-Vice Chairman, and Residency
    Program Director
Department of Otolaryngology—Head and Neck
    Surgery
University of Kansas Medical Center
Kansas City, Kansas

Ralph P. Tufano, M.D.
Assistant Professor
Department of Otolaryngology—Head and Neck Surgery
Johns Hopkins University School of Medicine
Baltimore, Maryland

David E. Tunkel, M.D., F.A.A.P., F.A.C.S.
Associate Professor
Department of Otolaryngology—Head and Neck Surgery
Department of Pediatrics
Director
Division of Pediatric Otolaryngology
Department of Otolaryngology—Head and Neck Surgery
Johns Hopkins University School of Medicine
Baltimore, Maryland

Ravindra Uppaluri, M.D., Ph.D.
Assistant Professor
Department of Otolaryngology—Head and Neck Surgery
Washington University School of Medicine
St. Louis, Missouri

Mark L. Urken, M.D.
Professor
Derald H. Ruttenberg Cancer Center
Professor and Chair
Department of Otolaryngology—Head and Neck Surgery
Mount Sinai School of Medicine
New York, New York

Michael F. Vaezi, M.D., Ph.D.
Staff
Center for Swallowing and Esophageal Disorders
Department of Gastroenterology and Hepatology
Cleveland Clinic Foundation
Cleveland, Ohio

Thierry Van Den Abbeele, M.D.
Chief
Department of Otolaryngology—Head and Neck Surgery
Hôpital Robert Debré
Paris, France

Jason F. Vollweiler, M.D., Ph.D.
Chief Fellow
Department of Gastroenterology and Hepatology
Cleveland Clinic Foundation
Cleveland, Ohio

Phillip A. Wackym, M.D., F.A.C.S.
Chief
Division of Otology and Neurotologic Skull Base Surgery
Medical Director Koss Hearing and Balance Center
Residency Program Director
John C. Koss Professor and Chairman
Department of Otolaryngology and Communication
    Sciences
Medical College of Wisconsin
Milwaukee, Wisconsin

David L. Walner, M.D., M.S.
Assistant Professor
Department of Otolaryngology and Bronchoesophagology
Rush Presbyterian St. Luke's Medical Center
Chicago, Illinois

Edward J. Walsh, Ph.D.
Staff Scientist
Developmental Auditory Physiology Laboratory
Boys Town National Research Hospital
Omaha, Nebraska

Tom D. Wang, M.D., F.A.C.S.
Professor
Division of Facial Plastic and Reconstructive Surgery
Department of Otolaryngology—Head and Neck Surgery
Oregon Health and Sciences University
Portland, Oregon

Randal S. Weber, M.D.
Professor and Chair
Department of Head and Neck Surgery
MD Anderson Cancer Center
Houston, Texas

Harrison G. Weed, M.S., M.D., F.A.C.P.
Associate Professor
Division of General Internal Medicine
Department of Internal Medicine
The Ohio State University Medical Center
Columbus, Ohio

Richard O. Wein, M.D.
Assistant Professor
Department of Otolaryngology and Communicative Sciences
University of Mississippi Medical Center
Jackson, Mississippi

Gregory S. Weinstein, M.D., F.A.C.S.
Associate Director
Center for Head and Neck Cancer
Associate Professor
Department of Otorhinolaryngology
University of Pennsylvania Medical Center
Philadelphia, Pennsylvania

Ralph F. Wetmore, M.D.
Professor
Department of Otorhinolaryngology—Head and Neck Surgery
University of Pennsylvania Medical Center
Director
Pediatric Otolaryngology Fellowship Program,
Attending Surgeon
Department of Otolaryngology
The Children's Hospital of Pennsylvania
Philadelphia, Pennsylvania

Ernest A. Weymuller, Jr., M.D.
Professor and Chairman
Department of Otolaryngology—Head and Neck Surgery
University of Washington Medical Center
Seattle, Washington

Brian J. Wiatrak, M.D.
Clinical Associate Professor
Department of Surgery and Pediatrics
Chief
Department of Pediatric Otolaryngology
Pediatric ENT Associates
Children's Hospital of Alabama
Birmingham, Alabama

J. Paul Willging, M.D.
Associate Professor
Department of Pediatric Otolaryngology
Cincinnati Children's Hospital Medical Center
Cincinnati, Ohio

Michael A. Williams, M.D.
Co-Chair
Ethics Committee and Consultation Service
The Johns Hopkins Hospital
Faculty Associate
The Johns Hopkins University School of Nursing
Assistant Professor
Departments of Neurology and Neurosurgery
The Johns Hopkins University School of Medicine
Baltimore, Maryland

Franz J. Wippold II, M.D., F.A.C.S.
Chief
Neuroradiology Section
Professor of Radiology
Division of Diagnostic Radiology
Department of Radiology
Mallinckrodt Institute of Radiology
Washington University School of Medicine
St. Louis, Missouri

Matthew Wolpoe, M.D.
Fellow
Department of Otolaryngology—Head and Neck Surgery
Johns Hopkins University School of Medicine
Baltimore, Maryland

Gayle Ellen Woodson, M.D.
Professor and Residency Program Director
Division of Otolaryngology
Southern Illinois University School of Medicine
Springfield, Illinois

Audie L. Woolley, M.D., F.A.C.S.
Associate Professor
Department of Surgery
Associate Professor
Department of Pediatric Otolaryngology
Medical Director
Cochlear Implant Program
Children's Hospital of Alabama
Birmingham, Alabama

Charles D. Yingling, Ph.D., D.A.B.N.M.
Department of Otolaryngology—Head and Neck Surgery
Stanford University School of Medicine
Yingling Neurophysiology Associates
Sausalito, California

Bevan Yueh, M.D., M.P.H.
Associate Professor
Department of Otolaryngology—Head and Neck Surgery
Department of Health Services
University of Washington
VA Puget Sound Health Care System
Seattle, Washington

Rex Yung, M.D., F.C.C.P.
Assistant Professor
Medicine and Oncology
Director
Bronchology and Pulmonary Oncology
Division of Pulmonary and Critical Care Medicine
Johns Hopkins University School of Medicine
Baltimore, Maryland

George H. Zalzal, M.D.
Professor
Departments of Otolaryngology and Pediatrics
The George Washington University Medical Center
Chairman
Department of Otolaryngology—Head and Neck Surgery
Children's National Medical Center
Washington DC

David S. Zee, M.D.
Director
Vestibular/Eye Movement Testing Laboratory
Professor
Department of Neurology, Otolaryngology, Ophthalmology,
    and Neuroscience
Johns Hopkins School of Medicine
The Johns Hopkins Hospital
Baltimore, Maryland

Jacob W. Zeiders, M.D.
Resident
Department of Otolaryngology—Head and Neck Surgery
University of South Florida
Tampa, Florida

Marc S. Zimbler, M.D.
Attending
Department of Otolaryngology—Head and Neck Surgery
Director
Facial Plastic and Reconstructive Surgery
Beth Israel Deaconess Medical Center
Associate Adjunct Professor
New York Eye and Ear Infirmary
New York, New York

S. James Zinreich, M.D.
Professor
Department of Otolaryngology—Head and Neck Surgery
Professor
Department of Radiology and Radiological Science
Division of Neuroradiology
The Johns Hopkins Hospital
Baltimore, Maryland

Teresa A. Zwolan, Ph.D.
Associate Professor
Department of Otolaryngology—Head and Neck Surgery
University of Michigan Medical Center
Director
Cochlear Implant Program
Hearing Rehabilitation Center
Ann Arbor, Michigan

Preface

Otolaryngology—Head & Neck Surgery was created to fill the need for a contemporary, definitive textbook on the specialty of otolaryngology—head and neck surgery. The scope of the fourth edition is a testimonial to the tremendous expansion of knowledge in this specialty. Our desire is to record this expansion in a retrievable fashion so that these volumes become indispensable reference works. The fourth edition builds on the success of the past three editions. The reader will note the continued use of algorithms and boxed lists, which serve to enhance learning.

The field of otolaryngology—head and neck surgery is represented in all of its diversity; the extensive interrelationship of its various components provided the skeleton for the table of contents. These volumes are intended as a detailed reference text and not as a surgical atlas; a definitive work, not an introductory overview. It is designed for residents and practitioners alike. We hope that our quest to document significant and up-to-date information in the specialty has been successful.

Another of our goals throughout the pages of this textbook is to acknowledge all those who have contributed to the specialty. Since significant medical expertise has no geographic boundaries, there are contributors from countries all over the world.

To ensure continuity at the editorship level, Drs. Paul Flint, Bruce Haughey, K. Thomas Robbins, and J. Regan Thomas have assumed editorship roles in this expanded effort. It is hoped that the ecumenicism which combines the effort of all the contributors will further the excellence of those now associated with otolaryngology—head and neck surgery and provide the foundation for continued progress by the generations to follow. This fourth edition builds on the success of the first three. It is more comprehensive, is of broader scope, and continues the tradition established 18 years ago.

Acknowledgment

I would like to acknowledge my father for enabling me to survive comfortably during my seemingly endless years of education. As well, my wife, Jane, and my family who have recognized the importance of and supported the mission that resulted in this resource for *Otolaryngology—Head & Neck Surgery*. I would also like to acknowledge the students and residents who are constant sources of motivation and the patients who served as the fuel that energized this project. Through their coping with illness, we are constantly aware that our search for resolution of illness must continue.

Charles W. Cummings

For those individuals privileged to serve and train under Dr. Charles Cummings, we recognize him as mentor, colleague and friend, physician and healer; we are grateful for his leadership and everlasting imprint on our mission in academic medicine.

Charlie, thank you. From your student, colleague, and friend,

Paul W. Flint

Scientific knowledge is only contemporary; a portion of what we know today is true, but much will soon be disproven or rendered obsolete. Galen was as right in his day as we are in ours. The authors have done a superb job of presenting today's knowledge. My contribution is dedicated to my wife Jill and our children Elizabeth, Robert, and Alexa.

Lee Harker

It has been a distinct honor and pleasure to be part of the editorial and publishing team assembled for this edition of *Otolaryngology—Head & Neck Surgery*. The authors have been tireless in their efforts and have worked strongly to produce chapters that are truly comprehensive in scope and depth. My sincere thanks go to each one of them and their families, who inevitably have put up with liberal amounts of "burning the midnight oil." My loyal assistant of 14 years, Debbie Turner, has kept us up to our deadlines and liaised with both authors and publishers in a highly organized way, while my office nurses Shannon Daut, Fernanda Polesel, Teresa Bieg, and Joan Martin have provided generous amounts of patient care to cover for my time away from the front lines during this textbook's creation. The residents and fellows at Washington University in St. Louis have similarly "held the fort" when necessary in the interests of this publication.

The ability to purvey knowledge starts, and continues, with one's education, for which thanks go to my parents, the late Thomas, and Marjorie Haughey, my teachers, medical professors, Otolaryngology residency mentors in Auckland, New Zealand and the University of Iowa, and colleagues in the specialty, from whom I have and will continue to learn.

My family has unswervingly endorsed the time required for this project, so heartfelt love and thanks go to my wife, Helen, as well as Rachel, Jack, Chris, Will, and Gretchen.

Finally, as we enjoy the teaching of this book and its ensuing online updates, readers are encouraged to keep in mind the source of all knowledge and truth: in the words of Proverbs 2 v.6 "... the Lord gives wisdom and from his mouth come knowledge and understanding." My sincere hope is that the readers everywhere will benefit from this textbook, better accomplishing our specialty's common goal of top quality patient care.

Bruce H. Haughey

The process of learning is truly lifelong. Participating in the creation of this text allows another way for me to continue to become invigorated and inspired by my specialty field. To my invaluable support mechanism, my wife, children, and family. Thank you.

Mark Richardson

It is a great honor to serve as an editor of this important textbook. I am deeply appreciative for this opportunity and the support of my co-editors. While there are many individuals who have influenced my career, I want to acknowledge the mentoring of John Fredricksen, Douglas Bryce, the late Sir Donald Harrison, Robert Byers, Oscar Guillamondegui, Helmuth Goepfert, Robert Jahrsdoerfer, Charles Cummings, and Edwin Cocke. Also, I would like to remember and honor my parents, the late Elizabeth and Wycliffe Robbins, for the values they instilled in me. Finally, and most of all, I cherish the love and support of my wife Gayle Woodson and the children, Phil, Nick, Greg, and Sarah, who together provide the caring background for making it all meaningful.

K. Thomas Robbins

I have had the privilege of being involved with this textbook since its inception. The quality of this fourth edition reflects the talent and hard work of the numerous authors and the editorial staff of Elsevier. However, special gratitude is expressed to Charlie Cummings and the other editors for their strong leadership and ability to recruit this spectacular group of authors. These projects involve a huge effort and, once again, my great family has continued to be supportive of the effort necessary to turn this project into reality. Carole, Rebecca, and Mike, you are my primary motivators. You understand the need to be supportive of this multiprong attack using patient care, research, and education to expand our ability to help our patients. Our love for one another makes this effort worthwhile.

David E. Schuller

I am pleased to thank and acknowledge the great help and assistance provided by the administrative staff in the Department of *Otolaryngology—Head & Neck Surgery* at the University of Illinois at Chicago in editing this section. I would also like to thank my co-editor, David Schuller, M.D., with whom it was a genuine pleasure to work.

J. Regan Thomas

Table of Contents

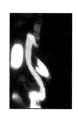

PART SEVEN

LARYNX/TRACHEA/BRONCHUS

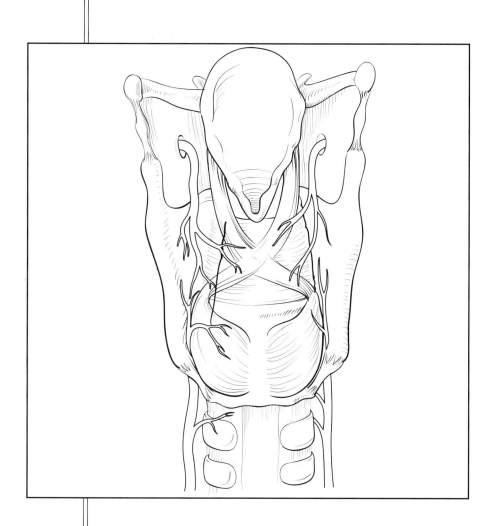

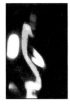

CHAPTER EIGHTY FIVE A

LARYNGEAL AND PHARYNGEAL FUNCTION

‖ Gayle E. Woodson

INTRODUCTION

The upper aerodigestive tract serves the competing functions of respiration and swallowing and, in humans, the added role of speech. Eating and breathing cannot be conducted simultaneously. Swallowing requires total collapse of the pharynx, whereas breathing requires active support to maintain its patency. During a swallow, the airway must be protected and the ingested material should be directed into the appropriate channel. The aspiration of food or foreign material can lead to serious consequences, such as asphyxia or lung infection. This complicated and potentially hazardous configuration results from embryology and reflects evolution.

The lower respiratory tract has evolved as an offshoot of the digestive tract, first appearing in the lungfish as a simple muscle sphincter to protect the lungs from water.[32] During embryologic development, the foregut is the common origin of the larynx and trachea. The nose is the primary respiratory orifice and the mouth is the portal for ingestion of food; both open into a common cavity, the pharynx. In infants and in all nonhuman mammals, the pharynx is functionally compartmentalized into separate passages for breathing and alimentation. The epiglottis interdigitates with the uvula to form a respiratory channel from the nose into the larynx and two lateral pathways from the mouth to the esophagus through the pyriform sinuses.[23] During postnatal development in humans, enlargement of the cranium with flexion of the base of the skull results in a downward displacement of the larynx. This displacement elongates the pharynx and distracts the uvula and epiglottis so that they are no longer in contact, resulting in a common pharyngeal cavity for breathing and swallowing (Figure 85A-1).[24,40] The larynx begins its descent at the age of about 18 to 24 months. The common chamber complicates functions that are vital to survival, although there are two positive outcomes. Vocal power is greater because of increased resonance, and articulatory diversity is expanded.[25]

Normal function of the larynx and pharynx requires precise timing and coordination of competing functions. The treatment of diseases and disorders of this region may have an impact on more than one system. It is imperative for otolaryngologists to understand the function of the upper aerodigestive tract as a unit and not just as the sum of the activities of component organs.

LARYNGEAL MOTION
Applied Anatomy

Until recent years, only limited information was available about the motions of the larynx because observation was primarily obtained by mirror laryngoscopy and fluoroscopy with contrast. Consequently, models of laryngeal motion have been primarily two-dimensional. Illustrations of the glottis in many textbooks are based on observations of mirror laryngoscopy. Vocal folds are depicted as opening and closing as though they were rigid linear structures, pivoting at the anterior commissure and moving solely in the axial plane. Details of motion in the posterior commissure have been largely ignored. These common misconceptions of laryngeal motion are at odds with the anatomy of the larynx as presented in anatomic descriptions dating back for hundreds of years.

Flexible endoscopy, stroboscopy, and computerized imaging have revealed that laryngeal motion is more complex than previously recognized. Commonly used terms for vocal fold position, such as *cadaveric* and *paramedian* are inadequate to reflect the three-dimensional configuration of the glottis.[46] Rather than merely opening and closing within a single plane, the vocal folds move in three dimensions, and length and shape may be actively altered (Figure 85A-2).[18]

Moreover, segmental compartmentalization within intrinsic laryngeal muscles suggests the capability for intricate fine control. For example, the human posterior cricoarytenoid muscle is divided into two compartments.[48] These are supplied by separate nerve

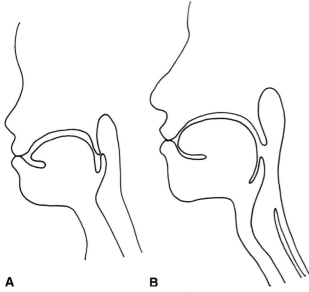

Figure 85A-1. Postnatal descent of the larynx. Migration of epiglottis away from the uvula results in loss of pharyngeal compartmentalization for breathing and feeding. **A,** Sagittal view through the head and neck of a neonate. **B,** Sagittal view through an adult head and neck.

branches; they differ in fiber type composition, and they insert on opposing sides of the muscular process (Figure 85A-3).[6,36] The human thyroarytenoid muscle has long been regarded to have a separate medial compartment, the "vocalis" muscle.

The specific mechanisms responsible for each motion of the larynx are not known, although certain fundamental principles of laryngeal motion are apparent. The actively moving parts of the larynx are the arytenoids. Vocal fold abduction and adduction result from movement of the vocal processes of the arytenoids relative to the anterior commissure. The anterior ends of the vocal folds are stationary, being fixed to the thyroid cartilage at the anterior commissure. The posterior ends are attached to the arytenoids, which articulate with the cricoid cartilage via shallow ball-and-socket–type joints. Motion of the vocal process, and hence the vocal fold, results from contraction of muscles directly attached to the arytenoid or from force transmitted from other structures. As with any muscle, the specific action of a laryngeal muscle depends on its origin and insertion and on the mechanics of the involved joint or joints. For example, contraction of the posterior cricoarytenoid muscle pulls the muscular process posteriorly and caudally. The structure of the cricoarytenoid joint prevents the entire arytenoid from being pulled along this vector. Instead, the arytenoid rotates, displacing the vocal process upward and laterally, abducting the vocal fold (Figure 85A-4).[6] Conversely, the lateral cricoarytenoid muscle pulls the muscular process of the arytenoid anteriorly and caudally, which rotates the arytenoid, moving the vocal process medially and adducting the vocal fold. Contraction of the cricothyroid muscle increases the distance between the anterior commissure and the cricoid, increasing tension in the vocal fold and, consequently, pulling anteriorly on the arytenoid cartilage. Cervical strap muscle activity affects glottic function, and downward traction on the trachea with inspiration results in vocal fold abduction.[9,47] A second basic type of laryngeal motion is alteration of the shape of the membranous vocal fold.

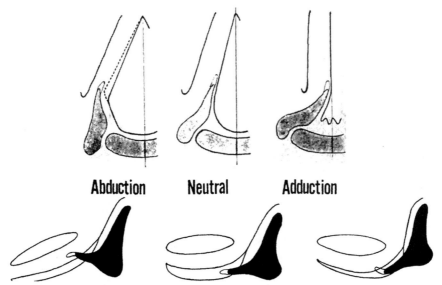

Figure 85A-2. Three-dimensional motion of the arytenoid cartilage and vocal fold. (From Hirano M: *Anatomy and behavior of the vocal process.* In Baer T, Sasaki C, Harris K, editors: *Laryngeal function in phonation and respiration,* Boston, 1987, College-Hill Press.)

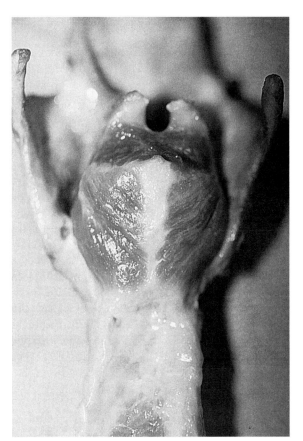

Figure 85A-3. Compartmentalization of the human posterior cricoarytenoid muscle. Posterior view of a cadaver larynx.

Cricothyroid muscle contraction can stretch the vocal fold and make it thinner. Active contraction of the thyroarytenoid muscle results in a shorter, thicker vocal fold (Figure 85A-5).

LARYNGEAL FUNCTION IN BREATHING

The primary and most primitive function of the larynx is to protect the lower airway. In evolution, the larynx first appeared as a sphincter to prevent the ingress of water into the airway of the lungfish.[32] Subsequently, dilator muscles evolved to permit active opening of the larynx. In more evolved animals, the larynx is not just an open or shut valve, but rather a variable resistor, capable of regulating airflow. Other laryngeal functions include the Valsalva maneuver and coughing. The larynx is also a sensory organ, providing information about airway function and the purity of inhaled air and serving in the afferent limb of many reflexes.

Protection

When the larynx is mechanically stimulated, the larynx closes abruptly and respiration ceases. Apnea can also occur in response to such diverse chemical agents as ammonia, phenyl diguanide, and cigarette smoke.

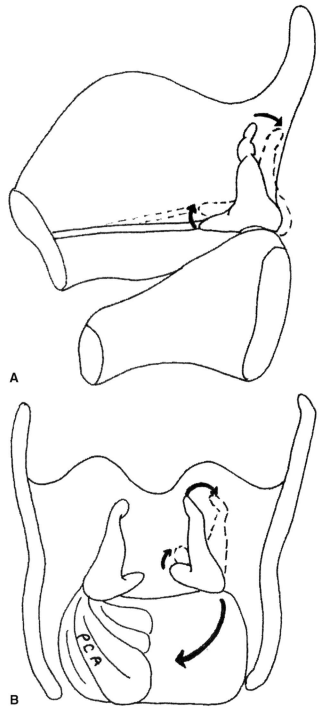

Figure 85A-4. Three-dimensional effects of posterior cricoarytenoid muscle contraction. **A,** Sagittal view. **B,** Posterior view.

These are appropriate and beneficial responses that prevent the entry of foreign matter into the lower airway, although strong laryngeal stimulation may result in responses that appear to be maladaptive, such as laryngospasm or prolonged bronchoconstriction.[27] These reflexes may be produced in experimental animals by electrical stimulation of the superior laryngeal nerve

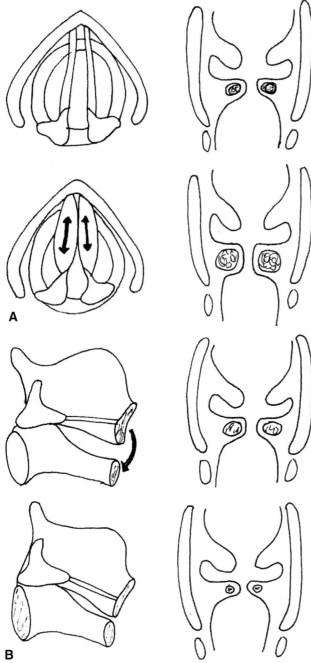

Figure 85A-5. Effects of **(A)** thyroarytenoid and **(B)** cricothyroid muscle contraction on the thickness of the vocal fold.

and probably represent an oversaturation of pathways that serve a useful function at lower levels of input.

The larynx occupies a protected position in the body, and it is rarely subject to direct stimulation. Therefore, laryngospasm and apnea are not everyday occurrences. Severe laryngeal reflexes are most often encountered in patients in the operating room in response to direct stimulation during intubation, endoscopy, or extubation. These reflexes most likely

occur in patients during light anesthesia and in those who are well oxygenated.

Recurrent paroxysmal laryngospasm is occasionally encountered in clinical practice. In some patients, this is caused by gastroesophageal reflux, which responds to acid-suppressing medication. In other patients, the pathophysiology appears to be a hypersensitive laryngeal closure reflex because patients report some triggering event such as eating or inhaling steam or odors. The onset frequently occurs during an upper respiratory infection, but it also can occur after surgical trauma to the recurrent laryngeal nerve. Most often, the condition resolves spontaneously within a few months, but it may become a permanent and debilitating problem. The laryngeal closure reflex is particularly sensitive in infants and can be elicited by a stimulus as weak as water. During early infancy, the strength of this reflex increases, then decreases, along a time course similar to that of the incidence of sudden infant death syndrome, suggesting that laryngeal reflexes may play a role in its cause.[39]

Cough

Another important protective reflex involving the larynx is the cough, which ejects mucus and foreign material from the lungs.[21] Cough can be a voluntary action or a reflexive response to stimulation of the larynx or receptors in the lungs. The cough reflex is suppressed during sleep, so that a greater stimulus is required with progressive stages of sleep. During deep sleep, a cough cannot be elicited unless the stimulus first results in arousal to a lighter level of sleep.

The first phase of a cough is inspiratory. The larynx opens widely to permit rapid and deep inhalation. In voluntary cough, the degree of inspiratory effort is varied according to the intended strength of the cough. The second phase is compressive, involving tight closure of the glottis and strong activation of expiratory muscles. The effectiveness of the cough is impaired by glottic incompetence. Finally, the larynx suddenly opens widely, resulting in a sudden and rapid outflow of air, at speeds of as much as 10 L/second. Cough plays an important role in cleaning the tracheobronchial tree and in maintaining patency of the lower airways. Abnormal cough can be a serious clinical problem that interferes with normal daily function and impairs quality of life.

Control of Ventilation

The role of the larynx as an active organ of respiration is not widely recognized. Abduction and adduction of the larynx in phase with respiration has been acknowledged for many years.[12,29] It has been postulated that all respiratory motion of the larynx is passive, resulting from biomechanical coupling of the larynx to the tracheobronchial tree.[9,44] There is some evidence that downward traction on the larynx dilates the glottis.[47] But clinical observations and experimental evidence indicate that the larynx moves actively in respiration and in fact plays an important role regulating respiration. The larynx is located at the entrance into the trachea and is capable not only of rapid opening and closure but also of sudden alterations in resistance. Hence, the larynx is better adapted than any other portion of the respiratory tract for regulating airflow. The resistance changes resulting from laryngeal responses to respiratory stimuli, such as negative airway pressure or blood gas changes, have a beneficial effect on ventilation.[37]

Widening of the glottis during inspiration is a primary action of ventilation that only ceases during deep anesthesia or sleep. The posterior cricoarytenoid muscle (PCA), the only active dilator of the larynx, begins to contract with each inspiration before activation of the diaphragm.[4,15,32]

The level of PCA activity, and hence laryngeal movement with breathing, varies. Laryngeal motion may be imperceptible during unlabored, quiet breathing. With increasing respiratory drive, peak inspiratory PCA activity increases proportionately with diaphragmatic activity. There are important differences between PCA and diaphragmatic behavior (Figure 85A-6). When the upper airway is partially occluded, inspiration generates negative airway pressure, which is a potent stimulus to the PCA and the several other upper airway muscles that dilate the upper airway.[26,37] In contrast, the diaphragm responds by actually decreasing inspiratory force and by increasing the duration of inspiration.[27] This response occurs because, during partial airway obstruction, the PCA and the diaphragm have opposing effects on patency of the lumen. Increasing diaphragmatic force increases the negative pressure, favoring airway collapse. To inspire the same volume, the diaphragm extends the duration of inspiration. PCA contraction dilates the airway, opposing the effects of the diaphragm. During strong respiratory demand, the PCA continues contracting during expiration after the diaphragm has relaxed, thus delaying expiratory adduction and facilitating the outflow of air. During panting, the glottis sustains an abducted posture, assuring maximal airflow. Because of these physiologic differences, the phrenic nerve is not an ideal choice for reinnervation of the PCA in patients with laryngeal paralysis.

There has been some controversy in the literature as to whether laryngeal adduction during expiration is an active or passive process. Some electromyographic (EMG) studies have failed to confirm any expiratory

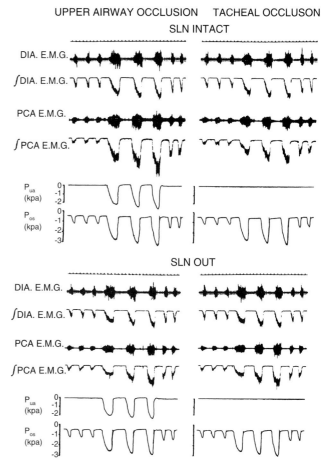

Figure 85A-6. Effects of upper airway and tracheal occlusions in an anesthetized dog, before and after a section of the superior laryngeal nerve (SLN). In each panel, the top trace is time in seconds, and the second and third traces are integrated electromyographic activity of the diaphragm and posterior cricoarytenoid muscle. The lower two traces in each panel are pressure in the upper airway and esophagus (intrathoracic pressure). Tracheal occlusion affects only intrathoracic pressure, whereas upper airway occlusion also affects upper airway pressure, which is sensed by the SLN. (From Sant'Ambrogio and others: *J Appl Physiol* 58:1298, 1985.)

activity of laryngeal adductor muscles, suggesting that expiratory narrowing of the glottis is passive, a result of relaxation of the PCA.[3,30] Other researchers have documented phasic expiratory activity of laryngeal adductors.[31,41] These conflicting observations have been reconciled by the finding that respiratory activity of laryngeal adductor muscles is much less consistent than that of the PCA. Expiratory adduction of the larynx is either active or passive, depending on breathing strategy. During baseline conditions, such as sleep, laryngeal adductor muscles are silent. During consciousness, expiratory activation of laryngeal adductor muscles is frequently detected, but at highly variable levels. Correlations of laryngeal adductory muscle activity with expiratory airflow, ventilatory pattern, and transglottal resistance suggest that this is an important mechanism for controlling the rate of breathing (Figure 85A-7).[22] Glottic adduction increases expiratory resistance to airflow, prolonging exhalation. During normal breathing conditions, respiratory rate is primarily controlled by varying the rate of exhalation.[13] Exhalation is slowed by partial contraction of the diaphragm during expiration. Abdominal muscle pushing increases the rate of exhalation, although during tidal breathing under baseline conditions, the larynx appears to be the primary mechanism for controlling the ventilatory pattern.

Laryngeal regulation of breathing is not essential for life, as evidenced by the fact that patients ventilate satisfactorily through a tracheotomy, although the inability to breathe and speak normally through natural orifices has a devastating impact on quality of life. Optimal function of the upper aerodigestive tract requires normal laryngeal function.

Sensory Receptors

The larynx is not only a motor organ. It also is the location of a variety of sensory receptors that exert influences on breathing and cardiovascular function. The larynx is densely supplied with sensory receptors; sensory fibers from the larynx are several times more numerous than those from the lungs. This is remarkable, considering that the internal surface area of the lungs is several square meters, whereas the larynx is a small orifice. Single nerve fiber recordings from the superior laryngeal nerve have identified three major types of laryngeal respiratory receptors: negative pressure, airflow, and "drive."[38] These receptors are activated by the process of breathing and have an influence on the central control of breathing. Airflow receptors actually respond to a decrease in temperature because the larynx is cooled by inspired air. Thus, flow receptors do not respond to air that has been warmed and humidified by the nose. They are activated by air that comes in through the mouth, particularly in cold and dry weather. "Drive" receptors are probably proprioceptors that respond to the respiratory motion of the larynx. Laryngeal sensation of touch and chemical stimuli are not activated during normal breathing conditions, but stimulation can profoundly affect ventilation.

Circulatory Reflexes

Stimulation of the larynx can alter heart rate and blood pressure. During induction of general anesthesia, endotracheal intubation can result in bradycardia. The direct result of experimental laryngeal stimulation on blood pressure is hypertension,[42] although in the clinical situation, the effects of bradycardia or ectopy usually prevail, resulting in hypotension. In patients with obstructive sleep apnea, negative airway pressure may stimulate receptors in the larynx so strongly that cardiac arrhythmias occur. Animal experiments show that the afferent limb is the superior laryngeal nerve because transection of this nerve abolishes cardiovascular responses (Figure 85A-8). The efferent limb for bradycardia is the vagus nerve, and the efferent limb for blood pressure elevation is via sympathetic nerve fibers, but intervening central connections have not been identified.[14]

PHARYNGEAL FUNCTION IN BREATHING

The upper airway is a conduit with several points wherein the shape and cross-sectional area can be dynamically altered. The pharynx is the largest but most compliant region, and it is susceptible to passive collapse. Maintenance of patency requires the action of striated upper airway muscles in coordination with the activity of respiratory pump muscles. Upper airway muscles also determine whether air is inspired through the nose or the mouth. The anatomy and intrinsic properties of upper airway muscles indicate that they are primarily adapted for nonrespiratory functions but can be used in respiratory tasks. Most of the muscles acting on the pharynx show no respiratory activity during awake, tidal breathing, but they are recruited by increased respiratory drive or upper airway obstruction (Figure 85A-9).[45]

In healthy patients, the nose is the preferred route of breathing because the relaxed position of the mandible

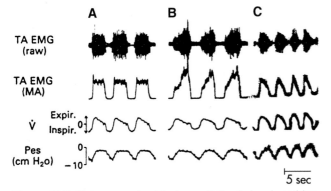

Figure 85A-7. Laryngeal adductor activity during breathing. TA EMG, Electromyography of thyroarytenoid muscle, raw, and averaged (MA). V̇, Aairflow; Pes, esophageal (intrathoracic) pressure. **A,** Plateau in TA activity correlates with decreasing flow. **B,** Progressive increase in TA activity correlates with flattened airflow trace and longer exhalation. **C,** Decreasing activity during expiration correlates with shorter exhalation. (From Kuna ST, Insalaco G, Woodson GE: *J Appl Physiol* 63:1332, 1988.)

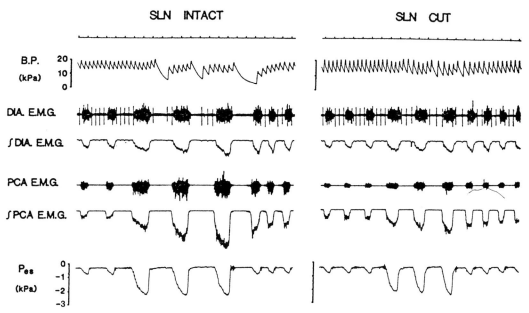

Figure 85A-8. The effects of upper airway occlusion on arterial blood pressure in an anesthetized dog before and after transection of the superior laryngeal nerve (SLN). (From Sant'Ambrogio and others: *J Appl Physiol* 58:1298, 1985.)

closes the mouth, and the relaxed palate occludes the oropharyngeal inlet. Furthermore, the nose warms, humidifies, and filters inspired air.[7] The selection of oral or nasal breathing is primarily accomplished by the soft palate, which is a band of moveable soft tissue suspended from the posterior bony palate. Oral breathing requires activation of the levator veli palatine to elevate the soft palate as well as activation of the musculus uvula. Nasal breathing is favored by con-

striction of the oropharyngeal passage, which is primarily accomplished by activation of the palatoglossal muscles, medialization of the faucial arches, and elevation of the base of tongue. This activity is most active during forced nasal breathing with the mouth open.[10]

Little objective information is available regarding the respiratory function of the pharyngeal constrictors. It is widely assumed that some degree of active tone in these muscles increases the stiffness of these muscles, thereby decreasing the tendency of the pharynx to collapse with the negative pressure generated during inspiration. Conversely, flaccidity of the constrictors is considered to destabilize the airway, promoting collapse, although there are no physical data to support this concept.[32] On the contrary, contraction of the constrictor muscles actively collapses the pharyngeal lumen. Spontaneous activity in the respiratory cycle has been detected in the superior constrictor muscle, but this activity occurs during the expiratory phase and disappears with bronchoconstriction, suggesting it plays a role in modulating expiratory airflow resistance.[8]

The dilator muscles of the pharynx are located anteriorly and laterally. The best-studied and probably most important pharyngeal dilator is the genioglossus (GG), a fan-shaped muscle that originates from the anterior mandible and spreads out to insert into the tongue. Although no studies have

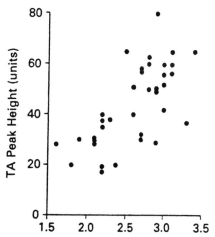

Figure 85A-9. The peak electromyography activity of the thyroarytenoid muscle (TA peak height) as a function of expiratory time in an awake human. Correlation coefficient = 0.680. (From Kuna ST, Insalaco G, Woodson GE: *J Appl Physiol* 63:1332, 1988.)

conclusively established what muscles are responsible for pulling the base of the tongue forward to dilate the airway, evidence strongly supports the role of the GG. In animal experiments, increased EMG activity of the GG is associated with a greater capacity of the pharynx to withstand negative collapsing pressure.[5] GG EMG activity reflexively increases in response to negative upper airway pressure (Figure 85A-10).[26,27] In humans with obstructive sleep apnea, decreased GG EMG activity has been noted during obstructive events, whereas obstruction is relieved with recovery of GG activity.[34]

The hyoid bone supports the hypopharynx. In humans, as in other primates, the hyoid does not articulate with any other skeletal element, but rather, it is suspended by muscles and ligaments. Contraction of muscles attached to the hyoid has been shown in animal experiments to increase the size and stability of the upper airway.[35] Muscles attached to the hyoid are also believed to resist the downward traction exerted on the airway by the trachea during inspiration.[1,10]

FUNCTION IN SPEECH

Human speech requires coordinated interaction of the mouth, pharynx, larynx, lungs, diaphragm, and abdominal and neck muscles. There are three fundamental components in the processes: phonation, resonance, and articulation. *Phonation* is the generation of sound by vibration of the vocal folds. *Resonance* is the induction of vibration in the rest of the vocal tract

to modulate laryngeal output. *Articulation* is the shaping of the voice into words.

Phonation

The role of the larynx in sound production has been recognized for centuries,[11] although the mechanism of how the larynx generates sound from exhaled air has not been clear until recently. In 1950, Husson[19] presented the neurochronaxic hypothesis, which held that glottic vibrations were caused by rhythmic impulses in the nerves to the larynx, synchronous with the frequency of the sound produced, so that each vibratory cycle was caused by a separate neural impulse. This hypothesis is physiologically impossible. It is currently accepted that the interaction of aerodynamic forces and the mechanical properties of the laryngeal tissues are responsible for generating vocal sound.[43]

Normal phonation requires that five conditions be satisfied, as listed in Box 85A-1. There should be adequate breath support to provide power, and the vibratory edges of the vocal folds should be aligned and separated by an appropriately small gap. The physical properties of the vocal fold should be conducive to vibration, and its three-dimensional contour should be favorable. Finally, a normal voice requires volitional control of glottic length, tension, and shape.

The process of phonation begins with the inhalation of air, and then glottic closure, to position the vocal folds near the midline. A simplified explanation of phonation is that exhalation causes subglottic pressure to increase until the vocal folds are displaced laterally, producing a sudden decrease in subglottic pressure. The forces that contribute to the return of the vocal folds to the midline include this pressure decrease, elastic forces in the vocal fold, and the Bernoulli effect of airflow. When the vocal folds return to the midline, pressure in the trachea builds again, and the cycle is repeated. Vocal fold structure determines whether the resulting vibration is periodic or chaotic.

Actual phonation is more complex than the previous model because the vocal fold is not a homogenous structure and also because it vibrates in three

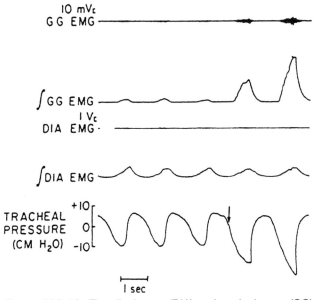

Figure 85A-10. The diaphragm (DIA) and genioglossus (GG) muscle response to nasal occlusion (beginning at arrow) in an anesthetized vagotomized rabbit. (From Mathew OP, Abu-Osba YK, Thach BT: *J Appl Physiol* 52:483, 1982.)

BOX 85A-1
REQUIREMENTS FOR PHONATION

Adequate breath support
Approximation of vocal folds
Favorable vibratory properties
Favorable vocal fold shape
Control of length and tension

dimensions.[2] Moreover, the pattern of vibration varies with pitch and vocal register. The "body-cover" concept of phonation is that vibration of the mucosa does not correspond directly to that of the rest of the vocal fold.[17] Instead, the "body" of the vocal fold is relatively static, whereas the wave is propagated in the mucosal "cover." This mucosal wave begins on the inferomedial aspect of the vocal fold and moves rostrally (Figure 85A-11). As the superior edges of the vocal fold begin to separate, the lower edges close, and this temporal relationship is accounted for by Ishizaka's two-mass model.[20] As the superior edges of the vocal folds separate, airflow through the divergent glottis generates greater negative pressure at the lower edge of the vocal folds, accelerating closure of the inferior glottis. The body-cover theory and two-mass model are consistent with most of the observed motion during modal phonation (e.g., chest register, in the middle range of pitch), although the mucosal wave decreases at higher pitches and is not visible during falsetto, suggesting that motion of the mucosa and the underlying tissue becomes coupled. In this mode, elastic recoil, rather than the Bernoulli effect, is the primary force driving the closing phase of phonation. The closing phase is much shorter, and only the superior edges of the vocal folds make contact. The vibratory characteristics of falsetto have been attributed to increased tension and decreased thickness of the vocal fold. During phonation at low pitches, the vocalis muscle is relaxed so that the "body" of the fold participates in oscillation.

Expiratory Force

The force available to drive phonation depends on the volume of air in the lungs, the elastic recoil in the chest wall and diaphragm, and the strength in abdominal and intercostal muscles. Normally, passive expiration is sufficient to power conversational speech. Shouting and singing require deeper prephonatory inspiration for larger lung volume and for active expiratory effort. Because the amount of breath support required for normal voice use is small compared with lung capacity, voice loss generally is not a presenting complaint of pulmonary disorders. Breath support available for phonation becomes a clinical issue in two situations: In patients with functional dysphonia there is insufficient prephonatory inspiration, so that excessive glottic pressure is required to produce an acceptable volume, which may lead to stress-induced injury of the vocal folds. In the second situation, a patient has an organic voice disorder, and impaired pulmonary function limits the capacity to compensate for the glottic defect. For example, a patient with laryngeal paralysis is more symptomatic when there is

coexisting emphysema. An important component of vocal training is instruction on control of breathing to maximize the power of vocal output.

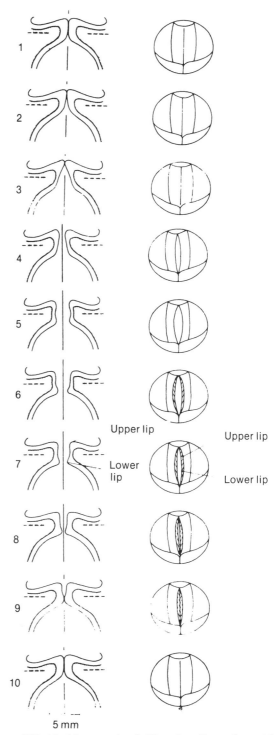

Figure 85A-11. Movements of different portions of vocal folds during one cycle of vibration shown schematically in coronal plane *(left)* and from above *(right).* Mucosal upheaval begins caudally and then moves rostrally. The lower portion is closing as the upper margin is opening. (From Hirano M: *Clinical examination of voice*, New York, 1981, Springer-Verlag.)

Vocal Fold Positioning

Phonation requires a critical relationship between the gap between the medial surface edges of the vocal folds and the expiratory airflow. The folds should be close enough together so that airflow entrains oscillations. If the gap is too wide, the voice is breathy, or aphonic, with only turbulent airflow noise and no periodic sound. The gap may be wider if airflow is greater; conversely, low airflow requires a narrower gap. If the vocal folds are too tightly apposed, excessive pressure is required, and phonation sounds strained or might not even be possible. An analogy to phonation is the sound generated by air released from a toy balloon. The pitch and volume may be varied by adjusting the tension across the neck of the balloon. The sound is louder with more air in the balloon. If pressure on the neck is sufficient to interrupt airflow, then sound ceases. With decreasing closing pressure, the sound becomes increasingly turbulent.

Vibratory Capacity of the Vocal Folds

The physical properties of the vocal folds are crucial in determining vocal function. During normal modal phonation, the mucosa undulates freely over the underlying vocal ligament and vocalis muscle. Hirano's[16] important histologic studies showed that this is possible because the mucosa and muscle are separated by a specialized layer of connective tissue that serves as a shock absorber. This highly specialized tissue is characterized by stratified concentrations of elastin and collagen. The most superficial layer is made up of loosely connected fibers of collagen and elastin. This layer also is known as Reinke's space. The intermediate layer is predominantly composed of elastic fibers, and the deep layer is constructed of densely arranged collagen fibers. Together, the intermediate and deep layers form the vocal ligament.

Vocal Fold Shape

In falsetto mode, only the superior edges of the vocal folds contact during the closing phase, although during modal phonation, which is more efficient, the mucosal wave begins on the inferior surface of the vocal fold. This requires a favorable configuration of the glottis in the coronal plane, with the medial surfaces of the vocal folds nearly parallel. If the vocalis muscle is atrophic or paralyzed, then the medial surface of the vocal fold is convex, and the glottal tract is too convergent for optimal phonation. A divergent glottis is also unfavorable.

Pitch Control

Changes in vocal fold length and tension are used to control the fundamental frequency of vocal fold vibration to produce dynamic inflections of the voice. Such adjustments involve fine motor control. In the lower vocal range, contraction of the thyroarytenoid results in a lowering of pitch because it decreases tension in the vocal cover. During contraction of the cricothyroid muscle, which increases length and tension, increasing thyroarytenoid muscle contraction results in rising pitch. Contraction of the cricothyroid muscle in the absence of thyroarytenoid muscle activity is generally accepted to be the mechanism of falsetto.

The size and physical properties of a larynx determine the range of pitch that can be produced. A child has a smaller larynx and a higher pitch range than an adult. During puberty in boys, the rapid increase in size of the larynx results in unstable pitch control until adaptation to the new anatomy occurs. Size is not the only determinate of pitch range, as age-related loss of elasticity and increasing ossification of the thyroid lamina result in an elevation of pitch. The lowest pitches are produced by young men, whose vocal folds are longer and heavier than those of women and more compliant than those of older men.

Resonance

The raw sound produced by the glottis in isolation from the rest of the vocal tract does not sound like human voice but is harsh and sounds something like a goose call. Phonated sound acquires the characteristics of a human voice because of the resonance of the chest, upper airway, and skull. Resonance is the prolongation, amplification, and filtering of sound by the induction of sympathetic vibration. The vocal frequencies that are enhanced by resonance are termed *formants*. The pharynx itself does not resonate because its walls are too compliant to support sympathetic vibration. The primary resonating structure is actually the air column contained in the pharynx. The length of the vocal tract and the locations of constricted segments confer characteristic resonant frequencies, which are excited by any sound fed into the tract, whether from the glottis or from an artificial larynx. These resonant frequencies are called *formants*. Resonance is controlled by altering the shape and volume of the pharynx, by raising or lowering the larynx, by moving tongue or jaw position, or by varying the amount of sound transmission through the nasopharynx and nose. Vocal training for singing, acting, or public speaking concentrates heavily on refining and maximizing resonance. The goal is to produce the loudest and most pleasing sound possible with minimal strain or pressure on the larynx.

Articulation

The source-filter hypothesis of speech states that the larynx is the source of a constant sound, which is shaped into words by the upper vocal tract. In this generally accepted model, consonants and vowels are formed by the action of the lips, tongue, palate, and pharynx. Participation of the larynx during articulation is generally considered to be limited to the onset and offset of phonation, coordinating with upper articulators to produce voiced and unvoiced sounds. In computerized simulation, this model seems to account for speech fairly well, although recent evidence suggests that the position and shape of the glottis may actually vary with production of different vowels, suggesting that the contribution of the larynx to phonation is more complex than previously recognized.[28]

Sensory Input to Speech Control

One obvious mechanism for controlling phonatory output during speech is auditory feedback. This sensory input is most important while one is learning speech and is not essential for everyday use. Prelingually, deaf persons never develop completely normal-sounding speech, although those who become deaf after language acquisition are able to maintain fairly normal speech patterns, in part because of ballistic speech production but also probably because of the use of nonauditory cues for feedback. An example of the importance of nonauditory cues in voice control is the ability of well-trained singers to perform with good control of pitch and loudness even when they cannot hear their own voices. Tactile sensation of induced vibration in the face, throat, and chest are important cues. There are many sensory receptors in the larynx, responding to such cues as air pressure and flow and joint motion, but the degree to which laryngeal sensation influences vocal control is not known.

REFERENCES

1. Andrew BL: The respiratory displacement of the larynx: a study of the innervation of accessory respiratory muscles, *J Physiol Lond* 130:474, 1955.
2. Baer T: *Investigation of the phonatory mechanism.* In Ludlow, O'Conell, editors: *Proceedings of the conference on the assessment of vocal pathology,* vol 11, no 38. Rockville, Maryland, 1979, ASHA Reports.
3. Bartlett D: Effects of hypercapnia and hypoxia on laryngeal resistance to airflow, *Resp Physiol* 37:293, 1979.
4. Brancatisano TP, Dodd DS, Engel LA: Respiratory activity of the posterior cricoarytenoid muscle and vocal cords in humans, *J Appl Physiol* 57:1143, 1984.
5. Brouillette RT, Thach BT: A neuromuscular mechanism for maintaining extrathoracic airway patency, *J Appl Physiol* 46:772, 1979.
6. Bryant NJ and others: Human posterior cricoarytenoid muscle compartments: anatomy and mechanics, *Arch Otolaryngol* 122:1331, 1996.
7. Cole P: *Modification of inspired air.* In Proctor D, editor: *The nose: upper airway physiology and the atmospheric environment.* Amsterdam, 1982, Elsevier Biomedical Press.
8. Collett PW, Brancatisano AP, Engel LA: Upper airway dimensions and moments in bronchial asthma, *Am Rev Resp Dis* 133:1143, 1986.
9. Fink RB, Demarast RJ: *Laryngeal biomechanic.* Cambridge, Massachusetts, 1978, Harvard University Press.
10. Fritzell B: Electromyography in the study of the velopharyngeal function: a review, *Folia Phoniatr* 31:93, 1979.
11. Galen: *On the usefulness of the parts of the body,* translated by May MT. Ithaca, New York, 1968, Cornell University Press.
12. Garcia M: Observations of the human voice, *Proc R Soc Lond* 7:399, 1855.
13. Gautier H, Remmers JE, Bartlett D Jr.: Control of the duration of expiration, *Resp Physiol* 18:205, 1973.
14. Gerber U, Polosa C: Some effects of superior laryngeal nerve stimulation on sympathetic preganglionic neuron firing, *Can J Physiol Pharmacol* 57:1073, 1979.
15. Green JH, Neil E: The respiratory function of the laryngeal muscles, *J Physiol Lond* 129:134, 1955.
16. Hirano M: *Phonosurgical anatomy of the larynx.* In Ford CN, Bless DM, editors: *Phonosurgery.* New York, 1991, Raven Press.
17. Hirano M, Kakita Y: *Cover-body theory of vocal fold vibration.* In Daniloff RG, editor: *Speech science.* San Diego, Calif, 1985, College-Hill Press.
18. Hirano M and others: *Anatomy and behavior of the vocal process.* In Baer T, Sasaki C, Harris K, editors: *Laryngeal function in phonation and respiration.* Boston, 1987, College-Hill Press.
19. Husson R: Etude des phenomenes physiologiques et acoustiques fondamentaux de la voix chantee, *These Fac Sc Paris* 1950.
20. Ishizaka K, Flanagan JL: Synthesis of voiced sounds from a two-mass model of the vocal cords, *Bell Syst Tech J* 51:1233, 1972.
21. Korpas J, Tomori S: *Cough and other respiratory reflexes.* Basel, Karger, 1979.
22. Kuna ST, Insalaco G, Woodson GE: Thyroarytenoid muscle activity during wakefulness and sleep in normal adults, *J Appl Physiol* 63:1332, 1988.
23. Laitman JT, Crelin ES: Developmental change in the upper respiratory system of human infants, *Perinatol Neonatol* 4:15, 1980.
24. Laitman JT, Crelin ES: *Postnatal development of the basicranium and vocal tract region in man.* In Bosma JF, editor: *Symposium on development of the basicranium.* Washington, DC, 1976, U.S. Government Printing Office.
25. Laitman JT, Reidenber JS: Advances in understanding the relationship between the skull base and larynx with comments on the origins of speech, *Hum Evol* 3:99, 1988.
26. Mathew OP, Abu-Osba YK, Thach BT: Influence of upper airway pressure changes in genioglossus muscle respiratory activity, *J Appl Physiol* 52:438, 1982.
27. Mathew OP, Abu-Osba YK, Thach BT: Influence of upper airway pressure changes in respiratory frequency, *Resp Physiol* 49:223, 1982.
28. Maurer D, Hess M, Gross M: High-speed imaging of vocal fold vibrations and larynx movements within vocalizations of different vowels, *Ann Otol Rhinol Laryngol* 105:975, 1996.
29. Mayo H: *Outlines of human physiology,* London, Burgess & Hill, 1829.

30. Murakami Y, Kirchner JA: Respiratory movements of the vocal cords: an EMG study in the cat, *Laryngoscope* 82:454, 1972.

31. Nakamura F, Uyeda Y, Sonoda Y: EMG study on respiratory movements of the intrinsic laryngeal muscles, *Laryngoscope* 68:109, 1958.

32. Negus V: *The comparative anatomy and physiology of the larynx*, London, Heinemann, 1949.

33. Olson T, Woodson GE, Heldt G: Upper airway function in Ondine's curse, *Arch Otolaryngol Head Neck Surg* 118:310, 1992.

34. Remmers JE and others: Pathogenesis of upper airway occlusion during sleep, *J Appl Physiol* 44:931, 1978.

35. Roberts JL, Reed WR, Thach BT: Pharyngeal airway-stabilizing function of sternohyoid and sternothyroid muscles in the rabbit, *J Appl Physiol* 57:1790, 1984.

36. Sanders I and others: The innervation of the human larynx posterior cricoarytenoid muscle: evidence for at least two neuromuscular compartments, *Laryngoscope* 104:880, 1994.

37. Sant'Ambrogio FB and others: Laryngeal influences on breathing pattern and posterior cricoarytenoid muscle activity, *J Appl Physiol* 58:1298, 1985.

38. Sant'Ambrogio G and others: Laryngeal receptors responding to transmural pressure, airflow, and local muscle activity, *Resp Physiol* 54:317, 1983.

39. Sasaki CT: Development of laryngeal function: etiologic significance in the sudden infant death syndrome, *Arch Otol* 103:8, 1977.

40. Sasaki CT and others: Postnatal descent of the epiglottis in man: a preliminary report, *Arch Otolaryngol Head Neck Surg* 103:169, 1977.

41. Sherry JH, Megirian D: Spontaneous and reflexly evoked laryngeal abductor and adductor muscle activity in cat, *Exp Neurol* 43:487, 1974.

42. Tomori Z, Widdicombe JG: Muscular, bronchomotor and cardiovascular reflexes elicited by mechanical stimulation of the respiratory tract, *J Physiol Lond* 200:25, 1969.

43. Van de Berg J: Myoelastic theory of voice production, *J Speech Hear Res* 1:227, 1958.

44. Van de Graff WB: Thoracic influence on upper airway patency, *J Appl Physiol* 65:2124, 1988.

45. van Lunteren E, Strohl KP: *Striated respiratory muscles of the upper airways*. In Mathew O, Sant'Ambrogio G, editors: *Respiratory function of the upper airway*. New York, 1988, Marcel-Dekker.

46. Woodson GE: Configuration of the glottis in laryngeal paralysis I: clinical study, *Laryngoscope* 103:1227, 1993.

47. Woodson GE and others: Effects of cricothyroid muscle contraction on laryngeal resistance and glottic area, *Annal Otol Rhinol Laryngol* 98:119, 1989.

48. Zemlin WR, Davis P, Gaza C: Fine morphology of the posterior cricoarytenoid muscle, *Folia Phoniat* 36:233, 1984.

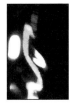

CHAPTER EIGHTY FIVE B

EVALUATION AND MANAGEMENT OF HYPERFUNCTIONAL DISORDERS

‖ Andrew Blitzer

INTRODUCTION

Patients are classified as having movement disorders if they have a disorder of motor programming resulting in a paucity of movement (akinesia or bradykinesia), excessive or hyperfunctional movement (hyperkinesia), or a combination of both. The hyperkinetic motor programming errors can produce spasms, tremors, jerks, or tics, and symptoms related to the body part involved.

Patients with movement disorders associated with the larynx are ideally evaluated by an otolaryngologist and by a neurologist specializing in movement disorders. Evaluation should include a complete head and neck examination, neurologic examination, and videotaping of the functional disability for documentation. Electromyography (EMG), magnetic resonance imaging (MRI), and blood analysis are performed as indicated by the initial evaluation. A multidisciplinary approach including the involvement of an otolaryngologist, a neurologist, and a speech pathologist is key to successful diagnosis and management of hyperfunctional disorders of the larynx.[33,131]

DYSTONIA

Many patients with hyperfunctional conditions of the larynx have dystonia, a syndrome dominated by sustained muscle contractions that frequently causes twisting and repetitive movements or abnormal postures that may be sustained or intermittent. Dystonia can involve any voluntary muscle. Because the condition is rare and the movements and resulting postures are often unusual, dystonia is among the most frequently misdiagnosed neurologic conditions.[45] The prevalence is unknown, but there are an estimated 50,000 to 100,000 cases of idiopathic dystonia in the United States.[95]

Patients can be classified according to clinical symptomatology, age at onset, and cause. Classification may be important because it can provide clues about prognosis and the approach to management. The classification scheme is outlined in Box 85B-1.

Dystonia can begin at nearly any age. Presenting signs have occurred as early as 9 months and as late as 85 years. In general, age at onset has a bimodal distribution, with peaks at ages 8 and 42 years. Patients are classified as having early onset dystonia when the presenting signs occur before age 26 years, and late onset when the signs present at older ages. Other classifications include infantile onset when the presenting signs occur before age 2 years; childhood onset, between ages 2 and 12 years; adolescent onset, between ages 13 and 20 years; and adult onset at older ages.[33] Patients are categorized as having focal, segmental, or generalized symptoms according to distribution. Focal dystonia symptoms involve one small group of muscles in one body part, segmental disease involves a contiguous group of muscles, and generalized dystonia is widespread. Common examples of focal dystonia are listed in Box 85B-2.[33]

Based on history, examination, or laboratory studies, patients may have no identifiable cause for the dystonic symptoms (idiopathic dystonia). Therefore, there should be a normal perinatal and early developmental history; no history of neurologic illness or exposure to drugs known to cause acquired dystonia (e.g., phenothiazines); normal intellectual, pyramidal, cerebellar, and sensory examinations; and normal diagnostic studies. The clinical phenomenology is often a clue to the cause. Primary dystonia is typically action induced; symptoms are enhanced with use of the affected body part, and the region may appear normal at rest. Secondary dystonia frequently results in fixed dystonic postures. The presence of extensive dystonia limited to one side of the body (hemidystonia) suggests a secondary cause.[33,45,95]

In one study of dystonia patients with primary laryngeal involvement, the disorder had spread to

---

BOX 85B-1
CLASSIFICATION OF DYSTONIA

Primary
  Without hereditary pattern
  With hereditary pattern
    Autosomal dominant
    Autosomal recessive
    X-linked recessive
    Undefined

Secondary
  Associated with other hereditary neurologic disorders
    (e.g., Wilson's disease, Huntington's disease, ceroid
    lipofuscinosis, progressive supranuclear palsy,
    Hallervorden-Spatz disease, olivopontocerebellar
    atrophy, acquired hepatocerebral degeneration,
    Tourette's syndrome)
  Environmental
    Posttraumatic
    Postinfectious
    Vascular
    Neoplastic
    Toxic
      Post–antipsychotic drugs (phenothiazines,
        piperazines, butyrophenones, malindone,
        thioxanthines)
      Antiemetics (prochlorperazine, promethazine,
        metachlopramide)
      Antiparkinsonian drugs (levodopa, bromcriptine,
        lisaride, pergolide)
  Associated with parkinsonism
  Hysterical

BOX 85B-2
DISTRIBUTION OF DYSTONIA

Focal
  Blepharospasm (forced, involuntary eye-closure)
  Oromandibular dystonia (face, jaw, or tongue)
  Torticollis (neck)
  Writer's cramp (action-induced dystonic contraction of
    hand muscles)
  Spasmodic dysphonia (vocal cords)
Segmental (cranial, axial, or crural)
Multifocal
Generalized (ambulatory, nonambulatory)

---

another body part in 16%. These data suggest that patients should be advised of the potential for spread and should be followed up and reexamined on a regular basis for signs of other dystonic involvement. Approximately 10% of patients with primary laryngeal dystonias have a family history of dystonia.[43]

In most cases of childhood-onset idiopathic dystonia, family studies show an autosomal dominant inheritance with reduced penetrance. A marker for some cases of childhood-onset dystonia has been found on chromosome 9.[97] There are heterogenous genetic patterns among patients with idiopathic dystonic symptomatology, including a linkage to the X chromosome and parkinsonism,[47,77,128] a DOPA responsive form.[96]

Family and linkage studies have identified several subtypes with different genetic bases, including an autosomal dominant dopamine-responsive dystonia,[96] X-linked Filipino torsion dystonia[47,77,128]; autosomal dominant (non–dopamine-responsive) idiopathic torsion dystonia (ITD) related to the *DTY1* gene mapped to chromosome 9q34. Both dopamine and X-linked torsion dystonia are rare forms of ITD associated with parkinsonism.[26,28,97,98]

The *DTY1* gene was first identified in a large non-Jewish family with multiple members who had dystonia.[98] Since that time, the *DTY1* gene has been identified in 12 Ashkenazi Jewish families with dystonia. Jewish and non-Jewish families presented with the same symptom complexes. The dystonia characteristically began in childhood or adolescence and started in a limb. The penetrance was greater in the non-Jewish family (0.75) compared with the Jewish families (0.30). It has been postulated that mutations in the *DTY1* gene may be responsible for the difference.[76] Ozelius and others[98] reported linkage dysequilibrium between halotype ABL-ASS at the 9q loci and the *DTY1* gene in the Ashkenazi Jewish population, suggesting that a single mutation in the *DTY1* gene is responsible for many ITD cases. In contrast, late-onset ITD in Ashkenazi Jews did not seem to be related to this mutation but rather to other mutations or genes.[26] Linkage dysequilibrium has not been reported in non-Jewish families.[28]

Nygaard and others[96] reported that the Segawa variant of the dystonia gene (*DRD*) was on chromosome 14. Ichinose and others[64] further refined this observation and reported that a guanosine triphosphate–cyclohydroxylase gene mutation was mapped on chromosome 14q.

Younger onset is associated with initial involvement of an arm or leg and a higher probability of spread to another body part. As the patient ages, onset is more likely in the neck, larynx, arm, or cranial muscle, and the dystonia tends to remain in a more focal distribution.[27,29]

SPASMODIC DYSPHONIA

Laryngeal dystonia (spasmodic dysphonia) is an action-induced, laryngeal motion disorder. Most cases represent manifestations of primary dystonia, but many result from other neurologic entities.

In 1871, Traube[124] coined the term *spastic dysphonia* when describing a patient with nervous hoarseness. Schnitzler[110] used the terms *spastic aphonia* and *phonic laryngeal spasm* to describe such patients. Nothnagel called the condition *coordinated laryngeal spasm.*[56] Fraenkel[53] used the phrase *mogiphonia* for a slowly developing disorder of the voice characterized by increasing vocal fatigue, spasmodic constriction of throat muscles, and pain around the larynx. He compared the laryngeal disorder with mogigraphia (occupational writer's cramp) or dystonic cramping of the arm when writing. In 1899, Gowers[58] described functional laryngeal spasm whereby the cords were brought together too forcibly while speaking (adductor spasmodic dysphonia). He contrasted this to phonic paralysis, whereby the vocal cords could not be brought together while speaking (abductor spasmodic dysphonia). In addition, as Gowers[58] reported, "The affection has been compared to writer's cramp . . . a case reported by Gerhardt, in which the patient had actually suffered from writer's cramp, and, at the age of 50, learned to play the flute. The act of blowing the flute brought on laryngeal spasm and an unintended voice sound, accompanied by muscular contractions in the arm and angle of the mouth."

Thus, the focal dystonia of spasmodic dystonia is being compared with dystonia involving other segments of the body (mouth, arm). Critchley[39] described the voice pattern as a condition in which the patient sounds as though he or she is "trying to talk whilst being choked." Bellussi[10] described the condition as "stuttering with the vocal cords."

In 1968, Aronson and others[6] reviewed the disorder in detail. At that time, there were approximately 122 cases in the literature. The Minnesota Multiphasic Personality Inventory and psychiatric interviews did not discriminate between patients with spasmodic dysphonia and healthy patients when distinguishing patients with spasmodic dysphonia from those with psychogenic dysphonias, helping establish spasmodic dysphonia as an organic or nonpsychiatric condition. Nevertheless, many patients are referred to psychiatrists for management because the correct diagnosis is elusive and not made when the patient initially presents for management. Aronson[5] later distinguished and reviewed two types of spasmodic dysphonia: adductor, caused by irregular hyperadduction of the vocal folds, and abductor, caused by intermittent abduction of the vocal folds. Patients with adductor spasmodic dysphonia exhibit a choked, strained-strangled voice quality, with abrupt initiation and termination, resulting in short breaks in phonation. The voice is generally reduced in loudness and monotonal. Vocal tremor is frequently observed, along with a slow speech rate and decreased smoothness of speech. Speech intelligi-

bility is generally decreased. Occasionally, patients with adductor spasmodic dysphonia exhibit compensatory pseudoabductor spasmodic dysphonia, compensating for severe adductor laryngeal spasms by whispering.

Patients with abductor spasmodic dysphonia exhibit a breathy, effortful voice quality with abrupt termination, resulting in aphonic whispered segments of speech. The voice is reduced in loudness, and vocal tremor is often observed. Speech intelligibility is generally decreased. Some patients display a combination of adductor and abductor signs and have been classified as "mixed."[33,56]

Aronson and Hartman[9] later noted that spasmodic dysphonia has tremor characteristics similar to those found in essential tremor. The differential diagnosis between spasmodic dysphonia caused by essential tremor vs that caused by dystonic tremor can be difficult. Blitzer and others[23] noted that spasmodic dysphonia is not a spastic disorder; electromyographic characteristics were inconsistent with those seen in pyramidal disorders. An irregular tremor was found in 25% of patients vs the regular tremor of essential tremor. The findings were comparable with those of patients who had generalized dystonia with laryngeal involvement and therefore supported the concept that spasmodic dysphonia was a focal dystonia. Schaefer and others[109] used EMG to further establish that spasmodic dysphonia is a disorder of vocal motor control. Because the condition is not a spastic disorder, the authors favor the term *spasmodic* dysphonia over *spastic* dysphonia.

Dystonia is characterized by abnormal involuntary movements that are typically action induced. In spasmodic dysphonia, the vocal apparatus is usually normal at rest but functions abnormally with speaking. Adductor spasmodic dysphonia is characterized by abnormal involuntary co-contraction of the vocalis muscle complex, resulting in inappropriate adduction of the vocal folds.[16] As an action-induced, task-specific, or functional movement disorder, spasmodic dysphonia shows muscles and anatomic structures that are normal at rest but move inappropriately with action.[33] The authors avoid using the word *functional*, which implies a psychogenic etiology.

Most authors who have performed vocal analysis on patients with spasmodic dysphonia have concluded that most patients have a dysphonia characterized by a strain-strangle–type voice that is often harsh, and is usually accompanied by a tremor, inappropriate pitch or pitch breaks, breathiness, and glottal fry.* Conversely, abductor spasmodic dysphonia is

---

*References 17, 22, 33, 99, 125, 132.

characterized by action-induced inappropriate co-contraction of the posterior cricoarytenoid muscles during speaking, resulting in inappropriate abduction of the vocal cords. In 1968, Aronson and others[6] thought that a group of patients with whispering dysphonia or aphonia and with breathy breaks had a psychogenic cause. This may be the earliest report of the true abductor spastic dysphonia. Many of these patients may be misdiagnosed as having a vocal cord paralysis because of the breathy character of the voice.[17,21,22]

Two other variations of presentation have been identified. The compensatory abductor dysphonia is found in the group of adductors that produce a breathy voice by not contracting the vocal cords to prevent the spasms and the broken speech pattern. Compensatory adductor dysphonia is a much more rare entity in which the abductors try to prevent the breathiness by tightly contracting the vocal cords.[17,18,22] In nearly 900 patients with laryngeal dystonia, 87% had adductor vocal involvement (spastic dysphonia), 12% had abductor vocal involvement (whispering dysphonia), and 1% had adductor breathing dystonia.

The authors have also described 12 individuals with respiratory adductor laryngeal dystonia.[17,18,25,31,59] These patients had abnormal involuntary adduction of the vocal cords on respiration but grossly normal function with speech. Eight were idiopathic. Two began with onset in the upper face (blepharospasm) progressing to involve the laryngeal and diaphragmatic muscles, one began with laryngeal symptoms, and one was tardive and began with laryngeal symptoms that progressed to involve the lower face and jaw.

Spasmodic dysphonia can occur with other cranial forms of dystonia. In 1910, Meige[90] described a syndrome of spasms of the eyelids and contractures of the pharynx, jaw muscles, and muscles of the floor of mouth and tongue. Meige described muscle spasms of prolonged duration with an irregular, repetitive pattern. Jacome and Yanez[67] in 1980 and Marsden and Sheehy[84] in 1982 associated spasmodic dysphonia with Meige's disease or segmental-cranial dystonia. In the authors' experience, about 25% of patients with Meige's disease have laryngeal involvement.

Dystonic movements can be rapid and repetitive, and tremor may be seen in dystonia affecting any segment of the body. Dystonic tremors are typically irregular and have a directional preponderance; symptoms increase when the patient postures the affected body part in a position opposed to the primary dystonic contractions. For instance, patients with torticollis often have a head tremor that can be diminished by placing the head into the preferred posture. Many patients with spasmodic dysphonia have an irregular vocal tremor that is audible and can be recorded electromyographically. Similar to the dystonic tremor that occurs in persons with arm or neck dystonia, the irregular tremor of spasmodic dysphonia can be caused by posturing of dystonic muscles in a position in which the agonist contractions do not fully neutralize those of the antagonists. This tremor needs to be differentiated from the regular tremor that occurs in benign essential voice tremor. The clinical distinction can be difficult in many cases, particularly when a patient presents with symptoms of essential tremor in other body parts. In many cases, the clinical distinction cannot be made.[8a]

Patients with spasmodic dysphonia have reported that symptoms momentarily improve when one pinches the nares, presses the hand against the back of the head, presses the hand into the abdomen, pulls on an ear, or touches the clavicular notch (personal experience). Many patients observe that they speak better after a yawn or sneeze or when they sing or yell; these sensory tricks are also common for patients with other craniocervical dystonias.[29,45] In patients with cranial dystonia, involuntary hissing or humming can be present. It is difficult to know whether these noises are primarily associated with the disorder or are secondary tricks to relieve symptoms.[122] Numerous patients with laryngeal dystonia hum before speaking, as if to initiate vibration of the vocal cords to prepare for vocalization.

Laboratory investigations are typically normal in idiopathic dystonia and in spasmodic dysphonia. Detailed studies by Finitzo and Freeman[51] support an organic basis for the condition: 35% of patients had abnormal brainstem auditory-evoked responses, 47% had an abnormal gastric acid secretory response to sham feeding (an index of vagal nerve function), 46% had reduced or absent vagally mediated fluctuations in heart rate during deep inspiration; women with spasmodic dysphonia had abnormal limb motor control, 23% had brain lesions on MRI, 56% had abnormal brain electric activity mapping scans, 76% had abnormal brain hypoperfusion on single photon emission computed tomography, and some patients had an abnormal electrophysiologic blink reflex.

Clinical features, such as improvement of symptoms with alcohol, sedatives, and tranquilizers and worsening while under stress or on the telephone, have been used as evidence that patients presenting with symptoms of spasmodic dysphonia have a psychogenic basis for their condition. However, these clinical features are common among the dystonias. Similar to torticollis,[54,70] spasmodic dysphonia remissions can occur and relapse. Such cases have been diagnosed as psychiatric until relapse. Psychogenic spasmodic dysphonia is very rare, and speech-language pathologists usually describe such cases.[33]

Systemic pharmacotherapy provides little relief of symptoms. Dedo and Izdebski[41] described dramatic relief of symptoms by sectioning the recurrent laryngeal nerve. The initial favorable reports were temporized by a review of 33 patients by Aronson and De Santo[7,8] that addressed surgical management. Three years later, only 36% of patients had some persistent improvement, and only 3% achieved a persistent normal voice. Adverse effects included breathiness, hoarseness, diplophonia, and falsetto. Of the 64% with failed voices at 3 years, 48% were worse than before surgery. Failures were more common among women (77%) than men (36%).

More recent surgical approaches have focused on selective denervation and reinnervation using the ansa cervicalis nerve. In a report based on preliminary experience with bilateral selective adductor denervation-reinnervation, favorable responses were observed in 19 or 21 patients.[11] Not all patients undergoing this procedure were included in the report, and data was subjective based on telephone survey by the authors. The mean follow-up period was 31.4 months (range, 12–68 months), and additional therapy was required in four patients including Botox injection (one patient), collagen injection (one), thyroarytenoid myotomy (one), and voice therapy (one). In a second study of patients undergoing selective adductor denervation-reinnervation, improvement in patient satisfaction, untrained and trained listener perception of voice quality, and rate of aphonic voice breaks were observed in five of six patients.[1] Although the rationale for selective adductor denervation-reinnervation is sound, caution regarding surgical approaches must be considered given the prior experience with denervation procedures. Long-term follow-up with objective data analysis in a blinded format will be required to prove the efficacy of these surgical approaches.

The authors began using Botox for the management of focal and segmental dystonias in April 1984.[34] Improvement in symptoms of spasmodic dysphonia with local injections of botulinum toxin has been dramatic. The American Academy of Neurology,[3] American Academy of Otolaryngology–Head and Neck Surgery,[2] and the National Institutes of Health Consensus Panel[94] have reviewed the clinical usefulness of botulinum toxin and found it to be safe and effective. The clinical application and technical aspects of botulinum toxin therapy for spasmodic dysphonia are considered in this chapter in the section titled "Botulinum toxin therapy."

Botulinum toxin therapy in patients with adductor spasmodic dysphonia has been demonstrated to improve speaking by 60% to 100% of normal function, with a mean of 90%; the duration of effect was between 3 and 4 months. Adverse effects include a mild breathy dysphonia for less than 2 weeks (45%), mild choking on fluids for the first several days (22%), hyperventilation and dizziness when trying to speak while hypophonic, a sore throat or coughing up blood-tinged sputum, and itching (without rash).[14,15,17]

In abductor laryngeal dystonia patients, botulinum toxin injection into the posterior cricoarytenoid muscle produces marked improvement with a return to mean maximal functional performance of 70% of normal. Adverse effects include mild dysphagia without aspiration and mild stridor on exertion. No significant breathing difficulties have been reported, even in cases in which both posterior cricoarytenoid muscles were injected.[14,15,21]

Local injection of botulinum toxin into laryngeal muscles is a safe and effective therapy for laryngeal dystonia. In contrast to surgery, botulinum toxin injections have the advantage of being administered on an ambulatory basis, both vocal cords can be managed, and the toxin is given under EMG control for precise localization of the most active part of the muscle complex. Graded weakening can be achieved using low doses and by repeating the injections to achieve optimal weakness. If too much weakness is produced, the strength gradually returns with time. The procedure is very acceptable to patients, with very satisfactory vocal results. It is too soon to tell whether patients will become refractory to this form of therapy. To date, no one has become refractory with laryngeal injections or has sustained a disability from laryngeal toxin injections.[17,31,35]

TREMOR

Tremor is an involuntary, purposeless rhythmic movement of a part of the body.[42] The proposed underlying neural bases for tremor include a central[42,62,126] and peripheral mechanism.[103] Tremors have been classified by their cause or clinical appearance and are characterized by their frequency, amplitude, distribution over the body, and exacerbating and relieving factors.[68] Marsden and others[83] described four types of human action tremors: a fast (8–10 Hz), fine postural tremor similar to enhanced physiologic tremor; classical essential tremor, with a postural tremor of slower frequency and greater amplitude than physiologic tremor; a classical essential tremor, which is disabling in degree; and symptomatic essential tremor, which is associated with other neurologic disorders (e.g., polyneuropathy, parkinsonism, dystonia).[81] Of patients with essential tremor, 60% have a family history of tremor, and 30% of these had voice involvement.[72]

The involuntary, rhythmic, oscillatory movements that affect the distal musculature in patients with tremulous diseases can also affect the muscles of speech production and generate rhythmic alterations in pitch and loudness, termed *vocal tremor*. Vocal tremor can result in rapid decreases and increases in loudness and pitch or in complete phonation stoppages. Intelligibility and rate of speech may be decreased. Vocal tremor has been described perceptually as "tremulous voice,"[30,36] "wavy voice,"[61] or "tremulous, quavering speech"[61] and has been associated with neurologic disorders such as essential tremor, Parkinson's disease, cerebellar ataxia, and flaccid dysarthria.[5,123] Analysis of vocal tremor can make important contributions to the early and differential diagnosis of neurologic diseases and consequently to management decisions. The primary noninvasive quantification of vocal tremor has been through acoustic analysis. Most acoustic data on vocal tremor have been obtained from visual inspection of oscillographic displays of wave form data[36,60] or graphic level recorder displays of amplitude contours[61,88] of sustained vowel phonation. Consequently, the bulk of acoustic data on vocal tremor includes only visually quantifiable amplitude oscillations.

Essential tremor is typically absent at rest, maximal during maintenance of a posture, attenuated during movement, and often accentuated at the termination of movement.[33,48,86] It is present at rest only occasionally; differentiation from parkinsonism can be difficult in these patients.[33,49] Vocal tremor occurs in approximately 10% to 20% of patients with essential tremor.[79] It may be the first[36] or only sign of the disease,[101] or it may accompany tremors in other body parts.[50] Vocal tremor may parallel the onset of other symptoms or have a sudden onset and cause rapid deterioration in speech intelligibility.[36,50] It has been reported that vocal tremor is greater with emotional stress or fatigue.[4] Pitch breaks (octave breaks to a lower frequency) and phonation arrests have been reported in some cases of essential tremor[79,80] and have been associated with visible vertical oscillations of the larynx.[87]

The effect of medication on reducing vocal tremor is equivocal. Certain researchers have reported reductions in vocal tremor with administration of propranolol;[79,80] primidone;[4,129] and clonazepam, propranolol, and diazepam in combination.[107] Limited clinically significant changes in vocal tremor have been found with administration of propranolol[61,73] and primidone.[55] One report describes a better than 70% improvement of vocal tremor with thalamotomies.[57] Preliminary studies have also shown reduction of tremor with chronic electric stimulation of the thalamic nucleus through surgically implanted neuropacers.[112] Local injection of botulinum toxin in the management of essential vocal tremor has shown a dramatic benefit in preliminary studies. The injections are given into the muscles that seem to be most tremulous. In many cases, the most active muscles are the sternohyoid and sternothyroid muscles, which rhythmically elevate and lower the larynx in the airway (resonator), causing oscillations and producing a tremulous voice quality. In these cases, injecting botulinum toxin into the strap muscles will diminish the up and down motion of the larynx, thereby diminishing the amplitude of the tremor and making speech more fluent. Generally, 5 units in 2.5-unit aliquots are injected on each side. If the vocal folds are tremulous, they are injected at a second session.

STUTTERING

Stuttering is a neurologic disorder. Because the phenomenology includes abnormal, involuntary, and inappropriate use of the muscles of speech production resulting in dysfluency, it might best be considered a movement disorder. The abnormal involuntary movements are task specific, and the movements may be repetitive and stereotyped. Stuttering occurs in three subsystems of speech: respiratory, phonatory, and articulatory. Stuttering is a result of increased muscle tension in these three subsystems, causing the muscles to move too quickly and too far.[127] This increased muscle tension results in postures that are sustained for longer than expected or in quick repetitive movements of the same posture. Patients may have primarily focal systems (phonatory, respiratory, articulatory) or segmental symptomatology involving two or three regions. In addition, other cranial musculature may inappropriately contract, including the eyelids and other muscles of facial expression.[102,104,117] One report[121] describes stuttering followed by the development of jaw opening dystonia.

Competing stimuli, such as emotional arousal, sensory stimuli, motor actions (e.g., walking), or the use of rhythmic patterns (e.g., a metronome), increase fluency. Novel modes of speaking such as singing, speaking in a sing-song voice, using a monotone, shouting, using a foreign accent, and using clear or slurred articulation also increase fluency for a period of time. Communicative pressures such as audience size, listener reactions, concern about social approval, time pressure, and the degree to which the stutterer is responsible for conveying a meaningful message to a listener are found to increase stuttering.[92]

The use of antidepressants does not improve fluency.[118] Most persons with a stuttering disorder respond to traditional speech therapy and training. Some adults, despite a long history of therapy, still have stuttering with glottal block. Management of the thyroarytenoid muscles in a group of patients with stuttering and glottal block achieved promising results.[121] Giving small doses of botulinum toxin (1 unit or less, bilaterally) has produced improvement in 50% of patients. The number of glottal blocks and the duration of the glottal blocks significantly diminish with management.

The most significant advances in treatment of stuttering have been achieved with altered auditory feedback in-the-ear devices.[71,119,120] Using both delayed and frequency-altered auditory feedback, significant improvement in fluency and normalcy of speech has been demonstrated. The in-the-ear canal device provides a frequency shift of +500 Hz in combination with delayed auditory feedback of 60 msec. Improvement was demonstrated for both youth and adult subjects and is currently marketed under the trademark "SpeechEasy."

MYOCLONUS

Myoclonus refers to sudden, brief, shock-like involuntary movements caused by muscular contractions (positive myoclonus) or inhibitions (negative myoclonus, asterixis) arising from the central nervous system.[46,82,133] The muscle twitches of fasciculations caused by lesions of the lower motor neuron are excluded from this definition. Phenomenologically similar muscle jerks may be produced by peripheral nerve or plexus lesions.[85]

Branchial or *oculopalatal myoclonus* refers to myoclonic symptoms affecting cranial structures. In the oral cavity, involuntary—usually unconscious—movement of the soft palate and pharynx is seen.[78] Further exploration often documents synchronous jerks affecting the eyes, face, palate, larynx, diaphragm, neck, shoulder, and arm. A patient complaint of clicking in the ears, thought to be caused by involvement of the eustachian tube and tensor veli palatini muscles, was first noted in the 19th century by Muller and then Politzer.[105] The clicking can often be heard by family and examiners. Laryngeal involvement may produce a broken speech pattern, simulating that heard in laryngeal dystonia or tremor (personal observation). Examination of the vocal cords often shows slow rhythmic adduction and abduction of the vocal cords at the same timing and frequency as the palatal, pharyngeal, and occasional diaphragmatic contractions. This causes the broken speech pattern and a respiratory dysrhythmia. Ventilatory dysfunction has been documented.[4]

Although usually unresponsive to pharmacotherapy, isolated cases have reportedly responded to serotonin,[4,129] carbamazepine,[107] clonazepam,[55,69] tetrabenazine,[69] and trihexyphenidyl.[65,66] Several symptomatic patients who were unresponsive to drug therapy have been managed with local injection of botulinum toxin into the thyroarytenoid muscles.

TIC DISORDER

Tourette's syndrome is considered to be the most severe form of tic disorder; involuntary vocalizations are the hallmark of the disease. Additional features include onset in childhood or adolescence, multiple tics of several body parts, variations in the intensity of the symptoms over weeks or months, suppressibility, and presence for more than 1 year. Obsessive-compulsive behavior is common.[100] Vocalizations can be articulate words or inarticulate sounds. Patients frequently present to an otolaryngologist for evaluation of laryngeal tics manifesting as inappropriate coughing, barking, throat clearing, hooting, and grunting. The voice may be harsh because of the effects of chronic voice abuse with polypoid changes of the vocal mucosa. Lingual tics present as hisses and nasal tics as sniffs and snorts. Phenothiazines (e.g., haloperidol) appear to offer the greatest amount of relief.[38] However, tardive dyskinesia and tardive dystonia, severely disabling movement disorders, may occur as secondary effects of phenothiazine administration[37,38,93,111]; this therapy should be reserved for resistant cases. Clonidine, an α_2-adrenergic agonist, and clonazepam, a benzodiazepine, have been helpful in managing many cases.[111] Brin and others[34] have used local injections of botulinum toxin to manage rapid facial tics and dystonic tics in selected patients with a dramatic relief of symptomatology. This form of therapy may be appropriate for patients with severe, persistent tics involving one group of muscles. Blitzer and Brin[18] used botulinum toxin to control refractory loud barking sounds in one patient.[108]

BOTULINUM TOXIN THERAPY

The bacteria *Clostridium botulinum* produces seven immunologically distinct toxins that are potent neuroparalytic agents: A, B, C_1, C_2, D, E, F, and G.[114,115] Although antigenically distinct, the seven neurotoxins possess similar molecular weights and have a common subunit structure.[40] The toxins are synthesized as single-chain polypeptides with a molecular mass of approximately 150,000 D. In this form, the toxin molecules have relatively little potency as neuromuscular blocking agents. The single-chain toxin can be cleaved by certain bacterial enzymes or by trypsin to yield a di-chain molecule in which a heavy chain (approximately 100,000 D) is linked by a disulfide bond to a light chain (approximately 50,000 D). It is in this form that the molecule paralyzes neuromuscular transmission. Reduction of the disulfide bond that links the two chains causes complete loss of toxicity. The amino acid sequences for the various serotypes of botulinum toxin have not been reported. Partial amino acid sequences have been determined for types

A, B, C$_{1\&2}$, D, E, and F and show that regions of structural homology exist.[40]

When botulinum neurotoxin is isolated from bacterial cultures, it is normally associated with nontoxic macromolecules. The associated molecules may be proteins or nucleic acids; a protein hemagglutinin associates noncovalently with type A toxin. When administered parenterally, nontoxic proteins do not enhance the toxicity of the neurotoxin and may even interfere slightly. However, when administered orally, nontoxic proteins can enhance toxicity greatly, possibly by protecting the neurotoxin from proteolytic enzymes in the gut.[106]

Botulinum toxin exerts its effect at the neuromuscular junction by inhibiting the release of acetylcholine, causing a flaccid paralysis.[12,13,101,116] Three steps involved in toxin-mediated paralysis are (1) binding, (2) internalization, and (3) inhibition of neurotransmitter release. Toxin binding to peripheral and central nerves is selective and saturable. In vitro studies with synaptosomal preparations suggest heterogeneity of acceptor sites with high- and low-affinity sites and some specificity for toxin type.[44,74,130] The heavy chain determines cholinergic specificity and is responsible for binding.[44,75] The light chain is the intracellular toxic moiety. The light chain is responsible for the proteolytic activity and, depending on the serotype, has a specific affinity for VAMP/synaptobrevin-2, SNAP-25, or syntaxin. Cleavage of any of these proteins interferes with the proper binding and fusion of a vesicle to the plasma membrane, therefore impeding exocytosis-mediated neurotransmitter release.[63]

It is likely that the clinical effect of toxin is caused primarily by the peripheral effect; the degree of improvement correlates with weakness appropriate to blockade of neuromuscular transmission. Clinically, there is typically a 24- to 72-hour delay between administration of toxin and onset of clinical effect. This delay may be secondary to the time necessary for adequate enzymatic disruption of the synaptosomic release process of botulinum toxin.

The mouse assay has been the standard when measuring potency of commercially available toxin. One unit of botulinum toxin is equivalent to the amount of toxin found to kill 50% of a group of 18- to 20-g female Swiss-Webster mice (i.e., the median lethal dose).[35]

Although botulinum toxin has been used therapeutically in humans since the mid-1970s without evidence of a direct effect on uninjected muscles, the long-term consequences of chronic injections are unknown. Weakness or routine EMG changes in muscles distal to the site of injection have not been reported. However, there are detectable abnormalities on single-fiber EMG.[35] It is not known how long these abnormalities persist or whether they have any clinical significance. There is a paucity of data regarding use during pregnancy. Currently, injection should be avoided in pregnant or lactating patients. Caution is warranted when managing patients with conditions such as myasthenia gravis, Eaton-Lambert syndrome, and motor neuron disease, particularly when large doses are required (e.g., in the management of cervical dystonia). However, the amount of toxin entering the circulation after injection is thought to be minute, and this theoretic concern should be balanced against the severity of the hyperkinetic symptoms.[35]

Botulinum toxin type A (Botox; Allergan, Inc., Irvine, Ca) and type B (Myobloc; Elan Pharmaceuticals, Inc, San Francisco, Ca) are currently available for clinical application. A standard vial of Botox contains 100 units of toxin. Toxin is shipped from the manufacturer on dry ice and stored at −20°C. Frozen lyophilized toxin is reconstituted with sterile saline to various concentrations, depending on the indication. For laryngeal injections, a volume of 0.1 mL is typically delivered. Initial dilutions to 50 units/mL (2 mL saline added to the vial) or 25 units/mL (4 mL saline added to the vial) are generally used for clinical application. Further dilution to 12.5 units/mL or lower concentrations may be needed for very low doses. For administration of higher doses (i.e., 20 units) occasionally used in unilateral injections, a vial is diluted with 0.75-mL saline, giving a concentration of 133.3 units/mL, and 0.15 mL is administered.[35]

Experience with Myobloc for laryngeal injections is less extensive as it has only recently been available for clinical use. Myobloc is shipped in solution in concentrations of 5000 units/mL and may be stored in a refrigerator up to 2 years. Based on experience with application in other dystonias, the relative strength of Myobloc to Botox is 50:1. Therefore, a starting dose of 50 units/0.1 mL of Myobloc would be equivalent to 1.0 unit/0.1 mL of Botox.

The effective treatment dose is variable for each patient and for each muscle injected; therefore, injections are individualized. The dose range for adductor spasmodic dysphonia is 0.05 to 30 units of Botox, with an average dose of less than 1 unit per vocal fold.[17,18,24,31,32] In general, a starting dose of 1.25 units in 0.1 mL of saline is used for bilateral thyroarytenoid injections. Subsequent doses are varied according to clinical response and adverse effects. A trend toward lower doses has been observed and may be useful in reducing adverse effects.[19] Injections are given using a tuberculin syringe with a 27-gauge monopolar polytef-coated hollow EMG recording needle. Adductor laryngeal injections are performed percutaneously through the cricothyroid membrane and into the thyroarytenoid-vocalis muscle complex using EMG guidance for optimum placement (Figure 85B-1).

After an injection, patients will typically report improvement in voice within 24 hours followed by a breathy, hypophonic period lasting 1 to 2 weeks (45%), occasionally causing hyperventilation and dizziness when trying to speak. Mild choking on fluids for the first several days (22%) is also common; in addition, sore throat or coughing up blood-tinged sputum may occur in the first 1 to 2 days after injection.[14,15,17]

The abductor patients are also managed with an EMG-guided percutaneous injection. The larynx is manually rotated away from the side of intended injection, and the hollow EMG needle with syringe is placed posterior to the posterior edge of the thyroid lamina (Figure 85B-2). The needle is advanced to the cricoid cartilage and moved out under EMG guidance to the optimum position in the posterior cricoarytenoid muscle. When the patient is instructed to sniff, which maximally uses the posterior cricoarytenoid muscle, there is a burst of activity on the EMG, and the toxin is administered.[14,15,21,23]

Some abductor patients cannot tolerate manual rotation of the larynx; thus, injections are performed

transcricoid.[91] This technique begins with a small amount of anesthetic agent injected in the subglottic airway via the cricothyroid membrane. After an adequate level of anesthesia has been achieved, the 27-gauge polytef-coated needle is placed through the cricothyroid membrane, traversing the airway until it engages the posterior wall of the airway, the cricoid cartilage. The needle is aimed slightly laterally and slowly advanced through the cartilage under EMG control. Once the needle has gone through the cartilage, the posterior cricoarytenoid muscle is encountered and there is a burst of electric potentials. The patient is asked to sniff to confirm the position and activity, and the toxin is injected as previously described.

Injections for abductor spasmodic dysphonia typically require dosages in the range of 2.5 to 10 units of Botox in 0.1 mL of saline per posterior cricoarytenoid muscle. Unilateral injections are recommended initially to minimize the risk of airway obstruction. After the initial injection, if no response is obtained, flexible fiberoptic examination should be performed to assess the degree of abduction on the treated side. If no impairment in motion is detected, repeat injection should be performed. If limitation in motion is

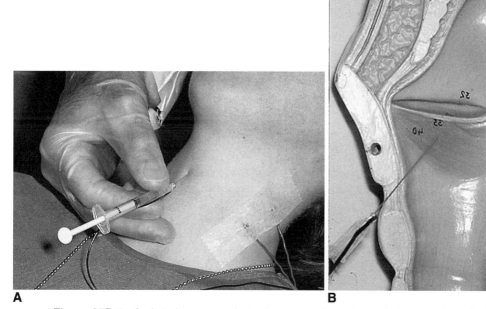

A **B**

Figure 85B-1. A, Anterior approach to the thyroarytenoid muscle through the cricothyroid membrane. The injection needle is passed into the airway and directed laterally and superiorly into the thyroarytenoid muscle. **B,** Model depicting placement of 27-gauge injection needle into the thyroarytenoid-vocalis muscle. An acute angle will place the injection into the anterior belly of the thyroarytenoid muscle.

Continued

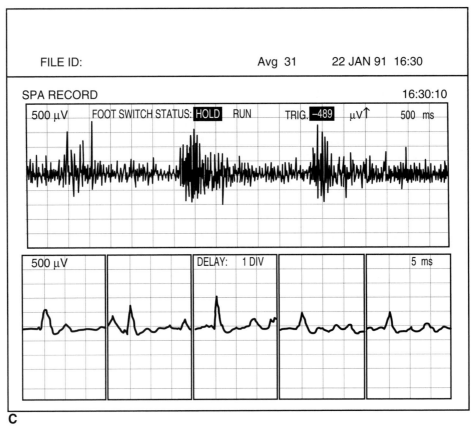

Figure 85B-1, cont'd C, EMG obtained during injection of the thyroarytenoid muscle. The patient is asked to say "E," resulting in recruitment and increased motor unit activation and confirming accurate placement of the electrode before injection.

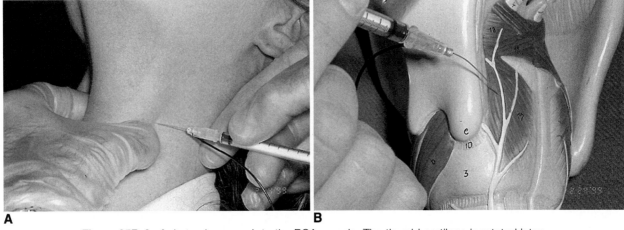

Figure 85B-2. A, Lateral approach to the PCA muscle. The thyroid cartilage is rotated laterally with simultaneous anterior displacement, exposing the posterior lateral border of the thyroid cartilage. The 27-gauge injection needle is inserted into the posterior lateral aspect of the cricoid cartilage. **B,** Model depicting placement of the injection needle into the PCA muscle using a posterior lateral approach.

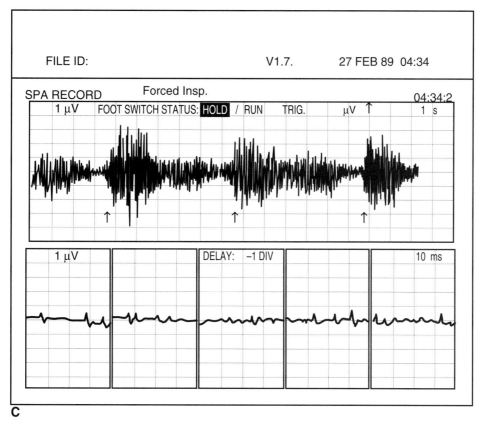

C

Figure 85B-2, cont'd C, EMG obtained during injection of the PCA muscle. Upward arrows indicate volitional "sniff" maneuver with recruitment of PCA motor units.

observed, without clinical response, bilateral injections may be required; however, the contralateral injection should be performed only after return of function is noted on the injected side (usually after 3–4 months). Occasionally, clinical response may be side dependent. Simultaneous bilateral injections may be performed, however, if the patient experiences airway compromise with unilateral injections, bilateral injections should be staged 1 to 2 months apart and lower dosages (1.0–2.0 units/0.1 mL) administered.

Onset of action after PCA injections may be delayed several days. Adverse reactions include dysphagia without aspiration, belching and regurgitation due to a weakening of the cricopharyngeus muscle, and mild stridor on exertion. Although no significant breathing difficulties have been reported, a cautious staged approach to bilateral injections is recommended.[14,15,21]

For adductor spasmodic dysphonia, Ford and others[52] reported an indirect laryngoscopic approach for injecting the toxin into the vocal fold. They reported that the technique has the advantage of being "familiar to the otolaryngologist and requires no special EMG equipment or training." The onset of response to

toxin appears delayed (mean, 9.1 days), but the degree of benefit and duration of efficacy appear comparable with EMG techniques. Nevertheless, when the patient is initially managed, the muscle appears to be electrically active at multiple sites throughout the course of the muscle. On follow-up, the electric recruitment pattern, an index of muscle contraction, may be patchy. EMG guidance has the advantage of controlled administration into the more actively contracting regions of the muscle.[17,33]

Regardless of technique, botulinum toxin injections have several advantages over surgical therapy in the management of intractable disease. The patient is awake for the procedure, and there is no risk of complications that would be involved with anesthesia. Graded degrees of weakening can be achieved by varying the dose. Most adverse effects are transient and are caused by an extension of the pharmacology of the toxin. If the patient has a strong response to therapy and too much weakness occurs, strength gradually returns. Follow-up therapy is carefully individualized. The response to therapy should be carefully documented.[35]

REFERENCES

1. Allegretto M and others: Selective denervation: reinnervation for the control of adductor spasmodic dysphonia, *J Otolaryngol* 32:185-189, 2003.
2. American Academy of Otolaryngology–Head and Neck Surgery policy statement: botox for spasmodic dysphonia, *Am Acad Otolaryngol Head Neck Surg Bull* 9:8, 1990.
3. American Academy of Neurology: Assessment: the clinical usefulness of botulinum toxin-A in treating neurologic disorders: report of the Therapeutics and Technology Assessment Subcommittee of the American Academy of Neurology, *Neurology* 40:1332, 1990.
4. Andrews J and others: Ventilatory dysfunction in palatal myoclonus, *Respiration* 52:76, 1987.
5. Aronson AE: *Clinical voice disorders*, New York, Thieme, 1985.
6. Aronson AE and others: Spastic dysphonia: II. comparison with essential (voice) tremor and other neurologic and psychogenic dysphonias, *J Speech Hear Disord* 33:219, 1968.
7. Aronson AE, DeSanto LW: Adductor spastic dysphonia: 1½ years after recurrent laryngeal nerve resection, *Ann Otol Rhinol Laryngol* 90:2, 1981.
8. Aronson AE, De Santo LW: Adductor spastic dysphonia: three years after recurrent laryngeal nerve resection, *Laryngoscope* 93:1, 1983.
9. Aronson AE, Hartman DE: Adductor spastic dysphonia as a sign of essential (voice) tremor, *J Speech Hear Disord* 46:52, 1981.
10. Bellussi G: Le disfonie impercinetiche, *Atti Labor Fonet Univ Padova* 3:1, 1952.
11. Berke GS and others: Selective laryngeal adductor denervation-reinnervation: a new surgical treatment for adductor spasmodic dysphonia, *Ann Otol Rhinol Laryngol* 108:227-231, 1999.
12. Black JD, Dolly JO: Interaction of ^{125}I-labeled botulinum neurotoxins with nerve terminals: I. ultrastructural autoradiographic localization and quantitation of distinct membrane acceptors for types A and B on motor nerves, *J Cell Biol* 103:521, 1986.
13. Black JD, Dolly JO: Interaction of ^{125}I-labeled botulinum neurotoxins with nerve terminals: II. autoradiographic evidence for its uptake into motor nerves by acceptor-mediated endocytosis, *J Cell Biol* 103:535, 1986.
14. Blitzer A, Brin MF: *Botulinum toxin for abductor spasmodic dysphonia*. In Jankovic J, Hallet M, editors: *Therapy with botulinum toxin*, New York, 1994, Marcel-Dekker.
15. Blitzer A, Brin MF: Botulinum toxin in the management of adductor and abductor spasmodic dysphonia, *Oper Techn Otolaryngol Head Neck Surg* 4:199, 1993.
16. Blitzer A, Brin MF: The dystonic larynx, *J Voice* 6:294, 1992.
17. Blitzer A, Brin MF: Laryngeal dystonia: a series with botulinum toxin therapy, *Ann Otol Rhinol Laryngol* 100:85, 1991.
18. Blitzer A, Brin MF: *Spasmodic dysphonia*. In Fried M, editor: *The larynx: a multidisciplinary approach,* ed 2, St Louis, 1995, Mosby.
19. Blitzer A, Brin MF, Stewart CF: Botulinum toxin management of spasmodic dysphonia: a 12-year experience in more than 900 patients, *Laryngoscope* 108:1435-1441, 1998.
20. Blitzer A, Sulica L: Botulinum toxin: basic science and clinical uses in Otolaryngology, *Laryngoscope* 111:218-226, 2001.
21. Blitzer A and others: Abductor laryngeal dystonia: a series treated with botulinum toxin, *Laryngoscope* 102:163, 1992.
22. Blitzer A and others: Clinical and laboratory characteristics of laryngeal dystonia: a study of 110 cases, *Laryngoscope* 98:636, 1988.
23. Blitzer A and others: Electromyographic findings in focal laryngeal dystonia (spastic dysphonia), *Ann Otol Rhinol Laryngol* 94:591, 1985.
24. Blitzer A and others: The use of botulinum toxin in the treatment of focal laryngeal dystonia (spastic dysphonia), *Laryngoscope* 98:193, 1988.
25. Braun N and others: Dyspnea in dystonia: a functional evaluation, *Chest* 107:1309, 1995.
26. Bressman SB and others: Dystonia in Ashkenazi Jews: clinical characterization of a founder mutation, *Ann Neurol* 36:771, 1994.
27. Bressman SB and others: Idiopathic tortion dystonia among Ashkenazi Jews: evidence for autosomal dominant inheritance, *Ann Neurol* 26:612, 1989.
28. Bressman SB and others: A study of idiopathic torsion dystonia in a non-Jewish family: evidence for genetic heterogeneity, *Neurology* 44:283, 1994.
29. Brin MF: *Dystonia: genetics and treatment with botulinum toxin.* In Smith B, Adelman G: *Neuroscience year.*
30. Brin MF, Blitzer A, Stewart C: *Vocal tremor.* In Findley LJ, Koller WC, editors: *Handbook of tremor disorders*, New York, 1994, Marcel-Dekker.
31. Brin MF and others: Adductor laryngeal dystonia (spastic dysphonia): treatment with local injections of botulinum toxin (BOTOX), *Mov Disord* 4:287, 1989.
32. Brin MF and others: Adductor laryngeal dystonia: treatment with local injections of botulinum toxin (BOTOX), *Neurology* 38(Suppl 1):244, 1988.
33. Brin MF and others: *Laryngeal motion disorders.* In Blitzer A and others, editors: *Neurological disorders of the larynx*, New York, 1992, Thieme.
34. Brin MF and others: Localized injections of botulinum toxin for the treatment of focal dystonia and hemifacial spasm, *Mov Disord* 2:237, 1987.
35. Brin MF and others: *Treatment of spasmodic dysphonia (laryngeal dystonia) with injections of botulinum toxin: review and technical aspects.* In Blitzer A and others, editors: *Neurological disorders of the larynx*, New York, 1992, Thieme.
36. Brown JR, Simonson J: Organic voice tremor: a tremor of phonation, *Neurology* 13:520, 1963.
37. Caine ED, Polinsky RJ: Tardive dyskinesia in a person with Gilles de la Tourette's syndrome, *Arch Neurol* 38:471, 1981.
38. Caine ED and others: Gilles de la Tourette's syndrome, tardive dyskinesia and psychosis in an adolescent, *Am J Psychiatry* 135:241, 1978.
39. Critchley M: Spastic dysphonia ("inspiratory speech"), *Brain* 62:96, 1939.
40. DasGupta BR, Foley JJ: C botulinum neurotoxin types A and E: isolated light chain breaks down into two fragments. Comparison of their amino acid sequences with tetanus neurotoxin, *Biochimie* 71:1193, 1989.
41. Dedo HH, Izdebski K: Intermediate results of 306 recurrent laryngeal nerve sections for spastic dysphonia, *Laryngoscope* 93:9, 1983.
42. DeJong RN: *The neurologic examination*, New York, 1967, Hueber.
43. De Leon D and others: Genetic factors in spastic dysphonia, *Neurology* 40(Suppl 1):142, 1990.
44. Evans GM and others: Botulinum type B: its purification, radioiodination and interaction with rat-brain synaptosomal membranes, *Eur J Biochem* 154:409, 1986.

45. Fahn S: The varied clinical expressions of dystonia, *Neurol Clin* 2:541, 1984.

46. Fahn S, Marsden CD, Van Woert MH: Definition and classification of myoclonus, *Adv Neurol* 43:1, 1986.

47. Fahn S, Moskowitz C: X-linked recessive dystonia and parkinsonism in Filipino males [abstract], *Ann Neurol* 24:179, 1988.

48. Findley LJ: *The pharmacology of essential tremor.* In Marsden CD, Fahn S, editors: *Movement disorders*, ed 2. London, 1987, Butterworths.

49. Findley LJ, Cleeves L: The relation of essential tremor to Parkinson's disease [letter], *J Neurol Neurosurg Psychiatry* 48:192, 1985.

50. Findley L, Gresty M: Head facial and voice tremor, *Adv Neurol* 49:239, 1988.

51. Finitzo T, Freeman F: Spasmodic dysphonia, whether and where: results of seven years of research, *J Speech Hear Res* 32:541, 1989.

52. Ford CN, Bless DM, Lowery JD: Indirect laryngoscopic approach for injection of botulinum toxin in spasmodic dysphonia, *Otolaryngol Head Neck Surg* 103:752, 1990.

53. Fraenkel B: Ueber die beschaeftigungsschwaeche der stimme: mogiphonie, *Dtsch Med Wochenschr* 13:121, 1887.

54. Friedman A, Fahn S: Spontaneous remissions in spasmodic torticollis, *Neurology* 36:398, 1986.

55. Gauthier S, Young SN, Baxter DW: Palatal myoclonus associated with a decrease in 5-hydroxy-indole acetic acid in cerebrospinal fluid and responding to clonazepam, *Can J Neurol Sci* 8:51, 1981.

56. Gerhardt P: Bewegungsstoerungen der stimmbaender, *Nothnagels spezielle pathologie und therapie* 13:307, 1896.

57. Goldman MS, Kelly PJ: Stereotactic thalamotomy for medically intractable essential tremor, *Stereotact Funct Neurosurg* 58:22, 1992.

58. Gowers WR: *Manual of diseases of the nervous system*, London, Churchill, 1899.

59. Grillone G, Blitzer A, Brin MF: Treatment of adductor breathing dystonia with botulinum toxin, *Laryngoscope* 104:30, 1994.

60. Hachinski VC, Thomsen IV, Buch NH: The nature of primary vocal tremor, *Can J Neurol Sci* 2:195, 1975.

61. Hartman DE, Overholt SL, Vishwanat B: A case of vocal cord nodules masking essential (voice) tremor, *Arch Otolaryngol Head Neck Surg* 108:52, 1982.

62. Hunker C, Abbs J: *Physiological analysis of parkinsonian tremors in the oral facial system.* In *The dysarthrias.* San Diego, 1984, College-Hill Press.

63. Huttner WB: Snappy exocytoxins, *Nature* 365:104, 1993.

64. Ichinose H and others: Hereditary progressive dystonia with marked diurnal fluctuation caused by mutations in the GTP cyclohydrolase I gene, *Nature Genet* 8:236, 1994.

65. Jabbari B and others: Effectiveness of trihexyphenidyl against pendular nystagmus and palatal myoclonus: evidence of cholinergic dysfunction, *Mov Disord* 2:93, 1987.

66. Jabbari B and others: Treatment of movement disorders with trihexyphenidyl, *Mov Disord* 4:202, 1989.

67. Jacome DE, Yanez GF: Spastic dysphonia and Meige disease, *Neurology* 30:349, 1980.

68. Jankovic J, Fahn S: Physiologic and pathophysiologic tremors: diagnosis, mechanisms, and management, *Ann Int Med* 93:460, 1980.

69. Jankovic J, Pardo R: Segmental myoclonus: clinical and pharmacologic study, *Ann Neurol* 43:1025, 1986.

70. Jayne D, Lees AJ, Stern GM: Remission in spasmodic torticollis, *J Neurol Neurosurg Psychiatry* 47:1236, 1984.

71. Kalinowski J: Self-reported efficacy of an all in-the-ear-canal prosthetic device to inhibit stuttering during one hundred hours of university teaching: an autobiographical clinical commentary. *Disabil Rehabil* 25:107-111, 2003.

72. Koller WC, Busenbark K, Miner K: The relationship of essential tremor to other movement disorders: report on 678 patients. Essential Tremor Study Group, *Ann Neurol* 35:717, 1994.

73. Koller WC, Royse VL: Efficacy of primidone in essential tremor, *Neurology* 36:121, 1986.

74. Kozaki S: Interaction of botulinum type A, B, and E derivative toxins with synaptosomes of rat brain, *Naunyn Schmiedebergs Arch Pharmacol* 308:67, 1979.

75. Kozaki S, Sakaguchi G: Binding to mouse brain synaptosomes of Clostridium botulinum type E derivative toxin before and after tryptic activation, *Toxicon* 20:841, 1982.

76. Kramer PL and others: Dystonia gene in Ashkenazi Jewish population is located on chromosome 9q32-34, *Ann Neurol* 27:114, 1990.

77. Kupke KG, Lee LV, Muller U: Assignment of the X-linked tortion dystonia gene to Xq21 by linkage analysis, *Neurology* 40:1438, 1990.

78. Lapresle J, Ben Hamida M: The dentato-olivary pathway: somatotopic relationship between the dentate nucleus and the contralateral inferior olive, *Arch Neurol* 22:135, 1970.

79. Lebrun Y and others: Tremulous speech, *Folia Phoniatr* 34:134, 1982.

80. Magnussen I and others: Palatal myoclonus treated with 5-hydroxytryptophan and decarboxylase-inhibitor, *Acta Neurol Scand* 55:251, 1977.

81. Marsden CD: *Origins of normal and pathological tremor.* In Findley LJ, Capildeo R, editors: *Movement disorders: tremor.* New York, 1984, Oxford University Press.

82. Marsden CD, Hallett M, Fahn S: *The nosology and pathophysiology of myoclonus.* In Marsden CD, Fahn S, editors: *Movement disorders,* London, 1982, Butterworths.

83. Marsden CD, Obeso JA, Rothwell JC: *Benign essential tremor is not a single entity.* In Yahr MD, editor: *Current concepts in Parkinson's disease,* Amsterdam, 1983, Excerpta Medica.

84. Marsden CD, Sheehy MP: Spasmodic dysphonia, Meige disease, and tortion dystonia, *Neurology* 32:1202, 1982.

85. Marsden CD and others: Muscle spasms associated with Sudek's atrophy after injury, *BMJ* 1:173, 1984.

86. Marshall J: Observations on essential tremor, *J Neurol Neurosurg Psychiatry* 25:122, 1986.

87. Massey EW, Paulson GW: Essential vocal tremor: clinical characteristics and response to therapy, *South Med J* 78:316, 1985.

88. Massey EW, Paulson G: Essential vocal tremor: response to therapy, *Neurology* 32:113, 1982.

89. Meeuwis CA, Baarsma EA: Essential (voice) tremor, *Clin Otolaryngol* 10:54, 1985.

90. Meige H: Les convulsions de la face: une forme clinique de convulsions faciales, bilaterale et mediane, *Rev Neurol (Paris)* 21:437, 1910.

91. Meleca RJ, Hogikyan ND, Bastian RW: A comparison of methods of botulinum toxin injection for abductor spasmodic dysphonia, *Otolaryngol Head Neck Surg* 117: 487-492, 1997.

92. Miller S, Watson BC: The relationship between communication attitude, anxiety, and depression in stutterers and non-stutterers, *J Speech Hear Res* 35:789, 1994.

93. Mizhari EM, Holtsman D, Tharp B: Haloperidol-induced tardive dyskinesia in a child with Gilles de la Tourette's syndrome, *Arch Neurol* 37:780, 1980.

94. Clinical use of botulinum toxin. Reprinted from *NIH Consens Dev Conf Consens Statement*, 1990.

95. Nutt JG and others: Epidemiology of focal and generalized dystonia in Rochester, Minnesota, *Mov Disord* 3:188, 1988.

96. Nygaard TG, Marsden CD, Fahn S: Dopa-responsive dystonia: long-term treatment response and prognosis, *Neurology* 41:174, 1991.

97. Ozelius L and others: Human gene for tortion dystonia located on chromosome 9q32-34, *Ann Neurol* 27:114, 1990.

98. Ozelius LJ and others: Strong allelic association between the tortion dystonia gene (DTY1) and loci on chromosome 9q34 in Ashkenazi Jews, *Am J Hum Genet* 50:619, 1992.

99. Parnes SM, Lavarato AS, Myers EN: Study of spastic dysphonia by video fiberoptic laryngoscopy, *Ann Otol Rhinol Laryngol* 87:322, 1978.

100. Pauls DL and others: Tourette syndrome and neuropsychiatric disorders: is there a genetic relationship, *Am J Hum Genet* 43:206, 1988.

101. Philippbar SA, Robin DA, Luschei ES: *Limb, jaw and vocal tremor in Parkinson's patients.* In Yorkston K, Beukelman D, editors: *Recent advances in clinical dysarthria,* San Diego, 1991, College-Hill Press.

102. Prins D: Personality, stuttering severity, and age, *J Speech Hear Res* 15:148, 1972.

103. Rack PM, Ross HF: The role of the reflexes in the resting tremor of Parkinson's disease, *Brain* 109:115, 1986.

104. Riley GD: A stuttering severity instrument for children and adults, *J Speech Hear Disord* 37:314, 1972.

105. Rondot P, Ben Hamida M: Myoclonies du voille et myoclonies squelettiques: etude clinique et anatomique, *Rev Neurol (Paris)* 119:59, 1968.

106. Sakaguchi G, Kozaki S, Ohishi I: *Structure and function of botulinum toxins.* In Alouf JEF, editor: *Bacterial protein toxins.* London, 1984, Academic Press.

107. Sakai T, Murakami S: Palatal myoclonus responding to carbamazepine, *Ann Neurol* 9:199, 1981 (letter).

108. Salloway S and others: Botulinum toxin for refractory vocal tics, *Mov Disord* 11:746, 1996.

109. Schaefer S and others: Vocal tract electromyographic abnormalities in spasmodic dysphonia: preliminary report, *Trans Am Laryngol Ass* 108:187, 1987.

110. Schnitzler J: Klinischer *Atlas der Laryngologie nebst Anleitung zur Diagnose und Therapie der Krankheiten des Kehlkopfes und der Luftrohre,* Wien, 1895, Braumuller.

111. Shale HM, Greene P, Fahn S: Tardive movement disorders in tic patients treated with dopamine receptor blocking agents, *Neurology* 39(Suppl 1):202, 1989.

112. Siegfried J, Lippitz B: Chronic electrical stimulation of the VL-VPL complex and of the pallidum in the treatment of movement disorders: personal experience since 1982, *Stereotact Funct Neurosurg* 62:71, 1994.

113. Simpson LL: Kinetic studies on the interaction between botulinum toxin type A and the cholinergic neuromuscular junction, *J Pharmacol Exp Ther* 212:16, 1980.

114. Simpson LL: Molecular pharmacology of botulinum toxin and tetanus toxin, *Ann Rev Pharmacol Toxicol* 26:427, 1986.

115. Simpson LL: The origin, structure, and pharmacological activity of botulinum toxin, *Pharmacol Rev* 33:155, 1981.

116. Simpson LL, DasGupta BR: Botulinum neurotoxin type E: studies on mechanism of action and on structure-activity relationships, *J Pharmacol Exp Ther* 224:135, 1983.

117. Smith A and others: Spectral analysis of activity of laryngeal and orofacial muscles in stutterers, *J Neurol Neurosurg Psychiatr* 56:1303, 1993.

118. Stager SV and others: Fluency changes in persons who stutter following a double blind trial of clomipramine and desipramine, *J Speech Hear Res* 38:516, 1995.

119. Stuart A and others: Investigations of the impact of altered auditory feedback in-the-ear devices on the impact of altered auditory feedback in-the-ear devices on the speech of people who stutter, *Int J Lang Commun Disord* 39:93-113, 2004.

120. Stuart A and others: Self-contained in-the-ear device to deliver altered auditory feedback: applications for stuttering, *Ann Biomed Eng* 31:2333-2337, 2003.

121. Sveinbjornsdottir S, Pakkenberg H, Werdelin L: Developmental stuttering followed by intermittent jaw opening dystonia, *Mov Disord* 8:396, 1993.

122. Tolosa ES: Clinical features of Meige's disease (idiopathic orofacial dystonia): a report of 17 cases, *Arch Neurol* 38:147, 1981.

123. Tomoda H and others: Voice tremor: dysregulation of voluntary expiratory muscles, *Neurology* 37:117, 1987.

124. Traube L: *Zur Lehre von den Larynxaffectionen beim Ileotyphus.* Berlin, 1871, Verlag Von August Hirschwald.

125. Van Pelt F, Ludlow CL, Smith PJ: Comparison of muscle activation patterns in adductor and abductor dysphonia, *Ann Otol Rhinol Laryngol* 103:192, 1994.

126. Walsh EG: Beats produced between the rhythmic applied force and the resting tremor of parkinsonism, *J Neurol Neurosurg Psychiatry* 42:89, 1979.

127. Webster RL: *Empirical considerations regarding stuttering therapy.* In Gregory HH, editor: *Controversies about stuttering therapy.* Baltimore, 1979, University Park Press.

128. Wilhelmsen KC and others: Genetic mapping of the "Lubag" (X-linked dystonia-parkinsonism) in a Filipino kindred to the pericentromeric region of the X chromosome, *Ann Neurol* 29:124, 1991.

129. Williams A, Goodenberger D, Calne DB: Palatal myoclonus following herpes zoster ameliorated by 5-hydroxytryptophan and carbidopa, *Neurology* 28:358, 1978.

130. Williams RS and others: Radioiodination of botulinum neurotoxin type A with retention of biological activity and its binding to brain synaptosomes, *Eur J Biochem* 131:437, 1983.

131. Woodson GE, Blitzer A: *Neurologic evaluation of the larynx and pharynx.* In Cummings CW and others, editors: *Otolaryngology—head and neck surgery: update I,* ed 2, St Louis, 1995, Mosby.

132. Woodson GE and others: Use of flexible laryngoscopy to classify patients with spasmodic dysphonia, *J Voice* 5:85, 1991.

133. Young RR, Shahani BT: Asterixis: one type of negative myoclonus, *Adv Neurol* 43:137, 1986.

CHAPTER EIGHTY SIX

VISUAL DOCUMENTATION OF THE LARYNX

Randall L. Plant
Robin A. Samlan

INTRODUCTION

In this chapter, the authors describe the equipment and techniques of video documentation of the larynx and how to analyze and interpret the images obtained. Laryngeal videoendoscopy with or without stroboscopy is used to diagnose and document voice and laryngeal disorders, track changes over time, and to provide biofeedback for voice and breathing therapy; it is a clinical tool that is also used in the office setting to examine vocal fold structure and gross function. Stroboscopy is a lighting technique that helps clinicians examine the body-cover relationship and vibration patterns, and it is valuable for describing mucosal disease and its effect on vocal-fold vibration. Stroboscopy is necessary to determine glottic closure and mucosal pliability, to make inferences about tension, and, sometimes, to identify lesions. Rigid and flexible endoscopes can be used with both continuous and stroboscopic light sources. The decisions to use continuous or strobe light and rigid or flexible endoscope are largely based on whether the examiner is more interested in gross structure and function or mucosal health and vibration patterns. Often, both rigid and flexible examinations are necessary to thoroughly assess laryngeal function during a variety of voicing conditions and therapy probes.

Laryngeal videoendoscopy and stroboscopy (LVES or videostroboscopy) can be performed by either an otolaryngologist or a qualified speech-language pathologist, in most states.[1] Each professional brings a different perspective and training to the process, and the most thorough examinations are typically conducted in a team setting. The otolaryngologist is responsible for assessing mucosal health and diagnosing laryngeal pathology; the speech pathologist is interested in the vocal-fold vibratory patterns during various voicing conditions, the behavior of the laryngeal and supralaryngeal structures during phonation, and how treatment probes alter phonatory physiology. As team

members work together over time, they often learn from one another and develop common skill sets.[28]

The advantages and disadvantages of rigid and flexible endoscopes are described in the first section of this chapter, with recommendations for technique and troubleshooting. The second section details the assessment process for endoscopy and stroboscopy. The final section discusses equipment for laryngeal imaging.

ENDOSCOPES
Rigid Endoscopes
Advantages

Rigid endoscopes used with LVES are usually 70- or 90-degree scopes. As stated in the "Equipment" section, rigid scopes have the advantage of higher resolution with brighter, clearer pictures. Contrast is better, there is a large selection of viewing angles, and the image is more accurately magnified than with a flexible endoscope. The examination is simple and does not usually require topical anesthetic.[17,18,28]

Disadvantages

The primary limitation of the rigid endoscope is that phonation is limited to sustained vowels. Because visualization with a 70-degree rigid endoscope usually requires an extended neck and protruded tongue, the size of a glottic gap might appear exaggerated with the rigid endoscope.[31] To counteract this problem, Rammage, Morrison, and Nichol[28] suggest a lateral approach to the larynx to decrease neck extension during the examination. Alternatively, a 90-degree endoscope does not require the same degree of neck extension as the 70-degree endoscope does.

Technique

The laryngeal examination with a 70-degree rigid endoscope is conducted with the patient bending slightly forward from the waist while maintaining a straight back. The neck is extended, and the tongue is protruded. The examiner wraps the tongue in gauze and holds it gently with the thumb on the underside and the middle finger on the surface. The index finger is used to protect the upper teeth and guide the endoscope during placement. The endoscope is advanced just under the uvula or between the uvula and faucial pillars until the epiglottis is visualized. Using a sustained vowel /ei/ will lower the tongue base and facilitate placement; the wrist is then flexed so that the endoscope tip tilts inferiorly. The angle can be varied for differing degrees of magnification and differing fields of view. The patient is then guided through the examination tasks listed in the "Assessment" section below. Examination with the 90-degree endoscope is similar, but the patient does not to need to bend forward or extend the neck. Another difference is the angle; the tip of the 90-degree scope is positioned with minimal tilt so that the light is parallel to the surface of the vocal folds. This type of endoscope is often preferable for viewing the larynx when a wider viewing angle is desired. A longer lens or a zoom lens might be necessary for adequate vocal-fold detail.

Defogging the endoscopes can be a challenge, because sterilizing beads can cause damage. Alternatives include liquid defogger, soap film, surgical wax, and holding the endoscope lens briefly against the cheek or the side of the tongue. The examination is generally tolerated without topical anesthetic, but a small amount of benzocaine topical spray or a similar product is sometimes useful and does not appear to affect examination results.[25]

Troubleshooting

A good quality examination means that the image is in focus, that it is large enough to show small lesions, and that it is bright enough to show details (but not so bright as to obscure them). Contrasting color is important for differentiating subtle lesions and vascular changes. Ideally, an examination includes a both a wide-angle view of the larynx and close-up view of the vocal folds. The stroboscopic portion of the examination should include several complete stroboscopic cycles at normal pitch and loudness in addition to the rest of the protocol (see "Assessment"). Common imaging problems and solutions are listed in Table 86-1.

TABLE 86-1

COMMON PROBLEMS ENCOUNTERED DURING LARYNGEAL VIDEOENDOSCOPY AND STROBOSCOPY WITH A RIGID ENDOSCOPE, ALONG WITH POSSIBLE SOLUTIONS

Problem	Solutions
Foggy image	• Warm the endoscope. • Apply a defogging agent. • Clean the endoscope lens; there may be mucous or dried disinfectant obscuring the image.
Fuzzy image	• Check or adjust the focus. Whenever possible, set the focus on the endoscope (if there is one) before connecting it to the camera, and then leave it alone. • Clean the endoscope lens.
Dark image	• Clean the lens of the endoscope, the eyepiece, or the camera. • Increase the light. Different techniques are used for different light sources and cameras. For some systems, decreasing the shutter speed or turning the electronic light control on or off can increase brightness. • Change the position of the endoscope; the light might not be directly over the vocal folds or the area of interest. • If it is the xenon light that is too dark, check the number of hours on the bulb. The brightness of the xenon light fades with use, whereas the halogen bulb burns out all at once.
Grainy image	• Decrease the gain. • Set the endoscope slightly out of focus. • Consider a shorter camera lens.
Tilted image, or the vocal folds appear to be different widths	• Modify the alignment of the endoscope and camera. • Be sure that your arm and wrist are approaching the patient straight on that that they are not tilted. • Have a third party hold the laryngeal microphone to the patient's neck, or attach it to a Velcro® strap.

TABLE 86-1

COMMON PROBLEMS ENCOUNTERED DURING LARYNGEAL VIDEOENDOSCOPY AND STROBOSCOPY
WITH A RIGID ENDOSCOPE, ALONG WITH POSSIBLE SOLUTIONS—cont'd

Problem	Solutions
Image of mostly the valleculae and the epiglottis	• Insert the endoscope further into the oropharynx. • Tilt the tip of the endoscope.
Image of mostly the arytenoids and the posterior vocal folds	• Withdraw the endoscope slightly from the oropharynx. • Tilt the tip of the endoscope. • Have the patient phonate in a high pitch. • Request that the sound be more "ee-like."
Base of tongue is high	• Ask the patient to produce sustained "hey" or "a." • Ask the patient to allow the back of the tongue and jaw to release and be "floppy." • Have the patient hold his or her own tongue.
Uvula is "in the way"	• Direct the endoscope around the uvula. • Have the patient breathe through the mouth, not the nose. • Ask for the sound to be more "ee-like." • Have the patient plug his or her nose or use nose clips.
Abnormal color	• This depends on the imaging system; color can often be adjusted by controls on the monitor, camera, or printer. • Check the brightness settings. • Check the focus; the image may need to be slightly out of focus.
Omega-shaped epiglottis	• Use a 90-degree endoscope. • Have the patient bend further forward so that the elbows rest on the knees, then have him or her extend the neck as much as possible. • Try a lateral approach.
Strobe is "not tracking"	• Modify placement of the laryngeal microphone or electroglottograph (EGG) electrodes; they should be placed flat on the neck, over the thyroid laminae. • Have the patient phonate more loudly. • Try the other fundamental frequency extractor (i.e., use the laryngeal microphone if the Fo is not tracking with the EGG). • The vibration might be aperiodic; try other vocalization tasks, such as high pitch, low pitch, quiet voice, phonation on inhalation, and instruction to take a bigger breath and relax the shoulders. • Some systems allow the examiner to select an approximate fundamental frequency as an override. If your system does not have that feature, the examiner can phonate at the approximate fundamental frequency to trigger the strobe light.
Plica ventricularis; the ventricular folds are closed, so the true vocal folds cannot be seen	• Ask the patient to produce a soft, gentle, breathy "hhheee," almost like a sigh. Model such a production. • Ask patient to laugh: "hee hee hee." • Have the patient phonate on inhalation. • Have the patient undergo voice therapy, followed by repeat evaluation.
Gagging	• First, educate the patient about the examination. It is sometimes helpful to use a model to show that the vocal folds are in view, with the endoscope placed far above them. • Talk the patient through the examination in a calming voice, reminding him or her to breathe slowly through the mouth and to start phonating in a relaxed, breathy voice. • Distract the patient by having him or her focus on a certain spot, think the alphabet backwards, or try not to blink (attenuation of the blink reflex will suppress the gag reflex). • Have the patient hold his or her own tongue. • Alter the approach (e.g., lateral versus anterior; elevate the endoscope tip or lower it). • Use a topical anesthetic. • Use a flexible endoscope.

Flexible Endoscopes
Advantages

The primary advantage of the flexible endoscope is the ability to view the larynx during speech and singing. Glottic gap can be more accurately described than with rigid endoscopy because of the neutral tongue and neck positions.[31] Flexible endoscopy also allows the clinician to assess the nasal cavity and velopharyngeal port during the same examination. Flexible endoscopy is preferred when the question is one of movement rather than structure or mucosal health. It is particularly useful for disorders such as spasmodic dysphonia, where the voice problem is more obvious during speech than sustained vowels, and vocal-fold motion impairment, where having the patient sniff through the nose allows the examiner to assess subtle motion changes.

Disadvantages

The primary limitation of the technique is that light transport and magnification of the image are inferior to the rigid endoscope. There is also a distortion of the periphery of the image. Figure 86-1 shows the differences in clarity and distortion between the rigid and flexible endoscopes. There is often a trade-off between adequate focus and light fiber mismatch so that, when the image in focus, there is a moiré or honeycomb effect that is enhanced by the edge-detection software of digital imaging systems (Figure 86-2). Although technology is improving, the examinations are still not equivalent. In addition, many patients find the flexible examination to be more invasive than the rigid; it carries with it the risks of nosebleed, adverse reactions to the anesthetic, and vasovagal reaction.

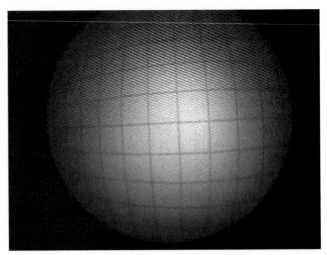

Figure 86-2. Moiré effect seen with a flexible endoscope.

Technique

The flexible endoscope is typically inserted after the application of a topical anesthetic and a vasoconstrictor. It can be passed through the middle meatus or along the floor of the nose. The higher path is preferred when examining the velopharyngeal port, but the paths are equivalent for visualizing the larynx.

Troubleshooting

As with the rigid endoscope, a good quality examination means that the image is in focus, large enough to see small lesions, bright enough to see details, and not so bright that details are obscured. It is easy to vary the field of view using the flexible endoscope, but it is sometimes challenging to bring the endoscope close enough to the vocal folds for optimal light and vibra-

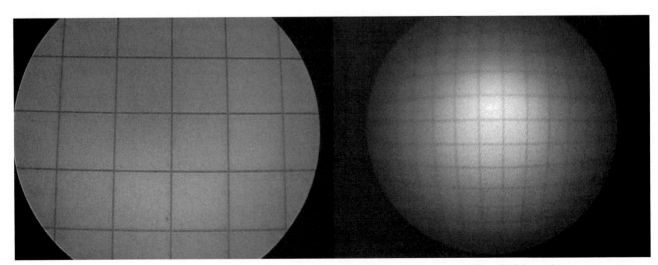

Figure 86-1. Distortion and image quality using **A,** a rigid endoscope, and **B,** a flexible endoscope.

tory detail. Patients generally allow a more complete examination when they are fully informed about the procedure, have some feeling of control (e.g., they know you will respond if they say they have had enough), and have had adequate anesthetic.

ASSESSMENT
Assessment Using Continuous Light
Introduction

Endoscopic parameters that require only continuous light (not stroboscopy) include laryngeal structure, arytenoid and vocal-fold motion, color and quantity of mucous, vascularity, change in laryngeal height or position with phonation, supraglottic activity or compression, and deformation of vocal-fold edges. The tasks during this portion of the examination include rest breathing, deep breathing, easy cough or throat clear, and laryngeal diadochokinesis (DDK), which consists of rapid repetitions of "ee" with glottal stops between productions. Repetitions of a short "ee" followed by a quick sniff through the nose are elicited if a flexible endoscope is used. Laryngeal DDK is a useful measure, and production rates of four to six syllables per second are considered normal.[9] Difficulty with accurately and rhythmically producing the voice onset/offset gesture has been found in patients with neurologic impairment.[3,40] A sample protocol is outlined in Box 86-1.

Laryngeal Structure

The valleculae, pyriform sinuses, epiglottis, aryepiglottic folds, ventricular folds, and posterior glottic rim should be examined. Abnormalities and asymmetries of laryngeal structure are noted. An omega-shaped epiglottis is a common variant in men, but it is rare in women.[9,34] Signs of laryngeal irritation or possible extraesophageal reflux are noted; these primarily include edema, erythema, surface irregularities, and lesions of the posterior larynx.[13,14,15,39] The specificity of these signs for reflux is still being evaluated. In par-

ticular, interarytenoid bar, arytenoid medial wall erythema, and posterior pharyngeal wall cobblestoning have been found in a substantial number of "normal" volunteers.[15]

Arytenoid and Vocal-Fold Motion

Movement and position of the arytenoids informs the examiner about the integrity of the cricoarytenoid joint and the recurrent laryngeal nerve. Arytenoids are typically described as upright or rotated, mobile or immobile, and symmetric or asymmetric. Immobility is further described by position: median, paramedian, intermediate, or lateral. Sometimes the arytenoid is mobile but the vocal fold is not. Mobility is rated as patients phonate then breathe, during laryngeal DDK, when they are coughing, and, sometimes, when they are sniffing. Vocal-fold motion impairment has many potential causes, including paralysis, paresis, arytenoid dislocation, fibrosis, or tumor invasion of the cricoarytenoid joint. The etiology of the motion impairment—along with the particular characteristics of arytenoid position, gap size and shape, and so on—can change management strategy, as described in the chapters about phonosurgical procedures.

Color and Quantity of Mucous

Thickened mucous often adheres to the vocal-fold edges or superior surface. The presence of thick mucous generally relates to a lack of hydration or chronic irritation. Mucous pooling in the pyriform sinuses can indicate poor laryngeal sensation, weak lateral pharyngeal walls, or inefficient swallow. Thickened mucous adhering to the vocal folds can masquerade as a lesion or mask an abnormality. Patients should be instructed to try to clear the mucous by swallowing or with a brief cough or throat clear to differentiate mucous from underlying structures or lesions.

Vascularity

The vocal folds are generally pearly white on examination. A blush throughout the tissue is considered erythema or hyperemia. If capillaries are visible, they are generally aligned parallel with the free edge. Abnormally dilated and tortuous vessels are called *capillary ectasias* or *microvarices,* and they might represent areas of stiffness or risk for hemorrhage. Hemorrhage occurs when enough blood cells have escaped from a vessel to lend a diffuse coloring to the vocal fold.

Change in Laryngeal Position or Height

Change in lateral position or tilting to one side can be the result of a mass displacing the larynx, muscle imbalance, trauma, or superior laryngeal nerve injury.

BOX 86-1

SAMPLE PROTOCOL FOR LARYNGEAL VIDEOENDOSCOPY WITH CONTINUOUS LIGHT. THE ITEMS MARKED WITH AN ASTERISK (*) ARE COMPLETED ONLY IF USING A FLEXIBLE ENDOSCOPE

Rest breathing
Deep breathing
Easy cough or throat clear
Laryngeal diadochokinesis "ee"
Laryngeal diadochokinesis "hee"
Sustained "ee," then quick sniff through the nose*

Change in laryngeal height is also noted. Some people raise or lower the larynx with talking or singing; this can be either a normal variant or a manifestation of altered laryngeal muscle tension. Pemberton and colleagues[24] found that the larynx tends to rise with ascending pitch glides and lower with descending pitch glides. There is no clear rule for differentiating normal from excessive vertical change with speaking or singing; it remains a decision based on clinical experience and tradition.

Supraglottic Activity

Supraglottic activity includes tremor of the laryngeal complex or pharynx, other involuntary contractions (e.g., myoclonic movements), or compression of the supraglottic structures. Supraglottic movements help tease apart neurologic and functional voice disorders; tremor and myoclonic movement are evidence of a neurologic disorder, whereas sustained compression is more typically found in functional disorders. Compression is often categorized by direction (anteroposterior or lateromedial) and frequency (constant or intermittent). Anteroposterior (AP) compression during phonation is shown in Figure 86-3, and lateromedial compression is shown in Figure 86-4. In the Stroboscopy Evaluation Rating Form, Poburka[26] displays a superior view of the vocal folds with superimposed concentric circles. Raters estimate the degree of constriction by selecting the circle that best approximates the degree of constriction. The frequency and severity of supraglottic constriction in subjects without voice disorders is still somewhat uncertain, although it is clear that both anteroposterior and lateromedial constriction are sometimes normal variants.[4,24,33] Stager and others[33] found that abnormal supraglottic movements in normal controls were present at the initiation of phonation as short compressions with connected speech and as static compression during specific tasks. The degree of supraglottic constriction may help differentiate normal cases from pathologic cases. Behrman and others[4] showed a greater severity of AP constriction in dysphonic subjects than in normal controls. At the extreme of lateromedial compression, the ventricular folds touch and may even vibrate (this was formerly called *plica ventricularis*). Ventricular fold closure is not considered a normal variant and can be the primary disorder[28] or compensation for another problem, such as incomplete glottic closure or a lesion.[5,21] Voice therapy maneuvers should be used to reduce the amount of compression, and visualization should be repeated.

Other supraglottic activity can occur in subjects with normal voices. Lateral wall constriction is frequently observed with increasing pitch. Anteroposterior narrowing of the epilaryngeal space without lateromedial constriction during singing might be a desired pattern that helps to create the singer's formant.[35]

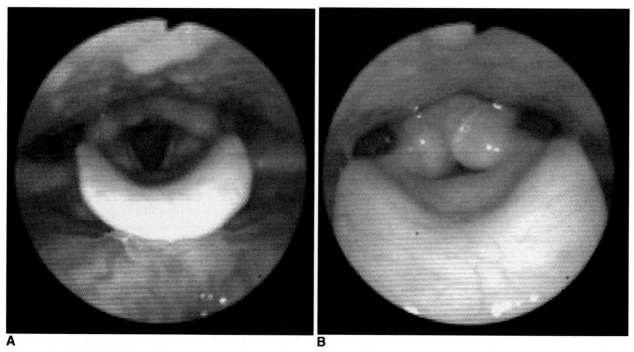

A **B**

Figure 86-3. A, Vocal folds during respiration. **B,** Vocal folds with anteroposterior constriction during phonation.

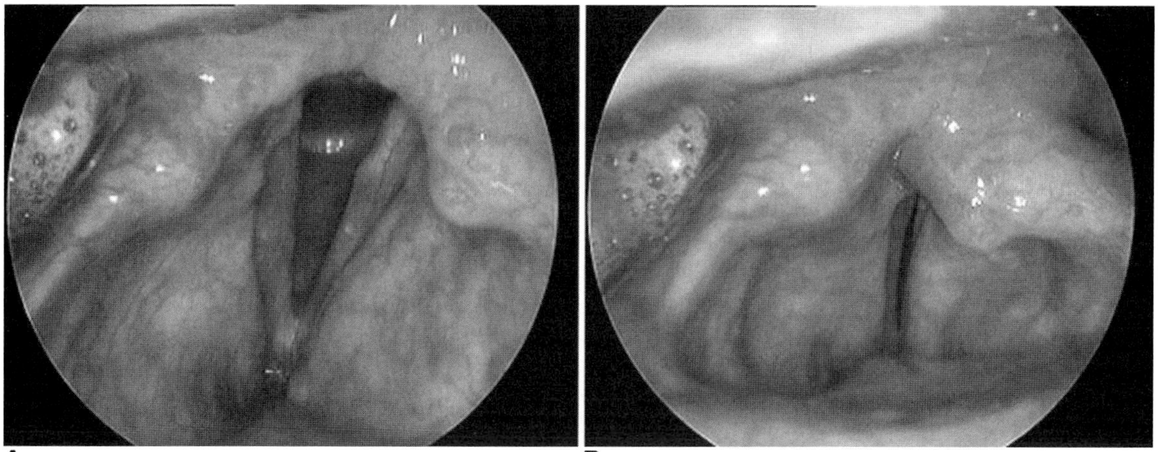

Figure 86-4. A, Vocal folds during respiration. **B,** Vocal folds with lateromedial constriction during phonation.

Vocal-Fold Edges

Vocal-fold edge shape can be rated on two scales: straight/smooth and rough/irregular.[26] Along the straight/smooth continuum, abnormalities should be further described as convex or concave, along with degree of deviation. Concavity is frequently described as "bowing."

Assessment Using Stroboscopy
Introduction

A stroboscope is defined as "an instrument for determining the speed of cyclic motion (as rotation or vibration) that causes the motion to appear slowed or stopped."[23] Videostroboscopy is not slow-motion photography; it is an illusion of slow motion created using a strobe light to illuminate the vocal folds at different points of different vibration cycles. The illusion is possible because images linger on the retina for 0.2 seconds, and only five distinct images can be viewed per second. If more than five per second are presented, the viewer perceives the images as connected and sees the result as a smooth motion; this phenomenon is referred to as Talbot's law. To use videostroboscopy for the analysis of vocal-fold vibration, the light must flash at specific points in the glottic cycle, or the illusion of slow motion vibration will crumble. Extraction of the vocal-fold fundamental frequency (rate of vibration) facilitates the process. The strobe light can be used to create two effects: the running phase (often called *strobe*) and the stop or locked phase. In the running phase (the more frequently used mode), the light flashes slightly faster or slower than the frequency of vibration, thereby creating the illusion that the vocal folds are vibrating in slow motion. In the stop phase, the light flashes at a rate

that is matched with the frequency of the vocal-fold vibration, thereby creating the illusion that the vocal folds are not moving at all. Because each image is from a different glottal cycle, the cycles must be fairly regular to show the smooth motion of a stroboscopic cycle during the running phase.

Videostroboscopy is used to assess vocal-fold vibration patterns, mucosal pliability, the underlying layered structure of the vocal folds, and the undersurface of the vocal-fold edges. When performed in the office, it can sometimes prevent the need for direct microlaryngoscopy. It is particularly valuable when assessing stiffness, scar, or submucosal injury; detecting small vocal-fold lesions; estimating the depth of invasion of a tumor; identifying asymmetric mass or tension; or determining the resumption of voicing activities after phonosurgery.

Understanding normal vocal-fold physiology for different modes of phonation is essential to interpreting stroboscopic examinations, although a thorough review is beyond the scope of this chapter. Chapters that detail vocal-fold vibratory physiology can be found in Rammage, Morrison, and Nichol,[28] Titze,[37] and Hirano and Bless.[17] In brief, it is helpful to think of the vocal folds as having three functional divisions. The cover is comprised of the epithelium and the superficial layer of the lamina propria; the transition is made up of the intermediate and deep layers of the lamina propria (also known as the vocal ligament). Stiffness increases through these layers as the proportion of dense collagen fibers increases and that of elastin fibers decreases. The body of the vocal fold is the thyroarytenoid muscle, which is even less pliable.[12,16,17] During vibration, the vocal folds close, and subglottic air pressure builds until it separates the folds. They return to a closed position by a combination of aerodynamic, muscular, and elastic forces. During a typical cycle at modal pitch, the glottis passes through several shapes that are determined by their variable mass and stiffness. The inferior vocal-fold edges separate before the superior edges, and they return to midline in the same order; this is called the *vertical phase difference*. The folds are less pliable at their anterior and posterior attachments.[12,17] During vibration, they separate at the anterior aspect before the posterior aspect, and they close in the same order; this is called the *horizontal phase difference*. The variations in stiffness likely create, in part, the potential for the complex vibratory patterns that influence voice quality.[28,37]

Many voice disorders and laryngeal pathologies affect the stiffness of the vocal fold cover, the transition, or the body and, consequently, the vocal fold's ability to vibrate in the typical manner. Vibration patterns are different for high and low pitch as well as loud and quiet phonation. For example, the vocal folds are stretched during high-pitch phonation, thereby increasing stiffness of the cover. During low-pitch phonation, they are contracted, and the cover is lax. This variation leads to different vibration patterns, which are discussed in more detail in the following sections.

Stroboscopic parameters include closure pattern, amplitude of vibration, mucosal wave, adynamic segments, vertical closure level, phase closure, symmetry, and regularity. Although it is tempting to consider judgments of these parameters as objective data, they are visual perceptual ratings and subject to reliability and validity errors. The protocol for stroboscopy includes several productions of sustained "ee" at normal pitch, normal loudness (NPNL); phonation on inhalation; pitch glide from mid-range to high, sustaining the high note; pitch glide from mid-range to low, sustaining the low note; quiet "ee," loud "ee"; "ee" at NPNL with locked phase; and, possibly, physical manipulation of the larynx or trial therapy. These tasks are listed in Box 86-2.

Each task contributes unique data to the assessment puzzle. During the examination, it is important to monitor the patient's voice so that all of the necessary information is recorded. For example, the patient may initially sustain phonation quietly and at a high pitch rather than at NPNL. Most vibratory parameters are rated from "ee" at NPNL, and the examiner should attempt to elicit several of these productions so that the vibration patterns can be accurately analyzed. At other times, the patient complains of roughness when talking, but the sustained vowel during stroboscopy is clear and normal. The examination would be most useful if the examiner can also elicit some productions that are similar to the patient's typical patterns or

---

BOX 86-2

SAMPLE PROTOCOL FOR LARYNGEAL VIDEOSTROBOSCOPY. THE ITEMS MARKED WITH AN ASTERISK (*) ARE COMPLETED ONLY IF USING A FLEXIBLE ENDOSCOPE.

Sustained "ee" at normal pitch, normal loudness (several)
Sustained "ee" on inhalation
Glide, mid-range to high, sustaining the high note
Glide, mid-range to low, sustaining the low note
Quiet "ee"
Loud "ee"
Sustained "ee" at normal pitch, normal loudness, using locked mode
Trial therapy or laryngeal manipulation, as needed
Consensus Auditory Perceptual Evaluation for Voice sentences*
  The blue spot is on the key again.
  How hard did he hit him?
  We were away a year ago.
  We eat eggs every Easter.
  My mama makes lemon muffins.
  Peter will keep at the peak.
Singing tasks, as needed*
Humming or other trial therapy tasks, as needed*

---

symptoms. The equipment should be monitored as well; it is quite frustrating to complete a difficult examination and find that the audio or video was not recorded.

Phonation on inhalation is useful when supraglottic constriction interferes with visualization of the vocal folds.[28] It also shows edema or lesions of the inferior compartment of the vocal-fold edge.

The pitch glides are used to evaluate vibration patterns at different points in the frequency range. Ascending pitch glides and high-pitch phonation highlight mid-membranous edema and stiff or scarred segments along the edge. Bilateral and symmetric lengthening of the folds confirms that gross cricothyroid muscle function is intact.

The locked phase is useful for assessing the regularity of vibration, which is the extent to which one vibration cycle is a similar length to the next. It is also useful for highlighting lesions of the vocal-fold edge. Most stroboscopy systems have foot-pedal control of the phase so that the examiner can select the point in the cycle that best shows the lesion.

When the flexible endoscope is used, connected speech should be an examination task. The sentences included in the Consensus Auditory Perceptual Evaluation for Voice[2] are a good standard sample, because each sentence has different characteristics. "The blue spot is on the key again" contains all of the vowel sounds in English; "How hard did he hit him?" emphasizes easy onset; "We were away a year ago" is all-voiced; "We eat eggs every Easter" elicits hard glottal onsets; "My mama makes lemon muffins" uses nasal sounds; "Peter will keep at the peak" is loaded with voiceless plosive sounds. If the patient's concern is related to the singing voice, that should also be assessed during the examination using glides, vocal eases, and songs.

Trial (probe) therapy techniques are often used during a flexible examination to "unload" the larynx or change vibration patterns for a more accurate diagnosis; they are also helpful to assess potential for change and to guide therapy. There are many such techniques, and some of the most useful are listed here. Pitch and loudness changes and phonation on inhalation were described earlier. Humming can alter glottic closure, symmetry, and regularity or decrease supraglottic activity. Twang, sighs, or descending glides with high airflow can alter laryngeal tilt or change the closure pattern. Trills, breathy voice, coughing, pushing, abdominodiaphragmatic onsets, and visual feedback are also useful probes. Leonard and Kendall[21] describe the combination of a traditional voice evaluation and flexible endoscopy as a "phonoscopic" evaluation. In a retrospective study of 100 cases, the findings from the phonoscopic evaluation differed from the findings of the referring physician in 42 cases. In an additional 32 cases, the findings were consistent with the referral diagnosis, but the phonoscopic examination provided additional detail (e.g., there was indeed hyperfunction, but it appeared as a result of an underlying pathology such as bowing or a lesion).

Closure Pattern

Closure pattern is described by the shape of the glottic gap at maximum closure during stroboscopy. Typical patterns are complete (Figure 86-5, *A*), posterior gap (Figure 86-5, *B*), incomplete anterior gap (Figure 86-5, *C*), spindle gap (Figure 86-5, *D*), hourglass (Figure 86-5, *E*), irregular, and variable. With complete closure, there is no space between the folds; this is the most common closure pattern for men,[30] and it occurs in some women at NPNL or with increased loudness.[30,31,32]

A posterior glottic gap can vary from small to large, and the extent of the gap should be indicated. Posterior glottic gap is the one of the most common closure patterns for women,[8,22,30] and it might be a normal variant for men.[30] The gap is typically limited to the space between the cartilaginous folds during NPNL, but it can extend into the membranous folds during quiet productions.[30] Rammage, Morrison, and Nichols[28] categorize extended glottic gap as a laryngeal isometric pattern of muscle tension dysphonia.

An incomplete closure pattern occurs when the gap extends for the entire length of the folds. Incomplete

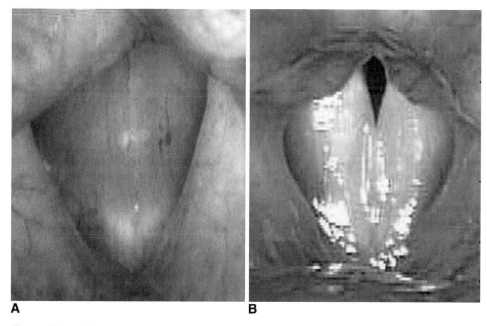

A   **B**

Figure 86-5. Glottal closure and gap patterns. **A,** Complete closure; **B,** posterior glottic gap;

Continued

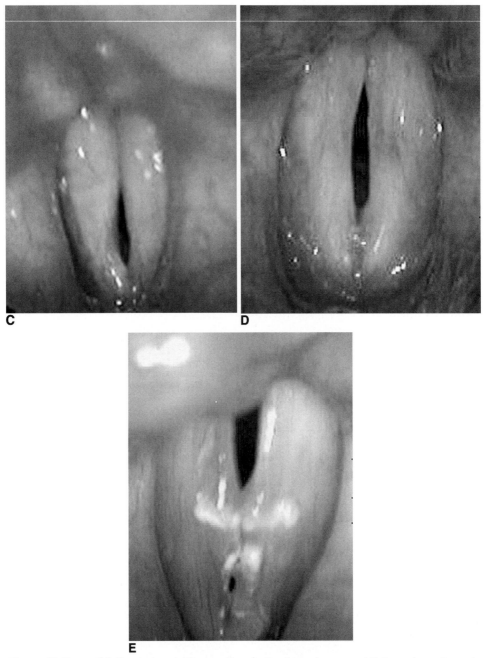

Figure 86-5, cont'd C anterior glottic gap; **D,** spindle-shaped gap; and **E,** hourglass-shaped gap.

closure most often occurs with vocal-fold motion impairment and a muscle tension dysphonia/aphonia variant in which the patient does not fully adduct the folds for phonation.

An anterior gap is a condition in which there is closure of the arytenoids and cartilaginous folds but a gap between part or all of the membranous folds. Anterior gaps occur as a normal variant in men of any age and

older women.[8,9] They are also present in patients with disordered voices and can occur with tissue deficit of the membranous folds as a result of scarring, prior surgery, bowing, superior laryngeal nerve deficit, or sulcus vocalis; at other times, they appear because of edematous posterior folds. A spindle-shape gap refers to a condition in which there is closure of the arytenoids but where there is otherwise a gap that is the length of the folds. In a way that is similar to anterior gaps, spindle-shaped gaps occur as normal variants in men of all ages and older women[9]; they also occur with bowing as a result of vocal-fold motion impairment, superior laryngeal nerve injury, sulcus vocalis, or tissue deficit due to aging or prior surgery.

Hourglass closure refers to a pattern of an anterior gap and a posterior gap with a point of closure in between. This pattern is typical for bilateral lesions (e.g., nodules) or a cyst or polyp and a contralateral nodule; it can also occur with large unilateral lesions. Irregular closure is a pattern that involves multiple gaps or that does not quite classify as another pattern. Irregular closure is most common with multilobular lesions or rough lesions.

Many times the closure alternates between two or more patterns; it is then called *variable,* with the multiple patterns delineated. The closure pattern is rated at NPNL. For most people, vocal-fold vibration patterns change as pitch and loudness change. With increasing pitch, the vocal folds lengthen, and only the medial edge is involved in vibration. Closure pattern can become incomplete, and the amplitude of vibration and mucosal wave can decrease. When describing glottic closure, it is often helpful to describe multiple conditions. For example, the closure pattern for a patient with bilateral lesions may be described as follows: "Closure pattern is variable at NPNL; it is sometimes hourglass shaped, and, at other times, a posterior gap extends to the mid-membranous folds. At higher pitch, closure is always hourglass. At low pitch and loud voice, glottic closure becomes complete."

Amplitude of Vibration

Amplitude of vibration refers to the fold's horizontal excursion from midline. Normal is defined as approximately one-third of the width of the fold[17]; this is demonstrated in Figure 86-6. Amplitude can be rated as a percentage of the width of the fold[26] or on a five- or seven-point equal-appearing interval scale from normal to reduced.[17] Amplitude is typically smaller in women than men; it generally covaries with loudness, and it varies inversely with pitch.[34] Decreased amplitude of vibration can be the result of glottic incompetence, tight glottic closure, or increased vocal fold mass or stiffness. Decreased amplitude is common in lesions such as firm polyps, cysts, papilloma, carcinoma, Reinke's edema, scarring, or hyperfunction.[17]

Mucosal Wave

Mucosal wave is the vertical upheaval of the cover over the body. It occurs because of the vertical phase shift (the timing difference between the upper and lower margins of the vocal folds) that appears to be vital to the self-oscillation of the folds.[38] Mucosal wave arises from the medial vertical surface of the vocal fold and is observed as it moves laterally from the vocal-fold edge along the superior surface of the fold. The velocity of the mucosal wave is linked to the amount of pressure that is needed to establish phonation[36,41]; normally, this wave moves approximately half of the width of the vocal fold during phonation at NPNL.[10] Increased mucosal wave is observed when mucosa is abnormally pliable, such as for polypoid degeneration or when there is increased subglottal air pressure. As such, it is normally greater than half of the width of the fold for loud phonation, when subglottal air pressure is increased. Mucosal wave is decreased or even absent when the mucosa is stiff or there is minimal differentiation of the vocal-fold layered structure; this occurs normally with increasing pitch[17] and aging.[8] In pathologic conditions, decreased or absent mucosal wave is seen with some lesions, scarring, or sulcus vocalis. Incomplete glottic

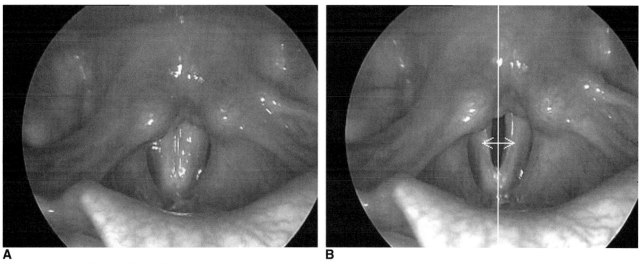

A   **B**

Figure 86-6. A, Complete glottic closure. **B,** Maximum amplitude of vibration/excursion.

closure resulting from aging or motion impairment can also lead to decreased amplitude of vibration and decreased or absent mucosal wave.[8,20]

Adynamic Segments

Adynamic segments refer to nonvibrating areas of the fold (i.e., segments that have minimal lateral amplitude of excursion and over which mucosal wave does not travel). They are described by location and by the percentage of the superior surface of the vocal fold that they cover. These stiff areas are generally related to a lesion or to a scarred segment.

Phase Closure

During vibration at NPNL, the vocal folds are typically open (opening, closing, or fully open) for approximately two-thirds of one vibratory cycle and maximally closed for the remaining third. This parameter is typically rated by counting "frames" using the jog/shuttle wheel of a video cassette recorder or clicks of a computer mouse. Closed time generally decreases with higher pitches and in older women; it increases in older men.[34] Phase closure is useful when a patient sounds breathy but achieves complete closure or during hyperfunctional patterns when the vocal folds open only briefly.

Symmetry

Symmetry refers to the degree with which the vocal folds appear as mirror images of one another during vibration. This parameter is used to describe the symmetry of the timing of opening, closing, and closed[10]; the vocal folds should arrive and depart from midline at the same time. The asymmetry should be described whenever possible; for example, "the excursion of the right fold lags behind that of the left," or "the folds are asymmetric at the end of tasks." Depending on the rating scale, the parameter can be rated as either the percentage of the examination during which vibration was asymmetric or the degree of asymmetry. Asymmetric vibration raises questions about differences in mechanical properties or neurologic status between the folds.[17] Differences between the vocal folds in position, mass, tension, elasticity, or viscosity should be further assessed.

Regularity

Regularity (or periodicity) refers to the degree to which one phonatory cycle is similar in both amplitude and time to the next phonatory cycle.[17] It is best assessed in the locked or stop mode, but it can be estimated from the running phase as well. In the stop mode, the image will appear static if the vibration is regular, and it will appear to quiver or shake if the vibration is irregular. In running mode, the strobe light cannot adequately track fundamental frequency and adjust the illumination rate if vibration is irregular, and so quiver or shimmer appears. Vibratory regularity is rated just like symmetry, either by describing the percentage of time that the vibration was regular or irregular or by describing occurrences of irregularity. It is difficult to assess degree from stroboscopy; this would require acoustic analysis. Incidence of aperiodicity increases with age. Biever and Bless[8] found that 85% of geriatric women demonstrated aperiodicity as compared with 30% of young women. Regular vibration depends on a steady balance between pulmonary pressure and the vocal folds. Irregular vibration can be caused by asymmetry of the mechanical properties of the vocal folds, interference with the homogeneity of the vocal folds, flaccidity, unsteady tonus, or inconsistent force. Some examples of the above would be paralysis (asymmetry); a small cyst or carcinoma (homogeneity); paralysis or edematous lesion (flaccidity); spasmodic dysphonia (SD) or another neuromuscular disease (tonus); and functional pulmonary disease (inconsistent force).[17]

Vertical Closure Level

Whether the vocal folds meet on the same plane is typically rated as on-plane or off-plane. When the vocal folds' vertical closure level is off-plane, it is typically because of neuromuscular differences between the folds (paralysis or paresis) or as a result of trauma.

INSTRUMENTATION
Introduction

Diagnosis and treatment of laryngeal disorders is enhanced with clear video and photographic documentation. Video recordings allow careful analysis, both in real time and in slow motion, of subtle abnormalities in vocal-fold vibration. Findings can be shown easily. During difficult examinations, the ability to record the procedure for more careful review after removal of the laryngoscope reduces patient discomfort. Finally, patients gain a better understanding of their condition if they can see images of their larynx.

When designing a system for documentation of the larynx, the clinician must consider how the information will be used; the intended use can have a strong effect on the choice of equipment. For example, will there be a need to rapidly review past video files (perhaps in the midst of an examination), or will they be stored as archives with slower access requirements? Will the examinations be integrated into other aspects of an electronic medical record? Will the recordings be edited for use in educational or scientific presentations? What level of expertise will be required of the end user?

Medical imaging, like other forms of photography and video, has been transformed by the development of digital imaging technology. Charged-coupled device (CCD) chips and digital storage media are rapidly replacing photographic film and videotape. Images and video clips can now be easily edited, enhanced, and manipulated by computer software. The large consumer market has also accepted this same technology, thereby guaranteeing further reductions in cost.

Improvements, innovations, and introduction of new features continue to occur in digital imaging. Because state-of-the-art technologies quickly become outdated, this section will not concentrate on specific products. Instead, important concepts underlying these technologies and their application in laryngology will be described.

It should be noted that changes have occurred much more slowly in the "front end" of the imaging system (i.e., the various flexible and rigid endoscopes themselves). There have been improvements in the optical components within the telescope and in fiberoptic technology, but these changes are minor as compared with innovations in digital imaging. Similarly, cost reductions have also been much more dramatic in imaging electronics than in optical components.

Laryngoscopes

The decision about whether to use a flexible or a rigid endoscope is often influenced by the laryngologist's preference and the goal of the examination. Each technique has its advantages and disadvantages. Rigid endoscopy offers a much clearer and brighter image. Because the imaging is done entirely with lenses, there is none of the degradation seen with fiberoptic imaging endoscopes. Rigid endoscopy is clearly supe-

rior when one is looking at the structural detail of the larynx. On the other hand, fiberoptic laryngoscopy sometimes is more easily tolerated than rigid endoscopy and may be the only option is some cases (e.g., a patient with a strong gag reflex, a young child); it also allows for examination during speech and other normal laryngeal tasks. The light transmission of optical fibers has also improved so that stroboscopy can often be done using a flexible scope. The most significant disadvantage of fiberoptic laryngoscopy is the loss of resolution due to the fiber bundle. There also is a "fisheye" effect that produces panoramic views but distorts the image and decreases illumination intensity as the scope is moved backward from the tissue (Figure 86-7).

Many companies, including Olympus (Tokyo, Japan), Fujinon (Saitoma City, Japan), Pentax (Tokyo, Japan), and Machida (Orangeburg, NY), manufacture flexible laryngoscopes. Laryngoscopes intended for adult patients typically have a diameter between 3.4 and 4.8 mm; the narrower size is near the minimum that will allow for worthwhile stroboscopy using the most strobe light sources. Unless the nasal anatomy is perfectly straight, fiberoptic scopes with diameters of more than 4.8 mm can be uncomfortable and may not allow the patient to relax during the examination. Some flexible scopes of this diameter or slightly larger also are available with separate channels that admit a biopsy wire.

Video Cameras

CCD cameras have been used for many years in video systems for the office and the operating room; similar CCD chips are now also used in digital still cameras. These electronic chips have an array of individual photodetectors. The chip is exposed to an image for a short period of time, and each photodetector records a voltage proportional to the amount

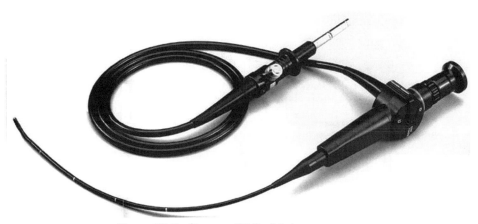

Figure 86-7. Olympus P4 flexible laryngoscope.

of light shining on it. The array elements are then sampled in a sequential shift-and-register fashion, once for still cameras and many times a second for video cameras.

Until recently, most CCD cameras operated in an analog mode. Although the image was captured from discrete photodetector elements, the signal itself was converted to an analog video signal. The camera output could then be displayed on a standard monitor or recorded onto videotape (see below). Newer digital video cameras have as their output a digital signal that can be directly sent into a computer or stored on digital videotape.

The display on a video monitor is produced when electrons are swept across the back face of the screen. The electrons strike phosphors, thereby emitting light and producing the image we see with our eyes. To reduce a flicker effect, alternating lines are scanned in an interlacing fashion. Standards have been established by the broadcast industry for the scanning parameters. In the United States and Canada, a National Television Standard's Committee (NTSC) format is used, with 525 lines per frame scanned at 29.97 frames per second. Two other international standards are PAL (used mostly in Europe) and SECAM (used mostly in Africa and some European countries). There are slight differences in the scan rate and management of color, so none of these standards is compatible with the others. Recordings must be converted to the appropriate standard if they are to be played in other countries.[27]

Another consequence of this scan display is a bothersome moiré pattern. This pattern develops when there is an overlap of linear features in an image (in this case, the fibers of the scope and the scan lines of the display). The typical moiré pattern has fringes of multiple colors. The effect can be reduced by slightly defocusing the camera lens or by an anti-moiré filter.

Standard CCD cameras only record light intensity (black, white, or shades of gray), so color signals are captured in one of two ways. In single-chip CCD, a grid pattern of red, green, and blue filters is placed over the chip so that light of just one color strikes each pixel. Four pixels are then spatially combined to produce the color image. There is a loss of resolution with this process, and there can be aliasing of color (i.e., the appearance of false colors) at rapid transitions between light and dark regions.

A much better image is obtained with a three-chip camera. In these cameras, a prism refracts the light into its three separate color components. A separate CCD records light from each of the colors, and the signals from these three chips are then combined to produce the final image. Resolution is much higher, and there is no aliasing.

One of the new improvements now being developed for flexible laryngoscopy is the integrated scope and camera. These systems have until now been used mostly in gastroenterology endoscopy. The eyepiece is replaced with a direct connection to the camera and results in superior optics (Figure 86-8).

Laryngoscopes have also been developed in which the CCD chip is at the distal end of the flexible endoscope, thereby completely eliminating the fiberoptic bundle. Because of size limitations, only a single-chip CCD camera can be used. Color images are produced either with a standard grid pattern or with a rotating wheel containing red, green, and blue filters. The latter technique allows for a smaller chip, but it cannot be used with stroboscopy.[19]

Another new development made possible with CCD electronics is the ability to rapidly turn image acquisition on and off. The CCD camera can then act as its own strobe device, thereby eliminating the need for expensive stroboscopic light sources. Both Kay Elemetrics (Lincoln Park, NJ) and Jedmed (St. Louis, Mo) have camera systems that offer this application, although the current models are not sensitive enough to allow for stroboscopy through flexible laryngoscopes.

Videokymography is another development that makes use of the rapid scanning properties of CCD

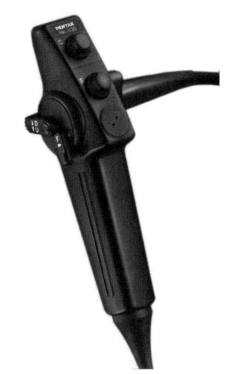

Figure 86-8. Integrated Pentax videolaryngoscope. The eyepiece has been replaced by a direct connection to the video camera.

cameras. With this technique, a single line of pixels perpendicular to the direction of the vocal folds is scanned at 8000 times per second. Each scan line is displayed in succession, thus producing an image that shows the time history of the glottic cycle. Very minor asymmetries in mucosal wave vibration are readily apparent with this technology.[29]

Video Recorders

Analog video recorders range from consumer-level VHS recorders up to professional grade Betamax systems. Digital technology has been making inroads here as well with DVD recorders that are now well within the budget of many speech clinics. DVD recording media are especially useful for the rapid retrieval of patient data. Digital video files in their raw form are huge and are usually compressed before storage onto DVD or other recording media. New capture boards and software allow this to be done in real time.

When choosing a video recording medium, it is important to select a format that will not quickly become outmoded. One should be especially cautious when using proprietary formats, because technical support may not be available if the original company that authored the software is no longer in business; the same holds true for uncommon types of storage media.

Except for very simple examinations, commercial grade VHS is too poor in quality for clinical laryngeal recordings. It is especially poor for frame-by-frame analysis, and it suffers significant degradation when copies are made. Standard VHS is a composite signal in that the luminance or brightness signal (called Y) is combined with the color chrominance signal (called C) before transmission. In S-video (sometimes also referred to as S-VHS or Y/C), these two signals are transmitted separately, and, therefore, the quality is greater.[11]

Even higher quality can be obtained with commercial grade Betamax tapes. However, recording now is often done using digital imaging technology. As with analog tapes, there are many different digital formats. The most popular format for the consumer is the DV format, which is also used on semiprofessional recorders. Other formats, which are more often seen in professional video cameras, include DVCAM and DVCPRO. Unlike analog recordings, examinations stored in a digital format can be copied multiple times with no degradation in image quality.

High-quality recorders place a time code on the videotape either during the recording or during an initial formatting run. This feature allows the user to place the recorded tape into the VCR and know its exact position. Some companies offer computer-con-trolled systems in which the name of a patient can be entered and the tape will automatically advance to the start of that patient's examination. These features typically come at an additional cost, but they greatly simplify the review of old examinations. Time coding is not necessary with DVD, because there is rapid access to all data on the disk.

Audio recordings are obviously crucial when documenting laryngeal examinations in patients with voice disorders. High-quality video recorders typically have a second input for the audio signal, which is sufficient for basic archiving of the patient's voice. However, the audio quality of videotapes is not that high, and, if quantitative analysis of the voice is expected, a separate recording should be made. Small digital recorders are now available that can make near–professional-level recordings at low cost. The setting of the examination should be as quiet as possible, and the same protocol for microphone placement should be used for all patients.

Light Sources

Bright light sources are essential for laryngeal examinations, especially stroboscopy. There are three basic types of light sources used for most medical imaging. Halogen filament light sources are the least expensive, but they offer several disadvantages. The color temperature for halogen is about 3200°K, which is lower than the natural sunlight temperature of about 5600°K. Lower light temperature has two effects. First, the light is slightly yellow. Second, our eyes' ability to resolve worsens as the light temperature decreases. Halogen filaments are also large (approximately 8 mm), so it is difficult to focus the beam down to a small spot size before transmission through an optical fiber.

Xenon light sources are more expensive, but they overcome some of these disadvantages. The light originates from an arc source that is 1 to 2 mm in diameter, so a smaller spot size can be achieved. The arc burns at a higher color temperature (4200°K), so the light is closer to that of natural sunlight.

One of the newest light sources used for medical illumination is the metal halide system. This light source has a color temperature of 5600°K, and the bulbs have three times the efficiency of xenon and offer more light for less cost. There may be a slight shift to a bluer light as the bulb ages, but they retain 70% of their original output (vs 50% with xenon bulbs).

Strobe light sources use special electrical and electronic components to produce an extremely short bright flash of light in synchronization with vocal-fold vibration. A contact microphone placed against the patient's neck detects the vocal-fold frequency. Some strobe light sources use halogen light for continuous viewing and switch to xenon when the operator switches to the strobe mode. Others, such as the Nagashima unit (Nagashima, Tokyo, Japan), strobe a xenon light at a constant rate (usually about 200 Hz) during continuous mode and then switch to the vocal-fold frequency when a signal is detected by a contact microphone (Figure 86-9).

Monitor

The monitor is the final link in the video system, and its quality should match that of the other components. Most current displays involve a cathode ray tube, but the new flat-screen liquid crystal and plasma displays will undoubtedly become more affordable and more popular. Monitors for clinical examinations do not need to be large, and, for most applications, a diagonal size of 17 to 20 inches (43–51 cm) should be adequate. It is, however, important to have high resolution. Resolution is measured with a parameter called the *dot pitch*. In a standard cathode ray tube, there is a metal shield called an aperture mask immediately behind the phosphor screen; this screen has many small holes through which the electrons pass, and the dot pitch is the distance between the holes. In Sony's Trinitron system, a linear grill of fine wires is used as the aperture mask; the dot pitch is the distance between the wires. Smaller dot pitch means better resolution, and a typical high-resolution monitor has a value of about 0.22 mm.

The monitor should have the capability to accept multiple formats (e.g., S-video [Y/C]) as well as composite signals. Higher-quality monitors may also have an RGB input (seen more commonly in computer monitors) and BNC jacks.

Video Editing

One of the most useful developments in the last several years has been the ability to edit video on the computer. These digital tools eliminate the need for expensive tape-editing equipment, and they allow for the rapid production of videos for presentation. These are very user-friendly tools, and they require only a modest investment of time to become proficient at producing high-quality video presentations. Currently available examples of such software include iMovie, iDVD, Final Cut Pro, and Avid Express.

To digitally edit video, the clip must first be converted to a form that the computer can process, (i.e., a digital format). Several companies offer hardware that will take an NTSC signal and convert it to a digital signal. Because these files are large (DV files with audio require about 36 megabits per second), newer computers have Firewire ports (IEEE 1394) that speed the transfer from videotape to hard disk. With the new digital cameras and digital recorders, the files can be directly transferred through a firewire cable to the computer.

After editing, video files can then be burned onto DVDs, converted back to NTSC signals for storage on

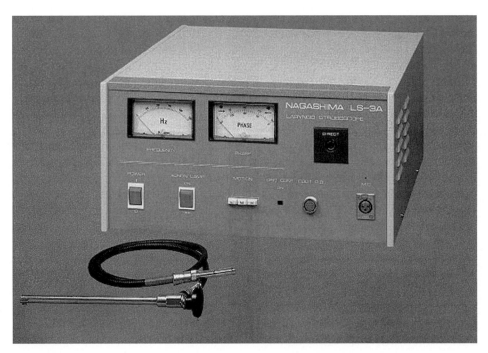

Figure 86-9. Nagashima light stroboscopic light source and rigid laryngeal telescope.

analog videotape, or converted into formats for posting on the internet or for use in multimedia presentations.

Manufacturers also offer various image processors that can improve the image quality; these may adjust the contrast or sharpen the edges of the image. It is difficult to make a general statement about whether these additional features are necessary. The results are usually subjective, and each user will therefore need to check the end result to determine if such a processor is worth its cost.

System Comments

The proliferation of digital image products makes it much easier to develop a powerful studio for documenting laryngeal examinations. However, compatibility problems and difficulties with driver software can develop when assembling a system in a piece-by-piece fashion. Unless someone is very proficient with imaging hardware and software, most equipment dealers recommend that these systems be purchased as a "turnkey" package. The initial cost may be higher, but the user has a much better chance of obtaining a trouble-free system.

It is also extremely useful to have a single cart for storage of the individual pieces of equipment. The cart should have a rear door to allow access to the cables that connect the various components. Users should be familiar with the cabling sequence, because unplugged or incorrectly placed cables are common causes of picture failure (Figure 86-10).

Still Photography

Digital cameras are also rapidly becoming the norm for capturing still images of the larynx, both in the operating room and during office examinations. A key advantage of digital still photography is the ability to instantly see the image and make any adjustments that may be necessary. Light and shutter speed, for example, can be difficult to optimize, even with through-the-lens (TTL) shutter meters. Some digital cameras have built-in macro modes that eliminate the need for separate expensive lenses when photographing smaller items. In addition—and most importantly—digital cameras offer much more flexibility when it comes to image management.

Couplers are available that allow a camera to be connected to the end of a standard endoscope eyepiece (Figure 86-11). These can be used to photograph through rigid telescopes or fiberoptic endoscopes. Most couplers have a C-ring attachment to screw into the filter ring on a standard 35-mm single-lens reflex camera. Various adapters are available to convert from one ring diameter to another. However, not all digital cameras have threading to accommodate such a coupler (also called a *lens*

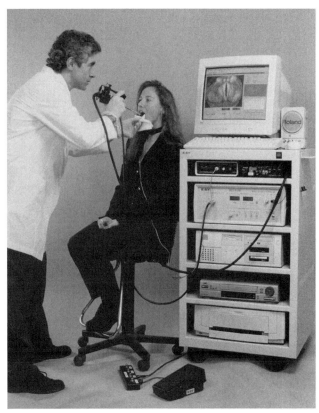

Figure 86-10. Example of a well-organized single cart containing the equipment necessary for documentation of a laryngeal examination. Photograph courtesy of Kay Elemetrics.

adapter tube). When purchasing a digital camera for endoscopic photography, make sure that this threading is present.

A dedicated electronic flash unit that is triggered by the camera shutter produces the best illumination for still photography. The Karl Storz model 610 (Karl Storz, Tuttlingen, Germany) works well in this capacity, although it is quite expensive. Newer non-flash light units (e.g., the metal halide light source described earlier) are now available that often provide sufficient light using digital or film cameras. Even with TTL meters, it is often necessary to bracket the shutter speed or the aperture to ensure proper exposure.[6]

Many digital cameras are now sold with simple image-processing software for improving contrast, color adjustment, cropping, and so on. More powerful programs, such as Adobe Photoshop (Adobe, San Jose, Ca), offer many more tools for image enhancement. When combined with a high-resolution digital camera, images can also be magnified with software instead of with expensive lenses.

For traditional single-lens reflex cameras and 35-mm film, greater care must be taken, because the picture will not be seen until long after it has been taken. Best

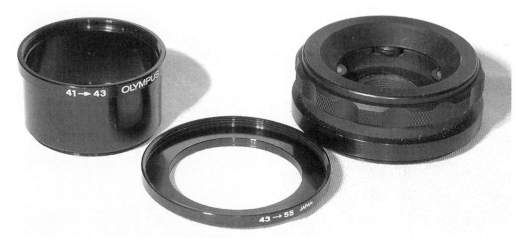

Figure 86-11. Adapter rings and coupler for attaching endoscopes to a digital camera. *Left to right,* lens adapter tube for digital camera, 43- to 55-mm adapter ring, and endoscope coupler.

results in these cases are obtained with a variable zoom lens attached to the endoscope adapter, a dedicated electronic flash unit, and TTL metering of exposure time.[7]

Video cameras have improved to such an extent that high quality still images can also be captured from the video recording. Video processing software usually allows a displayed frame to be saved in a standard image format. These images can be printed for immediate display or converted to a digital form that allows for storage or processing.

CONCLUSION

Video endoscopy and stroboscopy are important components of a voice evaluation, providing essential information about vocal-fold structure and function. Proper documentation of laryngeal examination is an important component of overall patient care. New developments in digital technology have introduced powerful features that simplify the acquisition of still and video images. An understanding of the basic concepts that underlie these technologies is extremely helpful when selecting the proper system and using it in the clinical setting.

REFERENCES

1. American Speech-Language-Hearing Association: The roles of otolaryngologists and speech-language pathologists in the performance and interpretation of strobovideolaryngoscopy, *ASHA* 40(Suppl 18):32, 1998.
2. American Speech-Language-Hearing Association, Special Interest Division 3, Voice and Voice Disorders: Consensus Auditory-Perceptual Evaluation of Voice (CAPE-V), 2003: Instrument in preparation. Available at: *www.asha.org/about/membership-certification/divs/div_3.htm.* Accessed December 30, 2003.
3. Bassich CJ, Ludlow CL, Polinsky RJ: Speech symptoms associated with early signs of Shy Drager syndrome, *J Neurol Neurosurg Psychiatry* 47:995, 1984.
4. Behrman A and others: Anterior-posterior and medial compression of the supraglottic: signs of nonorganic dysphonia or normal postures? *J Voice* 17:403, 2003.
5. Belafsky PC and others: Muscle tension dysphonia as a sign of underlying glottal insufficiency, *Otolaryngol Head Neck Surg* 127:448, 2002.
6. Benjamin B, Baker DC Jr.: Memorial lecture. Art and science of laryngeal photography, *Ann Otol Rhinol Laryngol* 102:271, 1993.
7. Benjamin B: Indirect laryngeal photography using rigid telescopes, *Laryngoscope* 108:158, 1998.
8. Biever DM, Bless DM: Vibratory characteristics of the vocal folds in young adult and geriatric women, *J Voice* 3:120, 1989.
9. Bless DM and others: *Stroboscopic, acoustic, aerodynamic, and perceptual attributes of voice production in normal speaking adults.* In Titze IR, editor: *Progress Report 4,* Iowa City, Iowa, 1993, National Center for Voice and Speech.
10. Bless DM, Hirano M, Feder R: Videostroboscopic evaluation of the larynx, *Ear Nose Throat J* 66:48, 1987.
11. Browne SE: *Video editing: a post production primer,* ed 4, New York, 2002, Focal Press.
12. Gray SD, Hirano M, Sato K: *Molecular and cellular structure of the vocal fold tissue.* In Titze I, editor: *Vocal fold physiology: frontiers in basic science,* San Diego, 1993, Singular Publishing Group.
13. Habermann W and others: Ex juvantibus approach for chronic posterior laryngitis: results of short-term pantoprazole therapy, *J Laryngol Otol* 113:734, 1999.
14. Hanson DG and others: Outcomes of antireflux therapy for the treatment of chronic laryngitis, *Ann Otol Rhinol Laryngol* 104:550, 1995.
15. Hicks DM and others: The prevalence of hypopharynx findings associated with gastroesophageal reflux in normal volunteers, *J Voice* 16:564, 2002.
16. Hirano M: Morphological structure of the vocal cord as a vibrator and its variations, *Folia Phoniatr (Basel)* 26:89, 1974.
17. Hirano M, Bless DM: *Videostroboscopic examination of the larynx,* San Diego, 1993, Singular Publishing Group.

18. Izdebski K, Ross JC, Klein JC: Transoral rigid laryngovideostroboscopy (phonoscopy), *Semin Speech Lang* 11:16, 1990.

19. Kawaida M, Fukuda H, Kohno N: Digital image processing of laryngeal lesions by electronic videoendoscopy, *Laryngoscope* 112:559, 2002.

20. Kokesh J and others: Correlation between stroboscopy and electromyography in laryngeal paralysis, *Ann Otol Rhinol Laryngol* 102:852, 1993.

21. Leonard R, Kendall K: Phonoscopy—a valuable tool for otolaryngologists and speech-language pathologists in the management of dysphonic patients, *Laryngoscope* 111:1760, 2001.

22. Linville SE: Glottal gap configurations in two age groups of women, *J Speech Hear Res* 35:1209, 1992.

23. Merriam-Webster Online Dictionary: Definition of "stroboscope." Available at *http://www.m-w.com/cgi-bin/dictionary?book=Dictionary&va=stroboscope&x=16&y=13* Accessed April 8, 2004.

24. Pemberton C and others: Characteristics of normal larynges under flexible fiberscopic and stroboscopic examination: an Australian perspective, *J Voice* 7:382, 1993.

25. Peppard RC, Bless DM: The use of topical anesthetic in videostroboscopic examination of the larynx, *J Voice* 5:57, 1991.

26. Poburka BJ: A new stroboscopy rating form, *J Voice* 13:403, 1999.

27. Poynton CA: *A technical introduction to digital video,* New York, John Wiley and Sons, 1996.

28. Rammage L, Morrison M, Nichol H: *Management of the voice and its disorders,* ed 2, San Diego, Singular Publishing Group, 2001.

29. Schutte HK, Svec JG, Sram F: First results of clinical applications of videokymography, *Laryngoscope* 108(8 Pt 1):1206, 1998.

30. Södersten M, Lindestad P-Å: Glottal closure and perceived breathiness during phonation in normally speaking subjects, *J Speech Hear Res* 33:601, 1990.

31. Södersten M, Lindestad P-Å: A comparison of vocal fold closure in rigid telescopic and flexible fiberoptic laryngostroboscopy, *Acta Otolaryngol (Stockh)* 112:144, 1992.

32. Södersten M, Hertegård S, Hammarberg B: Glottal closure, airflow, and voice quality in middle-aged women as related to changes in loudness, *Phoniatric and Logopedic Progress Report* 9:3, 1994.

33. Stager SV and others: Incidence of supraglottic activity in males and females: a preliminary report, *J Voice* 17:395, 2003.

34. Sulter AM, Schutte HK, Miller DG: Standardized laryngeal videostroboscopic rating: differences between untrained and trained male and female subjects, and effects of varying sound intensity, fundamental frequency, and age, *J Voice* 10:175, 1996.

35. Titze IR: Acoustic characteristics of resonant voice, *J Voice* 15:519, 2001.

36. Titze I: Phonation threshold pressure: a missing link in glottal aerodynamics, *J Acoust Soc Am* 91:2926, 1991.

37. Titze IR: *Principles of voice production,* Englewood Cliffs, California, 1994, Prentice-Hall.

38. Titze IR, Jiang JJ, Hsiao T: Measurement of mucosal wave propagation and vertical phase difference in vocal fold vibration, *Ann Otol Rhinol Laryngol* 102:58, 1993.

39. Toohill RJ, Kuhn JC: Role of refluxed acid in pathogenesis of laryngeal disorders, *Am J Med* 103(5A):100S, 1997.

40. Verdolini K, Palmer PM: Assessment of a "profiles" approach to voice screening, *J Med Speech Lang Pathol* 6:217, 1997.

41. Verdolini-Marston K, Titze I, Druker D: Changes in phonation threshold pressure with induced conditions of hydration, *J Voice* 4:142, 1990.

CHAPTER EIGHTY SEVEN

VOICE ANALYSIS

‖ Robin A. Samlan

INTRODUCTION

Voice is a complex phenomenon that is produced by interactions among the respiratory, laryngeal, and resonance subsystems. Describing vocal function and evaluating voice problems are, likewise, complex tasks. The focus of this chapter is the perceptual, physical, and physiologic examination of the voice and its components. The patient history and videostroboscopy, which are the two other components of the voice evaluation, are detailed in other chapters.

Both research and clinical needs factor into decisions of whether and how to measure voice. From a research perspective, voice measurements can improve our understanding of voice production, help identify links between laryngeal disease and voice production, and document change with interventions. In the clinical arena, vocal function measures are used in both the diagnosis and treatment of voice disorders. Vocal function testing helps clinicians document the status of the glottal tone and the supraglottic vocal tract, characterize the type and severity of the voice disorder, and explain discrepancies between voice quality and stroboscopic evaluation by providing cycle-to-cycle information that is not available with stroboscopy. Vocal function measures can help the voice care team determine treatment goals and can be used as visual feedback during behavioral treatment. Repeated testing over time allows clinicians to monitor and document changes that result from treatment and also to monitor disease progression or recurrence.

Many of the instrument-based tests yield numbers, and it is therefore tempting to view the results as "objective," but the examiner influences results by selecting the stimulus, the token, the measure, and the equipment. Results of vocal function testing should therefore be interpreted in the light of these factors. To be considered reliable, measures must be made using standard protocols, recording procedures, patient instructions, and test environments. It would be simple if there was one measure that accurately categorizes all voices; however, voice quality is multidimensional, and attempting to describe it with one number would be simplistic. Generally the solution is to select a group of measures that capture various aspects of the voice, such as quality, loudness, and pitch.

In the discussion that follows, several voice measures are described. They are divided into three categories: patient scales, perceptual evaluation, and measures. Within each category, measures can reflect typical voice use or maximum performance capabilities.

PATIENT SCALES

Individuals have different requirements and expectations of their voices; it is therefore likely that the same degree of dysphonia will differentially affect peoples' abilities to function in their typical activities. Therefore, as part of a complete voice evaluation, the effect of the voice problem on each individual's life should be assessed. Patient measures are scales completed by the patient and sometimes a caregiver or significant other. These scales typically measure patient satisfaction, quality of life, general health, handicap or loss as a result of the voice disorder, and some aspect of voice production (e.g., ease of phonation, effort, quality). Reflecting a shift in society's expectations from healthcare, several scales specific to voice have been published over the last decade, including the Voice Handicap Index,[44] the Voice-Related Quality of Life scale,[41] the Voice Activity and Participation Profile,[53] the Voice Symptom Scale,[19] the Reflux Symptom Index,[9] the Patient Questionnaire of Vocal Performance,[15] and the Voice Outcome Survey.[23] The scales are all completed by the patient and reflect the patient's perception of the problem and its consequences; they vary in length, construction, and what they assess. A summary of each scale is included in the chapter; details and information about scale construction can be found in the reference articles listed. A synopsis of the scales can be found in Table 87-1.

Voice Handicap Index

The Voice Handicap Index (VHI)[44] was designed to assess handicap, defined as "a social, economic, or environmental disadvantage resulting from an impairment or disability."[94] The instrument consists of 30 statements that patients rate on a five-point equal-appearing interval scale that reflects the frequency of occurrence. The total possible score is 120, with higher scores reflecting greater handicap. The total scale can be divided into three subscales: functional, physical, and emotional. Since its publication in 1997, this instrument has been widely used to show voice handicap in specific groups of patients, comparisons between handicap and vocal function measures, and change with treatment.* The index can be found in Figure 87-1.

Voice-Related Quality of Life

The Voice-Related Quality of Life (V-RQOL) scale[41] comprises 10 items divided into physical functioning and social-emotional functioning subscales. Each item is scored on a five-point interval scale that reflects the degree of problem. For the subscales and the total score, 100 is the highest possible score and reflects the highest quality of life. The instrument is reprinted in Figure 87-2.

Voice Activity and Participation Profile

The Voice Activity and Participation Profile (VAPP)[53] was constructed in response to the World Health Organization's 1997 revision (ICIDH-2 Beta-1)[95] of the

---

*References 10, 42, 62, 63, 66, 68, 69, 74, 76.

International Classification of Impairments, Disabilities, and Handicaps 1980 framework.[94] The profile consists of 28 items that represent the severity of the voice problem and its effect on job, daily communication, social communication, and emotions. The three middle sections address 10 different speaking situations using a pair of questions about the extent of limitation in daily activities and the extent of restriction of participation in the corresponding activity. Each item is scored using a 10-cm visual analog scale on which the left end is labeled "never" and the right end "always." Several subscores can be calculated and reflect activity limitation and participation restriction for the different sections.

Voice Symptom Scale

The Voice Symptom Scale (VoiSS)[19] is an instrument in progress. In its current form, patients rate 43 items on a five-point equal-appearing interval scale that reflects frequency of occurrence. Questions represent five aspects (or domains) of voice pathology: communication problems, throat infection, psychosocial distress, voice sound and variability, and phlegm.

Other Patient Scales

The Reflux Symptom Index (RSI), the Patient Questionnaire of Vocal Performance (VPQ), and the Voice Outcome Survey (VOS) are more limited in scope. The RSI is made up of nine items and is designed to document patient symptoms of laryngopharyngeal reflux.[9] The VPQ is a 12-item scale designed to assess the physical, social, and emotional impacts of a nonorganic voice disorder.[14,15] The VOS is a five-item

---

TABLE 87-1

PATIENT SCALES

Scale	Abbreviation	Total Items	Domains
Voice Handicap Index[44]	VHI	30	Function, physical, and emotional
Voice-Related Quality of Life[41]	V-RQOL	10	Physical and social-emotional functioning
Voice Activity and Participation Profile[53]	VAPP	28	Severity, effect on job, daily communication, social communication, and emotion
Voice Symptom Scale[19]	VoiSS	43	Communication problems, throat infection, psychosocial distress, voice sound and variability, and phlegm
Reflux Symptom Index[9]	RSI	9	Symptoms associated with laryngopharyngeal reflux
Patient Questionnaire of Vocal Performance[15]	VPQ	12	Physical, social, and emotional
Voice Outcome Survey[23]	VOS	5	Symptoms associated with unilateral vocal fold paralysis

UPMC HEALTH SYSTEM | University of Pittsburgh Voice Center

Name: _____   Date: _____

I need active use of my speaking voice primarily for:
  ❑ A. my profession (teacher, minister, lawyer, salesperson etc.).
  ❑ B. activities outside of work (coaching, community
     organizations, etc).
  ❑ C. normal everyday conversation.

I need active use of my singing voice primarily for:
  ❑ A. my profession (singer-primary income, student of voice).
  ❑ B. activities outside of work (choir/chorus, singer/band
     member-secondary income).
  ❑ C. none of the above. I do not sing.

I would rate my degree of talkativeness as the following: (circle response)

1	2	3	4	5	6	7
Quiet Listener			Average Talker			Extremely Talkative

To be filled out by Voice Staff:

P Spk   ❑
NPV   ❑   VHI

NPV   F=_____
         P=_____
         E=_____

P Sing   ❑
R Sing   ❑   Total=____

Talkativeness: _____

VOICE HANDICAP INDEX

Instructions: These are statements that many people have used to describe their voices and the effects of their voices on their lives. Circle the response that indicates how frequently you have the same experience.

0 = Never 1 = Almost Never 2 = Sometimes 3 = Almost Always 4 = Always

Part I-F

1) My voice makes it difficult for people to hear me   0 1 2 3 4

2) People have difficulty understanding me in a noisy room   0 1 2 3 4

3) May family has difficulty hearing me when I call them throughout the house.   0 1 2 3 4

4) I use the phone less often than I would like to.   0 1 2 3 4

5) I tend to avoid groups of people because of my voice.   0 1 2 3 4

6) I speak with friends, neighbors, or relatives less often because of my voice.   0 1 2 3 4

7) People ask me to repeat myself when speaking face-to-face.   0 1 2 3 4

8) My voice difficulties restrict personal and social life.   0 1 2 3 4

9) I feel left out of conversations because of my voice.   0 1 2 3 4

10) My voice problem causes me to lose income.   0 1 2 3 4

Part II-P

1)	I run out of air when I talk.	0 1 2 3 4
2)	The sound of my voice varies throughout the day.	0 1 2 3 4
3)	People ask, "What's wrong with your voice?"	0 1 2 3 4
4)	My voice sounds creaky and dry.	0 1 2 3 4
5)	I feel as though I have to strain to produce voice.	0 1 2 3 4
6)	The clarity of my voice is unpredictable	0 1 2 3 4
7)	I try to change my voice to sound different	0 1 2 3 4
8)	I use a great deal of effort to speak.	0 1 2 3 4
9)	My voice is worse in the evening.	0 1 2 3 4
10)	My voice "gives out" on me in the middle of speaking.	0 1 2 3 4

Part III-E

1)	I am tense when talking to others because of my voice.	0 1 2 3 4
2)	People seem irritated with my voice.	0 1 2 3 4
3)	I find other people don't understand my voice problem	0 1 2 3 4
4)	My voice problem upsets me.	0 1 2 3 4
5)	I am less outgoing because of my voice problem.	0 1 2 3 4
6)	My voice makes me feel handicapped.	0 1 2 3 4
7)	I feel annoyed when people ask me to repeat.	0 1 2 3 4
8)	I feel embarrassed when people ask me to repeat.	0 1 2 3 4
9)	My voice makes me feel incompetent.	0 1 2 3 4
10)	I am ashamed of my voice problem.	0 1 2 3 4

The Voice Handicap Index (VHI): Development and Validation
Barbara H. Jacobson, Alex Johnson, Cynthia Grywalski, Alice Silbergleit, Gary Jacobson, Michael S. Benninger
American Journal of Speech-Language Pathology, Vol 6(3), 66-70, 1997

Figure 87-1, Voice Handicap Index (VHI). From Jacobson GH and others: The Voice Handicap Index (VHI): development and validation, *Am J Speech Lang Pathol* 6:70, 1997. Used with permission.

survey designed for patients with unilateral vocal fold paralysis.[23]

General Comments

Each published scale measures a different aspect of the voice. Some scales were constructed more carefully than others, so reliability and validity characteristics differ. Scale selection should be made according to variables of interest and reliability requirements. In general, patient scales are a wonderful addition to voice evaluation and provide novel information from the patient point of view. A patient scale can guide discussion between healthcare providers and patients and help the team to determine treatment goals.

PERCEPTUAL EVALUATION
Auditory Perceptual Assessment

Several formal measures and scales have been proposed to rate voice quality. Although auditory perceptual assessment often results in a number, the number

VOICE - RELATED QUALITY OF LIFE (V-RQOL) MEASURE
UNIVERSITY OF MICHIGAN

NAME: _____   DATE: _____

We are trying to learn more about how a voice problem can interfere with your day to day activities. On this paper, you will find a list of possible voice-related problems. Please answer all questions based upon what your voice has been like over the past **two weeks**. There are no "right" or "wrong" answers.

Considering both how severe the problem is when you get it, and how frequently it happens, please rate each item below on how "bad" it is (that is, the amount of each problem that you have). Use the following scale for rating the **amount** of the problem:

1 = None, not a problem
2 = A small amount
3 = A moderate (medium) amount
4 = A lot
5 = Problem is as "bad as it can be"

Because of my voice,   How much of a problem is this?

1. I have trouble speaking loudly or being heard in noisy situations.   1 2 3 4 5

2. I run out of air and need to take frequent breaths when talking.   1 2 3 4 5

3. I sometimes do not know what will come out when I begin speaking.   1 2 3 4 5

4. I am sometimes anxious or frustrated (because of my voice).   1 2 3 4 5

5. I sometimes get depressed (because of my voice).   1 2 3 4 5

6. I have trouble using the telephone (because of my voice).   1 2 3 4 5

7. I have trouble doing my job or practicing my profession (because of my voice).   1 2 3 4 5

8. I avoid going out socially (because of my voice).   1 2 3 4 5

9. I have to repeat myself to be understood.   1 2 3 4 5

10. I have become less outgoing (because of my voice).   1 2 3 4 5

Figure 87-2. Voice-Related Quality of Life (V-RQOL). From Hogikyan ND, Sethuraman G: Validation of an instrument to measure voice-related quality of life (V-RQOL), J Voice 13:69, 1999. Used with permission.

represents a perceptual judgment rather than a measurement and should be treated accordingly. The three auditory perceptual scales described below are listed in Box 87-1.

GRBAS

GRBAS is a well-known standard scale that was developed by the Committee for Phonatory Function of the Japanese Society of Logopedics and Phoniatrics. As described by Hirano,[33] the "G" represents grade or overall quality. The other four letters represent dimensions of voice quality: "R" for roughness, "B" for breathiness, "A" for asthenia, and "S" for strain. Descriptions of each parameter are given in Table 87-2. Each parameter is rated on a 4-point scale: 0 means that there is no deficit in this parameter, 1 is for a mild deficit, 2 is for a moderate deficit, and 3 refers to a severe deficit.

BOX 87-1

AUDITORY PERCEPTUAL SCALES

GRBAS: Grade, Roughness, Breathiness, Asthenia, and Strain
CAPE-V: Consensus Auditory-Perceptual Evaluation—Voice
VPA: Vocal Profile Analysis

CAPE-V

The Consensus Auditory-Perceptual Evaluation—Voice (CAPE-V) is a modification of the GRBAS scale that was developed from a consensus conference sponsored by the American Speech-Language-Hearing Association Special Interest Division 3, Voice and Voice Disorders.[1] Six core and optional examiner-selected parameters are rated on a visual analog scale. The clinician uses a tick mark to rate function on a 100-mm line and then measures the distance from the left end of the line to establish a score; higher scores reflect a more severe handicap. iHiThe core parameters are overall severity, roughness, breathiness, strain, pitch, and loudness. The judged parameters are identified as consistent or intermittent, and resonance differences are noted. The CAPE-V is to be scored from two sustained vowels, six standard sentences, and at least 20 seconds of natural running speech. Recommendations about testing and recording environments are included. A copy of the rating form is reprinted in Figure 87-3.

VPA

The Vocal Profile Analysis (VPA) system represents an entirely different perspective and framework for assessing voice quality. Developed by John Laver and Janet MacKenzie-Beck,[50,51] the VPA approaches voice quality

TABLE 87-2

Grbas Scale For Auditory Perceptual Assessment

Parameter	Hirano Definition[33]	Definition from NCVS Summary Statement[81]
Grade (G)	Overall severity	
Rough (R)	Psychoacoustic impression of irregular vocal fold vibration	An uneven, bumpy quality that appears to be unsteady for the short term but stationary over the long term; acoustically, the waveform is often aperiodic, with the modes of vibration lacking synchrony, but voices with subharmonics can also be perceived as rough.
Breathy (B)	Psychoacoustic impression of air leakage through the glottis	A quality of containing the sound of breathing (expiration) during phonation; acoustically, breathy voice, like falsetto, has most of its energy in the fundamental, but a significant component of noise is present due to turbulence in the glottis; in hyperfunctional breathiness, air leakage may occur in various places along the glottis, whereas, in normal voice, air leakage is usually at the vocal processes.
Asthenic (A)	Weakness or lack of power in the voice	A voice that appears too low in effort, weak; hypofunction of laryngeal muscles is apparent.
Strained (S)	Psychoacoustic impression of a hyperfunctional state of phonation	A voice that appears effortful; visually, hyperfunction of the neck muscles is apparent; the entire larynx seems compressed.

from a phonetic perspective. The voice is profiled according to 18 supralaryngeal (e.g., "raised larynx," "close jaw") and eight phonatory (e.g., "whispery voice," "creaky voice") settings. Each setting is first determined to be neutral or nonneutral. All nonneutral settings are then scaled according to degree of variance from neutral.

Other Aspects of Speech Production

Imprecise articulation, resonance, and prosody disturbances should be noted, because they often indicate structural or neurologic disorders that affect the voice. Resonance is described as hypernasal, hyponasal, or cul-de-sac. Prosody refers to rate, repeated or prolonged syllables, rushes of speech, decreased intonation (i.e., monopitch or monoloudness), and stress patterns, which are described as reduced, equal, or excess stress.

General Comments

Auditory perceptual ratings are appealing because the ultimate goal of voice treatment is to improve voice quality. Unfortunately, voice quality is difficult to define, no standard definitions exist, definitions are frequently circular and/or invalid, it is difficult to differentiate between related qualities, people have different internal representations of parameters and severity, and univariate ratings do not often correlate well with global ratings or measurements (for a detailed discussion, see Kreiman and Gerratt[48]). In addition, the perceptual judgments of quality do not provide information about how the larynx works to

produce voice,[11] and they do not differentiate between structure and function.

Ratings can be influenced by the listener's expectation, training, and frame of reference. Listener expectations become an obvious problem when the rater is the same person who treated the patient. For most auditory perceptual rating systems, "normal" is defined by the individual listener. The listener compares a voice to an internal representation of normal and then judges the degree of deviation. In many research studies, an anchor is presented to the listener and then other samples are judged in comparison with this anchor. Using an anchor and training raters generally improve interjudge reliability.[16,48] Ratings of overall quality tend to be more reliable than unilateral dimensions such as breathiness or strain. To decrease potential bias, perceptual judgments can be made from randomized recordings rather than in person. This solution is imperfect, because it is time consuming and rarely feasible in a busy clinical environment. In fact, judgments made from recordings can have their own sources of error; they are influenced by the quality of the recording, the recording environment, and the listening environment.

Visual Perceptual Evaluation

Voice evaluation must include the documentation of visible aspects of voice production and physical factors that can relate to etiology, maintenance, or effect of dysphonia. Koschkee and Rammage[47] have divided

Consensus Auditory-Perceptual Evaluation of Voice (CAPE-V)

Name:_____   Date:_____

The following parameters of voice quality will be rated upon completion of the following tasks:
1. Sustained vowels, /a/ and /i/ for 3-5 seconds duration each.
2. Sentence production:
    a. The blue spot is on the key again.   d. We eat eggs every Easter.
    b. How hard did he hit him?   e. My mama makes lemon muffins.
    c. We were away a year ago.   f. Peter will keep at the peak.
3. Spontaneous speech in response to: "Tell me about your voice problem." or "Tell me how your voice is functioning."

```
Legend: C = Consistent I = Intermittent
        MI = Mildly Deviant
        MO = Moderately Deviant
        SE = Severely Deviant
```

SCORE

Overall Severity _____ C I   ___/100
                    MI   MO   SE

Roughness   _____ C I   ___/100
                    MI   MO   SE

Breathiness   _____ C I   ___/100
                    MI   MO   SE

Strain   _____ C I   ___/100
                    MI   MO   SE

Pitch   (Indicate the nature of the abnormality): _____
                 _____ C I   ___/100
                    MI   MO   SE

Loudness (Indicate the nature of the abnormality): _____
                 _____ C I   ___/100
                    MI   MO   SE

_____   _____ C I   ___/100
                    MI   MO   SE

_____   _____ C I   ___/100
                    MI   MO   SE

COMMENTS ABOUT RESONANCE: NORMAL   OTHER (Provide description):_____
_____

ADDITIONAL FEATURES (for example, diplophonia, fry, falsetto, asthenia, aphonia, pitch instability, tremor, wet/gurgly, or other relevant terms):

                                    Clinician: _____

Figure 87-3. CAPE-V. From American Speech-Language-Hearing Association, Special Interest Division 3, Voice and Voice Disorders: *Consensus Auditory-Perceptual Evaluation of Voice (CAPE-V), 2003: Instrument in preparation.* Available at: *http://www.asha.org/about/membership-certification/divs/div_3.htm.* Accessed March 3, 2004.

the visual perceptual examination into five categories: general appearance; posture, breathing, and musculoskeletal tension; neurologic dysfunction; physical dysmorphology; and clinical manifestations of disease. A brief description of each follows, and more complete descriptions of each area can be found in the reference chapter.[47] The categories are summarized in Box 87-2.

General Appearance

General appearance includes such factors as age; height and weight; facial expression; skin, hair, and nails; per-

VISUAL PERCEPTUAL EVALUATION

General appearance
Posture, breathing, and musculoskeletal tension
Neurologic dysfunction
Physical dysmorphology
Physical manifestations of disease

sonal hygiene and dress; and head and neck observations. An overall examination of the patient's physical status can help the examiner identify potential areas of concern. The patient's chronologic age is compared with their apparent age, and voice and speech factors that contribute to differences are noted. The patient's physical stature can also be a consideration. When patients are overweight, underweight, or have experienced rapid weight change, an underlying physical or psychological condition may be responsible for the change in voice quality. Facial expression can indicate affective state, pain, or some neurologic disorders (e.g., the "masked face" of Parkinson disease). Changes in skin, hair, and nails can indicate systemic disease that may affect voice quality. Inattention to personal hygiene and dress can be indicative of an emotional disorder or dementia. Head and neck observations include the presence of staining on the teeth as a result of smoking or coffee consumption and evidence of previous surgeries that may affect either voice or resonance.

Posture, Breathing, and Musculoskeletal Tension

Posture, breathing, and musculoskeletal tension are key components of a voice evaluation. Posture includes alignment of the head, neck, torso, pelvis, and legs. Patients may not present to a clinic using their typical posture, but they can usually demonstrate it when asked. To examine breathing, observe repeated breaths during rest and speech production. Very little motion of the neck, shoulders, and upper chest should take place. Musculoskeletal tension can be identified through limited jaw motion, jutting the chin forward, neck extension, bulging of the neck muscles while talking, or raised shoulders.

Neurologic Dysfunction

Neurologic dysfunction can affect movement, including speech and voice production. Unsteadiness, asymmetry, rigidity, hesitation, slowness, weakness, incoordination, inconsistency, and extraneous movements are clinical features that should trigger a complete neurologic assessment in addition to the voice evaluation. Weakness, asymmetry, and incoordination of the tongue, jaw, lips, or soft palate are especially noteworthy. The presence of focal dystonias, such as

writer's cramp, blepharospasm, torticollis, or oromandibular dysphonia may prompt the examiner to consider a neurologically based voice disorder, such as spasmodic dysphonia.

Physical Dysmorphology

Physical dysmorphologies are common in patients with congenital disorders and patients who have undergone head and neck surgery. Both groups can have voice and speech problems either as a result of the underlying disorder or from compensatory movements.

Physical Manifestations of Disease

Physical manifestations of systemic illness or disease are important to note, because many diseases can affect vocal fold structure or function. A few examples include hypothyroidism, lupus, rheumatoid arthritis, scleroderma, and Sjögren's syndrome. Medications used to treat these disorders can also have significant effects on vocal function.

Tactile Perceptual Evaluation

The tactile perceptual evaluation includes the palpation of extrinsic laryngeal muscle tension and the physical examination of the breathing apparatus.

Extrinsic Laryngeal Muscle Tension

The manual examination of laryngeal musculoskeletal tension includes the palpation of the suprahyoid muscles, the major horns of the hyoid bone, the superior cornu and the lateral aspects of the thyroid cartilage, the thyrohyoid space, and the anterior border of the sternocleidomastoid. It is useful to assess suprahyoid tension and thyrohyoid space both at rest and during phonation. Lateral displacement of the thyroid cartilage is attempted.[2,65,67] Box 87-3 lists the key palpation points, and Figure 87-4 depicts this evaluation. Rammage, Morrison, and Nichol propose a slightly different protocol that includes palpating the suprahyoid, thyrohyoid, cricothyroid, and pharyngolaryngeal (inferior constrictor and posterior cricoarytenoid) muscles.[4,61] Normal findings include space between

TACTILE PERCEPTUAL EVALUATION: PALPATION SITES

Suprahyoid muscles
Major horns of the hyoid bone
Superior cornu of the thyroid cartilage
Lateral aspects of the thyroid cartilage
Thyrohyoid space
Anterior border of the sternocleidomastoid
Lateral displacement of the thyroid cartilage

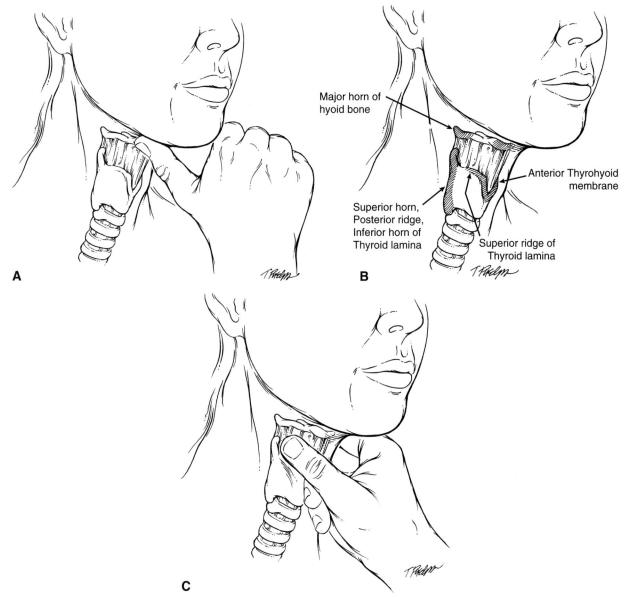

Figure 87-4. Manual musculoskeletal tension evaluation. **A,** Palpation of suprahyoid muscu-lature. **B,** Palpation of major horns of the hyoid bone, superior cornu of the thyroid cartilage, and lateral aspects of the thyroid cartilage. **C,** Palpation of the thyrohyoid space.

the hyoid bone and the superior border of the thyroid cartilage and laryngeal complex mobility. Findings indicative of excessive musculoskeletal tension include pain with palpation (frequently more severe on one side), decreased or absent thyrohyoid space at rest or with phonation, muscle "knots," high carriage of the hyoid bone and thyroid cartilage, and difficulty rotating the larynx.[2,4,61,65,67]

Diagnostic therapy to assess the effects of perturb-ing the larynx by changing configuration of the vocal tract is undertaken *during voicing* with several maneuvers: (1) pushing back of the suprahyoid mus-culature, hyoid bone, superior border of thyroid carti-lage, thyroid notch, thyroid prominence, or anterior cricoid ring; (2) manual lowering of the thyroid carti-lage with downward traction applied to the superior border of the thyroid cartilage; (3) manual lowering with medial compression of the thyroid cartilage; and (4) circumla-ryngeal massage using a circular motion over sites of focal tenderness or tautness.[2,65,67] Box 87-4 lists and Figure 87-5 show these maneuvers.

A drawback to the examination is that it is subjec-tive, and examiner skill and experience likely affect ratings. In addition, there are currently no intra- or

TACTILE PERCEPTUAL EVALUATION: TRIAL THERAPY MANEUVERS

Pushing back of suprahyoid muscles, hyoid bone, and thyroid cartilage
Manual lowering of thyroid cartilage
Manual lowering with medial compression
Circumlaryngeal massage

---

interexaminer reliability data for the technique, and the sensitivity and specificity of abnormal findings are unknown. Even with these apparent limitations, tactile perceptual evaluation is a powerful technique to use to rapidly assess the contribution of muscle tension to the observed voice quality. Trial therapy with these techniques demonstrates to the patient and clinician the potential for improved voice quality with voice therapy, thus achieving "buy in" to a behavioral remediation approach. Teasing apart the muscle tension component from the other components of the dysphonia can help ensure proper diagnosis and management. In many instances, this technique becomes the method of therapy, and patients achieve substantial and lasting improvement in one session.[65,67]

Physical Examination of the Breathing Apparatus

Physical examinations of the diaphragm,[38] the abdominal wall,[39] the and ribcage wall[40] have been described as components of the breathing apparatus assessment. The three reference articles thoroughly describe the contribution of each component to voice production and propose protocols for the evaluation of the structure, movement, and force-production capabilities during performance activities. To complement physical examination of the apparatus, the contribution of respiratory factors to speech can be assessed by measuring airflow, changes in lung volumes with phonation, or chest wall motion during speech.*

MEASURES

Measuring voice is accomplished using acoustic analysis, aerodynamic assessment, and source measures.

Acoustic Analysis

The acoustic signal produced as speech is quite complex. The components of this signal can be isolated and studied using a variety of techniques. Components of interest include the dimensions of frequency, amplitude (intensity), and time. Several commonly used techniques are described below. They are listed, along with their perceptual correlates, in Table 87-3.

---

*References 36, 37, 56, 57, 71, 73.

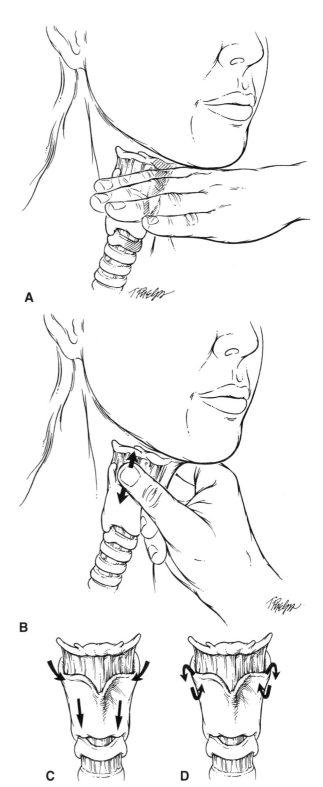

Figure 87-5. Trial therapy maneuvers. **A,** Pushing back of the suprahyoid, hyoid, thyrohyoid space, thyroid notch, thyroid prominence, and anterior cricoid ring. **B,** Lowering of the thyroid cartilage. **C,** Lowering, with medial compression. **D,** Circumlaryngeal massage.

TABLE 87-3

ACOUSTIC MEASURES AND THEIR PERCEPTUAL CORRELATES

Measure	Perceptual Correlate
Frequency	Pitch
Intensity	Loudness
Voice range profile	Interaction of pitch and loudness ranges
Variability measures	Quality (e.g., roughness, breathiness, timbre)
Spectral displays	Quality
Fast Fourier transform	Quality
Linear predictive coding	Quality
Long-term average spectrum	Quality
Cepstral peak prominence	Quality
Nasalance	Hyper/hypo nasality

Frequency

One basic measure used for voice analysis is frequency. Frequency refers to the repeating cycles of vibration in the acoustic waveform. It is measured in cycles per second, also called Hertz (Hz). The perceptual correlate of frequency is pitch. In truth, there are many additional factors that contribute to perception of pitch, but frequency is the most salient one. A longer cycle of repeat (lower frequency) is perceived as a lower pitch, and a shorter cycle of repeat (higher frequency) is perceived as a higher pitch. Altered pitch and restricted pitch range are common symptoms of voice disorders and can represent a significant concern for patients. Average speaking fundamental frequency and maximum phonational frequency range are the most common clinical tasks used to examine frequency. Normative values are influenced by intensity, speech sample, vowel type, age, and gender.[7,75] Baken and Orlikoff[7] summarize results of frequency measures from many acoustic studies. On the basis of their summary tables, average speaking fundamental frequency ranges from approximately 100 to 125 Hz for normal adult men into their 70s and 190 to 225 Hz for normal adult women. The maximum phonation frequency range is frequently reported using a semitone scale, whereby perceived changes in pitch are equalized across the frequency range. The semitone scale corresponds with the musical scale, with 12 semitones in an octave.[7] Maximum phonational frequency range for men and women is typically two and a half to three octaves, or approximately 29 to 36 semitones.

Intensity

Intensity is the acoustic correlate of loudness. Again, many factors influence the perception of loudness, but intensity is the primary one. Intensity is measured as sound pressure level in decibels (dB) using a sound level meter or acoustic analysis equipment. Measurements are affected by frequency, vowel, speech sample, equipment, mouth-to-microphone (or sound level meter) distance, and ambient noise.[75] The most common measures are average speaking intensity and minimum and maximum intensities. Average adult men and women speak at approximately 70 dB,[7] although there can be a large variability in conversational speech; the range is typically less than 60 dB to at least 110 dB.[11,12] Intensity measures are useful to document patient and family concerns about decreased loudness level, which is common for patients with Parkinson's disease or vocal fold motion impairment, and they help identify patients who have difficulty speaking quietly, which is common for patients with vocal fold scarring or lesions.

Combined Frequency and Intensity

A frequency-by-intensity plot for an individual's total range is called a phonetogram or a voice range profile (VRP). The "low-tech" version requires a sound level meter and a keyboard.

The minimum and maximum intensities an individual can produce are plotted for every frequency in that person's range. "High-tech" versions are possible using computer programs. There is a typical shape to the plot, which is demonstrated in Figure 87-6. Visual inspection of the VRP highlights the interaction between frequency and intensity, with the highest frequencies generally produced at greater intensities than the lowest frequencies. The middle of the frequency range is usually the location of the individual's maximum intensity range.[82] There is no standard for analyzing the VRP, but several authors have proposed methods of quantifying the plot.* Even given the limitations of analysis, the VRP shows the physiologic limits of the system and is very useful for tracking changes. Singers in particular often present with difficulty with specific pitch and loudness combinations (e.g., trouble singing quietly for particular notes), and the phonetogram helps document their concerns.

Variability Measures

Acoustic measures include those associated with cycle-to-cycle variability of the acoustic signal (perturbation) and ratios of harmonic energy to noise energy. The most well-known perturbation measures

---

*References 3, 8, 28, 43, 79, 83.

Fundamental frequency in Hz

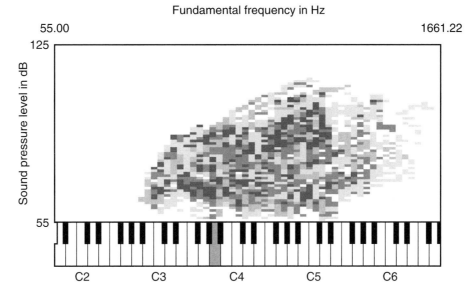

Figure 87-6. Sample Voice Range Profile (VRP).

are jitter and shimmer. *Jitter* is the cycle-to-cycle variation in frequency, whereas *shimmer* is the cycle-to-cycle variation in intensity. Various measures of harmonics or signal to noise have been proposed, and many other measures have been suggested through the years. An excellent review of acoustic measures and algorithms can be found in a chapter by Buder.[13] Theoretically, measures that document variability in the sound wave should correspond well with perceived roughness or hoarseness. Unfortunately, how well the measures relate to voice quality ratings remains uncertain,* and no particular measure or group of measures has emerged as indispensable for the diagnosis of voice disorders.

The National Center for Voice and Speech published a summary statement in 1995 that reflected recommendations for how to perform and interpret perturbation analyses. Among the recommendations is the caution that acoustic waveforms should be visually inspected before analysis and rated according to the nature of qualitative changes of the signal.[81] Type 1 signals are nearly periodic, with no qualitative changes. Type 2 signals either do not have an obvious single fundamental frequency or have qualitative changes in the signal. Type 3 signals have no apparent periodic structure. According to Titze,[81] perturbation analysis has utility and reliability only for Type 1 signals. Type 2 signals should be analyzed using visual displays and Type 3 signals with perceptual ratings. Both high vowels (/i/ or /æ/) and low vowels (/ɑ/ or /—/) should be used for perturbation analysis, collecting multiple tokens, and a variety of stimuli, such as sustained vowels, sustained consonants, pitch and loudness glides, adductory glides, register glides, counting,

sentences, reading, picture description, parent-child speech, dramatic speech, and singing.

Spectral Displays

According to the source-filter theory of vowel production,[20] the vocal folds produce a signal with a fundamental frequency and multiples of that frequency, called harmonics. This source signal is modified by attenuation or amplification as it passes through the supraglottic vocal tract, which is called the filter. The vocal tract structures change position for different vowels, thus changing the shape of the filter. Therefore, each vowel has a unique pattern of resonant peaks of the vocal tract, which are commonly called formants.[7] Because the voice people hear is a combination of source and filter characteristics, the harmonics and the formants each tell part of the story of voice production.

A spectrogram is the most common visual depiction of an acoustic wave. It displays time on the x axis, frequency on the y axis, and amplitude on a gray scale. Changing the bandwidth of the analysis window allows us to view details of either the source or the filter. A narrow-band spectrogram, with its greater frequency resolution, emphasizes the fundamental frequency and the harmonics. A wide-band spectrogram, with its greater time resolution, highlights the formants.[7] Figure 87-7 is a narrow-band spectrogram and a wide-band spectrogram of /a ɛ i o u/. Spectrograms clearly show noise versus harmonic structure, tremor, phonation breaks, and pitch breaks. The relative amplitude of the first harmonic has been shown to correlate with ratings of breathiness.[30,31] Spectrograms are useful for tracking change and can be used in real time during voice therapy for visual feedback.

---

*References 5, 29, 32, 45, 54, 60, 75, 90, 91.

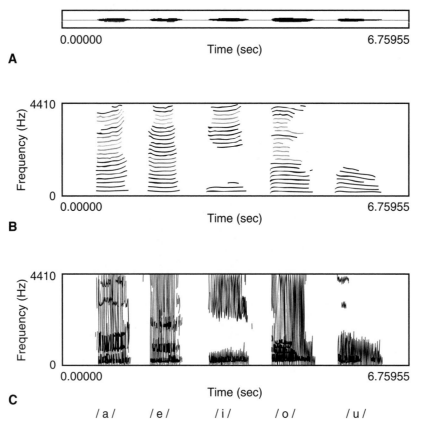

Figure 87-7. A, Audio signal, **B,** narrow-band spectrogram, and **C,** wide-band spectrogram for /ɑ ɛ i o u/.

Additional Acoustic Measures

FFT and LPC Spectra. A Fast Fourier Transform (FFT) analysis converts the signal so that the individual frequencies that make up the sound of a narrow time band can be identified. The display shows frequency on the x axis and intensity on the y axis. A linear predictive coding (LPC) spectrum shows a smoothed line that highlights the formant structure but that again reveals the amplitude of a frequency for a narrow band of time. Figure 87-8 shows the FFT and LPC spectra for the marked location in the audio signal of a sustained /i/.

LTAS. Long-term average spectra (LTAS) show the amount of energy at each frequency over a long period of time (e.g., a standard reading). Because the meas-

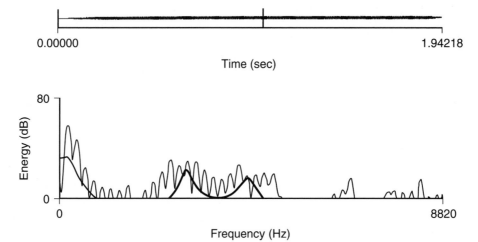

Figure 87-8. A, Audio signal of sustained /i/. **B,** FFT (jagged) and LPC (smooth line) spectra from the marked portion of the /i/.

ure is averaged over such a long sample, the effects of speech context are minimized. Measurements of the LTAS typically compare the amount of energy in different frequency bands. The resultant values, which are often referred to as spectral tilt, indicate whether low or high frequencies dominate the spectrum.[49]

CPP. Cepstral peak prominence (CPP) has recently garnered some attention.[25–27,59] It is a measure of signal periodicity that does not rely on fundamental frequency extraction, and it has been found to correlate with breathiness.[30,31] A cepstrum is a log power spectrum of a log power spectrum (i.e., a Fourier transformation of a spectrum), and it corresponds with the regularity of harmonic peaks.[30,31] The time at which the predominant cepstral peak appears (frequency) corresponds with the fundamental period of the signal, and the amplitude corresponds with the harmonic organization. The measure CPP reflects the amplitude of the predominant cepstral peak that has been normalized for the signal amplitude.[30,31] A lower CPP reflects aperiodic vibration. A CPP-smoothed (CPPS) is a modification of the CPP whereby the individual cepstra are smoothed before calculating the CPP. The CPPS is reportedly a better predictor of perceived breathiness than the CPP.[31] A recent study found the CPPS to be useful for predicting overall dysphonia as well.[27]

Acoustic assessment of velopharyngeal function.

Oronasal resonance balance can be assessed acoustically using a commercial program such as the Nasometer (Kay Elemetrics, Lincoln Park, NJ). This instrument is comprised of two microphones that are separated by a plate. The plate is pressed against the upper lip so that one microphone is positioned in front of the nose and the other in front of the mouth. A measure called *nasalance* is computed by dividing the nasal sound energy by the total (oral plus nasal) sound energy and multiplying by 100. There has been some debate about the validity of the measures because of variable correlation between nasalance and the perceptual evaluation of hypernasality. Proposed hypernasality cutoff scores have varied according to testing center and raters but appear to range from 25% to 33% for a standard passage without nasal consonants (zoo passage).[17,28,24,58] That is, mean nasalance scores of 25% to 33% or greater are generally associated with perceived hypernasality; hyponasality is generally perceived when mean nasalance falls below 50% for nasal sentences.[17,18,24,58] There is evidence to suggest that regional normative data should be collected, because resonance patterns vary according to dialect.[17]

General Comments

Acoustic analysis is appealing because it uses non-invasive techniques to analyze the voice. Examination of the acoustic signal can provide a clinician or researcher with information about how a disease is affecting vocal function and voice quality. Several factors influence all of the measures, however, including age, gender, interactions between parameters, equipment, recording environment, vowel, speech sample selected for analysis, and number of tokens. To maximize reliability, standard equipment, instructions, and protocols are recommended. When interpreting results, the examiner should take into account whether the task was connected speech or sustained sound and whether it was representative of a typical performance or a maximum performance task.

Aerodynamic Assessment

Aerodynamic evaluation involves measuring air pressures and airflows. Many calculations from these measures appear to be useful for vocal function analysis. Equipment can range from "low tech" to "high tech." Techniques are listed, along with perceptual correlates, in Table 87-4.

Maximum Phonation Time

Maximum phonation time (MPT) has long been used as a measure of both breath support and phonatory efficiency. The maximum length of time a patient can sustain phonation, however, is not fully explained by either vital capacity or laryngeal function.[71] Multiple factors influence MPT, such as respiratory capacity and function, phonatory function (especially efficient valving of the airstream), resonance, practice, frequency, intensity, instructions, and, potentially, vowel choice.* It can take as many as nine to 15 trials for adults[77] and

TABLE 87-4

AERODYNAMIC MEASURES AND THEIR PERCEPTUAL CORRELATES

Measure	Perceptual Correlate
Subglottic air pressure	Phonatory effort
Phonation threshold pressure	Effort to initiate phonation
Airflow	Breathiness
Laryngeal airway resistance	Phonatory effort, vocal strength, strain
Velopharyngeal measures	Nasal emission, strength of pressure consonants

---

*References 11, 71, 80, 84, 85, 96, 97.

20 trials for children[52] to achieve MPT. No standard instructions exist for the task, but the longest of three trials is often used clinically.[7] No group is homogenous. Even for healthy young adults, a range of 6.6 to 69.5 seconds is reported in the literature.[7] Because of the variety of influences and the differences between system demands for MPT and connected speech, the usefulness and accuracy of the measure are suspect,[71] especially if considered in isolation.[46] In general, it is preferable to measure laryngeal valving using other techniques (e.g., mean airflow, laryngeal airway resistance, videostroboscopy, and to measure respiratory capabilities using spirometry or chest wall measurements.

Subglottic Air Pressure

Subglottic air pressure (Ps) is a variable of interest, both in its own right and as a component of the laryngeal airway resistance calculation. A relatively constant Ps is required to sustain vocal fold vibration. For speech, air pressure is measured in cm H_2O (i.e., the amount of pressure necessary to elevate a column of water by a particular number of centimeters). Intraoral air pressure (Po) during a voiceless consonant (when the glottis is open) is an excellent estimate of Ps and can be measured noninvasively.[70] Intraoral air pressure is analyzed by visual inspection of the shape of the pressure peak and the length and magnitude of the peak. The Po should fall sharply with release of the consonant. The magnitude of a normal pressure peak varies with loudness, age, gender, consonant, and speech context.[7] Normative values of 6.43 cm H_2O (standard deviation, 1.07) for adult men and 7.52 cm H_2O (standard deviation, 2.17) for adult women are reported.[78] Abnormal values can indicate a lack of driving pressure, an incompetent or insufficient velopharyngeal or laryngeal valve, or increased vocal fold mass or stiffness. Intraoral air pressure is useful to document clinician perceptions of weak pressure consonants, such as with velopharyngeal incompetence or dysarthria.

Phonation Threshold Pressure

The minimum amount of Ps necessary to cause the vocal folds to vibrate is called phonation threshold pressure (PTP).[82] Procedures for collecting and measuring PTP have been described in detail by Verdolini and colleagues.[86–89] In brief, repetitions of the syllable /pæ/ or /pi/ are produced as quietly as possible without whispering. The maximum values of several serial pressure peaks from /p/ are averaged to estimate the minimum Ps necessary to cause the vocal folds to vibrate. The measure is often collected at various percentages of the maximum fundamental frequency range, with PTP at high pitches showing sensitivity to increasing viscoelasticity of the vocal folds. Phonation threshold pressure has been helpful in the evaluation of subtle changes such as hydration/dehydration, vocal fatigue, and changes with vocal warm up.[21,55,72,86–89] The measure is useful for documenting a patient's perception of increased effort required to phonate, which is common with many voice disorders, including lesions, muscle tension dysphonia, and adductor spasmodic dysphonia.

Airflow

Airflow is a change in volume of air over a specific amount of time, and is measured as quantity (mL or L) per time (second or minute).[7] Mean airflow is commonly assessed during sustained phonation, although sometimes it is measured during connected speech. Airflow is typically measured using a pneumotachograph connected to a differential pressure transducer system; the pressure drop across a known resistance is then measured. Another common measurement system is the Rothenberg mask, which is a circumferentially vented mask with 1-cm holes that are covered with fine-mesh screens to act as resistance.[64] Airflow is measured using strain gauge differential pressure transducers. Airflow measures are influenced by gender, age, fundamental frequency, and intensity. Normal values for adult women range from 91 to 156 mL per second, with a standard deviation range of 16 to 71 mL per second.[7] Mean values for normal adult men range from 101 to 183 mL per second, with a standard deviation range of 16 to 77 mL per second.[7] Mean airflow is typically increased when there is poor vocal fold closure, such as for vocal fold motion impairment.[33,34] The shape of the airflow trace can also be useful; it is common with motion impairment to see a burst of air at the beginning of phonation and low airflow by the end.[11] With hyperfunction, mean airflow might be reduced.[11]

Laryngeal Airway Resistance

Laryngeal airway resistance (R_{law}) is the ratio of translaryngeal air pressure to translaryngeal airflow.[7] Smitheron and Hixon[70] demonstrated that it can be estimated using Po and mean airflow from repetitions of the syllable /pi/ at a rate of 1.5 syllables per second. Higher R_{law} can occur with increased intensity, a long closed phase, or an increased force of closure.[11]

Aerodynamic Assessment of Velopharyngeal Function

The velopharyngeal system can be assessed aerodynamically using an airflow mask that covers only the nose to measure nasal airflow (Vn). Intraoral air pressure is measured during anterior stop consonants, as described earlier. Comparing the Vn and Po traces during a transition between nasal and stop consonants (e.g., "mp" in the word "pamper") shows the timing of the velopharyngeal closure. If the nasal cavity pressure is also measured, velopharyngeal orifice area can be calculated.[92,93]

Source Measures
Electroglottography

Electroglottography (EGG) measures the conductance of a low-frequency electric signal across the neck between two surface electrodes.[7,11,22] The conductance of the signal varies with the vibration of the vocal folds; when the vocal folds contact one another, conductance increases, and the resultant trace has a positive slope. As vocal folds separate, conductance decreases, and the trace has a negative slope. The traces display the degree of contact relative to the rest of the signal so that maximum contact does not indicate complete vocal fold closure. The waveform's shape is potentially meaningful for describing the pattern of vocal fold vibration. Baken and Orlikoff[7] summarize a variety of EGG shapes and the corresponding glottic cycles. Specific measures of increasing contact, decreasing contact, and speed quotients have been proposed over the years, but some researchers question their validity.[6]

In EGG, abnormalities in the signal are not always the result of abnormalities in vocal fold motion; the signal can be affected by the placement of electrodes, movement of the larynx during phonation, irregularities of neck tissue, and mucous bridges. Even given its limitations, EGG is an excellent measure of fundamental frequency and offers a unique opportunity to study the vocal fold vibration without any influence of supraglottic structures or shaping. It is noninvasive, relatively inexpensive, and can be used at the same time as other measures (e.g., airflow, videostroboscopy).

Inverse Filtered Flow

In inverse filtered flow, the effects of the vocal tract (resonances) are filtered out of either the acoustic or aerodynamic waveform, and the glottic source signal is left. From this trace, several measures can be made, including skewing quotient (the ratio of the positive slope to the negative slope) and open quotient (the ratio of the time open to the period of the waveform).[82] Inverse filtered airflow presents the advantage of assessing individual glottal cycles. The primary disadvantages are that it can only be measured on a sustained sound and that the validity of the measure relies on correctly setting the filters, which can be a technically challenging task.

SUMMARY

Voice evaluation and measurement should be multidimensional, reflecting the complexity of the voice and communication. Voice analysis includes patient scales, perceptual evaluation, and measures. Individual measures are influenced by many factors that need to be understood by the clinician or researcher before interpreting. Each of the measures addresses a piece of the puzzle, and none stands alone as the perfect measure for all questions. A set of measures should be selected that documents the patients' particular concerns or that parallels the question that is of interest to the examiner. The development of standard protocols and testing conditions across centers will improve the ability of clinicians and researchers to communicate and hasten further understanding of the human voice.

REFERENCES

1. American Speech-Language-Hearing Association, Special Interest Division 3, Voice and Voice Disorders: *Consensus Auditory-Perceptual Evaluation of Voice (CAPE-V), 2003: Instrument in preparation.* Available at *http://www.asha.org/about/membership-certification/divs/div_3.htm.*
2. Aronson AE: *Clinical voice disorders: an interdisciplinary approach,* ed 3, New York, 1990, Thieme.
3. Airainer R, Klingholz F: Quantitative evaluation of phonetograms in the case of functional dysphonia, *J Voice* 7:136, 1993.
4. Angsuwarangsee T, Morrison M: Extrinsic laryngeal muscular tension in patients with voice disorders, *J Voice* 16:333, 2002.
5. Askenfelt A, Hammarberg B: Speech waveform perturbation analysis: a perceptual-acoustic comparison of seven measures, *J Speech Hear Res* 29:50, 1986.
6. Baken RJ: Electroglottography, *J Voice* 6:98, 2002.
7. Baken RJ, Orlikoff RF: *Clinical measurement of voice and speech,* ed 2, San Diego, 2000, Singular Publishing Group.
8. Behrman A and others: Meaningful features of voice range profiles from patients with organic vocal fold pathology: a preliminary study, *J Voice* 10:269, 1996.
9. Belafsky PC, Postma, GN, Koufman JA: Validity and reliability of the reflux symptom index (RSI), *J Voice* 16:274, 2002.
10. Benninger MS and others: Assessing outcomes for dysphonic patients, *J Voice* 12:540, 1998.
11. Bless DM: *Assessment of laryngeal function.* In Ford CN, Bless DM, editors: *Phonosurgery: assessment and surgical management of voice disorders,* New York, 1991, Raven Press, p 95.
12. Bless DM and others: *Stroboscopic, acoustic, aerodynamic, and perceptual attributes of voice production in normal speaking adults.* In Titze IR, editor: *Progress Report 4,* Iowa City, 1993, National Center for Voice and Speech, p 121.
13. Buder EH: *Acoustic analysis of voice quality: a tabulation of algorithms 1902–1990.* In Kent RD, Ball MJ, editors: *Voice quality measurement.* San Diego, 2000, Singular Publishing Group, p 119.
14. Carding PN, Horsley IA: An evaluation study of voice therapy in nonorganic dysphonia, *Eur J Disord Commun* 277:137, 1992.
15. Carding PN, Horsley IA, Docherty GD: Measuring the effectiveness of voice therapy in a group of forty-five patients with non-organic dysphonia, *J Voice* 13:76, 1999.
16. Chan KMK, Yiu EML: The effect of anchors and training on the reliability of perceptual voice evaluation, *J Speech Lang Hear Res* 45:111, 2002.

17. Dalston RM, Neiman GS, Gonzalez-Landa G: Nasometric sensitivity and specificity: a cross-dialect and cross-culture study, *Cleft Palate Craniofac J* 30:285, 1993.

18. Dalston RM, Warren DW, Dalston ET: Use of nasometry as a diagnostic tool for identifying patients with velopharyngeal impairment, *Cleft Palate Craniofac J* 28:184, 1991.

19. Deary IJ and others: VoiSS, a patient-derived voice symptom scale, *J Psychosom Res* 54:483, 2003.

20. Fant G: *Theory of speech production,* The Hague, 1960, Mouton.

21. Fisher KV and others: Phonatory effects of body fluid removal, *J Speech Hear Res* 44:354, 2001.

22. Fourcin A: *Voice quality and electrolaryngography.* In Kent RD, Ball MJ, editors: *Voice quality measurement,* San Diego, 2000, Singular Publishing Group, p 285.

23. Glicklich RE, Glovsky RM, Montgomery WM: Validation of a voice outcome survey for unilateral vocal cord paralysis, *Otolaryngol Head Neck Surg* 120:153, 1999.

24. Hardin MA and others: Correspondence between nasalance scores and listener judgments of hypernasality and hyponasality, *Cleft Palate Craniofac J* 29:346, 1992.

25. Hartl DM and others: Objective acoustic and aerodynamic measures of breathiness in paralytic dysphonia, *Eur Arch Otorhinolaryngol* 260:175, 2003.

26. Hartl DM and others: Objective voice quality analysis before and after onset of unilateral vocal fold paralysis, *J Voice* 15:351, 2001.

27. Heman-Ackah YD, Michael DD, Goding GS: The relationship between cepstral peak prominence and selected parameters of dysphonia, *J Voice* 16:20, 2002.

28. Heylen L and others: Evaluation of the vocal performance of children using a voice range profile index, *J Speech Lang Hear Res* 41:232, 1998.

29. Hill DP, Meyers AD, Scherer RC: A comparison of four clinical techniques in the analysis of phonation, *J Voice* 4:198, 1990.

30. Hillenbrand J, Cleveland RA, Erickson RL: Acoustic correlates of breathy vocal quality, *J Speech Hear Res* 37:769, 1994.

31. Hillenbrand J, Houde, RA: Acoustic correlates of breathy vocal quality: dysphonic voices and continuous speech, *J Speech Hear Res* 39:311, 1996.

32. Hillman RE and others: Phonatory function associated with hyperfunctionally related vocal fold lesions, *J Voice* 4:52, 1990.

33. Hirano M: *Clinical examination of voice,* Wien/New York, 1981, Springer-Verlag.

34. Hirano M: Objective evaluation of the human voice. Clinical aspects, *Folia Phoniatr (Basel)* 41:89, 1989.

35. Hirano M and others: Vocal function in patients with unilateral vocal fold paralysis before and after silicone injection, *Acta Otolaryngol* 115:553, 1995.

36. Hixon TJ, Goldman MD, Mead J: Kinematics of the chest wall during speech production: volume displacements of the rib cage, abdomen, and lung, *J Speech Hear Res* 16:78, 1973.

37. Hixon TJ, Mead J, Goldman MD: Dynamics of the chest wall during speech production: function of the thorax, rib cage, diaphragm, and abdomen, *J Speech Hear Res* 19:297, 1976.

38. Hixon TJ, Hoit JD: Physical examination of the diaphragm by the speech-language pathologist, *Am J Speech Lang Pathol* 7:37, 1998.

39. Hixon TJ, Hoit JD: Physical examination of the abdominal wall by the speech-language pathologist, *Am J Speech Lang Pathol* 8:35, 1999.

40. Hixon TJ, Hoit, JD: Physical examination of the rib cage wall by the speech-language-pathologist, *Am J Speech Lang Pathol* 9:179, 2000.

41. Hogikyan ND, Sethuraman G: Validation of an instrument to measure voice-related quality of life (V-RQOL), *J Voice* 13:557, 1999

42. Hsiung MW, Pai L, Wang HW: Correlation between voice handicap index and voice laboratory measurements in dysphonic patients, *Eur Arch Otorhinolaryngol* 259:97, 2002.

43. Ikeda Y and others: Quantitative evaluation of the voice range profile in patients with voice disorder, *Eur Arch Otorhinolaryngol* 256(Suppl 1):S51, 1999.

44. Jacobson GH and others: The Voice handicap index (VHI): development and validation, *Am J Speech Lang Pathol* 6:66, 1997.

45. Kempster G, Kistler DJ, Hillenbrand J: Multidimensional scaling analysis of dysphonia in two speaker groups, *J Speech Hear Res* 34:534, 1991.

46. Kent RD, Kent JF, Rosenbek JC: Maximum performance tests of speech production, *J Speech Hear Disord* 52:367, 1987.

47. Koschkee DL, Rammage L: *Voice care in the medical setting.* San Diego, Singular Publishing Group, 1997.

48. Kreiman J, Gerratt B: *Measuring vocal quality.* In Kent RD, Ball MJ, editors: *Voice quality measurement,* San Diego, 2000, Singular Publishing Group, p 73.

49. Löfqvist A, Mandersson B: Long time average spectrum of speech and voice analysis, *Folia Phoniatr (Basel)* 39:221, 1987.

50. Laver J: *Phonetic evaluation of voice quality.* In Kent RD, Ball MJ, editors: *Voice quality measurement.* San Diego, 2000, Singular Publishing Group, p 37.

51. Laver J, Mackenzie-Beck J: *Vocal Profile Analysis.* Edinburgh, University of Edinburgh, Queen Margaret College, 1991.

52. Lewis K, Casteel R, McMahon J: Duration of sustained /a/ related to the number of trials, *Folia Phoniatr (Basel)* 34:41, 1982.

53. Ma EP-M, Yiu EM-L: Voice activity and participation profile: assessing the impact of voice disorders on daily living, *J Speech Lang Hear Res* 44:511, 2001.

54. Martin D, Fitch J, Wolfe V: Pathologic voice type and the acoustic prediction of severity, *J Speech Hear Res* 38:765, 1995.

55. Motel T, Fisher KV, Leydon C: Vocal warm-up increases phonation threshold pressure in soprano singers at high pitch, *J Voice* 17:160, 2003.

56. Murdoch BE and others: Respiratory function in Parkinson's subjects exhibiting a perceptible speech deficit: a kinematic and spirometric analysis, *J Speech Hear Dis* 54:610, 1989.

57. Murdoch BE and others: Respiratory kinematics in speakers with cerebellar disease, *J Speech Hear Res* 34:768, 1991.

58. Nellis JL, Neiman GS, Lehman JA: Comparison of nasometer and listener judgments of nasality in the assessment of velopharyngeal function after pharyngeal flap surgery, *Cleft Palate Craniofac J* 29:157, 1992.

59. Olson DE, Goding GS, Michael DD: Acoustic and perceptual evaluation of laryngeal reinnervation by ansa cervicalis transfer, *Laryngoscope* 108:1767, 1998.

60. Rabinov C and others: Comparing reliability of perceptual ratings of roughness and acoustic measures of jitter, *J Speech Lang Hear Res* 38:26, 1995.

61. Rammage L, Morrison M, Nichol H: *Management of the voice and its disorders,* ed 2, San Diego, 2001, Singular Publishing Group.

62. Rosen CA, Murry T: Voice handicap index in singers, *J Voice* 14:370, 2000.

63. Rosen CA and others: Voice handicap index change following treatment of voice disorders, *J Voice* 14:619, 2000.

64. Rothenberg M: A new inverse-filtering technique for deriving the glottal waveform during voicing, *J Acoust Soc Am* 53:1632, 1973.

65. Roy N and others: Manual circumlaryngeal therapy for functional dysphonia: an evaluation of short- and long-term treatment outcomes, *J Voice* 11:321, 1997.

66. Roy N and others: An evaluation of the effects of two treatments for teachers with voice disorders: a prospective randomized clinical trial, *J Speech Lang Hear Res* 44:286, 2001.

67. Roy N, Leeper HA: Effects of the manual laryngeal musculoskeletal tension reduction technique as a treatment for functional voice disorders: perceptual and acoustic measures, *J Voice* 7:242, 1993.

68. Roy N and others: Three treatments for voice-disordered teachers: a randomized clinical trial, *J Speech Lang Hear Res* 46:670, 2003.

69. Roy N and others: Voice amplification versus vocal hygiene instruction for teachers with voice disorders: a treatment outcomes study, *J Speech Lang Hear Res* 45:625, 2002.

70. Smitheran JR, Hixon TJ: A clinical method for estimating laryngeal airway resistance during vowel production, *J Speech Hear Disord* 46:138, 1981.

71. Solomon NP, Garlitz SJ, Milbrath RL: Respiratory and laryngeal contributions to maximum phonation time, *J Voice* 14:331, 2000.

72. Solomon NP and others: Effects of a vocally fatiguing task and systemic hydration on men's voices, *J Voice* 17:31, 2003.

73. Solomon NP, Hixon TJ: Speech breathing in Parkinson's disease, *J Speech Hear Res* 36:294, 1993.

74. Spector BC and others: Quality-of-life assessment in patients with unilateral vocal cord paralysis, *Otolaryngol Head Neck Surg* 125:176, 2001.

75. Stemple JC, Glaze LE, Klaben BG: *Clinical voice pathology: theory and management,* ed 3, San Diego, 2000, Singular Publishing Group.

76. Stewart MG, Chen AY, Stach CB: Outcomes analysis of voice and quality of life in patients with laryngeal cancer, *Arch Otolaryngol Head Neck Surg* 124:143, 1998.

77. Stone RE J.: *Issues in clinical assessment of laryngeal function: contraindications for subscribing to maximum phonation time and optimum fundamental frequency.* In Bless DM, Abbs JH, editors: *Vocal fold physiology: contemporary research and clinical issues,* San Diego, 1983, College-Hill Press.

78. Subtelny JD, Worth JH, Sakuda M: Intraoral pressure and rate of flow during speech, *J Speech Hear Res* 9:498, 1966, as cited in Baken RJ, Orlikoff RF: *Clinical measurement of voice and speech,* ed 2, San Diego, 2000, Singular Publishing Group, p 315.

79. Sulter AM and others: A structured approach to voice range profile (phonetogram) analysis, *J Speech Hear Res* 37:1076, 1994.

80. Terasawa R, Hibi SR, Hirano M: Mean airflow rates during phonation over a comfortable duration and maximum sustained phonation, *Folia Phoniatr (Basel)* 39:87, 1987.

81. Titze IR: *Workshop on acoustic voice analysis: summary statement.* Iowa City, 1995, National Center for Voice and Speech.

82. Titze IR: *Principles of voice production,* Englewood Cliffs, 1994, Prentice-Hall, Inc.

83. Titze IR: Acoustic interpretation of the voice range profile (phonetogram), *J Speech Hear Res* 35:21, 1992.

84. Treole K Trudeau MD: Changes in sustained production tasks among women with bilateral vocal nodules before and after voice therapy, *J Voice* 11:462, 1997.

85. Trudeau MD, Forrest LA: The contributions of phonatory volume and transglottal airflow to the s/z ratio, *Am J Speech Lang Pathol* 6:65, 1997.

86. Verdolini K and others: Biological mechanisms underlying voice changes due to hydration, *J Speech Lang Hear Res* 45:268, 2002.

87. Verdolini K, Titze IR, Fennell A: Dependence of phonatory effort on hydration level, *J Speech Hear Res* 37:1001, 1994.

88. Verdolini-Marston K, Sandage M, Titze IR: Effect of hydration treatments on laryngeal nodules and polyps and related voice measures, *J Voice* 8:30, 1994.

89. Verdolini-Marston K, Titze IR, Druker DG: Changes in phonation threshold pressure with induced conditions of hydration, *J Voice* 8:30, 1994.

90. Wolfe V, Cornell R, Palmer C: Acoustic correlates of pathologic voice types, *J Speech Hear Res* 34:509, 1991.

91. Wolfe V, Fitch J, Cornell R: Acoustic prediction of severity in commonly occurring voice problems, *J Speech Lang Hear Res* 38:273, 1995.

92. Warren DW, Dalston RM, Dalston ET: Maintaining speech pressures in the presence of velopharyngeal impairment, *Cleft Palate J* 27:53, 1989.

93. Warren DW and others: The speech regulating system: temporal and aerodynamic responses to velopharyngeal inadequacy, *J Speech Hear Res* 32:566, 1989.

94. World Health Organization: *International classification of impairment, disability, and handicap.* Geneva, 1980, World Health Organization.

95. World Health Organization: *International classification of impairment, disability and handicap—beta-1: a manual of dimensions of disablement and participation,* Geneva, 1997, World Health Organization.

96. Yanagihara N, Koike Y: The regulation of sustained phonation, *Folia Phoniatr (Basel)* 19:1, 1967.

97. Yanagihara N, Koike Y, von Leden H: Phonation and respiration: function study in normal subjects, *Folia Phoniatr (Basel)* 18:323, 1966.

CHAPTER EIGHTY EIGHT

DIAGNOSTIC IMAGING OF THE LARYNX

II   Franz J. Wippold, II

INTRODUCTION

The opinions and assertions contained herein are the private views of the authors and are not to be construed as official or as reflecting the views of the Department of Defense.

The radiologist plays an important role in the evaluation of upper airway disorders in children and adults by providing unique and useful diagnostic information directly affecting the treatment of the patient.[99,149] In the past, evaluation of the airway included plain-film radiography, barium studies, and fluoroscopy. Now, computed tomography (CT) and magnetic resonance (MR) imaging have become the procedures of choice for defining mass lesions and traumatic abnormalities. These procedures can supplement the findings at laryngoscopy when additional diagnostic information is required to plan treatment.

NORMAL AIRWAY
Technique

Plain films remain an effective and inexpensive screening examination for acute airway obstruction. Except in rare circumstances, plain-film examination of the airway should include anteroposterior and lateral radiography of the pharynx and laryngotracheal air column. In cooperative patients, these films should be exposed during inspiration with the patient upright, because acute respiratory obstruction may be exacerbated in the recumbent position. Although conventional soft-tissue techniques are often adequate, a high-kilovoltage magnification technique with selective filtration better visualizes the airway with improved air/soft-tissue interfaces.[79,90,102] Xeroradiography has largely been abandoned in clinical practice.[35,131] When plain films are inconclusive, fluoroscopy and barium studies of the esophagus may be required for diagnosis. Abnormal vocal cord motion or swallowing mechanisms, vascular impressions, mass lesions, or nonopaque foreign bodies are best evaluated by these methods. Cross-sectional imaging may also be helpful in chronic airway disease.

Anatomy

Lateral radiography is excellent for identifying the tongue, adenoids, tonsils, epiglottis, aryepiglottic folds, pyriform sinuses, laryngeal ventricle, and subglottic trachea (Figure 88-1, A). The anteroposterior airway is superb for examining the glottic and subglottic areas (Figure 88-1, B). During quiet inspiration, the vocal cords are abducted, and the width of the upper airway almost equals that of the trachea. During phonation of the vowel "e," the vocal cords adduct, resulting in narrowing of the glottic area. However, narrowing of the subglottic area should be considered abnormal.

The airway may show considerable variability in children, unlike in adults. Therefore, knowledge of the normal airway anatomy is essential before attempting to recognize pathology. This requires that the patient be properly positioned for the study. Lateral airway radiography should be obtained as much as possible in full inspiration with the neck extended. If the study is performed during expiration or with forward flexion of the neck, the retropharyngeal soft tissue in children bulges anteriorly and may simulate a retropharyngeal mass (Figure 88-2).[13]

The size of the adenoids and tonsils in children and irregular cartilage ossification in adults can present significant problems in evaluation of the airway. In newborns and infants, the tonsils and adenoids are normally sparse; lymphoid tissue can be identified radiographically in all children at 6 months of age.[16] After age 6 months, the tonsils and adenoids vary considerably in size and may encroach on the nasopharynx or oropharynx, suggesting a pathologic soft-tissue mass. In most cases, these structures, even when large, are normal and are frequently noted as incidental findings on skull or spine radiography. Occasionally, however, they can be associated with airway obstruction (Figure 88-3).[44,94] The adenoids are largest at 7 to 10 years of age and then decline by the seventh decade.[168] In most instances, adenoidal size can be evaluated

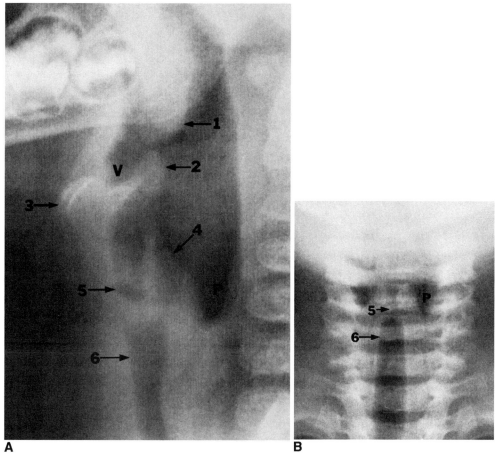

Figure 88-1. A and **B,** A healthy upper airway in a 20-month-old child. The following structures are well visualized: palatine tonsils *(1)*, epiglottis *(2)*, body of the hyoid bone *(3)*, aryepiglottic folds *(4)*, laryngeal ventricle *(5)*, subglottic airway *(6)*, vallecula *(V)*, and pyriform sinus *(P)*.

subjectively, but objective methods of assessing adenoidal size with an adenoidal/nasopharyngeal ratio have been described.[47,168] The final decision as to whether adenoid or tonsillar tissue is of symptomatic importance is clinical, not radiographic.

Cartilage of the neck may pose another problem, because in certain adults, normal thyroid and cricoid calcifications can be irregular and incomplete, thereby simulating a foreign body or neoplastic destruction.[121] These normal calcifications occasionally can be seen in older children, but as a rule, the only cartilage calcified routinely in the younger child is the hyoid bone. Any other radiopaque structure usually is abnormal.

Cross-sectional imaging also adequately shows the airway. Configuration of the airway on axial or transverse images varies, depending on the level of the image. At the level of the epiglottis and aryepiglottic folds, the airway is elliptical. Approaching the false cords, the airway narrows and assumes a teardrop shape. The airway becomes elliptical at the true

cords. The term *rima glottidis* refers to the airway at the level of the true vocal cords. The intermembranous portion of the rima glottidis (glottis vocalis) consists of the ventral 60% of the cords, and the dorsal intercartilaginous portion (glottis respiratoria) consists of the portion between the arytenoid cartilages.[101] Below the cricoid cartilage, the airway appears circular. The posterior membrane of the trachea may posteriorly flatten, and the normal esophagus occasionally indents the airway silhouette.[49] Nodular projections into the airway or asymmetric tracheal wall thickening should be viewed suspiciously as subglottic tumor involvement. Multirow detector CT imaging has recently allowed computer-generated three-dimensional (3D) visualization of the airway lumen and contiguous structures by reconstructing two-dimensional data. Named "virtual laryngoscopy," this technique offers noninvasive interactive evaluation of the tracheal lumen that correlates well with conventional rigid endoscopy (Figure 88-4).[45,61]

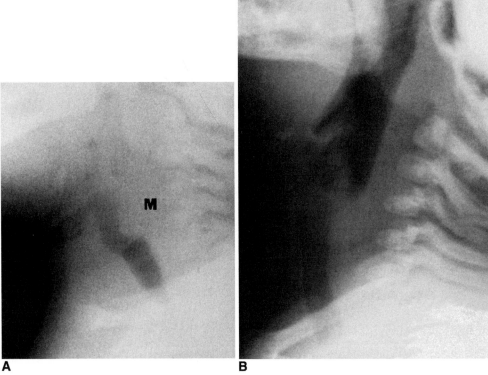

Figure 88-2. Pseudoretropharyngeal mass. **A,** A retropharyngeal mass *(M)* is suggested in this child, who was examined with the neck flexed and the airway only partially distended. **B,** Healthy retropharyngeal soft tissue is seen when the examination is repeated during inspiration with the neck extended.

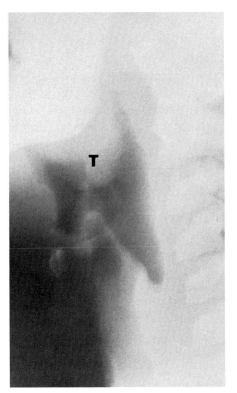

Figure 88-3. Tonsillitis. Lateral view shows enlarged palatine tonsils *(T).*

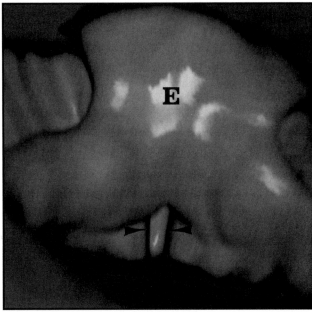

Figure 88-4. Volume-rendered three-dimensional image of the normal epiglottis *(E)* and normal vocal cords *(arrowheads)* derived from multirow detector spiral CT data. (Case courtesy of Dr. Elizabeth McFarland.) To view this image in color, please go to *www.ototext.com* or the Electronic Image Collection CD, bound into your copy of Cummings Otolaryngology—Head and Neck Surgery, 4th edition.

INFLAMMATORY DISEASE OF THE LARYNX
Epiglottitis

Epiglottitis is an inflammation of the epiglottis caused by the bacteria *Hemophilus influenzae.* The entire supraglottic airway may be involved, but the epiglottis and aryepiglottic folds are most extensively involved. These normally well-defined thin structures become edematous, enlarged, and unsharp, resulting in a rounded thumblike density in place of the epiglottis. The edema often encroaches on the vallecula and rarely may extend to the posterior pharyngeal wall. In addition, the hypopharynx and pyriform sinuses usually are mildly to moderately overdistended.[17,38,39,87] The remainder of the airway is fairly normal, although at least 25% of children with epiglottitis have subglottic narrowing.[138]

The changes in the epiglottitis are shown best on lateral radiography (Figure 88-5). Extensive manipulation of the patient should be avoided because of the possibility of inducing glottic spasm. Cross-sectional imaging is unnecessary.

Enlargement of the epiglottis may result from various other disorders, including irritation from a foreign body or burn, tumors such as epiglottic cysts or neoplasms (e.g., lymphoma), granulomatous disease (e.g., sarcoidosis, tuberculosis, Wegener's granulomatosis), and angioneurotic edema.[110,142] The radiographic findings should therefore be correlated with the patient's clinical history (Figure 88-6). On occasion, an omega epiglottis (a normal anatomic variant in children in

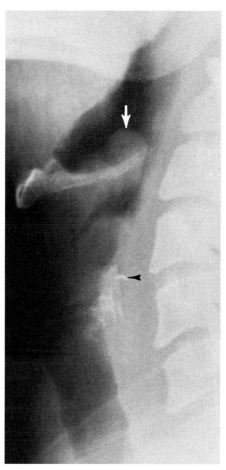

Figure 88-6. Sarcoidosis. Marked enlargement of the epiglottis *(arrow)* is present. *Arrowhead* points to normal calcification in the posterosuperior aspect of the cricoid cartilage.

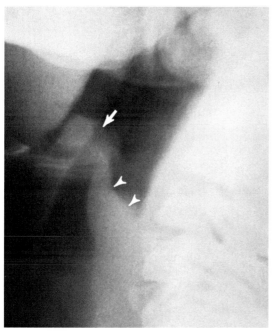

Figure 88-5. Epiglottitis. Marked thickening of the epiglottis *(arrow)* and aryepiglottic folds *(arrowheads)* is seen. Mild hypopharyngeal overdistention is also present.

which the epiglottis is floppy, vertically positioned, and resembles the capital Greek letter "omega") may be misdiagnosed as epiglottitis.[154] An important distinguishing feature is the absence of thickened aryepiglottic folds or other edematous changes.

Croup

Croup is an inflammation of the subglottic larynx usually caused by parainfluenza virus type 1. It typically occurs in young children. Radiographic studies are not indicated or obtained routinely in patients with croup, but are useful in confusing cases, primarily to exclude other causes of stridor. The radiographic changes are the result of inflammatory edema affecting the larynx and subglottic tissue. Radiographically, the frontal view is most helpful in the diagnosis (Figure 88-7). Symmetric subglottic airway narrowing or "pencilling" of the airway is the major radiographic finding.[17,38,39,87] In contrast to congenital subglottic stenosis, narrowing of the subglottic portion of the trachea is not fixed and may improve on expiration.[155] The lateral view of the neck seems less helpful,

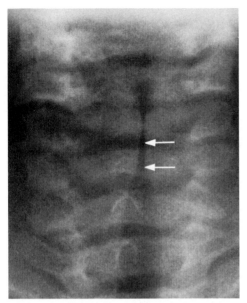

Figure 88-7. Croup. Frontal view shows typical funnel-shaped subglottic narrowing *(arrows)*.

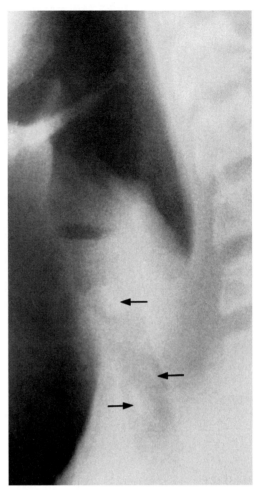

Figure 88-8. Membranous croup. Multiple irregular membranes *(arrows)* are present in the subglottic airway.

although the narrowing may be noted. This projection shows hypopharyngeal airway distention, but more importantly, it establishes that the epiglottis and aryepiglottic folds are normal.

Membranous or bacterial croup and viral croup may present with similar symptoms; however, membranous croup is characterized by diffuse inflammation of the larynx, trachea, and bronchi with adherent exudate and mucus on the surface of the upper tracheal mucosa.[66] Radiography shows subglottic narrowing and multiple tracheal soft-tissue excrescences (Figure 88-8). These intraluminal lesions can be mistaken for foreign bodies, so clinical correlation is required for diagnosis.

Retropharyngeal Abscess

The retropharyngeal space lies posterior to the larynx between the middle and deep layers of the deep cervical fascia. It extends from the base of the skull to the mediastinum and frequently serves as a conduit for spread of disease from the neck into the chest.[28,29] Retropharyngeal abscess results from suppuration of retropharyngeal lymph nodes in patients with upper respiratory tract infection or from perforation of the pharynx or upper esophagus by a foreign body. If the abscess compresses the larynx and upper trachea, symptoms of upper airway obstruction develop.

Lateral soft-tissue radiography of the neck will show fixed thickening of the retropharyngeal soft tissues, anterior displacement of the airway, reversal of normal cervical lordosis, and occasionally gas bubbles within the abscess (Figure 88-9).[17,39,155] The retropha-

ryngeal space should not exceed 7 mm as measured from the most anterior aspect of C2 to the posterior pharyngeal wall. At C6, the thickness of the retropharyngeal tissues should not be >14 mm in children and 22 mm in adults.[62] Fluoroscopy or barium esophagraphy may be necessary to confirm that the radiographic changes did not occur with expiration or with the head in a flexed position.

CT and MR imaging superbly evaluate the retropharyngeal space. Suppurative adenopathy is usually limited to the suprahyoid region of this space and spares the midline. As infection becomes extranodal, the entire width of the retropharyngeal space frequently becomes thickened. Inflammation can then easily track into the infrahyoid region. The full extent of the process can be imaged by CT or MR imaging before therapy.[28] Abscess will appear hypodense on CT, hypointense on T1-weighted, and hyperintense on T2-weighted MR images, reflecting the presence of liquefaction (Figure 88-10). Ring enhancement may

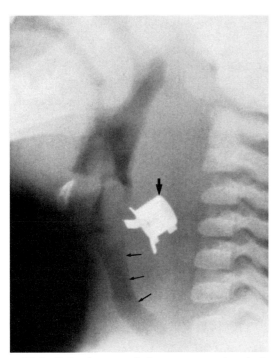

Figure 88-9. Retropharyngeal abscess secondary to foreign body perforation of the esophagus. The prevertebral soft tissues are markedly swollen, and the trachea is displaced anteriorly *(small arrows)*. *Large arrow* points to a metallic foreign body.

be seen after administration of intravenous contrast. Differentiation between retropharyngeal abscess and adenitis is difficult on CT, because both processes cause hypodense regions within the inflammatory mass. Some authors advocate the use of ultrasound in this evaluation.[56] If air bubbles or a foreign body are present within the mass, the diagnosis of a retropharyngeal abscess is more likely.

Thickening of the retropharyngeal soft tissues also can occur secondary to bleeding and edema from cervical spine trauma, lymphadenopathy (e.g., lymphoma, tuberculosis), or retropharyngeal tumors (e.g., cystic hygroma, neuroblastoma, hemangioma, retropharyngeal goiter, cancer).[68,109,155,170] The imaging findings should therefore be correlated with the clinical history.

LARYNGOMALACIA

Laryngomalacia or congenital flaccid larynx is one of the most common causes of inspiratory stridor in the neonate and infant.[39] Laryngoscopy shows flaccidity of the epiglottis, aryepiglottic folds, or the entire larynx, which collapses during inspiration. The corresponding radiographic findings are best shown with fluoroscopy. Hypopharyngeal overdistention with associated collapse of the aryepiglottic folds and epiglottis is observed on inspiration. Paradoxic narrowing of the subglottic portion of the airway may also

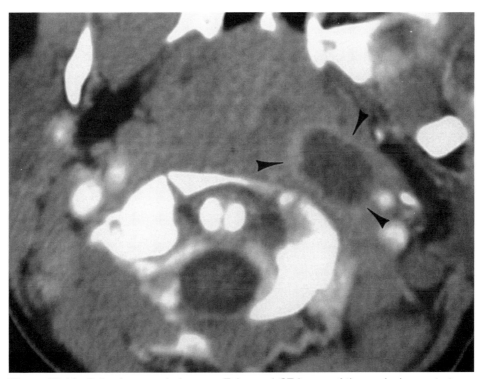

Figure 88-10. Retropharyngeal abscess. Enhanced CT image of the neck demonstrates a fluid collection in the left retropharyngeal space *(arrowheads)*.

be seen as the patient inspires. The primary reasons for laryngoscopy and radiography are to exclude other causes of congenital stridor (e.g., cysts, webs, tumors, stenoses). In most children, the symptoms disappear by 1 year of age.

VOCAL CORD PARALYSIS

Paralysis of the vocal cord may be caused by any process involving the vagus nerve or its recurrent laryngeal branch between the jugular foramen and its entrance into the larynx. Almost 75% of patients have unilateral paralysis.[158] Almost 90% of paralyses are caused by lesions that compress the nerve along peripherally located segments, and only 10% originate in the central nervous system or before the nerve exits the jugular foramen; central paralyses are accompanied by other cranial neuropathies.[1] The peripheral location of most lesions reflects the long and redundant routes of the recurrent laryngeal nerves. Specific causes include neoplasm (36%); post-

operative complications, such as from parathyroid and thyroid surgery (25%); and inflammation (13%). Some cases are idiopathic.[158] Congenital central nervous system anomalies are often associated with childhood vocal cord paralysis.[12] Although laryngeal cancers can paralyze the cord, direct infiltration of the recurrent or superior laryngeal nerves by local tumor is rare.[112]

Although plain-film radiography, fluoroscopy, and CT can evaluate vocal cord mobility, abnormal vocal cord motion is generally diagnosed by laryngoscopy (Figure 88-11).[50,172] However, in patients with vocal cord paralysis secondary to neoplasm, imaging helps show the extent of neoplasm and its relationship to the adjacent cartilaginous structures.[77,107] Radiologic evaluation of the isolated paralyzed cord should entail imaging of the entire vagus nerve from the skull base to the pulmonary hila. CT is excellent for evaluating the neck and chest; MR imaging is superior for the skull base (Figure 88-12).[58,78,158] Imaging signs of cord

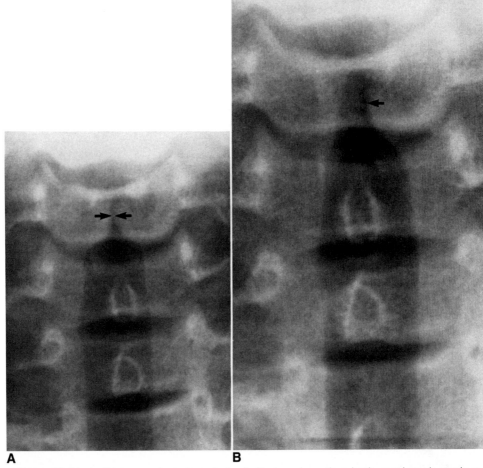

A   **B**

Figure 88-11. Left true vocal cord paralysis. **A,** During phonation, both vocal cords are in a paramedian location *(arrows)*. **B,** During inspiration, the left true vocal cord remains in a paramedian position *(arrow)*, whereas there is abduction of the normal right true vocal cord.

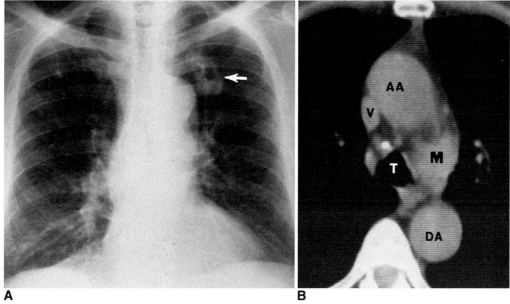

Figure 88-12. Left true vocal cord paralysis secondary to squamous cell carcinoma. **A,** Chest radiography shows an irregular cavitary mass *(arrow)* in the left upper lobe. **B,** Computed tomography shows a 3-cm mass *(M)* in the aortopulmonary window flattening the left side of the trachea *(T)*. The ascending aorta *(AA)*, descending aorta *(DA)*, and superior vena cava *(V)* are also seen. (From Glazer HS et al: Extralaryngeal causes of vocal cord paralysis: CT evaluation, *Am J Roentgenol* 141:529, F3A, B 1983.)

paralysis include paramedian position of the cords, displaced arytenoid cartilage, ipsilateral dilation of the pyriform sinus, tilting of the thyroid cartilage, and prominent laryngeal ventricle.[1]

BENIGN LARYNGEAL MASSES

Benign neoplasms can cause respiratory obstruction. Symptoms and radiographic features depend on tumor distribution and extent. Although good quality films of the larynx and upper trachea supplemented by a high-kilovoltage magnification technique are usually adequate in showing the intraluminal lesion, CT has largely replaced plain film evaluation because of its widespread availability and superior information.

Although rare in adults, subglottic hemangioma is the most common laryngeal and upper tracheal neoplasm in the newborn and infant. The lesion typically appears as a well-defined mass in the posterior or lateral portion of the subglottic airway (Figure 88-13).[142,153] The subglottic narrowing is usually eccentric; however, circumferential narrowing suggestive of croup may also be seen. Additional hemangiomas may occur on the skin or elsewhere in the body.

Squamous papillomas, the most frequent laryngeal tumors in children, have also been reported in adults.[43,63] The imaging appearance of papillomatosis is contingent on the size and location of the lesions. Generally, single or multiple intraluminal soft-tissue nodules are seen in the glottis or in the tracheal air column (Figure 88-14). Because papillomas may extend to the bronchial tree or pulmonary parenchyma, chest CT is extremely important in defining the extent of disease. Localized areas of atelectasis, air trapping, or pneumonia have been reported. Papillomas also may appear as well-defined discrete pulmonary nodules that eventually cavitate, forming multiple thin-walled cystic lesions.[85,143]

A laryngocele is an abnormal elongation and expansion of the saccule of the laryngeal ventricle and represents >20% of submucosal lesions of the larynx.[73,135] Almost 25% are bilateral.[167] Although laryngoceles usually are asymptomatic, large lesions may be associated with airway obstruction and vocal cord paralysis.[65] Laryngoceles within the paraglottic space and confined by the thyroid lamina are termed *internal*. These lesions may present on laryngoscopy as soft, localized bulges of the aryepiglottic fold and may be mistaken clinically for submucosal neoplasms.[57,145,163] Lesions that pierce the thyrohyoid membrane to present in the lateral neck are termed *external*. Most cases are a combination of external and internal lesions and are referred to as *mixed*. Regardless of position, laryngoceles usually are visualized as sharply defined air-containing structures on imaging (Figure 88-15).[96] A modified Valsalva's maneuver occasionally improves visualization of these lesions. Laryngeal mucocele is a fluid-filled laryngocele caused by obstruction of the

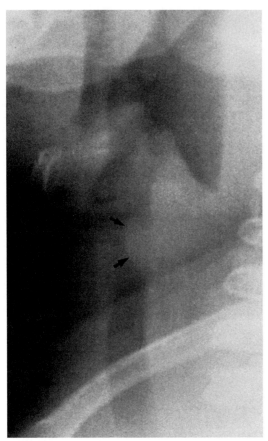

Figure 88-13. Subglottic hemangioma. Lateral view shows a soft-tissue mass *(arrows)* in the posterior portion of the subglottic airway.

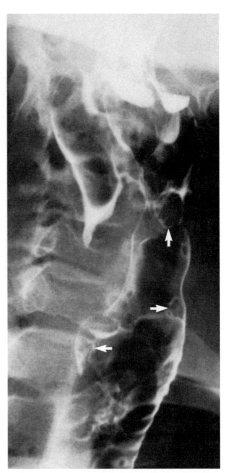

Figure 88-14. Laryngotracheal papillomatosis. Oblique view from a bronchogram shows multiple nodules *(arrows)* of varying sizes in the glottic and subglottic airway.

ostium of laryngeal saccule and may appear as a soft-tissue mass. These lesions are overwhelmingly benign; however, up to 15% may be associated with a small ventricular cancer.[64,145,160] Rarely, cystic lesions, such as cystadenomas, can mimic a laryngeal mucocele.[46]

CT can be helpful in showing fluid-containing and air-containing laryngoceles (Figures 88-16 and 88-17).[57] If the mass is of soft-tissue density because it contains either mucoid or purulent material, the distinction from neoplasm may be more difficult. However, its location and smooth surface in conjunction with a healthy mucosa on laryngoscopy should suggest a laryngocele. CT may also help show the external component of a laryngocele that is not apparent on physical examination. An enhancing wall usually indicates infection. The endolaryngeal origin of this lesion differentiates it from a lateral thyroglossal duct cyst.[145]

Congenital cysts of the larynx are rare causes of respiratory obstruction in infants. They most commonly arise in the region of the epiglottis or aryepiglottic fold. Plain-film examination of the airway will disclose a soft-tissue mass of varying size encroaching on and displacing the healthy airway.

LARYNGEAL CARCINOMA

Nearly all mucosal tumors are diagnosed by direct inspection and biopsy; imaging provides crucial information about involvement of deep structures, such as the paraglottic space, cartilage, and lymph nodes. CT is a proven imaging technique for evaluating patients with laryngeal carcinoma.[4,103,133,137,150] In most patients, CT shows more extensive disease than is initially appreciated by laryngoscopy. The cross-sectional imaging provided by CT allows evaluation of the intrinsic and deep soft tissues of the larynx and the cartilaginous skeleton.

MR imaging provides anatomic information on the neck that compares favorably with CT[74]; however, its superiority to CT has not been conclusively established.[26,100,162] Advantages of MR imaging include its excellent soft-tissue contrast, which is superior to CT. Multiplanar display enables coronal, transverse, and sagittal anatomic formatting, whereas CT is usually limited to the transverse plane. Newer multirow detector CT scanners allow for multiplanar reconstructions;

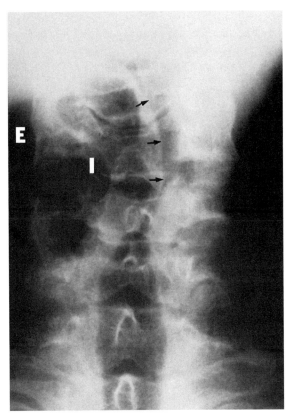

Figure 88-15. Mixed laryngocele. Frontal view shows the large internal *(I)* and external *(E)* components of the laryngocele with compression of the supraglottic airway *(arrows)*.

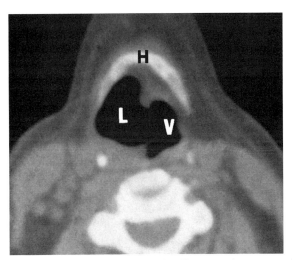

Figure 88-16. Internal laryngocele. Computed tomography shows the air-filled laryngocele *(L)* filling the right paraglottic space and compressing the laryngeal vestibule *(V)*. The hyoid bone *(H)* is also seen.

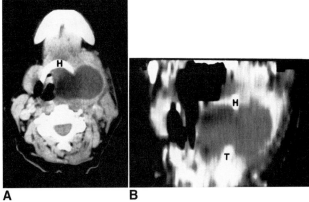

A   **B**

Figure 88-17. Bilateral mixed laryngoceles. **A,** Computed tomography (CT) shows a fluid-filled dumbbell-shaped cyst with intralaryngeal and extralaryngeal components on the left. Smaller air-filled laryngocele is seen on the right. **B,** Reformatted coronal CT shows both laryngoceles herniating through the thyrohyoid membrane. The hyoid bone *(H)* and thyroid cartilage *(T)* are also seen.

however, these views are derived from data obtained in the transverse plane. MR imaging uses no ionizing radiation and is not plagued by artifacts caused by beam hardening, dental amalgam, or poor beam pen-

etration of the shoulders. MR imaging does have limitations, however. It is slower than CT, and therefore motion artifacts from breathing, carotid artery pulsations, and swallowing may degrade images.[21,75,173] This should be considered when choosing a modality in patients with laryngeal cancer, who are often elderly and may have other medical debilities (e.g., chronic obstructive pulmonary disease).[75] MR imaging does not image cortical bone or calcifications well. Furthermore, MR imaging is contraindicated in patients with cardiac pacemakers, metallic cochlear implants, and cerebral aneurysm clips.[40,81,84,127]

The decision for selecting radiotherapy, conservation surgery, or total laryngectomy depends on an accurate delineation of tumor extent.[93,126] CT and MR imaging are excellent noninvasive methods capable of 3D anatomic display of portions of the larynx that are not well examined by laryngoscopy. Submucosal extension of tumor and cartilaginous destruction that are not suspected clinically can be assessed. Because imaging modalities have different strengths and weaknesses, the choice of CT or MR imaging should be tailored to the patient. Furthermore, imaging is not a substitute for, but is complementary to, laryngoscopy. Although imaging may show advanced mucosal abnormalities, minor mucosal abnormalities and abnormalities of intrinsic motion are best studied by laryngoscopy.[104]

Neoplasm is identifiable on CT as an area of increased soft-tissue density that alters the normal symmetric laryngeal anatomy. Similarly, the hallmark of an abnormal larynx on MR imaging is asymmetry. The superb soft-tissue contrast provides additional information. On T1-weighted images, fat signal is hyperintense and differs significantly from the mucosa and muscles in appearance. Signals from lymph nodes and infiltrating tumor, which are less intense than fat, are well visualized on T1-weighted images. On T2-weighted images, muscle signal is less intense than mucosa, fat, and many tumors. Carcinomas within the mucosa and muscles can be well delineated.[31] Neither CT nor MR imaging findings are histologically specific, and similar appearances can be produced with hemorrhage, edema, inflammation, or fibrosis. Therefore, examination should be correlated with the clinical history and should be performed before laryngeal biopsy or at least 48 hours after biopsy to avoid confusion with postbiopsy edema and hemorrhage.

Technique

Spiral (helical) CT is rapidly replacing conventional dynamic CT (slice-by-slice acquisition) in most medical centers.[80] Spiral CT permits rapid scanning of large volumes of tissues during quiet respiration.[152] Spiral images are less susceptible to patient motion than conventional CT, although image noise is slightly increased.[113,151] Thin sections can provide information about specific regions, such as the anterior commissure.[141] Moreover, volumetric spiral data permit multiplanar and 3D reconstructions.[67,151,179] The amount of intravenous contrast may be reduced compared with dynamic CT.[148] Iodinated contrast is administered intravenously to distinguish nonenhancing lymph nodes from enhancing vessels. Images are obtained during slow inspiration. If the images are performed during suspended inspiration, adduction of the true vocal cords may cause the airway to appear falsely narrowed. Scans occasionally are obtained during phonation or during modified Valsalva's maneuver to distend the pyriform sinuses and improve visualization of the aryepiglottic folds.

Three-dimensional CT is currently being used for radiotherapy planning. Slices are obtained in the conventional axial orientation. By use of special computer software, selected anatomic structures are then traced and reformatted into a 3D wire diagram depicting the tumor and key adjacent tissues that can then be manipulated to reveal the optimal radiation port. This technique limits extraneous collateral radiation to other organs, such as the salivary glands.[41,42] CT is also useful for guiding percutaneous biopsies.[51,52,119,176]

MR techniques may vary depending on scanner type and available hardware and software. Surface coils are essential to adequately image the larynx.[77,98] Sagittal, transverse, and coronal T1-weighted images best display anatomic relationships. T1-weighted and T2-weighted transverse images further define the signal characteristics of the tissues. Sections are usually 3 to 5 mm thick. Gradient moment nulling, flow compensation, cardiac gating, and presaturation pulses minimize motion artifacts.[75] The fast spin-echo T2-weighted technique has replaced the conventional spin-echo technique and offers relatively short acquisition times.[48,95,175,181]

Gadolinium-enhanced images improve delineation of margins in many lesions,[69,76,130,134,166] although lesions embedded in fat may be obscured.[7,181] Another potential pitfall is that healthy aerodigestive mucosa enhances, therefore possibly obscuring small mucosal tumor volumes.[167] Fat-suppression techniques improve conspicuity of soft-tissue lesions embedded in fat by selectively diminishing the hyperintensity of fat on T1-weighted images.[7,159] Gadolinium-enhanced, fat-suppressed T1-weighted images are especially useful in staging nodal disease.[132] Agents are typically well tolerated.[76,182] The use of double and triple doses of contrast, sometimes valuable in intracranial disease, has little value in neck imaging.[165]

Fat suppression may produce several annoying artifacts, however, such as signal loss at bone–air interfaces, in homogenous suppression at the base of skull compared with the infrahyoid regions, and frank failure of suppression at fat–air interfaces producing aberrant hyperintense signal.[2] Moreover, some techniques may be misleading, because nonfatty tissue with T1 values similar to fat (e.g., proteinaceous fluid, methemoglobin, intensely enhancing soft tissue) may also be suppressed.[86]

MR techniques and applications, such as magnetization transfer, improve the contrast between lesions and background tissue.[6,54,122,174,177] Reconstruction algorithms permit simultaneous 3D depiction of the tumor volume embedded within the surrounding soft tissues. This display facilitates the transformation of two-dimensional information into a 3D format and allows the examiner to "dissect" the display to a desired tissue depth.[97,164]

Open bore units are being used to guide biopsies.[91,111] These units are useful for the claustrophobic patient, who would otherwise be unable to tolerate the confining space of conventional magnets. Unfortunately, many of these scanners lack sufficient magnet strength to optimally display difficult or complex anatomic relationships.

Special applications, such as MR spectroscopy, have been evaluated for certain head and neck tumors.[19] MR spectroscopy measures and graphically displays tissue metabolites.[88] Choline (Cho), a precursor to phosphatidylcholine, is involved in membrane turnover. An elevation of the Cho spectral peak within tissue implies cellular turnover and may serve as a potential tumor marker.[117,118] MR spectroscopy may prove useful by using metabolic data to map tumors and complement anatomic data from conventional imaging.[114] Although MR spectroscopy has advanced rapidly on the intracranial application front, initial enthusiasm for head and neck lesions has dampened. Formidable technical issues such as artifacts from paranasal sinuses, airway, neck fat, and blood vessels have made consistently reliable spectra difficult. Therefore, widespread use in the head and neck awaits significant refinement.

Combined positron emission tomography (PET) CT is a new technique in which near simultaneously acquired PET and CT information is superimposed. This image fusion has the advantage of comparing superior sensitive functional PET data with the superior anatomic data offered by CT (Figure 88-18). Promising applications include evaluation of posttherapy patients for evidence of recurrent tumor, analysis of ambiguous lymph nodes and soft-tissue masses, and verification of biopsy sites (Broadbent LP and others: Combined PET/CT imaging for targeting fine needle aspirations to diagnose recurrent head and neck cancer, Personal communication, 2004).

Normal Anatomy

Accurate interpretation of scans of the larynx necessitates understanding of normal laryngeal anatomy as depicted on CT or MR images (Figures 88-19 through 88-26).[8] Some degree of normally occurring asymmetry should be recognized in patients with suspected laryngeal abnormalities to avoid misinterpretation of scans.

The laryngeal skeleton consists of the epiglottic, thyroid, arytenoid, and cricoid cartilages. The hyoid bone is considered part of the lingual apparatus, but relationships with the larynx are important. The unique appearance of the hyoid bone and laryngeal cartilages allows for easy orientation on CT. The degree of cartilaginous mineralization varies considerably. In particular, calcification of the thyroid cartilage may be irregular and incomplete, simulating neoplastic invasion. The calcified or ossified portions of the laryngeal skeleton are hypointense on MR scans and may be more difficult to identify than on CT. Noncalcified cartilage, such as the epiglottis, is intermediate in signal intensity. Fat within medullary spaces is hyperintense on T1-weighted sequences.

The intrinsic soft-tissue structures of the larynx include the aryepiglottic folds, true vocal cords, and false vocal cords. The aryepiglottic folds, which form the medial walls of the pyriform sinuses, extend obliquely from the top of the epiglottis toward the false cords inferiorly (see Figures 88-19 and 88-20). Although the aryepiglottic folds may be asymmetric during inspiration, distention of the pyriform sinuses during modified Valsalva's maneuver or phonation results in a more symmetric appearance.

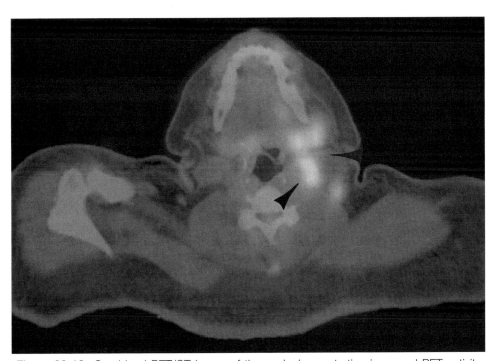

Figure 88-18. Combined PET/CT image of the neck demonstrating increased PET activity *(arrowheads)* superimposed on the corresponding CT image. The increased PET activity indicates hypermetabolic tumor. The CT image allows accurate anatomic localization of this tumor. To view this image in color, please go to *www.ototext.com* or the Electronic Image Collection CD, bound into your copy of Cummings Otolaryngology—Head and Neck Surgery, 4th edition.

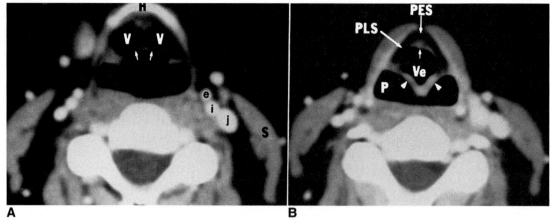

Figure 88-19. Normal anatomy on computed tomography showing supraglottic larynx after intravenous contrast injection. **A,** The two air-filled valleculae *(V)* separated by the median glossoepiglottic fold are seen anterior to the epiglottis *(arrows)*. The jugular vein *(j)*, internal carotid artery *(i)*, external carotid artery *(e)*, sternocleidomastoid muscle *(s)*, and hyoid bone *(H)* are also seen. **B,** Eight millimeters inferiorly, a fat-containing preepiglottic space *(PES)* anteriorly contrasts with the soft-tissue density of the epiglottis *(arrow)*. The fat in the preepiglottic space extends posterolaterally into the paralaryngeal (paraglottic) space *(PLS)*. The aryepiglottic folds *(arrowheads)* separate the air-containing pyriform sinuses *(P)* and the laryngeal vestibule *(Ve)*.

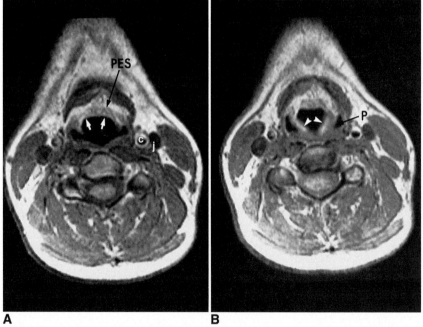

Figure 88-20. Normal anatomy of the supraglottic larynx on magnetic resonance imaging. **A,** A fat-filled preepiglottic space *(PES)* is anterior to the epiglottis *(arrows)*. The internal carotid artery *(c)* and internal jugular vein *(j)* are also seen. Fat on this sequence is higher in signal intensity than the epiglottis or muscle. **B,** Five millimeters inferiorly, the pyriform sinuses *(P)* are lateral to the aryepiglottic folds *(arrowheads)*.

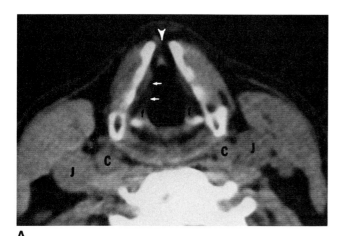

A

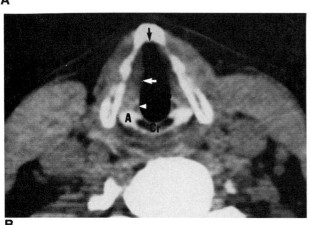

B

Figure 88-21. Normal anatomy of the false and true vocal cords on computed tomography. **A,** The false vocal cords *(arrows)*, medial to the fat-containing paraglottic space, lie at the level of the foot processes *(f)* of the arytenoid cartilages. The superior thyroid notch *(arrowhead)* is noted anteriorly between the thyroid laminae. The thyroid cartilage is incompletely calcified, which is a normal variation that should not be mistaken for cartilage destruction. The jugular vein *(J)* and carotid artery *(C)* are also seen. **B,** Four millimeters inferiorly, the true vocal cords *(white arrow)* are seen at the level of the vocal processes *(arrowhead)* of the arytenoid cartilages *(A)*, located superolateral to the upper posterior border of the cricoid cartilage *(Cr)*. Thyroid lamina join anteriorly to form the laryngeal prominence. The soft tissues at the anterior commissure *(black arrow)* are normally less than 2 mm in thickness.

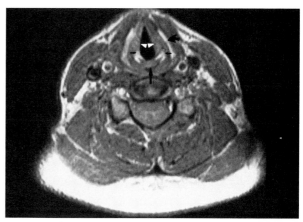

Figure 88-22. Normal anatomy of the true vocal cords on magnetic resonance imaging. The true cords *(arrowheads)* are soft-tissue intensity. The arytenoids *(small arrows)* and thyroid lamina *(curved arrow)* are seen as high-signal intensity on this sequence because of fatty marrow. The superior portion of the cricoid is also shown *(arrow)*.

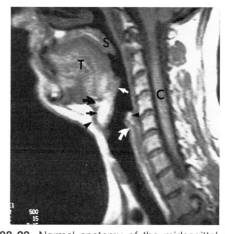

Figure 88-23. Normal anatomy of the midsagittal plane on magnetic resonance imaging. Epiglottis *(white arrow)*, fat-containing preepiglottic space *(black arrow)*, extrinsic strap muscles *(black arrowhead)*, arytenoid cartilages and muscles *(small black arrowhead)*, hyoid bone *(curved black arrow)*, and cricoid cartilage *(curved white arrow)* are shown. The soft palate *(S)*, tongue *(T)*, and spinal cord *(C)* are also seen.

The pyriform sinuses are bilateral air-containing structures bulging into the laterally positioned paraglottic spaces (see Figures 88-19 and 88-20). They are partially collapsed during quiet breathing but distend during modified Valsalva's maneuver or phonation. The pyriform sinuses are frequently asymmetric on scans, both in their size and their caudal extent.

The true vocal cords are visualized in an abducted position during slow inspiration (see Figures 88-21 and 88-22). They are triangular in shape and wider posteriorly, measuring about 9 mm in thickness. The posterior commissure is located in this area between the vocal processes of the arytenoids. Anteriorly at the anterior commissure, where the true vocal cords meet and attach to the thyroid cartilage, the thickness tapers to 1 mm. Only minimal soft-tissue thickening (1–2 mm or less) should be seen in the anterior or posterior commissure. If the cords are adducted, the soft tissues in the anterior and posterior commissures may appear falsely thickened. The rapid scanning times with spiral CT permit study of vocal cord motion and verification of questionable abnormalities detected with dynamic CT.

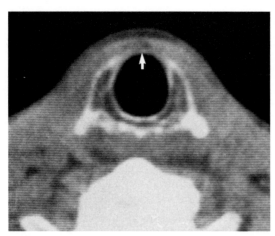

Figure 88-24. Normal anatomy of the subglottic level on computed tomography. The cricoid ring is almost complete, except in the area of the cricothyroid membrane anteriorly *(arrow)*. Note that the circular subglottic airway is in close apposition to the cricoid cartilage.

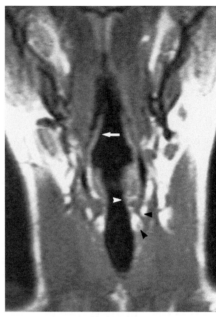

Figure 88-26. Normal anatomy of the coronal plane on magnetic resonance imaging. Cricoid cartilage *(large black arrowhead)*, thyroid cartilage *(small black arrowhead)*, true cords *(white arrowhead)*, and aryepiglottic folds *(white arrow)* are shown.

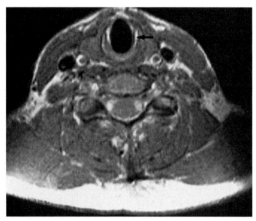

Figure 88-25. Normal anatomy of the subglottic level on magnetic resonance imaging. Fat-containing cricoid surrounds the airway *(arrow)*.

The false vocal cords appear as a thicker band of soft tissue at the level where the foot processes of the arytenoids are present (see Figure 88-21). In contrast to the region of the anterior commissure and true vocal cords, normally appreciable soft-tissue thickening occurs anteriorly behind the thyroid lamina, in part because of insertion of the thyroepiglottic ligament. The laryngeal ventricle separating the true and false vocal cords is visualized only in 10% of patients scanned in the axial plane because of partial volume averaging. On MR imaging, the ventricle is best identified in the coronal plane. The use of a reverse "e" maneuver may improve visualization of the laryngeal ventricle.

The soft tissue (preepiglottic and paraglottic spaces) deep to the endolarynx is well visualized on CT, because it is composed primarily of fat. Consequently, it is more hypodense than the true vocal cords or neoplasm (see Figure 88-19). On MR imaging, these spaces display relative hyperintensity on T1-weighted images, reflecting the fat composition. Sagittal MR images are especially useful in evaluating the preepiglottic space (see Figures 88-20 and 88-23).[55,89]

The laryngeal airway has different shapes at different levels. The laryngeal vestibule or supraglottic portion of the airway is elliptic with a long lateral axis. The anteroposterior dimension of the airway increases at the level of the true vocal cords. The subglottic region has a circular configuration with a flat posterior border at the level of the trachea. The cricoid ring indicates the level of the subglottic space. In this area, soft tissue should not be detectable on CT or MR scans between the inner surface of the cricoid cartilage and the airway (see Figures 88-24 through 88-26).

The jugular veins and carotid arteries can be clearly visualized posterolateral to the thyroid laminae. The right jugular vein, which is usually larger than the left, may be confused with lymphadenopathy on imaging and physical examination. In such cases, CT performed after administration of intravenous contrast improves identification of the normal vascular structures. Rapidly flowing blood within the jugular vein and carotid arteries is devoid of signal on MRI and therefore can be easily separated from soft-tissue structures.

Glottic Tumors

Carcinomas confined to a normally mobile true vocal cord may be treated with radiotherapy, laser, cordectomy, or partial laryngectomy.[104,126] In these cases, imaging may be normal or show nonspecific focal or diffuse vocal cord thickening (Figure 88-27). If the true cord is fixed in the midline, imaging shows deep infiltration of tumor before surgery.[107] CT cannot distinguish whether the cord is paramedian in position because of paralysis or direct involvement with tumor. MR imaging is helpful in this determination because of its superior soft-tissue contrast. Nevertheless, signal characteristics are often nonspecific. CT occasionally shows that vocal cord fixation or a laryngeal mass is secondary to prior occult trauma and that the laryngeal neoplasm is less extensive than suspected clinically.

Glottic tumors spread anteriorly, posteriorly, inferiorly, or laterally into the paraglottic space. The primary role of imaging true vocal cord neoplasms is evaluation of the anterior and posterior commissures, the paraglottic and subglottic spaces, and the thyroid and cricoid cartilages. CT and MR imaging reliably show tumor involvement at these sites. If involvement is >30% of the contralateral true vocal cord, thyroid cartilage invasion is evident, or subglottic extension of tumor is demonstrated, partial laryngectomy is generally contraindicated.[104,126]

Tumors can extend anteriorly to the anterior commissure and posteriorly to the arytenoid cartilage, posterior commissure, and cricoarytenoid joint (Figure 88-28). Identification of air abutting the thyroid carti-

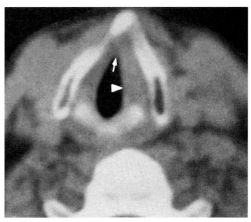

Figure 88-28. True vocal cord carcinoma with involvement of anterior commissure on computed tomography. Tumor of the left true vocal cord *(arrowhead)* extends anteriorly to involve the anterior commissure *(arrow)*.

lage at the anterior commissure on transverse images indicates tumor absence in this area. If soft-tissue thickening of the anterior commissure is >1 mm on imaging, tumor invasion is implied.[18,67,100] Tumor that has reached the anterior commissure can grow into the thyroid cartilage, preepiglottic space, opposite vocal cord, or subglottic space.[82] Care should be taken to avoid misdiagnosis of anterior tumor spread caused by various cord configurations that occur in different phases of respiration. Tumor that has reached the posterior commissure results in soft-tissue thickening over the arytenoid cartilages; rotation or displacement of the arytenoid cartilages may also occur.

Subglottic tumor is diagnosed on imaging by determining the relationship of the tumor mass to the level of the true cords (Figure 88-29). Exophytic tumor will distort the tracheal air column (Figure 88-30). If the extent of tumor caudad from the inferior margin of true vocal cords is >1 cm anteriorly and 6 mm posteriorly, total laryngectomy may be indicated.[82,126] However, the relationship between the subglottic tumor and the cricoid cartilage is more important than a standard measurement, because the cricoid cartilage supports the larynx. On CT and MR scans, no measurable soft-tissue thickness should be observed between the cricoid cartilage and the airway. MR imaging also can image the coronal plane, which allows tracing of tumor extension below the level of the conus elasticus.[26]

Imaging also shows spread of laryngeal carcinoma into the paraglottic space. Although a thin line of fat density may be seen medial to the thyroid cartilage at the level of the true vocal cords, the paraglottic space is wider in the area of the false vocal cord.[139] Therefore, extension into the paraglottic area is easier

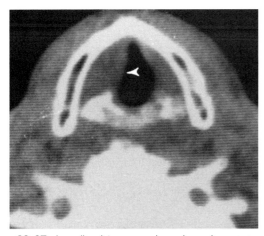

Figure 88-27. Localized true vocal cord carcinoma on computed tomography. A neoplasm diffusely thickens the right true vocal cord *(arrowhead)*. CT more interiorly showed no subglottic extension.

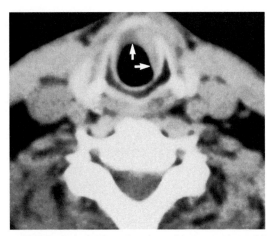

Figure 88-29. Subglottic extension of true vocal cord tumor on computed tomography. Soft-tissue thickening *(arrows)* is seen between the subglottic airway and the left anterior cricoid ring. (From Sagel SS: *Larynx.* In Lee JKT, Sagel SS, Stanley RJ (eds): *Computed Body Tomography,* New York, Raven Press, p48, F25, 1983.)

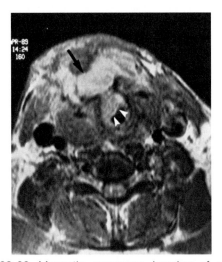

Figure 88-30. Magnetic resonance imaging of subglottic extension of carcinoma shows high signal in an extensive neck mass *(arrow)*. Subglottic extension *(arrowhead)* impresses the tracheal air column.

to show at this level. CT, however, may not be able to determine extension into the false vocal cord itself; this is better evaluated by laryngoscopy. Coronal MR images help document paraglottic extension.

CT and MR imaging are excellent methods for showing cartilaginous invasion by laryngeal carcinoma, although limitations exist.[3,21,101] Because the thyroid cartilage normally may have an irregular pattern of calcification and ossification, neoplastic involvement can be confidently diagnosed only when advanced. Frank destruction of the cartilage by an adjacent mass or demonstration of intramedullary cancer is the most

reliable imaging sign of cartilage invasion. On CT, marked destruction of the cartilage appears as fragmentation of the cartilage with lateral extension of soft-tissue tumor (Figure 88-31). Cartilage involvement may also be suggested by abnormal bowing of the thyroid cartilage. Because of its symmetry, sclerosis or destruction of the cricoid is easier to appreciate on CT than on MR scans.[18]

Ossified portions of cartilage are at higher risk for invasion possibly because of vascular channel penetration, whereas intact perichondrium surrounding avascular unossified cartilage resists tumor encroachment.[120,128,140,171] Almost 50% of pathologically sclerotic cartilages associated with a mass show invasion at surgery.[120,156] Nonmalignant causes of thyroid cartilage sclerosis include rheumatoid arthritis and polychondritis; however, these conditions can usually be differentiated from cancer by the presence of sore throat, difficult inspiration, subluxation of the arytenoid cartilages, and the absence of a mass.[120]

Many investigators contend that MR images detect cartilage invasion better than CT.[5,10,19,21,23,71,162] On MR scans, cortical bone and dense calcification have no signal on T1- or T2-weighted sequences. However, medullary fat is hyperintense on T1-weighted images. Invasion of fat lowers this signal and can be further differentiated from nonossified cartilage on T1-weighted and T2-weighted images because of the hyperintensity displayed by tumor (Figure 88-32).[24,77,128,162,178,180] Almost 10% of healthy thyroid cartilage may have focal areas of signal intensity; however, an associated mass increases confidence in the diagnosis, especially

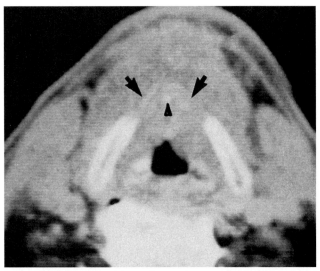

Figure 88-31. Thyroid cartilage destruction on computed tomography. A large neoplasm involving the anterior commissure destroys both thyroid alae anteriorly *(arrows)* and extends into the adjacent soft tissues. A small bony fragment can be seen within the tumor *(arrowhead)*.

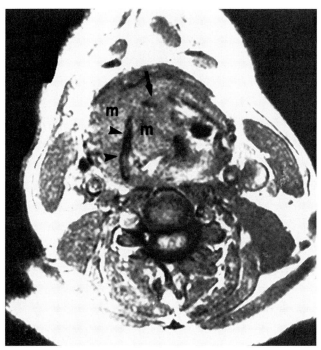

Figure 88-32. T1-weighted magnetic resonance imaging shows thyroid cartilage destruction. An extensive carcinoma *(m)* envelops the thyroid cartilage destroying anterior portions *(arrow)*. The invaded lateral cartilage has lost its hyperintensity because of tumor replacement *(arrowheads)*.

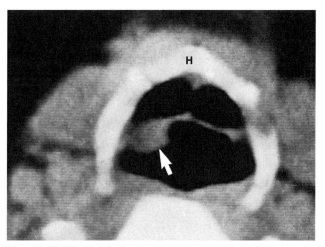

Figure 88-33. Epiglottic carcinoma on computed tomography. A tumor produces thickening of the right side of the epiglottis *(arrow)* at the level of the hyoid bone *(H)*.

if the mass exceeds 5 cm³ in volume.[22,77] If the imaging findings are equivocal, biopsy of the cartilage confirms the need for radical surgery.

Supraglottic Tumors

Imaging is extremely useful in staging supraglottic carcinoma and may discover more advanced disease than clinically suspected in up to 20% of patients.[37] Carcinoma of the epiglottis is seen on imaging as thickening of one of the margins of the epiglottis or as a large soft-tissue mass (Figures 88-33 and 88-34). Localized carcinoma of the epiglottis may be managed with radiotherapy or a supraglottic laryngectomy.[25] However, if there is invasion of the preepiglottic space, radiotherapy alone is considered inadequate.[83] Extension of epiglottic carcinoma to the preepiglottic space is frequently difficult to show clinically. CT and MR imaging help evaluate the preepiglottic and paraglottic spaces, because infiltrating tumors usually obliterate the normal appearance of fat in these areas (Figures 88-35 and 88-36).[9,26,180] T1-weighted sagittal MR imaging is especially useful for examining preepiglottic tumor invasion.[20,128] Transversely oriented CT or MR images are helpful when the vocal cords and the space immediately superior to the cords are normal. Similarly, transverse slices are use-

ful when the cords are unequivocally involved. In patients with supraglottic disease that approaches the ventricles but in whom transverse imaging does not clearly depict the ventricle, a coronal MR scan is the best study.[26] CT and MR scans can also show deep spread of tumor into the region of the anterior commissure. Spread of tumor into the base of the tongue is best evaluated by sagittal MR images.

Carcinoma of the aryepiglottic fold is recognizable by thickening of the aryepiglottic fold and is often better seen on scans obtained during phonation or a modified Valsalva's maneuver (Figure 88-37). The rapid scanning speed of spiral CT is ideally suited for such functional imaging. CT obtained during phonation shows distention of the pyriform sinuses and thinning of the healthy aryepiglottic fold, allowing for easier CT demonstration of tumor. If the tumor extends anteriorly across the midline, imaging studies may not determine whether the tumor originates in the aryepiglottic fold or in the epiglottis.

Neoplasms of the pyriform sinus generally are more aggressive than lesions of the endolarynx and have a high incidence of thyroid cartilage invasion. They may also spread to the true and false vocal cords, aryepiglottic folds, and preepiglottic space. CT or MR images can show tumor spread outside of the larynx between the thyroid and cricoid cartilages. This appearance usually is seen only with pyriform sinus tumors (Figure 88-38).[92]

In addition to the use of imaging appearances to evaluate stage of disease, quantitative methods may prove valuable. Calculated pretreatment tumor volumes using CT may predict local control after radiation or surgery.[70,106]

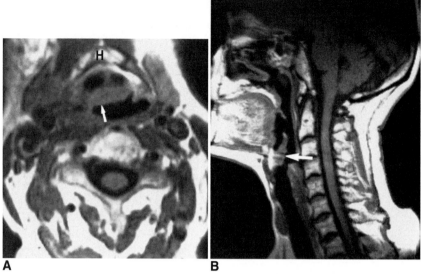

A   B

Figure 88-34. Magnetic resonance imaging of epiglottic carcinoma. **A,** Tumor thickens the right side of the epiglottis *(arrow)* at the level of hyoid *(H)*. **B,** Sagittal view shows nodular thickening of the epiglottis caused by tumor *(white arrow)*.

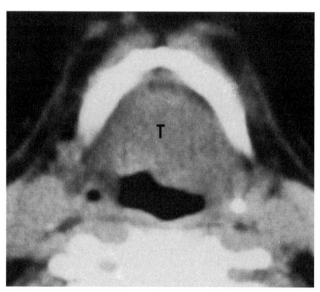

Figure 88-35. Epiglottic carcinoma on computed tomography. A large epiglottic tumor *(T)* infiltrates the preepiglottic space.

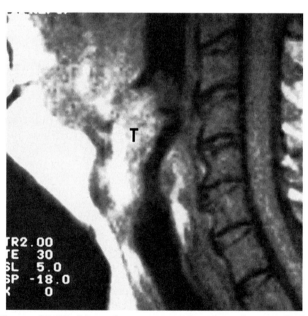

Figure 88-36. Magnetic resonance imaging of supraglottic carcinoma. Large mass *(T)* markedly thickens the epiglottis and invades the preepiglottic space.

Transglottic Tumors

Transglottic tumors extend across the laryngeal ventricle to involve the supraglottic, glottic, and often the subglottic portions of the larynx (see Figure 88-38).[18,161] This extension of tumor may be mucosal or submucosal. Transglottic tumors have a high incidence of thyroid cartilage destruction and extralaryngeal spread that may not be apparent clinically. Coronal MR scans may better show spread of tumor than axial images.

Lymph Nodes

Most enlarged lymph nodes identified on CT are clinically palpable, but occasionally CT may show enlarged lymph nodes that cannot be felt on physical examination.[108] Imaging also helps show the relationship of enlarged lymph nodes or tumor extension to adjacent vessels (Figure 88-39). Surgical salvage is less likely if the neoplasm totally encases or invades vascular structures.

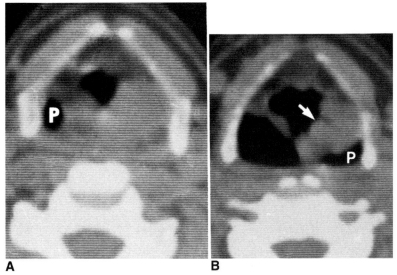

Figure 88-37. Aryepiglottic fold carcinoma on computed tomography. **A,** The left aryepiglottic fold and pyriform sinus are not well visualized. The right pyriform sinus is shown *(P)*. **B,** CT performed during a modified Valsalva's maneuver more clearly shows a tumor involving the left aryepiglottic fold *(arrow)* and compressing the left pyriform sinus *(P)*.

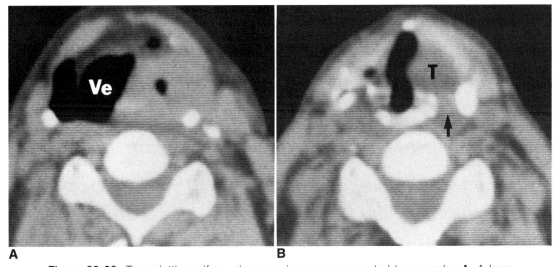

Figure 88-38. Transglottic pyriform sinus carcinoma on computed tomography. **A,** A large tumor is seen arising in the left pyriform sinus and displacing the laryngeal vestibule *(Ve)* to the right. **B,** Tumor extends inferiorly to involve the left true vocal cord *(T)* and widen the distance *(arrow)* between the left thyroid lamina and the arytenoid cartilage.

Posttherapy Larynx

Physical examination of patients who have undergone prior irradiation or surgery may be difficult because of altered normal laryngeal anatomy and swelling of the adjacent soft tissues. Although CT can define the anatomy of the postoperative larynx and assist laryngoscopy in the detection of recurrent neoplasm (Figure 88-40),[33,34,124,146] MR scanning is now preferred for posttherapy evaluation.[59]

In patients with previous vertical hemilaryngectomy, recurrent intralaryngeal cancer is suggested by increased width of the contralateral true vocal cord, convexity of the postsurgical pseudocord at the glottic level, mass in the subglottic region, or masses in the extralaryngeal neck.[34] In patients with supraglottic subtotal laryngectomy, recurrence is usually heralded by mass effect on the pharyngeal or laryngeal air column, obliteration of the adjacent soft-tissue planes,

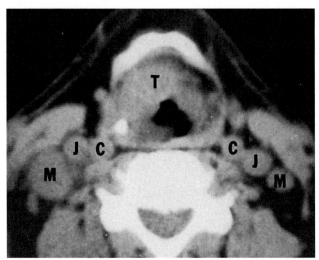

Figure 88-39. Epiglottic carcinoma with lymph node metastases on computed tomography. A large epiglottic tumor *(T)* infiltrates the preepiglottic space. Cervical lymph node metastases *(M)* are seen posterolateral to the internal jugular veins *(J)* and internal carotid arteries *(C)*. (From Sagel SS: *Larynx.* In Lee JKT, Sagel SS, Stanley RJ (eds): *Computed Body Tomography,* New York, Raven Press, p48, F25, 1983.)

destruction of cartilage, or development of lymphadenopathy.[124] Imaging signs of recurrence in patients who have undergone total laryngectomy include masses involving the internal jugular lymph node chain adjacent to the neopharynx or neurovascular bundle, masses within the mediastinum, thickening of the tracheal wall, or thickening of the soft tissues surrounding the tracheostomy.[33] Nodular

masses at the site of radical neck dissection are unusual and should prompt evaluation for tumor.[146] Care should be taken in radiographically evaluating the postoperative patient, because abscess or granulation tissue can mimic recurrent tumor.[34]

Regardless of the surgical procedure, hemorrhage and edema are usually evident on imaging during the early postoperative period and persist for 4 to 6 weeks. A baseline scan is therefore best postponed for at least 1 month and preferably for 6 to 8 weeks to avoid potentially confusing soft-tissue masses.[104] Scanning every 4 to 6 months for the first 3 years is recommended.[32,147] Examinations are then performed yearly unless an ominous change in clinical status prompts a more timely scan.[147]

Typically, cancer recurrence within the first 2 months after surgery is unusual if the specimen margins were free of tumor.[147] With time, tissue planes become more defined but remain somewhat obscured compared with the preoperative images. Scar tends to be less dense on CT but may be difficult to differentiate from fibrous tissue without biopsy. MR images usually cannot reliably distinguish recurrent tumor from edema, radiation necrosis, or inflammatory lesions.[128] Fibrosis tends to be hypointense on T2-weighted images, whereas recurrent tumor is hyperintense.[32] Growth of any soft-tissue density on imaging is another sign of recurrence, whereas scar remains stable or diminishes with time.[147]

Radiotherapy can also change the appearance of the neck on imaging.[125] The major and minor salivary glands are especially sensitive to radiation, and 1000

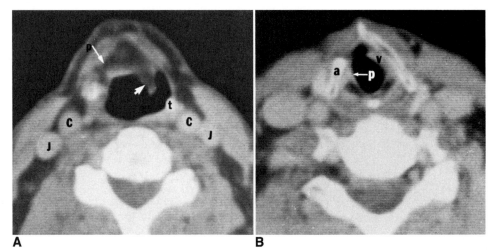

A　　　　　　　　　　　**B**

Figure 88-40. Computed tomography of normal anatomy after right vertical hemilaryngectomy. **A,** Level of superior cornua of the thyroid cartilage. *Arrow* points to residual aryepiglottic fold on the nonoperated side. The superior cornu of thyroid cartilage *(t),* preepiglottic space with diminution of fat content *(p),* carotid artery *(c),* and internal jugular vein *(J)* are also seen. **B,** Level of glottis. Note the normal tilt of the airway to the right. The residual right thyroid ala *(a),* surgically created pseudocord *(p),* and residual left true vocal cord *(v)* are also seen.

to 2000 cGy causes mucositis.[157] On CT, the major salivary glands enhance and eventually atrophy.[115] Three-dimensional radiation port planning shields the parotid glands and ameliorates posttherapy xerostomia.[41] The subcutaneous fat becomes thickened and streaked with linear soft-tissue densities at 6500 to 7000 cGy.[18,115] The skin also may become thickened. With doses approaching 7000 cGy, skin ulceration becomes increasingly likely.[157] At doses >7000 cGy, the pharyngeal walls and aryepiglottic folds become thickened as the paraglottic and preepiglottic spaces increase in CT density.[20,157] Higher doses of radiation weaken membranes and cartilage and may contribute to chondronecrosis and cartilage collapse.[18] Chondronecrosis is difficult to differentiate from recurrent tumor on CT. The soft tissues are thickened, and cartilage may be distorted or fragmented.[104] Radiated cartilage is also more prone to infection and may develop perichondritis if biopsied.[27]

Other organs may be affected by neck radiation. The adjacent skeleton may show hyperintense marrow signal on T1-weighted images because of posttherapy marrow fat infiltration, the mandible may succumb to osteoradionecrosis, and rarely, the radiated bone may give rise to sarcomas.[157] Osteoradionecrosis involves the devitalization of radiated bone and is caused by vascular damage and direct injury to osteoblasts augmented by xerostomia and resultant dental caries. The involved bone has focal demineralization, disorganized trabeculae, cortical thickening, patchy sclerosis, and occasionally pathologic fractures.[157] Periosteal reaction is unusual and should prompt consideration of infection.

Differentiating postradiation changes from recurrent tumor is difficult on imaging studies. Intralaryngeal edema may be symmetric or asymmetric and therefore offers no definitive criteria for tumor recurrence.[20,104,157] Residual tumor usually maintains high signal intensity on MR scans, and the signal intensity of successfully managed tumor tends to diminish with development of fibrosis.[60] However, similar nonspecific and occasionally confusing signal intensities can also be produced by edema, hyperplastic lymphadenopathy, infection, and hemorrhage.[14,59,60,157] Differentiation between fibrosis and early recurrent tumor often requires laryngoscopic biopsy. Complete or near complete resolution of the primary lesion on imaging is one of the best criteria for a successful radiation response. Residual mass >50% of the original tumor volume usually indicates therapy failure.[116] Finally, growth of associated soft-tissue mass suggests tumor recurrence. The appearance of new focal masses and ulcerations on barium pharyngography supports the clinical diagnosis of recurrence.[129] Other modalities, such as PET or single photon emission CT

(SPECT) with [22]fluorodeoxyglucose, may be more useful than conventional cross-sectional imaging.[20] Combined PET/CT merges PET and CT data into a single scan that couples functional metabolic information with precise anatomic localization. This information can be used for more confident diagnosis of recurrent tumor and for biopsy (Broadbent LP and others: Combined PET/CT imaging for targeting fine needle aspirations to diagnose recurrent head and neck cancer, Personal communication, 2004).

Postradiation sarcomas are rare and usually appear after a latent period lasting decades. Because of the age of the typical neck cancer patient, the associated multisystem debilities from chronic smoking, and the unfortunately high rate of recurrent tumor, sarcomas are usually not seen.

LARYNGEAL TRAUMA

Laryngeal trauma usually results from direct blunt injury to the anterior neck. The usual mechanism for the observed damage is the forceful impact of the larynx against the cervical spine. The thyroid cartilage may be fractured in almost 50% of cases. The cricoarytenoid joint may also be dislocated. The ring-shaped cricoid cartilage may also fracture. Because of its configuration, usually two or more sites are involved. Rarely, the epiglottis may be disrupted.[36] Hemorrhage and edema may spread into the paraglottic and preepiglottic spaces.[169] Nondisplaced fractures may be managed conservatively; however, displaced and comminuted fractures require surgery.[11,136]

Cross-sectional imaging permits easy and rapid evaluation of the extent of cartilaginous injury, adjacent soft-tissue changes (e.g., edema, hemorrhage), and the degree of airway compromise (Figures 88-41 and 88-42). Although conventional frontal and lateral radiography can provide useful information about the injured larynx, CT is preferred in the acutely injured patient because of its speed and ability to define calcified cartilages and soft-tissue damage.[53,105,136] Spiral techniques are well suited for this situation. A complete examination of the neck can be acquired within seconds. With the addition of intravenous contrast, the raw CT data can be used to reconstruct 3D images of the carotid and vertebral arteries in a technique known as CT angiography (CTA). CT also is useful in patients with marked supraglottic swelling that prevents adequate laryngoscopic evaluation. CT can accurately identify transverse or vertical fractures of the thyroid or cricoid cartilage, dislocation of the arytenoid cartilages at the cricoarytenoid joint, disruption of the cricothyroid joint, and extensive hemorrhage obliterating the airway. On occasion, the thyroid notch may be mistaken for a fracture, although contiguous sections usually provide the

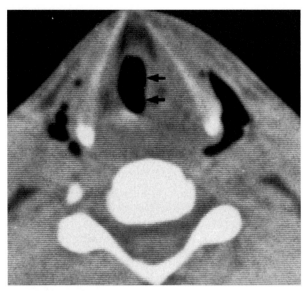

Figure 88-41. Soft-tissue swelling with intact cartilage on computed tomography. Marked soft-tissue thickening of the right paraglottic space is seen with compression of the airway *(arrows)*. Both thyroid alae are intact. Subcutaneous emphysema is secondary to a mucosal tear from an emergency tracheotomy.

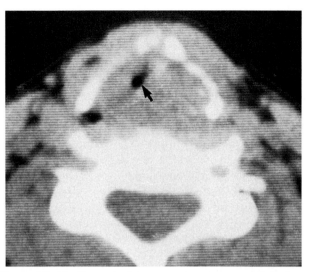

Figure 88-42. Computed tomography shows multiple fractures of the thyroid cartilage. Extensive hemorrhage and edema almost totally obliterate the airway *(arrow)*.

correct diagnosis. MR scans do not image calcified cartilage well and are, therefore, of no use in the initial evaluation of acute laryngeal trauma. After patient stabilization, MR imaging may be useful in evaluating adjacent soft tissue damage or spinal injury.

Pharyngeal perforation is a rare but known complication of endotracheal intubation.[30,72] Traumatic intubation may also cause severe soft-tissue damage, soft-tissue emphysema, and arytenoid cartilage dislocation. Radiography of the area often shows air within the retropharyngeal soft tissues or in the anterior mediastinum. Oral contrast studies of the esophagus may define the problems related to perforation, including subsequent development of a pseudodiverticulum.

FOREIGN BODIES

Foreign bodies in the larynx, trachea, or esophagus should be considered in patients, particularly children, with symptoms of acute or recurrent airway disease.[123,144] The radiopaque objects are readily diagnosed (Figure 88-43). With plain-film techniques, including high-kilovoltage radiography, nonopaque foreign bodies also may be identified at times. The radiographic findings of aspirated foreign bodies vary directly with the location and extent of obstruction. On occasion, calcification of a laryngeal cartilage or of the stylohyoid ligaments may be confused with aspirated foreign bodies, although oblique projections usually permit separation (Figure 88-44).[121]

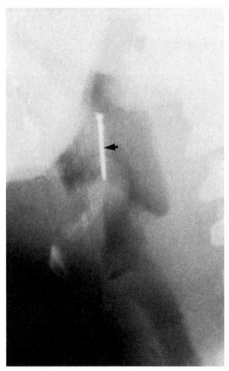

Figure 88-43. Foreign body. A straight pin *(arrow)* is lodged in the vallecula.

In patients with suspected aspiration of a foreign body and a normal examination of the upper airway, inspiratory-expiratory plain chest radiography or decubitus chest radiography should be performed. These may show regional obstructive emphysema resulting from aspirated foreign bodies in the

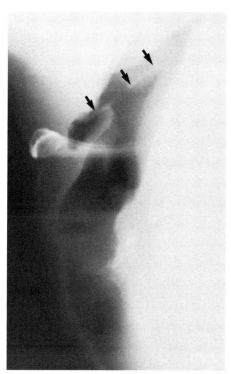

Figure 88-44. Stylohyoid ligament. Ossification of the stylohyoid ligament *(arrows)* can simulate a foreign body.

bronchi.[15,17] In uncooperative patients, fluoroscopic examination of diaphragmatic and mediastinal excursions may help determine whether air trapping is present.

Swallowed foreign bodies in the upper esophagus may produce airway obstruction by compressing the posterior wall of the larynx and trachea. Tracheal compression, appreciated best on lateral radiography, is the expected radiographic finding. A barium esophagram is the definitive procedure in disclosing the occult esophageal foreign body (Figure 88-45).[144] If the object erodes through the esophageal wall, a retropharyngeal abscess may form with resulting compression of the adjacent airway.

Various synthetic materials may be inserted into the larynx and neck. Teflon injected into the paraglottic space adds bulk to a paralyzed or reconstructed vocal cord. Stents ensure a patent airway in patients with laryngeal stenosis. Speaking tubes and valves help the laryngectomy patient use the esophagus when speaking. Tracheostomy tubes are inserted into the midcervical region in the patient with laryngeal stenosis, acutely compromised airway, or laryngectomy.[27] Some of these materials may be incidentally noted on scans in patients who have failed to mention past surgical procedures; these materials should not be misinterpreted as masses or traumatic foreign bodies.

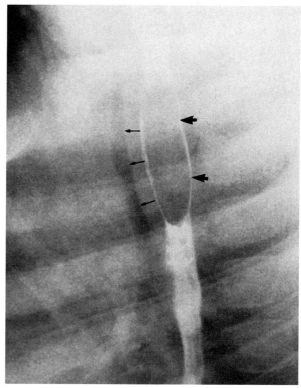

Figure 88-45. Esophageal foreign body in a child with stridor. Lateral view from a barium esophagram discloses a piece of meat *(large arrows)* in the upper esophagus compressing the posterior wall of the trachea *(small arrows)*.

REFERENCES

1. Agha FP: Recurrent laryngeal nerve paralysis: a laryngographic and computed tomographic study, *Radiology* 148:149, 1983.
2. Anzai Y and others: Fat-suppression failure artifacts simulating pathology on frequency-selective fat-suppression MR images of the head and neck, *Am J Neuroradiol* 13:879, 1992.
3. Archer CR, Yeager VL: Evaluation of laryngeal cartilages by computed tomography, *J Comput Assist Tomogr* 3:604, 1979.
4. Archer CR and others: Staging of carcinoma of the larynx: comparative accuracy of computed tomography and laryngography, *Am J Roentgenol* 136:571, 1981.
5. Atula T and others: Cartilage invasion of laryngeal cancer detected by magnetic resonance imaging, *Eur Arch Otorhinolaryngol* 258:272, 2001.
6. Balaban RS, Ceckler TL: Magnetization transfer contrast in magnetic resonance imaging, *Magn Reson Q* 8:116, 1992.
7. Barakos JA, Dillon WP, Chew WM: Orbit, skull base, and pharynx: contrast-enhanced fat suppression MR imaging, *Radiology* 179:191, 1991.
8. Barnstetter BF, Weissman JL: Normal anatomy of the neck with CT and MR imaging correlation, *Radiol Clin N Am* 38:925, 2000.
9. Becker M: Larynx and hypopharynx, *Radiol Clin North Am* 36:891, 1998.
10. Becker M and others: Neoplastic invasion of the laryngeal cartilage: comparison of MR imaging and CT with histopathologic correlation, *Radiology* 194:661, 1995.

11. Bent JP III, Porubsky ES: The management of blunt fractures of the thyroid cartilage, *Otolaryngol Head Neck Surg* 110:195, 1994.

12. Boey HP, Cunningham MJ, Webe AL: Central nervous system imaging in the evaluation of children with true vocal cord paralysis, *Ann Otol Rhinol Laryngol* 104:76, 1995.

13. Brenner GH: Variations in the depth of the cervical prevertebral tissues in normal infants studied by cinefluorography, *Am J Roentgenol* 91:573, 1964.

14. Briggs RJS and others: Laryngeal imaging by computerized tomography and magnetic resonance following radiation therapy: a need for caution, *J Laryngol Otol* 107:56, 1993.

15. Capitanio MA, Kirkpatrick JA: The lateral decubitus film: an aid in determining air-trapping in children, *Radiology* 103:460, 1972.

16. Capitanio MA, Kirkpatrick JA: Nasopharyngeal lymphoid tissue: roentgen observations in 257 children two years of age or less, *Radiology* 96:389, 1970.

17. Capitanio MA, Kirkpatrick JA: Upper respiratory tract obstruction in infants and children, *Radiol Clin North Am* 6:265, 1968.

18. Casselman JW, Biebau G: Imaging of laryngeal cancer, *Acta Otorhinolaryngol Belg* 46:161, 1992.

19. Castelijns JA: Diagnostic radiology of head and neck oncology, *Curr Opin Oncol* 3:512, 1991.

20. Castelijns JA and others: Imaging of the larynx, *Neuroimaging Clin North Am* 6:401, 1996.

21. Castelijns JA and others: Invasion of laryngeal cartilage by cancer: comparison of CT and MR imaging, *Radiology* 166:199, 1987.

22. Castelijns JA and others: Laryngeal carcinoma after radiation therapy: correlation of abnormal MR imaging signal patterns in laryngeal cartilage with risk of recurrence, *Radiology* 198:151, 1996.

23. Castelijns JA and others: MR findings of cartilage invasion by laryngeal cancer: value in predicting outcome of radiation therapy, *Radiology* 174:669, 1990.

24. Castelijns JA and others: MRI of normal or cancerous laryngeal cartilages: histopathologic correlation, *Laryngoscope* 97:1085, 1987.

25. Cocke EW, Wang CC: Part 1: Cancer of the larynx: selecting optimum treatment, *CA Cancer Clin* 26:194, 1976.

26. Curtin HD: Imaging of the larynx: current concepts, *Radiology* 173:1, 1989.

27. Curtin HD: *The larynx*. In Som PM, Curtin HD, editors: *Head and neck imaging*, ed 3, St. Louis, 1996, Mosby.

28. Davis WL and others: Retropharyngeal space: evaluation of normal anatomy and disease with CT and MR imaging, *Radiology* 174:59, 1990.

29. Davis WL and others: The normal and diseased retropharyngeal and prevertebral spaces, *Semin Ultrasound CT MR* 11:520, 1990.

30. Dawkes JDK: Traumatic perforations of the pharynx and esophagus, *J Laryngol Otol* 78:18, 1964.

31. Dillon WP: Applications of magnetic resonance imaging to the head and neck, *Semin Ultrasound CT MR* 7:202, 1986.

32. Dillon WP, Harnsberger HR: The impact of radiologic imaging on staging of cancer of the head and neck, *Semin Oncol* 18:64, 1991.

33. DiSantis DJ and others: The neck after total laryngectomy: CT study, *Radiology* 153:713, 1984.

34. DiSantis DJ and others: The neck after vertical hemilaryngectomy: computed tomographic study, *Radiology* 151:683, 1984.

35. Doust BD, Ting YM: Xeroradiography of the larynx, *Radiology* 110:727, 1974.

36. Duda JJ, Lewin JS, Eliacher I: MR evaluations of epiglottic disruption, *Am J Neuroradiol* 17:563, 1996.

37. Dullerud R and others: Influence of CT on tumor classification of laryngeal carcinomas, *Acta Radiol* 33:314, 1992.

38. Dunbar JS: Epiglottitis and croup, *J Can Assoc Radiol* 12:95, 1961.

39. Dunbar JS: Upper respiratory tract obstruction in infants and children, *Am J Roentgenol* 109:227, 1970.

40. Edelman RR, Shellock FG, Ahladis J: *Practical MRI for the technologist and imaging specialist.* In Edelman RR, Hesselink JR, editors: *Clinical magnetic resonance imaging*, Philadelphia, 1990, WB Saunders.

41. Emami B and others: 3-D Conformal radiotherapy in head and neck cancer, *Front Radiat Ther Oncol* 29:207, 1996.

42. Emami B and others: *Clinical experience with 3-D radiotherapy: the Washington University experience.* In Purdy JA, Emami B, editors: *3-D Radiation treatment planning and conformal therapy: proceedings of an international symposium*, Madison, Wis, 1995, Medical Physics Publishing.

43. Felson B: Neoplasms of the trachea and mainstem bronchi, *Semin Roentgenol* 18:23, 1983.

44. Fernbach SK and others: Radiologic evaluation of adenoids and tonsils in children with obstructive sleep apnea: plain films and fluoroscopy, *Pediatr Radiol* 13:258, 1983.

45. Fried MP and others: Virtual laryngoscopy, *Ann Otol Rhinol Laryngol* 108:221, 1999.

46. Friedman L and others: CT appearance of an oncocytic papillary cystadenoma of the larynx, *J Comput Assist Tomogr* 14:322, 1990.

47. Fujioka M, Young LW, Girdany BR: Radiographic evaluation of adenoidal size in children: adenoidal-nasopharyngeal ratio, *Am J Roentgenol* 133:401, 1979.

48. Fulbright R and others: MR of the head and neck: comparison of fast spin-echo and conventional spin-echo sequences, *Am J Neuroradiol* 15:767, 1994.

49. Gamsu G: *Computed tomography of the larynx and piriform sinuses.* In Moss AA, Gamsu G, Genant H, editors: *Computed tomography of the body*, Philadelphia, 1983, WB Saunders.

50. Gamsu G, Mark AS, Webb WR: Computed tomography of the normal larynx during quiet breathing and phonation, *J Comput Assist Tomogr* 5:353, 1981.

51. Gatenby RA, Mulhern CB, Strawitz J: CT-guided percutaneous biopsies of head and neck masses, *Radiology* 146:717, 1983.

52. Gatenby RA and others: CT-guided biopsy for the detection and staging of tumors of the head and neck, *Am J Neuroradiol* 5:287, 1984.

53. Gayler BW, Kashima HK, Martinez CR: Computed tomography of the neck, *Crit Rev Diagn Imaging* 23:319, 1985.

54. Gilliams AR and others: Magnetization transfer contrast MR in lesions of the head and neck, *Am J Neuroradiol* 17:355, 1996.

55. Giron J and others: Pre-therapeutic evaluation of laryngeal carcinomas using computed tomography and magnetic resonance imaging, *Isr J Med Sci* 28:225, 1992.

56. Glaser CM and others: CT and ultrasound imaging of retropharyngeal abscesses in children, *Am J Neuroradiol* 13:1191, 1992.

57. Glazer HS and others: Computed tomography of laryngocoeles, *Am J Roentgenol* 140:549, 1983.

58. Glazer HS and others: Extra-laryngeal causes of vocal cord paralysis: CT evaluation, *Am J Roentgenol* 141:527, 1983.

59. Glazer HS and others: Neck neoplasms: MR imaging part II. Posttreatment evaluation, *Radiology* 160:349, 1986.

60. Glazer HS and others: Radiation fibrosis: differentiation from recurrent tumor by MR imaging, *Radiology* 156:721, 1985.

61. Gluecker T, Lang F, Bessler S, Monnier P, Meuli R, Schnyder P, Duvoisin B: 2D and 3D CT imaging correlated to rigid endoscopy in complex laryngo-tracheal stenoses, *Eur Radiol* 11:50, 2001.

62. Goldenberg D, Golz A, Joachims HZ: Retropharyngeal abscess: a clinical review, *J Larngol Otol* 111:546, 1997.

63. Greenfield H, Herman PG: Papillomatosis of the trachea and bronchi, *Am J Roentgenol* 89:45, 1963.

64. Gregor RT and others: Saccular mucocele in association with laryngeal cancer, *Ann Otol Rhinol Laryngol* 103:732, 1994.

65. Griffen JL, Ramadan HH, Wetmore SJ: Laryngocele: a cause of stridor and airway obstruction, *Otolaryngol Head Neck Surg* 108:760, 1993.

66. Han BK: Membranous laryngotracheobronchitis (membranous croup), *Am J Roentgenol* 133:53, 1979.

67. Harnsberger HR: *The larynx and hypopharynx.* In Harnsberger HR, editor: *Handbook of head and neck imaging*, St Louis, 1995, Mosby.

68. Hasagawa Y, Matsuura H: Retropharyngeal node dissection in cancer of the oropharynx and hypopharynx, *Head Neck* 16:173, 1994.

69. Hasso AN, Brown KD: Use of gadolinium chelates in MR imaging of lesions of the extracranial head and neck, *J Magn Reson Imaging* 3:247, 1993.

70. Hermans R and others: Value of computed tomography as outcome predictor of supraglottic squamous cell carcinoma treated by definitive radiation therapy, *Int J Radiat Oncol Biol Phys* 44:755, 1999.

71. Hirano M and others: Computed tomography in determining laryngeal involvement of hypopharyngeal carcinoma, *Ann Otol Rhinol Laryngol* 97:476, 1988.

72. Hirsch M and others: Hypopharyngeal injury as a result of attempted endotracheal intubation, *Radiology* 128:37, 1978.

73. Holinger PH, Brown WT: Congenital webs, cysts, laryngoceles and anomalies of the larynx, *Ann Otol Rhinol Laryngol* 76:744, 1967.

74. Hoover LA and others: Magnetic resonance imaging of the larynx and tongue base: clinical applications, *Otolaryngol Head Neck Surg* 97:245, 1987.

75. Hudgins PA, Gussack GS: MR imaging in the management of extracranial malignant tumors of the head and neck, *Am J Roentgenol* 159:161, 1992.

76. Hudgins PA and others: Efficacy and safety of gadopentetate dimeglumine in the evaluation of patients with a suspected tumor of the extracranial head and neck, *J Magn Reson Imaging* 3:345, 1993.

77. Jabour BA, Lufkin RB, Hanafee WN: Magnetic resonance imaging of the larynx, *Top Magn Reson Imaging* 2:60, 1990.

78. Jacobs CJM and others: Vagal neuropathy: evaluation with CT and MR imaging, *Radiology* 164:97, 1987.

79. Joseph PM and others: Upper airway obstruction in infants and small children, *Radiology* 121:143, 1976.

80. Kaberle M, Kenn W, Hahn D: Current concepts in imaging of laryngeal and hypopharyngeal cancer, *Eur Radiol* 12:1672, 2002.

81. Kanal E, Shellock FG, Lewin JS: Aneurysm clip testing for ferromagnetic properties: clip variability issues, *Radiology* 200:576, 1996

82. Kirchner JA: Two hundred laryngeal cancers: patterns of growth and spread as seen in serial section, *Laryngoscope* 87:474, 1977.

83. Klein R, Fletcher GH: Evaluation of the clinical usefulness of roentgenologic findings in squamous cell carcinomas of the larynx, *Am J Roentgenol* 92:43, 1964.

84. Klucznik RP and others: Placement of a ferromagnetic intracerebral aneurysm clip in a magnetic field with a fatal outcome, *Radiology* 187:855, 1993.

85. Kramer SS and others: Pulmonary manifestations of juvenile laryngotracheal papillomatosis, *Am J Roentgenol* 144:687, 1985.

86. Krinsky G, Rofsky NM, Weinreb JC: Nonspecificity of short inversion time inversion recovery (STIR) as a technique of fat suppression: pitfalls in image interpretation, *Am J Roentgenol* 166:523, 1996.

87. Kushner DC, Harris GBC: Obstructing lesions of the larynx and trachea in infants and children, *Radiol Clin North Am* 16:181, 1978.

88. Kwock L: Localized MR spectroscopy: basic principles, *Neuroimaging Clin N Am* 8:713, 1998

89. Lakshminarayanan AV, Lee S, McCutcheon MJ: MR imaging of the vocal tract during vowel production, *J Magn Reson Imaging* 1:71, 1991.

90. Lallemand D, Sauvegrain J, Mareschal JL: Laryngo-tracheal lesions in infants and children, *Ann Radiol* 16:293, 1973.

91. Lambre H and others: Interventional magnetic resonance imaging of the head and neck and new imaging techniques, *Neuroimaging Clin North Am* 6:461, 1996.

92. Larrson S and others: Differentiation of pyriform sinus cancer from supraglottic laryngeal cancer by computed tomography, *Radiology* 141:427, 1981.

93. Lesinski SG, Bauer WC, Ogura JH: Hemilaryngectomy for T3 (fixed cord) epidermoid carcinoma of the larynx, *Laryngoscope* 10:1563, 1976.

94. Levy AM and others: Hypertrophied adenoids causing pulmonary hypertension and severe congestive heart failure, *N Engl J Med* 277:506, 1967.

95. Lewin JS and others: Fast spin-echo imaging of the neck: comparison with conventional spin-echo, utility of fat suppression, and evaluation of tissue contrast characteristics, *Am J Neuroradiol* 15:1351, 1994.

96. Lindell MM and others: Laryngocele, *Am J Roentgenol* 131:259, 1978.

97. Lofchy NM, Stevens JK, Brown DH: Three-dimensional imaging of the parapharyngeal space, *Arch Otolaryngol Head Neck Surg* 120:333, 1994.

98. Lufkin RB, Hanafee WN: Applications of surface coils to MR anatomy of the larynx, *Am J Neuroradiol* 6:491, 1985.

99. Macpherson RI, Leithiser RE: Upper airway obstruction in children: an update, *Radiographics* 5:339, 1985.

100. Madison MT and others: Radiologic diagnosis and staging of head and neck squamous cell carcinoma, *Radiol Clin North Am* 32:163, 1994.

101. Mafee MF and others: Computed tomography of the larynx: correlation with anatomic and pathologic studies in cases of laryngeal carcinoma, *Radiology* 147:123, 1983.

102. Maguire GH, Beigue RA, Rotenberg AD: Selective filtration: the practical approach to high-kilovoltage radiography, *Radiology* 85:343, 1965.

103. Mancuso AA, Hanafee WN: A comparative evaluation of computed tomography and laryngography, *Radiology* 133:131, 1979.

104. Mancuso AA, Hanafee WN: *Computed tomography and magnetic resonance imaging of the head and neck*, Baltimore, 1985, Williams & Wilkins.

105. Mancuso AA, Hanafee WN: Computed tomography imaging of the injured larynx, *Radiology* 133:139, 1979.

106. Mancuso AA and others: Preradiotherapy computed tomography as a predictor of local control in supraglottic carcinoma, *J Clin Oncol* 17:631, 1999.

107. Mancuso AA, Tamakawa Y, Hanafee WN: CT of the fixed vocal cord, *Am J Roentgenol* 135:529, 1980.

108. Mancuso AA and others: CT of cervical lymph node cancer, *Am J Roentgenol* 136:381, 1981.

109. McCook TA, Felman AH: Retropharyngeal masses in infants and young children, *Am J Dis Child* 133:41, 1979.

110. McCook TA, Kirks DR: Epiglottic enlargement in infants and children: another radiologic look, *Pediatr Radiol* 12:227, 1982.

111. Merkle EM and others: Percutaneous magnetic resonance image-guided biopsy and aspiration in head and neck, *Laryngoscope* 110:382, 2000.

112. Million RR: The larynx...so to speak: everything I wanted to know about laryngeal cancer I learned in the last 32 years, *Int J Radiat Oncol Biol Phys* 23:691, 1992.

113. Mukherji SK and others: Comparison of dynamic and spiral CT for imaging the glottic larynx, *J Comput Assist Tomogr* 19:899, 1995.

114. Mukherji SK, Chong V, Castillo M: *Magnetic resonance spectroscopy of the extracranial head and neck*. In: Mukherji SK, Castelijns JA, editors: *Modern head and neck imaging*, Berlin, Springer-Verlag, 2000, p 31.

115. Mukherji SK and others: Radiologic appearance of the irradiated larynx. Part I. Expected changes, *Radiology* 193:141, 1994.

116. Mukherji SK and others: Radiologic appearance of the irradiated larynx. Part II. Primary site response, *Radiology* 193:149, 1994.

117. Mukherji SK, Schiro S, Castillo M: Proton MR spectroscopy of squamous cell carcinoma of the upper aerodigestive tract: in vitro characteristics, *Am J Neuroradiol* 17:1485, 1996.

118. Mukherji SK and other: Proton MR spectroscopy of squamous cell carcinoma of the head and neck: in vitro and in vivo studies, *Am J Neuroradiol* 18:1057, 1997.

119. Mukherji SK and others: A technique for core biopsies of head and neck masses, *Am J Neuroradiol* 15:518, 1994.

120. Muñoz A and others: Laryngeal carcinoma: sclerotic appearance of the cricoid and arytenoid cartilage. CT-pathologic correlation, *Radiology* 189:433, 1993.

121. Muroff LR, Seeman WB: Normal anatomy of the larynx and pharynx and the differential diagnosis of foreign bodies, *Semin Roentgenol* 9:267, 1974.

122. Nelson KL, Runge VM: Basic principles of MR contrast, *Top Magn Reson Imaging* 7:124, 1995.

123. Newman DE: The radiolucent esophageal foreign body: an often-forgotten cause of respiratory symptoms, *J Pediatr* 92:60, 1978.

124. Niemeyer JH, Balfe DM, Hayden RE: Neck evaluation with barium-enhanced radiographs and CT scans after supraglottic subtotal laryngectomy, *Radiology* 162:493, 1987.

125. Nömeyr A and others: MRI appearance of radiation-induced changes of normal cervical tissues, *Eur Radiol* 11:1807, 2001.

126. Ogura JH, Heeneman H: Conservation surgery of the larynx and hypopharynx: selection of patients and results, *Can J Otolaryngol* 2:11, 1973.

127. Pavlicek W and others: The effects of nuclear magnetic resonance on patients with cardiac pacemakers, *Radiology* 147:149, 1983.

128. Phelps PD: Carcinoma of the larynx: the role of imaging in staging and pretreatment assessments, *Clin Radiol* 46:77, 1992.

129. Quillin SP, Balfe DM, Glick SN: Pharyngography after head and neck irradiation: differentiation of postirradiation edema from recurrent tumor, *Am J Roentgenol* 161:1205, 1993.

130. Robinson JD and others: Extracranial lesions of the head and neck: preliminary experience with Gd-DTPA–enhanced MR imaging, *Radiology* 172:165, 1989.

131. Rosenfield NS, Peck DR, Lowman RM: Xeroradiography in the evaluation of acquired airway abnormalities in children, *Am J Dis Child* 132:1977, 1979.

132. Ross MR and others: MR imaging of head and neck tumors: comparison of T1-weighted contrast-enhanced fat-suppressed images with conventional T2-weighted and fast spin-echo T2-weighted images, *Am J Roentgenol* 163:173, 1994.

133. Sagel SS and others: High resolution computed tomography in the staging of carcinoma of the larynx, *Laryngoscope* 91:292, 1981.

134. Sakai F and others: MR evaluation of laryngohypopharyngeal cancer: value of gadopentetate dimeglumine enhancement, *Am J Neuroradiol* 14:1059, 1993.

135. Saleh EM, Mancuso AA, Stringer SP: CT of submucosal and occult laryngeal masses, *J Comput Assist Tomogr* 16:87, 1992.

136. Schaefer SD, Close LG: Acute management of laryngeal trauma: update, *Ann Otol Rhinol Laryngol* 98:98, 1989.

137. Scott M and others: Computed tomographic evaluation of laryngeal neoplasms, *Radiology* 140:141, 1981.

138. Shackelford GD, Siegel MJ, MacAlister WH: I: Subglottic edema in acute epiglottitis in children, *Am J Roentgenol* 131:603, 1978.

139. Shulman HS, Noyek AM, Steinhardt MJ: CT of the larynx, *J Otolaryngol* 11:395, 1982.

140. Silverman PM and others: Carcinoma of the larynx and hypopharynx: computed tomographic-histopathologic correlations, *Radiology* 151:697, 1984.

141. Silverman PM and others: Work in progress: high-resolution, thin-section computed tomography of the larynx, *Radiology* 145:723, 1982.

142. Slovis TL and others: *Current problems in diagnostic radiology: noninvasive visualization of the pediatric airway*, Chicago, 1979, Mosby.

143. Smith A, Gooding CA: Pulmonary involvement in laryngeal papillomatosis, *Pediatr Radiol* 2:161, 1974.

144. Smith PC, Swischuk LE, Fagan CJ: An elusive and often unsuspected cause of stridor or pneumonia: the esophageal foreign body, *Am J Roentgenol* 122:80, 1974.

145. Som PM: Cystic lesions of the neck, *Postgrad Radiol* 7:209, 1987.

146. Som PM, Biller HF: Computed tomography of the neck in the postoperative patient: radical neck dissection and the myocutaneous flap, *Radiology* 148:157, 1983.

147. Som PM and others: Imaging the postoperative neck, *Radiology* 187:593, 1993.

148. Spreer J and others: Spiral versus conventional CT in routine examinations of the neck, *J Comput Assist Tomogr* 19:905, 1995.

149. Strife JL: Upper airway and tracheal obstruction in infants and children, *Radiol Clin North Am* 26:309, 1988.

150. Sulfaro S and others: T staging of the laryngohypopharyngeal carcinoma, *Arch Otolaryngol Head Neck Surg* 115:613, 1989.

151. Suojanen JN, Mukherji SK, Wippold FJ: Spiral CT of the larynx, *Am J Neuroradiol* 15:1579, 1994.

152. Suojanen JN and others: Spiral CT in evaluation of head and neck lesions: work in progress, *Radiology* 183:281, 1992.

153. Sutton TJ, Nogrady MB: Radiologic diagnosis of subglottic hemangioma in infants, *Pediatr Radiol* 1:211, 1973.

154. Swischuk LE: *Emergency radiology of the acutely ill or injured child*, Baltimore, 1979, Williams & Wilkins.
155. Swischuk LE, Smith PC, Fagan CJ: Abnormalities of the pharynx and larynx in childhood, *Semin Roentgenol* 9:283, 1974.
156. Tart RP and others: Value of laryngeal cartilage sclerosis as a predictor of outcome in patients with stage T3 glottic cancer treated with radiation therapy, *Radiology* 192:567, 1994.
157. Tartaglino LM, Rao VM, Markiewicz DA: Imaging of radiation changes in the head and neck, *Semin Roentgenol* 29:81, 1994.
158. Terris DJ, Arnstein DP, Nguyen HH: Contemporary evaluation of unilateral vocal cord paralysis, *Otolaryngol Head Neck Surg* 107:84, 1992.
159. Tien RD and others: Improved detection and delineation of head and neck lesions with fat suppression spin-echo MR imaging, *Am J Neuroradiol* 12:19, 1991.
160. Towler CR, Young SW: Magnetic resonance imaging of the larynx, *Magn Reson Q* 5:228, 1989.
161. Tucker GF: The anatomy of laryngeal cancer, *Can J Otolaryngol* 3:417, 1974.
162. van den Brekel MWM, Castelijns JA, Snow GB: The role of modern imaging studies in staging and therapy of head and neck neoplasms, *Semin Oncol* 21:340, 1994.
163. van Vierzen PBJ, Joosten FBM, Manni JJ: Sonographic, MR, and CT findings in a large laryngocele: a case report, *Eur J Radiol* 18:45, 1994.
164. Vogl T and others: 3D MR imaging with Gd-DTPA in head and neck lesions, *Eur Radiol* 1:151, 1991.
165. Vogl TJ and others: MR diagnosis of head and neck tumors: comparison of contrast enhancement with triple-dose gadodiamide and standard-dose gadopentetate dimeglumine in the same patients, *Am J Roentgenol* 163:425, 1994.
166. Vogl T and others: MR imaging with Gd-DTPA in lesions of the head and neck, *J Otolaryngol* 22:220, 1993.
167. Vogl TJ and others: MRI of the hypopharynx, larynx and neck, *Eur Radiol* 2:391, 1992.
168. Vogler RC, Wippold FJ II, Pilgram TK: Age-specific size of the normal adenoid pad on magnetic resonance imaging, *Clin Otolaryngol* 25:392, 2000.
169. Ward MP and others: Traumatic perforation of the pyriform sinus: CT demonstration, *J Comput Assist Tomogr* 9:982, 1985.
170. Watarai J and others: CT of retropharyngeal lymph node metastasis from maxillary carcinoma, *Acta Radiol* 34:492, 1993.
171. Weissman JL, Curtin HD: Benign erosion of laryngeal cartilage: report of two cases, *Am J Neuroradiol* 11:1215, 1990.
172. Williams JL, Capitanio MA, Turtz MG: Vocal cord paralysis: radiologic observations in 21 infants and young children, *Am J Roentgenol* 128:649, 1977.
173. Wippold FJ II, Balfe D: *Postoperative pharynx.* In Gore RM, Levine MS, editors: *Textbook of gastrointestinal radiology*, 2 ed, Philadelphia, 2000, WB Saunders.
174. Wolff SD, Balaban RS: Magnetization transfer contrast (MTC) and tissue water proton relaxation in vivo, *Magn Reson Med* 10:135, 1989.
175. Yousem DM, Hurst RW: MR of cervical lymph nodes: comparison of fast spin-echo and conventional spin-echo T2W scans, *Clin Radiol* 49:670, 1994.
176. Yousem DM, Sack MJ, Scanlan KA: Biopsy of parapharyngeal space lesions, *Radiology* 193:619, 1994.
177. Yousem DM and others: Head and neck neoplasms: magnetization transfer analysis, *Radiology* 192:703, 1994.
178. Yousem DM, Tufano RP: Laryngeal imaging, *Magn Reson Imaging Clin North Am* 10:451, 2002.
179. Zeiberg AS and others: Helical (spiral) CT of the upper airway with three-dimensional imaging: technique and clinical assessment, *Am J Roentgenol* 166:293, 1996.
180. Zinreich SJ: Imaging in laryngeal cancer: computed tomography, magnetic resonance imaging, positron emission tomography, *Otolaryngol Clin North Am* 35:971, 2002.
181. Zoarski GH and others: Head and neck: initial clinical experience with fast spin-echo MR imaging, *Radiology* 188:323, 1993.
182. Zoarski GH and others: Multicenter trial of gadoteridol, a nonionic gadolinium chelate, in patients with suspected head and neck pathology, *Am J Neuroradiol* 14:955, 1993.

CHAPTER EIGHTY NINE

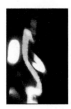

NEUROLOGIC EVALUATION
OF THE LARYNX AND THE PHARYNX

Gayle Ellen Woodson
Andrew Blitzer

INTRODUCTION

The upper aerodigestive tract serves the diverse purposes of breathing, eating, and communicating. These activities require some orthogonal functions. For example, pharyngeal patency should be maintained during respiration, but the pharynx should be forcibly constricted during swallowing. In addition, the anatomic structure of the upper aerodigestive tract is precarious, with ingested food and inspired air traversing the same space. Precise coordination of motor activity and appropriate response to sensory feedback are essential for normal function. Neurologic disorders may impair upper aerodigestive tract function by diverse mechanisms, including motor weakness, incoordination, or impairment of sensation.[16,25]

The diagnosis of disorders in patients with neurologically impaired function of the upper aerodigestive tract often is elusive, particularly when the problem is isolated to that region. This is because the ability of the throat and larynx to function cannot be directly observed. Patients with complaints of hoarseness, dysarthria, dysphagia, aspiration, or airway obstruction often are seen by otolaryngologists, whose training emphasized morphologic rather than functional evaluation. Neurologists, whose forte is functional assessment, generally confine their evaluations to structures that are more accessible, such as limbs. If the anatomy is normal and if no functional deficit is noted in a traditional neurologic examination, a patient who actually has a neurologic impairment often is incorrectly assumed to have a functional or psychiatric disorder. Thus, the diagnosis of a generalized neurologic disorder, such as myasthenia gravis or amyotrophic lateral sclerosis (ALS), may be delayed until the disease process is more widespread and apparent. As a result, patients may receive well-intentioned but ineffective therapy instead of potentially effective treatment.[8,28,34]

In patients whose neurologic diagnosis has been established, assessment of laryngeal and pharyngeal function is an important component and may be life saving. Optimal treatment and rehabilitation of patients with swallowing, speech, or phonation disorders requires identification of the precise pathophysiology of the problem so appropriate therapy may be designed.

The diagnosis of neurologic impairment of the upper airway requires an awareness of the possibility of neural dysfunction, familiarity with the signs and symptoms of neural dysfunction, and a systematic approach to the examination of the throat and pharynx. Box 89-1 lists some symptoms that suggest neurologic impairment. The patient's interests are best served by the collaborative efforts of the otolaryngologist, who is highly skilled in visualizing the throat and larynx, and the neurologist, who is knowledgeable in the pathophysiologic processes. This chapter reviews normal physiology and salient features of specific neurologic diseases that affect function, outlines the approach to the history and physical examination of these patients, and discusses how ancillary tests may be useful.

NORMAL FUNCTION

Phylogenetically, the most important function of the larynx is protective; the larynx prevents ingested food and drink from entering the lungs. To fulfill this role in humans, the larynx should be open during breathing and tightly closed during swallowing. Phonation is a more advanced evolutionary function. Glottic closure during forced exhalation results in an effective cough to clean the lungs and prevent atelectasis. Laryngeal closure is required to generate positive intrathoracic pressure for defecation, childbirth, and lifting heavy objects and for the stabilization of the thorax. The larynx also seems to play a sophisticated role in controlling airflow and pressure during breathing. The vocal folds open just before respiration and close gradually, during exhalation, braking expiratory

SYMPTOMS SUGGESTING NEUROPATHOLOGY

Speech Problems

Lack of volume
Breathiness
Instability of pitch or volume
Lack of voice inflection
Abnormal resonance
Dysarthria

Swallowing Problems

Oral incompetence
Velopharyngeal incompetence
Inability to initiate a swallow
Aspiration

Breathing Abnormalities

Fluctuating inspiratory stridor
Weak breathy cough
"Gurgly" breathing noises

airflow and thereby influencing the rate of breathing. The sensory feedback loops that control these respiratory functions of the larynx are not well understood, but it is clear that feedback from a variety of receptors is involved.[9,16,25]

Swallowing is a deceptively simple function. Food prepared in the mouth is ejected into the pharynx and then rapidly propelled downward around the glottis, through the pyriform sinus, and into the esophagus. During the swallow, the same pharynx that remains patent during breathing is responsible for constricting tightly in an organized sequence from top to bottom. Regurgitation into the nose or reflux into the mouth is prevented by actions of the soft palate, tonsillar pillars, and base of the tongue. The larynx is pulled upward and forward, away from the flow of the bolus. This action also decompresses the sphincter between the pharynx and esophagus. Flexion of the epiglottis and closure of the glottis prevent the entry of any errant material into the airway. After this complex and coordinated activity, the cricopharyngeal muscle should be relaxed when the bolus reaches the caudal end of the pharynx to permit passage into the esophagus. If pharyngeal peristalsis is inadequate or if the upper esophageal sphincter is insufficiently opened, residual material in the pharynx could penetrate the airway during the next inhalation. The unique anatomic configuration in humans after infancy renders swallowing more difficult. In all other mammals, the feeding and breathing channels are offered a degree of separation by interdigitation of the epiglottis and uvula. In humans, these structures are sepa-

rated during early development by the descent of the larynx relative to the palate.[18,19,21]

Speech is audible communication that results from phonation, resonance, and articulation. The production of sound (phonation) requires several conditions. Expired airflow and pressure should be sufficient to induce oscillation of the vocal folds. The vocal folds should be appropriately approximated. If they are closed tightly, excessive expiratory force is required, resulting in a strained, harsh voice, or complete aphonia. If the vocal folds are too far apart, increased expiratory airflow volume is required, so that the voice becomes weaker, breathier, or even fades to a whisper. The three-dimensional shape of the vocal fold also is important in imparting favorable aerodynamic features to the glottis. Atrophy of the vocal fold causes concavity in the axial and coronal planes. The former results in incomplete glottal closure, even during tight approximation of the vocal processes. Concavity in the coronal plane results in a convergent airflow tract. Control of length and tension is required to produce normal inflections in pitch and tone. In the absence of such control, the voice may be flat and expressionless, or it may be distorted by uncontrolled pitch breaks. The mucosa of the vocal folds should be supple to permit free vibration. All but the last of these requirements for phonation are susceptible to derangement by neurologic dysfunction.[1,3]

Resonance is the modification of phonation to produce voice. Pure phonated sound as produced by the vocal folds does not sound like a human voice; it is a strident and unpleasant noise. This sound is modified by resonance of the head, neck, and chest so that component frequencies are selectively amplified or dampened. Vocal resonance is largely determined by anatomy, but it also is significantly modulated by motor activity of the pharynx, soft palate, and oral cavity. This principle may be used in speech therapy to achieve stronger voices in patients with impaired function. Certain neurologic disorders, such as ALS, stroke, and Guillain-Barré syndrome, result in altered vocal resonance. The characteristic sound of the voice in patients with these disorders may be a valuable physical sign to aid in early diagnosis.[1,3]

Articulation is the shaping of voice into words by actions of the lips, tongue, palate, pharynx, and larynx and is highly susceptible to neurologic impairment. Whereas dysarthria in children is most often caused by a hearing deficit, acquired dysarthria in adults usually indicates neurologic impairment. Dysarthria may be a result of impaired motor output, such as weakness, paralysis, or incoordination. Dysarthria also may result from cognitive or language defects or from apraxia of speech.[1,3]

IDENTIFICATION OF LESION SITE

The list of neurologic lesions that may impair speech and swallowing encompasses a wide spectrum. It would be difficult for an otolaryngologist to be familiar with every possible disease process, although it is possible to identify symptoms and signs that correlate to abnormal conditions in specific components of the nervous system, and this is a great aid in diagnosis. The types of disorders that may be identified are motor deficits, because sensation is a subjective process that is not readily apparent to the examiner. Although clinical testing techniques of sensation are advancing, it remains true that the clinical signs that are observed and that patients experience are predominantly disruptions of motor acts (Box 89-2). These changes may reflect abnormal sensory feedback and coordination of signal. Therefore, the site of lesion is best identified by the type of motor disruption.[9,28]

Cortical Lesions

Cortical lesions, which may result from strokes, tumors, or trauma, impair memory and the planning and execution of actions. Because of the diffuse and bilateral representation of laryngeal structures in the cortex, cortical lesions, such as those caused by tumors or strokes, do not produce flaccid or spastic paralysis. Some patients experience aphasia or apraxia of speech. Diffuse emboli, such as those that occur after cardiac bypass surgery, may result in sustained abduction, and this may cause aphonia. Inappropriate vocal-fold adduction with inspiration may have the symptom of inspiratory stridor.[11,27]

Extrapyramidal System Defects

Extrapyramidal system defects are characterized by abnormal motor control such as inappropriate or excessive muscle tension, tremor, and involuntary spasmodic muscle contractions. For the otolaryngologist, this translates into such problems as vocal strain, voice arrests, pitch breaks, and pitch instability. The dysfunction may be focal, regional, or generalized. In addition to problems caused by tumors or trauma, the extrapyramidal system also is disrupted by conditions of uncertain etiology such as Parkinson's disease, tremor, and dystonia.[8]

Cerebellar Lesions

Cerebellar lesions impair coordination of motor activities. Patients' problems are generalized rather than focal. "Scanning speech" is regarded as characteristic of cerebellar involvement. Patients also may have vocal strain that sounds somewhat like spasmodic dysphonia, but they always have problems associated with dysarthria. The diagnosis is established by the presence of attendant physical signs such as intention tremors, dysdiadochokinesia, dysmetria, ataxia, and nystagmus.[12]

Brainstem Lesions

Brain stem lesions result in flaccid paralysis. Because of the close proximity of motor nuclei in this area, lesions do not result in isolated involvement of individual cranial nerves. Strokes and tumors of the brainstem produce severe dysfunction related to paralysis of the larynx, pharynx, or tongue and are associated with sensory deficits.[27]

Peripheral Nerve Injuries

Peripheral nerve injuries may result in paralysis and paresis. Until recently, it generally was believed that a specific nerve lesion could be determined by characterizing the position of the paralyzed vocal fold and detecting rotation of the larynx. It is now clear that the traditional terms of vocal-fold position (e.g., intermediate, paramedian, and cadaveric) do not adequately characterize glottic configuration and that the distance of the vocal fold from the midline is not a reliable indicator of lesion site.[29] The effect of an isolated superior laryngeal nerve lesion on the level of

---

BOX 89-2

SIGNS INDICATING LESION SITE

Cortex
Aphasia
Aphonia
Dysarthria
Dysphonia
Stridor

Extrapyramidal System
Vocal strain and pitch breaks
Tremor
Spasmodic movements
Focal, regional, or generalized dystonia

Cerebellar Lesions
Ataxia
Dysmetria
Tremor
Incoordination

Brainstem Lesions
Flaccid paralysis
Never isolated

Peripheral Nerve Lesion
Vagus nerve: flaccid, cadaveric position
Recurrent laryngeal nerve: position variable, partial lesions, and aberrant regeneration common

the vocal fold and rotation of the glottis also is controversial. Some authors report rotation of the glottis to the side of the lesion in patients with unilateral cricothyroid muscle paralysis, although the preponderance of the evidence indicates that the cricothyroid muscle does not appreciably influence the spatial orientation of either the vocal fold or the glottis as a whole. Clinically observed variations in glottal configuration are chiefly determined by the extent of the nerve lesion (complete or incomplete) and the extent and accuracy of nerve regeneration. Recent information on the cricothyroid joint structure indicates that the two cartilages interact in a visor fashion, similar to a bucket handle, with little translational movement. Thus, a unilateral cricothyroid muscle paralysis may decrease the strength of motion along the arc of rotation, but has no differential effect on one vocal fold.[31]

Other Peripheral Processes

Other peripheral processes include myopathies and neuromuscular joint dysfunction. Patients with these problems experience fatigue and weakness, and symptoms depend on the extent of muscle involvement. In general, these result from systemic diseases, such as diabetes.

Diffuse Central Nervous System Lesions

Diffuse central nervous system (CNS) lesions result from specific neurologic disorders, such as multiple sclerosis and ALS, and have a myriad of signs and symptoms.

LARYNGOLOGIC MANIFESTATIONS OF NEUROLOGIC DISEASES

There are a few important generalized neurologic disorders that are characterized by specific patterns of involvement of the larynx and pharynx. In early stages of involvement, patients with these disorders may consult otolaryngologists because symptoms are located in the head and neck region. If the otolaryngologist is aware of these disorders and their involvement patterns, an earlier diagnosis is possible. At any stage of these disease processes, otolaryngologic consultation may be vital to differentiate manifestations of the disease from problems caused by other concurrent disorders and to ensure appropriate management. The neurologic disorders affecting the larynx are best understood when characterized as hypofunctional, hyperfunctional, and mixed.

Hypofunctional
Vocal Fold Paralysis/Paresis

Laryngeal paralysis is most often the result of distal nerve injury in the neck or chest. Possible causes include surgery, trauma, tumors, and aneurysms.

More central disorders that may produce vocal fold paralysis/paresis are syringobulbia, Arnold-Chiari malformations, stroke (including Wallenberg's lateral postmedullary syndrome, PICA occlusion), and other lower motor neuron disorders.

Neuromuscular Junction Disorders

These include myasthenia gravis (MG) and, less commonly, Eaton-Lambert disease. Muscles fatigue quickly with use. The incidence of MG is less than 10 per 100,000 people. Specific patient complaints may vary, depending on the distribution of muscles involved. Many patients have ptosis or double vision, because ocular muscles are most commonly affected. General fatigue is also a frequent complaint. Sometimes the disease is localized to the throat, and patients have difficulty speaking, breathing, or swallowing. Careful examination of the larynx and palate in such patients may reveal fatigue as a result of repetitive movements. For example, asking the patient to repeat "ee-ee-ee" can elicit laryngeal fatigue. Electromyography and an edrophonium (Tensilon) test are used for rapid diagnosis and treatment. Blood testing is used to detect antibodies against acetylcholine. Early detection of this disorder is invaluable, because medical treatment is effective and may be lifesaving.[26,34]

Poliomyelitis

Poliomyelitis is essentially nonexistent today, thanks to vaccination programs. However, there are survivors of polio who experienced postpolio syndrome with a recurrence of motor weakness. The exact cause of postpolio syndrome is unknown, but it is thought that the syndrome may be derived from the natural loss of motor neurons during the aging process. Patients who have recovered from polio function by virtue of a small pool of surviving neurons that sprout to supply expanded numbers of muscle fibers. Thus, these patients are particularly susceptible to the loss of even a small number of neurons. Acute bulbar polio causes pharyngeal and laryngeal paresis but spares the cricopharyngeus muscle. The resulting symptoms are hoarseness, dysphagia, and aspiration. Because the cricopharyngeus retains tone, cricopharyngeal myotomy often is helpful with recent onset of polio; however, in those with postpolio syndrome, the effectiveness of myotomy has not been established.[34]

Myopathies

Examples of myopathies include dermatomyositis, muscular dystrophy, and metabolic myopathies. Dermatomyositis presents with dermatitis in conjunction with muscle weakness. This disorder may be associated with lung cancer, lupus, or poliomyelitis. The muscular dystrophies vary in age of onset and anatomic distribution of involvement. The infantile variety often presents with oculopharyngeal weakness. Metabolic myopathies may result from abnormalities in acid maltase, brancher enzyme, and cytochrome *c*-oxidase. There are also some episodic myopathies with periodic paralysis that are drug induced.

Medullary Disorders

Medullary disorders that affect motor neurons include ALS, primary lateral sclerosis, postpolio syndrome, Arnold-Chiari malformations, and medullary strokes. ALS (also known as Lou Gehrig's disease) is an idiopathic and progressive degeneration of upper and lower motor neurons and results in muscle wasting, fasciculations, and weakness. Incidence in the United States has been estimated at 1 to 2 per 100,000 people. As many as 25% of these patients initially have complaints related to speech and swallowing. In many patients, limb symptoms predominate. The clinical course varies in its rate of progression, but it is inevitably downhill. Approximately 25% of patients survive from 5 to 10 years after the onset of the disease. Death most often is related to respiratory insufficiency caused by weak breathing muscles and aspiration pneumonia. Therefore, prognosis for a more rapid demise is increased in patients with throat involvement.[7]

When ALS involves the upper airway, the voice is monotonous and raspy with abnormal hypernasal resonance. Speech is commonly dysarthric and labored and has velopharyngeal incompetence. The dysarthria is related to tongue involvement. Patients have slurred speech as a result of weakness and slowed activity of the tongue. The tongue often has visible fasciculations. There also is weakness in the palate, pharynx, and larynx, and there is an inability to make rapid muscle adjustments or repetitive motions. Secretions pool in the hypopharynx, and aspiration often occurs during swallowing. Certain characteristics distinguish ALS from myasthenia gravis. Symmetric facial weakness is common in patients with ALS, although extraocular motion is preserved. This contrasts with the proclivity of myasthenia to involve the eyelids and extraocular muscles. ALS results in muscle wasting and fasciculations that are most easily observed in the tongue and the intrinsic muscles of the hand. Tongue fasciculations have a classic "bag of worms" appearance.[7,24]

Therapeutic options for patients with ALS are essentially limited to supportive care. In some patients, a palatal-lift prosthesis may improve speech intelligibility and decrease nasal regurgitation during speech. In most patients, nothing can be done to improve speech. Eventually, the only options for avoiding aspiration are nasogastric feeding or gastrostomy. Tracheostomy often is necessary for airway protection and assisted ventilation.[7,24]

The lower motor neuron disorders that affect the laryngopharynx include progressive spinal muscular atrophy (PSMA) and progressive or pseudobulbar palsy (PBP). PBP results from bilateral lesions of the corticobulbar tracts. Patients have muscle spasticity and hyperreflexia of the pharynx, palate, lips, tongue, and larynx. The voice in these patients is harsh, strained, and strangled and may sound like patients with spasmodic dysphonia. These patients are easily distinguished clinically, because they have associated signs of hypernasality and slow labored articulation and emotional lability and subcortical cognitive impairments.

Parkinson's Disease

The criteria for diagnosis of Parkinson's disease require at least two of the following: a resting tremor, rigidity, bradykinesis, and/or a loss of postural reflexes. Parkinson's disease is an extrapyramidal syndrome caused by cell death in the substantia nigra. It may be idiopathic or secondary and caused by drugs, encephalitis, stroke, toxins, tumors, or head trauma. The patients typically have a flat facial expression and abnormal posture. Tremor is often present in the distal parts of the extremities and the lips when patients are at rest. "Pill-rolling" tremor of the hands is typical. Speech abnormalities in Parkinson's disease are nearly universal. This is manifest by defects in articulation and voicing. The patients have a hypokinetic dysarthria (45% of patients) with a reduced range of articulation for linguals and labials. They also have decreased loudness, monopitch, and prosodic insufficiency because of poor air presentation to the vocal apparatus (sound generator) caused by decreased airflow from a bradykinetic bellows mechanism. The vocal folds may be adynamic and/or bowed. On testing, these patients show an increased shimmer and jitter, a decreased harmonic/noise ratio, and a tremor. Less often, patients with Parkinson's disease experience a predominant effect of rigidity of the larynx and produce a strained voice with frequent breaks that are similar to the voice of those with spasmodic dysphonia. Swallowing usually is not noticeably impaired in patients with this syndrome, but patients may drool because of the inability to voluntarily swallow.[8,13,23,35]

Parkinson's disease may also be accompanied by autonomic nervous system dysfunction or failure of supranuclear functions. The Parkinson's plus syndromes include progressive supranuclear palsy (PSP) and multiple system atrophy (MSA). In MSA, there is an autonomic nervous system failure with orthostatic hypotension, impotence, sphincter dysfunction, and anhidrosis. One form of MSA is known as Shy-Drager syndrome. These patients have failure of vocal fold abduction with inspiration, which is worse during sleep. Many require tracheotomy for maintenance of their airway. The progression of MSA may be rapid and lead to death.[8]

Psychogenic, Malingering, and Mixed

Psychiatric voice disorders can mimic all of the preceding and hence are very difficult to distinguish from neurogenic voice disorders. Complete aphonia is most often due to a conversion disorder.

Hyperfunctional Disorders
Dystonia

This is a movement disorder that involves uncontrolled contractions of any voluntary muscle group of muscles and results in torsional posture or repetitive movements. The clinical signs are varied and depend on the specific muscles involved and on whether the contractions are continuous or intermittent. Dystonias may be focal, regional, or generalized, and they are classified as primary (idiopathic) or as a result of injury, toxicity, stroke, tumor, or a variety of hereditary neurologic syndromes. Idiopathic dystonia is not associated with any other neurologic abnormality. Therefore, the discovery of any other neurologic signs should prompt a thorough investigation for an underlying abnormal condition.[8]

Spasmodic dysphonia seems to be an idiopathic focal dystonia of the larynx. Patients with more generalized dystonia that also involves the larynx have vocal dysfunction, which is clinically indistinguishable from idiopathic spasmodic dysphonia. Meige's syndrome is a regional dystonia of the head and neck and may be evident in those with blepharospasm, oromandibular dystonia, torticollis, or spasmodic dysphonia. Laryngeal dystonia usually results in spasmodic closure of the vocal folds during speech, which in turn results in a strained and strangled voice or adductor dysphonia. Fewer patients have abductor dysphonia, with intermittent or sustained opening of the larynx during speech.[5] Abductor dysphonia causes breathy voice breaks or a whispering voice. Another form of laryngeal dystonia is adductor breathing dystonia, in which patients adduct their vocal cords while inspiring. This causes stridor and dyspnea, but these patients do not become hypoxic and do not need tracheostomy. Localized injection of botulinum toxin into involved muscles is an effective way to decrease the symptoms of patients with dystonia, particularly for patients with adductor spasmodic dysphonia.[1,4,6,22,30]

Pseudobulbar Palsy

Pseudobulbar palsy results from bilateral lesions of the corticobulbar tracts. Patients have muscle spastic-ity and hyperreflexia of the pharynx, palate, lips tongue, and larynx. The voice in these patients is harsh, strained, and strangled, and it sounds somewhat like those with spasmodic dysphonia. These patients are easily distinguishable clinically, because they have associated signs of hypernasality and slow, labored articulation and emotional lability and subcortical cognitive impairments.[27]

Myoclonus

Oculopalatolaryngopharyngeal myoclonus is an uncommon disorder consisting of rhythmic contractions of the soft palate, pharynx, and larynx at a rate of one or two contractions per second.[10] This condition may affect only the palate or all of the laryngopharynx, and even eyes, and is caused by a lesion in the central tegmental tract. It may result in a speech that sounds like a choppy voice with intermittent hypernasality. The palate and vocal folds may be treated with injections of botulinum toxin to decrease the severity of the contractions, and thereby decrease the symptom.

Essential Tremor

This disorder is a common neurologic disorder affecting those in middle to late adulthood. It causes a 6- to 8-Hz shaking of the hands, head titubation, and a tremulous voice. The vocal symptoms are related to tremor in the muscles in the larynx, pharynx, soft palate, and the strap muscles of the neck. Most patients with essential tremor are treated with systemic agents; however, in our experience, the voice tremor does not respond well. Injections of botulinum toxin may be very useful in controlling the symptom. The toxin does not eliminate the tremor but decreases the amplitude, thereby decreasing the severity of the symptom. Tremor commonly accompanies spasmodic dysphonia and other focal dystonias.[8]

Muscle Tension Dysphonia

In this disorder, which is functional, a patient postures their vocal folds. This hyperfunction causes tightness and dysphonia, with harshness, breathiness, choppy vocal production, or tremor. The patients are best treated with speech therapy to have the patients use their voice in a less-strained manner.

Mixed Disorders
Multiple Sclerosis

Multiple sclerosis is a diffuse demyelination process, with an incidence of approximately 3 per 100,000 people in the United States. The signs and symptoms are protean but basically consist of relapsing and remitting sensory and motor deficits. Visual problems, numbness, and limb weakness are common. As many as 50% of patients with multiple sclerosis have problems that lie in the domain of the otolaryngologist. These problems include vertigo, tremor, scanning speech, and dysphagia. The clinical course in some patients is intermittent and slowly progressive, whereas others experience a rapid and inexorable decline. Recently, there have been some promising developments in experimental drug therapy.[34]

Parkinson's Disease

Some patients with parkinsonism have hyperfunctional voice symptoms, with a strained and strangled voice.

NEUROLOGIC EXAMINATION OF THE MOUTH, LARYNX, AND PHARYNX

Listening to the patient is the first step of the examination in the voice patient. Often, it is possible within minutes to make a working diagnosis on the basis of the sound of the voice and the patient's description of the problem. The patient should be questioned carefully about vocal fatigue, pain with speaking, increased effort required for speech, glottal tightness, pitch breaks, and tremor.

The standard neurologic examination does not address the relatively inaccessible regions that are familiar to the otolaryngologist. The following protocol is suggested as a systematic approach to detecting neurologic dysfunction. The objectives are to assess the integrity of the lower cranial nerves and to seek signs of CNS disorders.[1]

Oral Cavity

Observe the lips, palate, and tongue for abnormal spontaneous movement. Spasmodic motions are characteristic of Meige's syndrome. Involuntary, slow, athetoid movements of the tongue occur in patients with tardive dyskinesia, which usually is a reaction to a major tranquilizer. A quivering, "bag of worms" appearance indicates fasciculations, a characteristic sign of ALS. Assess range of motion, strength, and symmetry of the mouth and palate muscles as usual. Ask the patient to purse his or her lips, to protrude his or her tongue and move it from side to side, and to open his or her mouth and say the traditional "ah" to test for palate motion and symmetry. The best way to assess tongue strength is to have the patient push his or her tongue against the buccal mucosa while the physician palpates the cheek externally.[1]

It is important to test not only the strength but also the central control of lip and tongue muscles. Rapid repetition of the syllable /Pa/ shows lip function. A healthy person is able to maintain a regular rhythm at a rapid rate. A lower motor neuron lesion decreases

the strength of this action. Upper motor neuron involvement decreases the rate at which the patient can repeat the syllable, but regular rhythm should be preserved. In patients with cerebellar dysfunction, the rhythm is erratic. Myasthenia gravis involvement results in fatigue with repetitive motion. Other syllables address other muscle groups. "Ta" tests the tip of the tongue, and "ga" tests the posterior tongue.[1]

Flexible Laryngoscopy

Neurologic function of the larynx is difficult to assess without the use of flexible laryngoscopy. This technique permits observation during quiet breathing and during a variety of tasks. The addition of a video camera is invaluable, because it produces an enlarged image on the monitor that may be recorded for detailed evaluation and saved for comparison with future evaluations.[32,33]

Attention is first directed to the soft palate. With the scope in the posterior choana, the soft palate is observed for any tremor or spasmodic movement at rest. The patient is instructed to swallow and say "kitty cat." These tasks show the symmetry and competence of velopharyngeal closure.[32,33]

The scope then is advanced to visualize the base of the tongue. Alternating phonation of /ee/ and /ah/ should result in first anterior and then posterior movement of the tongue. Assessment of the pharynx is more difficult, because during a normal swallow, the view through the flexible scope is totally obscured. In those with pharyngeal paralysis or paresis, closure is impaired, and impairment of motion on the involved side often may be detected. Pooling of secretions in the hypopharynx is indicative of poor swallowing function, which could be attributed to either sensory or motor impairment.[32,33]

The most detailed assessment is focused on the larynx. During quiet breathing, the vocal folds may appear motionless and partially abducted, but there usually is abduction just before inspiration and gradual adduction during exhalation. The degree of motion varies with the respiratory effort and with the degree of upstream resistance. With deep inspiration, the vocal folds abduct widely. During panting, the vocal folds remain fixed in an abducted position. Nasal breathing in most patients offers more resistance than mouth breathing, so the range of vocal fold movement usually is greater with the mouth closed.[32,33]

A vigorous voluntary cough is a good way to assess the strength and range of motion of the larynx. The vocal folds abduct during the inspiratory phase, close tightly for the compressive phase, and then suddenly open widely. The cough is a useful way to differentiate psychogenic stridor from true bilateral laryngeal paralysis.[32] During phonation, the vocal folds should adduct smoothly and symmetrically. Recurrent laryngeal nerve paralysis usually may be diagnosed by observing the vocal folds during breathing and phonation, although paresis may only become evident if the patient performs repetitive brief phonations. Repetitive phonations also will reveal fatigue in patients with MG. To assess the cricothyroid muscle, which is innervated by the superior laryngeal nerve, the patient is asked to perform a pitch glide, phonating from a low pitch to a high pitch and back down. The pitch should rise as the vocal folds become longer and thinner.[32,33]

It is sometimes difficult to differentiate a functional or psychiatric voice problem from a neurologic disorder. It is helpful if the physician is familiar with characteristic distortions of the larynx in hyperfunctional dysphonia. Some common distortions are compression of the glottis in the anteroposterior dimension, contraction of the aryepiglottic folds, and false vocal-fold adduction, which may be severe enough to totally obscure the true vocal folds. These patients also characteristically elevate the larynx and speak with a low lung volume. Such dysfunction usually is amenable to voice therapy. It is important to remember that neurologic and functional conditions commonly coexist, and some patients may use hyperfunction to compensate for a neurologic defect.

Video recording of the endoscopy may enhance the examination, because the record can be reviewed repeatedly or viewed by other consultants. An objective record also is provided for monitoring the progress of the disorder or the patient's response to therapy. Transoral telescopic laryngoscopy with a rigid-rod quartz lens system provides a clear, magnified view of the larynx. This is the best technique for demonstrating laryngeal morphology and documenting even minute laryngeal lesions. The use of the telescope has limitations. The patient's mouth should be open with anterior traction on the tongue, although this position prevents examination of the larynx during speech or swallowing. The examination also requires topical anesthesia in many patients.[32,33]

The stroboscope provides a flashing light to simulate a slowed vocal-cord vibration. The stroboscope has a microphone to sense the fundamental frequency of the vibrations and to coordinate the flashing light to the same frequency. If the light flashes at the fundamental frequency, the stroboscope will freeze one image in the vibratory cycle. The slowed motion allows the most accurate assessment of the mucosal wave, which may be impaired by scarring, edema, or subtle defects in the mucosa. Lesions such as subtle edema, vocal cord cysts, or early carcinoma may be best seen as an adynamic segment of the vocal cord

on stroboscopy. Stroboscopy also allows accurate evaluation of the closing and opening pattern of the larynx and may be able to indicate the probable underlying cause of a faulty closure. Probable causes that can be detected with a stroboscope include vocalis muscle atrophy, posterior laryngeal edema, and faulty vocal technique. The stroboscope has limitation in patients in whom an unstable voice will not allow for a steady frequency to slow motion. This occurs in patients with vocal cord paralysis or vocal cord scarring and in some patients with spasmodic dysphonia.[15]

ANCILLARY TESTS
Acoustic Analysis

Voice is not a simple sine wave; rather it is a complex group of waves of varying frequency. In a pure periodic waveform, all frequencies above the fundamental frequency (f_0) are multiples of f_0 called harmonics. Lack of periodicity is perceived as noise and described as frequencies between the harmonics. A Fournier analysis is a computational method of simplifying complex waveforms into component parts. Transmission of sound through the vocal tract with its characteristic resonant properties alters the sound by enhancing the resonant frequencies. An acoustic analysis generally measures f_0, perturbation (shimmer [loudness] and jitter [pitch]), and spectral analysis.[3]

Aerodynamic Assessment

Phonation is a function not only of the vocal muscles but also of the respiratory system. Measurements of airflow and air pressure provide important information regarding airway dynamics. One important measurement is the maximum phonation time or the maximum time that a patient can sustain a vowel after a maximum inhalation. This is technically not an aerodynamic measurement, because it measures time and not airflow or pressure. Phonatory and respiratory airflow can be easily measured directly and are useful in monitoring the effects of therapy. Accurate interpretation of airflow data requires concurrent measurement of subglottic pressure—the driving force for phonation. Direct measurement of subglottic pressure requires invasive procedures, such as transglottic placement of a transducer or tracheal puncture. More commonly, phonatory subglottic pressure is estimated from measures of intraoral pressure during repetitions of the syllable /pi/.

Other means of assessing aerodynamic ability include body plethysmography (measurements of chest wall movement), spirometry, and airflow measurement with a hot wire anemometer (to determine rapid changes in airflow).[3,17]

Photoglottography and Electroglottography

Photoglottography and electroglottography are important tools for the neurolaryngologist. Photoglottography is performed by shining a light on the larynx. The amount of light that passes through the glottis is proportional to the size of the glottic opening. The light transmission may be measured by a photosensor overlying the subglottic neck skin. Electroglottography is a technique based on a change in electrical resistance and related to movement of the vocal cords. Low-voltage electrical current is applied through surface electrodes that have been placed on the skin over the thyroid alae. The electrodes then measure a change in the electrical resistance that is representative of the surface area of contact of the vocal folds. Changes in the electroglottography amplitude and duration of the opening-and-closing phase may characterize abnormal function. The electroglottography suggests an abnormal condition by variance from normal rather than by a pathognomonic sign.[3,14]

Electromyography

Electromyography (EMG) has been available for many years and is a well-established means of assessing function in limb and facial muscles, although the use of EMG in the larynx has not been widespread. There may be technical difficulties caused by electrode placement and recording from very small muscles. Spontaneous EMG signals may be analyzed to assess resting activity and the interference pattern, which is the summation of individual motor units during voluntary muscle contraction. Evoked EMG is not a practical clinical test, because it is difficult to locate and selectively stimulate the motor nerves. Kinesiologic analysis quantifies muscle activation across tasks to study motor control. This is primarily a research tool, because it is a complex technique.[20]

The most common application of laryngeal EMG is the assessment of laryngeal nerve integrity, which differentiates between recurrent laryngeal nerve paralysis and mechanical fixation of the vocal fold. EMG also is used to detect lesions of the superior laryngeal nerve. EMG is essential in the preoperative examination of a patient for a laryngeal reinnervation procedure. A muscle that is not denervated will not accept a donor nerve. Clinical experience has shown that the results of EMG often are inconclusive. When a nerve is completely severed, voluntary activation of the muscle is abolished. After 2 weeks, fibrillation potentials may appear, but they are difficult to detect, because the muscle is so small and because there is competing noise from neighboring muscles. In such patients, recovery is extremely unlikely, and early surgical intervention is prudent. Most patients with recurrent laryngeal nerve paralysis do not have electrical silence, because the lesion was not complete or because reinnervation has occurred. The voluntary interference pattern may seem normal, despite the lack of observable motion. In patients in whom the interference pattern is reduced or in whom polyphasic action potentials are detected, a nerve lesion can be diagnosed with certainty, although the likelihood of recovery cannot be predicted. If the nerve regenerates synkinetically so that nerve fibers do not connect with the functionally appropriate muscles, the vocal fold may remain immobile despite recovery of a vigorous interference pattern. In some patients, synkinesis may be detected during EMG when muscles contract during inappropriate phases of respiration. For example, EMG is useful if there is increased contraction of the posterior cricoarytenoid muscle during expiration or if there is activation of the thyroarytenoid or lateral cricoarytenoid muscles predominantly during inspiration.

An important clinical use of laryngeal EMG is in the treatment of spasmodic dysphonia. It is used to localize muscles for injection of botulinum toxin.[20] Laryngeal EMG makes use of standard equipment. Recording is most easily accomplished by the percutaneous placement of concentric bipolar needles. For short-duration recording to verify nerve integrity, this is sufficient. Hooked-wire electrodes are more difficult to place, but they will remain at a fixed site in the muscle during various motor tasks. Electrodes also may be placed transorally. The stability of signal afforded by hooked wires is essential for prolonged or quantitative recording such as that used in kinesiologic analysis. Local anesthesia of the skin may be used to minimize discomfort, but care should be taken to ensure that the anesthetic does not diffuse into underlying muscles.[20]

The thyroarytenoid muscle, supplied by the recurrent laryngeal nerve, is most commonly sampled because of its accessibility. The needle is introduced between the thyroid and cricothyroid cartilages and directed superiorly. One approach is to enter the subglottic air space in the midline and then to divert the needle into the right or left vocal fold. This frequently stimulates coughing, because sensory receptors in the vocal fold mucosa are activated. An alternative approach is to enter the cricothyroid space off the midline so the muscle may be entered without violating mucosa. To verify needle location, the patient is asked to phonate. The thyroarytenoid muscle is normally active throughout phonation. A brief burst of activity at the onset of phonation followed by relaxation is characteristic of lateral cricoarytenoid activity. Either muscle may be activated by inspiration. Patients may have abnormal patterns of activation, which may complicate interpretation of the signal.[20]

The cricothyroid muscle is more difficult to test, because it is a small muscle in close proximity to the larger strap muscles. The authors' favorite technique is to insert the needle in the midline, down to the superior edge of the cricoid cartilage. The tip of the needle is then "walked" over the cartilage, superiorly and laterally. There usually is a palpable pop as the needle enters the cricothyroid muscle. To verify needle placement, the patient is asked to begin phonating at a comfortable pitch and then glide to a higher, falsetto pitch. The cricothyroid may be active or silent at the comfortable pitch, but it is activated at higher pitches. The cricothyroid may be silent or contract rhythmically with inspiration during quiet breathing. It is recruited with voluntary deep inspiration.[20]

The posterior cricoarytenoid muscle may be sampled to provide confirmatory information about the status of the recurrent laryngeal nerve and particularly to document synkinetic reinnervation. In those with abductor spasmodic dysphonia, EMG localization of the posterior cricoarytenoid also is used to direct the injection of botulinum toxin. The most direct means of electrode placement for this muscle is to rotate the larynx in the axial plane until the posterior cricoid is palpable through the cervical skin. The needle then may be passed down to the cartilage and retracted slightly.[20]

Edrophonium

Edrophonium is important in the diagnosis of MG. When symptoms are confined to the larynx or pharynx, this test may require observation of laryngeal and pharyngeal function before and after edrophonium is administered. To accomplish this, an intravenous tube is started, and the nose is topically anesthetized. The patient is asked to perform repetitive tasks to produce fatigue, and a baseline endoscopic video recording is made. A small test dose of edrophonium is administered, and if there is no adverse reaction, the full test dose is given. The patient is instructed to perform the same tasks, and a repeat recording is made.

Cineradiography

Cineradiography uses a modified barium swallow, and it is useful in assessing pharyngeal function and in planning therapy for patients with swallowing problems. It is most commonly performed with the collaboration of a radiologist and a speech pathologist.

Sensory Assessment

Laryngopharyngeal sensory testing is an exciting new method for evaluating the causes of aspiration. The sensory apparatus may be tested with a pressure-controlled and duration-controlled puff of air delivered to the anterior wall of the pyriform sinus (the area innervated by the superior laryngeal nerve). The air puff is delivered from the internal port of a flexible fiberoptic laryngoscope made especially for this purpose (Pentax Precision Instrument Corporation, Orangeburg, NY). To determine a patient's sensory pressure threshold, air pressure is varied according to the psychophysical method of limits, whereas the duration of the air puff is held constant at 50 ms.

The testing is carried out after a patient has had the opportunity to read a description of apparatus and procedure and has had the chance to feel an air puff on his or her cheek and comment on the sensation. The floor of the nose then is anesthetized with 1% lidocaine with epinephrine at a ratio of 1:100,000. The anesthetic is placed on a cotton-tipped applicator and inserted 1 cm from the nasal vestibule. Next, the flexible laryngoscope is inserted into the nasal passage, and the patient is given a 1-minute rest period to adapt to the laryngoscope and prepare for testing. Testing begins by orienting the patient to the supraglottic stimulus with a suprathreshold stream of air for 5 seconds. After a 15-second rest period, air puffs are presented. Six blocks of stimulus administration trials are given, and a threshold is obtained for each block. One stimulus is presented per trial. Trial duration is approximately 10 seconds with a 10-second intertrial interval. The air puff is administered after a verbal announcement of the beginning of the trial and at a random time from 2 to 8 seconds within the 10-second trial interval. Three blocks of descending pressure stimulus presentations and three blocks of ascending pressure stimulus presentations are randomly ordered for each subject. Within a block, air puffs are presented in sequential steps of 10 test-unit changes (each unit is equivalent to 7.5–10 mm Hg). The steps change from subliminal to supraliminal for ascending blocks and from supraliminal to subliminal for descending blocks. A detection response occurs when the patient raises his or her hand within 2 seconds of actual stimulus presentation. A 30-second rest period separates the blocks. The mean of the lowest detected pressures from the six blocks is used as that patient's sensory threshold. The right and left sides of the pharynx and supraglottic larynx are studied.[2]

SUMMARY

During the past decade, a greater understanding of neurologic disorders of the larynx has led to earlier diagnosis and treatment of these disorders. New technology and the collaboration of neurologists and laryngologists have created a better understanding of the neuromuscular physiologic abnormalities found in patients with motion disorders of the larynx. Because new treatment modalities are available, it is imperative to make accurate neurolaryngologic diagnoses.

REFERENCES

1. Aronson AE: *Clinical voice disorders*, New York, 1985, Thieme.
2. Aviv JE and others: Air pulse quantification of supraglottic and pharyngeal sensation: a new technique, *Ann Otol Rhinol Laryngol* 102:777, 1993.
3. Baken RJ: *Clinical measurements of speech and voice*, Boston, 1987, College-Hill Press.
4. Blitzer A, Brin MF: Laryngeal dystonia: a series with botulinum toxin therapy, *Ann Otol Rhinol Laryngol* 100:85, 1991.
5. Blitzer A and others: Abductor laryngeal dystonia: a series treated with botulinum toxin, *Laryngoscope* 102:163, 1992.
6. Blitzer A and others: The use of botulinum toxin in the treatment of focal laryngeal dystonia (spastic dysphonia), *Laryngoscope* 98:193, 1988.
7. Braun NMT: *Spirometry and flow volume loops.* In Blitzer A and others, editors: *Neurologic disorders of the larynx*, New York, 1992, Thieme.
8. Brin MF and others: *Movement disorders of the larynx.* In Blitzer A and others, editors: *Neurologic disorders of the larynx*, New York, 1992, Thieme.
9. Cooper DM, Lawson W: *Laryngeal sensory receptors.* In Blitzer A and others, editors: *Neurologic disorders of the larynx*, New York, 1992, Thieme.
10. Fahn S, Marsden CD, Van Woert MH: Definition and classification of myoclonus, *Adv Neurol* 43:1, 1986.
11. Gacek RR, Malmgren LT: *Laryngeal motor innervation-central.* In Blitzer A and others, editors: *Neurologic disorders of the larynx*, New York, 1992, Thieme.
12. Gilman S, Kluin KJ: *Speech disorders in cerebellar degeneration studied with positron emission tomography.* In Blitzer A and others, editors: *Neurologic disorders of the larynx*, New York, 1992, Thieme.
13. Hanson DG, Gerratt BR, Ward PH: Cinegraphic observation of laryngeal function in Parkinson's disease, *Laryngoscope* 94:348, 1984.
14. Hanson DG, Gerratt BR, Ward PH: Glottographic measurements of vocal cord dysfunction: a preliminary report, *Ann Otol Rhinol Laryngol* 92:413, 1983.
15. Hirano M: *Stroboscopic examination of the normal larynx.* In Blitzer A and others, editors: *Neurologic disorders of the larynx*, New York, 1992, Thieme.
16. Kirchner JA: The vertebrate larynx: adaptations and aberrations, *Laryngoscope* 103:1197, 1993.
17. Lofqvist A: *Aerodynamic measurements of vocal function.* In Blitzer A and others, editors: *Neurologic disorders of the larynx*, New York, 1992, Thieme.
18. Logemann JA: *Evaluation and treatment of swallowing disorders*, San Diego, 1983, College-Hill Press.
19. Logemann JA: Swallowing physiology and pathophysiology, *Otolaryngol Clin North Am* 21:613, 1988.
20. Lovelace RE, Blitzer A, Ludlow CL: *Clinical laryngeal electromyography.* In Blitzer A and others, editors: *Neurologic disorders of the larynx*, New York, 1992, Thieme.
21. Miller A: Neurophysiological basis of swallowing, *Dysphagia* 1:91, 1986.
22. Miller RH, Woodson GE, Jancovic J: Botulinum toxin in the treatment of spasmodic dysphonia, *Arch Otolaryngol* 113:81, 1987.
23. Ramig LO: *The role of phonation in speech intelligibility: a review and preliminary data from patients with Parkinson's disease.* In Kent R, editor: *Intelligibility in speech disorders: theory, measurements and management*, Amsterdam, 1992, John Benjamins.
24. Ramig LO and others: Acoustic analysis of voice in amyotropic lateral sclerosis: a longitudinal case study, *J Speech Hear Disord* 55:2, 1991.
25. Sasaki CT: *Electrophysiology of the larynx.* In Blitzer A and others, editors: *Neurologic disorders of the larynx*, New York, 1992, Thieme.
26. Schmidt-Nowara W, Marder E, Feil P: Respiratory failure in myasthenia gravis due to vocal cord paresis, *Arch Neurol* 41:567, 1993.
27. Tatemichi TK and others: *Pyramidal disease (strokes).* In Blitzer A and others, editors: *Neurologic disorders of the larynx*, New York, 1992, Thieme.
28. Ward P, Hanson DG, Berci G: Observations on central neurologic etiology for laryngeal dysfunction, *Ann Otol Rhinol Laryngol* 90:430, 1990.
29. Woodson GE: Configuration of the glottis in laryngeal paralysis I & II, *Laryngoscope* 103:1227, 1993.
30. Woodson GE and others: Functional assessment of patients with spasmodic dysphonia, *J Voice* 6:338, 1992.
31. Woodson GE and others: *Unilateral cricothyroid contraction and glottic configuration*, Presented at the Fourth International Phonosurgery Symposium, Philadelphia, June, 1996.
32. Woodson GE and others: Use of flexible laryngoscopy to classify patients with spasmodic dysphonia, *J Voice* 5:85, 1991.
33. Yanagisawa E: *Physical examination of the larynx and videolaryngoscopy.* In Blitzer A and others, editors: *Neurologic disorders of the larynx*, New York, 1992, Thieme.
34. Younger DS and others: *Neuromuscular disorders of the larynx.* In Blitzer A and others, editors: *Neurologic disorders of the larynx*, New York, 1992, Thieme.
35. Zwiner P, Murray T, Woodson GE: Phonatory function of neurologically impaired patients, *J Commun Disord* 24:287, 1991.

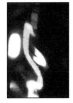

CHAPTER NINETY

INFECTIONS AND MANIFESTATIONS OF SYSTEMIC DISEASE OF THE LARYNX

II   Kim Richard Jones

INFECTIONS OF THE LARYNX

In general, infections of the larynx can be divided into acute and chronic infections. Most significant acute infections occur over a period of less than 7 days, present with airway distress and fever, and are more prevalent and problematic in children than in adults. In contrast, chronic infections generally have existed for weeks before presentation; in addition to airway distress, hoarseness and pain may predominate, systemic factors may be important, and the infections occur more frequently in adults than in children. Examples of chronic laryngeal infections include syphilis, tuberculosis, and various fungi.

The history is often the most important tool in the diagnosis. In acute and chronic infectious processes, the following should be ascertained: (1) the severity and progression of symptoms, especially as related to dyspnea; (2) associated regional or systemic signs and symptoms; and (3) precipitating factors. In acute infections, the critical point is the differentiation between run-of-the-mill viral laryngitis and the more serious diseases of croup and epiglottitis. For chronic infections, it is more important to distinguish infection from malignancy, because the two often appear similar on clinical examination and by history.

Acute Infections
Croup or Laryngotracheitis

Clinical features. *Laryngotracheitis*, or croup, can be defined as a viral illness characterized by fever, "barking" cough, and stridor. Parainfluenza viruses 1 and 2 and influenza A are the most common causes, but croup can also be caused by respiratory syncytial virus, adenovirus, and even enterovirus.[19] Croup usually occurs in the winter and rarely does a child have more than one episode per year. However, some children may have what is termed "spasmodic" or "recurrent" croup, which, as the name implies, occurs multiple times during the year. Spasmodic croup is also characterized by the acute onset of a barking

cough, dyspnea, and stridor, but was initially differentiated from "classic" croup by its recurrent nature, more rapid onset, and lack of fever. Also, spasmodic croup almost always resolves fairly rapidly with use of humidity and reassurance.

Although recurrent croup was initially thought to be allergy related, it is now believed that croup and recurrent croup are more similar than different and probably represent a spectrum of disease.[10] However, from an ear, nose, and throat standpoint, an important distinction should be made in that when a child is seen repeatedly with crouplike symptoms, other diagnoses should be considered, such as gastroesophageal reflux, acquired laryngotracheal stenosis, or congenital abnormalities.[20]

The seriousness of croup is the result of the amount of swelling in the subglottic area that can occur with this disease. The subglottis is the narrowest portion of the respiratory tract in children and is also the only part where a complete cartilaginous ring exists, so that all edema here occurs at the expense of the lumen. Stridor at rest, which is not uncommonly seen in the later stages of croup, does not occur before approximately 80% of the airway is compromised. Thus, it is not hard to imagine that a small increase in the amount of edema at this point, or a mucous plug, could be fatal. This scenario underscores the critical nature of this illness.

Differential diagnosis. The most important differential diagnosis in a child with suspected croup is epiglottitis. Fortunately, their clinical presentations are dissimilar enough that there is usually little trouble differentiating the two. First, patients with croup are usually younger, with a peak incidence at 2 years of age. Second, croup typically presents with a 12- to 72-hour prodrome consisting of cough and low-grade fever, even though patients with epiglottitis usually are seen with rapid onset of high fever, a muffled voice, and dysphagia.

Possible aspiration of a foreign body should be considered if there is rapid onset of respiratory symptoms such as cough and stridor without any viral prodrome. Radiography of the neck and chest can rule this out and may also show the tapered narrowing of the subglottis (steeple sign) that is associated with classic croup. However, the lack of a steeple sign does not rule out croup, because this finding is seen in only 50% of cases.[19] Finally, subglottic stenosis may be seen as recurrent croup. A narrowed subglottic airway, whether it be congenital or acquired, has much less tolerance for the viral edema that accompanies croup; thus, minor laryngotracheal infections, which would pass unnoticed in a healthy child, will cause the child with subglottic stenosis to become stridulous. Thus, a history of recurrent croup or a history of previous intubation is important to obtain.

Management. Historically, children with croup have been treated with humidified air, either from a humidifier or a steam shower. The presumed effect is to soothe the inflamed mucosa of the subglottis and liquefy secretions to allow expectoration.[62] Although there is strong anecdotal evidence that humidification helps, the two small studies that have looked at its effects showed no significant difference between treatment and nontreatment groups. However, as pointed out by Brown,[10] both studies had small numbers of patients, leaving open the possibility that a true difference may have been missed (beta error). Thus, the role of humidification is unclear at this point.

Racemic epinephrine is often given by way of a nebulizer to those children who are in some respiratory distress. It may be given with or without corticosteroids (see later), depending on the level of distress. Its effects are thought to be due to vasoconstriction of the airway mucosa and subsequent decrease in edema.[19] A number of clinical studies have demonstrated its efficacy.[10] Although initially it was thought that any child who required epinephrine treatment required overnight hospitalization because of a possible "rebound" effect, further research has shown that this rarely occurs.[10,19,62] It is now recommended that patients who require nebulized epinephrine be monitored in the emergency department for 3 hours, and if they are stable at that time, it is probably safe to discharge them.[10,19,62] Finally, although racemic epinephrine (a mixture of the D and L isomers) is typically used because it was believed that it caused fewer cardiovascular side effects, it has now been shown that the L form, which is cheaper and pharmacologically far more active, is equally effective and has no greater incidence of side effects.[68]

The use of corticosteroids in the management of croup is no longer controversial, although the mechanism of action for their beneficial effects is still unclear. Even though the known antiinflammatory effects of steroids may be important, the relatively rapid onset of action suggests a possible role of vasoconstriction with reduced vascular permeability.[19,62] Although intramuscular dexamethasone was traditionally the preferred route, oral dexamethasone or nebulized budesonide have been shown to be equally effective.[10,19,62] The most common treatment dose is 0.6 mg/kg for dexamethasone (either route) and 2 mg for nebulized budesonide.

When medical management fails, direct airway support through intubation or tracheostomy may be necessary. Indications for such support include rising carbon dioxide levels, a worsening neurologic status, or a decreasing respiratory rate in the face of poor gas exchange. Nasotracheal intubation is the procedure of choice for control of the airway in a child with severe croup. An endotracheal tube one size smaller than normal is used because of the narrowed subglottic airway. Elective extubation may be attempted once the child has become afebrile, secretions have diminished, and an air leak around the tube is present when positive pressure ventilation is given.[43] Most children only require intubation for 2 to 3 days. If a leak has not developed by 5 to 7 days or if a child has failed several attempts at extubation, endoscopy should be performed with consideration of a tracheostomy if significant edema, mucosal ulceration, or granulation tissue is present. If these criteria are followed, the incidence of acquired subglottic stenosis secondary to intubation is less than 3%.[43]

Bacterial Tracheitis

Bacterial tracheitis is a serious pediatric pulmonary infection characterized by signs of acute upper airway obstruction and purulent debris within the tracheal lumen. Especially in its early stages, bacterial tracheitis may be difficult to differentiate from croup, because its most common presenting symptoms are cough and stridor.[5] Patients who are initially seen with a high fever and leukocytosis are somewhat more likely to have tracheitis,[16] but the absence of these signs does not rule out the diagnosis. To further complicate matters, bacterial tracheitis frequently develops as a sequela of croup.[5,39] Soft-tissue lateral radiographs may be helpful, because a thick tracheal membrane may be seen on up to 80% of patients with bacterial tracheitis.[5]

Endoscopy is usually necessary to make the diagnosis. The epiglottis and larynx are normal in appearance, but the trachea is characterized by thick, purulent secretions. It has been suggested that any child with crouplike symptoms who does not improve after several days of medical management or who has a high fever or leukocyte cell count should undergo bronchoscopy to rule out the presence of such secretions.[39] Once the diagnosis is made and cultures obtained, patients with bacterial tracheitis should be started on cefuroxime or some other broad-spectrum antibiotic. Historically, the most common pathogens isolated were *Staphylococcus aureus* and *Haemophilus influenzae*,[15,17] but a more recent study also showed a significant percentage of *Moraxella catarrhalis*.[5]

The decision to intubate is based on the severity of symptoms at the time of bronchoscopy. Although earlier series reported intubation rates >80%,[39] the only large recent series reported a rate of only 57%. Reasons given for the decreased rate were a slightly older patient population, a less-virulent disease presentation, and a greater willingness to manage airway problems expectantly.[5] In addition, no child in the latter series underwent tracheostomy. Finally, although serious sequelae such as toxic shock syndrome, secondary-acquired pneumonia, and acute respiratory distress syndrome (ARDS) have been described secondary to bacterial tracheitis,[8,16] in the large series referenced previously,[5] all children recovered uneventfully.

Pediatric Epiglottitis

The rapid decline of pediatric epiglottitis caused by the development of a vaccine against *H. influenza* type B is well documented.[44,56] In fact, many otolaryngologists may go through their entire residency without ever seeing an example of this disease. However, there are now reports of *H. influenza* epiglottitis in children who have completed their full vaccination schedule.[44] The cause of these vaccine failures is unclear, but their existence underscores the need for otolaryngologists to remain up to date on the presentation and treatment of this life-threatening illness.

Clinical features. The onset of epiglottitis is acute, often in as little as 2 to 6 hours. The child has a high temperature, drools, and sits upright with greater inspiratory than expiratory stridor. A lateral extended soft-tissue radiograph is often diagnostic.

The inflammatory process occurs almost exclusively in the supraglottic larynx; a fiery, cherry-red epiglottis is the most impressive feature. However, aryepiglottic fold and false cord involvement also exist. Respiratory obstruction is probably caused by at least two factors: (1) a swollen epiglottis and aryepiglottic fold with supraglottic narrowing; and (2) excessive, tenacious oral and pharyngeal secretions that accumulate as a result of odynophagia. Sudden respiratory arrest may be caused by mucous plugging of the narrowed supraglottic airway, plugging of the supraglottic larynx during inspiratory efforts, or laryngospasm, to which these infants may be particularly susceptible if examined aggressively. The associated odynophagia from the marked inflammatory supraglottic process helps to distinguish this entity from croup.

Differential diagnosis. Croup and epiglottitis are usually easily distinguishable. As described, the child with epiglottitis classically is seen with a 2- to 6-hour history of stridor, sitting upright, and drooling. The child with croup has a several-day history of prodromal symptoms with worsening stridor and a seal-like (croupy) cough. A foreign body can mimic either condition, depending on its position in the upper respiratory tract.

Medical management. The cornerstone of epiglottitis management is antibiotics. A second- or third-generation cephalosporin, effective against β-lactamase–positive *H. influenza*, is the drug of choice. Ceftriaxone and cefuroxime are good examples. Corticosteroids are also commonly given,[42] although their efficacy has not been scientifically verified as is it has in the treatment of croup.

Airway management. Airway management of a child with suspected epiglottitis begins when the child is seen in the clinic or emergency department. The first step is to notify the otolaryngologist and anesthesiologist on call. Examination of the child is minimal and confined to visual inspection and auscultation of the heart and lungs. The child who is stable may be taken to the radiology department, accompanied by the otolaryngologist or anesthesiologist, for a single soft-tissue lateral radiograph. If a portable film can be taken in the emergency department, that is preferable. The child is then taken to the operating room, where mask induction is performed by the anesthesiologist while the otolaryngologist readies the appropriate laryngoscopes and rigid bronchoscopes. Once an appropriate level of anesthesia has been reached, an intravenous line is started, and preparations are made for intubation. The larynx is visualized, and the diagnosis confirmed. Either nasotracheal or orotracheal intubation is performed, usually with an endotracheal tube one size smaller than would ordinarily be used for the child. The tube is carefully secured and the patient taken to the intensive care unit (ICU). Intubation is usually maintained for 24 to 48 hours. Readiness for extubation is determined by applying positive pressure to the endotracheal tube and listening for an air leak. After extubation, the child is observed in the ICU for 4 to 6 hours and then may be transferred to a medical floor.

The use of a tracheostomy for airway control is of historic interest only. In the most recent large study,

94% of children admitted with epiglottitis were intubated, 6% were observed in the ICU while breathing spontaneously, and none underwent tracheostomy.[56]

Adult Supraglottitis

Supraglottitis in the adult is, in general, a different disease from that in children. The clinical course is less acute, the patients appear less toxic, and airway compromise is less common.[42,60] The most common presenting symptoms are sore throat and dysphagia.[11,60] An elevated leukocyte count is seen in about two-thirds of patients, and blood cultures are almost uniformly negative, unless the infecting organism is *H. influenzae*.[11,60] Cultures of the pharynx are also often negative, but of those that are positive, the most common pathogens are *H. influenzae* and β-hemolytic streptococcus.[11] Lateral soft-tissue neck radiographs may be obtained, but because they have a significant false-negative rate,[11,60] they are not particularly useful.

The preferred method of diagnosis is visualization of the epiglottis and other supraglottic structures. Unlike in children, there have been no reported incidents in adults of indirect laryngoscopy precipitating an airway emergency, so if the patient is not in respiratory distress, it is appropriate for the otolaryngologist to confirm the diagnosis in the emergency department or clinic with either mirror examination or flexible laryngoscopy. The epiglottis may not have the bright cherry-red appearance described in children but rather may be pale, boggy, and edematous. Also, other supraglottic structures, such as the aryepiglottic folds, may be involved.

Treatment depends on the severity of airway symptoms at the time of presentation. Emergent intubation or tracheostomy is rarely indicated in adults, with quoted rates between 9% and 16%.[42,60] However, all patients should be admitted for observation and intravenous antibiotics started after appropriate cultures are obtained. A second- or third-generation cephalosporin, active against ampicillin-resistant *H. influenzae*, is the drug of choice.[11]

Although most adult patients with epiglottis are in no acute distress, there is clearly a subgroup of patients who have a more rapid clinical course and go on to have significant respiratory compromise. Patients who are seen with stridor, tachycardia, or rapid progression of symptoms (<12 hours) are at greater risk to require airway intervention, and most of these patients will have blood cultures positive for *H. influenzae*.[42,60]

An epiglottic abscess is a rare complication of supraglottitis that is seen almost exclusively in adults.[27,60] The most common site of involvement is the lingual surface of the epiglottis, and significant airway obstruction may occur as a result of the expanding abscess and localized tissue edema. The most commonly isolated pathogens are *Streptococcus* and *Staphylococcus* species. Management consists of surgical drainage or admission to an ICU for careful observation and appropriate antibiotic and supportive measures. Recommended antibiotic coverage is the same as that for supraglottitis.

Whooping Cough

Whooping cough, caused by *Bordetella pertussis*, has been reported with increasing frequency in the United States.[2] Originally a disease of childhood, it is now more commonly seen in infants younger than 6 months and in adolescents and adults. Unlike other childhood diseases, such as measles, mumps, and rubella, there is apparently no passive immunity conferred by the mother to the child in utero, so that newborns are susceptible to *B. pertussis* infection until they receive their third immunization shot at 6 months. The reason for the increase in newborn infection is unclear. Widespread immunization for pertussis started in the 1940s, and there is some belief that there have been genetic changes in *B. pertussis* that have made the vaccine less effective. Others wonder if the potency of the vaccine itself has changed. On the other hand, there is evidence that much of the increase is simply because of greater awareness of the disease and better laboratory tests with which to diagnose it.[12] The reason for the increase in adolescents and adults is also unclear. Originally, it was believed that exposure to the natural disease conferred lifelong immunity, even though immunization with the *B. pertussis* vaccine provided a high degree of protection for only 3 years, after which resistance to infection gradually decreased. Thus, as a greater percentage of the population was vaccinated rather than exposed naturally to the disease, there would be more individuals who would become infected as adults. However, it has now been shown that acquiring pertussis naturally does not protect one from future infection any longer than vaccination.[12]

The clinical presentation of pertussis has also changed. Adults may only display a severe and protracted cough,[74] whereas newborns, who usually exhibit the catarrhal stage and subsequent fever and leukocytosis, may or may not exhibit episodes of paroxysmal whooping cough typical of the disease in children. Management is supportive, with frequent suctioning often necessary in infants.

The recommended treatment for pertussis has not changed in more than four decades. Erythromycin, although not changing the clinical course of the disease, causes patients to become noninfectious after 1 or 2 days and also has a clear prophylactic effect on persons who have been exposed to an infected patient but have not become symptomatic.[1] In either case, 50 mg/day of the estolate ester form in four divided doses for 14 days is recommended. Recently, similar results have also been achieved with azithromycin. Simple once-a-day dosing at 10 mg/kg on day 1 followed by 5 mg/kg/day on days 2 to 5 was sufficient to eradicate 97% of positive cultures by day 3 and 100% when tested again 3 to 4 weeks later.[51]

Other Acute Infections of Larynx

Mumps, measles, and chickenpox may cause localized laryngeal and tracheal inflammation. Mucous retention cysts of the larynx or even laryngoceles can become acutely infected, causing airway distress from local obstruction. Usually, indirect examination leads to the diagnosis, although occasionally axial computed tomography may help, especially with a laryngopyocele.

Conditions That May Mimic Acute Laryngeal Infections

In a child, a foreign body should always be considered in the differential diagnosis of acute epiglottitis or croup. In adults, an often overlooked cause of acute hoarseness or stridor is the swelling associated with cricoarytenoid arthritis. This symptom is most commonly seen in patients with rheumatoid arthritis but can also be a manifestation of other connective tissue disorders, such as systemic lupus erythematosus and Reiter's syndrome.[35] Management may include intraarticular injections of corticosteroids and systemic corticosteroids or other immunosupportive agents. The swelling may compromise the airway. Angioneurotic edema may occasionally be considered in the differential diagnosis of acute laryngeal swelling and erythema, but there is usually no associated fever or prodromal symptoms, and this entity is usually accompanied by associated oral, pharyngeal, or neck swelling.

Finally, generalized supraglottitis may also be associated with radiotherapy. However, it is important to know that various chemotherapeutic agents can exacerbate this reaction months to years after the initial management of the larynx with radiotherapy.[69]

Chronic Infections

Patients with chronic laryngeal infections often are seen with a history and symptoms similar to those of laryngeal carcinoma. The patient complains of hoarseness, dyspnea, or pain and may report a history of weight loss and tobacco or alcohol abuse. The diagnostic challenge is to first rule out cancer and then establish the correct diagnosis.

Physical examination is often unrewarding. Diffuse laryngeal edema and erythema may be the only patho-

logic findings, and a noninfectious cause, such as gastroesophageal reflux, must be ruled out. Even if a discrete lesion is visible, it may mimic the appearance of a laryngeal tumor. In the past, this sometimes led to radical surgery for what turned out to be benign disease, such as a total laryngectomy for blastomycosis.[63] On the other hand, an even more dangerous course of action is for the clinician to suspect a benign process without aggressively searching for a possible carcinoma.

Biopsy is thus the cornerstone of an appropriate workup. In addition to sending tissue for the usual tissue stains, the clinician also should send appropriately prepared specimens for special fungal stains, acid-fast bacilli smears, and fungal and acid-fast bacilli cultures. The possibility of sarcoidosis, relapsing polychondritis, and autoimmune disorders should also be considered. If a diagnosis is still not obtained, the patient should be closely observed, and additional biopsies should be done if the symptoms or physical examination changes.

Tuberculosis

Tuberculosis was once the most common disease affecting the larynx.[31,49] In the past, it commonly developed as a sequela of severe pulmonary tuberculosis. However, in the past 20 years, this pattern of involvement has changed, and many patients with laryngeal tuberculosis now are seen without pulmonary symptoms or a history of pulmonary tuberculosis.[31,49,53] Recently, it has been theorized that laryngeal involvement is now more commonly caused by hematogenous or lymphatic spread of the organism.[59] The most common presenting symptom of laryngeal tuberculosis is hoarseness, with a high percentage of patients also reporting dysphagia, odynophagia, cough, and weight loss.[31,49,53] Twenty percent to 40% of patients show no evidence of pulmonary involvement,[49,57] but purified protein derivative is usually positive.[31,48] Almost any area of the larynx can be involved, as well as supraglottic structures such as the aryepiglottic folds and epiglottis.[31,49,57,58] Lesions range from areas of nonspecific inflammation to a nodular, exophytic lesion or mucosal ulcerations.[31,49,57,58] Many patients with laryngeal tuberculosis are older men with a history of tobacco and alcohol use, and because of their history and the appearance of the lesions, some cases of laryngeal tuberculosis were at first thought to represent squamous cell carcinoma.[58] Diagnosis is usually made by the combination of positive sputum samples, characteristic findings on chest radiography, and positive biopsies for acid-fast bacilli. Histopathologic examination of biopsied tissue reveals tubercles consisting of a homogenous caseous center (staining red with eosin), a periphery of pale epithelial cells containing one or more giant cells, and an outer zone of lymphocytes. Management is essentially medical and is dictated by the sensitivities of the organism. Multidrug resistance is a growing problem, both in the United States and especially overseas.

Histoplasmosis

Histoplasmosis is caused by the dimorphic fungus *Histoplasma capsulatum*, which exists as a yeast at normal body temperature. The mycelial form is found in soil with a high-nitrogen content, such as is provided by large amounts of bird or bat feces. Endemic regions include the Ohio and Mississippi River valleys, where 80% to 90% of the population may be infected. Infection is through inhaled spores. The disease may present as an acute pulmonary infection or a more indolent disseminated form. In most cases of pulmonary histoplasmosis, the inoculum is usually small, in which case the patient is asymptomatic and spontaneous recovery occurs. Occasionally, a large inoculum will produce a symptomatic illness whose symptoms are fever, malaise, weight loss, and a nonproductive cough. Again, this is usually self-limited and requires no specific treatment. However, patients who have had either of the forms of pulmonary histoplasmosis may show small residual calcifications of the lungs and spleen.

The disseminated form of histoplasmosis occurs primarily in immunocompromised individuals such as patients with human immunodeficiency virus (HIV) and in those immunosuppressed because of organ transplant. It may manifest itself as an acute, subacute, or chronic illness. The acute form is rapidly progressive and often fatal. The subacute form presents with a less severe clinical picture and is associated with meningitis, endocarditis, hepatosplenomegaly, and anemia. It is the form most commonly seen in patients with HIV, and is an acquired immune deficiency syndrome (AIDS)–defining illness. Chronic disseminated disease has minimal systemic manifestations and tends to present as focal destructive lesions.

Otolaryngologic involvement has been reported to be 66% in chronic disseminated histoplasmosis, 33% in subacute, and 20% in acute.[25] However, because the acute form is usually rapidly fatal, most patients seen by the otolaryngologist have the subacute or chronic form of the disease. Mucosal ulcers of the upper aerodigestive tract (including the larynx) are the most common ear, nose, and throat manifestation. These lesions begin as flat, plaquelike nontender elevations or nodules that later ulcerate and become painful.[24] These ulcers may be found on any part of the larynx and may be mistaken for carcinoma or tuberculosis.[15,52] The diagnosis of laryngeal histoplasmosis can be somewhat difficult. The histologic appearance depends on the degree of immune responsiveness and may show chronic inflammation, granuloma formation, and even pseudoepitheliomatous hyperplasia.[4] However, multiple small calcifications on chest radiography are almost pathognomonic, and the intracellular yeast buds may be seen with periodic acid–Schiff (PAS) or silver stains. A complement fixation test for histoplasmosis can be useful if high titers are seen.[15] Treatment is typically intravenous amphotericin B, 0.3 to 0.6 mg/kg/day, up to a total dose of 2 to 4 g. Oral antifungals such as fluconazole and itraconazole have also been tried with some success.

Blastomycosis

Blastomycosis is caused by *Blastomyces dermatitidis,* a dimorphic fungus that is a natural soil saprophyte and is found throughout the United States. The mode of infection is presumed to be inhaled spores, and the lung is the most common site of involvement. Other organ systems are infected secondarily through hematogenous spread. The skin is by far the most common extrapulmonary site, followed at some distance by larynx and bone.[54] Although the larynx is infrequently affected, blastomycosis is important, because its appearance can mimic a neoplastic process, such as verrucous or squamous carcinoma (Figure 90-1). Several patients have been documented as having undergone surgery or radiation for squamous cell

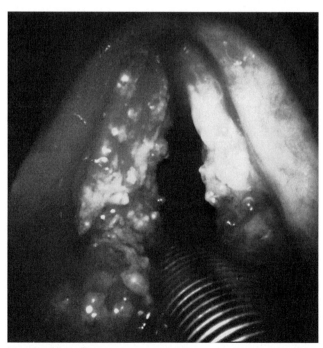

Figure 90-1. Blastomycosis of the larynx. A laser endotracheal tube is seen at the bottom, passing between the vocal cords. (Courtesy of Mark Weissler, M.D.)

carcinoma of the larynx when later review of their pathologic condition showed blastomycosis.[63]

Patients with laryngeal blastomycosis typically have hoarseness as their chief complaint.[46,54] Laryngoscopy typically shows scattered granular, exophytic masses, although ulcerative changes have also been noted. The true cords are by far the most commonly involved site, often with extension onto the false cords. Despite a presumed pulmonary route of infection, chest radiography of patients with laryngeal blastomycosis is usually normal.[46] Diagnosis is by biopsy, with acute and chronic inflammation, microabscesses, and giant cells being seen. However, the most important histologic finding is pseudoepitheliomatous hyperplasia, which can occasionally be misread as indicative of a neoplastic process. Fungal stains, such as PAS or Gomori stain, will almost invariably show the organism in its yeast form: a double-walled sphere 8 to 15 mm in diameter with single broad-based buds. The standard management is intravenous amphotericin B, given daily up to a total dose of 25 to 35 mg/kg. Ketoconazole or itraconazole, each taken daily for several months, have also been shown to be effective.[46]

Cryptococcosis

Cryptococcus neoformans is a budding yeast that is found in bird droppings and the surrounding soil. Human infection is through inhaled spores, and the resultant pulmonary disease is frequently mild, transitory, and unrecognized. However, hematogenous spread may subsequently occur, especially in immunocompromised patients, and the central nervous system becomes affected, resulting in meningitis, cranial nerve palsy, and the like. Most cases of laryngeal cryptococcus are seen in this patient population. However, rare cases of isolated laryngeal involvement have been reported.[30] The true cords are usually the only site affected, and hoarseness is the presenting complaint.[23,30] Findings on endoscopy are an erythematous vocal cord, sometimes with an exudative white lesion. Histologic findings show ovoid budding yeast and sometimes pseudoepitheliomatous hyperplasia. Treatment has ranged from no treatment to amphotericin B to 2 months of fluconazole.[30]

Coccidioidomycosis

Coccidioidomycosis, also called San Joaquin Valley fever, is a fungal disease endemic to the southwestern United States and northern Mexico. Infection is by way of inhaled spores, and the lungs are by far the most common site of involvement. Most long-term residents of endemic regions are exposed, usually as children, and persons traveling through these areas may sometimes acquire the disease. Extrapulmonary spread is rare, and only a few cases of laryngeal involvement have been reported.[7,70] Surprisingly, more than one-half of these cases have been in children.[26] The laryngeal lesions may appear as granulation tissue or ulceration and may cause airway compromise. Histologic findings often show only granulomas and an inflammatory infiltrate, so the diagnosis should be made by use of fungal stains to show the typical coccidioidal spherules filled with numerous endospheres. Management is intravenous amphotericin B.

Actinomycosis

Actinomycosis is an infection caused by any of several species of *Actinomyces*, a gram-positive, filamentous organism that is intermediate between bacteria and fungi. It is a commensal saprophyte of the normal mouth flora and is commonly found in tonsillar crypts and in the gingiva and oral mucosa. It is thought to become a pathogen when some form of trauma allows it to access an anaerobic environment, such as is provided by devitalized tissue, where it rapidly multiplies. The most common site of infection in the head and neck is the oral cavity, but occasional laryngeal infections have been described.[28,48] The presentation in the larynx is similar to that seen elsewhere; localized tissue induration progresses to an ulcer, which, if not managed, will form an abscess. Diagnosis is by histopathologic findings or culture and may be difficult. The presence of pathognomonic "sulfur granules" (actually a conglomeration of *Actinomyces* organisms) is variable, and many commensal microorganisms make identification of individual *Actinomyces* organisms difficult. Culture results are even less likely to confirm diagnosis; the organisms are fastidious, require an anaerobic culture medium, and may take up to 2 weeks to grow. The management of choice is penicillin. For deep-seated infection, intravenous penicillin, 10 to 20 million units/day for 4 to 6 weeks, followed by oral penicillin, 2 to 4 g/day for several months, is recommended. For early, superficial infections, the oral regimen alone may be sufficient. Clindamycin has also been used with some success.[48]

Candidiasis

Laryngeal candidiasis is usually seen as part of a more widespread pattern of disease also involving the oral cavity and esophagus. This clinical picture is typically seen in immunocompromised patients, such as those with AIDS or undergoing chemotherapy. However, isolated laryngeal disease has been reported in immunocompetent individuals.[22,64] Symptoms are hoarseness, pharyngeal discomfort, and dysphagia.[64] The appearance of the larynx in these patients may range from frank mucosal ulcerations and exudate[64] to more subtle findings, such as erythema and leukoplakia of the vocal cords.[22] Laryngeal biopsy with staining for fungi and yeast is often necessary for diagnosis. The most recently recommended treatment is fluconazole, 100 mg daily for 1 month.[22] Candida is also the most common organism cultured from tracheoesophageal voice prostheses. Its presence can cause early breakdown of the prosthesis. Recommended treatment is application of a miconazole gel, although there is some concern that resistance may be developing to this antifungal.[3]

Syphilis

Syphilis is an infectious disease caused by the spirochete *Treponema pallidum*. Most cases are acquired through sexual contact, although congenital syphilis has been described. Acquired syphilis may present in a primary, secondary, or tertiary form. The primary presentation is a painless ulcer or chancre at the point of primary contact, usually on the genital, oral, or anal mucosa. It usually heals in a few weeks. Secondary lesions may appear as the primary lesion is resolving and can present on any cutaneous or mucosal surface, most commonly as widespread erythematous plaques or nodules. The disease then becomes dormant for years to decades, until the gummatous lesions typical of tertiary-stage syphilis appear in almost any tissue of the body. These lesions are composed of granulomatous nodules containing plasma cells, lymphocytes, epithelial cells, and giant cells, with necrotic, avascular centers. Obliterative endarteritis is seen in the blood vessels surrounding and within the nodules. Occasionally, a diffuse, rather than nodular, granulomatous reaction is seen. Involvement of the larynx by syphilis is rare. Secondary syphilis may present as a diffuse laryngeal hyperemia, accompanied by a coalescing, maculopapular rash, usually of the supraglottic region. Tertiary laryngeal syphilis is usually in the form of a diffuse, nodular, gummatous infiltrate. The nodules may ulcerate or coalesce to form larger nodules.[45]

If not managed, syphilis of the larynx may progress to chondritis, fibrosis, and scarring. Management consists of high intramuscular doses of penicillin. Patients should subsequently be observed with repeat Venereal Disease Research Laboratory (VDRL) testing at 6- to 12-month intervals to detect any recurrence of infection.

Hansen's Disease

Hansen's disease, or leprosy, is rare in the United States. Even in areas where the disease is relatively common, most infected patients have a single acute lesion that heals spontaneously. The portal of entry is thought to be the nasal mucosa; thus, nasal ulceration with perforation is common. The larynx is the second most frequent site of involvement in the head and neck. The lepromatous form of Hansen's disease is the most debilitating and is most common in the head and neck. Laryngeal involvement presents initially as erythematous or nodular edema of the supraglottis and progresses secondarily to the glottis.[55] In the absence of definitive management, the nodules characteristically enlarge, ulcerate, and heal by scar formation. This scarring may occasionally cause laryngeal stenosis and airway obstruction. Despite the appearance of this lesion, the patient is often pain free. Diagnosis may be made on the basis of history, the presence of other clinical findings, and evaluation of a laryngeal biopsy or nasal smear. Histopathologic examination of tissue specimens reveals edema with a chronic inflammatory infiltrate and the presence of numerous large foam cells. Acid-fast staining can show an abundance of *Mycobacterium leprae* (Hansen's bacilli) in the foam cells. Management consists of the oral administration of dapsone or dapsone and rifampin, because dapsone-resistant strains of bacilli are being seen with increasing frequency in endemic areas. Management is continued for 1 to 2 years after the organism can no longer be seen on biopsy samples of affected areas. As many as 5 to 10 years of drug therapy may be required.

Differential Diagnosis

Chronic infections in the larynx are often difficult to diagnose, because physicians fail to suspect diagnoses other than squamous cell carcinoma. When pseudoepitheliomatous hyperplasia is found on microscopic study, blastomycosis, candidiasis, or histoplasmosis should be considered. In addition to bacterial, fungal, and acid-fast infections, other noninfectious diseases, such as granular cell tumors, relapsing polychondritis, rheumatoid arthritis, and Wegener's granulomatosis can also present as laryngeal lesions.

SYSTEMIC DISEASES AFFECTING THE LARYNX
Rheumatoid Arthritis

Rheumatoid arthritis is the most common autoimmune disease and affects 2% to 3% of the adult population. The usual age of onset is from 35 to 45, and women are affected three times as frequently as men.[9] Laryngeal involvement in patients with rheumatoid arthritis ranges from 26% to 53%.[9,40] Symptoms are numerous and include globus sensation, hoarseness, dyspnea, stridor, or dysphasia.[47] Diagnosis can be somewhat difficult, and the severity of laryngeal symptoms does not always correlate with the level of general disease activity. Computed tomography can sometimes be of benefit.[9] The mainstay of diagnosis remains direct or indirect laryngoscopy. Laryngeal findings have been described as depending on the stage of rheumatoid involvement. There is an initial acute phase in which the larynx may be tender and the mucosa over the arytenoids bright red and swollen and a chronic phase in which the arytenoid mucosa is thickened, the vocal cords bowed, and the arytenoids fixed to varying degrees.[9,40] Another finding on examination may be submucosal rheumatoid nodules. These most commonly involve the true cords but may also be seen in other parts of the larynx.[9,73] If symptomatic, these can be excised with standard microlaryngoscopy techniques.[73]

Systemic Lupus Erythematosus

Systemic lupus erythematosus is an autoimmune disease in which circulating immune complexes can cause blood damage to blood vessels, connective tissues, and mucosal surfaces. An antinuclear antibody test is usually positive.

The most commonly affected organs are the skin, joints, kidneys, and lungs. The most common otolaryngologic manifestation is ulcerative lesions of the oral cavity. The larynx is thought to be rarely involved, and laryngeal symptoms are usually seen in conjunction with other manifestations of the disease (e.g., skin or mucosal lesions, polyarthritis). Laryngeal symptoms may include hoarseness, throat pain, or dyspnea, depending on the site of involvement. Although the glottis and cricoarytenoid joints seem to be the most commonly affected areas, supraglottic and subglottic involvement have also been reported.[41,66] The appearance of the larynx may range from relatively normal to erythematous and swollen. Unilateral and bilateral vocal cord paralysis has been described.[66] Management of laryngeal lupus consists of high-dose intravenous or oral corticosteroids, usually with rapid resolution of symptoms.

Relapsing Polychondritis

Relapsing polychondritis (RP) is an idiopathic autoimmune disease of unknown cause. It is extremely rare, with an estimated annual incidence of 3.5 per million.[37] It occurs with equal frequency in men and women and is most common in middle-aged patients. Relapsing polychondritis usually presents with bilateral acute inflammation of the auricular cartilage. Because the lobule of the ear has no cartilage, it is usually spared. Other common clinical features are chondritis of the nasal cartilage, ocular inflammation, and polyarthritis. Other sites of involvement are the inner ear (sensorineural deafness, vertigo), the cardiovascular system (aortic incompetence, mitral regurgitation, and aneurysms), and skin.[29]

There is no laboratory test that is specific for RP. Two-thirds of patients will have antibodies to type II collagen, but this finding can be seen in other autoimmune diseases. The sedimentation rate is usually elevated, at least during acute attacks, but again, this is a very nonspecific finding. To make laboratory diagnosis even more difficult, approximately 25% of patients with RP will have another autoimmune disease. Because of these difficulties, the diagnosis of RP is usually based on the presence of clinical findings (see preceding), either alone or in combination with histologic results.[37]

Although the exact percentage of patients with laryngeal manifestations of RP is unknown, it is generally reported that approximately 50% of patients with RP will eventually have some degree of respiratory system involvement. In addition to the larynx, the trachea and bronchi are other common sites of inflammation.[61] Acute laryngeal involvement usually manifests itself as hoarseness, stridor, and dyspnea and presumably occurs as a result of laryngeal mucosal edema during acute attacks of the disease. Acute airway symptoms can be managed with an intravenous bolus of corticosteroids in combination with racemic epinephrine.[38] Repeated acute attacks of laryngeal chondritis may cause subglottic fibrosis and narrowing.[13] As a result, some patients require permanent tracheostomies because of airway stenosis or collapse. Oral corticosteroids, immunosuppressive drugs, and dapsone have been used with some success in long-term management.[29]

Sarcoidosis

Sarcoidosis is a chronic granulomatous disease that may involve any organ system. It usually presents in young adults and is more common in women and blacks. Its cause is unknown. Abnormal laboratory findings may include elevated serum and urine calcium and an elevated angiotensin-converting enzyme level.[14] Lymph nodes are the most common site of involvement, followed by the lungs, spleen, and liver. Many patients are asymptomatic, and their disease is discovered incidentally after routine chest radiography. Those patients who are symptomatic usually have respiratory complaints (e.g., cough, shortness of breath, hemoptysis) or more generalized symptoms (e.g., fever, weight loss, fatigue). Laryngeal involvement has been estimated to be between 1% and 5%.[14,72] The initial stages of laryngeal involvement may be relatively benign; the affected mucosa is often described as being covered with one or more white or brown nodules that eventually coalesce to produce a pale, edematous epiglottis, with lesser changes being seen in other supraglottic structures such as the arytenoepiglottic folds and false cords.[14] The true cords are usually described as rarely involved, possibly because of a lack of lymphatics, but one large series[6] reported a 24% incidence of glottic involvement. The lesions are rarely painful, and thus hoarseness or partial airway obstruction may be the first sign of laryngeal involvement.[6]

The microscopic appearance of sarcoidosis resembles that of miliary tubercles and consists of epithelioid cells, macrophages, and giant cells. These giant cells appear larger than those of tuberculosis and contain more nuclei. Inclusion bodies, such as asteroids and Schaumann's bodies, may be a striking feature of the giant cells. Lesions are conspicuous by their absence of caseation and lack of surrounding lymphocytic infiltration.

Management usually consists of long-term oral corticosteroids, but some success has been reported with intralesional corticosteroid injection,[32] which may be particularly useful in patients with partial airway obstruction who may otherwise require a tracheostomy. There have also been several case reports of patients whose disease was refractory to corticosteroids and who were managed with low-dose radiotherapy.[21]

Wegener's Granulomatosis

Wegener's granulomatosis is an idiopathic syndrome that is characterized by the triad of necrotizing granulomas of the respiratory system, a necrotizing vasculitis that may affect other organ systems, and glomerulonephritis. Its most common head and neck manifestations are chronic sinusitis and mucosal lesions of the nasopharynx, but laryngeal involvement can occur in up to 23% of patients.[33] Laryngeal manifestations of Wegener's are confined almost exclusively to the subglottis. Depending on the severity and progression of subglottic disease, initial endoscopy may show simply an isolated subglottic mass. Biopsy is often unrewarding, with nonspecific acute and chronic inflammation being the most common finding, and a definitive diagnosis of Wegener's made only approximately 5% of the time.[33] However, because most patients with laryngeal disease also have other organ system involvement, the diagnosis is usually presumptive. Management at this point may consist primarily of glucocorticoids alone or in combination with a cytotoxic agent.[71] However, in a number of patients, the subsequent granulomatous inflammation and scarring may lead to significant subglottic stenosis. Dyspnea and hoarseness are the most common symptoms.[33] Treatment at this stage may consist of repeated dilations with local injection of steroids[33] or various surgical techniques. Surgical treatments that have been shown to be of some benefit include laryngotracheal reconstruction[33, 34] or endoscopic longitudinal incisions through the area of stenosis followed by dilation and application of mitomycin-C.[18] Endoscopic CO_2 laser excision has not been shown to be effective, because it usually results in further scarring.[34]

Amyloidosis

Amyloidosis is an idiopathic disease that is characterized by the extracellular deposition of fibrillar proteins. Clinically, it can be divided into two categories: primary amyloidosis, in which there is spontaneous development of amyloid deposits, and secondary amyloidosis, in which the condition is found in conjunction with some other systemic disease, such as rheumatoid arthritis or tuberculosis. Primary amyloidosis can be broken down further into localized and generalized forms. In the former, the amyloid deposits are confined to a single organ system or even to a single location, whereas in the latter, as the name implies, the deposits are found to some extent in almost all tissues.

Deposition of amyloid in the larynx is rare, accounting for as little as 0.2% of benign tumors of the larynx.[67] Laryngeal amyloidosis is almost always of the localized type, with involvement confined to the respiratory system alone. Respiratory system amyloidosis most commonly affects the trachea (90%), with the larynx involved about 50% of the time.[36,50] Because multisite involvement is the rule rather than the exception, any patient with laryngeal amyloidosis requires complete endoscopy to rule out synchronous lesions.

Patients with laryngeal amyloidosis most often have hoarseness or stridor, because the most common sites of involvement in the larynx are the vocal cord, ventricle, and false vocal cord. Patients with deposits in the subglottis or lower airways typically have dyspnea or cough.[50] Although amyloid deposits have typically been described as smooth, pinkish gray masses lying under intact epithelium, other authors have described a cobblestone-like appearance or even circumferential thickening.[50] Under light microscopy, amyloid appears as amorphous, eosinophilic deposits and may show green birefringence under polarization after being stained with Congo red. The diagnosis can be confirmed with electron microscopy, which shows an interlacing mesh of nonbranching fibrils. Management of laryngeal amyloidosis is surgical excision. Because multiple managements for recurrent disease are often required,[36] it is important to use techniques that will minimize trauma to the larynx. To this end, several authors have reported good results with the carbon dioxide laser[65] or neodymium: yttrium–aluminum–garnet laser.[50]

REFERENCES

1. Bass JW: Erythromycin for treatment and prevention of pertussis, *Pediatr Infect Dis J* 5:154, 1986.
2. Bass JW, Stephenson SR: The return of pertussis, *Pediatr Infect Dis J* 6:141, 1987.
3. Bauters TG and others: Colonization of voice prostheses by albicans and non-albicans candida species, *Laryngoscope* 112: 708, 2002.

4. Bennett DE: Histoplasmosis of the oral cavity and larynx: a clinical, pathologic study, *Arch Intern Med* 120:417, 1967.

5. Bernstein T, Brilli R, Jacobs B: Is bacterial tracheitis changing? A 14-month experience in a pediatric intensive care unit, *Clin Infect Dis* 27:458, 1998.

6. Bower JS and others: Manifestations and treatment of laryngeal sarcoidosis, *Am Rev Respir Dis* 122:325, 1980.

7. Boyle JO, Coulthard SW, Mandel RM: Laryngeal involvement in disseminated coccidioidomycosis, *Arch Otolaryngol Head Neck Surg* 117:433, 1991.

8. Britto J and others: Systemic complications associated with bacterial tracheitis, *Arch Dis Child* 74:249–250, 1996.

9. Brooker DS: Rheumatoid arthritis: otorhinolaryngological manifestations, *Clin Otolaryngol* 13:239, 1998.

10. Brown, JC: The management of croup, *Br Med Bull* 61:189, 2002.

11. Carey MJ: Epiglottitis in adults, *Am J Emerg Med* 14:421, 1996.

12. Cherry JD: The science and fiction of the "resurgence" of pertussis, *Pediatrics* 112:405, 2003.

13. Clark LJ, Waheel RA, Ormerod AD: Relapsing polychondritis: two cases with tracheal stenosis and inner ear involvement, *J Laryngol Otol* 106:841, 1992.

14. Dean CM and others: Laryngeal sarcoidosis, *J Voice* 16:283, 2002.

15. Donegan JO, Wood MD: Histoplasmosis of the larynx, *Laryngoscope* 94:206, 1984.

16. Donnelly BW, McMillan JA, Weiner LB: Bacterial tracheitis: report of eight new cases and review, *Rev Infect Dis* 12:729, 1990.

17. Eckel HE, Widemann B, Damm M: Airway endoscopy in the diagnosis and treatment of bacterial tracheitis in children, *Int J Pediatr Otorhinolaryngol* 27:147, 1993.

18. Eliachar I, Chan J, Akst L: New approaches to the management of subglottic stenosis in Wegener's granulomatosis, *Cleveland Clin J Med* 69(SII):149, 2002.

19. Ewig JM: Lower respiratory tract infections, *Pediatr Ann* 31:125, 2002.

20. Farmer TL, Wohl DL: Diagnosis of recurrent intermittent airway obstruction ("recurrent croup") in children, *Ann Otol Rhinol Laryngol* 110:600, 2001

21. Fogel TD and others: Radiotherapy in sarcoidosis of the larynx: case report and review of the literature, *Laryngoscope* 94:1223, 1984.

22. Forrest LA, Weed H: Candida laryngitis appearing as leukoplakia and GERD, *J Voice* 12:91, 1998.

23. Frisch M, Gnepp DR: Primary cryptococcal infection of the larynx: report of a case, *Otolaryngol Head Neck Surg* 113:477, 1995.

24. Gerber ME and others: Histoplasmosis: the otolaryngologist's perspective, *Laryngoscope* 105:919, 1995.

25. Goodwin RA Jr and others: Disseminated histoplasmosis: clinical and pathological correlations, *Medicine* 59:1, 1980.

26. Hajare S and others: Laryngeal coccidioidomycosis causing airway obstruction, *Pediatr Infect Dis J* 8:54, 1989.

27. Heeneman H, Ward KM: Epiglottic abscess: its occurrence and management, *J Otolaryngol* 6:31, 1977.

28. Hughes RA, Paonessa DF, Conway WR Jr: Actinomycosis of the larynx, *Ann Otol Rhinol Laryngol* 93:520, 1984.

29. Irani BS and others: Relapsing polychondritis: a study of four cases, *J Laryngol Otol* 106:911, 1992.

30. Issacson JE, Frable MA: Cryptococcosis of the larynx, *Otolaryngol Head Neck Surg* 114:106, 1996.

31. Kandiloros DC and others: Laryngeal tuberculosis at the end of the 20th century, *J Laryngol Otolaryngol* 111:619, 1997.

32. Krespi YP and others: Treatment of laryngeal sarcoidosis with intralesional steroid injection, *Ann Otol Rhinol Laryngol* 96:713, 1987.

33. Langford CA and others: Clinical features and therapeutic management of subglottic stenosis in patients with Wegener's granulomatosis, *Arthritis Rheum* 39:1754, 1996.

34. Lebovics RS and others: The management of subglottic stenosis in patients with Wegener's granulomatosis, *Laryngoscope* 102:1341, 1992.

35. Leicht MJ, Harrington TM, Davis DE: Cricoarytenoid arthritis: a cause of laryngeal obstruction, *Ann Emerg Med* 16:885, 1987.

36. Lewis JE and others: Laryngeal amyloidosis: clinicopathologic and immunohistochemical review, *Otolaryngol Head Neck Surg* 106:372, 1992.

37. Letko E and others: Relapsing polychondritis: a clinical review, *Semin Arthritis Rheum* 31:384, 2002.

38. Lipnick RN, Fink CW: Acute airway obstruction in relapsing polychondritis: treatment with pulse methylprednisolone, *J Rheumatol* 18:98, 1991.

39. Liston SL and others: Bacterial tracheitis, *Am J Dis Child* 137:764, 1983.

40. Lofgren RH, Montgomery WW: Incidence of laryngeal involvement in rheumatoid arthritis, *N Engl J Med* 267:193, 1962.

41. Martin L and others: Upper airway disease in systemic lupus erythematosus: a report of 4 cases and a review of the literature, *J Rheumatol* 19:1186, 1992.

42. Mayo-Smith MF and others: Acute epiglottitis: an 18-year experience in Rhode Island, *Chest* 108:1640, 1995.

43. McEniery J and others: Review of intubation in severe laryngotracheobronchitis, *Pediatrics* 87:847, 1991.

44. McEwan J and others: Paediatric acute epiglottitis: not a disappearing entity, *Int J Ped Otohrhinolaryngol* 67:317, 2003.

45. McNulty JS, Fassett RL: Syphilis: an otolaryngologic perspective, *Laryngoscope* 91:889, 1981.

46. Mikaelian AJ, Varkey B, Grossman TW: Blastomycosis of the head and neck, *Otolaryngol Head Neck Surg* 101:489, 1989.

47. Montgomery WW: Cricoarytenoid arthritis, *Laryngoscope* 73:801, 1963.

48. Nelson ET, Tybor AG: Actinomycosis of the larynx, *Ear Nose Throat J* 71:79, 1991.

49. Nishiike S, Irifune M, Doi K: Laryngeal tuberculosis: a report of 15 cases, *Ann Otol Rhinol Laryngol* 111:916, 2002.

50. Piazza C and others: Endoscopic management of laryngotracheobronchial amyloidosis: a series of 32 patients, *Eur Arch Otorhinolaryngol* 260:349, 2003.

51. Pichchero ME, Hoeger WJ, Casey JR: Azithromycin for the treatment of pertussis, *Pediatr Infect Dis J* 22: 847, 2003.

52. Rajah V, Essa A: Histoplasmosis of the oral cavity, oropharynx and larynx, *J Laryngol Otol* 107:58, 1993.

53. Ramandan HH, Tarayi AE, Baroudy FM: Laryngeal tuberculosis: presentation of 16 cases and review of the literature, *J Otolaryngol* 22:39, 1993.

54. Reder PA, Neel HB: Blastomycosis in otolaryngology: review of a large series, *Laryngoscope* 103:53, 1993.

55. Sandberg P, Shum TK: Lepromatous leprosy of the larynx, *Otolaryngol Head Neck Surg* 91:216, 1983.

56. Senior BA and others: Changing patterns in pediatric supraglottitis: a multi-institutional review, 1980-1992, *Laryngoscope* 104:1314, 1994.

57. Shin J and others: Changing trends in clinical manifestations of laryngeal tuberculosis, *Laryngoscope* 110:1950, 2000.

58. Singh B and others: Laryngeal tuberculosis in HIV-infected patients: a difficult diagnosis, *Laryngoscope* 106:1238, 1996.

59. Soda A and others: Tuberculosis of the larynx: clinical aspects in 19 patients, *Laryngoscope* 99:1147, 1989.

60. Solomon P and others: Adult epiglottitis: the Toronto hospital experience, *J Otolaryngol* 27: 332, 1998.

61. Spraggs PD, Tostevin PM, Howard DJ: Management of laryngotracheobronchial sequelae and complications of relapsing polychondritis, *Laryngoscope* 107:936, 1997.

62. Stroud RH, Friedman NR: An update on inflammatory disorders of the pediatric airway: epiglottitis, croup, and tracheitis, *Am J Otolaryngol* 22:268, 2001.

63. Suen JY and others: Blastomycosis of the larynx, *Ann Otol Rhinol Laryngol* 89:563, 1980.

64. Tashjian LS, Peacock JE: Laryngeal candidiasis: report of seven cases and review of literature, *Arch Otolaryngol* 110:806, 1984.

65. Talbot AR: Laryngeal amyloidosis, *J Laryngol Otol* 104:147, 1990.

66. Teitel AD and others: Laryngeal involvement in systemic lupus erythematosus, *Semin Arthritis Rheum* 22:203, 1992.

67. Thompson LD and others: Amyloidosis of the larynx: a clinicopathologic study of 11 cases, *Mod Pathol* 1352, 2000.

68. Waisman Y and others: Prospective randomized double-blind study comparing L-epinephrine and racemic epinephrine aerosols in the treatment of laryngotracheitis croup, *Pediatrics* 89:302, 1992.

69. Wallenborn PA III, Postma DS: Radiation-recall supraglottitis: a hazard in head and neck chemotherapy, *Arch Otolaryngol Head Neck Surg* 110:64, 1984.

70. Ward PH and others: Coccidioidomycosis of the larynx in infants and children, *Ann Otol Rhinol Laryngol* 86:655, 1977.

71. Waxman J, Bose WJ: Laryngeal manifestations of Wegener's granulomatosis: case reports and review of the literature, *J Rheumatol* 13:408, 1986.

72. Weisman RA, Canalis RF, Powell WJ: Laryngeal sarcoidosis with airway obstruction, *Ann Otol Rhinol Laryngol* 89:58, 1980.

73. Woo P, Mendelsohn J, Humphrey D: Rheumatoid nodules of the larynx, *Otolaryngol Head Neck Surg* 113:147, 1995.

74. Wright SW and others: Pertussis infection in adults with persistent cough, *JAMA* 273:512, 1995.

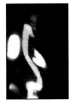

CHAPTER NINETY ONE

CHRONIC ASPIRATION

Steven D. Pletcher
David W. Eisele

INTRODUCTION

The three major functions of the larynx—respiration, phonation, and airway protection—are intimately related. Impairment of laryngeal protective function can result in aspiration; the laryngeal penetration of secretions such as saliva, ingested liquids or solids, and refluxed gastric contents below the level of the true vocal cords.

A certain amount of aspiration is known to occur normally. Scintigraphic evaluation of healthy persons during sleep reveals aspiration in nearly 50% of subjects.[46] A certain amount of aspiration can be tolerated without complications, provided that tracheobronchial clearance is normal and defense mechanisms are intact. Contamination of the respiratory tract associated with aspiration can result in a spectrum of bronchopulmonary complications. The severity of complications depends on the volume and the character (e.g., pH) of the aspirated material. Respiratory complications of aspiration include bronchospasm, airway obstruction, tracheitis, bronchitis, pneumonia, pulmonary abscess, sepsis, and death.[4,6,20] Significant aspiration results in a high mortality rate.[9]

Aspiration can be an isolated event related to temporary impairment of normal swallowing mechanisms and airway protection. Typically, isolated aspiration occurs because of neurologic dysfunction. This can result from a depressed state of consciousness related to drugs, alcohol, or metabolic derangement. In addition, seizure, injury, or infection can cause isolated aspiration. Elderly patients are more likely to experience aspiration, presumably related to physiologic and neurologic changes associated with age.[2,11,89] Patients with dentures experience impaired swallowing with decreased oral sensation and oral control, which may contribute to aspiration.

Chronic or intractable aspiration entails repeated episodes of aspiration. Patients with chronic aspiration require evaluation and effective management to prevent life-threatening complications. This chapter discusses the evaluation and management of patients with chronic aspiration and emphasizes surgical management.

ETIOLOGY

Chronic aspiration usually results from a severe loss of laryngeal protective function related to impaired motor activity or sensory loss. Chronic aspiration can occur despite healthy laryngeal function if dysfunctional swallowing is significant.

Box 91-1 lists causes of chronic aspiration. The most common cause is associated with cerebrovascular accidents, particularly those involving the brainstem with bilateral cranial nerve (CN) deficits.[45] In addition, degenerative neurologic diseases are frequently associated with chronic aspiration. Peripheral nerve disorders, particularly those involving the CNs as well as neuromuscular diseases and muscular disorders, can cause recurrent aspiration. Diffuse neurologic dysfunction from head injury, anoxic brain injury, infection, or drug toxicity can cause severe dysfunction and chronic aspiration.[16,40,58] Chronic aspiration can also result from disorders of the pharynx and the esophagus, including neoplasms, postsurgical and postirradiation dysfunction, Zenker's diverticulum, stricture, and severe gastroesophageal reflux.[67]

Chronic aspiration can occur in pediatric patients, in whom it is usually related to severe neurologic dysfunction resulting from cerebral palsy, anoxic encephalopathy, sequelae of neurologic trauma or surgery, tracheoesophageal fistula, and other severe congenital or acquired neurologic disorders.[57]

SYMPTOMS

Patients may be aware of recurrent aspiration and may describe episodes of coughing or choking during swallowing. Some patients, however, may experience silent aspiration, whereby cough does not occur after laryngeal penetration.[44,65,66] Fever and respiratory

---

BOX 91-1
CAUSES OF CHRONIC ASPIRATION

Cerebrovascular accidents
   Atherosclerotic thrombosis
   Embolism
   Intracranial hemorrhage
Degenerative neurologic diseases
   Parkinson's disease
   Amyotrophic lateral sclerosis
   Progressive supranuclear palsy
   Multiple sclerosis
Neuromuscular and muscular disorders
   Poliomyelitis
   Myasthenia gravis
   Muscular dystrophy
   Myopathies
Peripheral nerve disorders
   Cranial nerves
   Guillain-Barré syndrome
Intracranial neoplasms
   Primary dysfunction related to neoplasm
   Postsurgical dysfunction

Trauma
   Closed head injury
   Hematoma
Anoxic brain injury
Intracranial infection
Pharyngeal disorders
   Neoplasms
   Postsurgical dysfunction
   Postirradiation function
   Zenker's diverticulum
   Cricopharyngeal dysfunction
   Stricture
Esophageal disorders
   Reflux
   Achalasia
   Caustic injury
Miscellaneous
   Severe illness
   Multisystem disease
   Drug intoxication

---

symptoms such as productive cough with purulent sputum may occur, indicating an infectious complication. Patients may have weight loss, dysphonia, pain, dysphagia, odynophagia, or other symptoms depending on the cause of the underlying disorder.[45] Frequently, patients are severely ill because of their disease and secondary infectious complications.

EVALUATION

In the evaluation of a patient with chronic aspiration, a detailed medical history is important. Frequently, the cause of aspiration is apparent from the history. The medical history and history of prior surgery or injury should be thoroughly investigated.

A multidisciplinary approach to patients with chronic aspiration is important.[71] Frequently, an otolaryngologist–head and neck surgeon is consulted after complications of chronic aspiration have occurred. Once chronic aspiration has been identified, consultation with specialists in speech-language pathology, neurology, internal medicine, rehabilitation medicine, radiology, gastroenterology, thoracic surgery, and psychiatry may be beneficial. A cooperative effort in which each specialist provides his or her expertise ensures optimal care for the patient.

Physical examination should be thorough, with careful examination of the head and neck, including CN evaluation. Examination of the hypopharynx and larynx is performed by indirect mirror examination or fiberoptic nasopharyngoscopy. If these structures are not adequately visualized by these methods (e.g., in an endotracheally intubated patient), direct laryn-goscopy is recommended. Esophagoscopy is performed if an esophageal abnormality is suspected. Pulmonary function tests help assess pulmonary function and reserve.

Radiography provides important diagnostic information and should include chest radiography and swallowing evaluation. A videofluoroscopic swallowing study reliably provides information about the precise physiologic nature of aspiration and swallowing disturbance and about the degree of aspiration.[28,92] Logemann[68] described a modified barium swallow in which small amounts of barium are used because of the risk of aspiration. Different consistencies of contrast material are used to assess whether consistency alteration has any effect on aspiration reduction. A videofluoroscopic swallowing study performed in conjunction with a speech-language pathologist allows radiographic assessment of the effects of swallowing therapy and maneuvers on control of aspiration.[69,84]

Functional endoscopic evaluation of swallowing (FEES) was proposed by Langmore and colleagues[54] in 1988 as an alternative to videofluoroscopy for the evaluation of dysphagia. In this study, dyed pudding and liquids are swallowed by the patient, and nasopharyngeal fiberoptic observation is performed. The swallow is recorded and reviewed for evidence of oral leakage, pharyngeal stasis, laryngeal penetration, and aspiration. A assessment of FEES suggests that it has similar sensitivity and specificity to that of videofluoroscopic examination, with the advantages of lower cost, decreased radiation exposure, and bedside availability.[3,25,55,60,99] In general, the choice between videofluoroscopy and FEES is dependent on multiple factors, including physician and speech-language pathologist preferences and hospital availability.

Scintigraphy may help quantify the magnitude of aspiration,[77,90] but in general it adds little information beyond that obtained from a FEES or a videofluoroscopic swallowing study for the management of aspiration. Other imaging studies that may provide important information include computed tomography and magnetic resonance imaging of the head and neck and soft tissue radiography of the neck.

Comprehensive evaluation of the aspirating patient ideally determines the cause of the underlying disorder or disorders causing aspiration. A thorough search for any correctable cause of aspiration (e.g., obstructing lesion, Zenker's diverticulum, cricopharyngeal muscle dysfunction, esophageal motility disorder) is important to management.

Frequently, progressive functional deterioration can be anticipated for certain degenerative neurologic diseases and malignant neoplasms. It can be extremely difficult, however, to predict the time course of improvement and recovery for cerebrovascular accidents, head injuries, anoxic brain injuries, postsurgical dysfunction, and other disorders. Multispecialty input is helpful in planning management for these difficult cases.

NONSURGICAL MANAGEMENT

Initial management of a chronically aspirating patient should include appropriate antibiotics for any infectious complications. Aggressive pulmonary therapy is instituted. All oral intake is discontinued, and an alternative route of alimentation is provided. Enteral routes of alimentation include small, soft nasogastric feeding tubes, cervical esophagotomy, piriform sinusotomy, gastrostomy, and jejunostomy. Gastrostomy can easily be performed percutaneously with minimal morbidity. Patients with significant reflux may benefit from a tube passed through a gastrostomy into the small intestine or jejunostomy.

Depending on the cause of aspiration, nasogastric feeding tube alimentation decreases but does not eliminate the risk of aspiration.[23] Some researchers believe that nasogastric feeding tubes may actually predispose to aspiration.[1,38] In addition, nasogastric feeding tubes can be uncomfortable and aesthetically displeasing when used for long periods. Gastrostomy alone has been shown to not decrease aspiration in neurologically impaired patients.[42,49] Some patients may be candidates for parenteral hyperalimentation if gastrointestinal function is impaired (e.g., in patients with acute severe brain injury).[80]

Proper nursing care includes special positioning of the patient, such as elevation of the head of the bed for patients with severe reflux. However, one study showed no significant difference in aspiration with respect to patient position when the patient was endotracheally intubated.[38] Frequent suctioning of the oral cavity and oropharynx is also important.

TRACHEOTOMY

A tracheotomy tube with a low-pressure cuff provides comfortable airway control for patients requiring intubation and facilitates pulmonary toilet in patients with copious secretions. Tracheotomy also effectively reduces the pulmonary dead space. Despite these advantages, tracheotomy cannot be relied on to eliminate aspiration.[14,19] In addition, tracheotomy has been implicated as a causative factor for aspiration. The proposed mechanisms include esophageal compression via inflated tracheotomy cuff,[8,79] desensitization of the larynx from diversion of airflow through the tracheotomy,[39] impaired laryngeal elevation through tethering of the larynx by the tracheotomy tube,[13] disruption of the normally closed aerodigestive system,[78] disordered laryngeal reflexes due to chronic upper airway bypass,[47,86,88] reduced effectiveness of cough to clear secretions from the upper airway,[78,93] and an inability to generate subglottic air pressure.[30,76] However, in a study of 20 patients evaluated with FEES before and after tracheotomy (within 1 month), no causal relationship between tracheotomy and aspiration was demonstrated.[59] Nonetheless, use of a one-way valve (Passé-Muir valve) may improve the patient's ability to clear secretions from the airway by increasing subglottic pressure during swallowing and coughing.

In general, the use of a tracheotomy tube for aspiration control requires close attention and skilled care, particularly for a debilitated patient. Several studies have examined the effect of endotracheal and tracheotomy tube cuffs on the prevention of aspiration. Although low-pressure, high-compliance cuffs are the most effective in minimizing cuff leak, they do not prevent aspiration.[7,81,82]

VOCAL CORD MEDIALIZATION

Vocal cord paralysis can result in chronic aspiration, particularly when combined with a laryngeal sensory deficit (e.g., a high vagal lesion). Vocal cord injection with polytetrafluoroethylene (Teflon) paste or an absorbable material such as collagen, autologous fat, or collagen derivatives can be performed endoscopically or transcervically to achieve vocal cord medialization and to prevent aspiration related to vocal cord paralysis.[62,72,85] Bilateral vocal cord injection with Teflon, however, has been shown to be an unreliable method for the prevention of chronic aspiration.[61]

Alteration of the laryngeal framework by medialization laryngoplasty using an implant is another excellent technique for vocal cord medialization.[48,51] Carrau and colleagues[22] reported that 94% of patients with high vagal lesions experienced improved swallowing after medialization thyroplasty with or without arytenoid adduction. In the same study, 79% of patients who presented with tracheotomies underwent successful decanulation after laryngeal framework surgery.

SURGERY

Sometimes a correctable cause of chronic aspiration is not identified, and nonsurgical and minor surgical procedures (e.g., tracheotomy, vocal cord medialization) do not prevent chronic aspiration. In these cases, surgical separation of the upper digestive tract from the upper respiratory tract is necessary to prevent the morbidity and mortality of recurrent respiratory tract soilage. A reasonable probability of survival and duration of survival are necessary prerequisites for this surgery.

Clinical judgment should be used to determine the likelihood of recovery of laryngeal protective function and to identify patients who require prompt surgical intervention to separate the upper digestive and respiratory tracts to prevent death. The patient's general medical and mental status, severity of illness, and potential quality of life should be addressed.[12] Patients may have to sacrifice normal phonation and laryngeal respiration to ensure the restoration of airway protection. This difficult issue requires thorough discussions of management options and sequelae with the patient and family members.

"Ideal" Surgical Procedure for Chronic Aspiration

The ideal surgical procedure for chronic aspiration would be uniformly effective in preventing aspiration, would be simply achieved, and would have few complications and low morbidity. Ideally, the procedure could be performed with local anesthesia for debilitated patients. In addition, the ideal procedure would allow phonation and deglutition and would be reversible should the underlying cause of aspiration improve. Many surgical options have been described for the management of chronic aspiration (Table 91-1).

Laryngectomy

Before 1970, laryngectomy was considered the surgical management of choice for chronic aspiration. This procedure provides definitive separation of the upper digestive and respiratory tracts. Narrow-field laryngectomy (Figure 91-1) is used, in contrast to the total laryngectomy performed for malignancy. This proce-

TABLE 91-1

SURGICAL MANAGEMENT OF CHRONIC ASPIRATION

Reversible Procedures	Irreversible Procedures
Laryngotracheal separation	Subperichondrial cricoidectomy
Tracheoesophageal diversion	Narrow-field laryngectomy
Epiglottic flap laryngeal closure	Glottic closure
Endolaryngeal stent	
Double-barrel tracheostomy	
Partial cricoidectomy	
Vertical laryngoplasty	

dure preserves the hyoid, strap muscles, and as much hypopharyngeal mucosa as possible. Closure without tension and with reinforcement minimizes the potential postoperative complications of pharyngeal stenosis and fistula.[15]

Laryngectomy also is practical because of the low likelihood of recovery of most patients with chronic aspiration.[21,43] However, because of the negative psychosocial aspects of laryngectomy, most patients and family members are reluctant to consent to laryngectomy for chronic aspiration. Narrow-field laryngectomy can be performed with local anesthesia. Tracheoesophageal puncture and placement of a voice prosthesis can be used for vocal rehabilitation after laryngectomy in selected patients. Because of the disadvantage of irreversibility of laryngectomy and the observation that some patients with chronic aspiration recover, other surgical procedures have been developed since the 1970s for the surgical management of chronic aspiration.

Subperichondrial Cricoidectomy

An option for definitive surgical separation of the upper respiratory and digestive tracts when no chance of recovery of function is expected is subperichondrial cricoidectomy[34] (Figure 91-2). In this technique, the anterior aspect of the cricoid cartilage is exposed. The perichondrium of the anterior cricoid cartilage is divided vertically in the midline to expose the cricoid cartilage. The outer cricoid perichondrium is raised with an elevator to the posterior cricoid lamina, and the inner cricoid perichondrium is elevated from the cricoid cartilage circumferentially. The cricoid cartilage is then removed piecemeal bilaterally using biting forceps, and the posterior cricoid lamina is preserved. The inner perichondrium and subglottic mucosa are transected horizontally, inverted, and closed, creating a subglottic pouch. The closure is buttressed

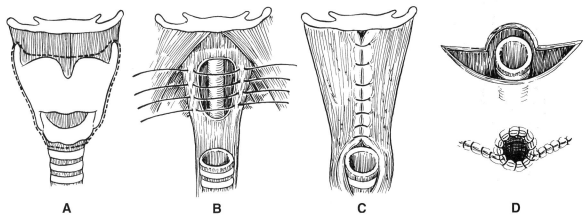

Figure 91-1. Narrow-field laryngectomy. **A,** Outline of larynx removal; the hyoid is preserved. **B,** Closure of the pharynx. **C,** Closure is reinforced with sternohyoid muscles. **D,** A tracheostoma is created.

by approximation of the strap muscles, and the wound is closed in layers over a drain. A tracheotomy is necessary.

The advantages of this technique include a high success rate, simplicity, and low morbidity. For these reasons, subperichondrial cricoidectomy is preferable to narrow-field laryngectomy and other procedures for chronic aspiration when recovery of laryngeal protective function is not expected. This procedure can be performed easily with the patient under local anesthesia. Disadvantages include the remote possibility of fistula into the upper trachea and the need for a tracheotomy. The procedure was not designed to be reversible, and no reversals have been reported.

Partial Cricoidectomy

Krespi, Pelzer, and Sisson[52] described subtotal and submucosal cricoid resection for the control of chronic aspiration after extensive surgical resection of pharyngeal and base-of-tongue tumors, particularly for patients undergoing myocutaneous flap reconstruction. The posterior cricoid perichondrium is elevated, and the posterior half of the cricoid lamina is removed without entering the mucosa. A cricopharyngeal myotomy is also performed. A tracheotomy is necessary. Partial cricoidectomy enlarges the pharyngeal inlet, facilitating deglutition, and narrows the laryngeal inlet, thereby reducing aspiration and preserving the voice.

Biller and Urken[10] described partial cricoid collapse for the prevention of aspiration after extended horizontal partial laryngectomy. Vertical segments of the hemicricoid are removed. The hemicricoid is then collapsed with stabilization of the cricoid segments to a midline position, narrowing the laryngeal opening and correcting glottic incompetence.

Endolaryngeal Stents

Several types of endolaryngeal stents have been used to prevent chronic aspiration. Weisberger and Huebsch[98] reported the use of a solid silicone laryngeal stent, which was placed endoscopically and secured transcervically with sutures (Figure 91-3). A tracheotomy tube was necessary. Aspiration was prevented and oral intake tolerated in three of seven patients with chronic aspiration. Perioperative mortality rates were high in this series, and this was thought to be related to tracheotomy tube obstruction. Endoscopic reversal of the stent procedure was reported in two patients; however, both required stent replacement for aspiration control.

Eliachar and others[36,37] reported two types of vented silicone laryngeal stents for control of aspiration (Figure 91-4). The newer of the two stents is inserted through a tracheotomy and secured by a flexible strap of silicone extending from the tracheotomy tract above the tracheotomy tube. Eliachar and Nguyen[36] reported aspiration control in 11 of 12 patients with chronic aspiration with the newer stent. For one patient in whom the initial procedure failed, placement of a larger stent achieved aspiration control. The stent was reportedly used for up to 9 months. Of three patients who survived and had successful stent removal, one experienced laryngeal granulation tissue requiring laser excision, and another developed an anterior subglottic web.

Laryngeal stents are easily introduced and, if properly sized for the patient, prevent aspiration.[36,74] Laryngeal stents, however, have the disadvantages of a lack of uniform success caused by leakage around the stent or extrusion. Because of the potential for endolaryngeal injury from the stent or tracheotomy tube displacement with airway occlusion by the stent, short-term use is recommended. Other

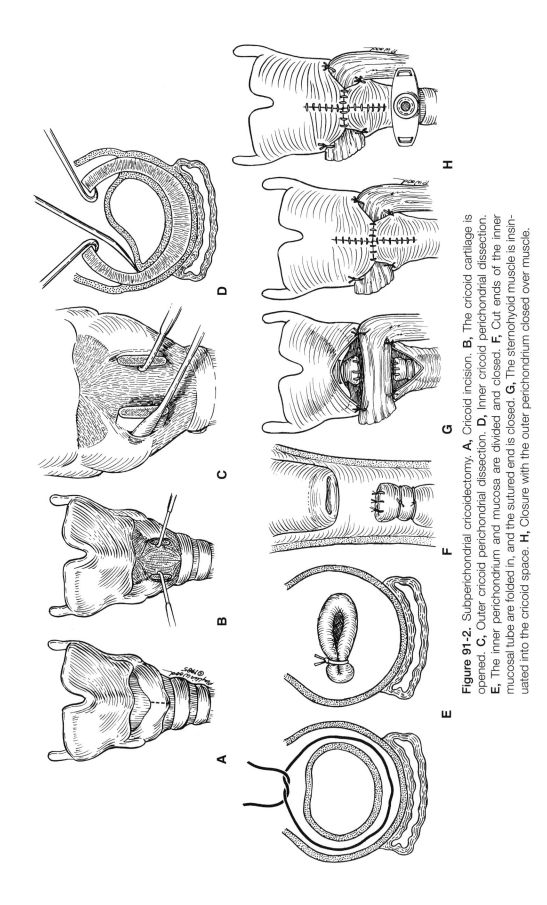

Figure 91-2. Subperichondrial cricoidectomy. **A,** Cricoid incision. **B,** The cricoid cartilage is opened. **C,** Outer cricoid perichondrial dissection. **D,** Inner cricoid perichondrial dissection. **E,** The inner perichondrium and mucosa are divided and closed. **F,** Cut ends of the inner mucosal tube are folded in, and the sutured end is closed. **G,** The sternohyoid muscle is insinuated into the cricoid space. **H,** Closure with the outer perichondrium closed over muscle.

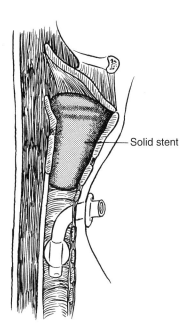

Figure 91-3. Endolaryngeal stent.

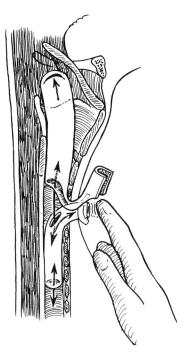

Figure 91-4. Vented endolaryngeal stent.

disadvantages of stents include patient discomfort, the need for stents of different sizes, and the potential for life-threatening complications such as stent dislodgement. At the present time, endolaryngeal stents failed to gain wide acceptance for chronic aspiration control.

Epiglottic Flap Closure of Larynx

Habal and Murray[41] described an epiglottic flap technique of glottic closure. With this technique, the supraglottic larynx is approached through an infrahyoid pharyngotomy. The supraglottic larynx is closed after denuding the edges of the epiglottis, aryepiglottic folds, and arytenoids (Figure 91-5). A tracheotomy is required.

Since this initial report, several modifications and refinements of this procedure have been described. Strome and Fried[94] described: (1) diminishing the tensile strength and elasticity of the epiglottic cartilage by morselization, linear striations, or wedge excision; and (2) severing of the hypoepiglottic and thyroepiglottic ligaments. These modifications lessened dehiscence of the flap posteriorly.[41,96,98] However, this frequent complication allowed speech in some patients.

A further modification of the epiglottic flap closure procedure purposefully leaves the posterior laryngeal inlet open to allow phonation.[18,96] Another modification of this procedure suspends the larynx to the mandible to provide additional laryngeal protection.[97]

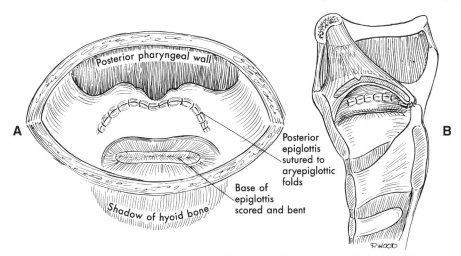

Figure 91-5. Epiglottic flap closure of larynx. **A,** Superior view. **B,** Lateral view.

Denuding the false vocal cords of the mucosa and approximating the false vocal cords provide an additional layer of closure for laryngeal inlet obliteration.[26]

Epiglottic flap closure of the larynx prevents chronic aspiration in only approximately 50% of the procedures reported, although failures can be successfully revised.[56] Although reports of reversal of epiglottic flap closure are uncommon, successful reversal with endoscopy has been reported.[94]

The advantages of epiglottic flap closure include reversibility, allowance of deglutition, and speech preservation if the posterior laryngeal inlet is left open or if dehiscence of the closure occurs. In addition, the true vocal cords are not injured by this procedure. Disadvantages of the epiglottic flap closure procedure include a high rate of flap dehiscence and failure and the need for a transcervical approach and tracheotomy. Supraglottic stenosis is a potential complication after reversal.[96]

Vertical Laryngoplasty

Biller, Lawson, and Baek[9] described vertical laryngoplasty for the prevention of aspiration in patients who required total glossectomy for advanced carcinoma of the tongue (Figure 91-6). In this technique, an incision is made along the outer borders of the epiglottis and is carried inferiorly and posteriorly along the aryepiglottic folds over the arytenoids and into the interarytenoid area. The epiglottis and supraglottic larynx are then closed vertically in two layers as a tube, leaving a small opening superiorly. This technique has also been applied to patients with chronic aspiration with satisfactory results, allowing deglutition and speech.[12] A modification of this procedure has been described in which the epiglottic cartilage is scored to eliminate the cartilaginous spring and thus minimize dehiscence of the closure.[73]

Glottic Closure

Glottic closure was described by Montgomery.[75] In this procedure (Figure 91-7), the larynx is closed at the level of the true and false vocal cords. A midline thyrotomy is performed initially, exposing the endolarynx. The true and false vocal cords, ventricles, and posterior commissure are denuded of mucosa. Nonabsorbable monofilament sutures are used to approximate the glottic surfaces to provide glottic closure. In addition, absorbable sutures are used to approximate the false vocal cord margins. A tracheotomy tube is necessary. Sasaki and others[50,87] modified glottic closure by adding a sternohyoid muscle flap to provide an additional layer of laryngeal closure.

The results of glottic closure for the prevention of aspiration are reported to be excellent (success rate, approximately 95%). There has been only one report of a successful reversal of the glottic closure procedure.[70]

The advantages of the glottic closure procedure include high success rate for prevention of aspiration, allowance of deglutition, and potential reversibility. Glottic stenosis, however, makes reversal difficult. The disadvantages of the glottic closure procedure include the need for a transcervical approach and thyrotomy, the loss of phonation, the need for a tracheotomy, and endolaryngeal injury involving the true vocal cords. Performing the procedure is technically challenging; the interarytenoid closure is the most difficult step. A preexisting laryngeal abnormality is a contraindication for this procedure.

A dynamic glottic closure technique using implanted electrodes to stimulate the recurrent laryngeal nerve at the time of swallow has been proposed as a new method of preventing aspiration without surgical manipulation of the endolarynx.[17]

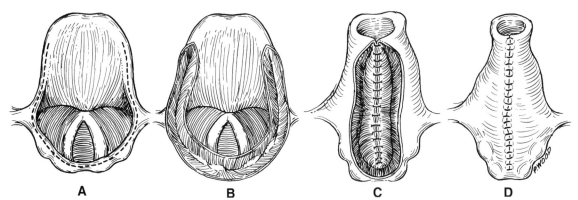

Figure 91-6. Vertical laryngoplasty. **A,** Incision along epiglottis, aryepiglottic folds, arytenoids, and interarytenoid area. **B,** Submucosal flaps are created. **C,** Inner layer closure. **D,** Outer layer closure.

A   B   C

Figure 91-7. Glottic closure procedure. **A,** Midline thyrotomy, removal of the glottic mucosa and transglottic sutures placed for closure. **B,** False vocal cords are approximated. **C,** The glottis is closed.

Along with the obvious benefit of preservation of respiration and phonation, a preliminary report of two stroke patients suggests efficacy in control of aspiration.

Tracheoesophageal Diversion and Laryngotracheal Separation

Lindeman[63] described tracheoesophageal diversion in 1975. This procedure for chronic aspiration was devised with the objective of controlling aspiration for an indefinite period while preserving the larynx and the integrity of the recurrent laryngeal nerves. The procedure was designed to be reversible, should healthy laryngeal protective function return.

Tracheoesophageal diversion (Figure 91-8) is performed by division of the trachea horizontally at the fourth and fifth tracheal rings. The proximal tracheal segment is anastomosed in an end-to-side fashion to an opening in the anterior esophagus. The distal tracheal segment is used to create a tracheostoma.

In 1976, a similar surgical procedure for chronic aspiration, laryngotracheal separation, was described.[64] Laryngotracheal separation was designed for patients with chronic aspiration who had previously undergone high tracheotomy, which prevents establishment of a tracheoesophageal anastomosis, as performed in tracheoesophageal diversion.

Laryngotracheal separation (Figure 91-9) is performed by division of the trachea horizontally between the second and third tracheal rings or at the level of an existing tracheotomy. The proximal tracheal edges are closed onto themselves anteroposteriorly as a blind pouch. The tracheal closure is buttressed with rotated sternothyroid muscles. The distal tracheal segment is used to create a tracheostoma.

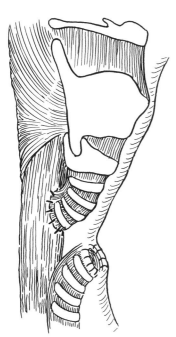

Figure 91-8. Tracheoesophageal diversion.

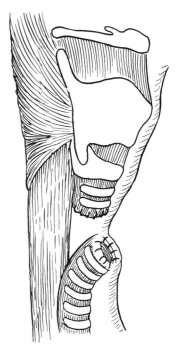

Figure 91-9. Laryngotracheal separation.

A modification of tracheoesophageal diversion (Figure 91-10) has been described; an anterior tracheal flap is created by removing the inferior half of the cricoid cartilage and the anterior aspects of the first and second tracheal rings.[53] This modification creates a soft flap, which allows tracheoesophageal diversion in patients who have undergone prior tracheotomy. This modification may jeopardize the reversibility of the procedure.

Tucker[95] proposed division of the trachea and externalization of the proximal trachea between the fibers of the sternocleidomastoid muscle to the cervical skin. It was theorized that sternocleidomastoid muscle compression would collapse the trachea, thus limiting external leakage of secretions. This procedure affects definitive separation of the respiratory tract and the digestive tract and prevents aspiration. Tracheal secretions draining onto the neck, however, are aesthetically displeasing and require local care.

Many authors have reported uniform success in chronic aspiration control with tracheoesophageal diversion and laryngotracheal separation.[5,31,35,40,90] Postoperatively in both procedures, most patients can tolerate a normal diet, depending on their neurologic function. In some instances, reversals of both procedures and resultant normal voice, swallowing, and respiration have been reported.[32,35,83,91] Both procedures can be performed with local anesthesia, if necessary.

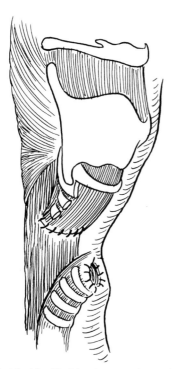

Figure 91-10. Modified tracheoesophageal diversion.

Tracheoesophageal diversion has been recommended for patients with chronic aspiration who have not undergone high tracheotomy.[33] Tracheoesophageal diversion allows secretions and oral intake that have penetrated the larynx to pass into the esophagus. However, laryngotracheal separation is technically easier to perform than tracheoesophageal diversion. These techniques are equally effective in controlling chronic aspiration. Complications are uncommon; they include postoperative fistula, which usually closes spontaneously with local care and antibiotics. Fistula formation is more common in patients with prior tracheotomy.[31]

Candidates for reversal of laryngotracheal separation or tracheoesophageal diversion must demonstrate neurologic improvement and should be evaluated with laryngoscopy and videofluoroscopic swallowing studies to confirm improved laryngeal protective mechanisms. Reversals of these procedures have been performed most commonly in patients who have recovered from cerebrovascular accidents or who have had resection of benign intracranial tumors.[31] Excellent long-term speech and swallowing capabilities have been demonstrated in patients who have undergone reversal procedures.[83] Tracheoesophageal diversion and laryngotracheal separation have the advantage of being the most dependable of the reversible techniques for preventing chronic aspiration. These procedures allow oral alimentation and are reversible because the endolarynx is avoided and the larynx is not injured. Also, the procedures are technically straightforward and can be performed from the bedside. Disadvantages include the need for a transcervical approach and the loss of capacity for air-powered speech. Most patients, depending on their neurologic function, communicate with an electrolarynx after these procedures. Tracheoesophageal puncture and placement of a Blom-Singer voice prosthesis with successful speech rehabilitation has been reported after laryngotracheal separation.[27] Careful criteria, including sufficient manual dexterity and visual acuity, are necessary to select candidates for this rehabilitative procedure after laryngotracheal separation.[27]

Tracheoesophageal diversion and laryngotracheal separation have also been successfully performed with satisfactory results in children with chronic aspiration.[24,29,57]

SUMMARY

Chronic or intractable aspiration is a serious problem that is usually related to severe neurologic dysfunction. Chronic aspiration requires thorough evaluation and management of any correctable causes. Surgical separation of the upper respiratory tract and upper digestive tract may be necessary to prevent repeated soilage of the respiratory system with recurrent infectious complications, as well as to avoid death.

If there is no change or recovery of neurologic function, surgical options for chronic aspiration control include subperichondrial cricoidectomy and narrow-field laryngectomy. If recovery is possible, laryngotracheal separation is an effective and reversible surgical technique that prevents chronic aspiration.

REFERENCES

1. Alessi DM, Berci G: Aspiration and nasogastric intubation, *Otolaryngol Head Neck Surg* 94:486, 1986.
2. Aviv JE and others: Age-related changes in pharyngeal and supraglottic sensation, *Ann Otol Rhinol Laryngol* 103:749, 1994.
3. Aviv JE and others: Cost-effectiveness of two types of dysphagia care in head and neck cancer: a preliminary report, *Ear Nose Throat J* 80:553, 2001.
4. Awe WC, Fletcher WS, Jacob SW: The pathophysiology of aspiration pneumonitis, *Surgery* 60:232, 1966.
5. Baron BC, Dedo HH: Separation of the larynx and trachea for intractable aspiration, *Laryngoscope* 90:1927, 1980.
6. Bartlett JG, Gorbach SL: The triple threat of aspiration pneumonia, *Chest* 68:560, 1975.
7. Bernhard WN and others: Adjustment of intracuff pressure to prevent aspiration, *Anesthesiology* 50:363, 1979.
8. Betts RH and others: Post-tracheotomy aspiration, *N Engl J Med* 273:155, 1965.
9. Biller HF, Lawson W, Baek SM: Total glossectomy: a technique of reconstruction eliminating laryngectomy, *Arch Otolaryngol Head Neck Surg* 109:69, 1983.
10. Biller HF, Urken M: Cricoid collapse, a new technique for the management of glottic incompetence, *Arch Otolaryngol Head Neck Surg* 111:740, 1985.
11. Blitzer A: Approaches to the patient with aspiration and swallowing disabilities, *Dysphagia* 5:129, 1990.
12. Blitzer A: Evaluation and management of chronic aspiration, *NY State J Med* 87:154, 1987.
13. Bonanno PC: Swallowing dysfunction after tracheostomy, *Ann Surg* 174:29, 1971.
14. Bone DK and others: Aspiration pneumonia: prevention of aspiration in patients with tracheostomies, *Ann Thorac Surg* 18:30, 1974.
15. Briant TD: Spontaneous pharyngeal fistula and wound infection following laryngectomy, *Laryngoscope* 85:829, 1975.
16. Brin MF, Younger D: Neurologic disorders and aspiration, *Otolaryngol Clin North Am* 21:691, 1988.
17. Broniatowski M and others: Dynamic laryngotracheal closure for aspiration: a preliminary report, *Laryngoscope* 111:2032, 2001.
18. Brooks GB, McKelvie P: Epiglottopexy: a new surgical technique to prevent intractable aspiration, *Ann R Coll Surg Engl* 65:293, 1983.
19. Cameron JL, Reynolds J, Zuidema GD: Aspiration in patients with tracheotomies, *Surg Gynecol Obstet* 136:68, 1973.
20. Cameron JL, Zuidema GD: Aspiration pneumonia: magnitude and frequency of the problem, *JAMA* 219:1194, 1972.
21. Cannon CR, McLean WC: Laryngectomy for chronic aspiration, *Am J Otolaryngol* 3:145, 1982.
22. Carrau RL and others: Laryngeal framework surgery for the management of aspiration, *Head Neck* 21:139, 1999.
23. Ciocon JO and others: Tube feedings in elderly patients: indications, benefits, complications, *Arch Intern Med* 148:429, 1988.
24. Cohen SR, Thompson JW: Variants of Mobius' syndrome and central neurologic impairment: Lindeman procedure in children, *Ann Otol Rhinol Laryngol* 96:93, 1987.
25. Coloeny N: Interjudge and intrajudge reliabilities in fiberoptic endoscopic evaluation of swallowing (fees) using the penetration-aspiration scale: a replication study, *Dysphagia* 17:308, 2002.
26. Cummings CW: *Epiglottic sewdown (epiglottopexy) procedure.* In Cummings CW: *Atlas of laryngeal surgery,* St Louis, 1984, Mosby.
27. Darrow DM, Robbins KT, Goldman SN: Tracheoesophageal puncture for voice restoration following laryngotracheal separation, *Laryngoscope* 104:1163, 1994.
28. Donner MW, Silbiger ML: Cinefluorographic analysis of pharyngeal swallowing in neuromuscular disorders, *Am J Med Sci* 251:600, 1966.
29. Eavey RD: Airway interruption in encephalopathic children: a clinical and histological analysis, *Laryngoscope* 95:1455, 1985.
30. Eibling DE, Gross RD: Subglottic air pressure: a key component of swallowing efficiency, *Ann Otol Rhinol Laryngol* 105:263, 1996.
31. Eibling DE, Snyderman CH, Eibling C: Laryngotracheal separation for intractable aspiration: a retrospective review of 34 patients, *Laryngoscope* 105:83, 1995.
32. Eisele DW: Surgical approaches to aspiration, *Dysphagia* 6:71, 1991.
33. Eisele DW, Yarington CT Jr, Lindeman RC: Indications for the tracheoesophageal diversion procedure and the laryngotracheal separation procedure, *Ann Otol Rhinol Laryngol* 97:471, 1988.
34. Eisele DW and others: Subperichondrial cricoidectomy: an alternative to laryngectomy for intractable aspiration, *Laryngoscope* 105:322, 1995.
35. Eisele DW and others: The tracheoesophageal diversion and laryngotracheal separation procedures for treatment of intractable aspiration, *Am J Surg* 157:230, 1989.
36. Eliachar I, Nguyen D: Laryngotracheal stent for internal support and control of aspiration without loss of phonation, *Otolaryngol Head Neck Surg* 103:837, 1990.
37. Eliachar I and others: A vented laryngeal stent with phonatory and pressure relief capability, *Laryngoscope* 97:1264, 1987.
38. Elpern EL, Jacobs ER, Bone RC: Incidence of aspiration in tracheally intubated adults, *Heart Lung* 16:527, 1987.
39. Feldman SA, Deal CW, Urquhart W: Disturbance of swallowing after tracheostomy, *Lancet* 1:954, 1966.
40. Gilbert RW and others: Management of patients with long-term tracheotomies and aspiration, *Ann Otol Rhinol Laryngol* 96:561, 1987.
41. Habal MB, Murray JE: Surgical treatment of life-endangering chronic aspiration pneumonia: use of an epiglottic flap to the arytenoids, *Plast Reconstr Surg* 49:305, 1972.
42. Hassett JM, Sunby C, Flint LM: No elimination of aspiration pneumonia in neurologically disabled patients with feeding gastrostomy, *Surg Gynecol Obstet* 167:383, 1988.
43. Hawthorne M, Gray R, Cottam C: Conservative laryngectomy (an effective treatment for severe aspiration in motor neurone disease), *J Laryngol Otol* 101:283, 1987.
44. Horner J, Massey EW: Silent aspiration following stroke, *Neurology* 38:317, 1988.
45. Horner J and others: Aspiration following stroke: clinical correlates and outcome, *Neurology* 38:1359, 1988.
46. Huxley EJ and others: Pharyngeal aspiration in normal adults and patients with depressed consciousness, *Am J Med* 64:564, 1978.

47. Ikari T, Sasaki CT: Glottic closure reflex: control mechanisms, *Ann Otol* 89:220, 1980.

48. Isshiki N, Okamura H, Ishikawa T: Thyroplasty type I (lateral compression) for dysphonia due to vocal cord paralysis or atrophy, *Acta Otolaryngol* 80:465, 1975.

49. Kadakia SC, Sullivan HO, Starnes E: Percutaneous endoscopic gastrostomy or jejunostomy and the incidence of aspiration in 79 patients, *Am J Surg* 164:114, 1992.

50. Kirchner JC, Sasaki CT: Surgery for aspiration, *Otolaryngol Clin North Am* 17:49, 1984.

51. Koufman JA: Laryngoplasty for vocal cord medialization: an alternative to Teflon, *Laryngoscope* 96:726, 1986.

52. Krespi YP, Pelzer HJ, Sisson GA: Management of chronic aspiration by subtotal and submucosal cricoid resection, *Ann Otol Rhinol Laryngol* 94:580, 1985.

53. Krespi YP, Quatela VC, Sisson GA: Modified tracheoesophageal diversion for chronic aspiration, *Laryngoscope* 94:1298, 1984.

54. Langmore SE, Schatz MA, Olsen N: Fiberoptic endoscopic examination of swallowing safety: a new procedure, *Dysphagia* 2:216, 1988.

55. Langmore SE, Schatz K, Olson N: Endoscopic and videofluoroscopic evaluations of swallowing and aspiration, *Ann Otol Rhinol Laryngol* 100:678, 1991.

56. Laurian N, Shvili Y, Zohar Y: Epiglotto-aryepiglottopexy: a surgical procedure for severe aspiration, *Laryngoscope* 96:78, 1986.

57. Lawless ST and others: The use of a laryngotracheal separation procedure in pediatric patients, *Laryngoscope* 105:198, 1995.

58. Lazarus C, Logemann JA: Swallowing disorders in closed head trauma patients, *Arch Phys Med Rehabil* 68:79, 1987.

59. Leder SB, Ross DA: Investigation of the causal relationship between tracheotomy and aspiration in the acute care setting, *Laryngoscope* 110: 641, 2000.

60. Leder SB, Sasaki CT, Burrell MI: Fiberoptic endoscopic evaluation of dysphagia to identify silent aspiration, *Dysphagia* 13:19, 1998.

61. Lewis WS, Wikholm RP, Passy V: Bilateral vocal cord Teflon injection: an ineffective treatment for recurrent aspiration pneumonia, *Arch Otolaryngol Head Neck Surg* 117:427, 1991.

62. Lewy RB: Glottic rehabilitation with Teflon injection: the return of voice, cough, and laughter, *Acta Otolaryngol* 58:214, 1964.

63. Lindeman RC: Diverting the paralyzed larynx: a reversible procedure for intractable aspiration, *Laryngoscope* 85:157, 1975.

64. Lindeman RC, Yarington CT, Sutton D: Clinical experience with the tracheoesophageal anastomosis for intractable aspiration, *Ann Otol Rhinol Laryngol* 85:609, 1976.

65. Linden P, Kuhlemeier KV, Patterson C: The probability of correctly predicting subglottic penetration from clinical observations, *Dysphagia* 8:1970, 1993.

66. Linden P, Siebens AA: Dysphagia: predicting laryngeal penetration, *Arch Phys Med Rehabil* 64:281, 1983.

67. Logemann JA: Aspiration in head and neck surgical patients, *Ann Otol Rhinol Laryngol* 94:373, 1985.

68. Logemann JA: Treatment for aspiration related to dysphagia: an overview, *Dysphagia* 1:34, 1986.

69. Logemann JA and others: Effects of postural change on aspiration in head and neck surgical patients, *Otolaryngol Head Neck Surg* 110:222, 1994.

70. Lulenski GC: Laryngeal closure and glottic reconstruction, *Ear Nose Throat J* 59:23, 1980.

71. Martens L, Cameron T, Simonsen M: Effects of a multidisciplinary management program on neurologically impaired patients with dysphagia, *Dysphagia* 5:147, 1990.

72. McCaffrey TB, Lipton R: Transcutaneous Teflon injection for paralytic dysphonia, *Laryngoscope* 99:497, 1989.

73. Meiteles LZ, Kraus W, Shemen L: Modified epiglottoplasty for prevention of aspiration, *Laryngoscope* 103:1395, 1993.

74. Miller FR, Eliachar I: Managing the aspirating patient, *Am J Otolaryngol* 15:1, 1994.

75. Montgomery WW: Surgery to prevent aspiration, *Arch Otolaryngol Head Neck Surg* 101:679, 1975.

76. Muz J and others: Aspiration in patients with head and neck cancer and tracheostomy, *Am J Otolaryngol* 10:282, 1989.

77. Muz J and others: Detection and quantification of laryngotracheopulmonary aspiration with scintigraphy, *Laryngoscope* 97:1180, 1987.

78. Muz J and others: Scintigraphic assessment of aspiration in head and neck cancer patients with tracheostomy, *Head Neck* 16:17, 1994 .

79. Nash M: Swallowing problems in the tracheotomized patient, *Otolaryngol Clin North Am* 21:702, 1988.

80. Norton JA and others: Intolerance to enteral feeding in the brain-injured patient, *J Neurosurg* 63:62, 1988.

81. Pavlin EG, VanNimwegan D, Hornbein TF: Failure of a high-compliance low-pressure cuff to prevent aspiration, *Anesthesiology* 42:216, 1975.

82. Petring OU and others: Prevention of silent aspiration due to leaks around cuffs of endotracheal tubes, *Anesth Analg* 65:777, 1986.

83. Pletcher SD, Mandpe AH, Block MI and others: Reversal of laryngotracheal separation: a detailed report with long-term follow-up. Presented at the Western Section of the Triologic Society, Indian Wells, California, Feb 1, 2003.

84. Rasley A and others: Prevention of barium aspiration during videofluoroscopic swallowing studies: value of change of posture, *Am J Roentgenol* 160:1005, 1993.

85. Rontal E and others: Vocal cord injection in the treatment of acute and chronic aspiration, *Laryngoscope* 86:625, 1976.

86. Sasaki CT and others: The effect of tracheostomy on the laryngeal closure reflex, *Laryngoscope* 87:1428, 1977.

87. Sasaki CT and others: Surgical closure of the larynx for intractable aspiration, *Arch Otolaryngol Head Neck Surg* 106:422, 1980.

88. Sasaki CT Fukuda H, Kirchner JA: Laryngeal abductor activity in response to varying ventilatory resistance, *Trans Am Acad Ophthamol Otolaryngol* 77:403, 1973.

89. Schindler JS, Kelly JH: Swallowing disorders in the elderly, *Laryngoscope* 112:589, 2002.

90. Silver KH, VanNostrand DL: The use of scintigraphy in the management of patients with pulmonary aspiration, *Dysphagia* 9:107, 1994.

91. Snyderman CH, Johnson JT: Laryngotracheal separation for intractable aspiration, *Ann Otol Rhinol Laryngol* 97:466, 1988.

92. Splaingard ML and others: Aspiration in rehabilitation patients: videofluoroscopy vs. bedside clinical assessment, *Arch Phys Med Rehabil* 69:637, 1988.

93. Stachler RJ and others: Scintigraphic quantification of aspiration reduction with the Passey-Muir valve, *Laryngoscope* 106:231, 1996.

94. Strome M, Fried MP: Rehabilitative surgery for aspiration, *Arch Otolaryngol Head Neck Surg* 109:809, 1983.

95. Tucker HM: Management of the patient with an incompetent larynx, *Am J Otolaryngol* 1:47, 1979.

96. Vecchione TR, Habel MB, Murray JE: Further experiences with the arytenoid-epiglottic flap for chronic aspiration pneumonia, *Plast Reconstr Surg* 55:318, 1975.

97. Warwick-Brown NP, Richards AES, Cheesman AD: Epiglottopexy: a modification using additional hyoid suspension, *J Laryngol Otol* 100:1155, 1986.

98. Weisberger EC, Huebsch SA: Endoscopic treatment of aspiration using a laryngeal stent, *Otolaryngol Head Neck Surg* 90:215, 1982.

99. Wu CH and others: Evaluation of swallowing safety with fiberoptic endoscope: comparison with videofluoroscopic technique, *Laryngoscope* 107:396, 1997.

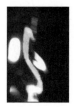

CHAPTER NINETY TWO

LARYNGEAL AND ESOPHAGEAL TRAUMA

|| Steven D. Schaefer

INTRODUCTION

Within the neck are the elements necessary to connect and coordinate the function of the head with the body. Injury to the neck can disrupt any of these vital functions and may involve bony, soft tissue, vascular, and central nervous system elements. Although many associated injuries may appear more impressive, correct management of the neck injury with immediate attention to securing the airway is always the first priority. A multidisciplinary approach is very useful because each member of the team contributes expertise in a particular area.

This chapter addresses the management of nonvascular soft tissue injuries of the neck, primarily laryngeal trauma. Experience in managing laryngeal trauma is limited because of the rarity of this injury. External laryngeal trauma accounts for only 1 in 30,000 emergency room visits.[35] Iatrogenic laryngeal injury had been becoming more frequent with the increased incidence of long-term endotracheal intubation. This may have stabilized or even declined with improved technique and preventive measures. Although these injuries are rare, their initial management has a tremendous impact on the immediate probability of survival of the patient and the patient's long-term quality of life.

MECHANISMS OF INJURY

Injury to the larynx is uncommon for several reasons. The inferior projection of the mandible affords significant protection from anterior blows. Posteriorly, the larynx is protected by the rigid cervical spine. Nonetheless, injuries occur, and the resultant damage to the larynx is usually characteristic of the mechanism of injury. The mechanisms of laryngeal injury can be divided into blunt trauma, including clothesline, crushing, and strangulation injuries; penetrating trauma; inhalation injuries; and injuries caused by caustic ingestions.

Anterior blunt injuries are most commonly the result of motor vehicle accidents (Figure 92-1).[26,29]

The incidence of this type of injury is declining, presumably because of mandatory seat belt laws, lower speed limits, and better education regarding drunk driving. The use of front seat air bags may reduce the incidence even further. If no seat belt is worn or if only a lap belt is used, the driver is thrust forward during rapid deceleration with the neck in a hyperextended fashion. This position removes the bony protection afforded by the mandible, exposing the larynx to anterior crushing forces. If the larynx then strikes the steering wheel or dashboard, it can be compressed between these objects and the cervical spine.[26]

Clothesline injuries occur when the rider of a vehicle such as a motorcycle or snowmobile encounters a fixed horizontal object, such as a clothesline, at neck level. This type of injury imparts a large amount of energy over a relatively small area, resulting in massive trauma.[4] Many of these injuries lead to immediate death resulting from a crushed larynx or separation of the cricoid from the larynx or trachea.

Strangulation injuries occur from manual compression, from assaults with strangulation by a soft object, or from attempted suicides by hanging. Typically, the initial finding may be hoarseness or abrasions on the skin of the overlying neck. However, these injuries may later (in 12–24 hours) be associated with marked edema of the larynx and resultant loss of airway.[38] The magnitude of the force sustained to the anterior neck should be considered in the course of managing such patients to avoid subsequent potential loss of the airway.[31] Overall, in blunt trauma to the anterior neck, fractures of the thyroid cartilage occur more frequently than do injuries of all other airway cartilages combined.[12]

Penetrating trauma, in contrast to trauma from motor vehicle accidents, had been increasing because of a rise in the number of personal assaults (Figure 92-2).[27] For example, in a review of 148 cases of penetrating neck trauma, injury to the larynx or trachea

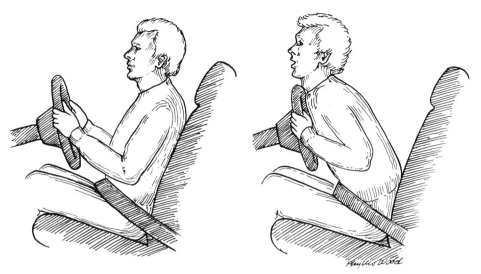

Figure 92-1. With a lap belt and without a shoulder harness, the neck is extended, removing protection that the mandible affords the neck. The larynx is crushed between the steering wheel and the cervical spine. (Redrawn from Schaefer S: *Ann Otol Rhinol Laryngol* 91:399, 1982.)

was noted in 12 cases.[30] The future incidence of such trauma will parallel the state of violence in America. Injury from a gunshot wound depends on the type of weapon used and the range from which it was fired. Gunshots at close range impart intense energy to the soft tissues and are usually fatal. From a long range, the damage may be minimal. Low-velocity handguns (commonly used in domestic assaults) generally have only a moderate blast effect on surrounding tissue; these injuries can be misleading on initial examination because of the bullet's erratic course in soft tissues. High-velocity weapons, such as hunting rifles and military assault weapons, impart a significant amount of kinetic energy to the tissues.[15] In these

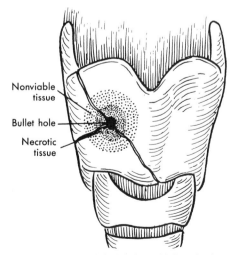

Figure 92-2. Penetrating injuries from high-velocity weapons. Tissue damage extends beyond the zone of obvious necrosis.

injuries, wide débridement of surrounding tissue is advisable at the time of repair because the injured area may necrose beyond the limit of the immediately evident nonviable tissue. Knife injuries do not destroy tissue distant to the path of injury, and their course can be accurately estimated based on the entrance and exit wounds.

The pediatric larynx is injured less often than the adult larynx. Situated higher in the neck than the adult larynx, the pediatric larynx is afforded greater protection from the caudal projection of the mandible. However, in injury of the pediatric larynx, increased soft tissue damage and decreased cartilaginous fractures likely occur because of the loose attachment of the overlying mucous membrane, lack of fibrous support, and increased elasticity of the cartilaginous framework. Also, the relative cross-sectional area of the pediatric larynx compared with that of the adult larynx is decreased. This combination of increased soft tissue injury and decreased cross-sectional area makes the pediatric airway especially vulnerable to embarrassment, particularly because attending medical personnel may not recognize the severity of the injury because of the lack of associated cartilage fractures.

Inhalation injuries are caused by superheated air, especially steam, with its increased capacity to carry thermal energy. On inhalation of heated air, the glottis reflexively closes. This limits the amount of thermal injury by stopping respiration, thus decreasing the amount of air inhaled, and limits the injury to the supraglottic larynx. This injury is usually associated with burns to other parts of the body, especially burn injuries sustained in closed areas. The initial presentation may be unremarkable except for erythema of the upper airway and occasionally carbon-stained sputum. An airway should be secured early in these injuries before fluid resuscitation of the associated burn injury begins because this will lead to marked edema of the injured mucosa with loss of airway and an inability to endotracheally intubate the patient. Injuries from caustic ingestion typically occur in the pediatric population and can result from various household products. In adults, inhalation injuries are usually the result of a suicide attempt, characteristically from ingestion of lye or hydrocarbons. Besides the usual oral, pharyngeal, and esophageal injuries, the larynx can be injured by direct contact during ingestion or regurgitation of the ingested substance. Reflex glottic closure limits these injuries to the supraglottic larynx.

EXTERNAL LARYNGEAL TRAUMA
Diagnosis

The signs and symptoms of external laryngeal trauma vary from obvious open fractures to subtle aberrations of laryngeal function. External examination of the neck may reveal an open fracture or laryngocutaneous fistula. The larynx should be palpated for any crepitance. Tenderness to palpation, although not specific, is often present in significant injury.[31] The skin of the neck may reveal contusions or abrasions from blunt trauma or a line pattern indicative of a strangulation injury.[28,38] Any penetrating injury is examined for an entrance and exit wound, and the most likely path of travel of the projectile is determined. Open wounds are not explored with instruments, nor are they probed for fear of dislodging a hematoma and initiating further bleeding. The cervical spine should be palpated for any bony stepoffs or tenderness. Hemoptysis may reveal an injury to the upper aerodigestive system, but this type of injury is often difficult to differentiate from bleeding caused by associated facial trauma.

External laryngeal trauma is often associated with a change in voice.[37] In severe trauma, the patient may be entirely aphonic. More commonly, the voice is present but is altered because of the change in architecture of the larynx. Hematomas of the true vocal folds add mass to this vibratory unit and lower the fundamental frequency of vibration. Paresis of the vocal fold from damage to the recurrent laryngeal nerve or from mechanical dislocation of the cricoarytenoid joint can cause a weak, breathy voice. Finally, any alteration in the larynx that changes the airflow patterns has the potential to alter the voice. The diagnosis of the more subtle injuries benefits from the application of videostroboscopy and selective electromyography.

Among the most serious alterations of laryngeal function is the abnormal flow of air through the upper airway. In instances of cricotracheal separation, the airway can be maintained via a cutaneous laceration that connects with the trachea or a bridge of mucous membrane between the cricoid and trachea. In a gunshot wound, the path of the missile serves as a laryngocutaneous fistula and allows respiration despite obstruction at the glottic or supraglottic level (Figure 92-3).[9] In this instance, airflow from the wound will be obvious, and no attempt should be made to cover, compress, or otherwise manipulate such a wound until the surgeon is ready to secure the airway. Stridor may occur from bilateral vocal fold paresis or disruption or may result from any combination of unilateral immobility and subglottic, glottic, or supraglottic edema. If severe enough, edema alone with healthy vocal fold function may cause stridor.

A third, more subtle form of laryngeal dysfunction is aspiration, which is usually caused by immobility of one or both vocal folds. Although not clinically apparent immediately after an injury, this may later become evident.

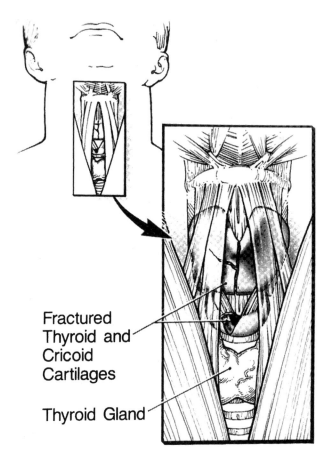

Figure 92-3. Various injuries can be encountered in the larynx. (From Schaefer SD: *Op Tech Otolaryngol Head Neck Surg* 1:65, 1990.)

Fractured Thyroid and Cricoid Cartilages

Thyroid Gland

After the initial examination and securing of the airway, examination of the endolaryngeal anatomy is attempted. In the past, this was only possible in the awake patient using the indirect mirror examination and was therefore not very useful in severely injured patients. Today, widespread use of direct fiberoptic examination allows for improved nonoperative evaluation of the injured larynx.[31,32] Care should be taken in the examination of a nonintubated patient because minor trauma associated with insertion of the fiberoptic laryngoscope can precipitate an airway emergency. After insertion of this instrument through the nares, the oropharynx and hypopharynx are examined for injury. The larynx is examined for hematomas, and their size and location are noted. The arytenoids are evaluated for full range of motion with phonation and respiration.[13] Partial limitation of range of motion indicates a structural deformity or dislocation of the arytenoid, whereas complete immobility is more suggestive of recurrent nerve injury. Failure of the true vocal folds to meet in the same horizontal plane may also be present, indicating a structural change in the laryngeal framework or superior laryngeal nerve injury. Finally, any exposed cartilage is noted along with the integrity of the surrounding mucosa.

Computed Tomography

The role of preoperative radiographic evaluation of the injured larynx has changed dramatically with the widespread availability of computed tomography (CT).[7,18,19,33] Before CT, plain soft tissue neck films, contrast laryngography, and tomography were available to assess the soft tissues of the larynx. Frequently, these studies added little information about the integrity of the larynx not already known by physical examination of the patient with direct fiberoptic laryngoscopy. Plain films can identify fractures but reveal the anatomy in only two dimensions. Laryngography is often impossible in an acutely injured patient because of the patient's inability to cooperate. Plain tomography lacks the three-dimensional analysis and clarity of CT. CT allows evaluation of the laryngeal skeletal framework in a noninvasive manner, thus avoiding unnecessary operative explorations by selecting patients who should do well without surgical intervention (Figure 92-4). Optimal imaging is performed using spiral technique and subsecond scan times, particularly when using two-dimensional sections for multiple projections or three-dimensional reconstructions.[17] In injured patients in need of open surgical repair, such as those with exposed cartilage or displaced fractures with overlying mucosal lacerations, CT adds little to the preoperative and surgical examination of the larynx.[33] Rather, CT should be reserved for patients in whom

laryngeal injury is suspected by history and physical examination without obvious surgical indications. This may include patients who have only one sign or symptom of laryngeal injury, such as hoarseness, and minimal findings suggestive of laryngeal injury. In this instance, CT may allow the surgeon to confirm the lack of injury in a noninvasive manner without direct laryngoscopy and the concomitant need for general anesthesia. CT can also be used to identify patients with minimally displaced midline and lateral thyroid cartilage fractures that are otherwise unremarkable and minimally symptomatic and that, if left unrepaired, would lead to long-term phonatory disturbances because of disruption of the laryngeal valving mechanisms.[37] When massive edema or hematomas are present, direct laryngoscopy may not be useful in determining the integrity of the laryngeal framework. In this instance, if CT does not show evidence of laryngeal fractures, the patient can be managed with a tracheotomy and observation, thus avoiding open exploration.

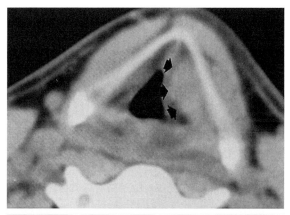
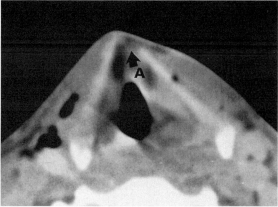

Figure 92-4. Computed tomography shows a hematoma involving the right vocal fold *(arrows)* with the thyroid cartilage intact. The injury was completely resolved with only medical management. Fracture of the right anterior thyroid lamina with angulation is seen. The management consisted of open reduction and internal fixation.

Initial Management

In a patient with neck injury who presents to the emergency department, the first priority is to establish an airway. This can be very difficult and often requires emergent tracheotomy or cricothyroidotomy. Care should be taken to avoid manipulation of the neck. Until a cervical spine injury has been excluded, no extension of the neck should be allowed during either orotracheal intubation or tracheotomy. After the airway is secured, venous access should be obtained with at least two large-bore cannulas. Isotonic fluids are administered as needed to maintain circulation. The patient is then disrobed and examined for other injuries. If the patient is unstable after these measures, immediate surgery is needed. However, if the patient is relatively stable after these measures, diagnostic assessment can proceed. The minimum radiographic evaluation consists of a cervical spine series and a chest radiograph. Subplatysmal penetrating injuries in the area of the carotid arteries should be evaluated with arteriography. After full assessment of all injuries, the various physicians involved should determine the order of management and proceed accordingly.

Management

Management of injuries to the larynx and esophagus is based on the mechanism and extent of injury found during the initial assessment (Figure 92-5). The first priority is always securing the airway.[14] If the patient is breathing well and the injury does not require surgical care, observation without tracheotomy or endotracheal intubation may be indicated. However, all injuries to this region carry a propensity for airway embarrassment. It is best to be cautious, especially in patients without prior trauma to this area, when determining the need for airway intervention.

Nonsurgical vs Surgical Management

The purpose of the extensive physical and radiologic evaluation is to identify the patients with injury and to select patients who are likely to do well without

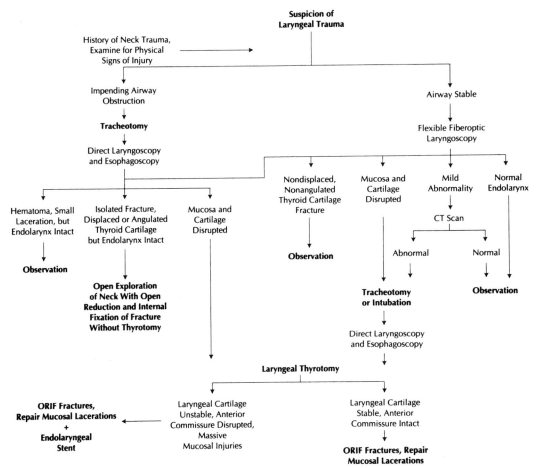

Figure 92-5. Management protocol for an acutely injured larynx. (From Schaefer SD: *Arch Otolaryngol* 118:603, 1992.)

surgical intervention.[31–33,41] Medical management assumes that the patient does not require a tracheotomy and has an otherwise stable airway. If the patient has only minor laryngeal mucosal lacerations not involving the anterior commissure or has single nondisplaced fractures of the thyroid cartilage without overlying mucosal lacerations or exposed cartilage, then management can be confined to close observation and elevation of the head of the bed. Corticosteroids can be useful if administered soon after injury. Minor hematomas stable in size and not causing respiratory embarrassment can be managed in a similar manner. Open surgical exploration and repair are the management of choice for all of the following injuries: those involving the anterior commissure, having exposed cartilage, having multiple or displaced fractures of the thyroid cartilage involving multiple fractures of the cricoid cartilage, causing vocal fold paralysis or airway compromise sufficient to require intubation or tracheotomy, or associated with an injury to another area of the neck that requires surgical intervention (Figures 92-6, 92-7, and 92-8).[31]

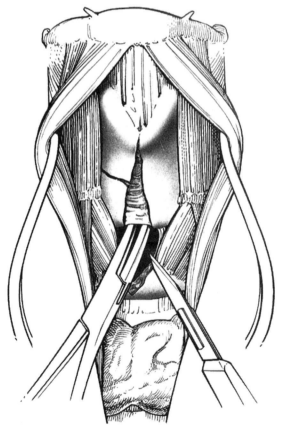

Figure 92-6. Exploration of the larynx is performed via a midline thyrotomy or via a paramedian vertical thyroid cartilage fracture. (From Schaefer SD: *Op Tech Otolaryngol Head Neck Surg* 1:65, 1990.)

Surgical Management

Repair of the larynx should be coordinated with all surgical teams involved and with an anesthesiologist. The person responsible for the airway at each stage of the procedure should be designated before the patient is brought to the operating room. Plans for emergently obtaining an airway and the instruments required for surgery should also be established.

The most conservative, reliable method of securing an airway in a patient with laryngeal injury is local tracheotomy while the patient is awake. Endotracheal intubation can further damage the larynx, can be exceedingly difficult, can interfere with subsequent examination and repair of the larynx, and may convert an urgent procedure to an emergent one (Figure 92-9). Endotracheal intubation is acceptable when the endolaryngeal mucous membrane is intact, the laryngeal skeleton is minimally displaced, and intubation is performed by a person highly skilled in such procedures.

After local tracheotomy or intubation in these limited situations, general anesthesia is induced, followed by direct laryngoscopy. The larynx is examined for exposed cartilage, hematomas, lacerations, and range of motion of the true vocal folds. The subglottis is evaluated for injury to the cricoid and trachea. Rigid esophagoscopy is performed to rule out injury to the esophagus.[14]

Pediatric patients warrant special consideration when obtaining a surgical airway. Endotracheal intubation in an injured pediatric larynx carries all of the same risks as in an adult larynx. The option of local tracheotomy is not feasible in a frightened, injured child. The time margin of error is also less because the arterial oxygen saturation drops more quickly than in an adult. In this instance, rigid bronchoscopy is performed to secure the airway under direct visualization. A tracheotomy can then be performed over the bronchoscope.

After direct laryngoscopy and examination with the patient under anesthesia and after review of the CT findings, the need for open exploration and repair is reevaluated. Microlaryngoscopy should also be considered, particularly in evaluating lesser injuries.[13] In patients with edema, hematomas, nondisplaced fractures of the thyroid cartilage, healthy true vocal fold motion, and no injury to the anterior commissure, no further surgery is usually indicated.[23,31,41] Anesthesia is discontinued, the head of the bed is elevated, and the patient is observed carefully. Serial flexible fiberoptic laryngoscopic examinations are performed to ensure proper healing, and the tracheotomy tube is removed as soon as this can be tolerated by the patient.

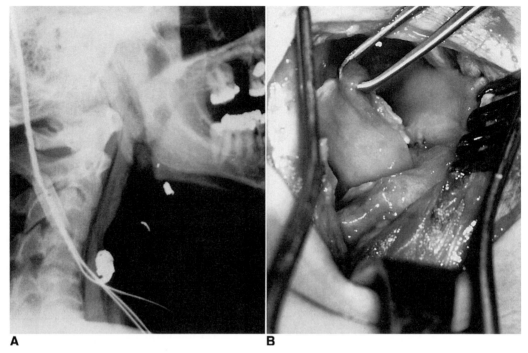

A   **B**

Figure 92-7. A, A soft tissue lateral radiograph of the neck shows a bullet in the pharynx and subcutaneous emphysema. The larynx of the same patient is exposed by midline thyrotomy. **B,** Right hemilarynx has been avulsed by intubation. A clamp is holding the mucosa of the right side of the larynx. (From Schaefer S: *Ann Otol Rhinol Laryngol* 91:399, 1982.)

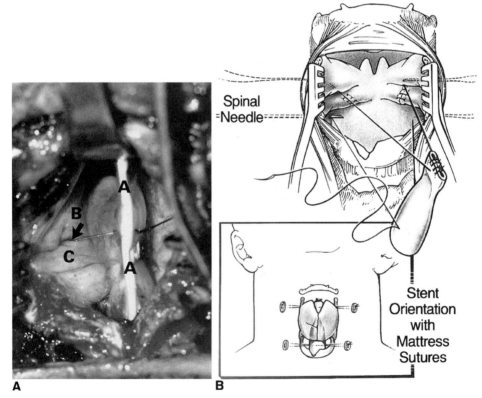

A   **B**

Figure 92-8. A, A Portex endotracheal tube stent in the larynx. **B,** The upper end of the modeled stent should be placed at the level of the aryepiglottic folds, and the lower limit of the stent should rest at the first tracheal ring. The stent is held in place by 0 Prolene or Mersilene sutures, which are passed through the laryngeal ventricle and cricothyroid membrane using an 18-guage spinal needle. The sutures are held in place using skin buttons. (From Schaefer SD: *Op Tech Otolaryngol Head Neck Surg* 1:65, 1990.)

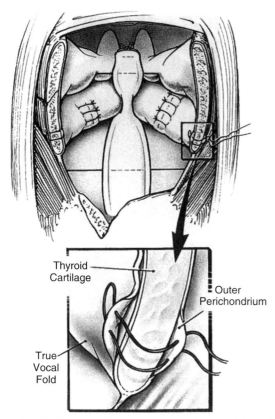

Thyroid Cartilage

Outer Perichondrium

True Vocal Fold

Figure 92-9. After endolaryngeal surgery is complete, with or without stenting, the scaphoid shape of the anterior commissure should be restored by suturing the most anterior aspect of the vocal folds to the outer perichondrium of the thyroid cartilage (see enlargement). This maneuver often avoids the need for stenting as long as the anterior commissure was intact before surgical exploration and no lacerations involve this site. (From Schaefer SD: *Op Tech Otolaryngol Head Neck Surg* 1:66, 1990.)

In patients with more severe injuries, surgical exploration is performed. Controversy exists as to the optimal time for repair.[16,22,27] Some authors advocate delay of repair for 3 to 5 days to allow edema to subside and for easier identification of mucosal lacerations. *However, the best results have been obtained with early repair, avoiding the morbidity of leaving open wounds in a contaminated field.*[13,25,31] In either case, surgical exploration begins with a subplatysmal apron flap that is elevated to the level of the hyoid bone. The strap muscles are divided in the midline and retracted laterally. A midline thyrotomy is used to enter the larynx. Laryngeal skeletal fractures are repaired using wire or nonabsorbable suture. To avoid further damage to the laryngeal mucosa and skeleton, no fracture site sutures are tightened until all fractures have been reduced. Simple nondisplaced fractures can be repaired by suturing the outer perichondrium with nonabsorbable sutures. An alter-

native to wire is internal fixation using absorbable or nonabsorbable plates.[1,6] For such plating to be effective the screws must be well anchored in the laryngeal skeleton, and this can be problematic in younger patients with minimal calcification of the larynx. All mucosal lacerations are meticulously repaired using fine absorbable sutures. A dislocated arytenoid is reduced. In most injuries, wounds can be closed using adjacent mucosa. In cases involving military weapons or other instances in which the loss of tissue is large, regional mucosal flaps or skin grafts can be used to complete the lining of the larynx.

The indications for stenting in these injuries are controversial.[16,22,31,39,41] The advantages of using a stent should be weighed against additional damage to the mucosa. Stents are recommended in the treatment of injuries involving the anterior commissure, comminuted fractures of the thyroid cartilage, and cases in which the architecture of the larynx is not maintained by open fixation of the fractures. The advantages of stenting in these instances are decreased web formation at the anterior commissure and better support of the laryngeal architecture during healing. This additional support can be useful in light of the movement of the larynx with phonation and swallowing during the healing process. Stenting alone without open reduction and the fixation of fractures and closure of lacerations is unsatisfactory.

The choice of stent ranges from finger cots filled with foam rubber to commercially manufactured polymeric silicone stents. All should be roughly the shape of the larynx and made of soft material to avoid further mucosal damage. The stent should extend from the false vocal fold to the first tracheal ring to add stability and prevent endolaryngeal adhesions. Ideally, the stent should be secured in such a manner as to be easily removed using endoscopic techniques. A 3.5-cm length of endotracheal tubing (Portex) can be used to create an easily available stent (Figures 92-10 and 92-11).[34] The superior end of the tube is sewn tightly closed to prevent aspiration, and smooth clamps are placed to approximate the true and false vocal folds. The stent is then autoclaved to 82°C, thereby reforming the tube to the desired shape. The stent is secured by two monofilament sutures passed through the laryngeal ventricle and cricothyroid membrane and tied to skin buttons. All stents should be removed as soon as possible to minimize mucosal damage. Usually a period of 10 to 14 days is adequate, even in the case of severe injury.

After repair of the injured larynx and placement of a stent, if indicated, the anterior commissure is reconstituted by suturing the true vocal fold to the outer perichondrium. Regardless of the need for stenting, reconstructing the anterior commissure is

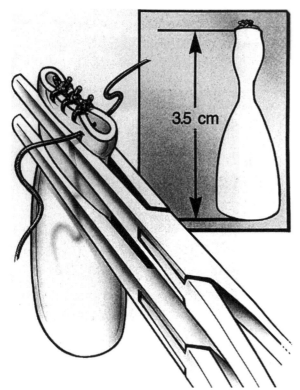

Figure 92-10. A laryngeal stent can be fabricated from a Portex endotracheal tube by using a 3.5- to 4-cm straight segment of the endotracheal tube that is cross-clamped with two parallel straight clamps. The first clamp is placed within 2 to 3 mm of the upper end of the tube, and the second clamp is positioned approximately 0.5 cm below the first clamp. The upper end of the tube is closed with 2-0 silk suture. The clamped tube is placed within a steam autoclave that is manually raised to 180°F and immediately decompressed. (From Schaefer SD: *Op Tech Otolaryngol Head Neck Surg* 1:65, 1990.)

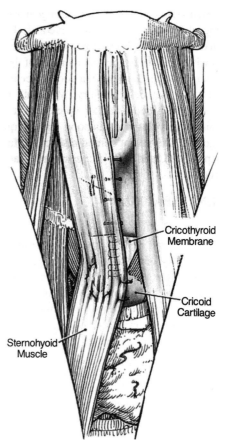

Figure 92-11. Anterior defects of the cricoid ring are repaired by mobilizing the sternohyoid muscle over the cricoid defect. The muscle is then sutured to the adjacent remnants of the cricoid cartilage and the cricothyroid membrane. (From Schaefer SD: *Op Tech Otolaryngol Head Neck Surg* 1:66, 1990.)

essential to maintain the scaphoid shape of this site and to preserve a normal voice. The thyrotomy is closed using permanent sutures or wire. The strap muscles are reapproximated, and the wound is closed over a drain.

Various other injuries can also be encountered during surgery. As much as one third of the anterior cricoid or trachea can be repaired using the sternohyoid muscle and its overlying fascia. Loss of the anterior third of the thyroid cartilage or hemiglottis can be repaired by closure of mucosal lacerations over a stent. If the recurrent laryngeal nerve is severed by the injury, a neurorrhaphy of the severed ends should be performed. Although the intricate abductor-adductor function of the larynx will not likely return, reinnervation can help maintain muscle tone and therefore voice quality. If open reduction and internal fixation with stenting are unsuccessful in restoring the laryngeal architecture because of massive trauma and

tissue loss, partial or total laryngectomy may be necessary. The decision for partial or total laryngectomy should be based on the defect, using the same guidelines used in oncologic reconstruction. However, total laryngectomy has not been necessary in large series of laryngeal trauma and is more likely to be considered acceptable management for military wounds.[31]

Postoperative Care

All patients with laryngeal trauma should continue to receive postoperative antibiotics for 5 to 7 days in an effort to reduce infection and granulation tissue. The head of the bed should be elevated, as tolerated, to minimize edema. The patient should be encouraged to ambulate as soon as this is bearable. If a tracheostomy is present, routine care should be provided. Stents placed at the time of surgery should be removed as soon as possible to prevent further mucosal damage, usually 10 to 14 days after surgery. Decannulation can be performed as soon as the stent is removed. Follow-up examinations should be scheduled periodically for at least 1 year to assess true vocal fold function return and to monitor the development of any subglottic stenosis. Antacids and H_2-blockers should be routinely used to prevent reflux, which may cause increased scarring of laryngeal tissues. The use of nasogastric tubes is avoided when possible to reduce reflux and to prevent erosion of the posterior cricoid mucosa associated with their use.

Complications

Complications after repair of external laryngeal trauma include impaired vocalization, respiration, and deglutition (Figure 92-12). Postoperative granulation tissue may be seen after removal of the stent. This is best managed by prevention with meticulous closure of all mucosal lacerations at the time of the surgery. Postoperative antibiotics and early removal of the stent may reduce the amount of granulation tissue. Profuse granulation tissue that persists can be debulked endoscopically.

Vocal fold immobility can cause a weak voice if it is unilateral, or aphonia and respiratory compromise if bilateral. Unless the recurrent laryngeal nerve was shown to be severed at the time of surgery, no procedures should be performed to compensate for the paralysis for at least 6 months because delayed recovery can occur. If after 6 months to 1 year no return is noted, a medialization procedure can be performed to strengthen the voice in the case of a unilateral paralysis or in the case of aspiration in the presence of a unilateral paralysis. If a bilateral paralysis is present and the patient desires an attempt at decannulation, an arytenoidectomy or cordotomy can be performed.

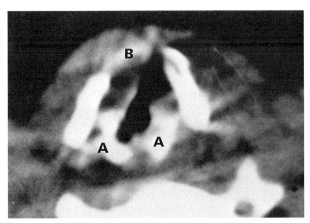

Figure 92-12. Computed tomography of initially unrecognized laryngeal fractures in a 23-year-old woman shows fixated arytenoid cartilages and fracture of the thyroid cartilage. The patient remained aphonic and tracheotomy dependent for 4 years until the larynx was reconstructed.

However, immobility caused by cricoarytenoid joint fixation should be ruled out before these other procedures are considered.[25] Subglottic stenosis may also be present and may cause a failure to decannulate. Again, no repair should be undertaken for 6 to 12 months to allow for scar maturation. After this time, direct laryngoscopy and bronchoscopy should be used to examine the lesion and plan the repair. If a short segment of tracheal stenosis is found with a healthy airway below, then an excision of the stenotic segment and primary reanastomosis can be performed, using a release of the suprahyoid suspensory system to gain further mobilization.[44] Additionally, mediastinal tracheal dissection and incision of the annular ligaments of the trachea can be used in combination with suprahyoid release to allow for excision and primary reanastomosis of lesions up to 12.5 cm in adults.[8] Longer stenotic segments can be repaired with anterior and, if needed, posterior cricotracheal cartilage grafts as popularized in the repair of subglottic stenosis in children.[43] In the very rare case of massive trauma with inability to decannulate the patient postoperatively and repeated problems with aspiration despite medialization procedures, a total laryngectomy may be necessary to prevent further aspiration. In this situation, the indications are the same as would be used for aspiration after partial laryngectomy.

Outcome

The outcome after laryngeal trauma depends on the extent of the original injury and the quality of subsequent repairs. In patients who do not require operative intervention, the prognosis for full return of function is excellent.[13,17,32,36] Patients requiring surgical intervention have an excellent chance of eventual decannulation with an adequate to good voice.[10,14,29,31,38] Long-term complications after repair are uncommon.

The results of airway and voice evaluations after laryngeal trauma are as follows. Group 1 patients had minor injuries managed without operative intervention. Group 2 patients were managed with tracheotomy and endoscopy, but their injuries did not warrant open exploration and repair. Patients in group 3 had displaced or multiple fractures of the laryngeal skeleton or endolaryngeal lacerations. Group 4 patients sustained massive injuries, and similar to group 3 patients, required open exploration, careful closure of lacerations, and internal fixation of fractures. However, management of the patients in group 4 also included endolaryngeal stenting because laryngeal fractures were massive enough so as to be unstable after internal fixation, or lacerations were so severe there was a danger of stenosis of the laryngeal lumen or loss of the scaphoid anterior commissure. In this report, a good voice was normal or comparable to that before injury. Moderate to marked hoarseness was described as a *fair* voice, and a voice just above a whisper was classified as *poor*. Airway quality was judged as *good* if the patient denied restriction, *fair* if some restriction persisted, and *poor* if permanent tracheostomy was required.

IATROGENIC TRAUMA
Intubation Injuries

Most endolaryngeal injuries result as a complication of intubation. This can occur as a result of technique or from trauma to the glottis or subglottis from the endotracheal tube. The type of endotracheal tube can also be significant. Polyvinylchloride (PVC) tubes have been shown to exert 7 to 10 times the force and pressure of silicone or armored tubes.[11] Laryngeal mask for administration of general anesthesia is relatively new and may present unique injuries in the future.[2] Other injuries to the larynx can result from surgical intervention, including tracheotomy, excision of laryngeal masses (e.g., papillomas, granulomas), or surgery to improve an already injured larynx (e.g., polytef injection of a true vocal fold).

The best management for intubation trauma is prevention. This is best accomplished by educating personnel who perform intubations as to the correct techniques of intubation, choosing a correctly sized endotracheal tube for the patient, and performing all intubations in a controlled manner. Possible complications of intubation include pharyngeal lacerations; cricoarytenoid dislocation; injury to the lingual, hypoglossal, superior laryngeal, or recurrent laryngeal nerves; and injury to the vocal folds from forceful manipulation and insertion of the tube or inserting a tube too large for the patient. Nerve injuries usually represent a neurapraxia and, unless an obvious or likely severing of the nerve has occurred, are best managed expectantly. Laryngeal electromyography is useful in differentiating vocal immobility due to alternation of the cricoarytenoid joint vs a neurapraxia. Minor pharyngeal lacerations are managed with a short course of antibiotics unless a severe injury has occurred (e.g., perforation of the pyriform sinus or esophagus), in which case the injury should be repaired surgically and drained, and the patient should be fed via a nasogastric tube for 5 to 7 days.[40] Cricoarytenoid dislocation results from traumatic intubation and is usually first noticed as a postintubation vocal fold paralysis. If diagnosed early, cricoarytenoid dislocation can be managed with endoscopic reduction of the dislocated joint.[5] Abrasion to the larynx from intubation is usually mild and can be managed in most instances with elevation of the head of the bed, cool mist humidification, and observation. Indications for operative intervention are the same as those for other forms of laryngeal trauma.

Another major source of iatrogenic laryngeal injury is prolonged intubation. Since the advent of low-pressure cuffed endotracheal tubes, long-term intubation is less hazardous. However, as the use of advanced intensive care for critically ill patients becomes more widespread, the incidence of long-term intubation and its subsequent complications have increased. The decision to convert endotracheal intubation to a tracheostomy should be based on several factors, including the risk of surgery in a critically ill patient and the likely need for further ventilatory support. In general, the risk of prolonged endotracheal intubation outweighs the risk of tracheotomy 7 to 10 days after intubation.[43] Conversion to tracheostomy should occur earlier in certain instances, including preexisting circumferential subglottic mucosal injuries, as it does with inhalation of supraheated air and patients with excessive movement and resultant increased trauma to the larynx from the endotracheal tube. Another complication of endotracheal intubation is accidental extubation. In situations of accidental extubation after which reintubation may be difficult or impossible because of edema of the airway or other reasons, early tracheotomy should be strongly considered to prevent a possibly fatal catastrophe.

Injuries During Tracheotomy

Tracheotomy may injure the larynx or trachea; similar to endotracheal intubation, the best means of avoiding this is to perform the procedure in a controlled situation under the supervision of experienced personnel. Injury to the larynx or trachea is more likely in an emergent situation in which hemostasis and identification of anatomic landmarks are difficult, and therefore compromise is accepted in an effort to rapidly secure an airway. These procedures can damage the larynx because of an incision made too high, causing injury to the cricoid, or from injury to the recurrent laryngeal nerve as a result of dissection too lateral on the trachea. Improper choice of tracheotomy cannula size can also damage the trachea because of poor fit and subsequent wear on the tracheal wall, causing erosion of the tracheal epithelium. Before the use of low-pressure endotracheal cuffs, tracheal erosion leading to subclavian artery hemorrhage was common even with relatively short periods of intubation. However, even with low-pressure cuffed endotracheal tubes, hyperinflation of the tracheal cuff or prolonged use can cause a similar type of injury.

Injury to the larynx from surgical excision in benign disease, such as papilloma or granulation tissue, usually results from overly aggressive removal of tissue or failure to follow standard principles of laryngeal surgery. When removing areas of benign disease, it is important to avoid exposing cartilage during the dissection because this can lead to a chondritis of the larynx, especially in irradiated tissue. It is also important not to denude the anterior commissure bilaterally at one time because this can lead to anterior webbing. During removal of tissue in the subglottic region, only one quadrant of the circumference should be addressed at each setting to prevent cicatricial scarring and its sequela of subglottic stenosis.

ESOPHAGEAL INJURIES

Esophageal injuries can be isolated or can occur in association with other trauma. Blunt trauma to the neck seldom causes esophageal injury, but it may result from severe laryngeal trauma and perforation of the esophagus by cartilage fragments. A review of 246 penetrating injuries to the neck that violated the platysma revealed 16 injuries to the esophagus.[30]

More common are injuries from ingestion of caustic substances.[42] These commonly occur in the pediatric population as a result of accidental ingestions and usually involve household products or hydrocarbons. In adults, these injuries are usually the result of attempted suicides.

Diagnosis

The diagnosis of esophageal injuries often relies on the history. The patient, witnesses, and paramedic personnel should be questioned regarding the possible substance ingested. Whenever possible, the container should be examined because the contents may not be accurately labeled. In the case of blunt or penetrating trauma, hematemesis might be present if the esophageal mucosa has been violated. Plain chest radiography may reveal pneumomediastinum in the presence of esophageal perforation. Pain is usually present to some degree. Physical examination will usually show oral cavity and oropharyngeal mucosal injury in the case of ingestion. Hoarseness may be present if the substance contacted the glottis through direct contact or regurgitation. Edema may be present and is occasionally severe enough to compromise the airway. External trauma to the esophagus is usually diagnosed radiographically via a barium swallow or with endoscopy. Rigid esophagoscopy is thought to be more sensitive than barium swallow for the diagnosis of esophageal injury but requires general anesthesia and personnel skilled in its use.[21] The indications for esophagoscopy in substance ingestion are controversial.[20] In cases in which the presumed ingested substance is especially tissue damaging, the amount large, or the airway compromised, or if the patient manifests signs or symptoms of shock from fluid redistribution, esophagoscopy is probably warranted.[45]

Management

Surgical therapy is indicated for all blunt and penetrating trauma showing injury to the esophagus. This should be undertaken as part of a complete exploration for other associated injuries. Any lacerations to the esophageal mucosa should be closed in several layers, and a drain should be placed. A nasogastric tube should be inserted, and the patient should be given nothing by mouth for 7 to 10 days.[40] Limited use of esophageal stents for minor iatrogenic perforations has been reported and awaits further applications.[24]

Management of caustic ingestion depends on the degree of tissue injury. If the larynx is involved at the time of endoscopy, tracheotomy is preferred over endotracheal intubation to prevent further laryngeal mucosal damage. Any obviously necrotic tissue in the esophagus or stomach is resected, and a feeding jejunostomy is placed. In less severe esophageal injuries, supportive care and fluid resuscitation may be the only management necessary.[42] Corticosteroids may be useful, but their use is controversial. If medical management is used, repeat endoscopy can be used to reassess tissue viability and dilate any strictures that form.

REFERENCES

1. Bhanot S and others: The efficacy of resorbable plates in head and neck reconstruction, *Laryngoscope* 112:890, 2002.
2. Braun U: A comparison of the proseal laryngeal mask to the standard laryngeal mask on anesthesized, non-relaxed patients, *Anasthesiol Intensivmed Notfallmed Schmerzther,* 12:727, 2002.
3. Bumpous JM and others: Penetrating injuries of the visceral compartment of the neck, *Am J Otolaryngol* 21:190, 2000.
4. Close DM: Traumatic avulsion of the larynx, *J Laryngol Otol* 95:1157, 1981.
5. Close LG and others: Cricoarytenoid subluxation, computed tomography, and electromyography findings, *Head Neck Surg* 9:341, 1987.
6. de Mello-Filho FV, Carrau R: The management of laryngeal fractures using internal fixation, *Laryngoscope* 110:2143, 2000.
7. Friedman WH and others: Computed tomography vs laryngography: a comparison of relative diagnostic value, *Otolaryngol Head Neck Surg* 89:579, 1981.
8. Grillo HC: Circumferential resection and reconstruction of the mediastinal and cervical trachea, *Ann Surg* 162:374, 1965.
9. Harrison DFN: Bullet wounds of the larynx and trachea, *Arch Otolaryngol Head Neck Surg* 110:203, 1984.
10. Hirano M, Kurita S, Terasawa R: Difficulty in high-pitched phonation by laryngeal trauma, *Arch Otolaryngol Head Neck Surg* 111:59, 1985.
11. Joo HS and others: PVC tracheal tubes exert forces and pressures seven to ten times higher than silicone or armoured tracheal tubes: an in vitro study, *Can J Anaesth* 49:986, 2002.

12. Khokhlov VD: Knitted fractures of the laryngopharynx framework as a medical legal matter, *Forensic Sci Int* 104:147, 1999.

13. Kleinsasser NH and others: External trauma to the larynx: classification, diagnosis, therapy, *Eur Arch Otorhinolaryngol* 257:439, 2000.

14. Krekorian EA: Laryngopharyngeal injuries, *Laryngoscope* 85:2069, 1975.

15. Lemay SR: Penetrating wounds of the larynx and cervical trachea, *Arch Otolaryngol Head Neck Surg* 94:558, 1971.

16. Leopold DA: Laryngeal trauma, *Arch Otolaryngol Head Neck Surg* 109:106, 1983.

17. Lupetin AR, Hollander M, Rao VM: CT evaluation of laryngeal trauma, *Semin Musculoskelet Radiol* 2:105, 1998.

18. Maceri DR, Mancuso AA, Canalis RF: Value of computed axial tomography in severe laryngeal injury, *Arch Otolaryngol Head Neck Surg* 108:449, 1982.

19. Mancuso AA, Hanafee WN: Computed tomography of the injured larynx, *Radiology* 133:139, 1979.

20. Meredith JW, Kon ND, Thompson JN: Management of injuries from liquid lye ingestion, *J Trauma* 28:1173, 1988.

21. Meyer JP and others: Mandatory vs selective exploration for penetrating neck trauma, *Arch Surg* 122:592, 1987.

22. Miles WK, Olson NR, Rodríguez A: Acute treatment of experimental laryngeal fractures, *Ann Otol Rhinol Laryngol* 80:710, 1971.

23. Miller LH: Laryngotracheal trauma in combat casualties, *Ann Otol Rhinol Laryngol* 79:1088, 1970.

24. Mumtaz H and others: Successful management of a nonmalignant esophageal perforation with a coated stent, *Ann Thorac Surg* 74:1233, 2002.

25. Nahum AM: Immediate care of acute blunt laryngeal trauma, *J Trauma* 9:112, 1969.

26. Nahum AM, Siegel AW: Biodynamics of injury to the larynx in automobile collisions, *Ann Otol Rhinol Laryngol* 76:781, 1967.

27. Olson NR: Surgical treatment of acute blunt laryngeal injuries, *Ann Otol Rhinol Laryngol* 87:716, 1978.

28. Olson NR, Miles WK: Treatment of acute blunt laryngeal injuries, *Ann Otol Rhinol Laryngol* 80:705, 1971.

29. Pennington CL: External trauma of the larynx and trachea, *Ann Otol Rhinol Laryngol* 81:546, 1972.

30. Saletta JD and others: Penetrating trauma of the neck, *J Trauma* 16:579, 1976.

31. Schaefer SD: Acute management of external laryngeal trauma: a 27 year experience, *Arch Otolaryngol Head Neck Surg* 118:598, 1992.

32. Schaefer SD: Primary management of laryngeal trauma, *Ann Otol Rhinol Laryngol* 91:399, 1982.

33. Schaefer SD, Brown OE: Selective application of CT in the management of laryngeal trauma, *Laryngoscope* 93:1473, 1983.

34. Schaefer SD, Carder HM: Fabrication of a simple laryngeal stent, *Laryngoscope* 40:1561, 1980.

35. Schaefer SD, Close LG: Acute management of laryngeal trauma, *Ann Otol Rhinol Laryngol* 98:98, 1989.

36. Schaefer SD, Close LG, Brown OB: Mobilization of the fixated arytenoid in the stenotic posterior laryngeal commissure, *Laryngoscope* 96:656, 1986.

37. Stanley RB, Cooper DS, Florman SH: Phonatory effects of thyroid cartilage fractures, *Ann Otol Rhinol Laryngol* 96:493, 1987.

38. Stanley RB, Hanson DG: Manual strangulation injuries of the larynx, *Arch Otolaryngol Head Neck Surg* 109:344, 1983.

39. Thomas GK, Stevens MH: Stenting in experimental laryngeal injuries, *Arch Otolaryngol Head Neck Surg* 101:217, 1975.

40. Tomaselli F and others: Management of iatrogenous esophagus perforations, *Thorac Cardiovasc Surg* 50:168, 2002.

41. Trone TH, Schaefer SC, Carder HM: Blunt and penetrating laryngeal trauma: a 13-year review, *Otolaryngol Head Neck Surg* 88:257, 1980.

42. Tseng YL and others: Early surgical correction for isolated gastric stricture following acid corrosion injury, *Dig Surg* 19:276, 2002.

43. Whited RE: A prospective study of laryngotracheal sequelae in long term intubation, *Laryngoscope* 94:367, 1984.

44. Williams MW: Suprahyoid release for tracheal anastomosis, *Arch Otolaryngol Head Neck Surg* 99:255, 1974.

45. Zargar SA and others: Ingestion of corrosive acids: spectrum of injury to upper gastrointestinal tract and natural history, *Gastroenterology* 97:702, 1989.

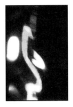

CHAPTER NINETY THREE

SURGICAL MANAGEMENT OF UPPER AIRWAY STENOSIS

David Goldenberg
Ramon Esclamado
Paul Flint
Charles W. Cummings

INTRODUCTION

This chapter discusses the surgical management of adult laryngeal and upper tracheal stenosis. The causes and pathophysiology of laryngotracheal stenosis are outlined, and the surgical options and controversies are evaluated and discussed in the context of selecting the appropriate techniques for specific problems.

Successful repair requires establishing an adequate airway while preserving the laryngeal functions of airway protection, phonation, and sustained glottic closure to increase intrathoracic pressure. Laryngotracheal injuries are rarely identical among patients. The injury may vary in location, severity, duration, cause, and degree of functional impairment. Selection of the appropriate surgical repair should consider these factors in conjunction with the patient's associated injuries, medical problems, and psychosocial milieu. The variety of techniques for a specific problem attests to the difficulty of obtaining consistent long-term results with any one specific repair and to the complexity of laryngotracheal stenosis.

PATHOPHYSIOLOGY

Adult laryngotracheal stenosis has many various etiologies (Table 93-1). The pathophysiologic processes that result in a stenosis should be taken into consideration, because they often affect management decisions in terms of the timing of surgical intervention, the surgical procedure chosen, and the outcome. For example, repair of a subglottic stenosis in a patient with active Wegener's granulomatosis would be deferred until systemic treatment has ameliorated the systemic symptoms, and it often requires multiple procedures because of exacerbation of the disease.[44] Similarly, caution should be used when managing a patient with a posterior glottic stenosis resulting from radiotherapy who has a marginal but adequate airway,

because the relative lack of blood supply may worsen the stenosis or result in chondroradionecrosis.

The most common causes of laryngotracheal stenosis continue to be external trauma to the neck and prolonged endotracheal intubation. Both can result in acute and chronic stenosis; however, the pathophysiologic processes that lead to chronic stenosis differ. The larynx and trachea can be considered as a semi-rigid tubular structure. When the laryngotracheal complex is injured by external trauma, disruption of the cartilaginous framework, hematoma in the laryngeal spaces, and mucosal disruption usually result. Resorption of the hematoma can cause cartilage loss and extensive deposition of collagen. Subsequent scar contracture will result in stenosis and loss of motility.

The location, mechanism, and severity of the laryngeal injury caused by external trauma vary.[82] By contrast, the injury from endotracheal intubation is usually initiated by ischemic necrosis of the mucosa by the endotracheal tube.[86,87] Mucosal ulceration in the presence of bacterial infection can lead to perichondritis and chondritis with cartilage resorption. Healing occurs by secondary intention with subsequent submucosal fibrosis and scar contraction. Injuries from endotracheal intubation occur primarily in the posterior glottis as a result of pressure exerted by the wall of the tube and tracheal injury from the pressure of the cuff on the tube tip. The latter injury has been reduced significantly with low-pressure, high-volume cuffs. Other factors, including tube size and composition, duration of intubation, and laryngeal movement, also contribute to the development of laryngotracheal stenosis. However, with the widespread acceptance and use of endotracheal intubation to provide ventilatory and airway support, preventive efforts have been directed toward modifying endotracheal tube design.[72,86]

TABLE 93-1

CAUSES OF ADULT LARYNGEAL AND UPPER
TRACHEAL STENOSIS

Trauma
    External laryngotracheal injury
        Blunt neck trauma
        Penetrating wound of the larynx
    Internal laryngotracheal injury
        Prolonged endotracheal intubation
        Posttracheotomy
        Postsurgical procedure
        Postirradiation therapy
        Endotracheal burn
            Thermal
            Chemical
Chronic inflammatory disease
    Bacterial Diphtheria
    Syphilitic
    Fungal histoplasmosis
        Tuberculosis
        Leprosy
        Sarcoidosis
        Scleroma
Benign neoplasms
    Intrinsic
        Papillomas
        Chondromas
        Minor salivary gland
        Neural
    Extrinsic
        Thyroid
        Thymus
Malignant neoplasms
    Intrinsic
        Squamous cell carcinoma
        Minor salivary gland
        Sarcomas
        Lymphoma
    Extrinsic
        Thyroid
Collagen vascular disease
    Wegener's granulomatosis
    Relapsing polychondritis
    Other

Patient-dependent processes may also influence tolerance to the endotracheal tube and the development of stenosis. Patients with diabetes mellitus, congestive heart failure, or a history of stroke have an increased incidence of severe acute laryngeal injury from intubation, thus prompting early tracheotomy.[85] In addition, gastroesophageal reflux should be considered as a cause and potentiator of laryngotracheal stenosis, which can be managed with H_2 blockers.[38]

CLASSIFICATION OF STENOSIS

Multiple staging systems exist for airway stenosis; these are based on function or location of the stenotic section. Perhaps the most common—albeit general—classification system divides laryngeal obstruction into four grades: Grade I, less than 50% laryngeal lumen obstruction; Grade II, 50% to 70% obstruction; Grade III, 71% to 99% obstruction, with minimal lumen present; and Grade IV, complete obstruction, with no lumen present.

In 1980, Bogdasarian and Olson[3] classified the extent of posterior glottic stenosis into the following four types: Type I, vocal process adhesion; Type II, posterior commissure stenosis, with scarring in the interarytenoid plane and internal surface of the posterior cricoid lamina; Type III, posterior commissure stenosis with unilateral cricoarytenoid joint ankylosis; and Type IV, posterior commissure stenosis with bilateral cricoarytenoid joint ankylosis. This classification for posterior glottic stenosis was proposed on the basis of a worsening degree of injury and poorer outcome.

McCaffrey[47] showed that, in a series of 72 patients, the site of stenosis most consistently predicted the time to decannulation in univariant and multivariant analyses, and he used this as a basis for a clinical staging system. In this classification system, Stage 1 lesions are confined to the subglottis or trachea and are less than 1 cm long. Stage 2 lesions are subglottic stenoses longer than 1 cm within the cricoid ring without extension into the glottis or trachea. Stage 3 lesions extend into the upper trachea but do not involve the glottis, and Stage 4 lesions involve the glottis with fixation or paralysis of one or both vocal folds.[47] This clinical staging system is highly predictive for successful decannulation. Ninety percent of Stage 1 and 2 patients, 70% of Stage 3 patients, and 40% of Stage 4 patients are successfully decannulated.[48]

SURGICAL PRINCIPLES
Goals and Assessment

The goal of any surgical procedure designed to correct laryngotracheal stenosis is to establish a satisfactory airway, which implies decannulation. To accomplish this goal for a patient, every effort should be made to preserve the other important laryngeal functions of phonation, airway protection, and glottic closure. When the stenosis involves the glottic or supraglottic larynx, surgical procedures designed to improve the airway often compromise other laryngeal functions. The anticipated overall function of the larynx and the impact on the quality of life of the patient after surgical intervention should be carefully discussed with the patient so that expectations are reasonable.

Several guidelines should be considered when determining the appropriate assessment and management in cases of airway stenosis. Accurate assessment of the stenosis in terms of location, dimensions, quality (soft vs fibrous), associated vocal fold motion impairment, and degree of functional impairment is essential. Initial evaluation should therefore include a history detailing the degree of subjective impairment perceived by the patient together with objective measures (e.g., observing the patient walking 200 feet and climbing a flight of stairs, pulmonary function testing [flow volume loop]).[9,13]

Indirect laryngeal examination followed by direct laryngoscopy and bronchoscopy is essential. High-resolution computed tomography of the larynx and trachea may be useful. Recently, three-dimensional computed tomography with volume rendering[25] (Figure 93-1) or virtual endoscopy[34] has been employed to evaluate the extent or severity of the stenosis. This is particularly useful for cases in which the airway cannot be adequately assessed by laryngoscopy or endoscopy.

An important consideration is the reestablishment of structural support, usually by repositioning existing cartilage or, more commonly, through the use of cartilage or bone grafts. Other important considerations are the preservation of existing mucosa and the judicious use of antibiotics, stents, and skin or mucosal grafts to minimize infection, granulation tissue formation, and subsequent collagen deposition.

Timing of Repair

The timing of repair of a chronic laryngotracheal stenosis is generally elective. The development of stenosis requires scar contracture; therefore, the onset of symptoms is more insidious. Patients with

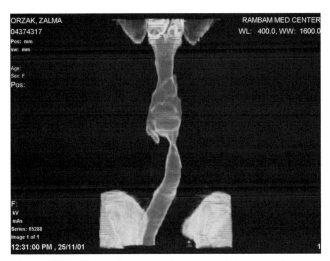

Figure 93-1. Three-dimensional computed tomography scan with volume rendering of patient with significant tracheal stenosis.

chronic laryngotracheal stenosis as a result of intubation usually fail several attempts at extubation and require tracheotomy. They subsequently cannot be decannulated, or, after a brief decannulation, they experience gradually progressive upper airway symptoms. Irreversible stenosis is usually diagnosed at this time, and repair can be performed electively after thorough evaluation. It is important to note that patients with inflammatory or autoimmune diseases require stabilization of their underlying disease processes before surgical management.

Endoscopic vs Open Repair

In the late 1940s, the endoscopic division of webs and subsequent keel placement were first described. Endoscopic techniques include manual or laser scar division that is occasionally followed by local mitomycin-C application, laser and microtrapdoor flaps, and the use of powered instrumentation. Evolution of laryngeal surgery has resulted in the development and improvement of microlaryngeal instrumentation and endoscopic laryngeal surgery. Better access to the supraglottis and glottis via refinements in laryngoscopes, coupled with enhanced visualization using telescopic digital imaging, has permitted many laryngeal lesions previously removed through open techniques to be resected endoscopically.

The technical refinements and widespread use of the carbon dioxide laser have resulted in more diversity in the endoscopic procedures used to manage glottic and subglottic stenoses. The theoretic advantages of the carbon dioxide laser are as follows: (1) delayed formation and maturation of collagen in laser wounds, thereby allowing reepithelialization before scar formation; (2) minimal deep-tissue injury; and (3) more precise control and hemostasis, thus facilitating preservation and the use of existing mucosa in the repair.[20,28] Because of these advantages, some authors have advocated the initial endoscopic management of chronic laryngotracheal stenosis, reserving open repair for cases that fail to resolve with endoscopic management.[11,20] The advantage of this approach is that an open surgical repair may be avoided in some instances; however, several endoscopic procedures may be required for long-term success. Proceeding directly with an open approach in patients with more severe stenosis is more likely to result in an early, successful outcome. Although the CO_2 laser is an important tool that has been used in many endoscopic laryngeal procedures, its use is not without risks and complications. There is the ever-present risk of an airway fire, and laser plume may be harmful to the surgeon and hospital staff if they are working with infectious lesions.[66] It is often difficult to control thermal injury, which may result in perioperative edema and postoperative scarring of the vocal folds.[18]

Microdébrider/Endoscopic Débridement

Powered instrumentation has been used with great success in many arthroscopic procedures. This technique combines the use of flexible forceps and a microdébrider.[45,46] These endoscopic procedures have employed the use of a powered microdébrider and video endoscopic control since 1985.[36] The powered rotating blade is combined with suction so that soft-tissue lesions are aspirated into the tip of the blade and cleanly cut. Adaptation of this instrumentation for endoscopic sinus surgery provided for more efficient and precise tissue removal, with reduced injury to normal mucosa.[50] A laryngeal microdébrider shaver was designed in 1996 in response to requests for better instrumentation and techniques for the removal of bulky, exophytic laryngeal papilloma in patients with recurrent respiratory papillomatosis,[51] obstructing carcinoma,[79] and Reinke's edema.[71] The microdébrider's laryngeal blade incorporates a suction device that enables the user to pull the obstructing granulation away from underlying tissue, thereby making it easier to remove the diseased mucosa.[68]

The laryngeal microdébrider eliminates the risk of airway fire. There is no laser plume, so the infectious risk to the operating room staff is minimized. Tissue injury is confined to the mucosa; therefore, laser burn and postoperative scarring may be minimized. Although objective data are not available, RRP patients previously treated with the laser have reported reduced postoperative pain and quicker return to a usable speaking voice. Decrease in operative time has also been observed, thus reducing the patient's exposure to a general anesthetic and overall operating room costs.[66,68]

The authors employ the use of the microdébrider for many laryngeal lesions (Table 93-2). Basic surgical technique in laryngeal shaver surgery employs the concept of "wedding" the rigid telescope and the laryngeal shaver; this promotes camera steadiness and good visualization of the blade tip relative to the lesion as it is removed. Subglottic and tracheal stenotic lesions are typically removed with the tricut (4-mm) subglottic blade to excise the fibrous scar. Softer, bulky lesions, such as laryngeal and tracheal papilloma, are rapidly removed with the 4.0-mm round window (skimmer) blade. Papillomas and other lesions involving the true vocal folds are removed with the 3.5-mm round window (skimmer) laryngeal blade (Figures 93-2 and 93-3).

Local Mitomycin C Application

The use of topical mitomycin-C may be useful for the treatment and prevention of subsequent restenosis

TABLE 93-2
INDICATIONS FOR LARYNGEAL USE OF A MICRODÉBRIDER

Internal laryngoceles
Tumor debulking
Supraglottic, glottic, subglottic, and tracheal lesions
Removal of Teflon granulomas
Subglottic and tracheal stenotic lesions
Excision of tracheostomal granulation tissue
Respiratory papillomatosis
Laryngeal cysts
Anterior commissure lesions (only in conjunction with CO_2 laser or monopolar suction cautery for hemostasis)
Relative contraindications for laryngeal use of microdébrider
Vascular lesions

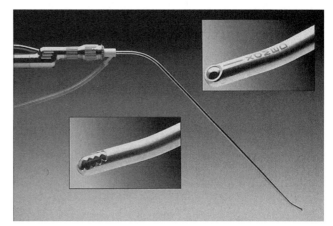

Figure 93-2. Powered instrumentation (microdébrider). Tricut blade *(upper),* for use in larynx, subglottis, and trachea, and skimmer blade *(lower),* for removal of mucosal lesions.

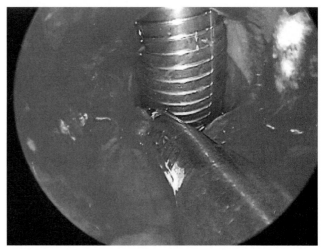

Figure 93-3. Endoscopic view of endolaryngeal lesion removal using the round blade of a microdébrider.

and scar formation in the larynx and trachea. Mitomycin-C is an antineoplastic antibiotic that acts as an alkylating agent by inhibiting DNA and protein synthesis. It can inhibit cell division, protein synthesis, and fibroblast proliferation.[69]

The use of local mitomycin-C is still controversial. Its usefulness is being evaluated, and long-term follow-up and controlled studies are necessary. In one study that followed 15 months of mitomycin application, all patients had clinical improvement of their airways and resolution of their preoperative symptoms, without recurrence.[69] Another study performed on the pediatric airway found no statistical difference between a single topical dose of mitomycin and isotonic sodium chloride after laryngotracheal reconstruction.[32]

A number of animal studies have been performed. In one study, topical mitomycin-C produced a statistically significant reduction in the rate of restenosis as compared with surgical lysis alone.[81] Correa and colleagues[5] performed a randomized prospective study of the efficacy of topical mitomycin-C in the inhibition of subglottic stenosis in a canine model. They found a statistically significant decrease in collagen formation in the subglottic scars of dogs treated with topical mitomycin-C and concluded that mitomycin-C favorably altered the clinical progression of subglottic stenosis, improved quantified airway patency, and reduced the amount of subglottic collagen formation.

Repair Requirements

The first requirement for the successful repair of acute or chronic laryngotracheal stenosis is the establishment of an intact, reasonably shaped skeletal framework to provide a scaffold for the airway. It is generally agreed that acute, blunt injuries to the larynx, in which cartilage is fractured and displaced, are best managed with open reduction and stabilization of the fragments. In chronic injuries, the cartilage is often absent as a result of resorption of devitalized segments or of chondritis and subsequent chondromalacia or necrosis. In either event, the absent cartilage is replaced by scar tissue. Therefore, cartilage or bone grafts are necessary to reestablish structural support and to provide luminal augmentation. The characteristics of an ideal mesodermal graft include the following: (1) rapid healing with minimal long-term graft resorption (which is best seen in vascularized grafts); (2) adequate strength, size, and pliability of the graft so that it may be contoured to the defect; (3) minimal donor site morbidity; (4) presence of an accompanying epithelial lining; (5) single-stage reconstruction, and (6) having the donor site within the same operative field. An ideal cartilage or bone graft does not exist as evidenced by the various grafts described, including the rib, iliac

crest, hyoid bone, epiglottis, thyroid cartilage, composite auricular cartilage, and nasal septal cartilage.*

Each of these grafts has various advantages, but they may be limited by size, lack of pliability, and variable resorption caused by lack of blood supply. The rib or costal cartilage graft is most commonly used because of its size, strength, and relative ease of harvesting. Vascularized hyoid and thyroid cartilage grafts have shown considerable success,[4,22,89] but they are limited by the amount of cartilage available. Composite auricular and nasal septal cartilage has the advantage of providing simultaneous epithelial repair, but it generally lacks adequate size and rigidity for cases in which large grafts are required. Free perichondrial and periosteal grafts have not gained widespread acceptance because of their lack of adequate strength and the need for prolonged stenting. Vascularized perichondrial grafts and periosteal grafts have been evaluated for their chondrogenic or osteogenic capabilities and show potential for providing a pliable, vascularized graft that generates viable rigid bone or cartilage. In a rabbit model, vascularized perichondrium was shown to form significantly more cartilage when placed in a subglottic defect, and it tolerated a two-hour ischemia time[31]; it was successfully tubed to reconstruct a segmental tracheal defect.[58] The sternocleidomastoid myoperiosteal flap has been successfully used for subglottic and tracheal reconstruction, with a low incidence of bony overgrowth on long-term follow-up.[19]

Use of Skin and Mucosal Grafts

The second requirement of the successful repair of acute and chronic laryngotracheal stenosis is the establishment of a completely epithelialized lumen of reasonably normal size and shape. In acute injuries, the ideal method is primary closure of mucosal lacerations after minimal débridement of nonviable tissue. In chronic stenosis, scar tissue should be excised, with the preservation of as much overlying mucosa as possible. Small mucosal defects can be left to remucosalize, with minimal detrimental effects.[61] The area of controversy lies in the use of epithelial grafts to resurface large defects in acute and chronic stenosis. In both cases, the principles of wound healing apply to the traumatic wound or the newly created surgical wound. Wounds that heal by secondary intention form granulation tissue and deposit collagen, which should later contract until covered by epithelium.[61] When the denuded area is secondarily infected—particularly after tracheotomy—epithelialization can be prolonged, and excessive granulation tissue and scar formation result.[74]

---

*References 4, 12, 15, 22, 49, 56, 63.

Epidermal grafts have been advocated to interrupt this process and result in healing similar to that of primary intention with minimal collagen deposition. When a stable cartilaginous framework is present, the tendency for the epidermal graft to contract is less, because the laryngeal skeleton acts as an external splint.[83] The indications, techniques, and results of skin grafting as an important adjunct in laryngotracheal reconstruction have been well described.[62]

The disadvantage of epidermal grafts in laryngotracheal reconstruction is that the larynx is not an ideal site to accept free epidermal grafts. The recipient bed is often not well-vascularized, particularly when a free cartilage or bone graft is used; the larynx is in constant motion with swallowing and neck movements; and the bed is potentially contaminated when a tracheotomy is present. A nonvascularized epidermal graft in the airway can become infected, thereby exacerbating the process of healing by secondary intention. An epidermal graft is useful when a large mucosal defect is present with adequate cartilaginous support. When cartilage or bone grafts that would require prolonged rigid internal stenting are used, epidermal grafts may be detrimental. In this instance, satisfactory results can be obtained by allowing healing and mucosalization around the stent and by not introducing a graft that, if infected, could jeopardize the skeletal reconstruction.

Use of Stents

Internal laryngeal and subglottic stenting is widely used with acceptable results; however, questions about the indications for stenting, the optimal type of stent, and the duration of stenting are largely unresolved. Internal stenting with soft or firm materials increases local infection, mucosal ulceration, and granulation tissue and is directly related to the duration of stenting.[83] Capillary blood flow ceases with pressure of 20 to 40 mm Hg in mucosa closely adherent to cartilage, which can initiate ischemic mucosal injury.[59] Therefore, several authors advocate avoiding internal stenting (unless absolutely necessary) and minimizing the duration of stenting. However, internal stenting is commonly used for specific indications: (1) to provide support for cartilage and bone grafts or to splint displaced cartilage fragments in the desired position; (2) to allow approximation and immobilization of epidermal grafts to a recipient site; (3) to separate opposing raw surfaces during healing; and (4) to maintain lumen in a reconstructed area that lacks adequate cartilaginous support and requires scar formation.

The optimal stent has not been determined, as evidenced by the various stents available. A tantulum[51] or umbrella silicone keel[55] is useful for anterior glottic webs, but, for more severe laryngotracheal stenosis, various stents are commonly used, including the Montgomery laryngeal stent (Figure 93-4), the Aboulker stent, the swiss roll siliconized rubber stent, and the finger cot stent; each has proponents who describe good results.[17,30,54,92] In general, a soft stent should be used to minimize pressure on mucosal surfaces when cartilaginous support is satisfactory and when the indication for stenting is to splint an epidermal graft or to separate opposing raw mucosal surfaces. A finger cot with a povidone-iodine–soaked sponge is an excellent soft stent; an alternative is a Montgomery laryngeal stent that is firm but conforms to endolaryngeal contours. A firm stent is required when the cartilaginous framework or graft requires splinting or when inadequate cartilage is present, thereby requiring that luminal support be achieved through collagen deposition and scar contraction. A solid stent is preferable to a hollow stent for minimizing aspiration. However, a soft, hollow stent such as the Montgomery T-tube allows phonation. This type of stent is commonly used for subglottic and upper tracheal stenosis; appropriate patient selection and education are essential, because this is a single-lumen tube with a greater risk of airway obstruction.[8,54] An Aboulker stent can be used for subglottic or combined subglottic and laryngeal stenosis. The advantage of this stent is that it is used with a double cannula metal tracheostomy tube, and it is secured to the tube, thus preventing removal.[92] Modifications of this technique that allow tracheotomy changes have recently been described.[52]

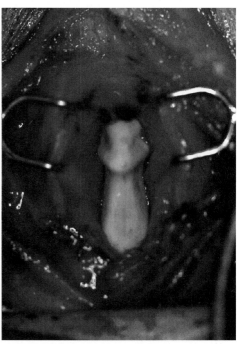

Figure 93-4. Thyrotomy with Montgomery stent in place.

There is no uniformly accepted optimal duration of stent placement. Most authors recommend 6 to 8 weeks, but the duration varies from 2 weeks to several months.[30,76] Usually 1 to 3 weeks are sufficient if only mucosal healing or epidermal graft take is required. If the laryngeal skeleton is adequate but requires splinting to maintain the appropriate position, 6 to 8 weeks is the generally accepted timeframe.

However, if the cartilaginous framework is deficient and mature scar is important for providing structural strength, prolonged stenting is indicated to allow scar contraction around an inert, firm object. Successful prolonged stenting has been reported for intervals of up to 14 months. In this situation, the problem arises in premature stent removal, usually before sufficient scar contraction has occurred.[76] The presence of a paratubal air envelope (manifested as linear air densities between the outside wall of the stent and the inside wall of the larynx and trachea) is reported to be a reliable indicator of laryngotracheal structural integrity and functional stability and a useful measure to determine optimal timing for stent removal.[23]

SURGICAL MANAGEMENT OF CHRONIC STENOSIS
Supraglottic Stenosis

Chronic hypopharyngeal stenosis usually results from unrecognized acute blunt injury to the hyoid and thyrohyoid membrane. The direction of force is posterosuperior and results in several discrete injuries: (1) the epiglottis can be adherent to the posterior or lateral hypopharyngeal walls; (2) the hyoid bone can be fractured and displaced posteriorly with the epiglottis, thereby producing laryngeal inlet stenosis; (3) a horizontal web of the posterior hypopharyngeal wall may form at the level of the superior aspect of the epiglottis; or 4) postcricoid stenosis may result in stenosis of the esophageal introitus.[54] The type and extent of the stenosis can be evaluated by indirect laryngoscopy, direct laryngoscopy, and barium swallow if the inferior extent is difficult to evaluate.

The surgical approach is through a transhyoid pharyngotomy. Tracheotomy is essential if it has not been previously performed. A horizontal skin incision is made over the hyoid bone, which is then identified. If the hyoid is fractured, attempts are made to reduce and wire it into its normal anatomic position; otherwise, the body of the hyoid can be excised. The vallecula is entered, and the mucosal incision can be extended to a lateral pharyngotomy, if needed, with care taken to preserve the superior laryngeal neurovascular pedicles and hypoglossal nerve. After satisfactory exposure has been provided, attention is directed to repair of the stenosis.

Adhesions of the epiglottis to the hypopharyngeal walls can be managed by division of the adhesion along its long axis, submucosal excision of scar tissue, and primary mucosal closure. When a horizontal web or shelf is present, a vertical incision is made through the web, and scar tissue is excised. Mucosal flaps are undermined to allow closure of the incision in a horizontal line. If necessary, superiorly based mucosal advancement flaps can be used. If the hypopharyngeal stenosis is so extensive that the division of bands and the excision of scar tissue result in an extensive denuded area over the constrictor muscle, consideration should be given to skin grafting these areas. Hollow silicone esophageal stents have also been used to assist in the healing of a skin graft.[54] If resection of scar tissue results in an extensive full-thickness pharyngeal defect, a radial forearm revascularized flap may be used to provide thin, pliable, soft tissue but it results in an adynamic hypopharyngeal segment.

Laryngeal inlet stenosis results from posterior displacement of the hyoid and epiglottic cartilage and can be accompanied by a fracture through the thyroid notch. This injury is approached through a laryngofissure; the thyrohyoid membrane is divided in the midline to excise the base of the epiglottis, which protrudes over the glottis. After the base of the epiglottis is identified, the anterior fascia, perichondrium, and epiglottic cartilage are incised in an inverted V fashion to the mucoperichondrium of the laryngeal surface of the epiglottis. The mucoperichondrium on the laryngeal surface of the epiglottis is elevated as a superiorly based flap, thereby allowing for the excision of this inverted V-shaped wedge of the base of the epiglottic cartilage, perichondrium, fascia, and scar. The mucoperichondrial flap is then incised in the midline, and the resultant flaps are turned outward and sewn to the free edge of the anterior epiglottic perichondrium. The thyrotomy is closed, and stenting is not required.[54]

Glottic Stenosis
Anterior Glottic Stenosis

Anterior glottic stenosis in adults can be caused by external trauma resulting in a thyroid cartilage fracture and mucosal disruption. Internal laryngeal trauma from endotracheal intubation or surgical removal of the mucosa from the anterior edges of both vocal folds simultaneously can cause the two opposing raw mucosal edges to heal together. A thin web that extends more than 3 to 4 mm posteriorly along the vocal fold can produce hoarseness; a thicker web or one that extends farther posteriorly can cause significant airway obstruction.[10] Hoarseness or airway compromise is an indication for surgical intervention. Excision of the anterior glottic scar will recreate the conditions that caused the original stenosis. Therefore, successful repair requires physical separation of the opposing edges until remucosalization is complete.

Endoscopic management of anterior glottic stenosis can be considered when the web does not extend below the inferior edge of the true vocal fold and when the posterior commissure is normal.[10,67] Division of the anterior webs can be performed by suspension microlaryngoscopy and with the use of either microlaryngeal instruments or CO_2 laser. Microlaryngeal instruments allow for the better development and preservation of mucosal flaps, if desired. Excess scar tissue is removed, and a keel is placed endoscopically and secured externally with wires or with a heavy suture placed through the thyrohyoid membrane. Alternatively, a mini cricothyrotomy may be performed to place the keel with endoscopic visualization. Different keel designs and compositions have been described. The principles of designing keels include the following: (1) the material used should be inert; (2) the length should be sufficient to extend from the cricothyroid membrane to at least 2 to 3 mm above the anterior commissure; (3) if the keel extends superiorly over the petiole of the epiglottis, the anterior edge of the keel should make a 120-degree angle (i.e., the angle of the epiglottis and the anterior tracheal wall) to minimize granulation tissue formation at the petiole of the epiglottis; and (4) the posterior wing of the keel should lie at the vocal processes and should not touch the posterior commissure.[10,67] The keel is removed after 2 to 4 weeks, and granulation tissue is removed concurrently.

An external laryngofissure approach should be considered when the anterior glottic stenosis extends more than 5 mm subglottically, when it accompanies a laryngeal inlet stenosis, when it is associated with a shortened anterior-posterior glottic aperture produced by a thyroid cartilage fracture, or when endoscopic approaches have failed. Resection of scar tissue should not be overzealous, and mucosa should be preserved whenever possible. When mucosa is deficient, Isshiki and others[37] described obtaining superior voice results by resurfacing the vocal fold with labial mucosa instead of split-thickness skin grafts and short-term stenting. Successful results have been achieved with the Montgomery umbrella silicone keel used for 2 to 3 weeks or with the McNaught tantalum keel.[10,54]

Posterior Glottic Stenosis

Posterior glottic stenosis is most commonly caused by endotracheal intubation, although mechanical fixation may also occur from cricoarytenoid joint arthritis. Posterior glottic stenosis can be confused clinically with bilateral vocal fold paralysis before direct laryn-goscopy. It should be considered when the history is appropriate and when there are indirect laryngoscopy findings of anteromedial displacement of the arytenoid cartilages (which often obscures the posterior commissure scar) with a pseudoforeshortening of the anterior-posterior length of the membranous folds or glottic aperture.

Mechanical fixation and neurogenic paralysis are differentiated by direct laryngoscopy. Palpation of the arytenoid to assess mobility is vital. Joint excursion should be uninhibited. Passive medial movement of the contralateral arytenoid when the ipsilateral arytenoid is displaced laterally suggests interarytenoid scar. Electromyography findings of denervation or action potentials of the vocalis muscle are very useful to document neurologic integrity, particularly when direct observation of the vocal fold movement is equivocal. These patients may have a preexisting tracheotomy, which decreases posterior cricoarytenoid muscle activity, thereby making active lateral vocal fold excursion difficult to visualize unless the tracheotomy is plugged temporarily.

The degree of injury is variable. Type III and IV posterior glottic stenoses are difficult to successfully manage, particularly when they are associated with subglottic stenosis.[3,48] The major therapeutic challenges are to reestablish a satisfactory airway and to preserve the voice, which is often normal.

Endoscopic repair of posterior glottic stenosis is successful in carefully selected patients. Those with an interarytenoid web and posterior sinus tract have been managed with a simple division of the web. Many patients restenose, particularly those who have had a tracheotomy.[11] A soft, sponge-filled finger cot stent has been advocated in this situation to separate the raw opposing surfaces; this can be placed endoscopically and remain for 2 weeks.[3]

Posterior commissure stenosis can be managed endoscopically with a CO_2 laser or a laryngofissure. Creation of a posterior microtrapdoor flap is successful when a posterior sinus or a 3- to 4-mm posterior interarytenoid scar is present.[11] This technique fails when there is arytenoid fixation or a scar that is more than 1 cm in height.[22] When posterior interarytenoid mucosa is insufficient to create a trapdoor flap (>3–4 mm), interarytenoid scar tissue is resected, with the mucosa preserved through a hockey-stick incision.

A 0.025-inch thick synthetic implantation fabric keel is placed endoscopically and left for 4 to 6 weeks. This is considered to widen the interarytenoid mucosa sufficiently to allow for a microtrapdoor flap. However, failures occurred in all patients who had arytenoid fixation.[11] Several authors recommend open repair through a laryngofissure approach.[3,8,53,80]

Repair is effected by developing a superiorly based mucosal flap, excising scar tissue and fibrosed interarytenoid muscle, and repositioning the mucosal flap to provide immediate epithelial coverage. Internal stenting is not required when both arytenoids are mobile. Care is taken to not enter the cricoarytenoid joints if both arytenoids are mobile. Successful surgical repair is an elusive goal.

Posterior glottic stenosis with arytenoid fixation has been traditionally managed through an external approach. If, after development of a mucosal flap and resection of scar, one arytenoid is freely mobile, resection of the fixed arytenoid is unnecessary. When bilateral arytenoid fixation exists, removal of the least mobile arytenoid is necessary to achieve a satisfactory airway. Denuded mucosal surfaces are covered with mucosal flaps, skin, or mucosal grafts. Stenting for 2 to 3 weeks is necessary with a conforming silicone laryngeal stent[50] or with a soft finger cot stent.[4] Posterior cricoid split with rib graft may also be considered (Figure 93-5).

In 1984, Ossoff, Karlan, and Sisson[64] first described complete arytenoidectomy via an endoscopic approach. Endoscopic laser arytenoidectomy is also useful for managing Type IV posterior commissure stenosis when subglottic involvement is limited. Although more frequently and successfully used for bilateral vocal fold paralysis, endoscopic laser arytenoidectomy avoids the complications of an external approach and allows for the immediate assessment of airway size (Figure 93-6). An excellent technical description of endoscopic laser arytenoidectomy is described;[64] this approach requires the removal of the entire arytenoid except for the muscular process. Care should be taken to preserve mucosal flaps while resecting the posterior commissure scar to attain as much primary mucosal coverage as possible to minimize additional scar formation and restenosis. Arytenoid perichondritis is a potential complication, and the administration of perioperative antibiotics and antireflux measures are recommended. The degree of vocal fold lateralization obtained is variable, and the use of

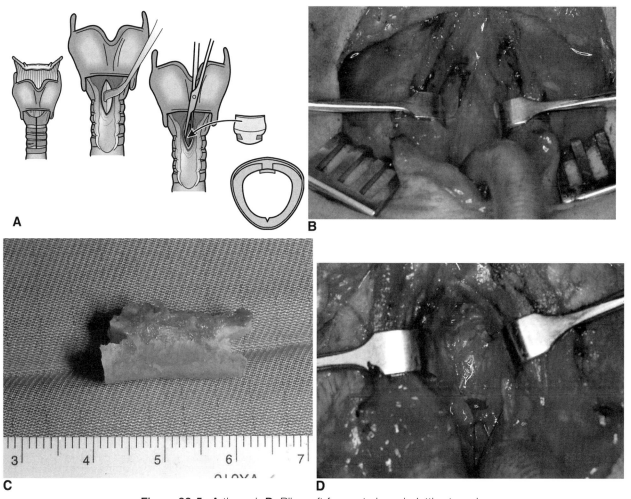

Figure 93-5. A through **D,** Rib graft for posterior subglottic stenosis.

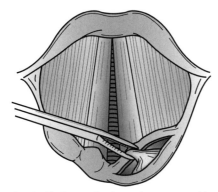

Figure 93-6. Endoscopic view of an arytenoidectomy.

a lateralization suture or a finger cot stent may improve the final result by controlling the degree of lateralization.

The external approaches for an arytenoidectomy are through a laryngofissure or a Woodman arytenoidectomy. This latter approach exposes the arytenoid cartilage through a posterolateral extralaryngeal dissection through the inferior constrictor muscle and by elevating the mucosa of the pyriform sinus and postcricoid area to expose the arytenoid cartilage. The entire arytenoid cartilage is resected, except for the vocal process. A submucosal suture is placed through the vocal process and anchored around the inferior thyroid cornu to lateralize the vocal fold (6 mm in males, 5 mm in females).[77,91] Other authors believe that tethering the vocal process around the inferior thyroid cornu may reposition the vocal fold inferior to the opposite fold; they recommend suturing to the thyroid lamina at the vocal fold level[5] or around the superior cornu[54] (success rate, 60%–80%). If the procedure is unsuccessful, completion arytenoidectomy through a laryngofissure approach with suture lateralization of the vocal fold can be performed.[70]

Exploration of the fixed cricoarytenoid joints with lysis of adhesions without arytenoidectomy has also been advocated. Fibrous bands on the medial aspect of the cricoarytenoid joints are divided, and the arytenoids are stented in full abduction for 2 to 3 weeks; stent removal and aggressive speech therapy follow. Return of vocal cord mobility has been described in 90% of patients managed in this way.[26,75]

Complete Glottic Stenosis

Complete glottic stenosis usually results from unrecognized severe extralaryngeal trauma. Injury limited to the glottis is unusual; there is often associated subglottic injury, which should be addressed concurrently. Endoscopic management is rarely indicated because of the severity and nature of the injury. However, isolated complete glottic stenosis has been

successfully managed by endoscopic incision and placement of a synthetic fabric keel.[43] The reported experience is limited to two patients, both of whom required a second procedure for the correction of a residual posterior glottic stenosis; further follow-up observation is required to evaluate the efficacy of this procedure. The mainstay of management involves an open laryngofissure approach. The stenosis should be divided at the midline and excessive scar tissue resected while preserving the mucosa and developing mucosal flaps from the aryepiglottic folds for coverage. If extensive areas are devoid of mucosa, epithelial grafts of buccal mucosa, grafts of nasal septal mucosa, or split-thickness skin grafts may be used. Large split-thickness skin grafts may cause excessive crusting. The grafts are sutured in place and stented with a form-fitting laryngeal stent for 4 to 8 weeks.[37,53] When the stent is removed, an umbrella keel is placed into the anterior commissure for 2 weeks.

An alternative approach is reconstruction with an epiglottic flap. This is indicated in severe glottic stenosis, with a more than 50% reduction in the anterior-posterior dimension of the glottis, in glottic-subglottic stenosis, or in glottic-supraglottic stenosis with an intact epiglottis.[12,41,63] The repair is approached through a midline thyrotomy, and the thick scar is transected in the midline. Submucosal excision of scar tissue can be attempted, and the mucosa can be repositioned and secured with 4-0 chromic suture. The base of the epiglottis is identified, and the median thyroepiglottic ligament is transected. The epiglottis is pulled inferiorly to reach the anterior cricoid arch. The epiglottic flap is sutured with 3-0 polyglactin 910 to the outer anterior edges of the thyroid cartilage laterally and the cricoid cartilage inferiorly. This results in an epithelialized, widened anterior commissure. Several cartilage-splitting incisions may be used to allow the petiole to be folded onto itself to make a sharper anterior commissure.[8]

Subglottic Stenosis

Endoscopic management of subglottic stenosis with the CO_2 laser and, more recently, with the laryngeal microdebrider, requires careful patient selection. The predictive factors for failure have been described and confirmed.[2,11,14,80]

CO_2 laser excision and repair with a microtrapdoor flap is moderately reliable for managing circumferential subglottic stenosis.[19] This technique requires laser incision of the superior surface of the scar and the submucosal excision of scar tissue. An inferiorly based rectangular mucosal flap is created by two lateral knife incisions. The preserved flap does not completely cover the lasered area, but it does divide the raw concave area into two flat lateral raw areas, which heal rapidly. A 90% success rate was reported in 10 patients, all of whom had scars that were less than 10 mm in height. A large flap that can potentially obstruct the airway through a ball-valve effect should not be created. Other authors[11] have confirmed the efficacy of this procedure in adults and emphasize that it is useful when the stenosis is less than 10 mm in height, but a tracheotomy should be performed if the flap is more than 4 mm in length. This procedure is uniformly unsuccessful in the pediatric population.[2] Failure also occurs if associated posterior glottic stenosis or arytenoid fixation is present.[14] An alternative method of radial incision of the stenosis at the 2, 3, 6, and 9 o'clock positions, followed by bronchoscopic dilation, has been proposed.[78] This series of patients was small, and follow-up observation involved 1 year; thus, success was not assumed.

The microdébrider is an excellent tool for treating subglottic stenosis and excising fibrous scar from this region. Subglottic and tracheal stenotic lesions are typically removed using a tricut (4-mm) subglottic blade. External repair is indicated when endoscopic techniques fail or when the extent of the stenosis is severe and factors are unfavorable for an endoscopic approach. Various techniques are available, and the selection of the appropriate repair technique should anticipate the amount of rigid support required for luminal augmentation and the possibility that scar resection requires epithelial grafting. Subglottic stenosis as a result of extensive mature scar (but with adequate cartilaginous support) can be approached by laryngofissure.

Subglottic scar is resected to cricoid perichondrium and is relined with the buccal mucosa or a split-thickness skin graft. The graft is preferably sewn around a stent that is fixed in place.[54] When cartilaginous support or luminal augmentation is also required, various autogenous cartilage grafts are available. The hyoid-sternohyoid muscle interposition graft has been extensively used, with a success rate of approximately 70% in adults.[4,89] This technique can be applied to isolated subglottic stenosis or subglottic stenosis in combination with anterior glottic or tracheal stenosis.

The procedure uses a vascularized segment of the body of the hyoid pedicle on the sternohyoid muscle and its adjacent periosteum. The length of bone can be tailored to the length of the stenosis; it is interposed vertically into the stenosis and secured with four-point fixation. A stent is not used unless an epidermal graft is required after scar excision to minimize possible graft resorption by pressure necrosis.

The advantages of this technique include immediate reconstruction with a single operative field, theoretically improved tissue survival with minimal graft remodeling, and versatility in augmenting glottic, subglottic, and upper tracheal stenosis. The long-term survival of the bone graft has not been conclusively shown; the graft is limited in the amount of augmentation it provides because of its narrow width and concave shape. Additional procedures are often required to remove granulation tissue. The thyroid-cartilage–sternothyroid pedicle composite graft was developed to overcome the limitation of the hyoid-sternohyoid graft.[22] A large central piece of thyroid ala attached to the sternothyroid muscle through its perichondrium is harvested. A flap of contralateral thyroid alar perichondrium is harvested in continuity with the ipsilateral perichondrium and serves as internal lining when the composite graft is transposed. Stenting for 1 to 6 weeks is required.

This technique offers the advantages of the hyoid-sternohyoid graft, except it cannot be used for glottic stenosis. A larger piece of cartilage, however, is available to reconstruct more extensive defects. The internal perichondrial transposition allows for remucosalization with minimal granulation tissue formation.

Various free autogenous cartilage grafts have been used for luminal augmentation. These grafts have variable amounts of resorption and require prolonged stenting to allow resorbed graft to be replaced by firm, mature scar tissue. Costal cartilage grafts have the advantage of providing large grafts that are easily sculpted. Specific details of graft tailoring have been well described.[80] Composite nasal septal cartilage grafts have been used successfully in 11 of 16 patients with stenosis of the larynx and upper trachea.[15] Stenosis of up to 3 cm in height can be repaired, and the respiratory epithelium is a theoretic advantage, because it provides immediate resurfacing with a match of epithelium from the stenotic area. In children, a stent is not used, and the graft is not used to prevent injury to nasal growth centers. Various other autogenous grafts, including auricular cartilage,[56] clavicular bone, and free hyoid bone, have been used but they have not received uniform acceptance.

A unique approach has recently been described that involves the use of vascularized clavicular periosteum pedicled in the sternocleidomastoid muscle.[19,21] This technique requires the harvesting of approximately 75% of the circumference of the clavicular periosteum that is left attached to sternocleidomastoid muscle that has intact blood supply. A vascularized periosteal graft of up to 8 × 4 cm can be obtained and rotated medially for the reconstruction of cricotracheal defects. A stent or T-tube is used until rigid bone forms. During long-term follow-up, 25 of 26 patients were ultimately decannulated, and bony overgrowth was not reported. Excessive granulation tissue formation was a problem that the authors thought could be prevented by lining the periosteum internally with split-thickness skin grafts. One case of osteomyelitis of the clavicle was reported, and subsequently the procedure was modified to include pectoralis muscle coverage of the denuded clavicle.

This technique has the advantage of providing a pliable graft that easily conforms to the defect, and the donor site is in the same field. The disadvantages are that it requires stenting until a rigid framework develops, the amount of periosteum is limited to 8 × 4 cm, and the blood supply to the sternocleidomastoid muscle should be intact, which limits its use in reconstruction after cancer resection when a neck dissection has been performed or radiotherapy has been given.

Division of the posterior cricoid lamina should be considered when severe subglottic stenosis is present with posterior glottic stenosis or for complete glottic and subglottic stenosis. This is approached through an anterior cricotracheal fissure, avoiding disruption of the anterior commissure. The entire posterior cricoid lamina is divided vertically in the midline to the level of the postcricoid submucosa. Scar tissue excision is not necessary, and the interarytenoid muscle is divided if it is fibrosed. Prolonged rigid internal stenting is required for at least 3 months. Interposition cartilage grafts with perichondrium can be harvested from the thyroid lamina for posterior support,[54] and anterior luminal augmentation can be performed.

Partial cricoid resection with thyrotracheal anastomosis is considered when other methods have failed. Several authors reported good results and specific technical details.[60] This procedure should only be performed in adults and is limited to stenosis involving the cricoid and upper trachea. There should be approximately 1 cm of normal lumen below the glottis. The main risks of this procedure are injury to the recurrent laryngeal nerves and anastomotic dehiscence with restenosis.

The procedure involves exposure of the involved laryngotrachea while preserving the recurrent laryngeal nerves. Identification of the nerves is often risky because of extensive scarring; therefore, dissection of the trachea is performed in the subperichondrial plane. The inferior resection line is immediately below the stenosis, beveling the anterior tracheal wall. The superior limit can include the cricoid up to the posterior lamina just below the cricothyroid joint. Care is taken to not injure the recurrent laryngeal nerves, which pass immediately posterior to the cricothyroid joints. The tracheotomy can be lowered if three of four tracheal rings can be interposed between the anastomosis and the tracheotomy; otherwise, the patient should be intubated and the anasto-mosis accomplished with 3-0 interrupted suture placed submucosally and tied extraluminally. Laryngeal release procedures are usually necessary, and the neck is kept in flexion for 7 to 10 days postoperatively to minimize tension on the anastomosis. If a tracheotomy is not used, the patient is extubated in the operating room in 3 to 4 days.

Grillo and others[37] refined this procedure to incorporate a posterior membranous tracheal wall flap to resurface the bared cricoid cartilage. In a series of 80 patients with subglottic and upper tracheal stenosis, failure was reported in only 2 out of 77 patients with at least 6 months follow-up; one perioperative death occurred. Of 77 patients, 66 had no restriction of their daily activities caused by dyspnea, and tracheotomy was required perioperatively only if the airway was of "borderline adequacy immediately after operation."

A sliding flap tracheoplasty has been described, which is a variation of the cricoid resection and thyrotracheal anastomosis.[24] The procedure involves resection of the anterior cricoid arch and the first two tracheal rings, with development of an inferiorly based anterior tracheal wall flap from the third through sixth ring; this is advanced and anastomosed to the thyroid cartilage superiorly. Patients selected for this procedure should have a subglottic stenosis involving only the anterior cricoid arch and the first ring, an intact posterior wall, mobile vocal folds, and an uninvolved segment of mucosa below the glottis.

Cervical Tracheal Stenosis

Cervical tracheal stenosis in adults most commonly results from trauma produced by intubation, trauma produced by tracheotomy, or blunt external trauma to the neck. Other causes include benign and malignant neoplasms, inflammatory diseases, and systemic autoimmune disease.

When surgical repair of tracheal stenosis is considered (Table 93-3), regardless of the cause, it is essential to determine the location, length, composition, extent of airway stenosis, and neurologic integrity of the larynx through indirect laryngeal examination, bronchoscopy, and radiography. In most instances, cervical tracheal stenosis can be categorized as cicatricial membranous stenosis, anterior wall collapse, or complete stenosis. Airway management should be considered preoperatively and discussed with the anesthesiologist. If a tracheotomy is not present or is not planned, it is safest to have the patient breathe spontaneously until the airway is secured. If a Montgomery T-tube is used as part of the reconstruction, patients should breathe spontaneously after the T-tube is inserted (Figure 93-7). If the airway is 5 mm or less at the time of reconstruction, dilation is performed initially under general anesthesia;

TABLE 93-3

TRACHEAL STENOSIS MANAGEMENT

Open resection and repair
Endoscopic dilatation/laser excision
Stent placement
Silicone stents (e.g., Dumon, Rusch Y)
Expandable stents (e.g., Gianturco Z, Wallstent, Nitinol)
Flexible silicone stents (e.g., PolyFlex)

microdébrider resection may also be performed. If the lumen is larger than 6 mm in diameter, intubation is carried out above the lesion, and dissection is performed carefully to prevent airway obstruction.[48] If a tracheotomy is planned postoperatively, it should be performed under local anesthesia at the onset of reconstruction.

Cicatricial Membranous Stenosis

Granular or fibrous stenosis of the cervical trachea with intact cartilage can initially be managed endoscopically. CO_2 laser excision of granular stenosis is useful because tracheotomy can be avoided, and the granular stenosis can be resected accurately with minimal bleeding. If the stenosis is circumferential, partial resections should be staged 2 to 4 weeks apart to prevent the formation of a circumferential denuded area of trachea that can re-stenose. Fibrous stenosis can be excised by a microtrapdoor technique.[11]

Open repair of a cicatricial membranous stenosis requires approaching the stenosis through a vertical midline incision through the anterior tracheal wall to expose the entire length of the stenosis. Care is taken to prevent lateral dissection, because the vascular supply to the cervical trachea from the inferior thy-

roid artery enters laterally. Submucosal excision of scar tissue is accomplished under direct visualization, and the tracheotomy may be lowered below the stenosis. An epidermal graft is useful to cover the denuded area, and it is usually fixed over a stent. Luminal augmentation is often required, and the type of graft used depends on the size of the graft needed and the surgeon's experience and preference. The pedicled thyroid-cartilage–sternothyroid graft or a composite septal cartilage mucoperiosteal graft seems to be reasonably successful.

Anterior Wall Collapse

Anterior wall collapse can result from anterior blunt neck trauma, but it more commonly results from tracheotomy. Montgomery[54] categorizes these injuries as suprastomal, stomal, or infrastomal. In this type of stenosis, a well-mucosalized posterolateral wall and residual cartilage in the area of the stenosis should be present.[8]

A suprastomal and stomal stenosis can be approached and managed as described for cicatricial membranous stenosis. However, restoration of the anterial wall is essential. This can be accomplished by stenting the lumen open with a T-tube or a firm stent of a tracheostomy tube (Aboulker stent) and repairing the anterior wall with a cartilage graft or by mobilizing the sternohyoid muscles and securing them together over the defect. Both instances require prolonged stenting.[8]

Wedge resection of an anterior tracheal wall stenosis can be considered if one of the following conditions is present: (1) the stenosis is limited to two or three rings, with significant loss of cartilage that would preclude stenting; 2) the posterior wall mucosa is intact; or 3) the stenosis is stomal or suprastomal. The procedure involves adequate exposure of the involved

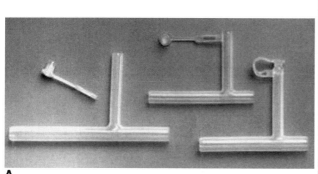
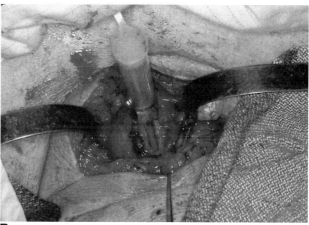

A   **B**

Figure 93-7. A, Silicone T-tube stents in tracheal stenosis. **B,** Open placement of T-tube.

trachea, including at least one ring above and below the stenosis. Subperichondrial dissection is carried out carefully around the involved trachea to prevent injury to the recurrent laryngeal nerves. The stenosis is resected, with care taken to preserve posterior tracheal wall mucosa. An oroendotracheal tube is passed through the anastomosis, and the cartilaginous trachea is reanastomosed with submucosal 3-0 polyglactin 910 sutures tied extraluminally. The patient is extubated when awake and alert, and granulation tissue is endoscopically excised as early as possible.[8]

Complete Tracheal Stenosis

Segmental resection and primary anastomosis provide optimal results for complete tracheal stenosis. The average length of the adult trachea is 11 cm (range, 10–13 cm), and there are 14 to 20 tracheal rings. With hyperextension of the neck, 50% of the trachea is cervical.[88] Approximately 50% of the trachea (5–7 cm) can be safely resected and anastomosed primarily with appropriate mobilization techniques. Other factors also should be considered when determining how much trachea can be resected. Older patients with calcification between tracheal rings may have less tracheal elasticity; a patient with a short, thick neck may have a deep trachea, with the cricoid at the level of the sternal notch. A patient with a decreased ability to extend the neck will limit tracheal mobilization. The procedure is essentially the same as a wedge resection except that dissection requires excision of the posterior membranous wall. The anterior cricoid arch and the posterior cricoid lamina have been resected to just

below the cricothyroid joints. An oroendotracheal tube is passed distal to the anastomotic site, and the anastomosis is performed with 3-0 submucosal sutures placed around a trachea ring and tied extraluminally. Adequate laryngeal and tracheal mobilization are required to relieve tension from the anastomosis. The neck is placed in extreme flexion, and a stay stitch is placed from chin to sternum.[8]

Segmental resection with primary anastomosis shows promise as the most efficacious procedure for managing near complete or complete tracheal stenosis (Figure 93-8). When the stenosis is limited to the trachea and subglottis and the glottis is normal, success rates in several large series are 95% to 97%.[29] When the stenosis also involves the glottis, resection with end-to-end anastomosis has been performed simultaneously with laryngofissure and decannulation repair of the glottic stenosis, which is achieved in approximately 95% of patients. In these instances, a Montgomery T-tube and prolonged stenting were uniformly used.

Extensive cervical and laryngotracheal stenosis not amenable to segmental resection and anastomosis can be managed with a multistaged trough reconstruction technique. The essential steps require the creation of a large tracheostoma by sewing cervical neck skin to residual tracheal mucosa. The second stage requires the formation of a rigid anterior wall by the insertion of Marlex mesh under adjacent cervical skin. Finally, the closure is obtained by tubing skin and Marlex mesh anteriorly to close the stoma and then advancing cervical neck skin as a second layer (success rate, 76%).

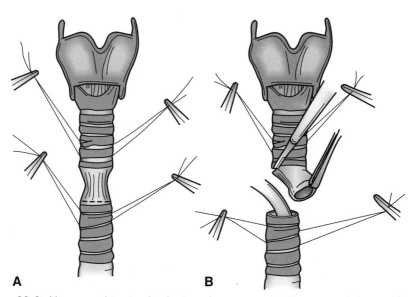

A   **B**

Figure 93-8. Near-complete tracheal stenosis managed with segmental resection with primary anastomosis.

Laryngeal Release Procedures

Tracheal mobilization and laryngeal release techniques are required when a gap greater than 3 cm in tracheal continuity occurs in young patients. Older patients lose elasticity of the annular ligaments of the trachea and therefore require release procedures when more than 1 to 2 cm is resected. Three techniques can gain extra length for end-to-end anastomosis. The first is incision of the annular ligaments, which can add up to 2.5 cm but is most useful in younger patients. Incisions should be placed on one side of the lateral trachea above the anastomosis and on the opposite side below the anastomosis to preserve the blood supply to both tracheal segments.[54] The second technique is superior mobilization of the distal trachea from the thorax,[38] which can result in the achievement of 6 cm of mobilization. This technique requires transection of the left mainstem bronchus and end-to-side anastomosis with the right mainstem bronchus, and it carries a risk of mediastinal dissection. The third technique involves laryngeal release procedures, which can gain 5 cm of tracheal mobilization. The infrahyoid release involves transecting the sternohyoid, omohyoid, and thyrohyoid muscles at the level of the superior border of the thyroid cartilage. The greater cornua of the thyroid cartilage are divided bilaterally, and the thyrohyoid membrane is sectioned. This procedure carries a risk of injury to the superior laryngeal nerve and is associated with prolonged dysphagia.

Suprahyoid laryngeal release is often preferred. This technique requires transecting the insertion of the mylohyoid, geniohyoid, and genioglossus muscles to expose the preepiglottic space. The stylohyoid insertions are transected, and the body of the hyoid is transected medial to the insertion of the digastric tendon. This allows the body of the hyoid, the thyroid cartilage, the cricoid cartilage, and the proximal trachea to drop inferiorly. Flexion of the neck allows an additional 1 to 2 cm of length.[54]

SPECIAL CONSIDERATIONS: EVALUATION AND MANAGEMENT OF BILATERAL VOCAL FOLD MOTION IMPAIRMENT

The predominant causes of bilateral vocal fold motion impairment have changed as medical care has become more sophisticated and as society has become more mechanized. Trauma to the larynx or to the recurrent laryngeal nerve as the result of a direct blow or traction is assuming a major role. Blunt and open trauma to the neck is far more common today than it was half a century ago, and the victims are more likely to survive. Indications for the surgical treatment of thyroid disease have diminished rather markedly as a result of improvements in the methods of diagnosis and management of thyroid disorders. Surgery usually is now indicated only when there is a high likelihood of malignancy. Furthermore, the otolaryngology–head and neck surgeon has become better versed in the anatomic vagaries of the recurrent laryngeal nerve as it courses through the neck, in addition to the current standard that the nerve is most always identified during surgery. Other cervical surgery may contribute to laryngeal nerve deficits, although bilateral involvement is very unlikely. These types of surgery include carotid endarterectomy, anterior cervical fusion, and cervical esophageal surgery—in short, any anterior cervical procedure in which traction and retraction play a role.

Trauma as a result of endotracheal intubation, especially in the chronic setting, has become more frequent and is a therapeutic challenge. Although vocal fold paralysis on the basis of pressure from the endotracheal tube may occur after brief periods of intubation, the most frequent pathologic finding is subglottic or interarytenoid fibrosis and cricoarytenoid ankylosis after prolonged intubation as described in the preceding section. Involvement of the cricoarytenoid joint by an arthritic process in rheumatoid arthritis occurs more frequently than is generally appreciated. Chronic arthritis of the cricoarytenoid or cricothyroid joint obviously would produce ankylosis rather than paralysis, a factor to be confirmed by direct laryngoscopy EMG before treatment.

Infiltrative disorders (amyloid), granulomatous diseases (tuberculosis, sarcoidosis), and neoplastic disease do play a role in the impairment of laryngeal function. Neoplastic disease is usually unilateral and may include squamous cell tumors from the upper aerodigestive tract or primary thyroid neoplasms, which are aggressively malignant. Benign infiltrative disorders and granulomatous disease are more commonly bilateral and result in the impairment of both abduction and adduction, despite intact neuromuscular function. Airway limitation and dysphonia tend to be more severe because of the decreased compliance associated with an infiltrative process.

Many of the etiologic processes are neurologic. Certainly the incidence of neuropathy in patients with longstanding diabetes and in those with small vessel peripheral vascular disease is higher. Parkinson's disease, Parkinson's-like disorders, and the progressive demyelinating processes (e.g., amyotrophic lateral sclerosis) may present with laryngeal involvement as one of the earliest signs. A complex form of laryngeal neuropathy may evolve as a result of trauma that affects the higher centers of the central nervous system. Closed head injury and stroke can cause abnormalities of laryngeal function that are particularly difficult to assess and treat, because the findings change as the lesion evolves.

The symptoms of bilateral vocal fold motion impairment are typically described as if there were a single deficit (either abduction or adduction), but this situation is rarely the case. In the individual with a predominance of abductor loss, the vocal folds tend to be near the midline and predispose the person to a compromised airway in the presence of a relatively good voice. The individual with a predominantly adductor deficit has a relatively good airway, a very breathy voice, and most likely a significant problem with aspiration. In the presence of bilateral paralysis without ankylosis, the compromised laryngeal inlet may close off completely during forced inspiration as the two cords are drawn together by the negative intratracheal pressure; this phenomenon is less likely to occur when the cricoarytenoid joints are ankylosed.

Patient Evaluation and Selection

A word of caution is appropriate at this point. Recall that a tracheotomy bypasses the larynx and thus diminishes the demands for the vocal cords to abduct during inspiration.[73] This situation may lead to an error in diagnosis if one assumes that, because there is no abductor muscle function during indirect laryngoscopy in the tracheotomized patient, there is a break in neural continuity. The tracheotomy tube must be occluded at the time of examination to properly assess abduction.

Indirect laryngoscopy either with the traditional laryngeal mirror or with the aid of a fiberoptic system is the best method for discerning vocal fold mobility on inspiration and phonation. EMG is becoming a more common means of evaluating the neural integrity of the laryngeal musculature. Neither test, however, allows for the absolute exclusion of fibrosis or cricoarytenoid ankylosis. Radiographic evaluation of the swallowing mechanism is an important part of the diagnostic workup to exclude previously inapparent, more general neurologic deficits.

The flow-volume loop (FVL) examination is a useful and easily obtained measurement of respiratory flow rate limitation.[35] The FVL documents air flow rate and volume, the site of obstruction, and the nature and severity of the obstructing lesion. Two distinct FVL patterns are seen with bilateral vocal fold motion impairment (Figure 93-9). Selective inspiratory limitation and normal expiratory flow rate (variable extrathoracic obstruction) are seen with bilateral vocal fold paralysis, cricoarytenoid ankylosis, interarytenoid fibrosis, and laryngeal webs.[13,39] Limitation of flow during inspiration and expiration (fixed obstruction) is seen with infiltrative disorders, either benign or malignant, as a result of mass effect and loss of compliance. FVL provides objective serial measures for the assessment of improvement or the progression of respiratory flow limitations and the assessment of treatment outcome. The minimal acceptable inspiratory flow rate for an average adult at midvital capacity is 1.5 L per second, and strong consideration for surgical intervention should be considered if flow drops below this level.

Finally, direct laryngoscopy should be used to ensure a correct diagnosis. Joint ankylosis becomes apparent on direct palpation of the vocal process and is evidenced by a lack of mobility; this is in contrast with the laxity in suppleness of the joint in the paralyzed state. Furthermore, lateral deflection of the arytenoid on one side should have no effect on the opposite arytenoid. If the contralateral arytenoid moves toward the midline as the other is deviated laterally, then interarytenoid fibrosis with tethering is likely (Figure 93-10).

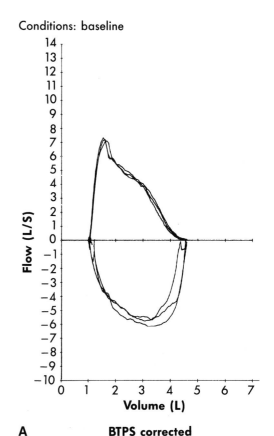

Conditions: baseline

A   **BTPS corrected**

Figure 93-9. Flow-volume loop for assessing adequacy of the upper airway. **A,** Normal examination shows expiratory flow indicated by positive deflection and inspiratory flow indicated by negative deflection.

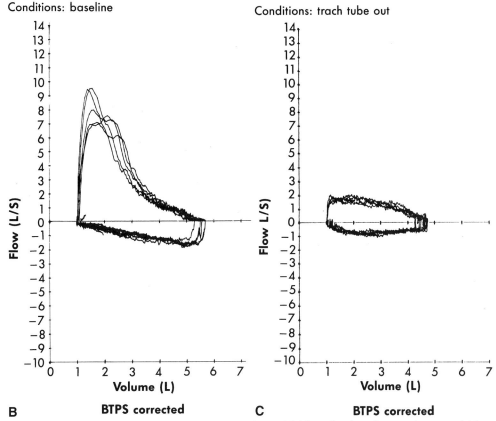

Conditions: baseline

Conditions: trach tube out

B   **BTPS corrected**   **C**   **BTPS corrected**

Figure 93-9, cont'd B, A patient with bilateral vocal fold motion impairment shows variable extrathoracic obstruction with a midvital capacity inspiratory flow rate (VI_{50}) of less than 1.5 L per second. **C,** A patient with an infiltrative tumor and a fixed obstruction.

Management of Bilateral Vocal Fold Motion Impairment with Airway Obstruction

The results of any surgical intervention should be compared with the results produced by tracheotomy alone, because the patient accepts the nuisance of a tracheotomy to gain assurance of a good airway and the probability of a good voice. Most procedures that enlarge the laryngeal airway—and thus eliminate the need for a tracheotomy—result in a voice of poorer quality and increase the possibility of aspiration.

The least invasive of the lateralizing procedures involves endoscopic surgery. An arytenoidectomy may be performed through the laryngoscope (Figure 93-11), but this is a difficult procedure for all but the

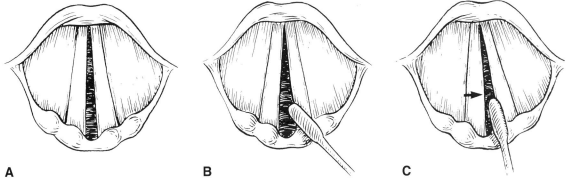

A   **B**   **C**

Figure 93-10. Assessment of arytenoid mobility and interarytenoid tethering by direct palpation. **A,** Endoscopic appearance of bilateral abduction paralysis. **B,** Palpation of the arytenoid cartilage to assess mobility. **C,** Diagnosis of interarytenoid tethering. From Cummings CW and others, editors: *Atlas of laryngeal surgery,* St. Louis, 1984, Mosby.

very experienced surgeon.[84] Lateralization of the vocal cord by suture placement is an alternative procedure (Figure 93-12).[42] Laser cordectomy has been suggested as a method for excising a portion of the vocal cord. Although cordectomy has proved successful for removing the anterior two thirds of the vocal cord, the posterior third represented by the arytenoid is more difficult to remove successfully with the CO_2 laser. Furthermore, partial arytenoidectomy may predispose the patient to a greater incidence of postoperative chondritis. If total arytenoidectomy is performed with the laser, significant scar formation ensues, which may bring the remaining ligamentous portion of the vocal cord medially rather than laterally, as intended. Comparison between cordectomy and arytenoidectomy has demonstrated comparable results with respect to airway improvement. Aspiration is more likely to occur after arytenoidectomy, and both procedures will adversely impact phonatory function.[16]

A simpler and more practical technique of laser cordotomy was introduced by Dennis and Kashima[13] and Kashima[39] as an alternative to cordectomy (Figure 93-13). Using the CO_2 laser, a transverse inci-

sion is made through the vocal fold immediately anterior to the vocal process, resulting in a wedge-shaped widening of the posterior glottis as a result of retraction of the divided thyroarytenoid muscle. Contracture of the thyroarytenoid muscle with secondarily increased anterior vocal fold mass minimizes the postoperative dysphonia associated with cordectomy. In selected cases, vestibulectomy (removal of the ipsilateral false vocal fold) may improve exposure and facilitate the cordotomy.[40]

The open technique for arytenoidectomy (the lateral external approach described by Woodman[90]) is depicted in Figure 93-14. A suture is used to fix the vocal process in a lateralized position at least until scar tissue forms, which must be confirmed by intraoperative endoscopy.[1,90]

Posterior commissure split and placement of a stent or rib graft to separate the vocal folds has also been advocated for the management of bilateral vocal fold motion due to posterior glottic fibrosis as well as bilateral vocal fold paralysis (see Figure 93-14).[26,27] The authors prefer a midline cricoid split and the placement of a posterior cartilage rib graft (Figure 93-15). The posterior graft approach is a nonablative procedure

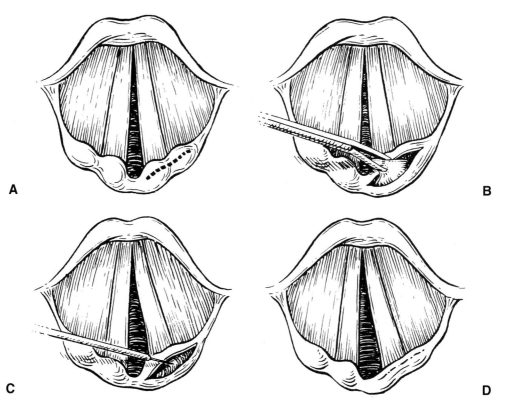

A

B

C

D

Figure 93-11. Technique for endoscopic arytenoidectomy. **A,** An incision is made on overlying arytenoid cartilage. **B,** Arytenoid cartilage is separated and removed. **C,** Needlepoint electrocoagulation is applied to the arytenoid bed. **D,** Vocal fold lateralization by cicatricial contraction. From Cummings CW and others, editors: *Atlas of laryngeal surgery,* Mosby, St. Louis, 1984.

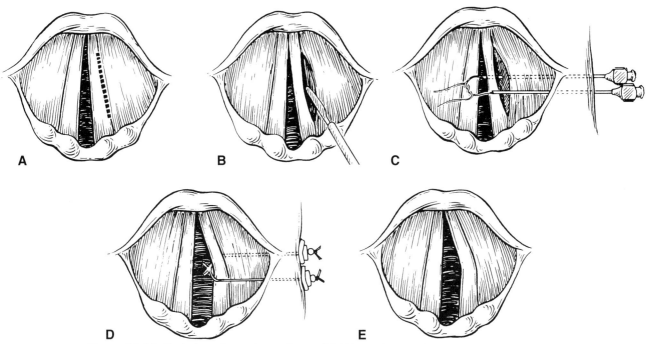

Figure 93-12. Technique for endoscopic vocal fold lateralization. **A,** An incision is made lateral and parallel to the vocal fold. **B,** A wedge of thyroarytenoid muscle is removed, and the base is cauterized. **C,** Placement of transcutaneous sutures. **D,** The vocal fold is lateralized by a temporary suspension suture. **E,** The site 6 weeks after sutures are removed. From Cummings CW and others, editors: *Atlas of laryngeal surgery,* St. Louis, 1984, Mosby.

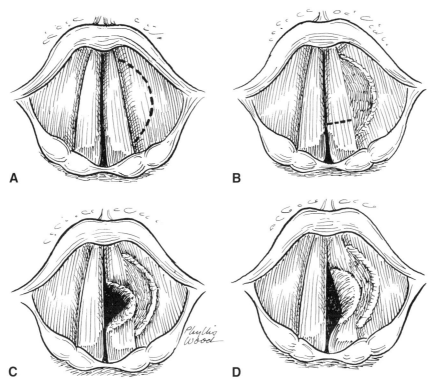

Figure 93-13. Endoscopic laser cordotomy. **A,** The site of the vestibulectomy incision is designed to improve access for cordotomy. **B,** The site of cordotomy is outlined anterior to the vocal process. **C,** Initial posterior glottal enlargement is obtained with cordotomy. **D,** Endoscopy result after the healing process.

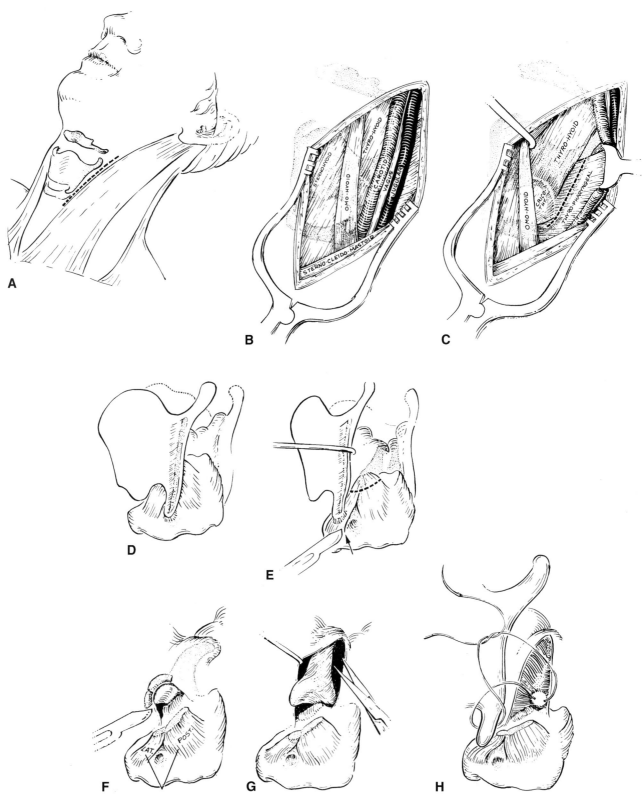

Figure 93-14. External approach for vocal fold lateralization. **A,** The line of incision is made medial to sternocleidomastoid muscle border. **B,** The sternocleidomastoid muscle retracts to reveal underlying structures. **C,** The thyropharyngeal constrictor muscles are separated. **D,** The cricothyroid joint is exposed. **E,** The cricothyroid joint is disarticulated. **F,** The posterior and lateral cricoarytenoid muscles are separated, and the cricoarytenoid joint is disarticulated. **G,** A vertical incision is made to remove arytenoid cartilage. **H,** A suture through the vocal process is stabilized around a cornu of thyroid cartilage.

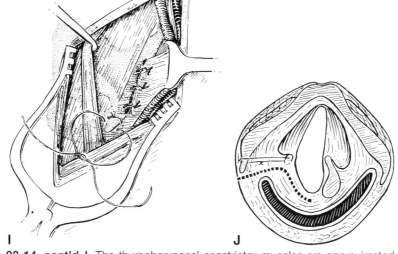

Figure 93-14, cont'd I, The thyropharyngeal constrictor muscles are approximated. **J,** The vocal fold is lateralized. From Cummings CW and others, editors: *Atlas of laryngeal surgery,* St. Louis, 1984, Mosby.

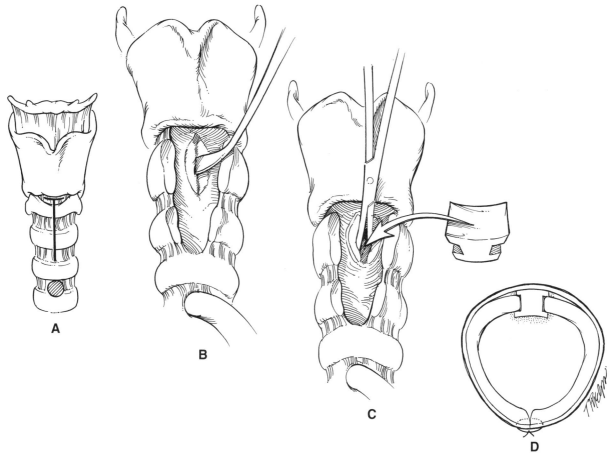

Figure 93-15. Inferior cricoid split with placement of posterior cartilage graft for laryngeal stenosis or bilateral vocal fold paralysis. **A,** Incision through the anterior cricoid and first tracheal ring provides exposure of interarytenoid region in the posterior aspect of the cricoid. **B,** The cricoid is split posteriorly, preserving the outer perichondrium; the outer perichondrium is elevated posteriorly on both sides, thereby creating a pocket to receive a cartilage graft. **C,** Rib cartilage is harvested and fashioned with inner and outer flanges to provide stabilization; grafts should provide 1 to 1.5 cm of displacement. **D,** Placement of a cartilage graft posteriorly with anterior and posterior flanges; the outer perichondrium and cartilage anteriorly are sutured with interrupted 3.0 Prolene sutures.

that preserves both the arytenoids and the vocal folds. The cricoid cartilage and the first and second tracheal rings are split anteriorly, thereby allowing access to the interarytenoid region. The thyroid cartilage and anterior commissure are left intact. The cricoid is split posteriorly, and the outer perichondrium is elevated, thereby creating a pocket to accept the cartilage graft. A rib graft is harvested and fashioned with anterior and posterior flanges. The body of the graft should provide approximately 1 to 1.5 cm of displacement of the cricoid posteriorly; the graft may be stabilized as necessary with 3-0 Vicryl suture. Stenting in not absolutely required if the graft is secure; however, tracheotomy should be performed. Further evaluation of outcome with respect to airway, phonatory function, and swallowing are necessary before this procedure is widely accepted.

The success rate for any of these procedures is generally no more than 70%, a point to be remembered when counseling the patient or making therapeutic decisions. If the patient has paralysis with a supple cricoarytenoid joint, one may consider a reinnervation procedure as a first option before performing a more irreversible operation. Tucker (1979) introduced the concept of neuromuscular pedicle transposition into the paralyzed posterior cricoarytenoid muscle to enhance the ability to abduct the vocal cord by establishing a reinnervated muscle (Figure 93-16); his high success rate of more than 80% (judged by the ability to decannulate the patient) has not been reproduced by others. Critics believe that, rather than reestablishing neuromuscular integrity in the posterior cricoarytenoid muscle by using the ansa cervicalis nerve pedicle, movement of the extralaryngeal

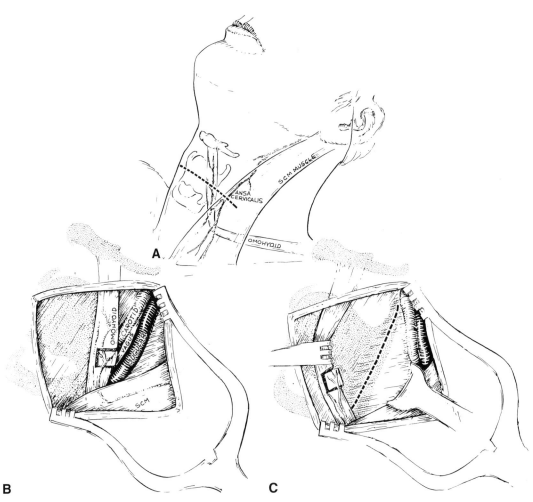

Figure 93-16. Neuromuscular pedicle reinnervation technique for vocal fold lateralization. **A,** A line of incision at the midthyroid cartilage level. **B,** The pedicle is formed with a segment of omohyoid muscle with accompanying nerve, artery, and vein. **C,** The thyropharyngeal constrictor muscles are incised.

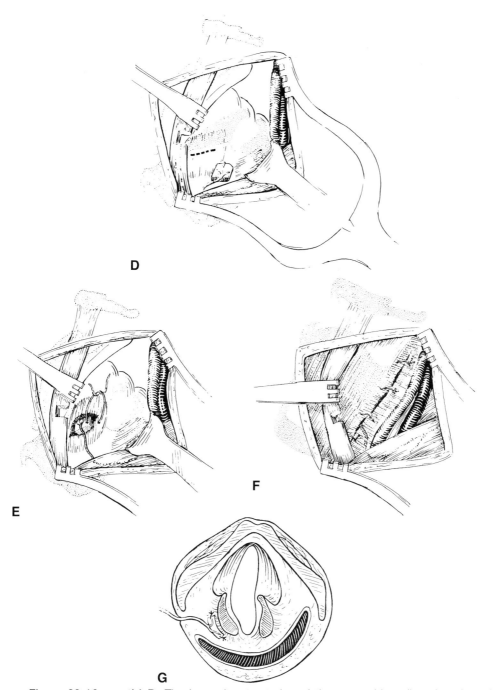

Figure 93-16, cont'd D, The larynx is retracted, and the arytenoid cartilage is palpated; myotomy is seen in the posterior cricoarytenoid muscle. **E,** The pedicle is sutured into the cricoarytenoid muscle. **F,** The thyropharyngeal constrictor muscles are approximated. **G,** The omohyoid pedicle is sutured to the posterior cricoarytenoid muscle. From Cummings CW and others, editors: *Atlas of laryngeal surgery,* St. Louis, 1984, Mosby.

muscles is transmitted to the arytenoid by scar tissue. Although still unresolved, the reinnervation concept has rekindled interest in therapeutic surgery for the paralyzed larynx (see the reinnervation section of Chapter 138 by G. S. Goding).

Management of Bilateral Vocal Fold Motion Impairment with Weak Voice and Aspiration

Bilateral adductor paralysis is a very unusual condition that is characterized by a weak voice and aspiration. During the acute phase (when there is still hope for the return of neural function), bilateral vocal fold augmentation with Cymetra can be used to close off the airway temporarily. Methods that are effective with unilateral adductor paralysis (specifically the injection of Cymetra and surgical medialization) may be applied at this point. The tradeoff between airway and phonatory function should be considered, along with tracheotomy. More specific surgical approaches to the laryngeal inlet may be indicated to confront the problem of severe, life-threatening aspiration. A narrow-field laryngectomy is the most effective method for the prevention of aspiration; however, it results in the elimination of the larynx as an organ of communication. Other surgical approaches, including the epiglottic sewdown procedure, surgical approximation of the vocal folds, and tracheal diversion procedures, have their place with conditions that are judged to be reversible. Management of intractable aspiration is discussed elsewhere in this text.

REFERENCES

1. Baker CH: Report of a case of abductor paralysis with removal of one vocal cord, *J Mich Med Soc* 15:485, 1916.
2. Beste DJ, Toohill RJ: Microtrapdoor flap repair of laryngeal and tracheal stenosis, *Ann Otol Rhinol Laryngol* 100:420, 1991.
3. Bogdasarian RS, Olson NR: Posterior glottic laryngeal stenosis, *Otolaryngol Head Neck Surg* 88:765, 1980.
4. Burstein FD, Canalis RC, Ward PH: Composite hyoid-sternohyoid interposition grafts revisited: UCLA experience 1974-1984, *Laryngoscope* 96:516, 1986.
5. Correa AJ and others: Inhibition of subglottic stenosis with mitomycin-C in the canine model, *Ann Otol Rhinol Laryngol* 1999:108(11 Pt 1), 1053.
6. Crumley RL: Endoscopic laser medial arytenoidectomy for airway management in bilateral laryngeal paralysis, *Ann Otol Rhinol Laryngol* 102:81, 1993.
7. Crumley RL: Phrenic nerve graft for bilateral vocal cord paralysis, *Laryngoscope* 93:425, 1983.
8. Cummings CW and others: *Tracheal stenosis.* In Cummings CW and others, editors: *Atlas of laryngeal surgery,* St Louis, 1984, Mosby.
9. Davidson J and others: Functional assessment after laryngotracheoplasty, *Otolaryngol Head Neck Surg* 97:294, 1987.
10. Dedo HH: Endoscopic Teflon keel for anterior glottic web, *Ann Otol Rhinol Laryngol* 88:467, 1979.
11. Dedo HH, Sooy CD: Endoscopic laser repair of posterior glottic, subglottic and tracheal stenosis by division or microtrapdoor flap, *Laryngoscope* 94:445, 1984.
12. Delaere PR and others: Epiglottoplasty for reconstruction of posttraumatic laryngeal stenosis, *Ann Otol Rhinol Laryngol* 100:447, 1991.
13. Dennis DP, Kashima H: Carbon dioxide laser posterior cordectomy for treatment of bilateral vocal cord paralysis, *Ann Otol Rhinol Laryngol* 98:930, 1989.
14. Duncavage JA and others: The microtrapdoor technique for management of laryngeal stenosis, *Laryngoscope* 97:825, 1987.
15. Duncavage JA, Ossoff RH, Toohill RJ: Laryngotracheal reconstruction with composite nasal septal cartilage grafts, *Ann Otol Rhinol Laryngol* 98:581, 1989.
16. Eckel HE and others: Cordectomy versus arytenoidectomy in the management of bilateral vocal cord paralysis, *Ann Otol Rhinol Laryngol* 103:852, 1994.
17. Evans JN: Laryngotracheoplasty, *Otolaryngol Clin North Am* 10:119, 1977.
18. Flint P: Powered surgical instruments for laryngeal surgery, *Otolaryngol Head Neck Surg* 122:263, 2000.
19. Friedman M, Mayer AD: Laryngotracheal reconstruction in adults with the sternocleidomastoid myoperiosteal flap, *Ann Otol Rhinol Laryngol* 101:897, 1992.
20. Friedman EM, Healy GB, McGill TJ: Carbon dioxide management of subglottic and tracheal stenosis, *Otolaryngol Clin North Am* 16:871, 1983.
21. Friedman M and others: Experience with the sternocleidomastoid myoperiosteal flap for reconstruction of subglottic and tracheal defects: modification of technique and report of long-term results, *Laryngoscope* 98:1003, 1988.
22. Fry TL, Fischer ND, Pillsbury HC: Tracheal reconstruction with pedicled thyroid cartilage, *Laryngoscope* 95:60, 1985.
23. Gallivan GJ: Laryngotracheal paratubal air envelope: a useful sign in voice and airway reconstructive surgery, *J Voice* 8:168, 1994.
24. Gates GA, Tucker JA: Sliding flap tracheoplasty, *Ann Otol Rhinol Laryngol* 98:926, 1989.
25. Goldenberg and others: *Third volume rendering CT in the diagnosis of subglottic stenosis.* Presented at the AAO-HNS Foundation Annual Meeting, San Diego, Califoring, 2002.
26. Goodwin WJ and others: Vocal cord mobilization by posterior laryngoplasty, *Laryngoscope* 98:846, 1988.
27. Grahne B and others: Surgical treatment of chronic laryngeal stenosis secondary to vocal cord paralysis: pre and postoperative evaluation of ventilatory function, *Laryngoscope* 93:163, 1983.
28. Hall RR: The healing of tissues incised by carbon dioxide laser, *Br J Surg* 58:222, 1971.
29. Har-El G and others: Resection of tracheal stenosis with end-to-end anastomosis, *Ann Otol Rhinol Laryngol* 102:670, 1993.
30. Harris HH, Tobin HA: Acute injuries of the larynx and trachea in 49 patients, *Laryngoscope* 80:1376, 1970.
31. Hartig GK, Esclamado RM, Telian SA: Chondrogenesis by free and vascularized rabbit auricular perichondrium, *Ann Otol Rhinol Laryngol* 103:901, 1994.
32. Hartnick CJ and others: Topical mitomycin application after laryngotracheal reconstruction: a randomized, double-blind, placebo-controlled trial, *Arch Otolaryngol Head Neck Surg* 127:1260, 2001.
33. Hoover WB: Bilateral abductor paralysis: operative treatment by submucous resection of the vocal cords, *Arch Otolaryngol* 15:339, 1932.
34. Hoppe H and others: Multidetector CT virtual bronchoscopy to grade tracheobronchial stenosis, *AJR Am J Roentgenol* 178:1195, 2002.
35. Hyatt RE, Black LF: The flow-volume curve, a current perspective, *Am Rev Respir Dis* 107:191, 1973.
36. Imhoff AB, Ledermann T: Arthroscopic subacromial decompression with and without the holmium: YAG-laser. A comparative study, *Arthroscopy* 5:549, 1995.
37. Isshiki N and others: Surgical treatment of laryngeal web with mucosa graft, *Ann Otol Rhinol Laryngol* 100:95, 1991.
38. Jindal JR and others: Gastroesophageal reflux disease as a likely cause of "idiopathic" subglottic stenosis, *Ann Otol Rhinol Laryngol* 103:186, 1994.
39. Kashima HK: Bilateral vocal fold motion impairment: pathophysiology and management by transverse cordotomy, *Ann Otol Rhinol Laryngol* 100:717, 1991.
40. Kashima HK: Personal communication, September 1, 1991.
41. Kennedy TL: Epiglottic reconstruction of laryngeal stenosis secondary to cricothyroidotomy, *Laryngoscope* 90:1130, 1980.

42. Kirchner F: Endoscopic lateralization of the vocal cord in abductor paralysis of the larynx, *Laryngoscope* 89:1179, 1979.
43. Langman AW, Lee KC, Dedo HH: The endoscopic Teflon keel for posterior and total glottic stenosis, *Laryngoscope* 99:571, 1989.
44. Lebovics RS and others: The management of subglottic stenosis in patients with Wegener's granulomatosis, *Laryngoscope* 102:1341, 1992.
45. Mayer HM, Brock M: Percutaneous endoscopic discectomy: surgical technique and preliminary results compared to microsurgical discectomy, *J Neurosurg* 78:216, 1992.
46. Mayer HM, Brock M: Percutaneous endoscopic lumbar discectomy (PELD), *Neurosurg Rev* 16:115, 1993.
47. McCaffrey TV: Classification of laryngotracheal stenosis, *Laryngoscope* 102:1335, 1992.
48. McCaffrey TV: Management of laryngotracheal stenosis on the basis of site and severity, *Otolaryngol Head Neck Surg* 109:468, 1993.
49. McComb H: Treatment of tracheal stenosis, *Plast Reconstr Surg* 39:43, 1967.
50. McGarry GW, Gana P, Adamson B: The effect of microdebriders on tissue for histological diagnosis, *Clin Otolaryngol* 22:375, 1997.
51. McNaught RC: Surgical correction of the anterior web of the larynx, *Laryngoscope* 60:264, 1950.
52. Mohr RM: A modification of the Aboulker stent for reduction of granulation tissue that allows tracheotomy changes, *Laryngoscope* 102:350, 1992.
53. Montgomery WW: Posterior and complete glottic stenosis, *Arch Otolaryngol Head Neck Surg* 98:170, 1973.
54. Montgomery WW, editor: *Surgery of the upper respiratory system,* vol 2. Philadelphia, Lea & Febiger, 1989.
55. Montgomery WW, Gamble JE: Anterior glottic stenosis, *Arch Otolaryngol Head Neck Surg* 92:560, 1970.
56. Morganstein K: Composite auricular graft in laryngeal reconstruction, *Laryngoscope* 82:844, 1972.
57. Myer CM and others: Use of laryngeal micro resector system, *Laryngoscope* 109:1165, 1999.
58. Naficy S, Esclamado RM, Clevens R: Reconstruction of the rabbit trachea with vascularized auricular perichondrium, *Ann Otol Rhinol Laryngol* 105:356, 1996.
59. Nordin U, Lindholm CE, Wolgast M: Blood flow in rabbit tracheal mucosa and the influence of tracheal intubation, *Acta Anesthesiol Scand* 21:84, 1977.
60. Ogura JH, Biller HF: Reconstruction of the larynx following blunt trauma, *Ann Otol Rhinol Laryngol* 80:492, 1971.
61. Olson NR: Wound healing by primary intention in the larynx, *Otolaryngol Clin North Am* 12:735, 1979.
62. Olson NR: Skin grafting of the larynx, *Otolaryngol Head Neck Surg* 104:503, 1991.
63. Olson NR, Sullivan MJ: Epiglottis in reconstruction of the larynx and trachea, *Ann Otol Rhinol Laryngol* 94:437, 1985.
64. Ossoff RH, Karlan MS, Sisson GA: Endoscopic laser arytenoidectomy, *Lasers Surg Med* 2:293, 1983.
65. Ossoff RH and others: Endoscopic laser arytenoidectomy for the treatment of bilateral vocal cord paralysis, *Laryngoscope* 94:1293, 1984.
66. Patel N, Rowe M, Tunkel D: Treatment of recurrent respiratory papillomatosis in children with the microdebrider, *Ann Otol Rhinol Laryngol* 112:7, 2003.
67. Parker DA, Das Gupta AR: An endoscopic silastic keel for anterior glottic webs, *J Laryngol Otol* 101:1055, 1987.
68. Pasquale K and others: Microdebrider versus CO_2 laser removal of recurrent respiratory papillomas: a prospective analysis, *Laryngoscope* 113:139, 2003.

69. Rahbar R, Valdez TA, Shapshay SM: Preliminary results of intraoperative mitomycin-C in the treatment and prevention of glottic and subglottic stenosis, *J Voice* 14:282, 2000.
70. Remsen K and others: Laser lateralization for bilateral vocal cord abductor paralysis, *Otolaryngol Head Neck Surg* 93:645, 1985.
71. Sant'Anna GD, Mauri M: Use of the microdebrider for Reinke's edema surgery, *Laryngoscope* 110:2114, 2000.
72. Santos PM, Afrassiabi A, Weymuller EA: Prospective studies evaluating the standard endotracheal tube and a prototype endotracheal tube, *Ann Otol Rhinol Laryngol* 98:935, 1989.
73. Sasaki CT, Fukuda H, Kirchner JA: Laryngeal abductor activity in response to varying ventilatory resistance, *Trans Am Acad Ophthalmol Otolaryngol* 77:403, 1973.
74. Sasaki CT, Horiuchi M, Koss N: Tracheotomy related subglottic stenosis: bacteriologic pathogenesis, *Laryngoscope* 86:857, 1979.
75. Schaefer SD, Close LG, Brown OE: Mobilization of the fixated arytenoid in the stenotic posterior laryngeal commissure, *Laryngoscope* 96:656, 1986.
76. Schuller DE: Long term stenting for laryngotracheal stenosis, *Ann Otol Rhinol Laryngol* 89:515, 1980.
77. Sessions D, Ogura JH, Henneman H: Surgical management of bilateral vocal cord paralysis, *Laryngoscope* 86:559, 1976.
78. Shapshay SM and others: Endoscopic treatment of subglottic and tracheal stenosis by radial laser incision and dilation, *Ann Otol Rhinol Laryngol* 96:661, 1987.
79. Simoni P and others: Use of the endoscopic microdebrider in the management of airway obstruction from laryngotracheal carcinoma, *Ann Otol Rhinol Laryngol* 112:11, 2003.
80. Simpson GT and others: Predictive factors of success or failure in the endoscopic management of laryngeal and tracheal stenosis, *Ann Otol Rhinol Laryngol* 91:384, 1982.
81. Spector JE and others: Prevention of anterior glottic restenosis in a canine model with topical mitomycin-C, *Ann Otol Rhinol Laryngol* 110:1007, 2001.
82. Stell PM and others: Chronic laryngeal stenosis, *Ann Otol Rhinol Laryngol* 94:108, 1985.
83. Thomas GK, Stevens MH: Stenting in experimental laryngeal injuries, *Arch Otolaryngol Head Neck Surg* 101:217, 1975.
84. Thornell WC: New intralaryngeal approach for bilateral abductor paralysis of vocal cords, *Trans Am Acad Ophthalmol Otolaryngol* 53:631, 1949.
85. Volpi D and others: Risk factors for intubation injury of the larynx, *Ann Otol Rhinol Laryngol* 96:684, 1987.
86. Weymuller EA: Laryngeal injury from prolonged endotracheal intubation, *Laryngoscope* 98:1, 1988.
87. Whited RE: Laryngeal fracture in the multiple trauma patient, *Am J Surg* 136:354, 1978.
88. Whited RE: A prospective study of laryngotracheal sequelae in long term intubation, *Laryngoscope* 94:367, 1984.
89. Wong ML and others: Vascularized hyoid interposition for subglottic and upper tracheal stenosis, *Ann Otol Rhinol Laryngol* 87:491, 1978.
90. Woodman DG: Bilateral abductor paralysis, *Arch Otolaryngol* 58:150, 1953.
91. Woodman D: A modification of the extralaryngeal approach to arytenoidectomy for bilateral abductor paralysis, *Arch Otolaryngol Head Neck Surg* 43:63, 1946.
92. Zalzal GH: Use of stents in laryngotracheal reconstruction in children: indications, technical considerations, and complications, *Laryngoscope* 98:849, 1988.
93. Zalzal GH, Cotton RT: A new way of carving cartilage grafts to avoid prolapse into the tracheal lumen when used in subglottic reconstruction, *Laryngoscope* 96:1039, 1986.

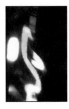

CHAPTER NINETY FOUR

THE PROFESSIONAL VOICE

Gregory N. Postma
Mark S. Courey
Robert H. Ossoff

INTRODUCTION

Care of patients who use their voices professionally requires knowledge and skills not easily mastered within the field of otolaryngology alone. It is part of the discipline of performing arts medicine. The laryngologist enlists the expertise of speech pathologists and singing voice scientists to retrain and rehabilitate the professional voice patient. A team approach is mandatory and has been strengthened over the past decade by the establishment of several multidisciplinary voice centers.

Professional voice patients are a diverse group. Limiting the definition to singers and actors is too narrow. Any person who depends on speaking or singing skills for employment (e.g., salesmen, receptionists, telephone operators, lawyers, clergy, teachers, politicians, public speakers, and most physicians) should be considered a professional voice user because all of these persons place diverse yet significant demands on their voices.

Singers and actors place the greatest demand on the vocal apparatus. The extraordinary amount of practice and performance stress these people are under exceeds that of any other type of vocal professional. They are often highly trained and push their voices to their physical limits. No other patients are as sensitive to subtle changes in their vocal abilities. Singers and actors with voice disorders often challenge the most experienced laryngologist. The knowledge and expertise gained from managing these patients can and should be generalized to care for other professional and nonprofessional patients with voice disorders.

ANATOMIC CONSIDERATIONS

Voice is an extremely sensitive indicator of emotional status and general health. Therefore, when evaluating the vocal professional with a voice disorder, the entire body and psyche should be considered. The body itself is the vocal instrument, and the larynx is the most sensitive part of the instrument. Altered function in nearly any area of the vocal professional's body can result in vocal changes. The larynx, therefore, should not be evaluated as an isolated entity.

Sound generation of any type requires a power source, a vibrator, and a resonator. The lungs are the power supply, the larynx is the vibratory source, and the supraglottal vocal tract (supraglottal pharynx, oral cavity, and potentially the nasal cavity) is the resonator that shapes the sound into words and song. The sound of the voice is affected by changes in any of these three systems, which should be considered as a unit during evaluation of the professional voice patient.

Laryngeal function depends on extrinsic and intrinsic laryngeal musculature. The extrinsic laryngeal muscles alter the position of the larynx. Classically trained singers use the extrinsic musculature to stabilize the larynx within the neck when singing.[92] The intrinsic laryngeal muscles allow delicate control of adduction, abduction, and tension of the vocal folds.

Within the larynx, the human vocal folds are unique structures with no correlates in another animal species. Hirano and others[46,47] have provided an understanding of the laminar structure of the human vocal fold and described the cover-body theory of vocal fold vibration. The vocal fold is covered by a layer of stratified squamous epithelium. The subepithelial tissue, the lamina propria, is divided into superficial, intermediate, and deep layers. The superficial layer, often called Reinke's space, is composed of fibroblasts, which produce proteins to form an extracellular matrix of loose connective tissue. The intermediate layer is composed chiefly of elastin fibers, and the deep layer is composed primarily of collagen fibers. Collagen fibers from the deep layer blend into the underlying thyroarytenoid muscle, which forms the main bulk of the vocal fold (Figures 94-1 and 94-2).

In the cover-body theory of vocal fold vibration, the cover is composed of the overlying epithelium combined with the superficial layer of the lamina propria. The intermediate and deep layers of the lamina propria, known as the vocal ligament, form a transition zone, and the body is composed primarily of the thyroarytenoid muscle. The contrasting masses and physical properties of the vocal fold cover and the body causes them to move at different rates as air passes between the vocal folds. This movement, or vibration, creates sound by chopping the airstream. The sound, a buzzing-like tone, is modulated by the supraglottal vocal tract into speech or song.

Blood vessels enter the vocal fold anteriorly and posteriorly. Vessels run parallel to the longitudinal axis of the fold. This arrangement allows the cover to vibrate over the body without placing excessive stretch or shearing forces on the vessels. Electron microscopy has shown that several arteriovenous shunts are

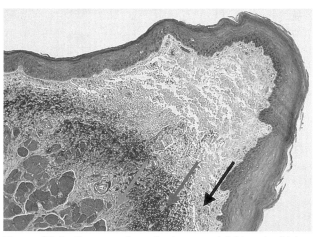

Figure 94-2. Cross section of a true vocal fold under higher magnification. Collagen with increased cross-linking appears deeper yellow (*blue arrow*) compared with less cross-linked collagen in the superficial portion of the lamina propria (*black arrow*) (Movat stain; ×100). To view this image in color, please go to *www.ototext.com* or the Electronic Image Collection CD, bound into your copy of Cummings Otolaryngology—Head and Neck Surgery, 4th edition.

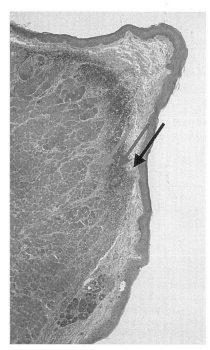

Figure 94-1. Cross section of a true vocal fold stained for elastin (*black*) and collagen (*yellow*). The trilaminar arrangement to the lamina propria is shown. Nonkeratinized squamous epithelium forms the mucosal layer over the superficial portion of the lamina propria. The black arrow indicates the superficial portion, the red arrow indicates the intermediate layer, which is rich in elastin, and the blue arrow is pointing to the deep layer, which is rich in collagen (Movat stain; ×40). To view this image in color, please go to *www.ototext.com* or the Electronic Image Collection CD, bound into your copy of Cummings Otolaryngology—Head and Neck Surgery, 4th edition.

present in the vocal fold microcirculation. These may allow autoregulation of blood flow to this area.[69]

Gray and others[41] have begun to identify the contents of the basement membrane zone and the lamina propria. The basement membrane zone is a complex area anchoring the epidermis to the superficial layer of the lamina propria (Figure 94-3). It is the site of tremendous sheering forces in the human vocal fold

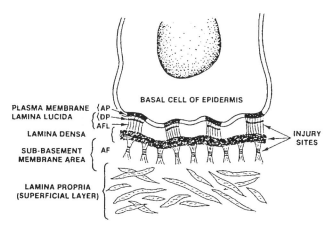

Figure 94-3. Arrangement of structures visible with the electron microscope from the basement cell to the fibers of the superficial layer of the lamina propria. AP, attachment plaques; DP, subbasal dense plate; AFL, anchoring filaments; AF, anchoring fibers. (From Gray SD and others, editors: *Molecular and cellular structure of vocal fold tissue.* In *Vocal fold physiology,* San Diego, CA, 1993, Singular Publishing Group.)

that occur during vocal fold vibration. Excessive sheer forces can lead to disruption of the basement membrane zone and the development of infiltrates in this area.[40] This process is important in vocal fold nodule formation. In the superficial layer of the lamina propria, collagen type III and VII fibers intertwine. This arrangement fixates the basement membrane zone to the superficial layer of the lamina propria, yet allows passive stretch during vibration (Figure 94-4).[29,39,41,42]

Immunohistochemical analysis has also been used to study the basement membrane zone and extracellular matrix of the lamina propria. In diseased states, which clinically correlate with vocal fold nodules, the basement membrane zone is widened significantly. In lesions that are clinically labeled polyps, collagen type IV within the basement membrane zone appears less pronounced than in the healthy state. Perhaps this relative weakness predisposes patients to polyp formation.[24,39]

VOICE PRODUCTION

Vocalization begins with the air or power supply. The lungs supply the essential energy for sound production by presenting the larynx (oscillator) with a stream of air. The diaphragm; intercostal, back, and abdominal musculature; and the elastic recoil of the chest wall work in concert during inspiration and expiration to control the release of air.[50,51] Classically trained singers use the abdominal and thoracic musculature to regulate exhalation; they tend to use a greater percentage of total lung capacity than non-classically trained singers to produce sound in a more efficient manner.[37,38] This enhanced efficiency of air propulsion to the larynx is a key difference between trained and untrained voice users.

As the diaphragm relaxes and the chest wall recoils to a resting state, air is pushed through the nearly closed vocal folds. Due to a reduction in the size of the air passage at the glottal level compared with the size of the air passage of the trachea and subglottis, pressure in the region of the glottis drops as the velocity of the air column increases. The vacuum, created by this drop in pressure, draws the pliable rima glottal tissue of the membranous vocal fold region together. After closure at the membranous glottal level, the air column from the lungs and trachea continues to flow into the subglottal region. The increasing subglottal air pressure forces the vocal folds back open. The vocal folds, or rima glottal tissues, open inferiorly to superiorly (inferior to superior lip), forming an alternating convergent and divergent glottal configuration. The aerodynamic forces of the air column and the inherent myoelastic properties of the vocal folds, particularly in the region of the vocal fold cover, are responsible for the repeated opening and closing of the rima glottal tissue that pulses the air column as it flows out of the glottis. These disruptions in the steady state of the tracheal air pressure by glottal activity result in sound production. The sound produced by the vibratory source has a buzz-like quality. In professional voice production, glottal sound production can be further complicated by voluntary muscular activity that can influence the intensity and frequency characteristics of the glottal sound before its presentation to the supraglottal vocal tract.

The intensity of the sound source is related directly to subglottic pressure. That is, as subglottal pressure increases, sound intensity also increases. Humans can alter subglottal pressure, and therefore sound intensity, by two methods. The first and probably most efficient method is to modify the force of the expelled air from the trachea. This is accomplished through activation of the abdominal and thoracic musculature to increase the amount of air inspired and then, partially through elastic recoil properties of the thoracic cavity and partially through voluntary muscular activity, controlling the rate of air egress. The varied regional schools of classical singing all emphasize different areas of muscular control to accomplish this phenomenon. However, the effect is the same in that the percentage of air used during singing is increased. The second method used to control subglottal pressure is to modify the force of vocal fold adduction. This method is somewhat less efficient. By increasing the force of laryngeal closure through thyroarytenoid (TA), lateralcricoarytenoid (LCA), and interarytenoid (IA) muscle activity, greater resistance to the glottal opening is achieved. This in turn increases subglottal pressure, which increases sound intensity. However, frequency of vocal fold vibration is directly related to tension within the vibratory system. Therefore, if sound intensity is controlled by the addition of tension into the vibrating system, the frequency of vibration can be inadvertently affected.

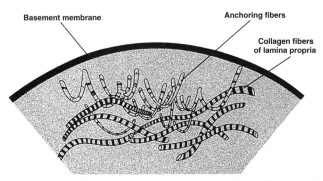

Figure 94-4. The basement membrane and basal lamina of cell anchoring fibers that attach to the lamina densa of the basement membrane, and type 111 collagen fibers passing through the loops of the anchoring fibers. (From Gray SD, Pianatni SS, Harding P: *J Voice* 8:48, 1994.)

Well-trained vocal professionals can independently modulate the frequency characteristic of the source signal from vocal fold vibration through voluntary behaviors. This is accomplished through adjustments in cricothyroid (CT), TA, LCA, and IA muscle activity. The CT muscle, when activated, elongates the vocal fold thus tensing the cover and elevating the frequency of vibration. Fine control of the degree of tension is accomplished by balancing these CT contraction forces against TA, LCA, and IA muscle forces to maintain the vocal folds in an appropriate position for phonation. Unopposed CT muscle contraction will lead to increases in the glottal width, which will negatively affect the vibratory cycle. In addition, fine control of this mechanism allows the blending of the registers of the singing voice for a smoother transition between what singers term the *chest* and *head voice regions.* Inappropriate or unbalanced changes lead to what is perceived as voice breaks. Although these breaks may be unappealing in a classically trained singer, they can be used for stylistic effects in commercial singing voice production. The yodel is probably the most commonly appreciated stylistic technique using the break in registers to produce a desired sound.

The sound source signals produced by vocal fold oscillation, has a fundamental vibratory rate termed the *fundamental frequency.* In addition, the oscillatory source produces a rich spectrum of harmonics. Each harmonic is a whole number multiple of the fundamental frequency. The supraglottal vocal tract, based on its physical characteristics of length, shape, and size of the opening at the distal end, amplifies or attenuates particular regions in the source harmonic spectrum. The harmonic frequencies that are amplified are referred to as *formant regions,* and they shape the output from the sound source into speech sounds appreciated as vocal communication. There are four or five formant regions significant in vocal sound production. The first two of these regions are primarily responsible for vowel determination, whereas the third, fourth, and fifth formant regions color the sound or provide timbre. Vocal professionals, particularly classically trained singers, are able to alter the characteristics of the vocal tract to modulate or shift these formant regions. When the third through fifth formant regions are brought closer together by the voluntary changes in characteristics of the vocal tract, they amplify each other and a ring, termed the *singer's formant,* is produced. This formant region, in the range of 2300 to 3200 cycles/second, is preferentially detected by the human auditory system over other frequencies and allows the singer to be heard and understood above the sound of an orchestra or other instruments.[88–90] Appropriate use of these principles may allow a professional voice user greater vocal efficiency, that is, greater radiated output with less physical effort. Again, by altering the length of the vocal tract through actions of the abdominal, thoracic, and cervical musculature; altering the shape of the vocal tract through the action of the pharynx, tongue, jaw, and lips; and altering the size of the distal opening primarily through the actions of the jaw and lips, a trained vocal professional can modulate the formant regions of the sound produced to provide an aesthetically pleasing sound quality for the listener. The purpose of all vocal training, either commercial or classical, is to teach the performer to control these vocal subsystems to produce the desired, and hopefully aesthetically pleasing, sound.

LARYNGEAL STROBOSCOPY

Although first reported by Oertel[70,71] in 1878, stroboscopic examination of the larynx has only recently become popular. Stroboscopy is necessary to evaluate the vibratory patterns of the vocal folds that occur too rapidly to be visualized by the unaided human eye.[80,82,83] According to Talbot's law, the retina is only able to resolve five images/second. Therefore, images presented to the retina for less than 0.2 seconds (five images/second) persist and are fused together by the ocular cortex to produce apparent motion. Because the vocal folds vibrate at rates of 75 to 1000 cycles/second, even the slowest vibratory patterns are not able to be visualized without assistance. During stroboscopy the larynx is visualized with a xenon light source. Characteristics of xenon light allow rapid on-and-off bursts. In this manner, the larynx is visualized for only brief periods in the range of 1/1000 of a second. These brief images, sampled from various points across many vibratory cycles, are then fused together to provide apparent slow motion of the laryngeal vibratory tissue. In modern stroboscopic equipment, the rate of laryngeal vibration is sensed by a microphone and used to control the rate of xenon light firing. When the rate of visually sampling the laryngeal image is out of phase with the rate of vibration, the laryngeal tissue appears to move. When the sampling rate is in phase with the vibratory rate, the laryngeal tissue appears to stand still.

Stroboscopy permits observation of the vibratory action of the vocal folds, which is not possible with still-light examination (Figure 94-5). As previously described, this vibratory action is responsible for sound production. Therefore, by using stroboscopy, the examiner can observe how small lesions alter the normal laryngeal vibratory pattern. The significance of a given lesion can then be determined.

In addition to providing information regarding vibratory status, examinations captured in video format can be reviewed for comparison with previous examinations and for consultation. This information improves accuracy in the diagnosis of vocal problems.

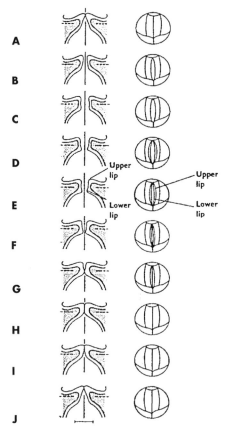

Figure 94-5. Vocal fold vibration. The frontal section (left column) and the view from above (right column). (From Hirano M, Bless DM: *Videostroboscopic examination of the larynx,* San Diego, CA, 1993, Singular Publishing Group.)

Ideally, each professional voice patient should have a baseline laryngeal stroboscopy performed while his or her health and voice are good. The findings can be compared with the vocal fold appearance during dysphonic states, and conclusions regarding the effects of vibration patterns on the cause of dysphonia can be made.

Recorded laryngeal stroboscopic examinations can be used to follow changes in the glottal vibratory pattern over days, weeks, and years. This process, known as interval examination, helps determine the effects of behavioral, medical, and surgical interventions on the larynx. Changes in laryngeal stroboscopy findings can be shown and documented on videotape, computerized formats, and still prints.

Interpretation of laryngeal stroboscopy requires knowledge of the stroboscopic appearance of the healthy larynx phonating at various frequencies and intensities. A regular format for evaluation also helps to provide a more objective interpretation of this subjective test. Standardized checklists for laryngeal stroboscopy interpretation are available.[13,46,49,83] Evaluation criteria include symmetry, amplitude, periodicity,

mucosal wave propagation, and glottal closure (Table 94-1). These vibratory characteristics are evaluated at a comfortable loudness level and modal speech frequency. In professional voice patients, it is beneficial to perform laryngeal stroboscopy under high and low pitch and loud and soft phonation. This provides additional data regarding the vibratory characteristics.

Symmetry refers to the paired appearance of the vocal folds, which are mirror images of each other during glottal vibration. Any difference in the mechanical properties of the vocal folds: mass, tension, pliability of the superficial layer of the lamina propria or mucosa, elasticity, position, or inflammation can alter symmetry. Asymmetry can result in dysphonia.

Amplitude of vibration refers to the lateral excursion of the midmembranous portion of the vocal fold during vibration. This is normally one third to one half of the width of the visible fold. Again, lesions that affect the mass, tension, or pliability of the vocal fold will alter amplitude.

Periodicity, or the regularity of successive glottal cycles, is ascertained by synchronizing the stroboscopic flash with the frequency. This "freezes" the image. Any perceived motion of the folds indicates a degree of aperiodicity. Any alteration in the balance of the vocal folds and the lungs can result in aperiodic vibrations. During a single phonation, vibratory cycles can range from periodic to aperiodic. Therefore, it is helpful to determine whether the vibratory pattern is completely periodic, mostly periodic, mostly aperiodic, or completely aperiodic.[94,100]

Mucosal wave propagation is visualized over the superior surface of the fold. It depends on the frequency and intensity of vocal fold vibration. Lesions that fill the superficial layer of the lamina propria and abut or infiltrate the vocal ligament tend to restrict or eliminate the mucosal wave. In contrast, small- to moderate-sized lesions limited to the mucosa or superficial portion of the superficial layer of the lamina propria usually allow propagation of the wave, although it may be decreased and asymmetric.[26,85] Finally, large and exophytic lesions may disrupt the mucosal wave by altering the glottal shape and impairing glottal closure. The mucosal wave should be separated from the vertical phase difference, which refers specifically to the time difference between closure of the upper and lower lips of the vocal folds.

Closure of the membranous glottis is vital to laryngeal efficiency. Men usually have complete glottal closure, whereas up to 70% of women normally show a small posterior glottal chink.[76] The type of closure can be described as complete, long or short, small or large posterior chink, slit, elliptic, and hourglass or asymmetric hourglass. It can be altered by a mass lesion, scarring, muscular tension, and neurologic abnormalities.

TABLE 94-1

LARYNGOVIDEOSTROBOSCOPY INTERPRETATION

Criteria	Result
Symmetry:	Normal
	Side to side
	Teeter-totter
	Vertical O not symmetric
Amplitude:	Right equals left
	Right is greater than left
	Left is greater than right
	Both decreased
Periodicity:	Yes, consistent
	Yes, inconsistent
	No, inconsistent
	No, consistent
Mucosal wave:	Right normal
	Right great
	Right abnormal pattern
	Right decreased
	Right adynamic (where)
	Left normal
	Left great
	Left abnormal pattern
	Left decreased
	Left adynamic (where)
Closure:	Complete, long
	Complete, short
	Small posterior chink
	Large posterior chink
	Slit
	Elliptic
	50% Elliptic
	Hourglass
	Asymmetric hourglass
	Other

RECORDING QUALITY (1 = Poor, 2, 3, 4 = Great)

Focus _____ Size _____ Brightness _____

Color _____ Notable feature _____

Videotape number: _____

Verbal diagnosis:

VOICE ANALYSIS

Several methods quantify voice or measure vocal vibration. No single test is considered the gold standard to document vocal fold function. All tests have significant limitations. In addition, intrapatient and interpatient variability exists. Therefore, in professional voice patients, perceptual analysis by a trained observer and patient satisfaction with vocal outcome are often the most useful indicators of a successful intervention. Most laryngologists consider objective and semiobjective voice analysis to be important, particularly regarding preoperative and postoperative voice documentation. Little agreement exists as to the optimal tests and their performance, relative importance, or interpretation.

Acoustic Measures

Acoustic analysis has been used to objectively document voice and to compare preoperative and postoperative surgical results. Acoustic measures include fundamental frequency, perturbation or cycle-to-cycle variation in frequency and amplitude, maximal phonation range, and others. Comparison of interval examinations requires a high-quality microphone and recording system with strict standardized recording techniques and patient tasks. Although several computer-integrated acoustic analysis systems are available, they are of limited benefit for the average patient. The reliability of acoustic measures, secondary to variation in patient effort, is limited. In addition, the validity of acoustic measures designed to evaluate periodic vibration is questionable in dysphonic voices because dysphonia results from aperiodic vibration.

Spectrometry

Spectrometry provides a visual display of vocal harmonics and noise plotting time, intensity, and frequency. It shows the impact of resonance (formant structure) and articulation on the laryngeal buzz. Spectral analysis can evaluate and compare resonance changes and may be useful in documenting vocal alterations after surgical procedures on the pharynx. Some laryngologists have found this to be valuable in singers and other professional voice patients.[5,78]

Electroglottography

Electroglottography measures the efficiency of glottal closure by graphically recording the contact time of the vocal folds. It shows the opening and closing rates of the vocal folds not well visualized by stroboscopy. Electroglottography is performed by passing a low-voltage, high-frequency current between two electrodes placed on either side of the patient's neck. It measures the electrical impedance that varies with opening and closing of the glottis. Some clinicians consider this measure objective and reproducible. Electroglottography may provide clinically useful information when combined with laryngeal stroboscopy or other vocal measures.[6,64,68]

Aerodynamic Measures

Aerodynamic studies are based on the fluid mechanics of airflow and involve the measure of airflow, volume, and pressure. Some are related to Ohm's law ($R = P/F$, in which R is laryngeal resistance, P is subglottal pressure, and F is airflow).

Normative aerodynamic data are very broad, making almost useless comparisons among patients. However, changes in measures after intervention in individual patients are quite useful, particularly when evaluating changes in laryngeal closure.

Standard pulmonary function testing may be used to objectively evaluate the lungs. Mild obstructive or restrictive pulmonary disorders can be found to be the basis of a patient's vocal fatigue or dysphonia. Bronchodilator trials and methacholine challenge may rule out cough variant asthma and other types of reactive airway disease.

Subglottal pressure is usually measured indirectly rather than by tracheal puncture or esophageal balloon. It is measured via oral pressure when the glottis is open. The oral pressure achieves equilibration with the subglottal pressure across the open vocal folds for voiceless stop consonants, such as /p/ or /t/.[87]

Maximum phonation time is an average of the (1) phonation length in one breath voicing the vowel /a/ at a comfortable pitch and (2) loudness after deep inspiration. It is highly variable but reasonably estimates laryngeal competence and glottal closure.

Mean airflow rate (airflow volume divided by phonation time) of a sustained vowel /a/ is occasionally tested. In general, low flow rates suggest laryngeal hyperfunction, obstruction, or primary pulmonary disorders. Increased values imply abnormalities in glottal competence, allowing air loss.

Perceptual Analysis

To evaluate the professional voice, the "trained" ear remains the most discerning instrument.[7,28,61] Perceptual improvement or degradation of the professional voice to the performer, manager, other performers, the laryngologist, speech language pathologist, and singing voice scientist is critical. To make perceptual vocal analysis more objective, vocal characteristics can be evaluated independently in a systematic manner. In addition, judges are trained in vocal evaluation to decrease subjective bias. However, agreement on the terminology of vocal characteristics is not universal. Hirano[48] proposed the GRBAS scale (grade, rough, breathy, asthenic, strained), which is widely used. However, Sundberg[91] and Kreiman and others[60] performed research in this area, and they concluded that the clinical application of perceptual analysis remains difficult at this time.[60,91]

Voice Outcomes

Because of daily variation in vocal measures, vocal quality is frequently best judged by measures of patient satisfaction or direct comparisons of voice at different times. Patient satisfaction can be assessed through direct questioning or specially designed questionnaires for rating perceived vocal problems. Voice can be directly compared using taped samples. By eliminating dates and other identifying factors, blinded analysis of vocal changes can be determined. A panel of judges can thus evaluate objective qualitative changes in a blinded manner over time. This is useful to determine the effect of a specific therapeutic intervention.

Outcomes research is becoming valuable in studying many disorders. A voice handicap index has been developed to quantify a patient's perception of his or her voice and its change in response to therapy.[12] This method of research should prove valuable for assessing professional voice patients.

EVALUATION
Medical History

A complete history of the present illness and past medical problems is necessary. Several laryngologists have developed patient questionnaires to obtain the most complete history possible and to streamline the evaluation process.[77]

Salient points regarding a patient's past medical history and general health include diseases that affect pulmonary status, posture, and hydration. Any underlying chronic or acute pulmonary condition can significantly affect a singer's voice. Asthma, emphysema, or chronic bronchitis, all of which impair pulmonary function, will decrease a singer's power supply to the voice. Musculoskeletal injuries will alter posture and impair a patient's ability to position the larynx within the neck, leading to vocal dysfunction. Prescription and nonprescription drugs alter the voice through effects on the autonomic nervous system and indirect effects on the larynx and vocal tract.[55,93] Drugs that alter a patient's emotional status affect the manner in which the patient approaches the vocal task. Drug-induced changes in hydration lead to poor laryngeal lubrication, which affects vocal fold vibration. History taking in a female singer should include questions regarding oral contraceptives and hormonal drugs (e.g., danazol), which may adversely effect the voice.[14,84,98]

A singer's personal habits should also be reviewed. Moderate use or abuse of alcohol is detrimental to the voice through dehydration and effects on judgment. Caffeine (a diuretic) and high-fat dairy products affect the voice by thickening mucous secretions and decreasing the efficiency of vibration. Certain foods and alcohol exacerbate gastroesophageal reflux.[55] Finally, all tobacco use should be evaluated. Inhaled smoke is particularly irritating to the mucosa acutely and is highly refluxagenic, which means it will lead to decreased vibratory efficiency. In addition, it can induce neoplastic changes.

A history of surgery is important to obtain in patients with laryngeal dysfunction. In addition to questions concerning head- and neck-related procedures, any history of endotracheal intubation should be identified because it can adversely affect the larynx. Recent abdominal or thoracic surgery could also greatly restrict a singer's capacity for inspiration or expiration for many weeks or months after the operation.

The identification of endocrine dysfunction is often useful. The laryngeal manifestations of hypothyroidism can lead to potentially dramatic edema in Reinke's space.[44] Even mild hypothyroidism can cause a muffling of the voice, decreased range, and vocal fatigue.

Less well understood are the vocal changes caused by hormonal fluctuations in women just before and during menstruation. Flach and others[34] stated that 75% of female singers show a premenstrual change in their voices manifested as decreased range and vocal fatigue[34] Using cytologic smears, Abitbol and others[2] objectively showed cyclical changes in vocal fold epithelial cells corresponding to the menstrual cycle. This has been termed *laryngopathia praemenstrualis*.[63] Vocal fold varices often increase in size before and during menstruation and have been associated with an increased incidence of submucosal vocal fold hemorrhage.[22,79] Vocal fold varices are most commonly found in female professional voice patients.[1,22,67,73]

The history should also address what type of formal vocal training the singer has had. Does the patient have a current vocal coach, or has the patient changed coaches recently? What are his or her long-term goals? A trained vocalist may be able to fix the vocal technique more easily than an untrained vocalist.

History of Present Illness

The exact nature of a singer's complaint should be reviewed with care. A vocal professional may simply complain of "hoarseness." This common term describes various vocal abnormalities, including (most frequently) loss of upper register, roughness, pitch instability, difficulty in transition between singing registers, and early vocal fatigue. These are frequently symptoms of laryngeal edema, muscle tension dysphonia, extraesophageal reflux, upper respiratory infections, nonneoplastic lesions, or poor vocal technique. Patients, therefore, should be questioned specifically about range, pitch breaks, anterior cervical discomfort, esophageal reflux, and stamina. The onset and offset of the vocal difficulty can often provide clues regarding the cause. Specifically, time of the difficulty throughout the day, situations that aggravate the dysphonia, events that immediately precede the onset of the difficulty, and the association between dysphonia and voice use are significant in determining the cause and may aid in management.

Professional activities that can contribute to these problems include air travel, performing on older indoor stages, exposure to chemicals and fumes, required use of the speaking voice, and overscheduling of performances. Air travel remains a problem for the serious voice user because the air on planes is very dry (5%–10% relative humidity) and affects the larynx; also, the high background noise tempts the patient to speak more loudly.[32] Performing on older stages, which may be dusty, and traveling in areas with a large amount of allergens can degrade a patient's voice. Exposure to other types of irritants, including tobacco smoke at parties or at performances in smoke-filled rooms, also affects the voice. Vocal professionals required to give multiple interviews often develop dysphonia of various degrees. A singer's schedule may make it difficult for the singer to drink large quantities of water to lubricate the vocal cords, and although a singer may complain of singing problems, the main difficulty is voice abuse caused by excessive speaking. Significant abuse of the speaking voice leads to eventual singing difficulties.

Often, a younger vocal professional will not seek help until the problem becomes significant or the performer is about to go on tour or has a performance in the near future. Management of the problem may vary depending on when the next performance is to take place. This should be considered when developing a management plan.

Physical Examination

Every voice patient presenting to the otolaryngologist or laryngologist should undergo complete examination of the head and neck. The physical evaluation of the vocal professional begins with observation of gait and posture as the patient walks into the physician's office. Does the patient stand comfortably erect with shoulders slightly back or slouched? Does the patient appear tense and anxious?

While taking the history, the physician should evaluate the quality of the patient's speaking voice. The frequency or pitch should be appropriate for the performer's age, gender, and body habitus. Intensity should be appropriate for conversational speech. The timing of voice onset should be studied, including speech breaks and the overall rhythm. Finally, vocal quality is evaluated for roughness, breathiness, asthenia, or constriction.

Certain areas of the nonlaryngeal examination are key. Jaw range of motion should be checked, and the temporomandibular joint should be palpated. Temporomandibular joint dysfunction can create significant muscular tension difficulties in a professional voice patient. Tenderness in the anterior neck or the cervical paraspinal musculature can be caused by laryngeal hyperfunction.

The ears should be examined for any abnormalities, and an audiogram should be obtained. Hearing loss, particularly if sensorineural, can cause a singer to sing too loudly, resulting in excessive trauma to the vocal folds.

The nasal examination can provide information about mucous membrane disease. Pale and edematous nasal mucosa suggests the presence of significant allergies. Evidence of a chronic infection with purulent discharge or crusting should be sought. Nasal obstruction can lead to chronic mouth breathing. The subsequent exposure of the larynx to unfiltered dry air can cause significant dysphonia by thickening the secretions and therefore increasing the phonation threshold pressure. In addition, the nature of the patient's secretions can be determined by noting their consistency in the nose and oral cavity. Cough resulting from chronic postnasal drip can also lead to vocal fold edema.

There are three ways to examine the larynx: with a laryngeal mirror, a rigid telescope, or a flexible fiberoptic laryngoscope. The first and classical method is with a laryngeal mirror. This gives the most natural color on examination and potentially allows a panoramic view of the entire larynx. This is optimal in determining subtle signs of old vocal fold hemorrhage.

Vocal professionals are evaluated with the rigid telescope and flexible fiberoptic laryngoscope. Single-point light sources, however, can distort color, and this should be considered when evaluating the larynx. Rigid indirect endoscopy and flexible laryngoscopy are complementary; each has certain advantages. By using both methods, the laryngologist can fully evaluate the professional voice patient. Use of the rigid telescope requires that the examiner gently grasp the patient's tongue and draw it forward. This maneuver alters the patient's normal use of the supraglottal vocal tract and articulators, making glottal closure and laryngeal hyperfunction difficult to interpret. The telescope, however, provides the best illumination and magnification, allowing an unparalleled view of the larynx and the opportunity for outstanding photodocumentation. Small lesions or areas of vascular abnormality in the larynx, which may be missed with the mirror or flexible fiberoptic laryngoscopy, can be identified with a 70- or 90-degree telescope. In addition, laryngovideostroboscopy is performed optimally through the rigid telescope compared with the flexible device. The picture is clearer, larger, and brighter and therefore allows the examiner to better evaluate the laryngeal vibratory pattern.

Flexible fiberoptic laryngoscopy allows examination of a vocal professional in more natural fashion. The patient can use connected speech or can sing during evaluation of the supraglottal vocal tract and larynx. This provides a better evaluation of vocal biomechanics, particularly in a hyperfunctioning larynx. Finally, the flexible fiberoptic scope is better tolerated in patients who cannot tolerate a rigid telescope because of an anatomic variant or a dramatic gag reflex. Drawbacks of the optical system include the well-known fisheye distortion of the peripheral image, decreased resolution, linear color stripe distortion on video imagery (moiré effect), and decreased illumination, which makes stroboscopy more difficult to interpret (Table 94-2).[17] This is less difficult than using flexible endoscopes with distal chip cameras.

The presence of a large mucosal lesion or paralysis of the vocal folds may be apparent to the examiner. Certain, sometimes subtle, laryngeal findings may be less apparent. The presence of thick, tenacious mucous secretions should be noted and compared with the usually seen watery lubrication, which is preferable. Evidence of vocal fold swelling, ventricular effacement, and erythema, swelling, or granular tissue in the posterior glottis may indicate extraesophageal reflux. Areas of vocal fold edema, particularly in the middle third of the fold, may be present in a vocal professional who complains of slight dysphonia. Evidence of hyperfunction should be sought. This can manifest in its most subtle form as widening of the posterior glottis. More severe hyperfunction could show closure of the false vocal folds (plica ventricularis) as well as anterior to posterior contraction of the supraglottis. If these are present, subtle vocal fold paresis should be considered.

The vocalist should be evaluated by a vocal pedagogue if examination does not reveal the cause of dysphonia. The singer's posture and general stance should be noted. The "singer's stance" is a fully upright position with the feet about shoulder width apart and the weight slightly forward on the balls of the feet. Frequently, commercial performers are required to play instruments while singing. In this instance, the patient should be observed holding the instrument. Facial, shoulder, or cervical tension should be noted if present when the patient is singing. Is the singer using the abdominal muscles appropriately to support the singing voice or breathing only with the use of chest and shoulders? The presence or absence of laryngeal elevation with increasing pitch should be recorded. This is considered poor technique in a classically trained singer and can lead to vocal fatigue caused by excessive muscular tension. In commercial singing, however, laryngeal elevation can often be used to achieve a desirable sound, and elimination of elevation causes an uncharacteristic vocal quality.

PROBLEMS IN SINGERS

Professional voice patients have the same maladies that affect the general population. However, because of the tremendous demands placed on their voices, these vocalists are highly sensitive to problems affecting the larynx and the associated areas involved in voice production.

Extraesophageal Reflux

Gastroesophageal reflux is a common problem often manifested by symptoms of heartburn, belching, or an acidic taste on waking. Patients can have significant reflux with no abdominal or chest complaints; this type is called *extraesophageal or laryngopharyngeal* reflux.* The symptoms are often frequent throat clearing, mild dysphonia, cough, a sensation of phlegm or a foreign body sensation in the throat (globus), vocal fatigue, cervical dysphagia, or

---

*References 36, 45, 55, 59, 72, 74.

TABLE 94-2

LARYNGEAL EXAMINATION

	Laryngeal Mirror	Flexible Fiberoptic Laryngoscope	Rigid Telescope
Operator ease	+++	+++	++++
Patient tolerance	+++	+++	++
Photographic quality	−−	++	++++
Magnification	−−	+	++++
Color	++++	++	+++
Laryngovideostroboscopy	−−	++	++++
Observation of speech/singing	−−	++++	−−−
Evaluation of vocal mechanics	−−	++++	−−−−

+, Advantageous; − disadvantageous.

decreased singing range.[8,10] Singers and other vocal professionals with extraesophageal reflux often have hoarseness in the morning and require longer vocal warm-up. Signs of reflux laryngitis should always be sought during the physical examination.[9,11] If signs or symptoms suggest extraesophageal reflux, conservative management directed at diet and general lifestyle is initiated. Adhering to these measures might be difficult for performers with a demanding travel schedule. Extraesophageal reflux is optimally managed with a proton pump inhibitor. This is undertaken 30 minutes to an hour before a meal and for extraesophageal reflux is often used twice daily. It is uncertain whether the addition of drugs to enhance gastric emptying makes any definite contribution in the management of extraesophageal reflux. Patients with a confusing clinical picture or those who are not responding well to maximal-dose proton pump inhibitors undergo 24-hour pH monitoring. Some patients may be resistant to omeprazole.[4,15,53,65]

Laryngeal Hygiene

Laryngeal hygiene can be problematic in professional singers. The key to good laryngeal hygiene is adequate hydration. Poor hydration causes a decrease in mucous viscosity, resulting in less efficient vocal fold vibration.[33,95,96] Singers should drink increased amounts of water. Van Lawrence stated that singers should "pee pale" (ingest so much water that they exhibit lightly colored urine), and vocal professionals should not drink a set amount of water but allow their kidneys to "tell" them how much to drink. At least eight glasses (64 ounces) of water per day appear to be needed and should be increased if the voice user is traveling by air, is ill, or has a demanding or excessive performance schedule. The use of caffeine is discouraged because of its diuretic effect. Dairy products also appear to increase the viscosity of secretions and hinder the healthy smooth vibratory function of the vocal folds. Guaifenesin can thin the secretions in some patients. The use of tobacco in the professional voice patient also contributes to poor laryngeal hygiene.

Vocal Abuse and Misuse

Vocal abuse describes vocal behaviors associated with normal voice quality that often lead to vocal fold abnormalities and resultant dysphonia. These behaviors often lead to visible manifestations of abuse on laryngeal examination. Vocal abuse can occur in two ways: patterns of abuse exist in the patient's singing or speaking voice. Vocal abuse is characterized by gradually wearing down the voice, primarily by (1) overrehearsing; (2) spending too much time working in the studio; (3) singing too loudly; or (4) singing outside of the singer's capable range. In addition, commercial singing frequently incorporates artificial roughness to render "validity" to the performance.

Vocal abuse behaviors can occur if performers give excessive interviews. Shouting or excessive talking in areas of loud background noise (e.g., restaurants, airplanes) is also common. The vocal professional should conserve the voice by limiting unnecessary speaking, exercising what is called *relative voice rest*. This is particularly important if the vocalist is having vocal difficulties or is ill. Punt[75] advises singers "not to say an unnecessary word unless they are paid for it," especially if they are ill or have an excessively demanding performance schedule.

Vocal misuse refers to dysphonia caused by abnormal function of anatomically normal structures. Chronic misuse can eventually lead to organic vocal fold changes. These changes most commonly appear as vocal nodules and will disrupt the normal laryngeal vibratory pattern causing dysphonia. Elimination of the inappropriate vocal behaviors lessens or eliminates the dysphonia. With time, the organic changes may reverse, and healthy vibratory patterns may return.

Such muscular tension dysphonia is not limited to vocal professionals. It can be the primary or secondary cause of dysphonia. Singers are not immune from this despite common misconceptions that vocal training should eliminate such difficulties. This problem is common, particularly as a maladaptive, compensatory behavior after an upper respiratory infection. The singer attempts to maintain a normal voice while the vocal folds or pharynx are swollen and develops inappropriate vocal behaviors. Patients often complain of hoarseness, vocal fatigue, loss of range, and neck or ear discomfort.

Koufman and Blalock[54,58] formulated a grading or classification system for muscular tension dysphonia. Class I muscular tension dysphonia is defined as an increase in muscular tension manifested by an enlarged posterior glottal chink, an elevated larynx, and palpable neck tension or tenderness. This may produce a breathy or strident voice and commonly occurs in patients with vocal nodules. Class II muscular tension dysphonia is a lateral to medial constriction of the larynx with the false vocal folds adducted. This causes increased vocal fatigue. In its most severe form, the false folds are used for phonation, so-called *plica ventricularis*. It is often seen as a compensatory maneuver after laryngitis or laryngeal surgery. Class III muscular tension dysphonia is an anterior to posterior constriction of the supraglottis when the epiglottis and the arytenoids obscure at least 50% of the laryngeal aditus. Class IV muscular tension dysphonia is present when the epiglottis and arytenoids contact one another, and lateral constriction is often seen.

Koufman[56] reviewed laryngeal biomechanics during singing. One hundred singers of various singing styles were evaluated with fiberoptic laryngoscopy. Koufman found that vocal training, warming up before singing, and singing classical musical styles decrease muscular tension. This study supports the belief that vocal training increases vocal efficiency and decreases muscular tension. Koufman also found that singers with asymptomatic vocal nodules had significantly higher levels of laryngeal muscular tension than those without nodules. The management of muscular tension dysphonia is directed by the speech language pathologist and the vocal pedagogue. It aims to retrain the patient to improve speaking and singing efficiency, thereby decreasing laryngeal tension and vocal fold trauma.

An interesting type of vocal misuse in professional voice patients is an inappropriately low-pitched speaking voice. This deepening of the voice gives it a more authoritative quality. It requires a significant degree of muscular tension to maintain.[57]

Laryngitis

Acute laryngitis (inflammation of the laryngeal mucosa) is common in adults and can be devastating to a professional voice patient. Inflammation of the vocal folds leads to irritation and edema and hinders the pliable motion of the mucosa, leading to dysphonia. To compensate for this, singers may exert extra effort to maintain their normal voice. Singers may correctly compensate by decreasing their volume, increasing their amplification, altering their repertoire, and other measures.

A very mild case of laryngitis can be managed conservatively, and a well-trained singer can continue to perform. A singer should be aware, however, of the risk of permanent damage to the vocal folds and the increased risk for submucosal hemorrhage. The performer is instructed to increase fluid intake and humidify the room. If cough is significant, an antitussive agent may be of benefit. Conservative voice use is key. The singer should speak little, if at all, before the performance and should warm up in a normal fashion. The performer should sing by feel and not by sound to avoid exacerbating the injury. He or she should speak in a normal, unforced voice without whispering. If a bacterial infection is present, antibiotics should be prescribed. The use of corticosteroids is beneficial in these patients but should only be used for a performance when there is objective evidence of vocal fold edema. Severe laryngitis should be managed similarly, but in this case the vocalist should be advised not to perform. Serial examinations will enable the physician to advise the vocal professional when it is safe to return to vocal activity.

Anxiety

Apprehension before a performance is normal. A few professional voice patients may have dramatic stage fright. Professional vocalists should learn to cope with this anxiety by working with a vocal coach and laryngologist. Several medications have been used, but all have potential adverse effects and none replace good training and the confidence that comes with repeated performance under such stress.

The use of β-blockers is common to decrease the tachycardia that often accompanies the anxiety, but this medication has adverse effects. Gates and others[35] stated that β-blockers decrease anxiety but also take some of the dramatic edge and excitement away from the singer. β-blockers should only be used on rare occasions (e.g., when a crisis occurs before a performance) and should never be used on a regular basis.

Pulmonary Disease

Any respiratory ailment alters the amount of power available for singing or phonation and limits the vocalist's ability to modulate it. Pulmonary health and good conditioning are important for proper voice support.[43,86]

An uncommon but well-documented type of exercise-induced asthma exists in some singers when they have been singing for a lengthy period. This airway reactivity–induced asthma in singers[18,81] can be diagnosed by pulmonary function testing before and after prolonged singing.

Vocal Fold Varices

A true vocal fold varix is a dilated, tortuous, or elongated vessel stemming from the microcirculation of the vocal fold; it occurs mainly in female professional vocalists. The cause of this relatively uncommon lesion is uncertain, but its preponderance in female singers suggests that hormones and vocal trauma are major factors.[22,30,52] The laryngologist should determine whether the patient's symptoms correlate with the menstrual cycle. Varices may enlarge premenstrually and menstrually and can increase a singer's dysphonia.

If a vascular lesion is found, its functional significance should be determined. This is best performed through laryngovideostroboscopy. The lesion's effect on the laryngeal vibratory pattern can be accurately determined, including whether the vascular lesion is the cause of the singer's problems. Nonsurgical management of vascular lesions involves improvement in vocal hygiene, particularly with increased water intake and the avoidance of caffeine. In addition, working with a speech pathologist and vocal pedagogue to improve vocal efficiency is important. Hormonal manipulation has been advocated by some but has not been proven to be beneficial. Indications for surgery include recurrent hemorrhage, an enlarging varix, or continued dysphonia despite maximal medical and behavioral management.

PERFORMANCE CANCELLATION

Possible cancellation of a performance can be very stressful for a professional singer and laryngologist. The performer and the manager have many concerns beyond the singer's health, for example, the singer's professional image, perceived reliability, and financial obligations. The musical style and the importance of the performance are also important variables; a slight vocal roughness in a contemporary rock or country performer would be unacceptable in an opera singer.

The physician's recommendations for performing are categorized by (1) conditions in which damage to the larynx will not be significant and (2) conditions that place the performer at significant risk for developing chronic vocal difficulties (Table 94-3). However, the decision to perform ultimately belongs to the performer. Singing will still be problematic during and after the performance. Examples of conditions that pose a mild risk to the performer are a mild viral upper respiratory infection or mild to moderate vocal fold edema. In an upper respiratory infection, the postnasal drip and generalized congestion can be managed, but the supraglottal vocal tract is altered and the singing voice will not be normal. To produce the usual perceived sound, the vocalist can exert significant extra effort, possibly resulting in the development of maladaptive singing behaviors that could take time for the vocal pedagogue and speech language pathologist to undo. The singer and manager should also decide whether a decrease in vocal quality would alter the performer's image or reputation.

Conditions that are likely to cause permanent vocal changes include submucosal vocal fold hemorrhage, enlarging varix, or a vocal fold mucosal break (see Table 94-3). Absolute voice rest is essential. In addition, the usual conservative care of the larynx should be undertaken. Aggressive antireflux therapy should be initiated in patients with laryngeal mucosal breaks. These individuals should be followed closely for the development of submucosal scarring, granulation tissue, or polyps.

MANAGEMENT
Medical Therapy

The mainstay of medical therapy for a singer is appropriate lifestyle change. This begins with maintaining adequate hydration. In addition, for many problems, a period of conservative voice use is the best remedy. A humidifier should be used when traveling or sleeping in rooms with inadequate humidity. Altering the diet and avoiding irritants are always important, particularly when the singer is ill. In general, these interventions improve laryngeal hygiene primarily because of their effect on lubrication and avoidance of further vocal trauma.

The special needs of vocal professionals require the avoidance of certain commonly used medications, including inhaled corticosteroids, antihistamines, decongestants, aspirin, topical analgesics, and mentholated preparations.

The use of topical corticosteroids on the larynx should be avoided. They directly irritate the laryngeal mucosa and are associated with an increased incidence of fungal infections of the larynx. In addition, there may be a slight analgesic effect on the larynx and vocal tract, affecting the performer's ability to regulate the voice.

Systemic corticosteroids are indicated for conditions in which there is little chance of permanent laryngeal damage (Table 94-4). They can be used when a patient with vocal fold edema has an upcoming performance. This approach is combined with improvements in laryngeal hygiene and conservative voice use. Laryngeal edema commonly occurs during repetitive recording sessions or after extensive rehearsals before major tours or performances. Corticosteroids are also beneficial when singers have mild viral laryngitis to decrease the vocal fold edema and to help control significant allergic reactions. Corticosteroids can be given for severe cases of laryngitis, but the vocalist will risk laryngeal damage by performing. Systemic corticosteroids are frequently given for vocal fold hemorrhage to decrease the deposition of scar tissue in the superficial layer of the

---

TABLE 94-3

CONDITIONS REQUIRING PERFORMANCE CANCELLATION

Submucosal hemorrhage
Enlarging vocal fold varix
Break in vocal fold mucosa
Significant systemic illness
Severe laryngitis

TABLE 94-4

INDICATIONS FOR SYSTEMIC CORTICOSTEROIDS IN THE PROFESSIONAL VOICE PATIENT

Edema from episodic abuse
Mild to moderate laryngitis
Allergic vocal fold edema
Vocal fold hemorrhage

lamina propria, to prevent polyp formation, and to decrease the overall inflammatory response. However, no scientific evidence exists that corticosteroids are beneficial in this clinical situation.

Management with corticosteroids varies depending on the severity of the problem. Dexamethasone (10 mg intramuscularly or intravenously) can be given if a performance is to be given within 24 hours. In subacute situations, stress-dose corticosteroids taken orally for 3 to 5 days with a rapid taper are appropriate.

Idiosyncratic reactions to corticosteroids can occur, in which case the performer's voice actually worsens rather than improves. In addition, corticosteroid-induced psychiatric changes may occur. Because of these reactions, systemic corticosteroids should not be used for the first time in any patient before a performance except in the most dire of circumstances. Corticosteroids are best used initially before routine studio recordings or song-writing sessions. This will allow the physician and the performer to gauge the response and will create a better understanding of how the patient will respond to corticosteroids in other situations. The singer should not depend on corticosteroids but only use them when required.

Most antihistamines have a significant drying effect on mucous membranes because of their anticholinergic effects. In patients requiring significant management of allergies, it is best to begin with topical nasal corticosteroids. These are effective for the relief of allergic rhinitis and do not adversely affect the voice. Some of the newer, nonsedating antihistamines may be useful.[19] For patients with more severe allergic symptoms, formal allergy testing should be performed early. After the identification of the specific allergens, avoidance or environmental therapy is attempted, but this can be difficult because of travel. If possible, the performer's travel schedule should be arranged to avoid certain environments where seasonal plants are in bloom. Allergic immunotherapy is very helpful in these patients.

Decongestants often provide symptomatic relief in a performer with an upper respiratory infection. Combination preparations that include an antihistamine should be avoided in professional voice patients because of the drying effects this medication has on mucous membranes.

Aspirin use is not advised in vocal professionals. Aspirin inhibits platelet function and can increase the risk of submucosal vocal fold hemorrhage. Professional voice patients should check the labels of nonprescription medications and should avoid those with aspirin.

Although once very popular with vocalists, topical anesthetic solutions for sore throats or laryngitis can harm the voice. By decreasing the sensitivity of the oropharynx or supraglottal larynx, these solutions allow the patient to overwork an injured area, which could lead to submucosal hemorrhage, mucosal tears, or a granuloma. If a performer believes that work is not possible without such an analgesic, he or she should not perform.

Patients complaining of a dry throat or a cough often initiate management with nonprescription cough or topical preparations. These frequently contain menthol, which is initially soothing. Menthol, however, is a drying agent and is habit forming in some patients.

Antibiotics are prescribed for singers in accordance with standard management indications. Overdispensing antibiotics, a major problem in our healthcare system, should be avoided. Antibiotics can be prescribed to a singer who is about to go out of town or on an extended tour. Written instructions outlining when to use the antibiotics should be given. The performer should contact his or her physician if he or she feels the need to use the medication.

Mucolytic agents (e.g., guaifenesin) are commonly use by singers as a pharmacologic adjunct to thin secretions, thereby improving the lubrication of the vocal folds. Although not proven to be effective, guaifenesin and similar agents appear to benefit some vocal professionals.

Role of the Speech Language Pathologist and Vocal Pedagogue

The speech language pathologist and vocal pedagogue work with patients to improve singing and speaking efficiency, to eliminate vocal abuse, to correct misuse, and to encourage vocal hygiene. Singers should understand that vocal abuse during speaking is intimately connected with the singing voice. They are taught to avoid cervical strain and they learn proper breathing patterns, improve posture, and develop a soft glottal attack when speaking. The goal is to improve laryngeal efficiency and thereby limit laryngeal trauma during singing and speaking.[20]

The role of the vocal pedagogue is complex. Classical vocalists should improve classical technique. Commercial singers, however, should optimize glottal efficiency when singing without producing a classical sound. Training, therefore, differs for classical vs commercial vocalists. Areas emphasized to classical artists include breath support, body alignment, stable laryngeal position low in the neck, and maintenance of a low subglottal pressure compared with other singing styles.[16] This enables the classical vocalist to produce the singer's formant, allowing greater voice projection with less vocal effort. Nonclassical or commercial singers should also concentrate on breath support and body alignment, but they do not incorporate the singer's formant. Therefore, these performers must sing more loudly to be heard over instruments and other singers. Commercial singers need to be educated on the proper use of electronic amplification, which is a substitute for loud singing. Other considerations for commercial singers include precise vowel integrity, phrasing similar to speech, and delayed onset of vibrato. Vocal efficiency should be improved without changing the performer's style or developing a classical sound. The use of full-length mirrors and videotaped recordings while performing help to educate the performer. Vocal efficiency is also improved with appropriate warm-up and range-building exercises.[31] Sabol and others[76] showed the benefit of vocal exercise in singers on objective aerodynamic testing.

Surgical Therapy

Before surgical intervention, behavioral and medical interventions should be maximized. Vocal hygiene, avoidance of vocal misuse, and resolution of vocal abuse should be accomplished. Patients failing to do these things will develop recurrent problems. Surgery is relatively contraindicated in patients who cannot comply with the recommendations of hygienic voice production from a speech language pathologist and vocal pedagogue. All patients learn to develop a soft glottal attack, which is vital for postoperative rehabilitation. The overall effect of maximizing medical and behavioral management is to improve the postoperative vocal outcome and shorten the postoperative recuperative time.

The decision to operate on the larynx of a vocal professional is often difficult. The singer should evaluate the risks and benefits and obtain a second opinion. It is important to realistically counsel the patient about the possible outcomes. The singer should understand that the singing or speaking voice may never be the same and that he or she may never perform at the same level again. Rehabilitation and healing after microsurgery of the larynx are long and often frustrating for the vocal professional. It is this period, working with the speech language pathologist and vocal pedagogue, during which the vocal professional needs the greatest amount of determination and encouragement. In most cases, surgery is only performed when it is apparent that the patient cannot perform at the required level to maintain an acceptable performance schedule. Recurrent vocal fold hemorrhage from a varix or an enlarging varix are other indications for surgery.

After the need for surgery has been determined, atraumatic establishment of the airway in the surgical suite is the next concern. This task should not be performed by an inexperienced physician but by the sur-

geon or an experienced anesthesiologist. Gentle intubation with the smallest possible caliber endotracheal tube should be performed. The laryngologist should consult with the anesthesiologist before a vocal professional is intubated for any procedure. If possible, the laryngologist should offer his or her services for the intubation. If local, regional, or spinal anesthesia is an alternative, it should be strongly considered.

Photographic documentation in the operative suite is performed immediately before and after the procedure. Zero-, 30-, 70-, and 120-degree telescopes can be used as needed to obtain optimal views of the pathology and examine poorly accessible areas such as the depths of the laryngeal ventricle.[3,21] The procedure is videotaped through the operating microscope.

The major determinants of a good postoperative result during laryngeal microsurgery are the conservation of normal mucosa, integrity of the vocal ligament, and the creation or maintenance of a straight vocal fold edge (see Figure 94-5).[84,99,101]

Superficial Vocal Fold Lesions

Vocal fold nodules that have not resolved with medical and speech therapy and polyps that cause dysphonia can be surgically excised. Bilateral vocal fold lesions are of significant concern. It is common to remove the larger lesion in the hope that the smaller lesion will resolve. However, reaction on the opposite fold may imply technical problems or hyperfunctional technique. Bilateral lesions predispose the patient to a less than optimal result; because bilateral lesions are more likely to be associated with hyperfunctional techniques, the resolution of the smaller lesion is the exception rather than the rule. Often, both lesions should be surgically removed.

Surgical therapy is always individualized. The choice of surgical approach is based on a thorough understanding of vocal fold anatomy and physiology. The goal of surgery is to restore the normal glottal configuration without the removal of uninvolved surrounding mucosa or excessive dissection in the superficial layer of the lamina propria. Superficial lesions represent a response to injury and reside almost exclusively in the superficial layer of the lamina propria. Therefore, surgery is limited to this region. A microflap approach with a medially placed incision is well suited to removal of these types of lesions.[25] After vasoconstriction of the laryngeal mucosa, an incision is made just over the lesion; the vocal ligament is identified using a combination of blunt and sharp dissection with microsurgical instruments. The mucosa and superficial layer of the lamina propria encompassing the lesion are freed from the underlying vocal ligament by dissecting in the superficial layer of the lamina propria, taking great care to remove only the involved mucosa. This often leaves a nearly imperceptible mucosal defect at the conclusion of the procedure (Figure 94-6).

Cysts

Vocal fold cysts are diagnosed and differentiated from nodules or polyps by laryngovideostroboscopy. Cysts that fill the superficial layer of the lamina propria are often tethered to the vocal ligament, frequently resulting in a loss of the mucosal wave over the lesion. More superficial lesions such as nodules tend to have a dampened yet perceptible mucosal wave.[85] Cysts and other lesions that do not separate easily from the vocal ligament on intraoperative palpation are approached via a lateral microflap technique.[23,26] The lateral microflap technique involves an incision along the superior aspect of the vocal fold lateral to the intracordal lesion. The vocal ligament is identified, and dissection occurs in the superficial layer of the lamina propria medially toward the lesion. The microflap is gently retracted medially, usually with a velvet eye microlaryngeal suction or with a flap elevator, and the cyst is sharply and bluntly removed from the vocal ligament and the overlying mucosal cover layer. After this is removed, the mucosal flap is redraped in place (Figure 94-7).

Vocal Fold Varix

Varices of the vocal fold are evaluated under high magnification, and palpation is used to alternately occlude and examine the feeding and draining vessels. After this, the vessels are vasoconstricted with chilled 1:10,000 epinephrine, and then an iced saline pledget is placed deep to the vocal fold to protect the endotracheal tube cuff. The carbon dioxide laser is slightly defocused and used at 1- to 2-W power. The feeding and then draining vessels are photocoagulated. The medial surface of the vocal fold is avoided. The vascular malformation is then coagulated. If still present, the mass is removed using the medial microflap approach.[22] Recent work using the pulsed-dye laser suggests that it may play a valuable role in the treatment of these lesions. A very large feeding vessel may require excision (Figure 94-8).

Postoperative Care

General laryngeal hygiene is reemphasized to the patient. In addition to hydration and the use of guaifenesin, perioperative antireflux medications are strongly recommended for most patients. Complete voice rest is instituted after surgery. In patients with minimal mucosal excision and limited disruption of the submucosal layer of the lamina propria, this period may last 5 to 7 days. Ten to 14 days of complete voice rest is recommended in cases in which extensive vocal fold dissection or revision surgery has been performed.

Healing after laryngeal microflap surgery can be divided into four phases (Table 94-5). The first phase in the immediate postoperative period lasts 5 to 14 days and consists of complete voice rest and hydration. Healing occurs between the vocal fold cover and the underlying vocal ligament. In cases in which mucosal excision was required, healing by secondary intention occurs.

The second phase begins 1 to 2 weeks after surgery. This is a stage of voice rehabilitation that occurs under the guidance and observation of a speech language pathologist. Laryngovideostroboscopy is usually performed after the second or third week. Pliability of the vocal fold and return of the mucosal wave is assessed. Rarely, vocal fold hemorrhage is noted and further voice rest required. This stage begins with graduated voice use. The first day, the patient speaks for 5 minutes. The phonation time is doubled each day until the patient is returned to full conversational speech. This usually occurs by the end of the third or fourth postoperative week. If voice use causes pain, the patient is asked to decrease his or her amount of speaking and contact the physician. The speech language pathologist stresses easy onset phonation, avoidance of vocal abusive behaviors, and the need to use appropriate pitch and vocal intensity. Biofeedback retraining is used during this time.

The third phase of healing occurs during the second and third months after surgery. The learned behaviors from the speech language pathologist are continued, and vocal and singing reeducation is begun under the guidance of a vocal pedagogue. All singers work with a vocal pedagogue regardless of their style of singing or previous vocal training. The patient relearns how to sing from the basic level. Maladaptive behaviors are noted early and addressed by the pedagogue.

After 3 months, the average patient can return to professional activity. Patients should be followed up with interval examinations for 24 months after surgery to assess for continued improvement or potential reoccurrence of the lesion.

RELATED SURGICAL PROCEDURES

Professional voice patients undergo many nonlaryngeal surgical procedures involving the upper airway. They should understand that any procedure that potentially alters the anatomy or function of the supraglottal vocal tract (e.g., tonsillectomy, septoplasty, sinus surgery, palatal surgery) can alter the vocal resonance. Professional voice patients should be counseled regarding this possibility.

A well-performed tonsillectomy should not cause vocal professionals significant long-term difficulty. It

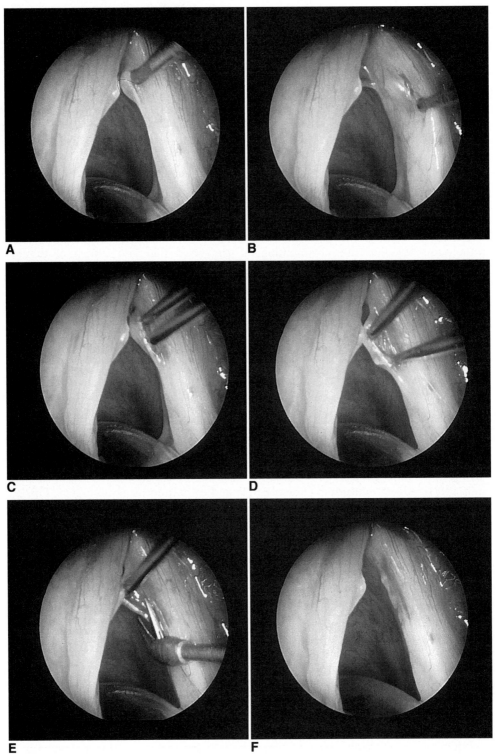

Figure 94-6. Intraoperative photographs of lesion excision through a medial microflap approach. **A,** The sickle knife is used to make an incision over the lesion on the medial surface of the vocal fold. **B,** A small angled probe, named a *flap elevator,* is used to elevate mucosa from the medial and superior surfaces of the vocal fold around the lesion. **C,** The lesion is bluntly dissected free from the underlying vocal ligament. **D,** The lesion is peeled off a portion of the overlying vocal fold cover. **E,** The lesion and a small portion of the cover are excised. **F,** The previously created flaps are redraped in position to cover the medial surface of the vocal fold. (From Courey MS, Garrett GG, Ossoff RH: *Laryngoscope* 107:340, 1997.)

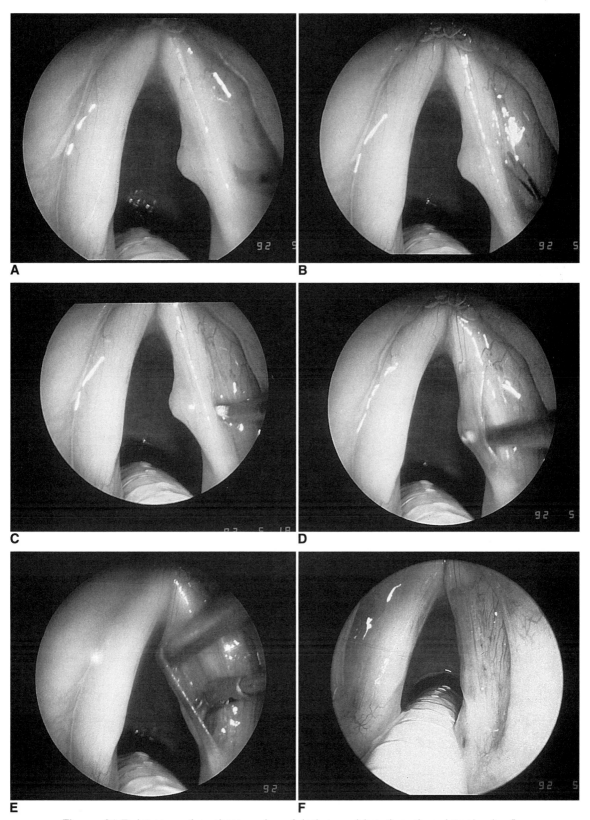

Figure 94-7. Intraoperative photographs of lesion excision through a lateral microflap approach. **A,** A sickle knife is used to make an incision on the superior surface of the vocal fold. **B,** The incision is further defined with upcutting scissors. **C,** A flap elevator is used to elevate the microflap. **D,** Dissection occurs between the vocal ligament and mucosa. **E,** The lesion is removed from the vocal ligament. **F,** The mucosal microflap is redraped into position. (From Courey MS and others: *Ann Otol Rhinol Laryngol* 104:267, 1995.)

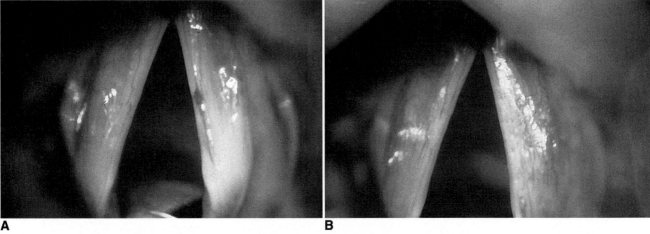

A   **B**

Figure 94-8. A professional singer with a microvascular lesion of the true vocal fold. **A,** Preoperative photograph. **B,** Postoperative appearance immediately after photocoagulation with the carbon dioxide laser at 1500 watts/cm². (From Rubin JS and others: *Diagnosis and treatment of voice disorders*, New York, 1995, Igaku-Shoin Medical Publishers.)

TABLE 94-5

POSTOPERATIVE RECOVERY

Phase	Time Period	Activity
I	7–14 days	Voice rest
II	7–28 days	Graduated voice use with speech language pathologist
III	4–12 weeks	Vocal reeducation (singing with pedagogue)
IV	3–18 months	Professional activity

will, at least transiently, affect the ability to modify that area of the resonator.[97] Tonsillectomy alters the frequency of the fourth formant in nonsingers but not in classically trained vocalists.[66] However, any significant palatal or faucial arch scarring could lead to laryngeal hyperfunction. This is caused by altered oropharyngeal sensation. The singer's vocal feel or sensory feedback is altered and results in a change in the singer's delivery.

Laser-assisted uvulopalatoplasty has become a popular management for snoring. This procedure should result in at least a temporary voice change. Compensation should be possible for well-trained vocalists, similar to posttonsillectomy patients. If the surgery is performed, the stages should be spread out over many months to allow the artist to compensate for the palatal changes.

Adenoidectomy, septoplasty, sinus surgery, or turbinectomy in a singer with a significant nasal obstruc-

tion should be done very conservatively, if at all. The development of even a small degree of hypernasality could significantly alter the patient's singing voice.[27,62]

Hearing is often neglected in singers. Classical singers are taught to sing by feel and not by what they hear. However, many singers have difficulty in doing so. Baseline audiometric evaluations are recommended on all professional and serious amateur singers. Ear-level monitors with selective input have been of benefit to commercial singers. These monitors deliver stage sounds, mixed by the sound engineer, back to the performer at a comfortable intensity. They allow singers to protect their hearing, sing at the proper intensity level, and not succumb to the tendency of oversinging in the concert environment (the Lombard effect).

CONCLUSION

A singer's body is a vocal instrument, and the larynx represents the most important portion of this instrument. Education and behavior modification can enable singers to maximize their gift. The maintenance of good vocal hygiene and regular reminders of abusive speaking and singing behaviors are part of this process. Even the most experienced singers may have to return to work with a vocal pedagogue after an upper respiratory infection or when they are busy recording or touring.

Professional vocalists are an interesting and challenging group of patients. Management should be undertaken by a coordinated team of professionals well versed in the care of such patients.

REFERENCES

1. Abitbol J: Vocal fold hemorrhages in voice professionals, *J Voice* 2:261, 1988.
2. Abitbol J and others: Does a hormonal vocal cord cyclic cyst in women? study of vocal premenstrual syndrome and voice performers by videostroboscopy-glottography and cytology on 38 women, *J Voice* 3:157, 1989.
3. Andrea M, Dias O: *Rigid and contact endoscopy in microlaryngeal surgery: technique and atlas of clinical cases.* New York, 1995, Lippincott-Raven.
4. Amin MR and others: Proton pump inhibitor resistance in the treatment of laryngopharyngeal reflux, *Otolaryngol Head Neck Surg* 125:374-378, 2001.
5. Baken RJ: *Clinical measurement of speech and voice,* Boston, 1987, College-Hill Press.
6. Bare T, Titze IR, Yoshioka H: *Multiple simultaneous measures of vocal fold activity.* In Bless D, Abbs JH, editors: *Vocal fold physiology: contemporary research and clinical issues,* San Diego, California, 1983, College-Hill Press.
7. Bassich CJ, Ludlow DL: The use of perceptual methods by new clinicians for assessing voice quality, *J Speech Hear Dis* 51:125, 1986.
8. Belafsky PC, Postma GN, Koufman JA: The association between laryngeal pseudosulcus and laryngopharyngeal reflux, *Otolaryngol Head Neck Surg* 126:649-652, 2002.
9. Belafsky PC, Postma GN, Koufman JA: Laryngopharyngeal reflux symptoms improve before changes in physical findings, *Laryngoscope* 111:979-981, 2001.
10. Belafsky PC, Postma GN, Koufman, JA: The validity and reliability of the reflux finding score (RFS), *Laryngoscope* 111:1313-1317, 2001.
11. Belafsky PC, Postma GN, Koufman JA: Validity and reliability of the reflux symptom index (RSI), *J Voice* 16:274-277, 2002.
12. Benninger MS and others: *New dimensions in measuring voice treatment outcomes.* In Sataloff RT, editor: *Professional voice: the science and art of clinical care,* ed 2, San Diego, California, 1996, Singular Publishing Group.
13. Bless DM, Hirano M, Feder RJ: Video stroboscopic evaluation of the larynx, *Ear Nose Throat J* 66:289, 1987.
14. Boothroyd CV, Lepre F: Permanent voice change resulting from danazol therapy, *Aust NZ J Obstet Gynaecol* 30:275, 1990.
15. Bough ID Jr and others: Gastroesophageal reflux laryngitis resistant to omeprazole therapy, *J Voice* 9:205, 1995.
16. Burns P: Acoustical analysis of the underlying voice differences between two groups of professional singers: opera and country and western, *Laryngoscope* 96:549, 1986.
17. Casper JK, Brewer DW, Colton RH: Pitfalls and problems in flexible fiberoptic videolaryngoscopy, *J Voice* 1:347, 1988.
18. Cohn JR, Spiegel JR, Sataloff RT: Vocal disorders in the professional voice user: the allergist's role, *Ann Allergy Asthma Immunol* 74:363, 1995.
19. Cohn J and others: Airwave reactivity-induced asthma in singers (ARIAS), *J Voice* 5:332, 1991.
20. Colton RH, Casper JK: *Understanding voice problems: a physiological perspective for diagnosis and treatment,* Baltimore, Maryland, 1990, Williams & Wilkins.
21. Courey MS, Garrett CG, Ossoff RH: The lateral microflap vs the medial microflap for excision of benign vocal fold lesions (unpublished observations).
22. Courey MS, Garrett CG, Ossoff RH: The medial microflap for excision of benign vocal fold lesions, *Laryngoscope* 107:340, 1997.
23. Courey MS, Ossoff RH: Art of intraoperative photo-documentation of laryngeal lesions. Transactions of the 1995 American Bronchoesphagological Association, *Ann Otol Rhinol Laryngol* 64–68, 1997.
24. Courey MS, Ossoff RH, Shohet JA: Immunohistochemical characterization of benign laryngeal lesions, *Ann Otol Rhinol Laryngol* 105:525, 1996.
25. Courey MS, Postma GN: Microvascular lesions of the true vocal folds, *Curr Opin Otolaryngol Head Neck Surg* 4:134, 1996.
26. Courey MS and others: Endoscopic vocal fold microflap: a three year experience, *Ann Otol Rhinol Laryngol* 104:267, 1995.
27. Croft CB, Shprintzen RJ, Ruben RJ: Hypernasal speech following adenotonsillectomy, *Otolaryngol Head Neck Surg* 89:779, 1981.
28. Dejonckere PH and others: Perceptual evaluation of dysphonia: reliability and relevance, *Folia Phoniatr (Base1)* 45:76, 1993.
29. Dikkers FG and others: Ultrastructural changes of the basic membrane zone in benign lesions of the vocal folds, *Acta Otolaryngol (Stockh)* 113:98, 1993.
30. Donchev C: Varicose veins of the vocal cords, *Folia Med (Plovdiv)* 25:24, 1983.
31. Elliot N, Sundberg J, Gramming P: What happens during vocal warm-up? *J Voice* 9:37, 1995.
32. Feder RJ: The professional voice and airline flight, *Otolaryngol Head Neck Surg* 92:251, 1984.
33. Finkelhor BK, Titze IR, Durham PL: The effect of viscosity changes in the vocal folds on the range of oscillation, *J Voice* 1:320, 1988.
34. Flach M, Schwickardi H, Simon R: Welchen Einfluss Haben Menstruation Ond Schwangerschaft Auf Die ausgabildete gesangsstimme? *Folia Phoniatr (Base1)* 21:199, 1968.
35. Gates GA and others: Effects of beta-blockade on singing performance, *Ann Otol Rhinol Laryngol* 94:570, 1985.
36. Gaynor EB: Otolaryngologic manifestations of gastroesophageal reflux, *Am J Gastroenterol* 86:801, 1991.
37. Gould WJ: The effect of voice training on lung volumes in singers, and the possible relationship to the damping factor of Pressman, *J Res Sing* 1:3, 1977.
38. Gould WJ, Okamura H: Static lung volumes in singers, *Ann Otol Rhinol Laryngol* 82:89, 1973.
39. Gray SD: *Basement membrane zone injury in vocal nodules.* In Gauffin NJ, Hammarberg B, editors: *Vocal fold physiology,* San Diego, California, 1991, Singular Publishing Group.
40. Gray SD, Hirano M, Sato K: *Molecular and cellular structure of vocal fold tissue.* In Titze IR, editor: *Vocal fold physiology,* San Diego, California, 1993, Singular Publishing Group.
41. Gray SD, Pignatari SSN, Harding P: Morphologic ultrastructure of anchoring fibers in normal vocal fold basement membrane zone, *J Voice* 8:48, 1994.
42. Gray SD, Titze I, Lusk RP: Electron microscopy of hyperphonated canine vocal cords, *J Voice* 1:109, 1987.
43. Griffin B and others: Physiological characteristics of the supported singing voice: a preliminary study, *J Voice* 9:45, 1995.
44. Gupta OP and others: Nasal pharyngeal and laryngeal manifestations of hypothyroidism, *Ear Nose Throat J* 56:10, 1977.
45. Hanson DG, Kamel PL, Kahrilas PJ: Outcomes of antireflux therapy for the treatment of chronic laryngitis, *Ann Otol Rhinol Laryngol* 104:550, 1995.
46. Hirano M: Morphological structure of the vocal cord as a vibrator and its variations, *Folia Phoniatr (Base1)* 26:89, 1974.
47. Hirano M: Phonosurgery: basic and clinical investigations, *Otologia Fukuoka* 21:239, 1975.
48. Hirano M: *Clinical examination of voice,* New York, 1981, Springer-Verlag.

49. Hirano M, Bless DM: *Videostroboscopic examination of the larynx,* San Diego, California, 1993, Singular Publishing Group.

50. Hixon TJ: *Respiratory function in speech and song.* London, Taylor and Francis, 1987.

51. Hixon TJ, Hoffman C: *Chest wall shape during singing.* In Lawrence V, editor: *Transcripts of the 7th annual symposium, Care of the professional voice,* vol 1, New York, 1978, Voice Foundation.

52. Kleinsasser O: Restoration of the voice in benign lesions of the vocal folds by endolaryngeal microsurgery, *J Voice* 5:257, 1991.

53. Klinkenberg-Knol EC, Meuwissen SGM: Combined gastric and oesophageal 24-hour pH monitoring and oesophageal manometry in patients with reflux disease, resistant to treatment with omeprazole, *Aliment Pharmacol Ther* 4: 485, 1990.

54. Koufman JA: Approach to the patient with a voice disorder, *Otolaryngol Clin North Am* 24:989, 1991.

55. Koufman JA: *Evaluation of laryngeal biomechanics by fiberoptic laryngoscopy.* In Rubin JS and others, editors: *Diagnosis and treatment of voice disorders,* New York, 1995, Igaku-Shoin.

56. Koufman JA: The otolaryngologic manifestations of gastroesophageal reflux disease (GERD): a clinical investigation of 225 patients using ambulatory 24-hour pH monitoring and experimental investigation of the role of acid and pepsin in the development of laryngeal injury, *Laryngoscope* 101(Suppl 53):1, 1991.

57. Koufman JA, Blalock PD: Functional voice disorders, *Otolaryngol Clin North Am* 24:1059, 1991.

58. Koufman JA, Blalock PD: Vocal fatigue and dysphonia in the professional voice user: Bogart-Bacall syndrome, *Laryngoscope* 98:493, 1988.

59. Koufman JA and others: Prevalence of esophagitis in patients with pH-documented laryngopharyngeal reflux, *Laryngoscope* 112:1606-1609, 2002.

60. Kreiman J and others: Individual differences in voice quality perception, *J Speech Hear Res* 35:512, 1992.

61. Kreiman J and others: Perceptual evaluation of voice quality: review, tutorial, and a framework for future research, *J Speech Hear Res* 36:21, 1993.

62. Kummer AW and others: Changes in nasal resonance secondary to adenotonsillectomy, *Am J Otolaryngol* 14: 285, 1993.

63. Lacina O: Der Einfluss Der Menstruation auf die Steimme der Sangerinnen, *Folia Phoniatr (Base1)* 20:13, 1968.

64. Leclure FLE, Brocaar ME, Verscheeure J: Electroglottography and its relation to glottal activity, *Folia Phoniatr (Base1)* 27:215, 1975.

65. Leite LP and others: Control of gastric acid with high dose H-2 receptor antagonists after omeprazole failure: report of two cases, *Am J Gastroenterol* 90:1874, 1995.

66. Lin PT, Stern JC, Gould WJ: Risk factors and management of vocal cord hemorrhages: an experience with 44 cases, *J Voice* 5:74, 1991.

67. Lin PT and others: Acoustic analysis of voice in tonsillectomy, *J Voice* 3:81, 1989.

68. Livesy JR and others: An assessment of the reproductability of combined glottography in a clinic setting, *Clin Otolaryngol* 18:500, 1993.

69. Nakai Y and others: Microvascular structure of the larynx, *Acta Otolaryngol Suppl (Stockh)* 486:254, 1991.

70. Oertel MJ: Das laryngo-stroboskop und die Laryngo-stroboskpische untersuchung, *Arch Laryngol Rhinol (Berl)* 3:1, 1895.

71. Oertel MJ: Ueber Eine Any Ue Laryngostroboskopiscag Unterschungs Methode, *Central F D Med Wiss* 16:81, 1878.

72. Olson NR: Laryngopharyngeal manifestations of gastroesophageal reflux disease, *Otolaryngol Clin North Am* 24:1201, 1991.

73. Postma, GN, Courey, MS, Ossoff RH: Microvascular lesions of the true vocal folds, *Ann Otol Rhino Laryngol* 107:472-476, 1998.

74. Postma GN and others: Esophageal motor function in laryngopharyngeal reflux is superior to that of classic gastroesophageal reflux disease, *Ann Otol Rhinol Laryngol* 110:1114-1116, 2001.

75. Punt NA: Applied laryngology: singers and actors, *Proc R Soc Med* 61:1152, 1968.

76. Sabol JW, Lee L, Stemple JC: The value of vocal function exercises in the practice regimen of singers, *J Voice* 9: 27, 1995.

77. Sataloff RT: Nonsurgical management of the professional voice, *Curr Opin Otolaryngol Head Neck Surg* 3:135, 1995.

78. Sataloff RT: *The professional voice.* In Cummings CW and others, editors: *Otolaryngology: head and neck surgery,* ed 2, St Louis, 1993, Mosby.

79. Sataloff RT: Vocal fold hemorrhage: diagnosis and treatment, *NATS J* May/June:45, 1995.

80. Sataloff RT, Spiegel JR, Hawkshaw M: Respiratory function and dysfunction in singers, *NATS J* 46:23, 1990.

81. Sataloff RT, Spiegel JR, Hawkshaw MJ: Strobovideolaryngoscopy: results and clinical value, *Ann Otol Rhinol Laryngol* 100:725, 1991.

82. Sataloff RT and others: Laryngeal mini-microflap: a new technique and reassessment of the microflap saga, *J Voice* 9:198, 1995.

83. Sataloff RT and others: Strobovideolaryngoscopy in professional voice users: results and clinical value, *J Voice* 1:359, 1988.

84. Schiff M: The pill in otolaryngology, *Trans Am Acad Ophthalmol Otolaryngol* 72:76, 1968.

85. Shohet JA, Courey MS, Ossoff RH: The value of videostroboscopic parameters in differentiating benign true vocal fold cysts, nodules and polyps, *Laryngoscope* 106: 19, 1996.

86. Slavit DH: *Role of the pulmonary laboratory in voice assessment.* In Rubin JS and others, editors: *Diagnosis and treatment of voice disorders,* New York, 1995, Igaku-Shoin.

87. Smitheran JR, Hixon TJ: A clinical method for estimating laryngeal airway resistance during vowel production, *J Speech Hear Dis* 46:138, 1981.

88. Sundberg J: The acoustics of the singing voice, *Sci Am* 236:82, 1977.

89. Sundberg J: Articulatory interpretation of the "singing format," *J Acoust Soc Am* 55:838, 1974.

90. Sundberg J: Perceptual aspects of singing, *J Voice* 8:106, 1994.

91. Sundberg J: *The science of the singing voice,* DeKalb, Illinois, 1987, Northern Illinois University Press.

92. Sundberg J, Nordstrom PE: Raised and lowered larynx: the effect on vowel format frequencies, *J Res Sing* 6:7, 1983.

93. Thompson AR: Pharmacological agents with affects on voice, *Am J Otolaryngol* 16:12, 1995.

94. Titze IR, Jiang JJ, Hsiao TY: Measurement of mucosal wave propagation and vertical phase difference in vocal fold vibration, *Ann Otol Rhinol Laryngol* 102:58, 1993.

95. Verdolini K, Titze IR, Pennell A: Dependence of phonatory effort on hydration level, *J Speech Hear Res* 37:1001, 1994.

96. Verdolini-Marston K, Sandage M, Titze IR: Effect of hydration treatments on laryngeal nodules and polyps and related voice measures, *J Voice* 8:30, 1994.

97. Wallner LJ and others: Voice changes following adenotonsillectomy: a study of velar function by cinefluorography and video tape, *Laryngoscope* 78:1410, 1968.

98. Wardle PG, Whitehead MI, Mills RP: Non-reversible and wide ranging voice changes after treatment with danazol, *B M J Clin Res Ed* 287:946, 1983.

99. Woo P: Quantification of videostroboscopic findings: measurements of the normal glottal cycle, *Laryngoscope* 106(Suppl 79):1, 1996.

100. Yumoto E, Kurokawa H, Okamura H: Vocal fold vibration of the canine larynx: observation from an infraglottic view, *J Voice* 5:299, 1991.

101. Zeitels SM: Premalignant epithelium and microinvasive cancer of the vocal fold: the evolution of phonomicrosurgical management, *Laryngoscope* 105(Suppl 67):1, 1995.

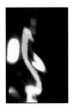

CHAPTER NINETY FIVE

BENIGN VOCAL FOLD MUCOSAL DISORDERS

|| Robert W. Bastian

INTRODUCTION

Benign vocal fold mucosal disorders (e.g., vocal nodules, laryngeal polyps, mucosal hemorrhage, intracordal cysts, mucosal bridges, glottic sulci) seem to be caused primarily by vibratory trauma (excessive voice use). In my experience, an expressive, talkative personality on the part of the patient correlates most consistently with most of these disorders. Occupational and lifestyle vocal demands are minor risks by comparison, unless these demands are truly extreme. Cigarette smoking and liberal voice use are cofactors in the formation of smoker's polyps, also termed *Reinke's edema* or *polypoid degeneration*. Other secondary influences (e.g., infection, allergy, acid reflux) also may increase the mucosa's vulnerability to vibratory trauma, leading to injury.

Nonsingers with benign vocal fold mucosal disorders present with a change in the sound or capabilities of the speaking voice. Singers with normal-sounding speaking voices may seek professional evaluation because of singing voice limitations, usually in the upper range. Benign vocal fold mucosal disorders are significant because of the importance of spoken or sung communication and the voice's contribution to identity.

Benign vocal fold mucosal disorders are common. More than 50% of patients with voice complaints have a benign mucosal disorder. Brodnitz[20] reported 45% of 977 patients had a diagnosis of nodules, polyps, or polypoid thickening, and Kleinsasser[53] (1964–1975) reported that slightly more than 50% of 2618 patients had one of these benign entities.

ANATOMY AND PHYSIOLOGY

The anatomy most relevant to the benign vocal fold mucosal disorders is the microarchitecture of the vocal folds, as seen on whole-organ coronal sections in a study of cancer growth patterns[26,62] or in the work of Hirano.[45] Medially to laterally, the membranous vocal fold is made up of squamous epithelium, Reinke's

potential space (superficial layer of the lamina propria), the vocal ligament (elastin and collagen fibers), and the thyroarytenoid muscle. Perichondrium and thyroid cartilage provide the lateral boundary of the vocal fold (Figure 95-1).

The vocal folds move as a whole between abducted and adducted positions for breathing and phonation, respectively. The mucosa (epithelium and superficial layer of the lamina propria [Reinke's potential space]), which covers the vocal folds, is the chief oscillator during phonation (continuous adduction); thus, one might speak of vocal fold *mucosal* vibration rather than vocal fold vibration. In a canine study that supports this idea, Saito and others[77] placed metal pellets at varying depths into the vocal fold (e.g., epithelially, subepithelially, intramuscularly) and used radiograph stroboscopy to trace their coronal plane trajectories during vibration. Mucosal pellet trajectories were far wider than those of the ligament or the muscle. Thus, primarily the vocal fold mucosa oscillates to produce sound.

Hirano's work[58] provides an explanation for Saito's observations. Hirano[58] described the vocal fold muscle as the body of the fold, the epithelium and superficial layer of the lamina propria (Reinke's potential space) as the cover, and the intermediate layers of collagenous and elastic tissue (vocal ligament) as the transitional zone (see Figure 95-1). Because of the different stiffness characteristics of these layers, they are somewhat decoupled mechanically from each other during phonation. Decoupling is graphically illustrated in Figure 95-2 (mucosa being stretched). This decoupling allows the mucosa to oscillate with a degree of freedom from the ligament and muscle. An analogy can be made to the relative freedom from the paddle experienced by the red rubber ball and elastic band in a child's paddleball toy. During phonation, pulmonary air power supplied to adducted vocal folds is transduced into acoustic power. To accomplish this, pulmonary air is passed

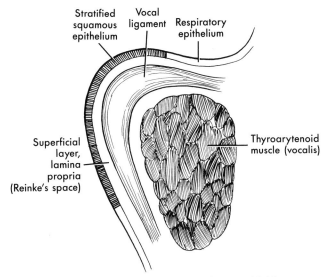

Figure 95-1. Cross section of the vocal fold.

between appropriately adducted vocal folds. At this point, the vocal fold (mucosa) vibrates passively according to the length, tension, and edge configuration determined by the intrinsic muscles and elastic recoil forces of the vocal fold tissues. Figure 95-3 shows the maximum open and closed phases of one vibratory cycle, as seen during laryngeal videostroboscopy. Further details concerning the mucosa's vibratory behavior can be found in the works of Baer[5] and Hirano[45] and in Chapter 98.

Other important microanatomy includes glands in the supraglottic, saccular, and infraglottic areas, which produce secretions that bathe the vocal folds during vibration.

EVALUATION OF PATIENT

The necessary and sufficient elements for diagnosis and management of benign mucosal disorders include (1) a skillful history; (2) a perceptual assessment of vocal capabilities and limitations, particularly through elicitation of vocal tasks designed to detect mucosal disturbances; and (3) a high-quality laryngeal examination (often including laryngeal videostroboscopy).

History

A detailed questionnaire may help in taking a complete history,[78,79] but basic lines of inquiry provide crucial information. Besides the usual items in the general medical history, the voice history should focus in particular on the following:

1. Onset and duration of vocal symptoms
2. Patient beliefs about causes or exacerbating influences
3. Common symptom complexes
4. Talkativeness (vocal personality or "push from within")
5. Vocal commitments or activities ("pull from without"), including voice type and training, if patient is a performer
6. Other risk factors
7. Patient perception of the severity of the disorder
8. Vocal aspirations and consequent motivation for rehabilitation

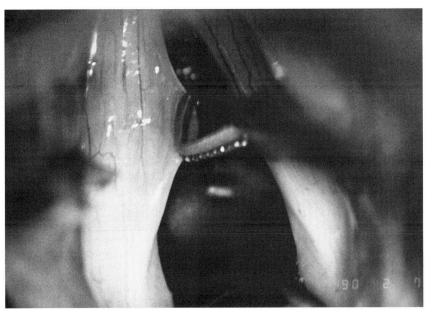

Figure 95-2. Gentle medial retraction shows the relative decoupling of the mucosa from the underlying, nondeformed vocal ligament.

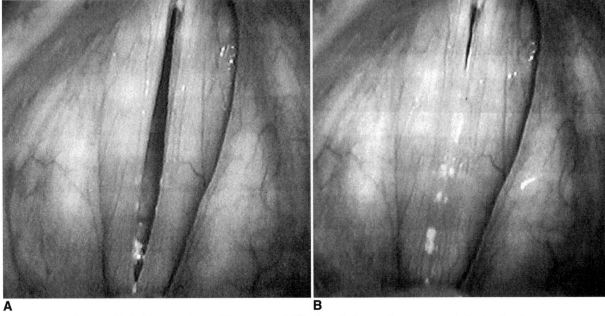

Figure 95-3. The maximum **(A)** open and **(B)** closed phase of an apparent single vibratory cycle as seen during videostroboscopy. The moving part is primarily mucosa, with little participation of ligament or muscle.

Onset

It is appropriate during history-taking to test the hypothesis that a patient who complains of frequently recurring bouts of vocal dysfunction may be experiencing exacerbations of a more chronic overuse disorder. Such a patient, who is often found to be living "at the edge" vocally based on assessment of vocal personality, lifestyle, vocal commitments, and voice production, may present because a small increase of vocal activity or an upper respiratory infection has thrown him or her "over the edge." In this situation, both the patient and clinician may focus only on the upper respiratory infection (e.g., providing management with antibiotics) rather than seeing past this acute issue to recognize the need for the more sophisticated behavioral therapy appropriate for a chronic vocal overdoer.

Patient Beliefs about Causes

It is prudent to maintain a degree of skepticism initially when patients with nodules or polyps suspect that their difficulties resulted from allergies or phlegm. Based on analysis of risk factors in a large group of patients with voice disorders, allergies usually play only a minor role at most compared with the behavioral causes of these mucosal injuries.

Common Symptom Complexes

As for many other types of voice disorders, a characteristic symptom complex accompanies benign mucosal disorders. Nonsingers, who often have moderate to large mucosal disturbances before they seek medical attention, usually describe chronic hoarseness with exacerbations at times of increased voice use. Singers may not note speaking voice symptoms but rather (1) exaggeration of day-to-day variability of singing capabilities; (2) increased effort necessary for singing; (3) reduced vocal endurance; (4) deterioration of high soft singing; and (5) delayed phonatory onset and air wastage (breathiness).

Talkativeness

The factor that correlates most strongly with the formation and maintenance of many benign vocal fold mucosal disorders appears to be personality. The clinician should pay close attention to this issue. For example, patients can be asked to rate themselves on a seven-point talkativeness scale, where one is very untalkative, four is averagely talkative, and seven is unusually talkative. (This scale deals with innate predisposition, not the demands of work or lifestyle.) Virtually all patients with nodules and polyps, and even cysts and sulci, rate themselves six or seven, except for persons who work in vocally extreme occupations (e.g., financial trading).

Vocal Commitments

To assess vocal commitments and activities, the clinician should inquire about occupation, voice type and level of training, and the nature and extent of vocal activities related to family life, childcare, politics, religion, athletics, and musical rehearsal and performance.

Other Risk Factors

Other risk factors include tobacco and alcohol use, acid reflux, insufficient fluid intake, certain drying medications, systemic illnesses, and allergies. Even when the history is positive for one of these factors, it is usually a secondary issue as compared with "sevenness."

Patient Perception of Severity and Consequent Motivation to Rehabilitate

Exploration of the patient's perception of severity of the voice problem, vocal aspirations, and motivation also is important. For example, the clinician may be confronted by a person who only wants to be reassured that the problem is not cancer. Even with a diagnosis of large smoker's polyps with severe dysphonia, management can appropriately be short-term and supportive, consisting primarily of education. However, therapy might be intense and long-term and may eventually include surgery for the patient with a normal speaking voice who, to pursue a competitive performing career, must be relieved of extreme upper singing voice limitations caused by small nodules.

Auditory-Perceptual Assessment of Vocal Capabilities and Limitations (What's Wrong with This Voice?)

Auditory-perceptual assessment of vocal capabilities and limitations is an often neglected part of the diagnostic process that provides the best means of understanding the nature and severity of the voice disorder. To be most efficient, this part of the diagnostic process is performed by the same clinician who takes the history and performs the laryngeal examination. Alternatively, a second clinician can perform this assessment, but for best results the findings of vocal capability elicitation should be immediately correlated with the other two components of the diagnostic process.

Vocal capability elicitation and interpretation require that the examiner have good pitch-matching abilities, a reasonably normal voice, extensive familiarity with his or her own vocal capabilities, intimate familiarity with normal singing voice capabilities according to age, sex, and voice classification, and the willingness to model and elicit with his or her own voice. Also needed is a frequency reference, such as a small electronic keyboard.

In voice clinics where expert vocal capability elicitation and assessment are not available or are not immediately correlated with history and laryngeal examination, clinicians may overlook or reject the power and centrality of this part of the evaluation. They may instead affirm various items of equipment that measure components of vocal output (e.g., acoustic, aerodynamic). Although useful for quantification, documentation, and some biofeedback applications, this equipment is cumbersome, expensive, time-consuming to interpret, and most importantly, weak diagnostically compared with the vocal capability battery that can answer far more quickly and holistically the question "what's wrong with this voice?"

A list of basic vocal capabilities and phenomena include the following: (1) average or anchor speech frequency; (2) maximum frequency range; (3) projected voice and yell; (4) ability to perform very high-frequency, very low-intensity tasks that detect mucosal disturbances[13]; (5) register use and phenomena; (6) maximum phonation time and (7) instability and tremors.

The ability to perform high-frequency, low-intensity tasks is most important for detecting benign mucosal disorders, which are suggested by a loss of expected range under these performance constraints; onset delays, air escape, and lack of tonal clarity all suggest a benign mucosal disturbance. The clinician should also search for inconsistencies between spoken and sung capabilities and note the patient's level of effort and overall vocal personality. Basic vocal capability testing requires only a few minutes to perform because the examiner focuses primarily on the extremes of physical capability and secondarily on vocal skill.

As stated, the **vocal capability battery** coupled with the **voice history** and **laryngeal examination** is crucial in diagnosing and directing subsequent management. For example, signs of a mucosal disturbance (e.g., detection of air escape, onset delays, loss of clarity and range) during assessment of the ability to perform high-frequency, low-intensity tasks minimize the possibility that a singer's normal-sounding speaking voice during history-taking will subconsciously bias the clinician to selectively perceive normal vocal folds when small vocal nodules are present. The vocal capability battery also provides insight into the severity of the patient's vocal limitations, which can then be correlated with the visual examination to help determine, along with the patient's needs and motivation, the intensity and direction of management.

Office Examination of the Larynx

The laryngeal mirror theoretically allows three-dimensional viewing and good color resolution, but in practice offers poor visualization in some cases. In other cases, visualization is good, but only during phonation, because the view obstructed by the epiglottis during respiration. In addition, no permanent image of the larynx results from this examination technique.

Because the physician must therefore remember the lesion or document it with a simple sketch, precise critique of the effectiveness of the therapy chosen may not be possible. Rigid laryngeal telescopes often allow a clearer view, particularly during respiration. With the naked eye, however, they have similar disadvantages to those of the mirror. The fiberoptic nasolaryngoscope or a newer video-endoscope is especially important when the patient is difficult to examine because of unusual anatomy or an exceptional gag reflex. Resolution of subtle-to-small mucosal changes may be limited (because the laryngeal image is brought to the examiner's eye fiberoptically) unless the larynx is topically anesthetized to allow a close approach of the tip of the fiberscope to the vocal folds. With topical anesthesia, the vocal folds, subglottis, and trachea can be examined easily (Figure 95-4).[10,11]

Strobe illumination added to any of these examining instruments allows mucosal vibratory dynamics to be evaluated in apparent slow motion (e.g., to understand mucosal scarring, to distinguish cysts from nodules). Adding a video camera and videocassette recorder to the rigid or fiberoptic scopes brings additional advantages; for example, patient understanding and motivation are facilitated by viewing the video documented examination. Other clinicians (otolaryngologists, speech pathologists, voice teachers) can participate more easily in assessment and management. Videotapes serve as permanent records that document the result of voice therapy or surgery. Teaching of residents is enhanced.

Direct Laryngoscopy

When videostroboscopy is available, lesions that are suspicious for cancer or papillomatosis can nearly always be easily distinguished from nodules, polyps, and cysts. Therefore, removal of these latter entities is appropriate only within a comprehensive plan for treatment/voice restoration and rarely, if ever, for tissue.

Objective Measures of Vocal Output

Skillful "triangulation" on the voice problem using the voice history, auditory-perceptual evaluation of vocal capabilities and limitations, and high-quality laryngeal examination, often with videostroboscopy, should lead to a clear diagnosis and description of the problem in virtually every case. By contrast, devices that analyze phonation aerodynamically and acoustically have little diagnostic value. However, aerodynamic and acoustic information is thought by some to be useful to quantify and document severity, to deepen understanding in the research arena, and to assist in some helpful biofeedback applications.

GENERAL MANAGEMENT OPTIONS
Hydration

Adequate hydration promotes lubrication, which helps the vocal fold mucosa withstand the rigors of vibratory collisions and shearing forces. Consistency supply of fluids seems to be particularly important. An expectorant, such as guaifenesin, may also help when secretions are viscid.

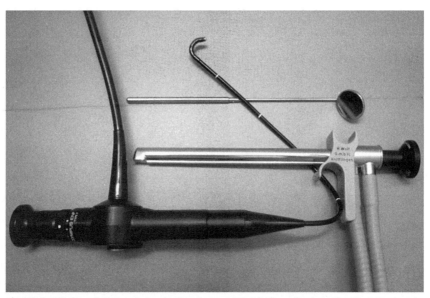

Figure 95-4. Three of the most commonly used tools for viewing the larynx: a mirror, a 90-degree telescope, and a flexible fiberoptic nasolaryngoscope.

Sinonasal Management

Patients often incorrectly attribute chronic hoarseness to sinonasal conditions. Existing sinonasal problems should be managed on their own merits; however, the clinician may need to help diminish the patient's perception of the contribution of these problems in favor of more convincing behavioral causes. When optimal laryngeal function is of concern, as in a vocal performer, nasal conditions should be managed locally (topically) when possible. This is because many systemic drugs (e.g., oral decongestants, antihistamine-decongestant combinations) dry not only nasal secretions, but also those in the larynx, where a continuous secretional flow is important for proper vibratory function and mucosal endurance, particularly under demanding phonatory conditions. Medications that affect voice minimally are the topical nasal decongestants, which should be used for only a few days before the nasal mucosa is allowed to rest, so as to avoid *rhinitis medicamentosa*. Profuse rhinorrhea that accompanies the common cold can also be managed with ipratropium bromide inhalations.[32,33] Corticosteroid inhalers are invaluable for the management of nasal allergies. Activating pump-action nasal inhalers without any inspiratory airflow will avoid the (undocumented) risk of nasally applied corticosteroid effects on the vocal folds.

Management of Acid Reflux Laryngopharyngitis

In a person with an incompetent lower esophageal sphincter or hiatal hernia, acid reflux into the pharynx and larynx during sleep can lead to chronic laryngopharyngitis. Such persons may or may not experience one or more of the following symptoms: a particularly bad taste in the morning; excessive phlegm; scratchy or dry throat irritation, which usually is worse in the morning; habitual throat clearing; and mild huskiness or lowered pitch of the voice in the morning. The larynx may show characteristic erythema of the arytenoid mucosa, interarytenoid pachyderma, or contact ulcers; laryngeal findings may, however, be subtle (Figure 95-5).

Basic management of this condition consists of avoiding caffeine, alcohol, and spicy foods; eating the last meal of the day (preferably a light one) no fewer than 3 hours before retiring; using bed blocks to place the bed on a mild head-to-foot slant; and taking at bedtime an antacid or H_2 blocker, or a proton pump inhibitor 1 hour before dinner.

Acute Mucosal Swelling of Overuse

Public speakers or singers may sometimes perform of necessity despite acute, noninfectious mucosal swelling resulting from recent overuse of the voice. A careful strategy of vocal rest is needed but sometimes not possible, and a preperformance warm-up, along with solid vocal technique, may be sufficient for the patient to "get through." A short-term, high-dose, tapering regimen of corticosteroids might also be useful in this context, as part of a larger strategy to help the patient through the performance.

Laryngeal Instillations for Mucosal Inflammation

In past years moreso than currently, laryngologists have used drugs such as mono-*p*-chlorphenol, topical anesthetics, mild vasoconstrictors, sulfur vapors, certain

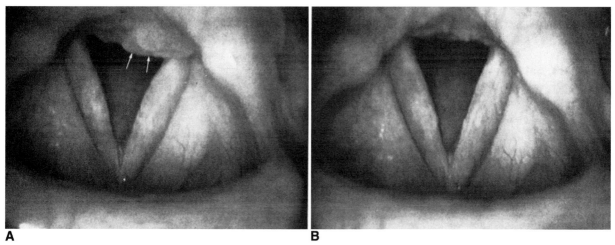

A **B**

Figure 95-5. Chronic laryngitis in a patient with severe acid reflux, a history of smoking, and excessive voice use. **A,** Note the interarytenoid pachyderma (*arrows*) and loss of normal color differential between true folds and supraglottic mucosa. Broad-based convexity of the true vocal fold margins suggests diffuse submucosal edema. **B,** Three weeks after institution of antireflux measures. Note the resolution of the interarytenoid pachyderma.

oils, and other substances for reduction of swelling, soothing effect, or promotion of healing. Although some physicians and patients believe in the efficacy of such management, it is supported only by anecdotal reports.

Systemic Medicines That May Affect the Larynx

Medicines that patients take for other reasons (e.g., antidepressants, decongestants, antihypertensives, diuretics) may dry and thicken normal secretions, thereby reducing their protective lubricating effect on the vocal folds and conceivably making the vocal fold mucosa more vulnerable to the development of benign disorders. History-taking should include inquiry about these medicines.

VOICE THERAPY

A course of therapy by a voice-qualified speech pathologist is frequently appropriate in patients with benign vocal fold mucosal disorders, which arise commonly with vocal overdoers. Vocal nodules in particular are expected to resolve, regress, or at least stabilize under a regimen of improved voice hygiene and optimized voice production. Although in some cases success is defined as having achieved a reliable, husky voice, without previously-experienced episodes of severe hoarseness or even aphonia, in other cases success may require complete resolution of all upper voice limitations. If surgery becomes an option because the mucosal disorder has not resolved completely and the patient regards residual symptoms and vocal limitations as unacceptable, voice therapy will have optimized the patient's surgical candidacy by decreasing the risk of recurrence postoperatively.

During evaluation, speech pathologists gather information on behavior that may adversely affect the voice and establish a program to eliminate injurious behavior. Voice-qualified speech pathologists also model and elicit a battery of spoken and sung vocal tasks to make an auditory-perceptual judgment of the type and degree of impairment and the efficiency of voice production for both speaking and singing. Depending on the results of this part of the evaluation, the speech pathologist may help the patient optimize the intensity, average pitch, registration, resonance characteristics, overall quality, general and vocal tract posture, and respiratory support for voice production. For singers, the singing teacher plays an invaluable role in this process, particularly with respect to singing voice production. Finally, some voice clinicians or technicians may document various aspects of vocal tract output, using acoustic analysis, spirometric measures to test respiratory adequacy, frequency and loudness measures, translaryngeal airflow rates, and other measures under various conditions.

(Information concerning what diagnostic information this adds to that already available from the history, vocal capability battery, and videostroboscopy appears to be lacking.) Speech pathologists may use this equipment for biofeedback (e.g., using a visual electronic frequency readout to modify average pitch for speech in a tone-deaf patient). For obligate false vocal fold phonation and intractable psychogenic disorders of voice production with visible vocal fold posture abnormalities, videoendoscopy can also be converted into an effective biofeedback tool[8,13] (Figure 95-6).

SURGERY

With some exceptions, vocal fold microsurgery should follow an appropriate trial of voice therapy. Patients are typically reexamined (vocal capability battery and videostroboscopy) at 8-week intervals after diagnosis. When a compliant patient does not improve on two or more successive examinations and remains unhappy with the voice's capabilities, surgery may be considered. Good surgical results are directly related to the accuracy of diagnosis, surgical judgment and precision, and the patient's compliance with proper voice care.

Although specific techniques vary for each disorder, the basic requirements for successful laryngeal microsurgery for all benign vocal fold mucosal disorders are the same. An understanding of vocal fold microarchitecture and vibratory dynamics is a prerequisite, and preoperative and postoperative videostroboscopic evaluation is necessary so that the patient and surgeon can see the results together, although this may initially be uncomfortable for the surgeon.

The first principle of surgery is that microlaryngoscopy (not direct laryngoscopy with the unaided eye) and extreme technical precision are required to disturb minimal mucosa. Because the disorder is benign and confined to the mucosa, including Reinke's potential space, the cancer concept of margins does not apply. Every case should be approached with the awareness that overly aggressive or imprecise surgery of the vocal fold mucosa can lead to disastrous results caused by scarring of regenerated or surgically manipulated mucosa to the underlying vocal ligament.

A full set of laryngoscopes, microlaryngeal forceps, scissors, dissectors, and knives should be on hand; Kleinsasser[53] noted that a relatively simple set suffices the experienced surgeon (Figure 95-7).

The carbon dioxide laser has become an important part of the surgeon's armamentarium, and many have discussed its application to benign laryngeal disorders. Tissue effects of the laser depend on spot size and focus, wattage, duration of beam activation, waveform mode (pulsed vs continuous), and perhaps most important, surgical precision. Microdissection may be

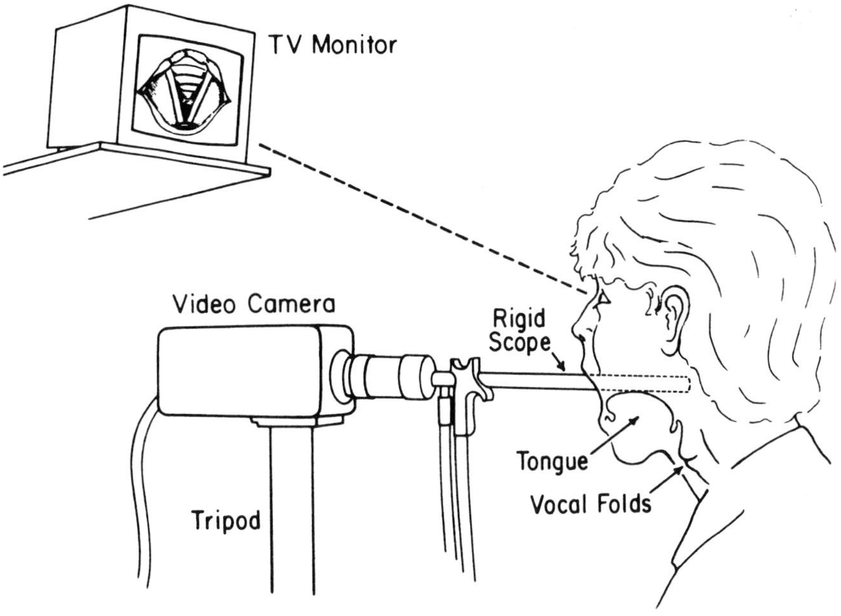

Figure 95-6. A patient learning to modify laryngeal posture by use of laryngeal image biofeedback. With a telescope rather than a fiberscope, pure vocal fold behavior is retrained initially (without speech gestures). Clearer optics and less mobility of the epiglottis permit a clearer and more stable view.

safer than laser techniques, provided the surgeon is equally proficient in both. Norris and Mullarky[73] compared continuous-mode carbon dioxide laser with cold scalpel for incising pig skin and reported that a short-term advantage resulted after laser incision with regard to the speed of reepithelialization; no long-term difference in healing was noted. However, although not noted in their article their histologic sections clearly showed a wider zone of tissue destruction beneath the epithelium with laser than with scalpel. Duncavage and Toohill[34] compared healing response in dogs after traditional fold stripping vs carbon dioxide mucosal vaporization. They concluded that, until late in healing, more edema, giant-cell reactions to bits of charred debris, and greater subepithelial fibrosis occurred with the laser technique than with the cup forceps alone. Manipulation of wattage, focus, and mode of laser irradiation of tissues may decrease thermal injury, charring, and other adverse effects of the laser.

The microspot laser[82,83] may also diminish these disadvantages, although a systematic comparison of functional results (including vocal capabilities and videostroboscopy) is not available to guide the surgeon in choosing between laser and microdissection methods.

After surgery, vocal quality, and more importantly, capabilities should show good to excellent improvement; however, patients should be counseled preoperatively that surgery may worsen the voice. For the experienced surgeon who uses dissection, rather than grab-and-pull techniques, along with preoperative and postoperative videostroboscopy as his or her "teacher," the question becomes not so much one of possibly making the voice worse, but rather, "Can I make this patient's speaking and singing capabilities normal, and if not, how close can I come?" Cornut's and Bouchayer's[25] experience operating on 101 singers and Bastian's[9] experience established a role for laryngeal microsurgery in restoring vocal capabilities and in diminishing or abolishing limitations.

SPECIFIC BENIGN VOCAL FOLD MUCOSAL DISORDERS
Vocal Nodules

The term *nodules* should be reserved for lesions of proven chronicity. Recent or acute mucosal swellings, which disappear quickly in response to simple voice rest and perhaps supportive medical management, are thus excluded when one is referring to nodules.

Epidemiology

Vocal nodules occur most commonly in boys and women. Such persons are almost always "vocal overdoers" (i.e., six or seven on the seven-point talkativeness scale.) A high push from within correlates more consistently than occupation, unless the occupation is extraordinarily demanding vocally (e.g., rock singer, stock trader). Comparatively, children with cleft palates

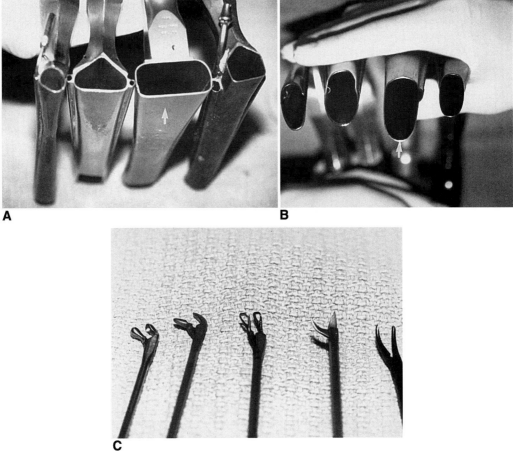

Figure 95-7. A, The viewing end (left to right) of the Holinger hourglass, Jako-Cherry, Bouchayer, and Dedo laryngoscopes. **B,** The distal end of the laryngoscopes (same order). The Bouchayer scope (*arrow*) is most useful for microsurgery. **C,** From left, the up-cup forceps, smaller biting forceps, Bouchayer microring forceps, curved scissors, and curved alligator forceps.

develop nodules frequently, presumably from using glottal stops to compensate for velopharyngeal incompetence.

Pathophysiology and Pathology

Only the anterior two thirds (membranous portion) of the vocal folds participates in vibration because the arytenoid cartilage lies within the posterior third of the glottic aperture. The mucosal shearing and collisional forces of each vibratory cycle can be viewed videostroboscopically. Thus, vibration that is too forceful or prolonged causes localized vascular congestion with edema at the midportion of the membranous (vibratory) portion of the vocal folds, where shearing and collisional forces are greatest. Fluid accumulation in the submucosa from acute abuse or overuse results in submucosal swelling (sometimes unwisely called *incipient* or *early nodules*). Long-term voice abuse leads to some hyalinization of

Reinke's potential space and possibly some thickening of the overlying epithelium. This pathophysiologic sequence explains the easily reversible nature of most acute nonhemorrhagic swellings vs slower or failed resolution of chronic vocal nodules. The change in mucosal mass, lessened ability to thin the free margin, and incomplete glottic closure caused by the nodules account for a constellation of vocal symptoms and limitations that is characteristic of mucosal swelling.[13]

Diagnosis

History. A pediatric patient with vocal nodules is usually described by the parent as vocally exuberant. An adult patient, virtually always a woman who describes herself as a six or seven on the talkativeness scale, describes experiencing chronic hoarseness or repeated episodes of acute hoarseness. Sometimes the initial onset is associated with an upper respiratory infection or acute laryngitis, after which the hoarseness never clears completely, leading the patient to incorrectly attribute the voice problem to the infection and to neglect higher-ranked ongoing behavioral causes. Singers with chronic nodules are usually relatively unaware of speaking voice limitations unless the nodules are at least moderate in size. More sensitive symptoms of vocal nodules include the following:

1. Loss of the ability to sing high notes softly
2. Delayed phonatory onset, particularly with high, soft singing
3. Increased breathiness (air escape), roughness, and harshness
4. Reduced vocal endurance
5. A sensation of increased effort for singing
6. A need for longer warm-ups
7. Day-to-day variability of vocal capabilities, which is greater than expected for the singer's level of vocal training

Vocal capability battery. In patients with moderate to large vocal nodules, the speaking voice is usually lower than expected, husky, breathy, or harsh. Patients with subtle to moderate swellings often have speaking voices that sound normal; the speaking voice is an insensitive indicator of mucosal disorders compared with the singing voice. In patients with subtle or small swellings (usually only singers present with small mucosal disturbances), vocal limitations (e.g., delayed phonatory onset with preceding momentary air escape, diplophonia, inability to sing softly at high frequencies) may become evident[12] only when high-frequency, low-intensity vocal tasks for detecting swelling are elicited. At high frequency, short-segment vibration may occur; in other words, the nodules stop vibrating and the short segments of mucosa anterior or posterior to them, or both, vibrates.

Many patients with nodules may have undergone indirect laryngoscopy and been told that their vocal folds were normal or given a nonspecific diagnosis such as "laryngeal irritation." Use of vocal tasks that detect swellings and videostroboscopy, when indicated (see Figures 95-3 and 95-4), will protect the laryngologist from missing the diagnosis of even subtle vocal fold swellings, a failure of diagnosis which can have serious consequences for the professional voice user.

Laryngeal examination. Nodules can vary in size, contour, symmetry, and color, depending on how long they have been present, the amount of recent voice use, and interindividual differences in mucosal response to voice abuse. Also, some variability exists in the correlation between size of nodules and their effect on vocal capabilities. Nodules do not occur unilaterally, although one may be somewhat larger than that on the other side. It is important to distinguish between nodules and cysts because management of these conditions differs. The correlation between the visually estimated softness or hardness of nodules and subsequent reversibility with voice therapy is imperfect. The larynx should be examined at high frequency (500–1000 Hz) to see subtle to small swellings, which can be poorly appreciated at lower frequencies.

Management

Medical. Medical management focuses on ensuring good laryngeal lubrication through general hydration, and, when appropriate, on managing the (usually secondary) contributions of allergy and nighttime reflux of stomach acid into the larynx.

Behavioral. Given the predominately behavioral etiology of vocal nodules, even for patients whose voice disturbance began with an upper respiratory infection, speech (voice) therapy should play a primary role initially. Typically, the nodules and the patient's more obvious symptoms will regress, particularly if the patient is not a singer. However, even when a highly skilled, voice-qualified speech pathologist is available, behavioral (voice) therapy sometimes fails to result in complete visual resolution of nodules that have been present for many months to years. The correlation among reduction of symptoms, decreased vocal limitations, and resolution of the visual findings is not exact. Sensitive singing tasks that detect impairment (not the size of persistent swellings) are generally more helpful for deciding whether to consider surgical removal.[11,12]

Surgical. Surgical removal becomes an option when nodules persist (even when they have regressed and are quite small), and the voice remains unacceptably impaired (from the patient's perspective) after an adequate trial of therapy (generally a minimum of 3 months, usually much longer). Some authors prefer precise removal using microdissection techniques (Figure 95-8). Vocal fold stripping has no place in the surgery of nodules. The proper duration of voice rest is controversial; some authors prefer a relatively short period. Typically, the patient is asked not to speak for 4 days, although sighing sounds begin 1 day after surgery. Beginning on the fourth day, the patient gradually progresses over 6 weeks to full voice use under a speech pathologist's supervision. Early return to nonstressful voice use as described in Box 95-1 seems to promote dynamic healing and preserve a degree of mucosal freedom from the underlying vocal ligament. The results of precision surgery are typically remarkably good, even in singers. Cornut and Bouchayer[25] stated, in their study of approximately 160 singers treated with surgery, "[As long as certain management

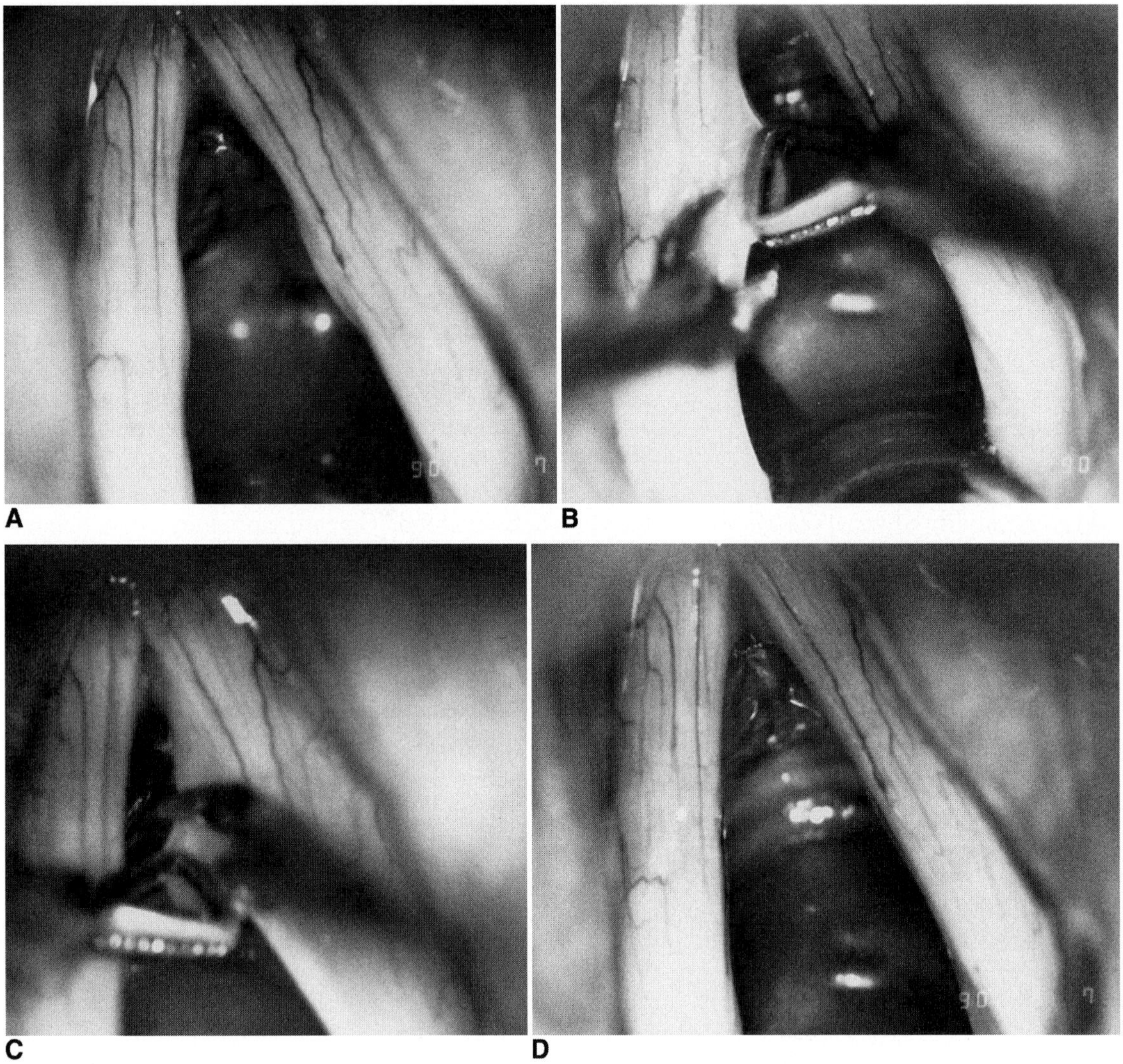

Figure 95-8. The operative sequence for a professional musical theater actress who had been experiencing vocal symptoms and limitations compatible with fusiform vocal nodules for more than 2 years. **A,** The operative view after many months of conservative management. Not all fusiform swellings are reversible with conservative measures alone. **B** and **C,** A polypoid nodule is grasped superficially and tented medially with Bouchayer forceps. Scissors, which curve away from vocal fold, are used for removal. The nodule is thus removed in a very superficial plane, thereby minimizing the risk of scarring of the remaining and regenerated mucosa to the underlying vocal ligament. **D,** The vocal fold appearance after excision. The patient experienced dramatic normalization of vocal capabilities and no evidence of scarring based on postoperative stroboscopic examination. The dilated capillaries may predispose to recurrent nodule formation and can be spot-coagulated with microspot laser.

principles are followed] in a majority of cases, laryngeal microsurgery enables the singing voice to regain the whole of its functioning."

Capillary Ectasia
Epidemiology

Capillary ectasia (Figures 95-9, 95-10, and 95-11) seems to happen most often with vocal overdoers. Because dilated capillaries occur more frequently in women, some authors have speculated about an estrogen effect.

Pathophysiology and Pathology

Repeated vibratory microtrauma can lead to capillary angiogenesis. In a circular fashion, abnormally dilated capillaries seem to increase the mucosa's vulnerability to further vibratory trauma. In particular, mucosal swelling, when present with capillary ectasia, always

BOX 95-1

GENERAL GUIDELINES FOR INITIAL VOICE USE AFTER VOCAL FOLD MICROSURGERY

Time after surgery*	Talking†	Singing (for singers)
Days 1 to 4–5	None	Gentle attempts at yawning or sigh for approximately 30 sec, 6–8 times per day‡
Week 1 (after first examination)	2	5 min twice per day
Week 2	3	10 min twice per day§
Week 3 (after second examination)	4	15 min twice per day
Week 4	4 or 5	20 min twice per day§
Weeks 5–8 (after third examination)	4 or 5	Up to 20 min three times per day‖

*After fourth examination, consider return to performance.
†Based on a seven-point talkativeness scale, in which 1 = very untalkative; 4 = average; and 7 = extremely talkative.
‡Accept what comes out, even if it is only air or is very hoarse.
§With emphasis on ease, clarity, and agility, not voice building. The entire expected range should be practiced in each session, with gentle insistence on high notes that do not want to sound. In general, practice, mostly a mezzo piano dynamic and only occasionally a mezzo forte.
‖Same as above footnote, but gradually increase the dynamic range and insistence.

appears to be larger on the side with greater ectasia. It seems that capillary ectasia predisposes to mucosal swelling, to a small incidence of vocal fold hemorrhage, and to hemorrhagic polyp formation.

Diagnosis

History. Capillary ectasia is diagnosed most often in female singers who complain that they become a little hoarse after relatively short periods of singing (reduced vocal endurance). When associated with mucosal swelling, additional symptoms reminiscent of nodules (e.g., delayed phonatory onset, loss of high soft singing, increased effort) may also be noted. The occasional singer with capillary ectasia may have experienced one or more episodes of acute vocal fold hemorrhage, which may precipitate the patient's first visit; capillary ectasia may be discerned only after the bruising has resolved.

Vocal capability battery. Without mucosal swelling, the voice's capabilities may be entirely normal. With swelling, vocal limitations may be similar to those

detected in the patient with nodules. If mucosal hemorrhage is recent, the speaking and singing voice may be very hoarse.

Laryngeal examination. Capillary ectasia may manifest as abnormal dilation of the long arcades of capillaries that proceed mostly anterior to posterior (see Figures 95-9, 95-10, and 95-11). However, aberrant clusters of dilated capillaries also may be seen. Occasionally, a virtual vascular dot may appear when a loop comes from within Reinke's space to the surface and doubles back down into the submucosa. Finally, some dilated capillaries are confluent or become so large as to almost resemble a chronic hemorrhage. This variant can be termed a *capillary lake*.

Management

Medical. Use of drugs that have anticoagulant effects (aspirin, nonsteroidal antiinflammatory drugs) should cease if medically appropriate. These drugs do not necessarily increase the risk of hemorrhage but may increase the severity of bruising. In addition, acid reflux may have an amplified effect on the mucosa when capillary ectasia is visible; thus, management of reflux is particularly important.

Behavioral. Many persons with capillary ectasia are vocal overdoers; therefore, the usual behavioral changes, which are also appropriate for persons with nodules, are advocated. In particular, patients are warned about sudden, explosive use of voice. The duration of voice use per practice session should also be reduced (e.g., three 20-minute sessions vs one 1-hour session).

Surgical. If the patient cannot accept residual vocal symptoms and limitations (e.g., decreased vocal endurance) after medical and behavioral management, laryngeal microsurgery is an excellent option.[95] Dilated capillaries are spot-coagulated to interrupt blood flow every few millimeters (see Figure 95-9, *C*). Capillaries proximal to each interrupted segment may subsequently dilate. Even so, not all visible dilations should be ablated; those that remain visible at the end of the procedure and even at the first postoperative visit routinely involute within a few weeks. If mucosal edema is minimal, management of the capillaries alone often leads to edema resolution.

Vocal Fold Hemorrhage and a Unilateral (Hemorrhagic) Vocal Fold Polyp
Epidemiology

The occurrence of vocal fold hemorrhage (see Figure 95-10) and a unilateral hemorrhagic vocal fold polyp is more common in men, particularly men who engage

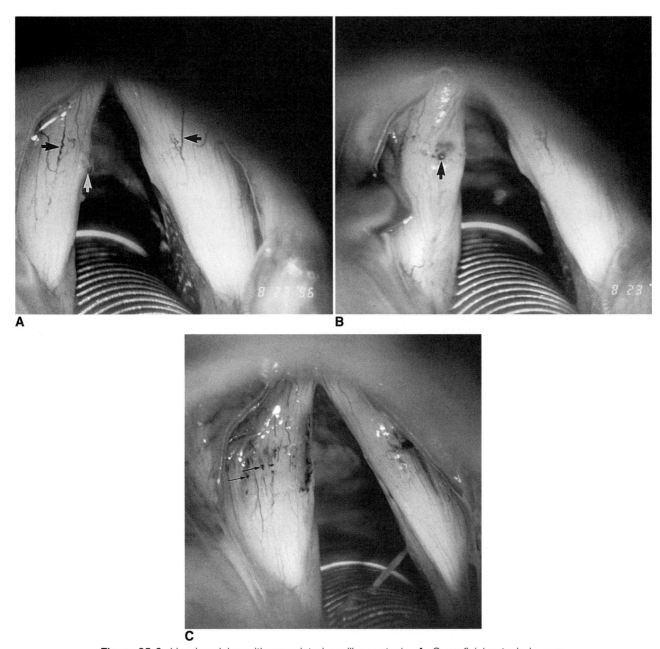

Figure 95-9. Vocal nodules with associated capillary ectasia. **A,** Superficial ectasia is seen (*black arrows*); the white arrow indicates deeper ectasia seen within left-sided nodule. **B,** The left vocal fold margin is rolled up onto the superior surface of the fold so that ectasia within the nodule can be seen more clearly (*arrow*), particularly the knuckle variant. **C,** Nodules have been removed (see Figure 95-8), but spot coagulation of dilated capillaries is present at approximately 2-mm intervals (*arrows*).

in intermittent severe voice abuse or who work in noisy environments. Some patients have a history of aspirin or other anticoagulant use.

Pathophysiology and Pathology

Shearing forces acting on capillaries within the mucosa during extreme vocal exertion lead to capillary rupture. Capillary ectasia seems to predispose to this sort of injury. Superficial capillary breakage may lead to a thin, widely suffused, superficial bruise without vocal fold margin convexity. This hemorrhage often may have little effect on mucosal oscillation. Resolution of the bruise may be complete within 2 weeks. However, extravasation of blood and accumulation of edema from a deeper capillary may lead to pooled blood, similar to a blood blister. This type of hemorrhage will alter

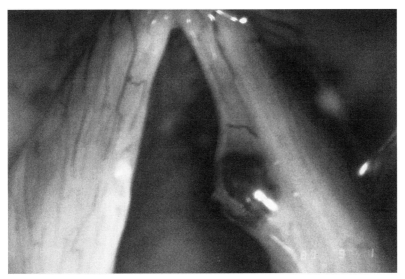

Figure 95-10. An operative view of a hemorrhagic polyp on the right true vocal fold of 14 months' duration. Note the capillary ectasia.

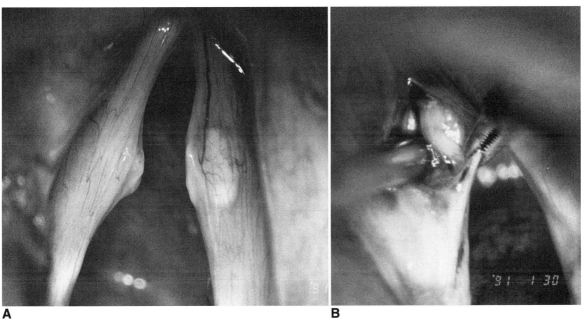

A   B

Figure 95-11. A, A large right epidermoid inclusion cyst with a characteristic dilated capillary. Note the large left nodule. **B,** An epidermoid inclusion cyst in another patient is delivered through a cordotomy incision.

the margin contour and stiffen the mucosa, as seen stroboscopically. It will cause significantly more and longer-lasting hoarseness and may even be the precursor of a hemorrhagic polyp. In this case, microscopic examination would reveal a relatively rich vascular stroma and areas of hyalinization, although a unilateral, nonhemorrhagic, often pedunculated polyp may also be seen as the end stage of a hemorrhagic polyp.

Diagnosis

History. The history of abrupt onset of hoarseness during extreme vocal effort, such as at a party or sporting event, or even after a loud sneeze, is classic but not universal in these patients.

Vocal capability battery. Vocal capabilities vary depending on the size, age, turgidity, and pedunculation of the polyp. Some patients have a normal-sounding speaking voice, except for intermittent subtle aberrant sounds. Other patients have a normal speaking voice but an impaired or nonexistent falsetto register. Some patients also manifest chronic vocal huskiness.

Laryngeal examination. Laryngeal examination reveals a largely unilateral lesion process in the node position, a contact reaction on the fold opposite the polyp, or a nodule if the person is a long-standing overdoer; the polyp represents an acute injury superimposed on chronic nodules. The hemorrhagic polyp usually is much larger than the typical nodule and may appear dark and hemorrhagic in early stages. If bleeding was recent, discoloration may be in any stage of bruise evolution. Long-standing, hemorrhagic polyps may lose their vascular appearance and become pedunculated, moving in and out of the glottis with inspiration and expiration, respectively. During phonation, this end-stage polyp may be displaced upward onto the fold's superior surface, interfering little with basic phonation.

Treatment

Medical. If possible, the intake of anticoagulant medications (e.g., aspirin, nonsteroidal antiinflammatory drugs, warfarin) should be stopped. Because acid reflux can increase hyperemia and dilate normal and abnormal capillaries, this condition should be controlled.

Behavioral. A short course of voice therapy is appropriate, mainly to instruct the patient in voice care. The occasional small, early hemorrhagic polyp will resorb completely with many months of conservative measures, but typically surgical removal is required to return the vocal fold to its normal appearance and vibratory function and to return the voice to normal capabilities.

Surgical. Evacuation of blood through a tiny incision in a recent large hemorrhage that looks like a blood blister may be appropriate. This is because one would expect a long wait for resorption (in the best case) and likely progression to a chronic hemorrhagic polyp. After microsurgical evacuation of the hematoma, care should be taken to detect the large capillaries within Reinke's space because these also should be interrupted, although a slightly deeper coagulation may be required to reach the level of the capillary. A long-standing polyp—whether hemorrhagic or end-stage and pale—should be trimmed away superficially at the time the spot coagulations take place. In the absence of associated limiting lesions beyond the polyp, progno-

sis for full return of vocal functioning after precision surgery is excellent.

Intracordal Cysts
Epidemiology

The most prominent epidemiologic finding is a history of vocal overuse. This is routine for the epidermoid cyst, but less so for the mucus retention variety.

Pathophysiology and Pathology

Histologically, intracordal cysts (Figures 95-11, 95-12, and 95-13) are classified as either mucus retention or epidermoid inclusion types. Mucus retention (ductal) cysts (see Figure 95-12) arise when the duct of a mucus gland becomes plugged and retains glandular secretions; epidermoid cysts (see Figure 95-13) contain accumulated keratin.[18,19,25,57,67] Two theories state that the epidermoid cyst results from a rest of epithelial cells buried congenitally in the subepithelial layer or from healing of mucosa injured by voice abuse over buried epithelial cells. Cysts may rupture spontaneously. If the resulting opening is small in relation the overall size of the cyst, some epidermoid debris may be retained and may create an open cyst; if the opening is as large as the cyst, the resulting empty pocket becomes a glottic sulcus.

Diagnosis

History. A patient with epidermoid cysts has many of the same symptoms and voice abuse factors as a patient with nodules. Mucus retention cysts can arise seemingly spontaneously.

Vocal capability battery. The vocal capability battery uncovers vocal limitations similar to those for a patient with vocal nodules. Patients with epidermoid cysts are more likely to experience diplophonia in the upper voice, and they may manifest an abrupt and irreducible transition to severe impairment at a relatively specific frequency rather than a more gradual transition to greater degrees of impairment, as often noted in patients with nodules. Mucus retention cysts often cause less vocal limitation than anticipated from the laryngeal appearance; epidermoid inclusion cysts often cause more limitation than expected.

Laryngeal examination. Mucus retention cysts often originate just below the free margin of the fold with significant medial projection from the fold. For this reason, mucus retention cysts are sometimes misdiagnosed as a nodule or polyp. Epidermoid cysts project less from the fold and are harder to diagnose when small. An inexperienced clinician may be more aware of what appear to be nodules than the faint cyst outline on the superior surface of the fold (see Figure 95-13).

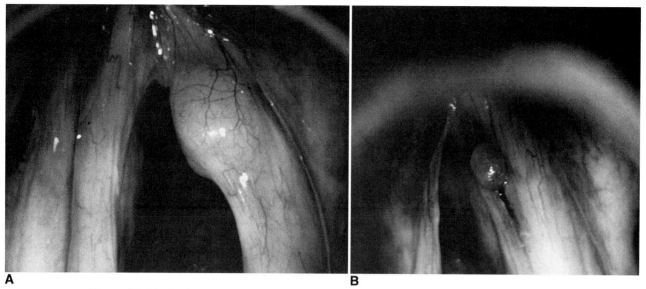

Figure 95-12. A, A mucus retention cyst of the right vocal fold. Note the relatively greater margin deformation compared with the epidermoid inclusion cyst. **B,** In another patient, a cyst is delivered through cordotomy incision.

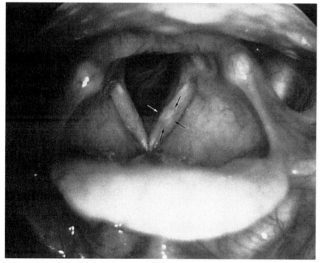

Figure 95-13. A 90-degree telescope view shows a faint spherical outline of a small epidermoid inclusion cyst (*arrows*).

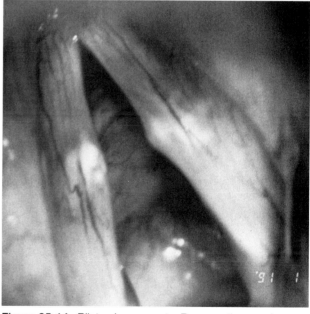

Figure 95-14. Bilateral open cysts. Because the openings are small in relation to the size of the cysts, partial emptying of the keratin contents causes a mottled appearance.

In an open cyst, the sphere may be less discrete and have a more mottled appearance on the superior surface of the vocal fold (Figure 95-14). Under strobe illumination, as the fundamental frequency of phonation increases, the mucosa overlying the cyst often stops vibrating before the mucosa anterior and posterior to the cyst. Even so, diagnosis can be confirmed in some patients only at the time of microlaryngoscopy.

Treatment

Medical. General supportive measures (e.g., hydration, potential acid reflux management) may be helpful.

Behavioral. Voice therapy is more appropriate for persons with epidermoid cysts than for those with the mucus retention variety. This is because persons with epidermoid inclusion cysts are more likely to be vocal overdoers than persons with mucus retention cysts. When the diagnosis is uncertain or when the surgeon and nurse provide little in the way of education, a course of voice therapy may also be warranted, even when a mucus retention cyst is found in a person without risk factors for mucosal reactive lesions. Postoperative voice therapy from a speech pathologist and singing teacher may facilitate healing.

Surgery. Patients with large mucus retention cysts and no history of voice abuse may be scheduled for surgery promptly. If under the edge of the vocal fold and extremely superficial and translucent (resembling a polyp), the cyst may be unroofed because its wall is so thin as to make its dissection from the overlying mucosa virtually impossible. In this case, mucosal oscillation may be normal after healing is complete. More typical mucus retention cysts are removed as described below.

A small, extremely shallow incision is made on the fold's superior surface. Careful dissection reveals that the swelling is indeed caused by a cyst. Taking care to avoid any injury to mucosa, other than that of the incision, the surgeon dissects the cyst free of the mucosa and vocal ligament (Figure 95-15). The opposite fold should be examined carefully because of the possibility of a more subtle cyst or sulcus. Results are not uniformly as good as for nodules and polyps. Considerable improvement is expected, however, and a percentage of patients achieve excellent results. Patients should also know that postoperative recovery takes longer than for nodule or polyp surgery (many months rather than a few weeks). Bouchayer and others[17] reported a series of 148 patients managed for cysts, sulci, or

mucosal bridges (very difficult surgical problems compared with nodules and polyps), of whom 10% had an overall excellent result, 42% a good result, 41% a fair result, and 5% a poor result. Follow-up supportive voice therapy from the speech pathologist or singing teacher assists vocal rehabilitation. A return to active voice use or training should occur within a few days of surgery because the amount of mucosal disturbance required leads to a greater tendency to mucosal adherence and stiffness.

Glottic Sulcus
Epidemiology

Although some believe sulci (Figures 95-16, 95-17, and 95-18) to be congenital, this entity occurs exclusively in vocal overdoers.

Pathophysiology and Pathology

Bouchayer and others[17] reviewed "acquired" vs "congenital" theories for these conditions. They described the appearance of the sulcus as an epithelium-lined pocket whose lips parallel the free edge of the folds and suggested that a sulcus may represent an epidermoid cyst that has spontaneously emptied, leaving the collapsed pocket behind to form a sulcus. In effect, a mucosal bridge (see Figure 95-18) is the result of two parallel sulci arising from a single cyst.

Diagnosis

History. A glottic sulcus patient often has a history of voice overuse and complains of chronic hoarseness.

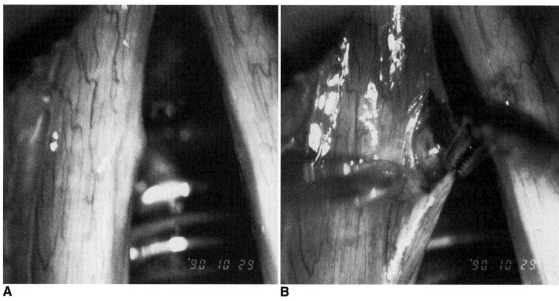

A   **B**

Figure 95-15. An operative sequence for removal of small mucus retention cyst in patient previously diagnosed as having vocal nodules. **A,** Initial operative view, left vocal fold. **B,** The cyst is exposed through an incision made on the superior surface of the fold.

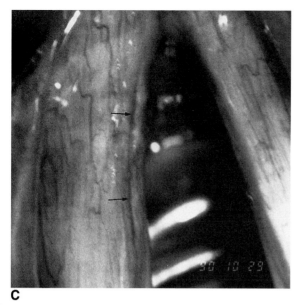

C

Figure 95-15, cont'd C, After removal of the cyst and redraping of undamaged overlying mucosa, only an incision line is seen (*arrows*). The patient's vocal fold was stiff under strobe illumination for several weeks postoperatively but ultimately regained full vibratory amplitude and mucosal wave as compared with unoperated cord. Vocal capabilities also returned to normal. With larger cysts, some stiffness can be recognized postoperatively on a permanent basis, particularly as the patient phonates at high frequencies.

Vocal capability battery. The voice is typically noticeably hoarse. Upper voice limitations, particularly diplophonia, are obvious. As for cysts, the transition between phonation and aphonia may occur abruptly, almost at a specific frequency, generally in the middle of the voice.

Laryngeal examination. Laryngeal examination may initially reveal fewer number of findings than expected to account for the abnormal speaking voice or reduced singing voice capabilities. Because the patient is likely a vocal overdoer, associated fusiform vocal fold margin swellings might also be seen. Stroboscopic evaluation reveals a segment of reduced vibration. The entire length of the mucosa may oscillate at lower frequencies; at higher frequencies, the midportion of the mucosa stops oscillating and short-segment vibration begins to occur. Microlaryngoscopy is required for definitive diagnosis because the lips of the sulcus are only occasionally faintly visible with inspiratory phonation during the office or voice laboratory examination.

Management

Medical. Medical management for glottic sulcus is supportive as appropriate.

Behavioral. A short preoperative course of voice therapy is indicated if the patient with glottal sulcus is a confirmed vocal overdoer, because the behavioral goal for patients with cysts is initially more selection

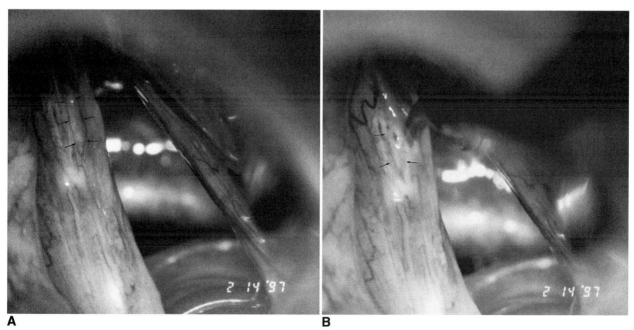

A   **B**

Figure 95-16. Sulcus of the left true vocal fold seen **(A)** undisturbed and **(B)** with forceps used to spread open its lips.

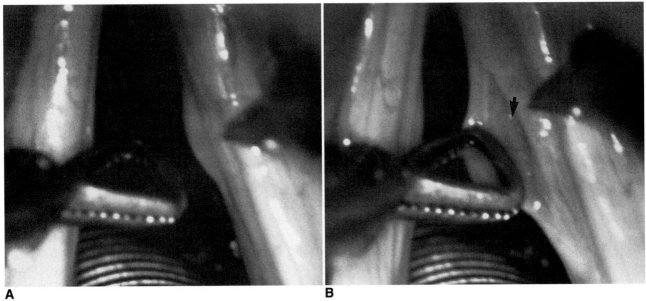

A **B**

Figure 95-17. A, An operative view of a chronic polypoid nodule. **B,** At the time of medial tenting of the mucosa preparatory to excision, a previously unsuspected sulcus is discovered (*arrow*). In this case, excision of the polypoid nodule alone without specifically addressing the sulcus resulted in marked improvement of vocal capabilities and eliminated this nonsinging patient's chronic hoarseness of the speaking voice.

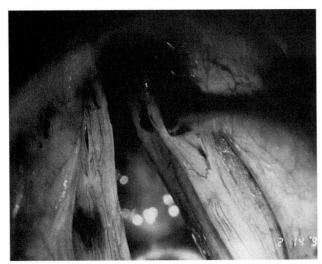

Figure 95-18. A mucosal bridge of the right vocal fold (with forceps passed under it) in the same patient seen in Figure 95-16.

and preparation for surgery rather than restoration of the mucosa to normal.

Surgical. Sulcus removal is technically demanding, and it involves considerable disturbance of the vocal fold mucosa compared with surgery for nodules.

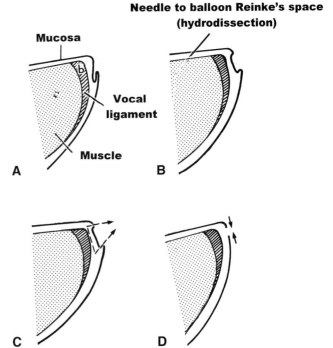

Figure 95-19. Removal of a glottic sulcus. **A,** A vocal fold coronal section shows the sulcus. **B,** Injection of 1% lidocaine with epinephrine into Reinke's space spreads the sulcus lips. **C,** Incisions at the sulcus lips and dissection off the vocal ligament. **D,** After removal of the sulcus.

Bouchayer and others[18] described the steps for removal of a glottic sulcus (Figure 95-19), including cordal injection to make the sulcus lips spread and the sulcus more shallow and to accomplish some hydrodissection. This is followed by circumcision of the lips of the sulcus and dissection of the invaginated mucosal pocket from the underlying fold without injuring the vocal ligament. Although the voice is typically better than before surgery, residual mucosal stiffness may occur even after optimal surgery.

Bilateral Diffuse Polyposis
Epidemiology

Voice change caused by bilateral diffuse polyposis (chronic Reinke's edema or smoker's polyps) (Figure 95-20) most often becomes noticeable enough to prompt a laryngeal examination in middle-aged women who have been long-term smokers.

Pathophysiology and Pathology

Smoking and a degree of talkativeness are required to develop this disorder. There also seems to be an individual susceptibility to this condition because only a small percentage of persons at risk (e.g., smokers who use their voices a lot) develop it. As detailed by several authors, chronic smoking and voice abuse result in edema, vascular congestion, and venous stasis.[53,55] These cause diffuse polypoid changes that become permanent, although the degree of edema may rise and fall with voice use.

Diagnosis

History. The combination of smoking and avid voice use is classic for this entity. A female patient with

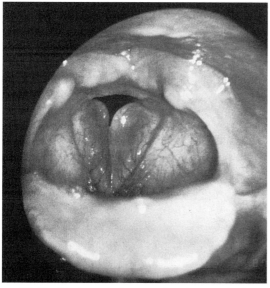

Figure 95-20. Moderately large unilocular smoker's polyps (inspiratory view through a rigid laryngeal telescope).

smoker's polyps may complain of being called "sir" on the phone, or she may have problems with increasing hoarseness during the day.

Vocal capability battery. The voice examination reveals lower pitch than would be expected, often well into the masculine range when the condition is seen in women. Upper voice is lost, and the female patient can often phonate through the range of a true bass singer. With large polyps, the voice may even be hypermasculine.

Laryngeal examination. Laryngeal examination usually reveals pale, watery bags of fluid attached to the superior surface and margins of the folds. Large smoker's polyps may cause an involuntary laryngeal snore on sudden inhalation. A to-and-from motion is often seen with respiration. In severe cases, clusters of polyps on polyps may be seen. Small smoker's polyps are easily overlooked unless the patient is instructed to phonate on inspiration, when the polypoid tissue is drawn from the superior surface of the folds into the glottic aperture and thereby made more visible as a greater-than-normal convexity of the margin. (The examiner will have been guided to elicit inspiratory phonation by having noted the virilization of the patient's singing range during vocal capability testing.)

Management

Medical. The patient with bilateral diffuse polyposis is encouraged to give up smoking. Thyroid function tests can be done if hypothyroidism is suspected. This latter entity has often been invoked, although Reinke's edema is extremely rare in the absence of smoking and avid voice use.

Behavioral. Short-term voice therapy may be appropriate to introduce optimal vocal behavior. These measures alone may reduce the polyps' turgidity, with a corresponding modest improvement in vocal functioning.

Surgical. Microsurgery for polyp reduction is necessary when the voice remains objectionable to the patient. The common practice of stripping the polyps away often results in aphonia for many weeks postoperatively, and the final voice achieved may sound unacceptably high and husky to the patient. Polyp reduction with mucosal sparing (Figure 95-21) is recommended for earlier and optimal return of voice (usually beginning within 10 days). It is better to leave the patient with a voice that still sounds rich (even with some residual polyposis and mild vocal virilization) than to strip the folds and leave the patient with a voice that sounds thin, insubstantial, and effortful.

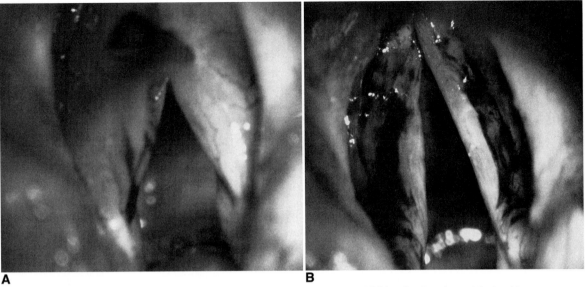

Figure 95-21. A, This operative view is seen after a left vocal fold polyp has been bivalved in the axial plane. Bouchayer forceps are holding the superior half of the polyp in preparation for removal. **B,** The final view after the upper part of polyp has been removed and myxoid material has been suctioned and dissected from between mucosal flap and vocal ligament; the resulting inferiorly based mucosal flap has been redraped over a free edge of the vocal fold. This female patient's speaking voice was markedly virilized preoperatively and considerably feminized postoperatively. The patient was aphonic for only 7 days postoperatively, whereas after traditional stripping, she may not have regained voice for many weeks.

Postsurgical Dysphonia
Epidemiology

Vocal fold surgery can lead to a stable dysphonia (Figures 95-22 and 95-23) that is worse than that which the surgery was designed to correct.[6,94] Commonly, the operative report describes vocal fold stripping or laser vaporization of the mucosa. The pathology report frequently describes a fairly large specimen that may contain fibrous tissue or even muscle, suggesting that the removal went too deeply into the vocal fold.

Pathophysiology and Pathology

Dysphonia can result from a scarred stiff vocal fold cover, phonatory mismatch of the vocal fold margins, or both. In the former case, the degree of freedom of the mucosa from the underlying vocal ligament has been lost where mucosa has adhered to the underlying ligament. In the latter case, the mismatch may arise from an iatrogenic irregularity or mass on the fold margin, such as a granuloma from surgery that exposed the fold's deeper mesenchymal tissues; a depression from too deep an excision; or pseudobowing, such as that from not sparing enough mucosa during smoker's polyp reductions. With few exceptions, postoperative dysphonia can be avoided by use of an appropriately precise surgical technique and by early graduated resumption of voice use after surgery (see Box 95-1).

Diagnosis

History. A history of prior surgery is common to all cases, but a clear understanding of the original lesion should be sought, as well as any history indicating continuing vocal abuse that might indicate recurrent mucosal injury, rather than scarring, as a possibility.

Vocal capability battery. The voice may vary from aphonia to a harsh whisper to a relatively normal speaking voice but with disastrous limitation of the upper singing voice with diplophonia and loss of expected upper range.

Laryngeal examination. Laryngeal videostroboscopy is essential for these patients. This technique allows careful analysis of mass lesions, areas of asymmetry, and the mucosa's vibratory pattern, from which a clear diagnosis and a therapeutic plan can be generated.

Management

Medical. General medical issues that relate to the voice should be optimized in the course of management.

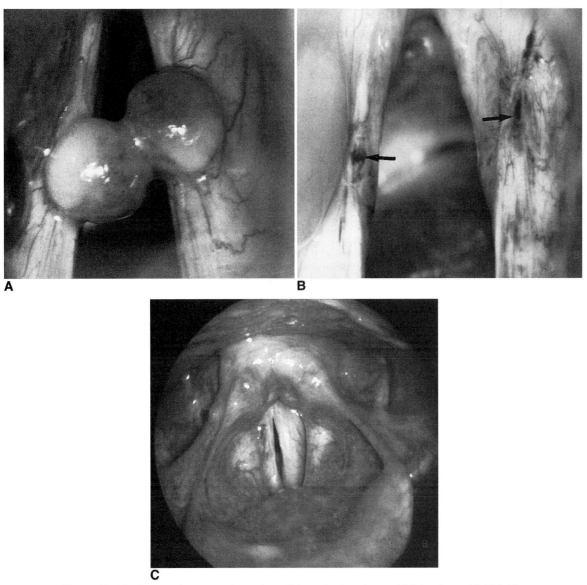

Figure 95-22. Iatrogenic mucosal scarring. This patient underwent bilateral vocal fold "stripping" elsewhere for persistent dysphonia, which was subsequently diagnosed as spasmodic dysphonia. The patient was reportedly aphonic for many weeks postoperatively. **A,** This operative photograph was taken 4.5 months after the original surgery. Granulomas are highly pedunculated and may have eventually detached or regressed spontaneously. Note the medial to lateral reorientation of vocal fold capillaries, a common finding after vocal fold stripping. **B,** The same patient after granuloma removal. Attachment points are marked at arrows. In this view, vocal folds are rolled superiorly, and considerable scarring is evident, particularly on right vocal fold. **C,** The same patient as viewed through a laryngeal telescope a few weeks later. The larynx shows pseudobowing caused by mucosal loss rather than by vocal fold atrophy. Under strobe illumination, these vocal folds were very stiff with minimal mucosal wave evident even at low frequencies. With a voice building regimen and scar maturation, a serviceable but limited voice was achieved.

Behavioral. If stiffness, scarring, and tissue loss are problems, voice therapy is tried first, using a voice-building approach. A person who is resting the voice should stop. Instead, the patient is advised to speak whenever they would otherwise and, in addition, sing with moderately great vigor for 10 minutes two or three times per day at all vocal frequencies of their ranges. Using the facilitating the vowel sound /oo/ is helpful in cases of severe dysphonia. When only a very narrow frequency range is available to a patient

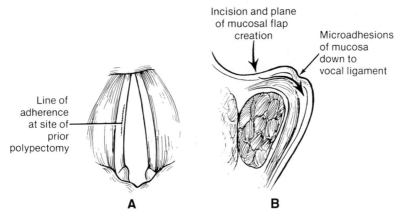

Figure 95-23. Postoperative dysphonia (severe diplophonia) from suspected overly aggressive polypectomy. **A,** The operative view from above shows a longitudinal scar. **B,** Cross-sectional view shows the surgical approach releasing microadhesion of mucosa down to vocal ligament. The patient experienced immediate and enduring relief of diplophonia.

because of postoperative scarring, the patient is asked to start phonating at a frequency that works (often quite high in the expected vocal range) and to coax the voice lower and higher from this small area of working frequencies. Some remarkable improvements may be seen from this approach. However, even with achievement of a serviceable speaking voice, the voice's singing capabilities will remain limited compared with a normal voice. Proof for this approach is difficult to procure. However, improvement does not seem to be only from spontaneous softening of scar tissue because improvement can occur with voice building in patients more than 1 year after surgery or another scarring event.

The rationale for this voice-building strategy may require some explanation for patients, whose voice abuse is what caused the problem for which they underwent surgery. Ideally, a speech pathologist or specialized singing teacher comfortable with teaching vigorous vocal output should monitor voice-building exercises initially. Some patients can work independently because of the short duration of exercise sessions and because the overall idea of the voice-building approach is not to yell or scream or to enhance vocal skills. Rather, the goals are to strengthen the laryngeal musculature to compensate for—overdrive—the damaged mucosa and to encourage the mucosa to oscillate more freely because of this sort of "phonatory massage" of the mucosa.

Reoperation is occasionally an option, although ample time (9–12 months) should pass before this idea is entertained because the voice may improve and iatrogenic lesions may diminish slowly for many months after the first surgery. A second surgery can be planned to correct the videostroboscopically identified defect in mucosal mass, mobility, or edge configuration.

For example, if an iatrogenic mass (granuloma) is causing poor phonatory closure, it should first be allowed to mature and possibly to resolve spontaneously. If it remains after a minimum of 6 months, it can be removed. Collagen injection into an area of depression has been advocated,[36] but this approach does not yield more than very modest results, and even these occur on an inconsistent basis. Incision and simple mucosal elevation across a limited line of adherence with early postoperative phonation may cure diplophonia or lessen dysphonia, occasionally to a surprising degree. It should be stressed, however, that in some instances little can be done beyond voice building, and avoidance of this problem altogether through precision surgery is the ideal. Some authors have written of fat injection or medialization thyroplasty, but these approaches remain to be systematically validated, and make sense theoretically where there is a significant gap between the folds, and not simply mucosal stiffness.

Contact Ulcer or Granuloma
Epidemiology

Contact granuloma or ulceration (Figure 95-24) is seen primarily in males—commonly in lawyers, ministers, teachers, and executives. Chronic coughing or throat clearing and reflux of acid from the stomach into the posterior larynx during sleep also seem to cause contact ulceration.[41] Some authors have also suggested that patients with this entity are experiencing psychological stress or conflict.

Pathophysiology and Pathology

The thin mucosa and perichondrium overlying the cartilaginous glottis become inflamed, perhaps as a result of overly forceful apposition (slamming together) of the arytenoids at the onset of voicing

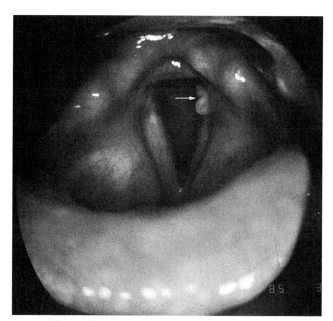

Figure 95-24. Contact granuloma, left. The general appearance and the cleft (*arrow*) where the opposite vocal process fits are typical.

(glottal stroke) or during chronic coughing or throat clearing. Acid reflux may also increase inflammation of the vocal process area. The traumatized area ulcerates or produces a heaped-up granuloma.

Diagnosis

History. Caffeine and alcohol use and late-night eating habits should be questioned, along with more specific acid reflux symptoms (e.g., acid eructations, raw throat in the morning with sour taste, unusually low-pitched gravelly morning voice, heartburn). Frequent symptoms include unilateral discomfort over the midthyroid cartilage, occasionally with referred pain to the ipsilateral ear. When contact granulation tissue becomes large, hoarseness can occur.

Vocal capability battery. The speaking voice of a patient with contact ulcer or granuloma may sound normal or only slightly husky. The patient may be noted to be speaking habitually in an overly low frequency range, often with a "held back" vocal quality but sometimes with a kind of "constrained emphasis." In particular, the voice characteristics of the held-back quality, habitual coughing or throat clearing, and low and monotone voice use are typical.

Laryngeal examination. A depressed, ulcerated area with a whitish exudate clinging to it or a bilobed, heaped-up lesion on the vocal process may be noted. At the instant of glottal closure, the vocal process of the uninvolved side can be seen to fit into the cleft

of a bilobed granuloma. Erythema is also usually apparent on the vocal process and coming upward on the medial surface of the arytenoid cartilage. A mature, soon-to-detach granuloma may be pedunculated and flip above and below the plane of the vocal fold margin with expiratory and inspiratory phonation, respectively (Figure 95-25).

Management

An antireflux regimen should begin on an empiric basis even for patients with no symptoms of reflux. The necessity of routine barium or pH monitoring studies remains controversial. Maturation and resolution of the granuloma can often occur spontaneously over 3 to 6 months. Thus, the role for voice therapy to abolish throat clearing, raise average pitch for speech, and so forth is indeterminate.

Significant but not universal success has been achieved with indirect injection of a depot corticosteroid directly into the lesion and the area around its base during indirect laryngoscopy. This can be accomplished in a videoendoscopy laboratory examining chair with a curved injection apparatus, topical anesthesia, and, for patients with excessive gag reflexes or high anxiety levels, a short-acting sedative administered intravenously.[11] Anecdotally, this technique has worked especially well for some granulomas but poorly for contact ulcers.

Surgery should be a last resort because postoperative recurrence of the ulcer or granuloma is predictable. Furthermore, when the lesion has a classic appearance and can be visually monitored, there is little need for tissue diagnosis. Microlaryngoscopy may be justified, however, if after a several-month trial of management an uninflamed, pedunculated lesion remains and is causing symptoms. Removal should be limited, leaving the base or pedicle undisturbed.

Intubation Granuloma
Epidemiology

Intubation granuloma (Figure 95-26) occurs in patients who have undergone endolaryngeal surgery affecting the arytenoid perichondrium, acute or chronic intubation, rigid bronchoscopy, or other direct laryngeal manipulations.

Pathophysiology and Pathology

Granuloma after intubation can occur because of direct abrasion of the arytenoid perichondrium, a break in the mucosa covering it as a result of coughing on an endotracheal tube, or long-term pressure necrosis of the vocal process area. The resulting reparative granuloma may initially progress from fairly sessile to large and pedunculated, but it may

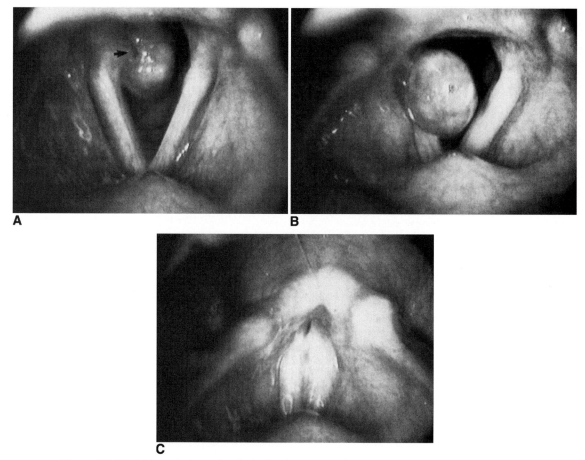

Figure 95-25. Video photographs through a laryngeal telescope of highly pedunculated right contact granuloma. **A,** The granuloma is drawn into the subglottis during sudden inspiration, thereby revealing more clearly its pedicle (*arrow*). **B,** Sudden exhalation blows the granuloma upward into the laryngeal vestibule. **C,** During phonation, the granuloma remains below the level of the vocal fold. Vocal fold closure is thus excellent, and speaking voice quality is remarkably undisturbed.

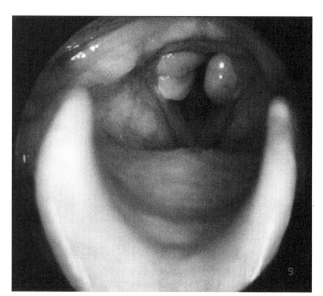

Figure 95-26. Postintubation granulomas.

then regress entirely with maturation over several months.

Diagnosis

History. The history of a patient with intubation granuloma reveals a fairly recent event during which the larynx was subjected to direct instrumentation or intubation.

Vocal capability battery. The speaking voice of a patient with intubation granuloma may not sound abnormal because the membranous (vibratile) portion of the vocal folds may be unaffected by the granuloma, which may sit above or below the vocal process during phonation. The laryngeal appearance, however, is characteristic. The granuloma can vary in size but is often large and spherical with some pedunculation. The granulomas are attached directly to the vocal process and are frequently bilateral. In cases of long-standing intubation, there may be associated findings such as tissue loss with resulting posterior glottic incompetence. In even more severe cases, there may be partial or complete fixation of one or both arytenoid cartilages. An interarytenoid synechium also may be noted on occasion.

Management

Regarding the management of intubation granuloma, if the history and physical examination are unequivocal, patience is recommended. Antibiotic coverage for several weeks seems to be helpful. Voice therapy may have a role on a highly individualized basis. With time and use of these measures, intubation granulomas usually mature and "fall off." If they become mature and persistent, however, surgery or a trial of indirect corticosteroid injection in the office may be an option. During microlaryngoscopy, corticosteroid injection into the base of the granuloma before removal is suggested. Any identifiable stalk should be left with the patient to minimize the size of the surgical wound More recently, topical application of mitomycin C has come into use to inhibit fibroblast proliferation that might lead to the reformation of granulation tissue.

Summary

The benign vocal fold mucosal disorders are important because of their impact on identity and communication and their commonness. For optimal results, diagnosis should include a skillful history, vocal capability elicitation, and laryngeal videostroboscopy. Intervention, whether medical management, voice therapy, surgery, or some combination of these, should match the diagnosis.

SACCULAR DISORDERS

At its anterior end, the normal laryngeal ventricle has a small outpouching called the *saccule* or *laryngeal appendix*. This structure is a blind sac that extends upward between the false vocal fold and thyroid cartilage, just posterolateral to the edge of the epiglottis. Containing many mucous glands, the saccule empties through an orifice in the anterior part of the ventricle. In a study of 100 random cadaver larynges, Broyles[21] found significant variation in the size of this normal structure, with 75% measuring 6 to 8 mm in length, 25% measuring 10 mm or greater, and 7% of the 25% measuring 15 mm or more. Although these structures may represent vestigial air sacs, their function is unknown in humans, besides perhaps to supply lubrication to the true folds.

Saccular disorders (laryngocele, saccular cyst, and laryngopyocele) involve abnormal dilation of the laryngeal saccule. In the laryngocele, the saccule is filled only with air through an orifice that remains patent, whereas the saccular cysts are filled with glandular secretions, and the orifice is obstructed. In laryngopyocele, the contents of a saccular cyst become infected, at which time radiographs can show the presence of both air and fluid. It should be noted that true laryngocele appears to be relatively rare; I have seen many saccular cysts, a single laryngopyocele, and also a number of cases of pharyngeal or buccal dilation in wind or brass instrument players, but never a true laryngocele. It appears that the term *laryngocele* is often used to describe a saccular cyst, however.

Laryngocele and Saccular Cyst

Classification

Most authors accept the classification for laryngoceles described by Holinger and others[49] or de Vincentiis and Biserni.[32] Laryngoceles are classified as internal alone (within the thyroid cartilage) and combined (internal and external) or internal, external, and combined (Figure 95-27). The cause of laryngoceles is uncertain. Some have cited an increase in transglottic pressure, such as that seen in trumpet players, glass blowers, and those using the voice in unusually forceful ways.[31,49] Others, such as Stell and Maran,[87] believe that the relationship of laryngocele to these activities may have been overstated because few reported patients in the world literature had hobbies or occupations requiring high transglottic pressures. A perhaps more clearly documented although uncommon cause for saccular cysts is laryngeal carcinoma, which causes obstruction of the saccular orifice.[63] Laryngocele formation also may be facilitated by the congenital presence of an abnormally large saccule. I have also seen saccular cyst months or years after excision of a large supraglottic carcinoma with the laser, leaving remnants of the saccule buried.

Clinical Information

Stell and Maran[87] found laryngocele to be most common among white men aged in their fifties, with few cases occurring among women or nonwhites. They also found that laryngoceles were mostly unilateral and of the combined internal/external variety.

Symptoms depend somewhat on whether the laryngocele is internal, external, or combined. The usual symptoms are hoarseness, possibly with a swelling in the neck, and (in decreasing order of frequency) stridor, dysphagia, sore throat, snoring, and cough.

Examination of the head and neck in a person with laryngocele reveals swelling of the false vocal fold and aryepiglottic fold to a degree commensurate with the laryngocele's size. If a component of the laryngocele extends through the thyrohyoid membrane, a mass is palpable in the lateral neck in that location.

The diagnosis is made primarily on the basis of the laryngeal and neck examination and confirmed by

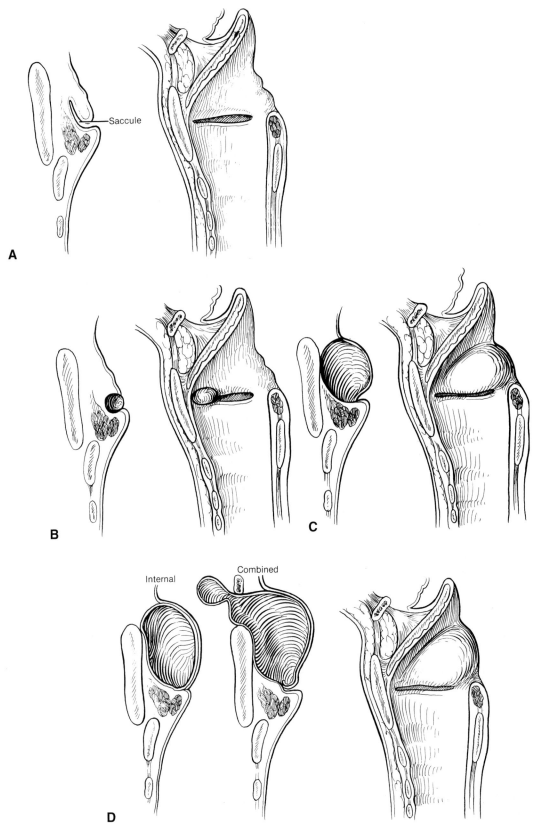

Figure 95-27. The classification scheme for a laryngocele or saccular cyst. **A,** Normal anatomy. **B,** Anterior saccular cyst. **C,** Lateral saccular cyst. **D,** Laryngocele types.

the finding of a fluid- or air-filled sac on plain radiography or computed tomography (CT).

Management

Management is surgical. Although some controversy exists in the literature on the merits of primary endoscopic marsupialization vs an external approach, most authors seem to prefer the external approach for definitive removal in adults, particularly when an external component is present. This approach involves following the external portion of the laryngocele sac through the thyrohyoid membrane. Some believe that removal of the upper portion of one side of the thyroid cartilage may be necessary to provide easier access to the endolarynx. The laryngocele is then transected as close as possible to the orifice of the saccule.[7,29,31,49,87] Many authors have cited the need for careful endoscopic examination and multiple biopsies to rule out laryngeal carcinoma in the ventricle as the cause for the laryngocele before definitive surgery. Removal of small internal laryngoceles, which are relatively rare, has been reported through laryngofissure or microlaryngoscopic techniques,[15,39] although these approaches are generally less favored than the external approach in much of the literature. Hogikyan and Bastian[47] recently reported on complete endoscopic removal of large or recurrent saccular cysts as their preferred approach, which has some applicability to the management of laryngoceles. Even more recently, I have succeeded in definitive endoscopic removal of saccular cysts that also include an external component, palpably beginning to protrude through the thyrohyoid membrane and into the neck.

Saccular Cysts

Laryngeal cysts and laryngoceles are actually disorders of the saccule. Knowledge of the saccule's anatomy is necessary to understand saccular cysts (Figures 95-27 through 95-30).

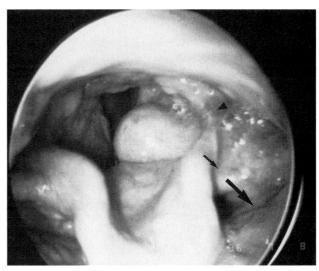

Figure 95-28. A saccular cyst, left, obscures most of the left vocal fold. A slightly larger cyst can be seen presenting at the medial wall of the pyriform (*arrowhead*), at the pharyngoepiglottic fold (*arrow*), or through the thyrohyoid membrane and into the neck (*large arrow*).

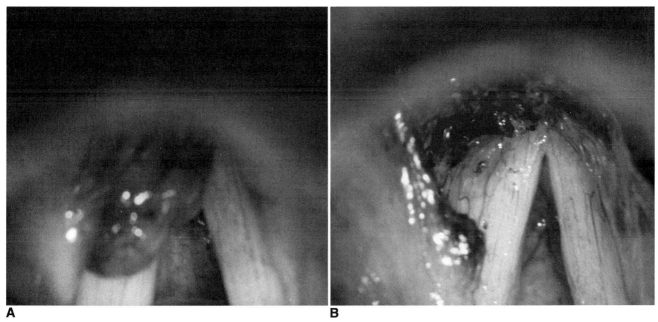

A   **B**

Figure 95-29. A, A moderate-sized anterior saccular cyst obscures the anterior left true vocal fold and is shown **(B)** after complete excision with laser (not marsupialization).

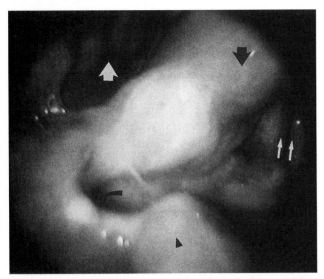

Figure 95-30. A voice laboratory view 1 week after complete endoscopic excision (*not marsupialization*) of a large lateral saccular cyst that had penetrated above the thyroid cartilage (direction of *curved arrow*) and outside the confines of the larynx. Parallel white arrows demarcate the vocal folds. The *fat white arrow* indicates the right pyriform sinus, and the *fat black arrow* shows the right arytenoid apex. The wall of the cyst was followed through the aryepiglottic fold, detaching it from the epiglottis (*arrowhead*).

Classification

DeSanto, Devine, and Weiland,[30] based on a comprehensive review of the literature, clinical experience, and extensive histologic study of the glandular elements within the larynx, helped propose the following classification:

1. Saccular cysts
   a. Anterior saccular cysts
   b. Lateral saccular cysts
2. Ductal cysts

Saccular cysts appear when the orifice of the saccule is obstructed, with resultant dilation by glandular secretions. Anterior saccular cysts are the smaller of the two types and tend to bulge medially from the ventricle into the laryngeal lumen, obscuring the anterior portion of the vocal fold, sometimes pressing down on the upper surface of the vocal fold, causing hoarseness.

DeSanto, Devine, and Weiland[30] reported that the lateral saccular cyst, the larger of the two types, is the same as a congenital cyst of the larynx. It tends to enlarge in a more superior and lateral direction, into the false vocal fold and aryepiglottic fold. In my experience, in addition to bulging the false and aryepiglottic folds within the laryngeal vestibule, large saccular cysts can extend into the lateral vallecula or bulge the medial wall of the pyriform sinus. If a saccular cyst enlarges sufficiently, it can herniate through the thyrohyoid membrane similar to a laryngocele and can appear in the neck.

Clinical Information

Holinger and others,[49] in their review of 46 patients with laryngocele or saccular cyst, found that in the 41 cases involving a saccular cyst, 10 occurred in infants and children and 31 occurred in adults. Of the 31 adult cases, 22 were anterior saccular cysts and nine were lateral saccular cysts. Four cysts in the infants and children were anterior, and six were lateral.

When a saccular cyst occurs in infancy, it usually appears early, even at birth, as respiratory distress with inspiratory stridor. The infant's cry is abnormal, and cyanosis and dysphagia can occur. In adults, hoarseness seems to be the most common complaint, although with large or infected lateral saccular cysts (laryngopyoceles), dyspnea, dysphagia, pain, and a neck mass can occur.[49]

Physical Examination

Indirect mirror, fiberoptic, rigid telescopic, or direct laryngoscopic examination of the larynx reveals an appearance similar to that of the laryngocele. The anterior saccular cyst is seen as a relatively smaller round swelling protruding from the anterior ventricle and overhanging the anterior part of the ipsilateral vocal fold (see Figure 95-29). The lateral saccular cyst appears as a smooth, mucosa-covered swelling of the false vocal fold and aryepiglottic fold. A large cyst can displace the medial wall of the piriform and the vallecula.[47] Note that even a large lateral saccular cyst can become almost invisible under the conditions of direct laryngoscopy with general anesthesia. In this case, this author has found that one can begin by excising the false fold, during which maneuver the wall of the cyst is invariably encountered. When an unusually large saccular cyst has protruded through the thyrohyoid membrane, palpable swelling in the lateral neck may result.

Workup

Holinger and others[49] implied that lateral soft tissue radiographs of the neck are helpful in addition to appropriate history and physical examination because the cysts were apparent radiologically in all infants and children on whom these studies were performed. In 1984, Shagets, Barrs, and Rugh[80] compared standard tomography to CT, concluding that CT gives more information about the cyst and its anatomic extent. Goldman[43] discussed the value of what has currently become a forgotten technique, xeroradiography.

Management

Infants with congenital lateral saccular cysts who have weak cry, stridor, and cyanosis should first have a good airway secured. This is followed by aspiration of cyst contents through a direct laryngoscope or by endoscopic marsupialization with or without stripping of the cyst lining. Abramson and Zielinski[1] described application of the carbon dioxide laser to incise the cyst and to vaporize its lining. Booth and Birck[15] reported on laryngocele and lateral saccular cyst in neonates and described using simple cup forceps to unroof both lesions, followed by a 3-day intubation to act as a stent and to maintain the infant's airway. A 5-year follow-up revealed no recurrences. Holinger and others,[49] in their report of 10 infants with saccular cysts, described direct laryngoscopy and aspiration of the cyst. They noted that a mean of 7.5 aspirations were required for each infant, five of whom later needed endoscopic marsupialization. One child had external excision of a persistent laryngeal cyst after 11 laryngoscopies. The authors also described the necessity for tracheotomy in 6 of 10 children, with a mean duration of tracheotomy of 17 months. Based on this report, earlier definitive removal or marsupialization seems like a better option.

DeSanto, Devine, and Weiland[30] reported on adult patients with saccular cysts and described endoscopic cyst avulsion for 29 cases of anterior cysts. Only one patient had recurrence, which was later removed via laryngofissure. These authors found anterior saccular cysts in association with laryngeal carcinoma in two additional cases, which again points to the need to rule out a small ventricular cancer in cases of saccular cysts or laryngoceles.

The experience of Holinger and others[49] concerning 22 adults with anterior saccular cysts involved direct laryngoscopy and endoscopic removal with cup forceps. With this method, no cyst recurred.

For patients with lateral saccular cysts, Holinger and others[49] suggested an external approach. They mentioned a case of tuberculous laryngitis and a case of epidermoid laryngeal carcinoma presenting as a lateral saccular cyst. DeSanto, Devine, and Weiland[30] approach large lateral saccular cysts through the thyrohyoid membrane without disturbing the thyroid cartilage. However, these authors do not criticize earlier midline or lateral thyrotomy approaches, and they treated seven smaller lateral laryngeal cysts with endoscopic excision without recurrence.

A recent report[47] concerning seven large saccular cysts in my caseload, is well documented with preoperative and postoperative CT scans and endoscopic photos. This article affirms complete endoscopic excision instead of endoscopic marsupialization or transcervical removal, even for large recurrent lateral saccular cysts. In this series, complete excision was possible on an outpatient basis for four of seven patients, whereas three were admitted for a single night's observation. None required tracheotomy, and none has recurred. (see Figure 95-30). Since the time of this publication, I have also removed two saccular cysts with palpable neck components completely via endoscopic methodology. This requires following the cyst wall over the top of the thyroid cartilage and into the neck.

Summary

Saccular disorders, whether laryngocele or saccular cysts, can be easily diagnosed after appropriate history, physical examination, and radiologic evaluation. Initial evaluation in adults should exclude the presence of an occult laryngeal carcinoma involving the ventricle, the region of the saccular orifice, or the saccule. The decision between an endoscopic or external approach depends on the classifications of laryngocele or saccular cyst, its size, patient factors, and, perhaps most of all, surgeon experience and preference.

BENIGN MESENCHYMAL NEOPLASMS

Compared with the benign vocal fold mucosal disorders (e.g., nodules, polyps, contact ulcers), neurologic disorders, scarring or stenosis problems, and malignant tumors of the larynx, benign tumors of the larynx are rare. The literature sometimes incorrectly includes nonneoplastic mucosal reactive disorders (i.e., response to chronic injury), such as polyps and nodules, under the heading of benign neoplasms.[49,72] Even when nonneoplastic reactive lesions are excluded (e.g., in a large series by Jones and others[52]), the numbers of cases are small when divided by the years included in the review. If papillomas are excluded, laryngologists can expect to see only a few nonmalignant neoplasms during their careers.

Epithelial Tumors
Recurrent Respiratory Papillomatosis

Squamous papillomas (Figures 95-31 and 95-32) are the most common benign neoplasms seen by laryngologists. Jones, Myers, and Barnes[51] found that 84% of the benign laryngeal tumors they managed were papillomas, and they noted that this statistic matches those of other large series. Based on physician questionnaires about patients with recurrent respiratory papillomatosis, it is estimated that this entity occurs at a rate of 4.3 per 100,000 children and 1.8 per 100,000 adults.[28]

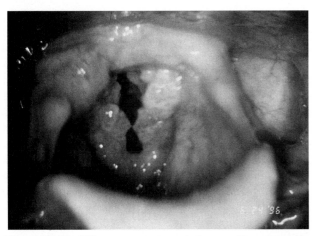

Figure 95-31. Diffuse recurrent respiratory papillomatosis distorts the contour of both true vocal folds and the right arytenoid apex. The dark dots (examples at *arrows*) represent the fibrovascular core within each papilloma.

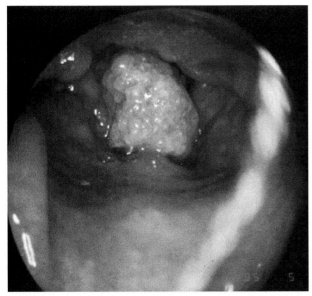

Figure 95-32. A large mass of papillomas obscures the vocal folds and airway. The patient has a tracheotomy tube.

Recurrent respiratory papillomatosis occurs in response to mucosal infection by human papillomavirus of the Papova class. An association between maternal genital condylomata and recurrent respiratory papillomatosis is known; however, the fact that only approximately 1 in 400 children at risk because of maternal infection will develop recurrent respiratory papillomatosis[80] suggests relatively low infectivity. This relatively small risk makes the question of whether to perform cesarean section in the context of maternal infection controversial.

Recurrent respiratory papillomatosis may commence in childhood or adulthood. The juvenile form, commonly designated *papillomatosis* because of diffuse involvement of the larynx, usually presents in infancy or childhood as hoarseness and stridor. This form of papillomatosis is often aggressive and rapidly recurrent, requiring frequent laryngoscopies for management. Rarely, papillomas may regress spontaneously, especially at puberty. On examination, exuberant tissue resembling miniature clusters of grapes may be seen, especially on the anterior part of the true vocal folds, the false folds, and the epiglottis (see Figure 95-32). The bulk of papilloma tissue can be so great as to obscure normal laryngeal landmarks.

Occasionally, the trachea and bronchi become involved with papillomas. Weiss and Kashima[92] reviewed 39 cases and reported that a history of tracheotomy, a high number of endoscopic procedures, and a long duration of the disease seem to correlate with an increased incidence of tracheal involvement.

Adult-onset papillomas are occasionally solitary, or at least more localized than juvenile-onset ones. There appears to be a variant I have come to call "carpet-variant" papilloma. These lesions do not show the typical exophytic growth pattern, instead causing a velvety appearance with little projection from the surface. The red "dots" on the surface representing the fibrovascular core of each papilloma are still visible, however. Behavior of adult-onset papillomatosis may also be less aggressive, and, rarely, a single removal alone is necessary for complete cure. However, adult-onset papillomatosis can also behave like the more aggressive juvenile-onset form.

The carbon dioxide laser remains the most widely accepted management for papillomas in the larynx; the number of laryngoscopies required to control these lesions during childhood can exceed 50. The laser is favored because of its hemostatic properties (papillomas tend to be friable and vascular). In addition, the precision of the micro-spot laser allows for vaporization of the lesion plane by plane to avoid harming the underlying vocal fold. The microdebrider is very useful in friable, exuberant cases that would require markedly more time to remove via laser excision or planar coagulation. That tool, however, is not very useful for the precise removal of the last "5%."

Many other management modalities have been tried. Options such as cryotherapy, radiation, photodynamic therapy, and vaccines are not yet validated.

Although dramatic responses have been observed in some cases, interferon's long-term role in the management of laryngeal papillomatosis is still being determined. In 1983, McCabe and Clark[60] reported a series of 19 patients with moderate to severe respiratory papillomatosis managed with interferon. They found that six patients were disease free by visual criteria, seven had a small amount of visible disease but not enough to require surgery, and two showed no response to interferon. These authors also noted that the papillomas tended to regrow on cessation of interferon therapy. Overall, they thought that interferon spared patients the need for multiple surgeries, although the duration of treatment necessary is being investigated. More recently, Leventhal and others,[56] using higher doses and longer duration of therapy, noted significantly higher response rate; some responses appeared to be long-term. Ogura and others[74] reported the recurrence of papilloma after a 6-year interval in a patient who seemed to have achieved a durable response to interferon. This author has used interferon using the Leventhal criteria in 12 adults. Three achieved long-term remission. Most of the rest had notable reduction of growth rate of the disease, sometimes on a durable basis, but not remission. Better understanding of the role of interferon awaits further study.

Another newer medical management modality uses indole-3-carbinol, a natural derivative of cruciferous vegetables such as cabbage and broccoli. Anecdotal reports suggest that a percentage of patients who take this medication experience significant benefit. An estimated 30 patients in my adult practice have used this nutritional supplement, but with disappointing results. One wonders if best result depends on more rapid growth than is often seen in adults.

Avidano and Singleton[4] reported the use of methotrexate in three patients with severe recurrent respiratory papillomatosis who failed to respond to interferon or cis-reninoic acid. All three experienced a prolonged surgical interval and reduced disease severity, but regression was not complete. Further study is needed.

European authors first wrote about the use of intralesional cidofovir—(S)-1-(3-hydroxy-2-phosphonyl-methoxypropyl) cytosine—as a treatment for deoxyribonucleic acid (DNA) viruses, including human papillomavirus.[2,72,85] At least one anecdotal report showed disappearance of a papillomatous lesion of the esophagus injected serially with HPMPC.[92] Subsequently, others have shown good results with this medicine, either for regression/remission of existing lesions,[14,68] or as an adjunct to surgery.[76,77] In my experience with over 30 patients, rapidly growing and focal lesions seem to respond best. Some durable remissions are indeed achievable, and pending further experience, long-term remission appears feasible in at least one in four adult patients when patients with slowly growing papillomas are included. The above authors and the present author have not seen scarring felt due to the use of cidofovir, except when an overly aggressive "bleb" was raised, depriving the mucosa of blood supply. Chhetri and others,[24] however, in a study using a canine model, found atrophy and scarring that appeared to be worse with number of times injected and with increasing concentration of cidofovir. In this model, use of concentrations higher than 20 mg/mL, in particular, seemed to have this effect. The same group found no change in leukocyte count or renal parameters in doses up to 4.26 mg/kg body weight.

McMillan and others[62] described use of the 585-nm pulsed dye laser on three patients in a pilot study.[61] As had previously been found by Tan and colleagues[89] for cutaneous warts, the hemoglobin in microvasculature selectively absorbed laser energy. In McMillan's study, either CO_2 or pulsed dye laser were used on different areas of papilloma growth. Papilloma response to both lasers appeared to be good, at least to the limited time of follow-up reported. Early edema seemed to be less on the side of the pulsed dye laser. This laser coagulates the microvasculature, due to red color of hemoglobin, but leaves the overlying epithelium uncoagulated. The mechanism of action for regression of papillomas was said to be deprivation of oxygen and nutrients to the lesions. Franco, Zeitels, and others[38] subsequently used this laser on 41 patients. In about half of these, papillomas were treated with the laser but not removed. This group also noted marked response, without evident scarring.

Some of these medical management modalities hold promise; all need further investigation and validation. Thus, optimal management is careful serial laser laryngoscopies with consideration of investigational use of interferon, indole-3-carbinol, cidofovir, or the 585-nm pulsed dye laser for selected patients.

Vascular Neoplasms
Polypoid Granulation Tissue

Fechner, Cooper, and Mills[35] reviewed 639 vascular lesions of the head and neck, 62 of which were found in the larynx or trachea, and found that polypoid granulation tissue is the most common vascular tumor in the larynx. They also noted that pyogenic granuloma does not occur in the larynx. Pyogenic granuloma, as seen most often on the tongue, consists of distinct lobules of capillaries separated by fibromyxoid stroma, whereas polypoid granulation tissue consists of radially arranged capillaries. These authors attribute formation of polypoid granulation tissue in the larynx to one of several forms of trauma (e.g., caused by laryngeal biopsy, intubation, direct external trauma to the larynx, or an external penetrating wound). Granulation tissue in the larynx should be handled primarily by conservative measures, including removal of the source of any ongoing irritation (e.g., from inappropriate voice use or acid reflux laryngitis) and intralesional corticosteroids. For non-response and continuing symptoms, careful endoscopic removal may be considered after the granulation tissue has been allowed to mature and become less active and vascular.

Laryngeal Hemangiomas

Infants with laryngeal hemangiomas often have associated cutaneous hemangiomas. These infants typically have respiratory symptoms of stridor or pseudocroup, usually within the first 6 months of life.

During direct laryngoscopy, a mucosa-covered mass with or without bluish coloration may be seen in the subglottis. Other suggestive findings include compressibility with palpation or shrinkage with administration of epinephrine.

In his review of the management of subglottic hemangioma in 1968, Calcaterra[22] addressed the then-prevalent practice of low-dose irradiation for subglottic hemangioma in infants. On the basis of an infant with a large cavernous hemangioma who did not respond to irradiation and on the basis of general knowledge of radiation's effect on vascular tissues, Calcaterra[22] suggested that this therapy was inadvisable. He suggested that tracheotomy be done when indicated for airway protection. This allows the tracheal lumen to enlarge with growth of the child and, more importantly, gives the hemangioma an opportunity to involute spontaneously, as most do if they are left alone.

More recent reports by Healy and others[44] and Mizono and Dedo[65] explored the usefulness of the carbon dioxide laser for the management of this lesion. Based on 11 cases in three centers, the authors concluded that for the usual capillary hemangioma in the infant subglottis, the carbon dioxide laser is clearly superior to radiotherapy or corticosteroid therapy. They described the procedure as beginning with removal of tissue for histologic examination followed by simple vaporization of remaining abnormal tissue. These authors also believe that if the tracheotomy was not required before the procedure for airway maintenance, it is probably unnecessary, provided intense humidification is supplied in the immediate postoperative period. None of the patients reported in this series had significant complications, although four required a second treatment with laser for a satisfactory final result. All patients with previously placed tracheotomy tubes were successfully decannulated.

Adult hemangiomas are usually found at or above the level of the vocal folds. Because they are more often the cavernous form and are usually covered by thinner mucosa than the congenital hemangioma, this type appears more often as a bluish, discolored mass.

Bridger, Nassar, and Skinner[19] reviewed literature on hemangioma in the adult patient, noting that in contrast to the congenital form, symptoms of this lesion may have been present for many years. Hoarseness is the expected symptom, and respiratory distress never occurs. Although hemorrhage may occur spontaneously, it is usually a surgical complication.

Bridger, Nassar, and Skinner[19] advised that adult laryngeal hemangiomas be left alone if at all possible. They recommended that corticosteroid or radiotherapy be used when necessary and that management of adult laryngeal hemangioma uses surgery when the hemangioma shows a tendency to involve progressively additional parts of the larynx, as occurred in one reviewed study. The carbon dioxide laser is not generally advised for adult cavernous hemangioma because the diameter of the vascular spaces exceeds this laser's coagulating ability.

Muscle Neoplasms
Rhabdomyoma

Most extracardiac rhabdomyomas are found in the head and neck region, especially in the pharynx and larynx. Winther[93] found 53 cases involving the hypopharynx or larynx in the literature up until 1976 and also supplied two case reports. He noted that none of these tumors recurred after local excision and advised that the approach be as conservative as possible for complete removal. He also noted that rhabdomyoma can be confused with a granular cell tumor or a rhabdomyosarcoma. Modlin[67] also stressed the need to differentiate between rhabdomyoma and granular cell tumor and noted that complete local excision is curative.

Neoplasms of Adipose Origin
Lipoma

Zakrzewski,[95] in his review of the literature through 1965, believed that only 70 of many cases reported as laryngeal lipomas actually involved the larynx and were sufficiently described to allow for analysis of this entity. He noted, however, that 23 of 70 cases had some other tumor characteristics, such as fibrolipoma, myxolipoma, nervous tissue, cyst fragments, and angiolipoma. Although sometimes seen among persons with numerous lipomas in other body areas, most laryngeal lipomas were isolated occurrences.

Of 70 cases, 54 were designated extrinsic, whereas only 16 were classified as true intrinsic laryngeal tumors. Because lipomas occurred more frequently in parts of the larynx in which fat was a normal part of the subepithelium, most tumors arose on the aryepiglottic fold and epiglottis (the periphery of the laryngeal vestibule). Of the intrinsic tumors, the most frequent site of origin was the false vocal fold. Only one case involved a true vocal fold.

Because lipomas are slow growing, symptoms were often present for many years before diagnosis. In general, respiratory symptoms were most common, and hoarseness was relatively infrequent.

Surgical management was successful. Procedures such as endoscopic removal, subhyoid pharyngotomy, lateral pharyngotomy, and laryngofissure were used according to tumor size and location. The guiding principle was conservative with complete removal or enucleation because incompletely removed lipomas regrow.

Benign Neoplasms of Glandular Origin
Benign Mixed Neoplasm

Benign mixed tumors (pleomorphic adenomas) are extremely uncommon in the larynx. Som and others[86] found only 27 cases of this tumor involving the larynx in the literature and supplied one case report. Most of these tumors involve the subglottic laryngeal region, and only six cases involved the supraglottis. These authors described the typical appearance as a smooth, ovoid submucosal mass. As is the case for most other benign laryngeal tumors, the approach to surgical excision depends on tumor size and location.

Oncocytic Neoplasms of Larynx

According to the literature, oncocytic tumors are actually oncocytic metaplasia and hyperplasia of the ductal cell portion of glandular tissue. Gallagher and Puzon[40] found that 18 of 19 cases in their series were cystic and concluded that these lesions represent duct metaplasia and hyperplasia rather than true neoplasia. One solid tumor in their series was considered to be an oncocytic adenoma, as seen in the parotid gland.

LeJeune, Putman, and Yamase[55] reported a case of a woman with numerous cystic oncocytic lesions of the epiglottis, aryepiglottic folds, false vocal fold, and right true vocal fold, supporting the opinion of Gallagher and Puzon. Lundgren, Olofsson, and Hellquist[59] presented a series of seven oncocytic cysts of the larynx and agreed that these lesions represent glandular duct metaplasia and hyperplasia rather than true neoplasia.

These authors seem to agree that simple excision, by whatever approach necessary according to lesion size and location, is the management of choice.

Cartilaginous Neoplasms
Chondroma

Although an attempt to differentiate histologically between chondroma and low-grade chondrosarcoma has been made, Mills and Fechner[64] believe that the behaviors of the chondromas and the low-grade chondrosarcomas are so similar that histologic distinction has little practical significance. Because neither grows quickly or metastasizes, the clinical approach to these entities can be the same. Neel and Unni,[70] in their experience with 33 patients, noted that most patients had an "obvious smooth rounded mass covered by mucous membrane in the subglottic region of the larynx," and in most cases this mass was situated posteriorly and laterally. Although plain radiography consistently revealed a soft tissue mass or calcification within the tumor, anteroposterior tomography of the larynx was the most helpful study.

Neel and Unni[70] did not tabulate symptoms separately between benign and malignant cartilaginous tumors; symptoms consisted mainly of hoarseness, dyspnea, neck mass, and dysphagia. These authors used laryngofissure most often for removal and total laryngectomy for high-grade malignant tumors.

Singh, Black, and Fried,[84] in a review of laryngeal tumors seen at four major hospitals between 1960 and 1977, found only two cartilaginous tumors of the larynx, but they found 177 cases reported in the English literature. Of cartilaginous tumors, 70% arose in the cricoid cartilage, primarily from the posterior plate. The growth of these tumors is mostly intralumenal, with a rare case appearing externally into the neck. These authors believed that because chondrosarcomas are usually indolent and rarely metastasize, local resection, if technically feasible, is adequate management. They described laryngofissure with submucosal resection as the most common approach to these tumors, unless the cricoid would be collapsed entirely by its subtotal removal.

Hyams and Rabuzzi,[50] in a series of 31 cartilaginous tumors of the larynx, found 15 chondromas and 16 chondrosarcomas. The chondromas occurred in a slightly younger age group than the chondrosarcomas. However, the chondromas included nine "chondromas of the true vocal cord," which probably represent metaplasia of the elastic connective tissue of the vocal fold rather than true chondromas.

Neoplasms of Neural Origin
Granular Cell Neoplasms

Mills and Fechner[64] noted evidence indicating that granular cell tumors originate in Schwann cells; these tumors had previously been called *granular cell myoblastomas* because they resemble muscle tissue with standard staining techniques. A notable characteristic of granular cell tumors is frequent association with overlying pseudoepitheliomatous hyperplasia of the mucosa. Insufficiently deep biopsy of this lesion can lead to an incorrect diagnosis of epidermoid carcinoma.

Although this tumor can involve any part of the larynx, the middle to posterior part of the true vocal fold is the most frequent site; hoarseness is thus the most common complaint. Conservative but complete local excision is considered definitive therapy.[2,3,16,37,90]

Neurofibroma

Chang-Lo[23] reviewed 19 previously reported cases of von Recklinghausen's disease with laryngeal involvement and supplied one case. Supance, Quenelle, and Crissman[88] reported that solitary neurofibromas of the larynx not associated with von Recklinghausen's disease were more common than those associated with the disease. The most common symptoms in patients with laryngeal involvement of von Recklinghausen's were hoarseness, dyspnea (most striking), and dysphagia. On physical examination, lobulated nodules ranging from less than 2 to 8 cm in diameter were noted, and the most common site of origin was the arytenoid or aryepiglottic fold.

Because these lesions are benign, the surgical approach should balance conservatism with the need for complete excision. For larger tumors, this may necessitate an external approach (e.g., lateral pharyngotomy, laryngofissure, lateral thyrotomy).[27]

Neurilemmoma

Neurilemmomas are less common than neurofibromas and usually involve the aryepiglottic fold and false vocal fold. Symptoms correspond with the slow growth of these lesions and can include a sensation of fullness in the throat, voice change, or slow development of respiratory distress. Management should consist of conservative but complete removal by an approach consistent with tumor size and location. Neurilemmomas are more encapsulated than neurofibromas; simple enucleation (e.g., by a lateral thyrotomy) with removal of a portion of the thyroid cartilage is believed to be adequate management.[43,69]

Summary

True benign neoplasms of the larynx do not include benign (reactive) vocal fold mucosal disorders. If papillomas are excluded, the number of persons with laryngeal neoplasms is small; busy laryngologists infrequently see these lesions. The basic management principles are similar for these tumors, regardless of the cell of origin. Removal should be complete but conservative (to spare the voice), with the approach determined primarily by tumor size and location.

REFERENCES

1. Abramson AL, Zielinski B: Congenital laryngeal saccular cyst of the newborn, *Laryngoscope* 94:1580, 1984.
2. Aduma P and others: Metabolic diversity and antiviral activities of acyclic nucleoside phosphonates, *Mol Pharmacol* 47:816, 1995.
3. Agarwal RK, Blitzer A, Perzin KH: Granular cell tumors of the larynx, *Otolaryngol Head Neck Surg* 87:807, 1979.
4. Avidano MA, Singleton GT: Adjuvant drug strategies in the treatment of recurrent respiratory papillomatosis, *Head Neck Surg* 112:197, 1995.
5. Baer T: *Observations of vocal fold vibration: measurement of excised larynges.* In Stevens KN, Hirano M, editors: *Vocal fold physiology,* Tokyo, 1981, University of Tokyo Press.
6. Baker BM and others: Persistent hoarseness after surgical removal of vocal cord lesions, *Arch Otolaryngol Head Neck Surg* 107:148, 1981.
7. Baker HL, Baker SR, McClatchey KD: Manifestations and management of laryngooceles, *Head Neck Surg* 4:450, 1982.
8. Bastian RW: Laryngeal image biofeedback for voice modification. Transcripts of the Fourteenth Annual Symposium for the Care of the Professional Voice, Denver, June, 1985.
9. Bastian RW: Vocal fold microsurgery in singers, *J Voice* 10:389, 1996.
10. Bastian RW and others: Indirect videolaryngoscopy versus direct endoscopy for larynx and pharynx cancer staging: toward elimination of preliminary direct laryngoscopy, *Ann Otol Rhinol Laryngol* 98:693, 1989.
11. Bastian RW, Delsupehe KG: Indirect larynx and pharynx surgery: a replacement for direct laryngoscopy, *Laryngoscope* 106:1280, 1996.
12. Bastian RW, Keidar A, Verdolini-Marston K: Simple vocal tasks for detecting vocal fold swelling, *J Voice* 4:172, 1990.
13. Bastian RW, Nagorsky MJ: Laryngeal image biofeedback, *Laryngoscope* 97:1346, 1987.
14. Bielamowicz S and others: Intralesional cidofovir therapy for laryngeal papilloma in an adult cohort, *Laryngoscope* 112:696-699, 2002.
15. Booth JB, Birck HG: Operative treatment and postoperative management of saccular cyst and laryngocele, *Arch Otolaryngol Head Neck Surg* 107:500, 1981.
16. Booth JB, Osborn DA: Granular cell myoblastoma of the larynx, *Acta Otolaryngol (Stockh)* 70:279, 1970.
17. Bouchayer M and others: Epidermoid cysts, sulci, and mucosal bridges of the true vocal cord: a report of 157 cases, *Laryngoscope* 95:1087, 1985.
18. Bouchayer M and others: Microsurgery for benign lesions of the vocal folds, *Ear Nose Throat J* 67:446, 1988.
19. Bridger GP, Nassar VH, Skinner HB: Hemangioma in the adult larynx, *Arch Otolaryngol Head Neck Surg* 92:493, 1970.
20. Brodnitz FS: Results and limitation of vocal rehabilitation, *Arch Otolaryngol Head Neck Surg* 77:148, 1963.
21. Broyles EN: Anatomical observations concerning the laryngeal appendix, *Ann Otol Rhinol Laryngol* 68:461, 1959.
22. Calcaterra TC: An evaluation of the treatment of subglottic hemangioma, *Laryngoscope* 78:1956, 1968.
23. Chang-Lo M: Laryngeal involvement in von Recklinghausen's disease: a case report and review of the literature, *Laryngoscope* 87:435, 1977.
24. Chhetri DK and others: Local and systemic effects of intralaryngeal injection of cidofovir in a canine model, *Laryngoscope* 113:1922-1926, 2003.
25. Cornut G, Bouchayer M: Phonosurgery for singers, *J Voice* 3:269, 1989.
26. Cummings CW and others: *Atlas of laryngeal surgery,* St Louis, 1984, Mosby.

27. Cummings CW, Montgomery WW, Balogh K: Neurogenic tumors of the larynx, *Ann Otol Rhinol Laryngol* 38:76, 1969.
28. Derkay CS: Task force on recurrent respiratory papillomas, *Arch Otolaryngol Head Neck Surg* 121:1386, 1995.
29. DeSanto LW: Laryngocele, laryngeal mucocele, large saccules, and laryngeal saccular cysts: a developmental spectrum, *Laryngoscope* 84:1291, 1974.
30. DeSanto LW, Devine KD, Weiland LH: Cysts of the larynx: classification, *Laryngoscope* 80:245, 1970.
31. de Vincentiis I, Biserni A: Surgery of the mixed laryngocele, *Acta Otolaryngol (Stockh)* 87:142, 1979.
32. Diamond L and others: A dose-response study of the efficacy and safety of ipratropium bromide nasal spray in the treatment of the common cold, *J Allergy Clin Immunol* 95:1139, 1995.
33. Dockhorn R and others: A double-blind, placebo-controlled study of the safety and efficacy of ipratropium bromide nasal spray versus placebo in patients with the common cold, *J Allergy Clin Immunol* 90:1076, 1992.
34. Duncavage JA, Toohill RJ: Wound healing of true vocal cord squamous epithelium following CO_2 laser ablation and cup forceps stripping. Paper presented at Laser Surgery Congress, Chicago, June, 1984.
35. Fechner RE, Cooper PH, Mills SE: Pyogenic granuloma of the larynx and trachea: a causal and pathologic misnomer for granulation tissue, *Arch Otolaryngol Head Neck Surg* 107:30, 1981.
36. Ford CN, Bless DM: Use of collagen for scarring problems on the vocal fold, *J Voice* 1:116, 1987.
37. Frable MA, Fischer RA: Granular cell myoblastomas, *Laryngoscope* 86:36, 1976.
38. Franco RA, Zeitels SM, Farinelli WA and others: 585-nm pulsed dye laser treatment of glottal papillomatosis, *Ann Otol Rhinol Laryngol* 111:486-492, 2002.
39. Frederick FJ: Endoscopic microsurgical excision of internal laryngocele, *J Otolaryngol* 14:163, 1985.
40. Gallagher JC, Puzon BO: Oncocytic lesions of the larynx, *Ann Otol Rhinol Laryngol* 78:307, 1969.
41. Goldberg M, Noyek AM, Pritzker KPH: Laryngeal granuloma secondary to gastro-esophageal reflux, *J Otolaryngol* 7:196, 1978.
42. Goldman NC: X-ray study of the month: laryngeal cyst, *Ann Otol Rhinol Laryngol* 90:522, 1981.
43. Gooder P, Farrington T: Extracranial neurilemmomata of the head and neck, *J Laryngol Otol* 94:243, 1980.
44. Healy G and others: Treatment of subglottic hemangioma with the carbon dioxide laser, *Laryngoscope* 90:809, 1980.
45. Hirano M: *Clinical examination of voice,* New York, 1981, Springer-Verlag.
46. Hirano M: Structure of the vocal fold in normal and disease states: anatomical and physical studies. In *Proceedings of the Conference on the Assessment of Vocal Pathology (ASHA Report II),* Rockville, Maryland, 1981, The American Speech-Language-Hearing Association.
47. Hogikyan ND, Bastian RW: Endoscopic CO_2 laser excision of large or recurrent laryngeal saccular cysts in adults, *Laryngoscope* 107:260, 1997.
48. Holinger B, Johnston K: Benign tumors of the larynx, *Ann Otol Rhinol Laryngol* 60:496, 1951.
49. Holinger LD and others: Laryngocele and saccular cysts, *Ann Otol Rhinol Laryngol* 87:675, 1978.
50. Hyams VJ, Rabuzzi DD: Cartilaginous tumors of the larynx, *Laryngoscope* 80:755, 1970.
51. Jones SR, Myers EN, Barnes L: Benign neoplasms of the larynx, *Otolaryngol Clin North Am* 17:151, 1984.
52. Kambic V and others: Vocal cord polyps: incidence, histology and pathogenesis, *J Laryngol Otol* 95:609, 1981.
53. Kleinsasser O: *Microlaryngoscopy and endolaryngeal microsurgery: technique and typical findings,* ed 2, Baltimore, 1979, University Park Press.
54. Kleinsasser O: Pathogenesis of vocal cord polyps, *Ann Otol Rhinol Laryngol* 91:378, 1982.
55. LeJeune JE, Putman HC, Yamase HT: Multiple oncocytic papillary cystadenomas of the larynx: a case report, *Laryngoscope* 90:501, 1980.
56. Leventhal BG and others: A longterm study of lymphoblastoid interferon in recurrent respiratory papillomatosis, *N Engl J Med* 325:613, 1991.
57. Loire R and others: Pathology of benign vocal fold lesions, *Ear Nose Throat J* 67:357, 1988.
58. Ludlow CL, Hart MO, editors: *Proceedings of the Conference on the Assessment of Vocal Pathology (ASHA Report II).* Rockville, Maryland, 1981, The American Speech-Language-Hearing Association.
59. Lundgren J, Olofsson J, Hellquist H: Oncocytic lesions of the larynx, *Acta Otolaryngol (Stockh)* 94:335, 1982.
60. McCabe BC, Clark KF: Interferon and laryngeal papillomatosis, *Ann Otol Rhinol Laryngol* 92:2, 1983.
61. McMillan K and others: A 585-nanometer pulsed dye laser treatment of laryngeal papillomas: preliminary report, *Laryngoscope* 108:968-972, 1998.
62. Michaels L: *Pathology of the larynx,* New York, 1984, Springer-Verlag.
63. Micheau C and others: Relationship between laryngoceles and laryngeal carcinomas, *Laryngoscope* 88:680, 1978.
64. Mills SE, Fechner RE: In *Pathology of the larynx (an atlas of head and neck pathology),* Chicago, 1985, American Society of Clinical Pathologist Press.
65. Mizono G, Dedo HH: Subglottic hemangiomas in infants: treatment with CO_2 laser, *Laryngoscope* 94:638, 1984.
66. Modlin B: Rhabdomyoma of the larynx, *Laryngoscope* 92:580, 1982.
67. Monday LA and others: Epidermoid cysts of the vocal cords, *Ann Otol Rhinol Laryngol* 92:124, 1983.
68. Naiman AN and others: Intralesional cidofovir and surgical excision for laryngeal papillomatosis, *Laryngoscope* 113: 2174-2181, 2003.
69. Nanson EM: Neurilemmoma of the larynx: a case study, *Head Neck Surg* 1:69, 1978.
70. Neel HB, Unni KK: Cartilaginous tumors of the larynx: a series of 33 patients, *Otolaryngol Head Neck Surg* 90:201, 1982.
71. New GB, Erich JB: Benign tumors of the larynx: a study of 722 cases, *Arch Otolaryngol Head Neck Surg* 28:841, 1938.
72. Neyts J, DeClercq E: Mechanism of action of acyclic nucleoside phosphonates against herpes virus replication, *Biochem Pharmacol* 47:39, 1994.
73. Norris CW, Mullarky BS: Experimental skin incision made with the carbon dioxide laser, *Laryngoscope* 92:416, 1982.
74. Ogura H and others: Persistence of human papillomavirus type 6e in adult multiple laryngeal papilloma and the counterpart false cord of an interferon-treated patient, *J Clin Oncol (Japan)* 23:130, 1993.
75. Pransky SM and others: Clinical update on 10 children treated with intralesional cidofovir injections for severe recurrent respiratory papillomatosis, *Arch Otolaryngol Head Neck Surg* 126:1239-1243, 2000.
76. Pransky SM, Albright JT, Magit AE: Long-term followup of pediatric recurrent respiratory papillomatosis managed with intralesional cidofovir, *Laryngoscope* 113:1583-1587, 2003.

77. Saito S and others: *X-ray stroboscopy.* In Stevens KN, Hirano M, editors: *Vocal fold physiology,* Tokyo, 1981, University of Tokyo Press.

78. Sataloff RT: Professional singers: the science and art of clinical care, *Am J Otol* 2:251, 1981.

79. Sataloff RT: Efficient history taking in professional singers, *Laryngoscope* 94:1111, 1984.

80. Shagets FW, Barrs DM, Rugh K: X-ray study of the month: computed tomographic study of laryngeal cyst, *Ann Otol Rhinol Laryngol* 93:410, 1984.

81. Shah K and others: Rarity of cesarian delivery in cases of juvenile-onset respiratory papillomatosis, *Obstet Gynecol* 68:795, 1986.

82. Shapshay SM and others: Benign lesions of the larynx: should the laser be used? *Laryngoscope* 100:953, 1990.

83. Shapshay SM and others: New microspot micromanipulator for carbon dioxide laser surgery in otolaryngology: early clinical results, *Arch Otolaryngol Head Neck Surg* 114:1012, 1988.

84. Singh J, Black MJ, Fried I: Cartilaginous tumors of the larynx: a review of literature and two case experiences, *Laryngoscope* 90:1872, 1980.

85. Snoeck R and others: Treatment of severe laryngeal papillomatosis with intralesional injections of cidofovir, *J Med Virol* 54:219-225, 1998.

86. Som PM and others: Benign pleomorphic adenoma of the larynx: a case report, *Ann Otol Rhinol Laryngol* 88:112, 1979.

87. Stell PM, Maran AGD: Laryngocele, *J Laryngol Otol* 89:915, 1975.

88. Supance JS, Quenelle DJ, Crissman J: Endolaryngeal neurofibromas, *Otolaryngol Head Neck Surg* 88:74, 1980.

89. Tan OT, Hurwitz RM, Stafford TJ: Pulsed dye laser treatment of recalcitrant verrucae: a preliminary report, *Laser Surg Med* 13:127-137, 1993.

90. Thawley SE, May M, Ogura JH: Granular cell myoblastoma of the larynx, *Laryngoscope* 84:1545, 1974.

91. Van Cutsem E and others: Successful treatment of a squamous papilloma of the hypopharynx-esophagus by local injections of (S)-1-(3-hydroxy-2-phosphonylmethoxypropyl) cytosine, *J Med Virol* 45:230, 1995.

92. Weiss MD, Kashima HK: Tracheal involvement in laryngeal papillomatosis, *Laryngoscope* 93:45, 1983.

93. Winther LK: Rhabdomyoma of the hypopharynx and larynx, *J Laryngol Otol* 90:1041, 1976.

94. Wolfe VI, Ratusnik DL: Vocal symptomatology of postoperative dysphonia, *Laryngoscope* 91:635, 1981.

95. Zakrzewski A: Subglottic lipoma of the larynx: case report and literature review, *J Laryngol Otol* 79:1039, 1965.

96. Zeitels, SM: Ectasias and varices of the vocal fold: clearing the striking zone, *Ann Otol Rhinol Laryngol* 108:10, 1999.

SUGGESTED READING

Alberti PW, Dykun R: Adult laryngeal papillomata, *J Otolaryngol* 10:463, 1981.

Barsocchini LM, McCoy G: Cartilaginous tumors of the larynx: a review of the literature and a report of four cases, *Ann Otol Rhinol Laryngol* 77:146, 1968.

Bloch CS, Gould WF, Hirano M: Effect of voice therapy on contact granuloma of the vocal fold, *Ann Otol Rhinol Laryngol* 90:48, 1981.

Cotalingam JD, Barnes L, Nixon VB: Pleomorphic adenoma of the epiglottis, *Arch Otolaryngol Head Neck Surg* 103:245, 1977.

El-Serafy I: Rare benign tumors of the larynx, *J Laryngol Otol* 85:837, 1971.

Goethals PL, Dahlin DC, Devine KD: Cartilaginous tumors of the larynx, *Surg Gynecol Obstet* 117:77, 1963.

Johnson JT, Barnes EL, Justica W: Adult onset laryngeal papillomatosis, *Otolaryngol Head Neck Surg* 89:867, 1981.

Naiman HB and others: Natural cytotoxicity and interferon production in patients with recurrent respiratory papillomatosis, *Ann Otol Rhinol Laryngol* 93:483, 1984.

Strong MS, Vaughn CW: Vocal cord nodules and polyps: the role of surgical treatment, *Laryngoscope* 81:911, 1971.

Suehs OW, Powell DB: Congenital cyst of the larynx in infants, *Laryngoscope* 77:651, 1967.

Thawley SE, Bone RC: Laryngopyocele, *Laryngoscope* 83:362, 1973.

Thomas RL: Non-epithelial tumors of the larynx, *J Laryngol Otol* 93:1131, 1979.

CHAPTER NINETY SIX

MEDIALIZATION THYROPLASTY

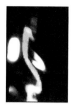

Paul W. Flint
Charles W. Cummings

INTRODUCTION

Since the first writing of this chapter, laryngeal phonosurgery has continued an evolution encompassing a variety of procedures designed to rehabilitate the dysfunctional larynx. Phonosurgical procedures can be classified into several categories, including the following: (1) microlaryngeal procedures for excision of benign or malignant disease; (2) vocal fold injection for augmentation and medialization; (3) laryngeal framework surgery; (4) laryngeal reinnervation procedures; and (5) reconstructive and rehabilitative procedures after tumor resection. Laryngeal framework surgery has been further categorized by Isshiki[28] into four types of surgical procedures based on functional alteration of the vocal folds: medial displacement (type I), lateral displacement (type II), shortening or relaxation (type III), and elongation or tensioning procedures (type IV).[22,25–27]

This chapter focuses on laryngeal framework surgery and vocal fold injection as applied to rehabilitation of the paralyzed larynx, while specifically addressing the management of glottal insufficiency from unilateral vocal fold motion impairment.

HISTORICAL ASPECTS

The predominate focus of phonosurgical procedures has been rehabilitation of the paralyzed larynx. With a few exceptions, primary repair by end-to-end anastomosis after injury to the recurrent laryngeal nerve has been universally unsuccessful.[51] Failure of primary repair is ascribed to a random process of axonal regeneration at the site of injury resulting in the simultaneous contraction of antagonistic muscle groups, otherwise known as *synkinesis*.[11,16] Alternative methods of reinnervation have been explored using ansa hypoglossus nerve-muscle pedicle implants into the posterior cricoarytenoid muscle and phrenic nerve to recurrent laryngeal nerve anastomosis for bilateral vocal fold paralysis.[4,5,13,52] Ansa hypoglossus nerve-

nerve anastomosis and nerve-muscle implant techniques have also been applied to unilateral vocal fold paralysis.[13,53] Despite significant efforts in establishing appropriate reinnervation and function after injury to the recurrent laryngeal nerve, debate continues about the efficacy of these procedures. Reinnervation procedures applied to laryngeal rehabilitation are covered in greater detail in this section by Goding.

The first report of a phonosurgical procedure appeared when Brunings[9] introduced the concept of vocal fold medialization by injecting paraffin within the body of the paralyzed fold. This was followed by Payr's[47] description of an external approach for medialization using a posterior vertical incision through the thyroid lamina, whereby the anterior flap is collapsed inward, resulting in limited medialization. Neither approach gained acceptance. Almost four decades later, Meurman[41] reported a series of patients with vocal cord paralysis in which external medialization procedures were performed using a vertical parasagittal incision in the anterior thyroid cartilage and autologous rib cartilage grafts placed between the thyroid ala and the inner perichondrium. Meurman's procedure resulted in a high incidence of complications, probably as a result of perichondrial and mucosal perforations occurring with the anterior midline approach. In the 1960s, Arnold[3] reintroduced vocal fold injection using an alloplastic material, Teflon. Over the ensuing years, experience with Teflon has demonstrated an increasing frequency of problems related to granuloma formation.[31a,44,46] Subsequently, an absorbable material (Gelfoam) was applied, allowing temporary vocal fold medialization by injection. Autologous fat has also been used to attempt permanent medialization.[8,42,57] However, the long-term effectiveness of autologous fat has been shown to be unpredictable with an overall success rate of 62% at 12 months.[36] Reports using bovine collagen injections for medialization were initially promising; however, soft tissue response resulted in variable results with respect to phonatory function.[17] More recently, micronized AlloDerm (Cymetra) has been applied for vocal fold injection with early reports indicating improved soft tissue response, increased tissue compliance, and overall improved phonatory function. Similar to bovine collagen, Cymetra may last 3 to 9 months and can be used for temporary medialization when recovery is likely to occur after RLN injury.[31,48]

Although numerous modifications of external approaches have been reported,[6,24,30,43,45] Isshiki[24] was the first to introduce the concept of alloplastic implant material for medialization. Using an external approach with Silastic implant, Isshiki is credited with the ultimate success and popularity of type I medialization thyroplasty. We are proponents of prefabricated implants with sizing systems. Two systems, VoCoM hydroxyapatite implants (Gyrus) and Montgomery Silastic implants (Boston Medical), are currently available.[10] More recently, Gore-Tex strips have been used to maintain vocal fold medialization with and without arytenoid adduction.[19,39,40]

Although type I medialization procedures result in dramatic improvement in glottal efficiency and sound production, a small group of patients continue to have difficulty during phonation as a result of a large posterior glottal chink or vocal folds at unequal levels. To address this problem specifically, Isshiki and colleagues[24] introduced the arytenoid adduction procedure for unilateral vocal cord paralysis. By using a suture placed around the muscular process of the arytenoid, traction in the direction of the lateral cricoarytenoid and thyroarytenoid muscles results in medial rotation of the arytenoid and downward displacement of the vocal process, thus closing the posterior gap and placing the paralyzed vocal folds at equal levels. Arytenoid adduction and related procedures are covered in greater detail in this section by Woodson (Chapter 97).

The advantages of an external approach to modify vocal fold tension and position without altering the structural components (mucosal fold and underlying muscle body) have expanded the role of laryngeal framework surgery. Isshiki and others[23,29] and Koufman[35] have reported their experience with medialization and tensioning procedures for the management of vocal fold bowing and dysphonia resulting from sulcus vocalis and soft tissue deficits.

MANAGEMENT OF GLOTTAL INSUFFICIENCY ASSOCIATED WITH UNILATERAL VOCAL FOLD MOTION IMPAIRMENT AND SOFT TISSUE DEFICITS

Several procedures are available to manage glottal insufficiency, including vocal fold injection for medialization, medialization thyroplasty, arytenoid adduction, adduction arytenoidopexy,[58] and a variety of reinnervation procedures. Selection of the appropriate procedure depends on the duration of symptoms, degree of impairment, presence of anatomic or surgical defect, and potential for recovery. In addition, the patient's overall condition and life expectancy should be considered before one embarks on a procedure that may predispose the patient to added morbidity.

Patient Evaluation and Selection

Degree of impairment can be determined by subjective criteria based on the patient's symptoms such as breathiness, aspiration, and exertional intolerance or on more objective criteria obtained through a variety of tests. Currently available studies for the objective assessment of laryngeal function include perceptual assessment, simple phonatory function tasks such as mean or maximum phonation time, acoustic parameters (i.e., spectrographic analysis, measurement of fundamental frequency, perturbation of frequency and amplitude, signal/noise ratio), and measurement of phonatory airflow. The objective assessment of laryngeal function is covered in greater detail in the chapter by Samlan (Chapter 87).

Videostroboscopy remains the most useful subjective and objective test for preoperative and postoperative evaluation of patients with unilateral vocal fold impairment, providing visual assessment of glottal closure and status of the mucosal wave. Reinnervation or denervation may be determined by the presence of abnormal or asymmetric mucosal wave patterns during stroboscopy; however, the absence of a mucosal wave does not necessarily imply denervation. Because the mucosal wave is a passive phenomenon established by adequate vocal fold tension and subglottal pressure, the presence of functional motor units is not a prerequisite for the development of the mucosal wave.[33]

Electromyography (EMG) is the only test available at this time for evaluating the integrity of the laryngeal motor unit in the presence of vocal fold motion impairment. Laryngeal EMG is useful for prognosticating and determining the presence of denervation or reinnervation potentials. EMG is assuming a more active role in the prognostication, timing of intervention, and choice of surgical procedures for the paralyzed larynx.[49,50] Despite normal voluntary electric activity, however, vocal fold immobility may be present as the result of laryngeal synkinesis, joint ankylosis, or cicatricial web formation. Distinction between these processes can be made only by palpation of the vocal process during direct laryngoscopy.

With documentation of denervation by EMG, medialization thyroplasty should be considered early in the presence of aspiration or severe dysphonia. If there is evidence of recovery visually or by EMG, medialization by injection using a resorbable material such as Cymetra can be considered as a temporizing procedure. Patients suffering from mild to moderate symptoms of dysphonia only may be counseled to allow spontaneous recovery to occur before considering permanent medialization procedures. Although type I thyroplasty is considered reversible, voice quality after the removal of implants has not been studied.

Prognosis, when combined with objective studies, will be useful for patient selection. Vocal fold paralysis with a favorable prognosis occurs after blunt trauma, endotracheal intubation, idiopathic vocal fold paralysis, and paralysis associated with viral pathogens (Ramsay Hunt syndrome). In this setting, severity of aspiration, dysphonia, and EMG findings can be used to determine the choice of procedure and timing of intervention, as outlined previously. Paralysis with poor prognosis for recovery includes those patients with injury after complete nerve section during surgical resection of tumor, invasion of cranial nerves by tumor, paralysis associated with thoracic aneurysm, and paralysis due to progressive neurologic disorders. Unlike peripheral recurrent laryngeal nerve injuries, high vagal injuries can result not only in loss of abductor/adductor function, but also loss of cricothyroid muscle function and deafferentation of sensory fibers. In this condition, vocal folds are more likely to be lateralized with marked bowing and atrophic changes. These patients generally have greater difficulty with dysphonia, dysphagia, and aspiration. Where denervation is documented or history portends a poor outcome, early medialization by thyroplasty is warranted.

Percutaneous medialization by injection should be considered in patients with short life expectancy and aspiration or severe dysphonia. In this situation, the time and expense of medialization thyroplasty or reinnervation procedures might not be justified.

Vocal Fold Medialization by Injection

Vocal fold medialization by injection remains a standard procedure for laryngeal rehabilitation. In the absence of arytenoid fixation and when adequate residual vocal fold structure remains to allow needle placement for augmentation, medialization of a paralyzed vocal fold by injection can be performed using a variety of materials. Autologous fat and Cymetra (human micronized AlloDerm) are the most common materials used today. Cymetra has been shown to provide excellent phonatory results lasting 6 to 12 months with little or no inflammatory response. The hyaluronic acid formulations such as Hylan B gel (Hylaform, Genzyme Biosurgery Inc.) used as an injectable material for medialization has also been shown to have favorable viscoelastic properties.[2] Collagen, although not specifically approved by the U.S. Food and Drug Administration for laryngeal injections, has been shown to be effective for management of vocal fold paralysis, sulcus vocalis, and soft tissue deficits.[7] Inflammatory changes associated with soft tissue response after bovine collagen injection can result in increased tissue stiffness and less than satisfactory results. Permanent adverse effects are unlikely to occur, however, since the collagen is ultimately resorbed. The use of Teflon paste (Polytef) for vocal fold injection is discouraged unless long-term patient survival is not anticipated. Adverse effects due to development of Teflon granuloma are well documented and include dysphonia caused by soft tissue reaction and airway obstruction from mass effect.[16]

Transoral and percutaneous approaches have added a new dimension to the management of vocal fold paralysis.[38,55] In most patients, medialization can be accomplished quickly and effectively in the office setting. These procedures are relatively simple and yield immediate results with little discomfort to the patient. If recovery of vocal fold function is likely, fat and Teflon are usually contraindicated, and alternative methods must be considered. Cymetra can be used as a temporizing measure in this setting. Percutaneous injections are performed without sedation using local anesthesia alone. Flexible fiberoptic laryngoscopy is required to visualize position and adequacy of injection. Given their advantages and ease of performance, percutaneous injections are becoming the preferred method in many centers. However, when airway management is a potential problem, injection in a controlled setting during direct laryngoscopy should be considered.

Percutaneous Injection

We prefer a lateral, percutaneous approach through the thyroid ala at the level of vocal fold determined by palpating the thyroid notch and inferior border of the thyroid ala anteriorly (Figure 96-1). The vocal fold lies perpendicular to this line at the midpoint. Alternatively, an anterior approach can be used through the cricothyroid membrane, approaching the vocal folds from below.[38,55] As the needle is inserted, it is angled superior and laterally under direct visualization using a flexible fiberoptic nasopharyngoscope.

When Cymetra is used for this procedure, it is reconstituted in saline and placed in a Luer Lock 1-cc syringe with a 1-inch, 23-gauge needle. Controlled pressure is required to pass the needle through the thyroid lamina. Visualization is best achieved with a flexible fiberoptic nasopharyngoscope with digital imaging system. The position of the needle can be visualized easily before entering the superficial layers

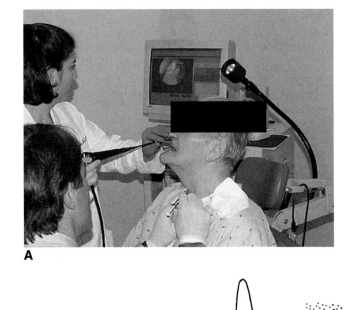

A

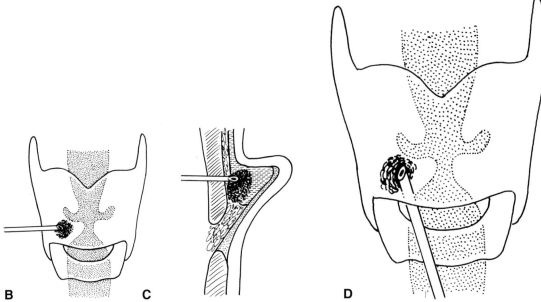

B   **C**   **D**

Figure 96-1. Percutaneous injection with fiberoptic visualization. **A,** Lateral approach is used with the needle passed through the thyroid cartilage. The needle is visualized in the paraglottal space anterior and lateral to the vocal process. **B,** A lateral percutaneous approach for vocal fold injection. **C,** Site of injection. **D,** An anterior percutaneous approach for vocal fold medialization. (D from Cummings CW and others: *Otolaryngology—head and neck surgery, update I,* St. Louis, 1989, Mosby.)

of the fold. Optimal results are obtained by placing the injection just anterior and lateral to the vocal process, and on a plane level with the lower border of the medial edge. This will build up the undersurface of the true fold and minimize the risk on injecting into Reinke's space. Using this technique, approximately 0.5 to 1.0 cc of Cymetra is adequate. In general, slight overinjection with Cymetra and autologous fat is preferred because resorption is anticipated. Patients should be counseled that voice change over time is expected.

Transoral Injection

Transoral injection can be performed in selected patients. Topical 4% lidocaine solution is applied to the pharyngeal and laryngeal mucosa. With the patient holding the tongue forward, allowing indirect visualization, the injection is performed using a curved laryngeal needle. Right and left needles are available so that the bevel is directed away from the midline to minimize the possibility of an intramucosal injection.

Laryngoscopic Injection

Laryngoscopic injection may be necessary in patients that do not tolerate the flexible fiberoptic examination by percutaneous or transoral approach. Injection via microlaryngoscopy is also used during ablative procedures in which recurrent laryngeal or vagal nerve resection is anticipated and temporary medialization is performed to minimize immediate postoperative symptoms. The injection can be performed with the patient under general anesthesia with spontaneous ventilation, controlled intermittent apnea, or jet ventilation using the Sanders device.

With the patient in the supine position, and after initiation of appropriate anesthesia, the laryngoscope is introduced and suspended using a suspension apparatus. Care is taken not to place unnecessary tension at the anterior commissure, which would result in distortion of the vocal folds. The arytenoid cartilages are palpated with a spatula to ensure mobility, and the false vocal fold is lateralized exposing the ventricle (Figure 96-2).

When injecting Cymetra, a 23-gauge butterfly needle is modified by removing the flange completely on one side and leaving a small flange on the other to grasp with a small alligator forceps. Visualization is best achieved using a 0- or 30-degree, 5-mm laryngeal telescope and digital video system. Telescopic visualization provides better assessment of the depth of injection. The needle is then inserted anterior and lateral to the vocal process approximately 2 mm deep or at the plane level with the lower margin of the true fold. Autologous fat is more viscous and may require an injection gun such as a Brunings syringe. After injection, a spatula or suction can be used to massage the vocal fold to distribute the injected material more evenly.

Laryngoscopy can also be performed with the patient under local anesthesia to monitor the changes in vocal quality during injection. Superior laryngeal nerve blocks with lidocaine should be avoided because they will alter vocal fold tension due to cricothyroid muscle paralysis and adversely affect voice quality. After the initial injection, the scope is relaxed and the patient is asked to phonate. Repeat injections are performed as necessary.

A distinction should be made between vocal fold medialization and intracordal injection. With injections for medialization, the material is placed in the paraglottal space lateral to the vocalis muscle, leaving the mucosa overlying the vocal fold unaltered. With intracordal injections for eliminating soft tissue defects, the injectable material (collagen or Cymetra) is placed more superficially into the area just deep to the lamina propria, avoiding Renke's space (Figure 96-3). Teflon is contraindicated for intracordal injections because granulomatous reactions to Teflon can increase vocal fold stiffness and mass, adversely affecting vocal fold vibration.[54,56]

Complications of vocal fold injection include underinjection requiring repeat procedures, overinjection with airway compromise, improper placement causing subglottal extension, and potential stenosis. Migration of Teflon particles, intracordal injection of Teflon impairing vibratory capability, and granuloma formation may occur (Figure 96-4). Management of

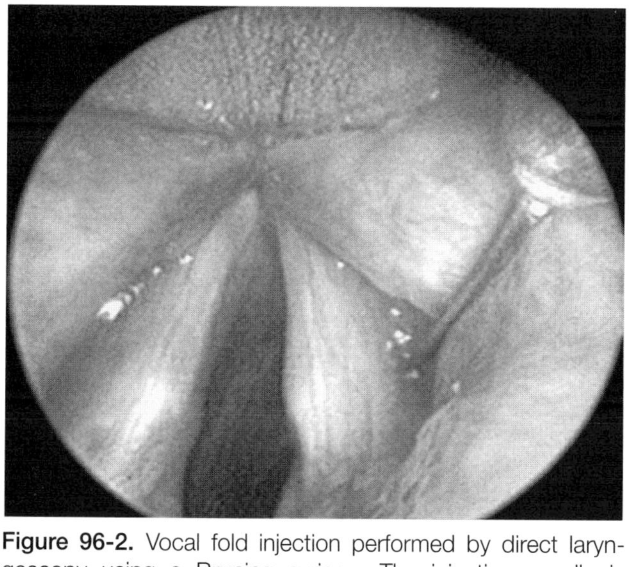

Figure 96-2. Vocal fold injection performed by direct laryngoscopy using a Bruning syringe. The injection needle is placed lateral to the vocal process and vocal ligament to prevent infiltration into Reinke's space.

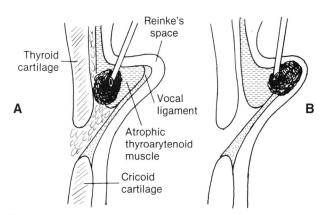

Figure 96-3. Types of vocal fold injection. **A,** Intrachordal injection for vocal fold paralysis showing the bevel of the needle directed away from the medial edge of the vocal fold. **B,** Intramucosal injection resulting from misplaced injection with the bevel of the needle directed toward the medial edge of the vocal fold. (From Cummings CW and others: *Otolaryngology—head and neck surgery, update I,* St. Louis, 1989, Mosby.)

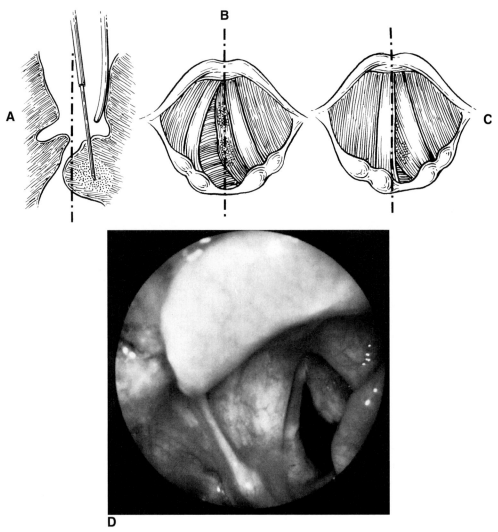

Figure 96-4. Complications of vocal fold injection. **A,** Excessive and incorrect placement of injected polytef. **B,** Inspiration with partial obstruction. **C,** Phonation with vocal fold overlap. **D,** Polytef granuloma developing 2 years after injection, resulting in dysphonia and airway obstruction. (From Cummings CW and others: *Atlas of laryngeal surgery,* St. Louis, 1984, Mosby.)

Teflon overinjection is a challenging problem and should be counteracted immediately by incising the mucosa over the site of injection and removing excess material by suction. Immediate removal is preferred because delayed removal is made difficult by migration of Teflon, granuloma, and scar formation. If necessary, delayed removal is generally attempted during microlaryngoscopy using cupped forceps or the carbon dioxide laser. Koch and others[32] evaluated the safety of using the carbon dioxide laser on Teflon and found no evidence or reports of untoward side effects. Endoscopic removal should be attempted initially, although open procedures (thyrotomy) may be required in cases of persistent granuloma.

Medialization Thyroplasty

Medialization thyroplasty is now considered by many in the surgical community to be the procedure of choice for management of the paralyzed vocal fold. The procedure can be performed alone or in conjunction with arytenoid adduction or reinnervation procedures. Also classified as a type I thyroplasty by Isshiki,[23,24] this procedure offers the following advantages: (1) it is performed with local anesthesia with minimal or no discomfort to the patient; (2) patient positioning is more anatomic, allowing better assessment of voice during the procedure; (3) it is potentially reversible; and (4) because the prosthesis is placed lateral to the inner perichondrium of the thyroid lamina, structural integrity of the vocal fold is preserved, allowing medialization with effective closure of the prephonatory gap—the end result being a decrease in oscillation threshold and improved vocal efficiency.[14,18,22] Disadvantages include the following: (1) the patient is subjected to an open procedure; (2) the procedure is technically more difficult; and (3) closure of the posterior glottis may be limited.

Medialization thyroplasty is currently used for management of vocal fold paralysis, vocal fold bowing resulting from aging or cricothyroid joint fixation, sulcus vocalis, and soft tissue defects resulting from excision of pathologic tissue.[28,34] Treatment for paralytic dysphonia is indicated when the likelihood of recovery is negligible. When recovery is anticipated, medialization thyroplasty may be considered for management of aspiration or severe dysphonia as an alternative to repeated injections with Cymetra. Generally, dysphonia by itself should be managed conservatively if recovery is anticipated; however, our experience has not revealed an adverse effect in those patients who have received a thyroplasty and subsequently recovered function.

Although modifications of Isshiki's description of medialization thyroplasty are abundant, the basic principles remain the same. Factors that affect outcome include size and shape of the implant, position of the implant, maintaining proper position of the implant, and limiting the duration of the surgical procedure. In our experience, the duration of the procedure is directly related to predictability of the end result. Carved Silastic implants, prefabricated Silastic implants (Montgomery)[43] and dense hydroxyapatite (VoCoM) implants are routinely used. Prefabricated implants with matched-sizing templates allow for more rapid determination of the correct implant position and size (Figure 96-5). Gore-Tex strips have also

been used with success, and in some situations may provide greater adaptability than prefabricated systems.[40] Gore-Tex is a Teflon product, and the potential for developing a granulomatous inflammatory response should be considered.

Technique

With the patient in the supine position and prepared for a sterile procedure, a paramedian horizontal incision is outlined over the middle aspect of the thyroid lamina. Local anesthesia is administered subcutaneously and in four quadrants over the ipsilateral lamina. A 5-cm incision is made through the platysma. Superior and inferior flaps are elevated in the subplatysmal plane exposing the thyroid notch and inferior border of the thyroid cartilage. The strap muscles are split in the midline and retracted laterally off the thyroid lamina, leaving the outer perichondrium intact. A single large skin hook is implanted in the anterosuperior aspect of the contralateral ala and retracted laterally, providing exposure of the ipsilateral lamina. The cartilage window is outlined by scoring the perichondrium sharply, or with electrocautery applied to a window template. For the VoCoM system, the window measures 6 mm (vertical) by 10 mm (horizontal) (Figure 96-6). The anterior aspect of the window is positioned 5 to 8 mm posterior to the ventral midline in females, and 8 to 10 mm in males. The superior aspect of the window should be placed at the level of the true fold. A point half the distance between the anterior-inferior border of the thyroid cartilage and the notch defines the level of the true fold. From this point, a line drawn posterior and parallel to the inferior border of the thyroid cartilage will approximate the level of the true fold. The outer perichondrium is incised and elevated from the thyroid cartilage within the confines of the window. Cartilage and osteoid material are removed precisely, preserving the dimensions of the window. Where ossification has occurred, the window can be drilled out or removed with a Kerrison punch. Care is taken to preserve the inner perichondrium, which is now elevated in circumferential fashion off the thyroid lamina using a laryngeal elevator.

Using the VoCoM system, one of five sizing prosthesis templates (3–8 mm) is inserted through the window and rotated 90 degrees with the bevel directed superiorly (Figure 96-7). This orientation is more likely to produce optimum voice quality; however, placing the bevel of the implant inferiorly or anteriorly in the horizontal plane can be tried. When using Silastic implants, pre-cut implants with progressively greater displacement (3–8 mm) may be used. Rarely are implants with displacement greater than 7 mm required. All retractors are removed and the

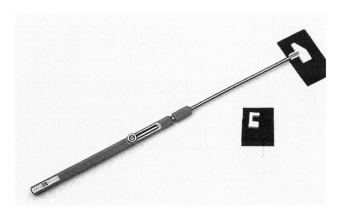

Figure 96-5. Prefabricated implant system made from hydroxyapatite. Implants vary from 3 to 7 mm of displacement. The implant is stabilized with a 0- to 3-mm offset shim (2-mm offset shim is shown with 6-mm displacement shim).

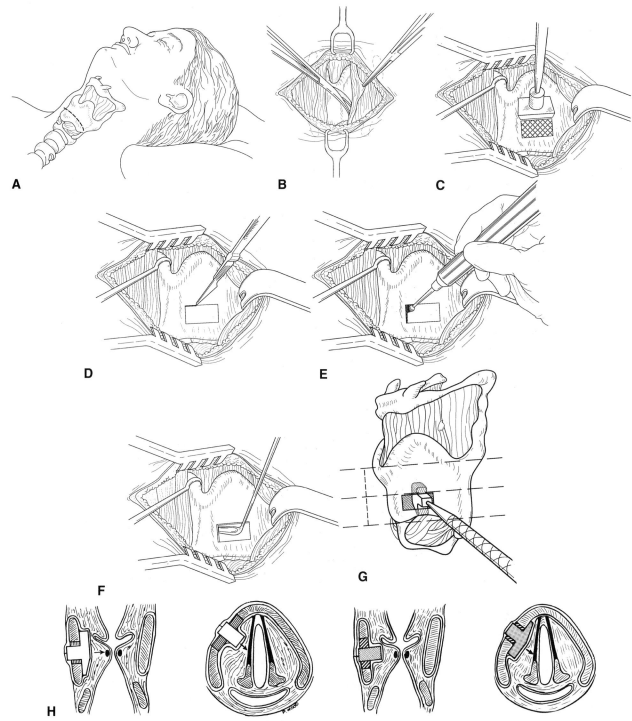

Figure 96-6. Medialization thyroplasty. **A,** Skin incision. **B,** Sternohyoid muscle is elevated off the thyroid cartilage. **C,** The muscle is retracted posterior to thyroid lamina, a cautery template marks the fenestra (6 × 10 mm); and the superior aspect of the window is at the vocal fold level. **D,** the outer perichondrium is incised and removed. **E,** A cutting burr, followed by a diamond burr, is used to remove cartilage and protect underlying periochondrium; a small Kerrison may facilitate removal of cartilage from the fenestra. **F,** The inner perichondrium is circumferentially elevated with a blunt dissector. **G,** A template or appropriately sized prosthesis is placed in the most effective position; the appropriate position of the fenestra is shown relative to the vocal fold level based on external landmarks. **H,** Variations in placement of the implant, showing vertical and horizontal implants relative to the plane of the true vocal fold.

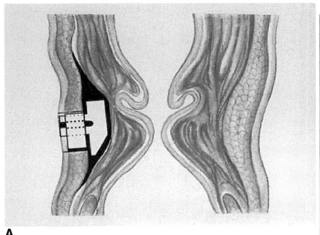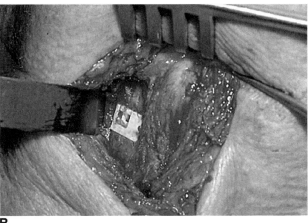

A   **B**

Figure 96-7. A, Schematic rendition of implant positioned within fenestra and secured with shim. **B,** Intraoperative view of hydroxyapatite implant (VoCoM system, Gyrus Inc., Wales) secured with shim.

patient asked to phonate while moving the template through all four quadrants of the window to determine the optimal position. Smaller or larger templates can be selected as needed. If medialization appears to be limited by the inner perichondrium and the thyroid cartilage is bowed outwards, the inner perichondrium can be incised, releasing tension and enhancing medialization. Once the appropriate size and position have been determined, the retractors are replaced and the implant is inserted and secured with the appropriate shim. If the window is fashioned correctly the shim will fit securely, preventing migration of the implant. If the shim is not stable, or the cartilage is thin, a suture is passed through the neck of the implant and tied over a titanium mini construction plate, thus, securing the shim. When using carved Silastic, the

implant can be secured by fashioning an implant with medial and lateral flanges to engage the thyroid cartilage (Figure 96-8). The wound is then irrigated with antibiotic solution. A small suction drain is placed deep to the strap muscles. Strap muscles and platysma are approximated with 4-0 absorbable suture and skin is closed with a running 5-0 subcuticular suture. Decadron is given preoperatively to minimize edema, and administration of prophylactic antibiotics is continued for 5 days.

We prefer to use the largest prosthesis possible while maintaining quality of voice. Overcorrection is supported by Isshiki and others,[28] who found deterioration in voice quality over time as intraoperative edema resolved in the postoperative period. When medialization is performed early after the onset of

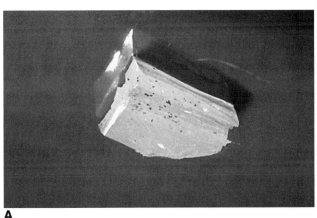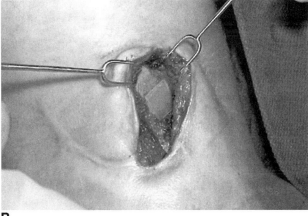

A   **B**

Figure 96-8. A, Carved Silastic implant with medial and lateral flange to engage the thyroid lamina. **B,** Implant secured within fenestra in thyroid lamina. To view this image in color, please go to *www.ototext.com* or the Electronic Image Collection CD, bound into your copy of Cummings Otolaryngology—Head and Neck Surgery, 4th edition.

paralysis, muscle atrophy can result in voice deterioration postoperatively. Minimizing operative time is critical in obtaining optimal results.[28] Fabricating implants before the procedure will facilitate determination of size and position intraoperatively and optimize the end result.

Thyroplasty performed with Gore-Tex as described by McCulloch and Hoffman is performed in a similar manner.[39] Window location and dimensions do not need to be as precise. The inner perichondrium is opened, and the implant material is simply layered into the paraglottal space (Figure 96-9).

Limitations of type I thyroplasty relate to the mechanical nature of the procedure. The procedure imparts static change to the laryngeal framework, with no influence on dynamic function. There is no effect on vocal fold muscle mass, innervation, or vocal fold mobility. Closure of the posterior glottis may be limited due to narrowing of the paraglottal space as the cricoid and thyroid cartilage converge posteriorly. Furthermore, type I thyroplasty may not affect vocal fold level in the vertical plane.

Complications associated with type I thyroplasty include penetration of the endolaryngeal mucosa, wound infection, chondritis, implant migration or extrusion, and airway obstruction. Airway compromise is the most serious potential problem and requires overnight inpatient observation.[1,37] Combined medialization thyroplasty and arytenoid adduction increases this risk.[1] Penetration of the endolaryngeal mucosa increases the risk of implant extrusion into the airway and infection. Before placement of the implant, the window should be assessed for air leak by filling the wound with saline while the patient phonates. If communication with the airway has occurred, as determined by air escape, the procedure should be terminated. Intubation soon after medialization can result in displacement of the prosthesis or mucosal erosion resulting from endotracheal tube pressure.

Although the overall complication rate with type I thyroplasty is less than 3%, incomplete glottal closure resulting from undercorrection or improper placement of the implant occurs in approximately 10% to 15% of patients. Incomplete glottal closure is more likely to occur in patients implanted acutely as a result of progressive vocal fold atrophy occurring after denervation. The surgical menu for management of incomplete closure includes revision thyroplasty, vocal fold injection with autologous fat or Cymetra, reinnervation procedures, and arytenoid adduction.

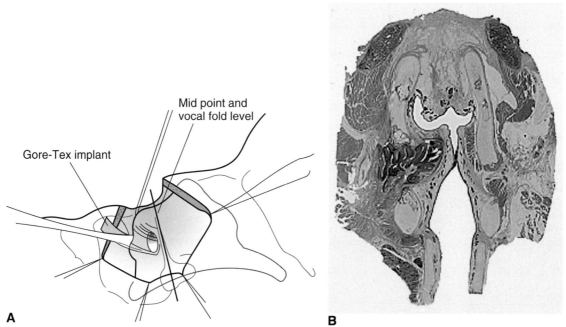

Figure 96-9. A, Schematic diagram of thyroplasty technique using Gore-Tex strip as described by McCulloch. The strip can be placed through a standard fenestra or, as shown in this figure, using an inferior approach. **B,** Postmortem whole organ section of human larynx obtained 6 months after Gore-Tex thyroplasty demonstrating medialization of implanted vocal fold. (Figure and Photomicrograph generously provided by Timothy McCulloch, M.D., University of Washington, Seattle, Washington.)

Revision thyroplasty is surgically feasible and provides a high yield of improvement over the preexisting condition. Silastic implants may be repositioned, or a larger prosthesis may be fashioned and reinserted through the previously created fenestra. However, removal of the implant with re-creation of the surgical envelope and reintroduction of a new prosthesis is more difficult than at the initial setting.

Medialization thyroplasty alone offers a simple solution to the management of unilateral laryngeal paralysis. Recognizing the limitations of this procedure, there are situations where more than one procedure will be required. Combining medialization thyroplasty with arytenoids adduction or reinnervation will, at times, be necessary. These surgical approaches are discussed in Chapters 97 and 98.

REFERENCES

1. Abraham MT, Gonen M, Kraus DH: Complications of type I thyroplasty and arytenoid adduction, *Laryngoscope* 111:1322, 2001.
2. Arnold GE: Dysplastic dysphonia: minor anomalies of the vocal cords causing persistent hoarseness, *Laryngoscope* 68:142, 1958.
3. Arnold GE: Vocal rehabilitation of paralytic dysphonia, *Arch Otolaryngol* 76:358, 1962.
4. Baldissera F and others: Recovery of inspiratory abduction of the paralyzed vocal cords after bilateral reinnervation of the cricoarytenoid muscles by one single branch of the phrenic nerve, *Laryngoscope* 99:1286, 1989.
5. Baldissera F and others: Restoring abduction of paralyzed vocal cords in the cat using selective laryngeal reinnervation by phrenic motoneurons, *Laryngoscope* 96:1399, 1986.
6. Beck C, Richstein A: Medianverlagerung einer paretischen Stimmlippe durch partielle Schildknorpelimpression, *Laryngol Rhinol Otol* 61:251, 1982.
7. Bless DM, Ford CN, Loftus JM: Role of injectable collagen in the treatment of glottic insufficiency: a study of 119 patients, *Ann Otol Rhinol Laryngol* 101:237, 1992.
8. Brandenburg JH, Unger JM, Koschkee MA: Vocal cord injection with autogenous fat: a long-term magnetic resonance imaging evaluation, *Laryngoscope* 106:174, 1996.
9. Brunings W: Uber eine neue Behandlungsmethode der Rekurrenslamung, *Verh Verl Deutsch Laryngol* 18:93, 1911.
10. Cummings CW, Purcell LL, Flint PW: Hydroxylapatite laryngeal implants for medialization: preliminary report, *Ann Otol Rhinol Laryngol* 102:843, 1993.
11. Crumley RL: Mechanisms of synkinesis, *Laryngoscope* 89:1847, 1979.
12. Crumley RL: Teflon versus thyroplasty versus nerve transfer: a comparison, *Ann Otol Rhinol Laryngol* 99:759, 1990.
13. Crumley RL, Izdebski K, McMicken B: Nerve transfer versus teflon injection for vocal cord paralysis: a comparison, *Laryngoscope* 98:1200, 1988.
14. D'Antonio LL, Wigley TL, Zimmerman GJ: Quantitative measures of laryngeal function following teflon injection or thyroplasty type I, *Laryngoscope* 105:256, 1995.
15. Flint PW, Corio RL, Cummings CW: Comparison of soft tissue response in rabbits following laryngea implantation with hydroxylapatite, silicone rubber, and Teflon, *Ann Otol Rhinol Laryngol* 106(5):399–407, 1997.
16. Flint PW, Downs DH, Coltrera MD: Laryngeal synkinesis following reinnervation in the rat; a neuroanatomic and physiologic study using retrograde fluorescent tracers and electromyography, *Ann Otol Rhinol Laryngol* 100:797, 1991.
17. Ford CN, Bless DM: Clinical experience with injectable collagen for vocal fold augmentation, *Laryngoscope* 96:863, 1986.
18. Gardner GM, Parnes SM: Status of the mucosal wave post vocal cord injection versus thyroplasty, *J Voice* 5:64, 1991.
19. Giovanni A and others: Medialization of paralysed vocal cord by expanded polytetrafluoroethylene implant (Gore-Tex), *Ann Otolaryngol Chir Cervicofac* 114:158, 1997.
20. Hallen L, Testad P, Sederhold E and others: DiHA (dextranomers in hyaluronan) injection for treatment of insufficient closure of the vocal folds: early clinical experiences, *Laryngoscope* 111(6):1063–1067, 2001.
21. Hertegard S and others: Cross-linked Hyaluronan used as augmentation substance for treatment of glottal insufficiency: safety aspects and vocal fold function, *Laryngoscope* 112:2211, 2002.
22. Hirano M: Phonosurgery, basic and clinical investigations, *Otologia* 21:239, 1975.
23. Isshiki N: *Phonosurgery: theory and practice.* Tokyo, 1989, Springer-Verlag.
24. Isshiki N, Okamura H, Ishikawa T: Thyroplasty type I (lateral compression) for dysphonia due to vocal cord paralysis or atrophy, *Acta Otolaryngol* 80:465, 1975.
25. Isshiki N, Taira T, Tanabe M: Surgical alteration of the vocal pitch, *J Otolaryngol* 12:335, 1983.
26. Isshiki N, Tanabe M, Sawada M: Arytenoid adduction for unilateral vocal cord paralysis, *Arch Otolaryngol* 104:555, 1978.
27. Isshiki N and others: Clinical significance of asymmetrical vocal cord tension, *Ann Otol Rhinol Laryngol* 86:58, 1977.
28. Isshiki N and others: Recent modifications in thyroplasty type I, *Ann Otol Rhinol Laryngol* 98:777, 1989.
29. Isshiki N and others: Thyroplasty as a new phonosurgical technique, *Acta Orolaryngol* 78:451–457, 1974.
30. Kamer FM, Som ML: Correction of the traumatically abducted vocal cord, *Arch Otolaryngol* 95:6, 1972.
31. Karpenko AN, Dworkin JP, Meleca RJ and others: Cymetra injection for unilateral vocal fold paralysis, *Ann Otol Rhinol Laryngol* 112(11):927–934, 2003.
31a. Kasperbauer JL, Slavit DH, Maragos NE: Teflon granulomas and overinjection of lefton: a therapeutic challenge for the otorhinolaryngologist, *Ann Rhinol Laryngol* 102:748, 1993.
32. Koch WM, Hybels RL, Shapshay SM: Carbon dioxide laser in removal of polytef paste, *Arch Otolaryngol Head Neck Surg* 113:661, 1987.
33. Kokesh J and others: Correlation between stroboscopy and electromyography in laryngeal paralysis, *Ann Otol Rhinol Laryngol* 102:852, 1993.
34. Koufman JA: Laryngoplasty for vocal cord medialization: an alternative to Teflon, *Laryngoscope* 96:726, 1986.
35. Koufman JA: Surgical correction of dysphonia due to bowing of the vocal cords, *Ann Otol Rhinol Laryngol* 98:41, 1989.
36. Laccourreye O and others: Intracordal injection of Autologous fat in patients with unilateral laryngeal nerve paralysis: long-term results from the patient's perspective, *Laryngoscope* 113:541, 2003.
37. Maves MD, McCabe BF, Gray S: Phonosurgery: indications and pitfalls, *Ann Otol Rhinol Laryngol* 98:577, 1989.
38. McCaffrey TB, Lipton R: Transcutaneous Teflon injection for paralytic dysphonia, *Laryngoscope* 99:497, 1989.

39. McCulloch TM, Hoffman HT: Medialization laryngoplasty with expanded polytetrafluoroethylene: surgical technique and preliminary results, *Ann Otol Rhinol Laryngol* 107:427–432, 1998.

40. McCulloch TM and others: Arytenoid adduction combined with Gore-tex medialization thyroplasty, *Laryngoscope* 110:1306, 2000.

41. Meurman Y: Operative mediofixation of the vocal cord in complete unilateral paralysis, *Arch Otolaryngol* 55:544, 1952.

42. Mikus JL, Koufman JA, Kilpatrick SE: Fate of liposuctioned and purified autologous fat injections in the canine vocal fold, *Laryngoscope* 105:17, 1995.

43. Montgomery WW, Blaugrund SM, Varvares MA: Thyroplasty: a new approach, *Ann Otol Rhinol Laryngol* 102:571, 1993.

44. Nakayama M, Ford CN, Bless DM: Teflon vocal fold augmentation: failures and management in 28 cases, *Otolaryngol Head Neck Surg* 109:493, 1993.

45. Netterville JL and others: Silastic medialization and arytenoid adduction: the Vandervilt experience, *Ann Otol Rhinol Laryngol* 102:413, 1993.

46. Ossoff RH and others: Difficulties in endoscopic removal of teflon granulomas of the vocal fold, *Ann Otol Rhinol Laryngol* 102:405, 1993.

47. Payr: Plastik am Schildknorpel zur Behebung der Folgen einseitiger Stimmbandlahmung, *Deutsche Medizinische Wochenschrift* 41:1265, 1915.

48. Pearl AW, Woo P, Ostrowski R and others: A preliminary report on micronized AlloDerm injection laryngoplasty, *Laryngoscope* 112(6):990–996, 2002.

49. Sataloff RT, Mandel S, Mann EA and others: Practice parameter: laryngeal electromyography (an evidence-based review), *Otolaryngol Head Neck Surg* 130(6):770–779, 2004.

50. Sulica L, Blitzer A: Electromyography and the immobile vocal fold, *Otolaryngol Clin North Am* 37(1):59–74, 2004.

51. Tashiro T: Experimental studies on the reinnervation of larynx after accurate neurorrhaphy, *Laryngoscope* 82:225, 1970.

52. Tucker HM: Human laryngeal reinnervation: long term experience with the nerve muscle pedicle technique, *Laryngoscope* 88:598, 1978.

53. Tucker HM: Reinnervation of the unilaterally paralyzed larynx, *Ann Otol* 86:789, 1977.

54. Varvares MA, Montgomery WW, Hillman RE: Teflon granuloma of the larynx: etiology, pathophysiology, and management, *Ann Otol Rhinol Laryngol* 104:511, 1995.

55. Ward PH, Hanson DG, Abemayor E: Transcutaneous Teflon injection of the paralyzed vocal cord: a new technique, *Laryngoscope*, 95:644, 1985.

56. Watterson T, McFarlane SC, Menicucci AL: Vibratory characteristics of Teflon injected and noninjected paralyzed vocal folds, *J Speech Hearing Discord* 55:61, 1990.

57. Zaretsky LS and others: Autologous fat injection for vocal fold paralysis: long-term histologic evaluation, *Ann Otol Rhinol Laryngol* 104:1, 1995.

58. Zeitels SM, Mauri M, Dailey SH: Adduction arytenopexy for vocal fold paralysis: indications and technique, *J Laryngol Otol* 118(7):508–516, 2004.

CHAPTER NINETY SEVEN

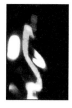

ARYTENOID ADDUCTION

|| Gayle Ellen Woodson

INTRODUCTION

The arytenoid adduction procedure (AA) addresses laryngeal incompetence in patients with unilateral laryngeal paralysis.[13] AA mimics the action of the lateral cricoarytenoid muscle (LCA) to close the glottis via rotation of the arytenoid cartilage, rather than direct displacement of the membranous vocal fold.[12] An adduction suture is placed in the muscular process of the arytenoid, which is the origin of the LCA. This suture is passed forward through the paraglottic space and secured to the inferior thyroid ala (Figure 97-1). This anterior traction pulls forward on the muscular process so that the arytenoid rotates. The vocal process, which is orthogonal to the muscular process, moves medially, dragging the membranous vocal fold with it. AA can be performed in conjunction with type I thyroplasty. Research in animal models indicates that a combination of the two is more effective than either procedure alone.[24]

AA is a more invasive procedure than type I thyroplasty and is technically more difficult. AA has been reported to carry somewhat greater surgical risks, including airway obstruction, joint dislocation, fistula, and carotid injury.[16,27] A recent study compared outcomes of type I thyroplasty alone or in combination with AA in 237 patients. The complication rate was 19% in patients undergoing AA vs 14% in those receiving thyroplasty alone. However, the difference in the complication rate was not statistically significant, and the two patients who required emergency tracheotomy for airway obstruction had thyroplasty alone.[1] AA does provide better closure of the posterior glottis, and research in animal models has objectively documented that acoustic and aerodynamic results for AA are better than for thyroplasty alone.[7,10] Thus, AA is a valuable component of the therapeutic armamentarium for rehabilitating patients with laryngeal paralysis, particularly those with significant glottal incompetence.

The clinical impact of laryngeal paralysis varies greatly.[35] Some patients with unilateral paralysis are completely asymptomatic. At the other end of the spectrum, some patients are aphonic and have severe problems with aspiration during swallowing. Such severe symptoms result from *laryngeal incompetence*—the inability of the glottis to close completely. Two key factors that influence glottal closure in patients with laryngeal paralysis are the configuration of the paralyzed vocal fold and the compensatory function of the contralateral fold.

Several theories have been proposed to explain variations in symptoms and vocal fold positions in patients with laryngeal paralysis, ranging from selective damage to abductor fibers[25] to adductor action of the cricothyroid muscle (Wagner-Grossman hypothesis).[15,23] However, it has been demonstrated that the cricothyroid muscle does not exert an adductor force on the vocal fold.[2,17,34] It is now generally accepted that a medial vocal fold position results from residual or regenerated innervation of laryngeal muscles.[3,8,11,29] When there is significant innervation of adductor muscles, the paralyzed fold is located near the midline, and compensatory activity of the normal side of the larynx can often close the glottis during phonation. In such cases, aspiration is rare, and hoarseness or breathiness responds well to surgical medialization of the membranous vocal fold performed by injection or thyroplasty. On the other hand, complete flaccid paralysis results in a cadaveric position of the vocal fold with more severe glottal incompetence, often referred to as a *posterior gap*.

It has long been recognized that vocal fold injection, such as with *polytetrafluoroethylene* (Teflon), cannot restore glottal competence when there is a large glottal gap.[9] There is some controversy regarding the efficacy of Ishiki type I thyroplasty in closing a posterior gap. It has been contended that a posterior extension of the thyroplasty implant can close a posterior gap, based on clinical observation.[20] However, other clinical reports as well as experimental studies

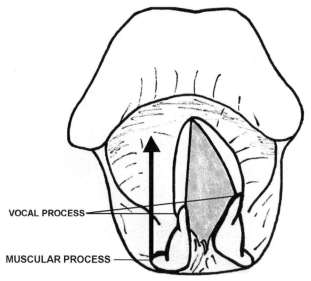

Figure 97-1. Arytenoid adduction procedure. Anterior traction on the muscular process rotates the arytenoid so that the vocal process moves medially.

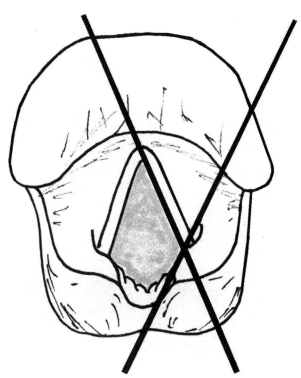

Figure 97-2. Vocal fold angle formed by membranous and cartilaginous portions of the vocal fold.

indicate that AA is much more effective than thyroplasty in closing the posterior glottis.[10,24]

The concept of a "posterior gap" is not entirely accurate because the maximal glottic opening is between the vocal processes. The open glottis actually converges posterior to the vocal processes because lateral displacement of the vocal process involves external rotation of the arytenoid cartilage, not lateral displacement of the arytenoid.[6] In other words, the angle between the membranous vocal fold and its posterior cartilaginous portion decreases as the vocal fold abducts[28] (Figure 97-2). Thus, the posterior portion of the cartilaginous vocal fold is medial to the vocal process in abduction, and it prevents glottic closure even with vigorous hyperadduction of the normal vocal fold (Figure 97-3). Procedures that medialize the membranous vocal fold may achieve some medial displacement of the vocal process; however, the force vectors created by such procedures are inadequate to effect significant internal rotation of the arytenoid cartilage.

Vocal fold injection and type I thyroplasty do not address differences in the level of vocal folds. The paralyzed vocal fold often lies in a different plane than the mobile vocal fold. Although both folds are firmly attached to the anterior commissure, the vocal process may sag on the paralyzed side or lie above the glottic plane, as it does in physiologic abduction. Thus, there can be a significant vertical gap between the edges of the vocal folds, even when they appear to be touching when viewed from above in a two-dimensional (2D) image. The paralyzed fold can lie either above or below the glottal plane. In cadaver specimens from subjects who had chronic vocal fold paralysis, the vocal fold has been reported to be caudally displaced with a wide ventricle and shift of the conus elasticus to a horizontal plane.[5,12] Other authors report superior displacement of the paralyzed vocal fold, essentially the same position assumed by an actively abducted vocal fold.[12,14,26]

A difference in the level of the vocal folds can often be appreciated with indirect mirror laryngoscopy, which permits binocular vision. In 1932, noting observations with mirror laryngoscopy, New and Childrey[23] stated, "In the absence of any innervation from the recurrent nerve fibers, the cord is somewhat relaxed or bowed; it is, therefore, shortened, somewhat narrowed and depressed, lying at a lower level than normal." In a 2D video image, a level difference is not apparent. What can be perceived is a difference in the apparent length of the vocal folds. Brewer and colleagues[4] noted that a paralyzed vocal fold generally appears shorter than its mobile mate. In patients with significant glottal incompetence, the apparent length of a paralyzed vocal fold during inspiration is approximately two-thirds that of the mobile side. During phonation, the mobile vocal fold appears to shorten to nearly the same length as its paralyzed mate (see Figure 97-3). Successful AA increases the apparent length of the paralyzed vocal fold.[31]

3D motion analysis in cadaver larynges indicates that the AA procedure does not actually lengthen the

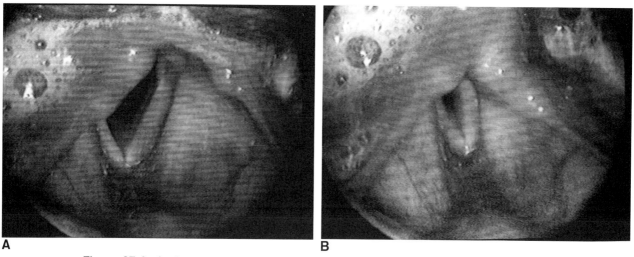

Figure 97-3. A, Apparent vocal fold shortening in laryngeal paralysis. **B,** Compensatory shortening of the mobile focal fold.

vocal fold but moves the vocal process caudally. It is this vertical component of motion that is endoscopically perceived as a length change; the visual image shortens due to rotation of the vocal fold out of the optical plane.[32] In AA, the arytenoid rotates about an oblique helical axis. As the vocal process moves medially, it is displaced caudally as well[22] (Figure 97-4). Conversely, when the posterior cricoarytenoid (PCA) muscle abducts the vocal fold, the vocal process moves laterally, rostrally, and caudally[6] (Figure 97-5). An abducted vocal fold appears shorter when viewed from above because the vocal process has moved rostrally; the vocal fold slopes upward, out of the plane of the image. In adduction and during AA the vocal process moves caudally, toward the level of the anterior commissure, so that the vocal fold is parallel to the image plane, and the apparent length is longer.[32]

The cricoarytenoid joint is a shallow ball and socket, and therefore, it is multiaxial. That is to say, vocal folds do not open and close along a fixed "track," and

the rostrocaudal level of the vocal process is not completely dictated by internal and internal rotation. Cadaver studies of simulated muscle contraction demonstrate that the axis of rotation for the posterior cricoarytenoid is quite different than that for the lateral cricoarytenoid muscle[6] (see Figure 97-5). This means that by varying the force of individual muscles, the rostrocaudal position of the vocal process can be varied independent of its medial/lateral position. This

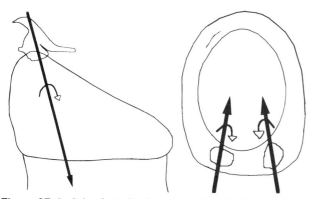

Figure 97-4. Axis of rotation in arytenoid adduction, as determined in 3D motion analysis in cadaver larynges.

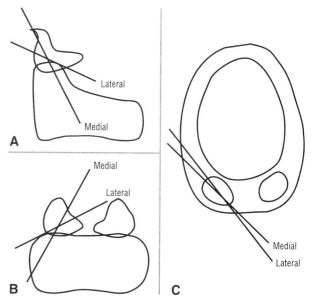

Figure 97-5. Axes of rotation with simulated individual contraction of the two bellies of the posterior cricoarytenoid muscle in cadaver larynges. **A,** Sagittal view. **B,** Posterior, coronal view. **C,** Axial view. This data, as well as those from the study depicted in Figure 97-5, illustrate the multiaxial nature of the cricoarytenoid joint.

is a likely mechanism of compensation by the active vocal fold in patients with laryngeal paralysis.

Because of the multiaxial nature of the cricothyroid joint, the vocal process of a paralyzed vocal is not necessarily located along the path of physiologic motion. In a normal larynx, the vocal process moves upward as the vocal fold is adducted. But in flaccid paralysis, the pull of the posterior cricoarytenoid muscle is lost, so that the arytenoid may "tip" forward (see Figure 97-3, *A*). The vector of the pull in the AA procedure is similar to that of the cricoarytenoid muscle, anteriorly and slightly inferiorly. Thus, AA cannot correct, and may exacerbate, anterior tip. One approach to correcting the "sagging" arytenoid is a posterior sus-

pension suture, which pulls posteriorly and inferiorly on the vocal process, to "rock" the arytenoid into a position that is nearer than that assumed during normal phonation[33] (Figure 97-6). Another approach to the sagging arytenoid is adduction arytenoidopexy.[36]

The membranous vocal fold is moved medially by AA. However, if the thyroarytenoid muscle is atrophic (which is frequently the case in cadaveric paralysis), there will still be a glottal gap anterior to the vocal process. This can be addressed by concomitant or subsequent medialization by injection or type I thyroplasty.

Dysphagia can be a significant problem when laryngeal paralysis is the result of a vagus nerve injury.

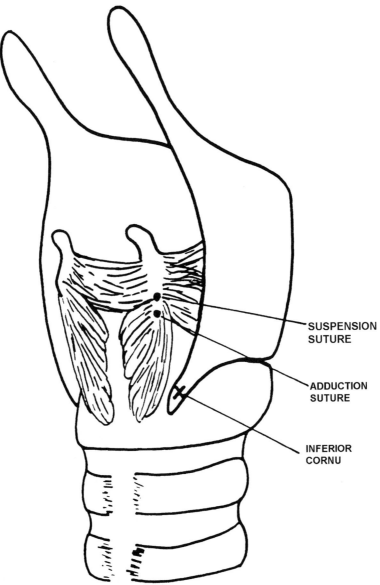

SUSPENSION SUTURE

ADDUCTION SUTURE

INFERIOR CORNU

Figure 97-6. Posterior view of larynx demonstrating muscular process attachment of the arytenoid adduction suture and the suspension suture. The suspension suture is anchored to the inferior cornu of the thyroid cartilage.

Pharyngeal propulsion is impaired due to ipsilateral paralysis of constrictor muscles. But the cricopharyngeal muscle retains tone because it is a continuous muscular sling that receives bilateral innervation. There is inadequate pharyngeal pressure to push the bolus into the esophagus, resulting in stasis of secretions and ingested food in the hypopharynx. In such cases, a cricopharyngeal myotomy can be effective in improving swallowing and reducing aspiration.[20] Cricopharyngeal myotomy is easily performed in conjunction with the AA procedure.[30]

AA is less effective in patients with long-standing laryngeal paralysis. This does not appear to be due to joint fixation because the arytenoid can be successfully internally rotated, with objective improvements in maximum phonation time and mean phonatory airflow. But the apparent length, and presumably the vertical position of the arytenoid, is not improved, so compensatory hyperfunction is still required for speech.[31] It is possible that contracture and fibrosis prevent correction of the vertical position of the vocal fold. The outcome of AA is also less favorable in patients with paralysis due to central neural lesions, such as tumor or stroke, because of other associated deficits.

OPERATIVE TECHNIQUE
Anesthesia

Local anesthesia is preferred for AA in most patients so that the changes in voice can be monitored intraoperatively. The correct degree of AA can be assured, and the potential need for a concomitant thyroplasty can be assessed, by transnasal flexible laryngoscopy. Moreover, glottic configuration can be adjusted without the confounding presence of an endotracheal tube. Finally, the risks of general anesthesia are avoided. Despite the fact that the larynx is rotated 90 degrees or more during the procedure, the airway is usually not appreciably compromised. Intraoperative swelling can compromise the airway and alter glottic closure, making intraoperative assessment less accurate. Therefore, preoperative steroids are recommended to minimize intraoperative swelling. Patients must be sufficiently alert during the procedure to cooperate. A patient who is overly sedated may actually become agitated during the procedure. Thus, sedation is recommended only during injection of local anesthesia. A field block provides adequate anesthesia at the outset; however, supplemental injections are required because the dissection proceeds posteriorly. An ipsilateral superior laryngeal nerve block will minimize coughing during intralaryngeal dissection.

General anesthesia can be used in uncooperative or very anxious patients or those in whom dissection is anticipated to be difficult, such as very obese patients or those with extensive scarring in the operative field. General anesthesia is also a good option for patients with an existing tracheotomy. When the procedure is performed under general anesthesia, direct laryngoscopy is used for intraoperative assessment. Obviously, this task is not precise when an endotracheal tube is present.

Surgical Procedure

The larynx is approached through a horizontal skin incision at the lower border of the thyroid cartilage, extending from the ipsilateral sternocleidomastoid muscle to approximately 1 cm past midline. It is most efficient to create a thyroplasty window at the outset of the procedure. This provides a route for the AA suture to be passed later in the case, and it also sets the stage for concomitant thyroplasty, should this be necessary.

After the thyroplasty window is created, the next objective is to expose the muscular process of the arytenoid. Several approaches have been described. I prefer to dissect lateral to the cervical strap muscles, rotating the larynx away from the opposite side. This displaces the larynx away from the carotid sheath, minimizing risk to those structures. Dissection should "hug" the strap muscles, continuing posteriorly to the inferior constrictor muscle and superiorly to identify the superior cornu of the thyroid cartilage. A sturdy cricoid hook should then be placed on the superior cornu of the thyroid cartilage to rotate the larynx away from the field (Figure 97-7). Dissection should then be continued inferiorly, medial to the thyroid gland, down to the level of the cricoid.

Next, the inferior constrictor muscle is transected over the posterior edge of the thyroid cartilage. Inferiorly, the cricopharyngeal muscle comes into view, and this muscle can then be resected, if needed. The muscle can be defined by blunt dissection just behind its attachment to the cricoid, and then a 1-to 2-cm segment of muscle is excised.

A critical step in the procedure is identification and displacement of the pyriform sinus mucosa, to expose the arytenoid cartilage and to avoid entry into the hypopharynx. The pyriform sinus is separated from the medial surface of the thyroid ala by blunt dissection. Identification of the posterior and inferior limits of the pyriform sinus is facilitated by having the patient utter plosive phrases (such as "puppy") that generate gentle positive intrapharyngeal pressure. This distends the pyriform sinus and makes its edges apparent. The sac is then reflected superiorly and anteriorly, exposing the posterior cricoarytenoid muscle. The fibers of this muscle are then followed to their convergence and insertion on the muscular process of the arytenoid. In males with a large thyroid cartilage,

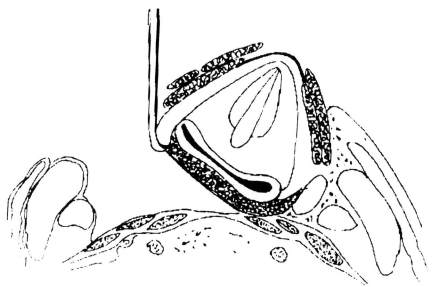

Figure 97-7. Surgical approach to the arytenoid, *lateral* to cervical strap muscles. The larynx is rotated to the opposite side, using traction on the superior cornu of the thyroid cartilage.

adequate exposure may require transaction of the thyrohyoid ligament to permit greater laryngeal rotation. Alternatively, a posterior portion of the thyroid cartilage could be resected, as described by Netterville and colleagues.[21] Maragos[19] has reported performing AA via a posterior thyroplasty window.

In their original description, Isshiki and colleagues[13] recommended transection of the cricothyroid joint as well as opening the cricoarytenoid joint to locate the muscular process. These steps potentially destabilized the larynx, and most subsequent authors have not found it necessary to compromise these structures.

The muscular process appears as a white prominence between the attachments of the anterior and posterior bellies of the posterior cricoarytenoid muscle (Figure 97-8). This is where the adduction suture is placed—a 4-0 permanent suture with a sturdy but small-radius curved needle. (I prefer a cardiac valve needle.) The muscle tendon is grasped near its insertion and the needle is passed from back to front through the cartilage process; care should be taken to not injure the pyriform mucosa. The suture should then be tugged while palpating the arytenoid, to assess the "purchase." If the entire arytenoid does not move with traction on the suture, the stitch was passed through soft tissue rather than the cartilage. The suture is then used to provide traction, to stabilize the arytenoid, and to ensure placement in the cartilage. When a satisfactory suture has been placed, it should be tied down securely, leaving two long ends.

The next step is to create a paraglottic tunnel, deep to cartilage and lateral to muscle, extending from the

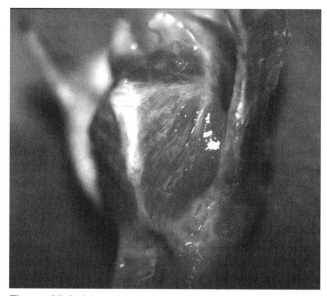

Figure 97-8. Muscular process of the arytenoid cartilage, located at the convergence of PCA muscle fibers.

site of the suture to the window that was previously created in the thyroid cartilage. One strand of the suture is then passed through this tunnel. At this point, the larynx should be observed endoscopically to detect arytenoid motion during alternate traction on the anterior and posterior ends of the AA suture. If appropriate rotation of the arytenoid is not observed, then the suture attachment is reassessed.

Once adequate rotation is ensured, the second, posterior end of the AA suture is passed forward through the tunnel, bringing it out under the thyroid cartilage rather than through the window. This allows the stitch to be secured by tying the suture over the inferior thyroid strut, at the posterior inferior corner of the window (Figure 97-9). In this position, a thyroplasty implant will not affect the sutures.

Next, the patient is asked to phonate with the vocal fold adducted so that the need for thyroplasty can be assessed. The thyroplasty can be performed in many ways, as covered in another chapter in this book.

If the arytenoid is tipped anteriorly, a posterior suspension suture should be considered. The suspension suture is placed in the arytenoid cartilage a few millimeters superior to the muscular process of the arytenoid, on the ridge that extends from the muscular process to the apex of the cartilage (see Figure 97-6). The suture is then passed through or around the inferior cornu of the thyroid cartilage, and then tied down to provide inferior traction. The larynx is observed endoscopically while tension is adjusted to rock the larynx posteriorly, without canceling out the adduction achieved by the AA suture.

In general, patients can resume oral intake within 1 to 2 hours after surgery. I keep patients admitted overnight after the procedure to observe for possible airway obstruction. Bleeding into the paraglottic space is the primary cause of postoperative airway obstruction. Thus, it is imperative to leave an adequate drain, suppress coughing, and control blood pressure. Maragos[18] has described postoperative airway obstruction due to herniation of pyriform mucosa into the airway. He reports that suture stabilization of pyriform mucosa at the close of the procedure is effective in preventing this complication.

FUTURE DIRECTIONS

AA is an effective means of altering the position of the arytenoid. However, the ideal position of the arytenoid has yet to be determined. Moreover, there are currently no means of precisely measuring the spatial displacement accomplished by AA in vivo. It is likely that the "ideal" position varies, not only among patients, but also with variation in vocal pitch, amplitude, and quality. Advances in 3D imaging will provide important information about laryngeal motion that will allow refinement of AA or development of better ways of restoring dynamic laryngeal function.

REFERENCES

1. Abraham MT, Gonen M, Kraus DH: Complications of type I thyroplasty and arytenoid adduction, *Laryngoscope* 111:1322–1329, 2001.
2. Amis TC and others: Effects of cricothyroid muscle contraction on upper airway flow dynamics in dogs, *J Appl Physiol* 72:2329–2335, 1992.
3. Blitzer A, Jahn AF, Keidar A: Semon's law revisited: an electromyographic analysis of laryngeal synkinesis, *Ann Otol Rhinol Laryngol* 105:764, 1996.
4. Brewer DW and others: Unilateral recurrent laryngeal nerve paralysis: a re-examination, *J Voice* 5:178–185, 1991.
5. Bridger GP: Unilateral laryngeal palsy: a histopathological study, *J Laryngol Otol* 91:303–307, 1977.
6. Bryant NJ and others: Human posterior cricoarytenoid muscle compartments: anatomy and mechanics, *Arch Otolaryngol Head Neck Surg* 122:1331–1336, 1996.
7. Chhetri DK and others: Combined arytenoid adduction and laryngeal reinnervation in the treatment of vocal fold paralysis, *Laryngoscope* 109:1928–1936, 1999.
8. Crumley RL: Laryngeal synkinesis revisited, *Ann Otolaryngol* 109:365–371, 2000.
9. Dedo HH: *Teflon injection of the vocal fold. In Surgery of the larynx & trachea.* Philadelphia, 1990, Dekker, p 25.
10. Green DC, Berke GS, Ward PH: Vocal fold medialization by surgical augmentation versus arytenoid adduction in the in vivo canine model, *Ann Ool Rhinol Laryngol* 100:280–287, 1991.
11. Hirano M and others: Electromyography for laryngeal paralysis. In Hirano M, Kirchner J, Bless D, editors: *Neurolaryngology: recent advances.* Boston, 1987, College-Hill, pp 232–248.
12. Isshiki N, Ishikawa T: Diagnostic value of tomography in unilateral vocal cord paralysis, *Laryngoscope* 86:1573–1578, 1976.
13. Isshiki N, Tanabe M, Masaki S: Arytenoid adduction for unilateral vocal cord paralysis, *Arch Otolaryngol Head Neck Surg* 14:555–558, 1978.
14. Kirchner JA: Atrophy of laryngeal muscles in vagal paralysis, *Laryngoscope* 76:1753–1765, 1966.
15. Konrad HR, Rattenborg CC: Combined action of laryngeal muscles, *Acta Otolaryngol* 67:646–649, 1969.
16. Koufman JA, Isaacson G: Laryngoplastic phonosurgery, *Otolaryngol Clin North Am* 1151–1173, 1991.

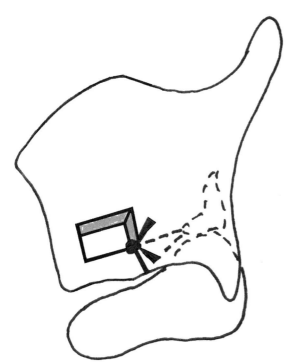

Figure 97-9. Position of arytenoid adduction suture in the posterior inferior corner of the thyroplasty window to allow simultaneous thyroplasty.

17. Koufman JA, Walker FO, Joharji GM: The cricothyroid muscle does not influence vocal fold position in laryngeal paralysis, *Laryngoscope* 105:368–372, 1995.

18. Maragos NE: Piriform sinus stabilization for prevention of postoperative airway obstruction in arytenoid adduction. Presented at the 124th Annual Meeting of the American Laryngological Association, Nashville, Tenn, May 3, 2003.

19. Maragos NE: The posterior thyroplasty window: anatomical considerations, *Laryngoscope* 109:1228–1231, 1999.

20. Montgomery WM, Hilman RE, Varvares MA: Combined thyroplasty type I and inferior constrictor myotomy, *Ann Otol Rhinol Laryngol* 103:858–862, 1995.

21. Netterville JL and others: Recurrent laryngeal nerve avulsion for treatment of spastic dysphonia, *Ann Otol Rhinol Laryngol* 100:10–14, 1991.

22. Neuman TR and others: Three-dimensional motion of the arytenoid adduction procedure in cadaver larynges, *Ann Otol Rhinol Laryngol* 103:265–270, 1994.

23. New GB, Childrey JH: Paralysis of the vocal cords: a study of 217 medical cases, *Arch Otol* 16:143–159, 1932.

24. Noordzij JP, Perrault DF, Woo P: Biomechanics of combined arytenoid adductionand medialization laryngoplasty in an ex vivo canine model, *Otolaryngol Head Neck Surg* 119:634–642, 1998.

25. Semon F: On the proclivity of the abductor fibers of the recurrent laryngeal nerve to become affected sooner than the adductor fibers or even exclusively, *Arch Laryngol* 2:197–222, 1881.

26. Von Leden H, Moore P: The mechanics of the cricoarytenoid joint, *Arch Otolaryngol* 73:541–550, 1961.

27. Weinman EC, Maragos NE: Airway compromise in thyroplasty surgery, *Laryngoscope* 110:1082–1085, 2000.

28. Woodson GE: Configuration of the glottis in laryngeal paralysis I: clinical study, *Laryngoscope* 103:1227–1234, 1993.

29. Woodson GE: Configuration of the glottis in laryngeal paralysis II: animal experiments, *Laryngoscope* 103: 1235–1241, 1993.

30. Woodson GE: Cricopharyngeal myotomy and arytenoid adduction in the management of combined laryngeal and pharyngeal paralysis, *Otolaryngol Head Neck Surg* 117: 339–343, 1997.

31. Woodson GE, Murry T: Glottic configuration after arytenoid adduction, *Laryngoscope* 104:965–969, 1994.

32. Woodson GE, Rosen CA, Yeung D: Changes in length and spatial orientation of the vocal fold with arytenoid adduction in cadaver larynges, *Ann Otol Rhinol Laryngol* 106:552–555, 1997.

33. Woodson GE and others: Arytenoid adduction: controlling vertical position, *Ann Otol Rhinol Laryngol* 109:360–364, 2000.

34. Woodson GE and others: Effects of cricothyroid contraction on laryngeal resistance and glottic area, *Ann Otol Rhinol Laryngol* 98:119–124, 1989.

35. Work WP: Paralysis and paresis of the vocal cords: a statistical review, *Arch Otolaryngol* 43:267–280, 1941.

36. Zeitels SM: Adduction arytenopexy: a new procedure for paralytic dysphonia with implications for implant medialization, *Ann Otol Rhinol Laryngol Suppl* 173:2–24, 1998.

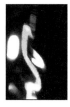

CHAPTER NINETY EIGHT

LARYNGEAL REINNERVATION

‖ George S. Goding, Jr.

INTRODUCTION

Complete recovery from laryngeal denervation can occur with spontaneous and appropriate regeneration of the recurrent laryngeal nerve (RLN). Surgical intervention cannot reliably provide appropriate vocal fold movement or the rapid and fine adjustments required for continuous vocal fold symmetry. Vocal fold medialization and augmentation allows for improved positioning of the paralyzed vocal fold. The RLN, however, supplies muscles with both abductor and adductor function. Reinnervation at the level of the RLN trunk can provide improvement in laryngeal muscle tone and mass. Reinnervation procedures designed to generate muscle movement must bypass the main trunk of the nerve and address individual muscles directly or at the most distal branches of the RLN.

In 1909, Horsley[67] reported the first successful vocal fold reinnervation. He performed a neurorrhaphy of the recurrent laryngeal nerve in a patient who had been shot in the neck with nearly complete recovery of laryngeal function. A number of authors[32,74] independently reported recurrent nerve repairs with return of function.

Most of the time after a RLN anastomosis vocal fold motion does not return. Instead, a laryngeal synkinesis occurs with adductor and abductor nerve fibers nonselectively innervating the laryngeal muscles.[34,63,70,113] The result of this neuromuscular mismatching is that counteracting forces are applied to the arytenoid by all the muscles innervated by the RLN and little or no functional movement occurs.[23] An inspiratory medial bulging is seen, which is thought to arise by the inappropriate activation of the thyroarytenoid muscle by abductor axons. The majority of RLN repairs, however, are incapable of producing abduction and adduction in functional coordination with the respiratory cycle.

The activity of the phrenic nerve during inspiration makes it an excellent candidate for reinnervation of the posterior cricoarytenoid (PCA) muscle.

A similar muscle fiber type profile between the diaphragm and the PCA also exists.[10] Abductor mobility of the vocal fold had been obtained in multiple animal models.[4,5,9,68,131] Experimental reinnervation with the phrenic nerve after a 9-month delay is successful, but the functional recovery is reduced.[130] Attempts to create vocal fold motion with phrenic nerve reinnervation in humans, however, were unsuccessful.[25]

Because of the inability to consistently obtain cyclical motion of the vocal folds in coordination with respiration, reinnervation at the level of the nerve trunk has not gained acceptance as a clinical modality in bilateral vocal fold paralysis.[46] Selective innervation of individual laryngeal muscles (in particular the posterior cricoarytenoid muscle) either by neuromuscular transfer technique,[18] selective anastomosis.[110,129] or direct nerve implantation[8,69] is required.

Although desirable, cyclical vocal fold motion is not mandatory for the successful rehabilitation of unilateral vocal fold paralysis. This has led to the successful use of vocal fold medialization techniques to improve the primary functions of the larynx (closure, respiration, and phonation). The vocal fold medialization techniques currently in use include thyroplasty, arytenoid adduction, and vocal fold injection. Laryngeal reinnervation at the level of the RLN can also take advantage of the resultant synkinesis to provide vocal fold position, bulk, and tone.

The two most common reinnervation techniques that have been applied to the problem of laryngeal paralysis in patients are the neuromuscular pedicle (NMP) and the ansa cervicalis-to-recurrent laryngeal nerve (ansa-RLN) anastomosis. Both take advantage of the same donor nerve (ansa cervicalis), but from there on the techniques differ.

The NMP procedure was developed in the 1970s and involves placement of the distal portion of the ansa cervicalis branch to the omohyoid muscle along with a small block of muscle into a denervated laryngeal muscle. The procedure is indicated in patients with either unilateral or bilateral vocal fold paralysis with different muscles being treated in each case. Depending on the success of reinnervation and the nature of the stimulus, there is a potential for recovery of vocal fold motion. In patients with unilateral vocal fold paralysis, the technique can be combined with thyroplasty.[119]

The ansa-RLN anastomosis was first reported by Frazier in 1924[41] and again in 1926[42] in an attempt to restore vocal fold movement. The current use of the technique was reported in 1986.[29] An end-to-end anastomosis of the proximal ansa cervicalis nerve to the distal stump of the RLN is performed. The procedure is indicated for unilateral paralysis because vocal fold motion is not restored. Instead, muscle tone is restored to the entire hemilarynx providing appropriate vocal fold position, bulk, and tone to the vocal fold. The result is the potential for a near normal vocal ability.

Physiologic and Anatomic Issues in Laryngeal Reinnervation

There is substantial evidence that reinnervated muscle takes on the characteristics of the donor nerve (see Talmadge[117] for review). This appears to happen by the reinnervating nerve imposing a pattern of activity on the muscle fibers it contacts. Thus, the selection of a donor nerve should ideally take into account the fiber type and contraction characteristics of the muscle to be reinnervated.

NERVE CHARACTERISTICS

The recurrent laryngeal nerve contains 1000 to 4000 motor axons, efferent axons, and sympathetic and parasympathetic secretomotor fibers depending on the level at which the count is made. The RLN gives off branches to the cricopharyngeal and inferior constrictor muscles as well as a sensory branch that communicates with the superior laryngeal nerve before entering the larynx. Five hundred to 1000 fibers are in the motor branches of the RLN.[58] Before branching within the laryngeal framework, the motor fibers to the various muscles are intermixed throughout the RLN nerve trunk, making selective reinnervation at this level impractical.[47] The anterior motor branch of the RLN enters the larynx posterior to the cricothyroid (CT) joint. The first branches that emerge from the RLN innervate the PCA muscle and often have connections to the midline interarytenoid muscle. The branch to the PCA has characteristics of a slow-twitch motor nerve with axons containing 200 to 250 muscle fibers in each motor unit.[56] The interarytenoid muscle also receives a separate branch from each RLN

resulting in bilateral innervation. The terminal branches of the RLN innervate the lateral cricoarytenoid (LCA) and thyroarytenoid (TA) muscles. The axons in this branch are more characteristic of fast-twitch fibers with motor unit sizes of 2 to 20 muscle fibers.[62] In some larynges, a connection between the SLN and the terminal fibers of the RLN can be seen within the TA.[105]

Except for proprioceptive fibers carried within the nerve, the ansa cervicalis is a purely motor derivative of the ventral rami of the cervical plexus. Fibers from the first cervical nerve (C1) join the hypoglossal nerve until it curves anteroinferiorly. At this point, the C1 fibers leave the hypoglossal nerve to form the superior root of the ansa cervicalis. The geniohyoid and thyrohyoid muscles are supplied entirely by C1 fibers. The branch to the superior belly of the omohyoid muscle typically originates from the superior loop of the ansa cervicalis. Because of its proximity to the thyroid ala and its infrahyoid position, this branch has been frequently used as a donor for reinnervation using the NMP technique. The other strap muscles receive motor fibers from second and third cervical nerves primarily via the inferior root of the ansa cervicalis. The lower portions of the sternothyroid and the sternohyoid muscles receive terminal nerves that branch off the loop of the ansa cervicalis as it passes deep to the omohyoid muscle.[20]

MUSCLE FIBERS IN GENERAL

The performance of a particular muscle depends on the character of the individual muscle fibers it contains. Based on their histochemical and contraction properties, the fibers of skeletal muscle can be classified as slow fatigue resistant (type 1), fast fatigue resistant (type 2A), or fast fatigable (type 2B). Several other classifications and subtypes exist (see Staron[115] for review). Type 1 fibers are characterized by a low peak tension, a slow contraction time, a low threshold of recruitment, fatigue resistance, and a dependence on aerobic metabolism. Muscles that are required to produce low tension over a prolonged period of time generally have a high proportion of type 1 fibers. Type 2 fibers are found to play a prominent role in muscles that can generate high tension for short periods. Type 2B fibers have a fast contraction time and can generate a higher tension. They are more easily fatigued, have a higher threshold of activation, and depend on anaerobic metabolism. Type 2A fibers are intermediate in tension, fatigability, and threshold, and they make use of both aerobic and anaerobic metabolism. The laryngeal muscles also have high-velocity, low-tension fiber types (2L or mixed fiber type) that may be similar to those found in extraocular and jaw-closing muscles.[109,111,112,133]

Most mammalian skeletal muscles are made up of multiple fiber types. Because of these combinations, the various whole muscles have a variety of contraction and relaxation characteristics. The peak contraction time of the extraocular muscles is the fastest, whereas the soleus is the slowest.

Laryngeal Muscles

Activity of the PCA muscle is synchronous with inspiration and precedes activation of the diaphragm by 40 to 100 msec.[51] The amount of activity varies directly with ventilatory resistance. Activity of the PCA produces lateral turning of the arytenoid, resulting in abduction of the vocal fold. Loss of PCA muscle tone results in instability of the arytenoid cartilage. Based on the gross anatomy[50] and innervation,[106] the PCA in humans can be divided into a horizontal compartment and a vertical/oblique compartment.[106] The PCA in laryngectomy specimens consists of nearly equal percentages of type 1 and type 2 fibers.[77] A similar ratio is seen in the primate PCA.[55] Other authors have found the PCA to have a higher percentage of type 1 fibers.[10] The remainder of the muscle fibers appears to be mostly of the intermediate (type 2A) variety. These findings are consistent with the peak contraction time of the PCA, which is approximately 40 msec.

Reinnervation occurs most easily at the sites of the original motor endplates. It is possible that placement of a reinnervating NMP near a large population of motor endplates could improve the end result.[48] The motor endplates of the human PCA muscle are distributed in a loosely arranged arc in the midportion of the muscle. The density of endplates is increased in the deeper portions of the PCA.

TA activity increases with phonation and reflex protection of the airway. Contraction of the TA is critical to the fine control of the mass and tension of the phonating edge of the vocal fold. Atrophy of the TA muscle results in a reduced vocal fold volume and glottal incompetence. LCA and TA muscle paralysis severely compromise the ability to adduct and stabilize the vocal process of the arytenoid. Bilateral innervation of the TA muscle is not sufficient to compensate for this loss.

The TA and LCA are faster muscles. Their peak contraction times of 14 msec (TA) and 19 msec (lateral CT) make them some of the more rapid muscles in the body.[55,102] The composition of muscle fibers in the TA is approximately 40% type 1, 55% type 2A, and 5% type 2B. The higher frequency of oxidative fibers characterizes this muscle as having aerobic metabolism, resistance to fatigue, and fast contraction.[52] The faster response characteristics of these muscles are appropriate for their phonatory and protective functions.

The pattern of motor endplate distribution in the TA and CT muscles is more diffuse than in the PCA. In the CT muscle, the majority of the motor endplates are in the medial two-thirds of the muscle,[31] whereas in the TA the endplates are scattered throughout the muscle.[100] Placement of an NMP in precise locations, therefore, can offer a limited advantage in reinnervating the PCA and CT muscles. These diffuse patterns differ from skeletal muscles elsewhere in the body where they form a narrow band at the midpoint of the muscle.[31]

Both adductor and abductor laryngeal muscles contribute to the position and stability of the arytenoid cartilage.[24] Restoration of adductor and abductor muscle tone should allow appropriate arytenoid position and stability.

The CT muscle participates in deep inspiration, expiration, and phonation. The CT is innervated by the superior laryngeal nerve and is not addressed by ansa-RLN reinnervation. CT contraction pulls the vocal process in an anterior and slightly medial direction. This anterior pull is offset by the stabilizing effect of PCA and LCA contraction.

Infrahyoid Muscles

The ansa cervicalis is the most commonly used donor nerve in laryngeal reinnervation. The peak contraction times of the thyrohyoid and sternothyroid are approximately 50 msec.[57] Approximately two-thirds of the muscle fibers are type 1.[64] The infrahyoid muscles have enzyme profiles similar to limb muscles and lack the presence of faster mixed fibers found in the laryngeal muscles.[65]

In the hope of obtaining vocal fold movement, the activity of the various infrahyoid muscles has been examined. The strap muscles extending below the larynx function as accessory muscles of inspiration in varying degrees. The sternohyoid muscle has consistently shown little to no consistent activity with respiration. In the canine a regular contraction of the sternothyroid muscle is seen with quiet respiration, but all strap muscles lacked phasic activity in the primate. With increased airway resistance and hypoxia, inspiratory activity was greatest in the omohyoid, followed by the sternothyroid, in the primate.[36] The sternothyroid in labored respiration can result in vocal fold lateralization even if the larynx is paralyzed by means of its effect on the laryngeal skeleton.[40]

The thyrohyoid muscle can similarly assist in adduction of the vocal folds. Medial positioning of the vocal folds is assisted by its action of displacing the thyroid cartilage upward. Based on activity relative to the respiratory cycle, the nerve supplies to the sternothyroid and omohyoid muscles would be acceptable candidates for reinnervation for laryngeal abduction. The thyrohyoid muscle activity makes its branch of the ansa cervicalis nerve an appropriate choice for laryngeal adduction. Because specific laryngeal muscles are not reinnervated in isolation with the ansa-RLN anastomosis, the activation patterns of the infrahyoid muscles become less meaningful with this technique. Denervation of an infrahyoid muscle does occur and can result in a change in vocal quality immediately after surgery. Sacrifice of the sternothyroid muscle can result in a decrease of lateral pull on the thyroid ala and a medialization effect. The opposite effect can occur with sacrifice of the thyrohyoid muscle.

The infrahyoid muscles are a less than perfect histochemical match to the recipient laryngeal muscles. After reinnervation for unilateral vocal fold paralysis with the ansa cervicalis, changes in the fiber type composition of the laryngeal muscles would be expected.

EFFECTS OF DENERVATION

With denervation, the area of sensitivity to acetylcholine, which is limited to the endplate region in the intact muscle, spreads out over most of the external membrane.[90] Denervation also eliminates both the trophic and activity-related influences on the muscle, resulting in muscle atrophy. Without reinnervation, there is progressive atrophy and eventual destruction of the muscle despite an adequate supply of all nutrients.

Reinnervation becomes less effective the longer a muscle is denervated. The different laryngeal muscles appear to atrophy at different rates, which vary with their fiber composition. In a study on primate larynges, the faster TA muscle showed a far greater reduction in fiber size than the slower CT or PCA muscles. By 8 weeks, however, all laryngeal muscles were fibrosed.[101] Muscle atrophy in human skeletal muscles apparently proceeds at a slower pace, with muscles surviving at least 3 years after denervation. Successful laryngeal reinnervation has been claimed as much as 50 years after the onset of laryngeal paralysis.[121] It is possible that some nerve sprouting occurs resulting in a low-grade but functionless innervation that preserves the muscle's ability to be reinnervated.[27] Innervation of laryngeal muscles can also come from misdirected reinnervation from autonomic nerves.[89]

REINNERVATION

Successful regeneration of injured nerves requires three conditions to be satisfied: (1) the neuron responds to the injury with the metabolic changes necessary to support axonal regrowth; (2) the environment of the injured axon permits axon growth; and (3) the environment provides guidance clues for restoration of function.

Neuron Response to Injury

Division of the axon results in a unique state for the neuron. A number of changes occur, including swelling of the cell body, displacement of the nucleus, and disappearance of cytoplasmic basophilic material. This process, termed *chromatolysis,* is a preparation for axon regeneration as well as an indicator of cellular trauma and is thought to be due to the loss of neurotrophic substances.[95] A portion of the neurons after axon division die.[39] Survival of the nerve cell is facilitated by a number of neurotrophic factors that include neurotrophins, neuropoietic cytokines, and fibroblast growth factors. The neurotrophin family includes nerve growth factor (NGF), brain-derived neurotrophic factor (BDNF), neurotrophin (NT)-3, NT-4/5, and NT-6. NGF plays an important role in sensory neuron survival.[44,135] BDNF, NT-3, and NT-4/5 support the survival of motor neurons.[60,134] Macrophages invading the area of injury release interleukin 1-β, which up-regulates the production of NGF.[86] This results in an increased expression of NGF in the nerve trunk after injury.[103] The neuropoietic cytokine ciliary neurotrophic factor, located primarily in the cytoplasm of myelinating Schwann cells,[43] also promotes the survival of motoneurons.[3] Cell death may be negligible with rapid reinnervation.

Axon Growth

Injury (pressure, cold, or section) leads to a breach in axon membrane, resulting in a breakdown of axonal internal structure associated with calcium entry and the activation of calcium-activated proteases.[108] Axonal disruption spreads proximally a variable amount (up to 2 mm). The entry of calcium ions into the injured axon is important for resealing the damaged membrane. In the distal axon, wallerian degeneration occurs. Macrophages invade the distal nerve segment and digest myelin debris and degrade axons. The process of wallerian degeneration creates an environment highly supportive of axonal growth. Schwann cells form Büngner's bands within the endoneurial tubes. NGF, BDGF,[82] insulin-like growth factor,[54] and ciliary neurotrophic growth factor[96] are produced by the Schwann cells in the injured nerve trunk.

Regenerating axon sprouts arise (mainly at nodes) up to 6 mm proximal to the injury site. Sprout formation is rapid. The ability to form sprouts is an intrinsic property of the axon and can occur before there are any changes in the cell body. Growth cones are found at the tip of the nerve sprouts. The growth cone consists of a swollen central core from which extend flattened, webbed processes called *lamellipodia* and numerous stiff, fine processes called *filopodia* (composed of actin). The growth cones interact with laminin, and fibronectin present in the basal lamina of the Schwann cells. These glycoproteins play a key role in promoting the growth and advancement of the regenerating axons.[78] Other molecules such as semaphorines, ephrins, netrins, and other extracellular matrix molecules provide important negative cues to axonal guidance.[19] Advancement of the axon appears to occur through the interaction of filopodia with a number of cell-adhesion molecules.[75]

Restoration of Function

Regeneration is pointless unless the regenerating axons grow back to reinnervate the original targets. Motor axons will preferentially reinnervate distal motor branches of a severed nerve. The specificity is gained primarily through pruning of misdirected fibers.[16] Some evidence for a neurotrophic mechanism for directional nerve regrowth exists,[72] but the usual outcome after nerve injury suggests the specificity is low. A major problem is that, after division of a nerve, a functional specificity in motoneuron regeneration for the original muscle does not exist.[7,17,118] The result, in a regenerating nerve supplying several muscles such as the RLN, is synkinesis.

Muscle fiber types can change under the influence of activation pattern[71] and altered innervation.[99] The changes following reinnervation with a different donor nerve may be related to a different pattern of activity imposed by the new nerve supply. Fiber type grouping is thought to be a result of this process.[73] Mechanisms for directing the regenerating motor axons within a single muscle leading slow- and fast-twitch axons to the appropriate muscle fibers have some influence on reinnervation.[132] The effect, however, is not enough to prevent changes in muscle fiber type. Reinnervation with a new donor nerve would be expected to be more likely to change the fiber type composition of the reinnervated muscle and thus its contraction characteristics.

NEUROMUSCULAR PEDICLE

The NMP technique attempts to transfer a nerve with a portion of its motor units intact to a denervated muscle. Preservation of motor units is brought about by including a small block of muscle at the distal end of the donor nerve. This distinguishes the technique from nerve anastomosis, implantation of a nerve stump, and direct electrical stimulation of muscle fibers.

Reinnervation with a Neuromuscular Pedicle

Successful reinnervation with an NMP depends partly on the ability of the transplanted axons to reach receptive sites on the recipient muscle fibers and partly on the ability of the muscle fibers to accept innervation from foreign nerves. With partial denervation of the transferred nerve, the remaining intact motor neurons develop sprouts that provide reinnervation preferentially at the original endplate sites of the denervated muscle fibers.[14,114] This phenomenon is important to successful transfer of the NMP because a portion of the nerve fibers in an NMP may have an intact motor unit.[127] Axon sprouting results in a larger number of motor fibers innervated by each nerve. Mature nerve terminals appear to be limited in functional expansion to three to five times the normal terminal field.[98]

Laboratory Investigations

In early experiments, a block of muscle containing the terminal branches of the recurrent laryngeal nerve was removed and reimplanted into the larynx.[126,127] A small portion of muscle was incorporated at the distal end of the transferred nerve to transfer intact nerve fibers. The short time to functional recovery (2–6 weeks) was thought to be caused by the avoidance of degeneration and regeneration before effective reinnervation.

In 1973, reinnervation of the canine larynx with an NMP derived from the ansa cervicalis nerve, and its insertion into the sternohyoid muscle was described.[61] The technique was modified because of the unavailability of the recurrent laryngeal nerve in most cases of laryngeal paralysis and the unsuitability of preserving a portion of the larynx in the presence of cancer.[120] A return of function was seen at approximately 6 weeks after surgery. Reinnervation could be successful up to 6 months after denervation.[76]

Evidence for reinnervation with the NMP has included muscle response to pedicel stimulation, demonstration of neural tracer in the central motor nuclei of the donor nerve,[1] and glycogen depletion in fiber of reinnervated muscles.[38] Successful use of the NMP technique in animal models has been reported by multiple authors.[18,49,53,81,107] In these studies, electrical stimulation of the transferred nerve or induction of increased respiratory effort was required to produce gross motion.

In other studies, the presence of vocal fold movement under hypercarbic conditions was not associated with evidence of reinnervation either by direct stimulation[22,87,97] or histologic evaluation.[97] Other maneuvers such as dividing the inferior pharyngeal constrictor[87] or dividing the superior laryngeal nerve or the strap muscles[22] were effective in eliminating the observed vocal fold motion. Postoperative scarring that could stabilize the arytenoid and lateral tethering of the arytenoid to the thyroid cartilage is a potential explanation for vocal fold motion not related to reinnervation.[28]

A modification of the NMP technique involves using a transferred NMP as a means of providing access to a denervated muscle for long-term electrical stimulation.[11-13] A cuffed electrode can be placed around the nerve component of an implanted NMP. This should prevent deterioration at the electrode-muscle interface. Successful pacing was accomplished for the sternothyroid[12] and PCA[13] muscles using tracheal motion with respiration as the triggering signal.

Indications
Bilateral Paralysis

The NMP can be considered for any patient with bilateral vocal fold paralysis that has persisted for 6 months[121] to 1 year.[123] In practice, however, only half of these patients are suitable candidates.[122] Fixation or limitation of the cricoarytenoid joint is the most common contraindication, composing approximately one third of cases.[123] Direct laryngoscopy and palpation of the arytenoids before proceeding with the NMP procedure is recommended.

The ansa cervicalis nerve and its insertion into the appropriate strap muscle must be available for this technique. Any prior surgery or trauma that may have injured the ansa cervicalis should be carefully reviewed. Other causes of airway obstruction should be resolved before reinnervation.[123]

Central nervous system disease resulting in vocal fold paralysis is a relative contraindication. Tucker[123] has reported only a 40% to 50% success rate in these patients. Such diseases can also disrupt the function of the ansa cervicalis nerve.

Finally, the laryngeal muscles must be able to accept reinnervation. Although successful reinnervation has been reported after 22 and 50 years of denervation, muscle atrophy probably plays a role in hampering the outcome. The incidence of cricoarytenoid fixation may increase with time,[124] but this finding has not been confirmed hstologically.[45]

Unilateral Paralysis

Consideration of reinnervation is usually delayed in patients with unilateral paralysis until enough time has passed to make spontaneous recovery unlikely. In patients who have difficulty with aspiration, vocal fold injection has been recommended. Prior injection of polytetrafluoroethylene (Teflon) into the vocal fold, however, has been associated with a poor vocal result.[79] The procedure also has been limited to patients who require above average vocal quality.

As for bilateral vocal fold paralysis, the patient must be able to tolerate the procedure, must have the ansa cervicalis nerve intact, must have the selected adductor muscle in suitable condition for reinnervation, and must have a mobile arytenoid on the paralyzed side. An inability to visualize the larynx by normal endoscopic methods precluding transoral injection is an additional indication for NMP reinnervation.[79]

Technique

The description of the NMP below is that described by Tucker[120,121,123-125] with modifications by other authors as noted (Figure 98-1).

Bilateral Paralysis

The procedure begins with laryngoscopy and palpation of the arytenoids with the patient under general anesthesia and paralyzed, with no endotracheal tube. Once it is determined the arytenoids are freely mobile, the patient is intubated and a tracheotomy is performed if one is not already present.

A horizontal incision is made near the lower border of the thyroid cartilage. The anterior border of the sternocleidomastoid muscle is exposed and retracted laterally. Demonstration of the anterior belly of the omohyoid muscle and the fascia overlying the internal jugular vein is completed. The branch of the ansa cervicalis supplying the anterior belly of the omohyoid muscle can be identified in two ways: first, the main trunk of the ansa cervicalis is found as it crosses the internal jugular vein and it is traced proximally and distally until the appropriate branch is recognized; second, the medial border of the omohyoid is mobilized near its attachment to the hyoid and dissected in a medial to lateral direction along the muscle. The nerve is usually accompanied by a small arterial vessel, which is preserved. If the nerve is injured, the branch to the sternothyroid is also acceptable.[28,128]

After the point of entry into the muscle is determined, dissection of the nerve is continued distally until its terminal branches are identified. This may require an additional 2 to 3 mm of dissection from the entrance of the nerve into the muscle. A block of muscle large enough to include the terminal branches (usually 2 to 3 mm on a side) is dissected free with the attached nerve. The muscle block is kept as small as possible since it will act as a free graft. The proximal portion of the omohyoid branch of the ansa cervicalis is mobilized, and care should be taken to preserve the accompanying vessel.

The lateral margin of the thyroid cartilage is identified and used to rotate the larynx toward the opposite side. Keeping the dissection close to the lateral edge of the thyroid ala, the fibers of the inferior constrictor are bluntly separated. Dissection is continued until either the pyriform sinus is encountered or the PCA muscle is seen. The mucosa of the pyriform sinus is bluntly displaced superiorly, if necessary. The PCA

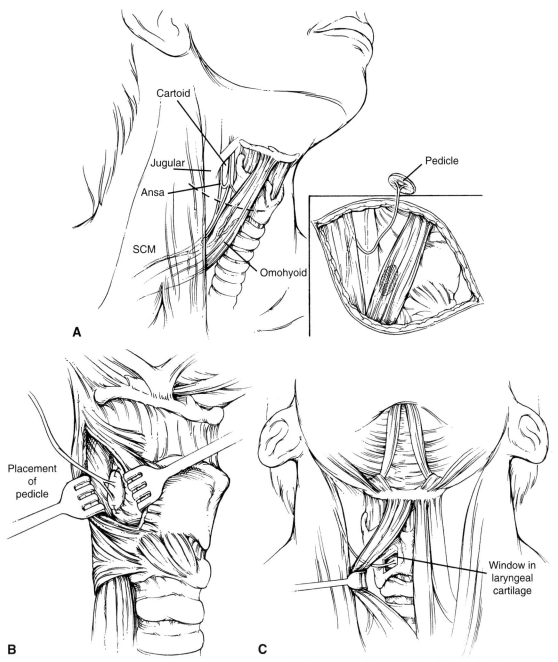

Figure 98-1. Neuromuscular pedicle (NMP). **A,** NMP harvested from omohyoid muscle. The branch of the ansa cervicalis nerve to the omohyoid is removed with a 2- to 3-mm attached block of muscle. **B,** NMP placed into PCA after rotating the larynx and separating the fibers of the inferior constrictor for the treatment of bilateral paralysis. **C,** NMP placed into LCA via a window in the thyroid ala for the treatment of unilateral paralysis.

muscle can be recognized by its fibers, which pass at right angles to those of the inferior constrictor.

The NMP is then sutured to the PCA with two or three sutures of 5-0 nylon. Abrasion of the surface of the PCA is not necessary for reinnervation to occur. Closure of the fibers of the inferior constrictor muscle is not necessary. A drain is placed, and the wound is

closed in layers. Postoperative antibiotics are not routinely used.

Unilateral Paralysis

When unilateral vocal fold paralysis is treated, the direct laryngoscopy and harvesting of the NMP is the same as with bilateral paralysis. No tracheotomy is performed. The recipient muscle in unilateral paralysis is the LCA, and the second portion of the operation varies accordingly.

The thyroid cartilage on the denervated side is exposed, and the lower half of the perichondrium of the thyroid cartilage is incised in the midline. A posteriorly based perichondrial flap exposing the lower half of the thyroid ala is created. A block of thyroid cartilage is removed from this area, leaving the underlying perichondrium and the inferior margin of the thyroid cartilage intact. The inner perichondrium is incised to expose the denervated LCA muscle and the NMP sutured in place with two or three sutures of 5-0 nylon. The outer perichondrial flap can be sutured back in place, and the wound is closed in layers with a drain. One modification includes placing two pedicles (each from a separate strap muscle) into the recipient muscle.[2]

Intravenous dexamethasone has been given to reduce laryngeal edema in the early recovery period.[128] Voice rest and postoperative antibiotics are not necessary.

Reported Results

In 1976, Tucker reported using the NMP in humans for bilateral vocal fold paralysis.[120] All five patients studied demonstrated vocal fold abduction with inspiration within 6 to 8 weeks after the procedure. In two patients with a marked improvement in exercise tolerance, vocal fold motion was not seen without an increased respiratory effort. In 1978, 45 cases of NMP laryngeal reinnervation for bilateral vocal fold paralysis were reviewed.[121] An 88.8% (40/45) success rate was reported. Follow-up ranged from 3 months to 4 years, and the duration of paralysis ranged from 6 months to 50 years. The time to return of function varied from 6 to 12 weeks.

The results of NMP reinnervation for bilateral vocal fold paralysis were divided into three categories by Tucker.[123] In approximately 40% of his cases, airway improvement was accompanied by visible motion of the vocal fold with inspiratory effort. Twenty percent of patients had no airway improvement. The remaining patients had airway improvement but little vocal fold motion. Most of these patients demonstrated vocal fold motion or tonic abduction only with increased respiratory demand. A second NMP procedure to the opposite PCA muscle has been performed successfully in patients with an inadequate result from the first procedure.[123]

A review of 214 patients with bilateral vocal fold paralysis demonstrated a 74% long-term success rate.[122] Forty-eight percent of patients had a tracheotomy performed at the time of reinnervation. Success was defined as decannulation with improved

airway that did not limit regular daily activities or exacerbate acute upper respiratory disease. The minimum follow-up was 2 years. Six-month results showed an 89% success rate, but 31 patients had subsequent deterioration of the airway. In a majority of late-failure patients that were evaluated, fixation of the cricoarytenoid joint was identified.

In 1977, Tucker reported the use of the NMP technique in nine patients with unilateral vocal fold paralysis.[125] Recovery of adductive function was seen in 2 to 12 weeks after surgery in all nine patients. Only six patients had a satisfactory improvement in vocal quality, and a subsequent Teflon injection was required in the other three. In a subsequent report on the use of the NMP in unilateral vocal paralysis, 25 of 27 patients receiving a NMP to the LCA were improved.[128]

In a 1989 report,[122] NMP procedures for unilateral paralysis had a success rate of 88%. Success was established by voice improvement, vocal fold adduction, and change in cord tension with elevated pitch. Voice results were noted to improve for several months and were aided by the addition of speech therapy.

May and others[80] reported their results with the NMP in 1980. Of eight patients with NMP reinnervation of the PCA for airway obstruction, the conditions of only three were improved. Thirteen of 15 patients with disordered phonation, deglutition, or both were improved by NMP reinnervation of the LCA. Applebaum and others[2] reported successful results in six of six patients with the NMP technique. Four of these patients had bilateral vocal fold paralysis with one requiring a tracheostomy. Dyspnea and stridor were relived in all four patients; vocal fold movement was seen only after physical exertion.

In isolated unilateral recurrent laryngeal paralysis, May and Beery[79] reported improvement in the voice in 19 of 20 (95%) patients treated with NMP implantation into the LCA muscle. Observable movement of the reinnervated cord was seen in only one patient, suggesting that enhanced muscle tone or a slight change in position was responsible for voice improvement. The degree of voice improvement was substantially less in patients with multiple cranial nerve deficits or vocal fold fixation.

Complications

The main complication of the NMP technique is failure to obtain a satisfactory result. Many of the patient selection factors listed above as contraindications are a result of these experiences. Relatively few operative complications associated with the NMP procedure are described. Of 214 patients undergoing a NMP for bilateral vocal fold paralysis, four complications were noted by Tucker and Rusnov.[128] Three of these were wound infections, and the other complication was related to the previously placed tracheotomy. No complications were reported in 73 patients undergoing an NMP procedure for unilateral paralysis. No operative complications were reported in other reported series.[2,79]

Future of the Neuromuscular Pedicle Technique

Despite successful use in a few authors' experience, widespread use of the NMP technique has not materialized. Reinnervation can occur with implantation of an NMP into denervated muscle, but the ansa cervicalis continues to be an imperfect source for neural input. Even in the absence of movement with respiration, the NMP can maintain muscular tone.

The NMP can provide a mechanism to access a denervated muscle for long-term pacing.[12,13] With electrical pacing, the options for a potential triggering source and the stimulus for muscle contraction are increased, providing a potentially more effective treatment of airway impairment resulting from bilateral vocal fold paralysis.

ANSA CERVICALIS-TO-RECURRENT LARYNGEAL NERVE ANASTOMOSIS

The current use of the ansa-RLN anastomosis is in unilateral vocal fold paralysis. No motion of the reinnervated vocal fold with respiration or phonation is expected. A variation of this technique involves a hypoglossal nerve-to-RLN anastomosis.[92,93] Use of the ansa cervicalis as a donor nerve has gained the widest acceptance because of the lower morbidity associated with the sacrifice of this nerve.

Advantages of Ansa-RLN Anastomosis

The procedure is relatively easy to perform in an unoperated neck by any surgeon familiar with head and neck anatomy. The primary difficulty is associated with identifying the appropriate nerves when excessive scarring is present. There is typically no "learning curve" with respect to the ultimate vocal result because fine adjustments of vocal fold position are not required. This is in contrast to vocal fold injection and thyroplasty, for which the ultimate vocal result is determined at the time of surgery and is dependent on the expertise of the surgeon.

The procedure provides tone, position, and bulk to the denervated muscles, resulting in less asymmetry between the normal and reinnervated vocal fold. This provides the opportunity for an outstanding rehabilitation of unilateral vocal fold paralysis. Improvement in vocal quality can also continue to occur after the initial improvement seen during the first year after surgery.

The sacrifice of the sternothyroid muscle is clinically insignificant and can theoretically improve vocal function. The resting tone of the sternothyroid muscle slightly lateralizes the normal vocal fold.[40] Loss of this tone can result in a slight medialization of the paralyzed vocal fold and an improvement in vocal quality soon after surgery.[27]

The procedure is primarily extralaryngeal and can be reversed by dividing the anastomosis at a later time. Because the thyroid ala and intrinsic muscles of the larynx are not violated in the course of the procedure, the subsequent use of vocal fold injection or thyroplasty is not limited.

The impact of the delay before reinnervation can be reduced when combined with the injection of absorbable material into the vocal fold at the time of surgery.

No permanent implant material is used. The potential for implant migration or foreign body reaction at the level of the vocal fold is eliminated.

Disadvantages of Ansa-RLN Transfer

The procedure requires a deeper level of dissection in the neck and typically takes longer to perform than thyroplasty or vocal fold injection. The time for completion of the ansa-RLN is estimated at 2 hours.[26] Whereas thyroplasty is typically performed with the patients under sedation and vocal fold injection can be performed in the clinic, ansa-RLN anastomosis must be performed with the patient under general anesthesia.

The possibility of spontaneous recovery of vocal fold function is eliminated with the division of the RLN before ansa-RLN anastomosis. It is important to wait until the possibility of spontaneous recovery is minimal.

There is a delay of 5 to 9 months before substantial improvement in the voice occurs. This may be added to a several month delay in waiting for the possibility of spontaneous recovery. Often an initial improvement can be seen as soon as 3 to 4 months after surgery. Improvement, however, can continue for several years.

The procedure requires one intact ansa and the intact distal stump of the RLN. This can be difficult after thyroid surgery or impossible after bilateral neck surgery when the ansa is sacrificed. In cases of unilateral neck surgery, the contralateral ansa cervicalis can be used. Unlike thyroplasty, the consequences of performing this procedure on the wrong (non-paralyzed) side are severe. With division of the only remaining intact RLN, a bilateral vocal fold immobility and resultant airway obstruction is a likely consequence.

Surgical Indications and Contraindications

Ansa-RLN anastomosis is indicated for the treatment of unilateral vocal fold paralysis with minimal chance for spontaneous recovery. The most commonly advised waiting period before consideration of reinnervation is 12 months. The distal stump of the RLN must be available for anastomosis. In the presence of extensive scarring, the RLN can be found behind the CT joint. A donor nerve must also be available. The ansa cervicalis, however, can be prepared from either the ipsilateral or contralateral side. The patient must be able to tolerate a general anesthetic and a delay for substantial improvement from reinnervation.

Absolute contraindications include glottal airway compromise, bilateral vocal fold paralysis, absence of the distal RLN, absence of the ansa cervicalis bilaterally, and poor general health.

The relative contraindications to ansa-RLN anastomosis include limitations of time, voice, and surgery. Time limitations primarily focus on the delay after surgery for the voice improvement. The physician must consider whether this is worthwhile for a patient who is able to wait for the result. Time can be limited either to social or work considerations or the patient's life expectancy. If the patent's life expectancy is less than 5 years, the delay for improvement with reinnervation may not be worthwhile. The procedure also appears to be less successful in the elderly and in those patients who have had paralysis for several decades. Voice limitations focus on the fact that ansa-RLN anastomosis fixes only the position, bulk, and tone of the paralyzed vocal fold. Other pathology that will limit the voice result might include dysarthria associated with multiple cranial nerve defects or stroke. Other vocal fold pathology that will limit the ultimate result such as the presence of a vocal fold scarring, web, or polyp must be considered. If a near-normal voice is not the anticipated result, the use of ansa-RLN should be considered carefully. Fixation of an arytenoid in a lateral position also has an adverse effect on the expected outcome.

Surgical considerations also come into play when prior surgery has occurred in the area of the RLN. Extensive scarring or atrophy of the nerve can have an effect. The possibility of not finding an adequate nerve for anastomosis must be considered, and alternative plans for intraoperative management should be reviewed with the patient.

Surgical Technique of Ansa-RLN Anastomosis

An incision in the natural creases of the neck is made below the level of the cricoid cartilage, often at the level of a thyroidectomy incision (Figure 98-2). The incision need not cross the midline, and 4 cm is usually adequate. The strap muscles are separated vertically in the midline and the RLN is identified in the tracheoesophageal groove. The nerve is dissected to its entrance into the larynx. In the presence of local scar

tissue, the RLN can be found behind the CT joint. A vessel loop can be placed around the nerve. The anterior border of the sternocleidomastoid muscle is identified. The ansa cervicalis nerve can be identified along the lateral border of the sternothyroid muscle, at the level of the omohyoid muscle, or along the internal jugular vein.

After both nerves are identified and the distal RLN is confirmed to be intact, the ansa and RLN are transected. Each nerve should be divided inferiorly enough to allow a tension-free anastomosis. A tunnel deep to the sternohyoid and sternothyroid muscles connects the two operative sites and facilitates the anastomosis. The anastomosis is performed using 9-0 or 10-0 nylon sutures. Two to three epineural sutures are adequate. Magnification can be performed with either a surgical microscope or loupes. The wound is closed in layers with an appropriate drain.

An absorbable material can be injected at the time of surgery to provide an initial improvement in vocal quality. After 2 to 3 months, the voice may deteriorate to the preoperative level. At 4 to 6 months after surgery, a gradual improvement in vocal quality begins. On laryngeal examination after ansa-RLN, transfer the reinnervated cord is immobile or demonstrates only minimal movement. The procedure produces a synkinesis that allows the mobile vocal fold to approximate the reinnervated fold in the midline.

Clinical Results

Ansa-RLN anastomosis has produced near-normal vocal quality according to most reports. The initial two reports by Crumley and colleagues[29,30] reported success in two and four patients. In one of these patients the contralateral ansa cervicalis nerve served as the donor nerve. No motion of the reinnervated vocal fold was seen in reinnervated patients. The vocal improvement was felt to be caused by precise positioning of the reinnervated vocal fold. Reinnervation of the of PCA, LCA, and TA muscles appears to provide the needed tone to stabilize and position the arytenoid properly.[24]

A series of 20 patients undergoing ansa-RLN anastomosis was reviewed by Crumley in 1991.[27] Vocal quality was judged to be normal or near normal in 18 of 20 cases. In the one failure, the identification of the RLN was in doubt because of local scar formation that resulted from multiple prior procedures. A second case demonstrated improvement, but to a lesser extent. In this case, lateralization of the arytenoid and the patient's age (65 years) were cited as possible factors contributing to the decreased result. Several patients with a delay between injury and reinnervation longer than 8 years had a successful result.

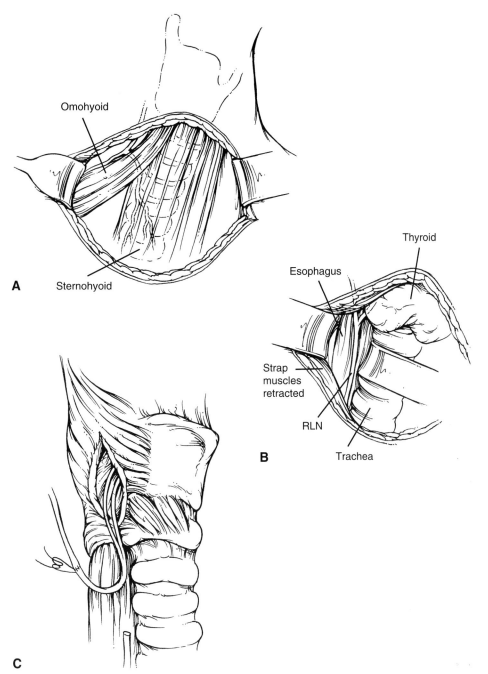

Figure 98-2. Ansa cervicalis to RLN anastomosis. **A,** Exposure of branch to sternohyoid muscle. **B,** Exposure of RLN in the tracheoesophageal groove. **C,** Ansa-RLN anastomosis.

Ansa-RLN anastomosis was successful in two elderly patients (66 and 71 years old) after resection of a mediastinal tumor with early reinnervation.[83]

Zheng and colleagues[136] presented eight cases with one disappointing result. The anterior branch of the RLN was used. A slight improvement was seen early after surgery with additional improvement seen at 2 to 3 months. Electromyographic confirmation was obtained in five patients. Passive arytenoid mobility was important in achieving good results and a lack thereof was related to the one substandard result.

Similar results in terms of mean phonation time and vocal fold position are seen after a direct anastomosis of the RLN, a free nerve graft reconstructing the RLN, a vagus to RLN anastomosis, and an ansa-RLN anastomosis when used during the course of thyroid surgery.[85] The ansa-RLN anastomosis has several advantages over other means of reconstruction of a divided RLN during the course of thyroid or other neck surgery. These include the requirement of only one anastomosis performed at a relatively accessible level in the neck, a relatively short time to recovery because the anastomosis is close to the larynx, and availability when the RLN is injured within the mediastinum. Performing the anastomosis behind the thyroid cartilage[85] as well as using the contralateral ansa cervicalis as a donor nerve[84] improves the percentage of cases that can be reconstructed successfully.

A quantitative analysis of 12 patients with ansa-RLN anastomosis for unilateral vocal fold paralysis was presented by Olson and others.[91] An improvement in vocal quality was demonstrated when compared with preoperative state. Postoperative results were similar to those of a control group of healthy subjects. Patients with isolated vocal fold paralysis achieved the best results.

The addition of ansa-RLN anastomosis to arytenoid adduction did not improve the acoustic results when compared with arytenoid adduction alone.[21] All patients had significant perceptual improvement in voice, but the relationship of surgical repositioning of the arytenoid and reinnervation in unilateral paralysis was questioned.

Direct Nerve Implant

Early in the 20th century, direct implantation of a nerve into a denervated muscle was shown to produce successful reinnervation in experimental models.[37,59,116] Insertion of a nerve ending into skeletal muscle results in the establishment of neuromuscular junctions.[94,104] Using multiple implants distributed over a wide area increases the effectiveness of reinnervation with the direct nerve implantation technique.[15] Direct nerve implants have been successfully used in patients with active muscle movement in 10 of 10 patients.[6] A short period of denervation, a healthy donor nerve, and a wide distribution of nerve fibers entering the muscle has a positive effect on the outcome.

Early experiments investigating direct nerve implantation also examined the value of the technique in laryngeal reinnervation.[66,88] Direct implantation of the RLN into the PCA muscle was successfully performed in the canine and proposed as a promising method for reinnervation.[32,33]

Comparisons of the NMP with direct implantation of the ansa cervicalis nerve into denervated muscle have shown mixed results. Meikle and others[81] showed no advantage of one method over the other, whereas Hall and colleagues[53] found the NMP to produce stronger evoked contractions and have a shorter time to return of function. Both authors felt their results were consistent with the NMP acting as a

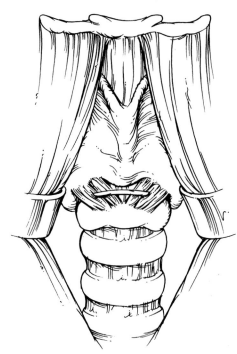

Figure 98-3. Muscle-nerve-muscle graft between the innervated and denervated cricothyroid muscle.

source for multiple direct nerve implants rather than a predominant reliance on transfer of intact motor units. Because of the need to support a distal muscle pedicle, the NMP was inferior to the direct nerve implant when the reinnervation procedure was extended with a cable graft.[49]

Direct nerve implantation of laryngeal muscles has not been reported in humans. A variant of this technique in which a nerve acts as a conduit from an innervated muscle to the contralateral, denervated muscle (muscle-nerve-muscle) has been successfully used.[35] Selective CT reinnervation with a muscle-nerve-muscle graft from the contralateral CT was used in combination with ansa-RLN anastomosis in three patients (Figure 98-3). All patients had improved voice and EMG evidence of CT muscle reinnervation.

REFERENCES

1. Anonsen CK and others: Reinnervation of skeletal muscle with a neuromuscular pedicle, *Otolaryngol Head Neck Surg* 93:48, 1985.
2. Applebaum EL, Allen GW, Sisson GA: Human laryngeal reinnervation: the Northwestern experience, *Laryngoscope* 89:1784, 1979.
3. Arakawa Y, Sendtner M, Thoenen H: Survival effect of ciliary neurotrophic factor (CNTF) on chick embryonic motoneurons in culture: comparison with other neurotrophic factors and cytokines, *J Neurosci* 10:3507, 1990.
4. Baldissera F and others: Innervation of the paralyzed laryngeal muscles by phrenic motoneurons: a quantitative

study by light and electron microscopy, *Laryngoscope* 102:907, 1992.

5. Baldissera F and others: Recovery of inspiratory abduction of the paralyzed vocal cords after bilateral reinnervation of the cricoarytenoid muscles by one single branch of the phrenic nerve, *Laryngoscope* 99:1286, 1989.

6. Becker M and others: Refinements in nerve to muscle neurotization, *Muscle Nerve* 26:362, 2002.

7. Bodine-Fowler SC and others: Inaccurate projection of rat soleus motoneurons: a comparison of nerve repair techniques, *Muscle Nerve* 20:29, 1997.

8. Brondbo K and others: Experimental laryngeal reinnervation by phrenic nerve implantation into the posterior cricoarytenoid muscle, *Acta Otolaryngol* 103:339, 1987.

9. Brondbo K and others: Functional results after experimental reinnervation of the posterior cricoarytenoid muscle in dogs, *J Otolaryngol* 15:259, 1986.

10. Brondbo K and others: The human posterior cricoarytenoid (PCA) muscle and diaphragm: a histochemical comparison as a basis for reinnervation attempts, *Acta Otolaryngol* 102:474, 1986.

11. Broniatowski M, Dessoffy R, Strome M: Long-term excitability and fine tuning of nerve pedicles reinnervating strap muscles in the dog, *Ann Otol Rhinol Laryngol* 107:301, 1998.

12. Broniatowski M and others: Laryngeal pacemaker: Part 1. electronic pacing of reinnervated strap muscles in the dog, *Otolaryngol Head Neck Surg* 94:41, 1986.

13. Broniatowski M and others: Laryngeal pacemaker: II. electronic pacing of reinnervated posterior cricoarytenoid muscles in the canine, *Laryngoscope* 95:1194, 1985.

14. Brown MC, Ironton R: Sprouting and regression of neuromuscular synapses in partially denervated mammalian muscles, *J Physiol (Lond)* 278:325, 1978.

15. Brunelli GA, Brunelli GR: Direct muscle neurotization, *J Reconstr Microsurg* 9:81, 1993.

16. Brushart TM: Motor axons preferentially reinnervate motor pathways, *J Neurosci* 13:2730, 1993.

17. Brushart TM, Mesulam MM: Alteration in connections between muscle and anterior horn motoneurons after peripheral nerve repair, *Science* 208:603, 1980.

18. Chang SY: Studies of early laryngeal reinnervation, *Laryngoscope* 95:455, 1985.

19. Chen H, He Z, Tessier-Lavigne M: Axon guidance mechanisms: semaphorins as simultaneous repellents and anti-repellents, *Nat Neurosci* 1:436, 1998.

20. Chhetri DK, Berke GS: Ansa cervicalis nerve: review of the topographic anatomy and morphology, *Laryngoscope* 107:1366, 1997.

21. Chhetri DK and others: Combined arytenoid adduction and laryngeal reinnervation in the treatment of vocal fold paralysis, *Laryngoscope* 109:1928, 1999.

22. Crumley RL: Experiments in laryngeal reinnervation, *Laryngoscope* 92:1, 1982.

23. Crumley RL: Laryngeal synkinesis: its significance to the laryngologist, *Ann Otol Rhinol Laryngol* 98:87, 1989.

24. Crumley RL: *Nerve transfer technique as it relates to phonatory surgery.* In Cummings CW and others, editors: *Otolaryngology–head and neck surgery: update II.* St Louis, 1990, Mosby–Year Book, p 100.

25. Crumley RL: Phrenic nerve graft for bilateral vocal cord paralysis, *Laryngoscope* 93:425, 1983.

26. Crumley RL: Teflon versus thyroplasty versus nerve transfer: a comparison, *Ann Otol Rhinol Laryngol* 99:759, 1990.

27. Crumley RL: Update: ansa cervicalis to recurrent laryngeal nerve anastomosis for unilateral laryngeal paralysis, *Laryngoscope* 101:384, 1991.

28. Crumley RL: *Update of laryngeal reinnervation concepts and options.* In Bailey BT, Biller HF, editors: *Surgery of the larynx.* Philadelphia, 1985, W.B. Saunders, p 135.

29. Crumley RL, Izdebski K: Voice quality following laryngeal reinnervation by ansa hypoglossi transfer, *Laryngoscope* 96:611, 1986.

30. Crumley RL, Izdebski K, McMicken B: Nerve transfer versus Teflon injection for vocal cord paralysis: a comparison, *Laryngoscope* 98:1200, 1988.

31. De Vito MA, Malmgren LT, Gacek RR: Three-dimensional distribution of neuromuscular junctions in human cricothyroid, *Arch Otolaryngol* 111:110, 1985

32. Doyle PJ, Brummett RE, Everts EC: Results of surgical section and repair of the recurrent laryngeal nerve, *Laryngoscope* 77:1245, 1967.

33. Doyle PJ, Everts EC, Brummett RE: Treatment of recurrent laryngeal nerve injury, *Arch Surg* 96:517, 1968.

34. Edwards TM: Progress in the surgical treatment of bilateral laryngeal paralysis, *Ann Otol Rhinol Laryngol* 61:159, 1952.

35. El-Kashlan HK and others: Selective cricothyroid muscle reinnervation by muscle-nerve-muscle neurotization, *Arch Otolaryngol Head Neck Surg* 127:1211, 2001.

36. Ellenbogen BG and others: Accessory muscle activity and respiration, *Otolaryngol Head Neck Surg* 89:370, 1981.

37. Erlacher P: Direct and muscular neurotization of paralyzed muscles, *Am J Orthop Surg* 13:22, 1915.

38. Fata JJ and others: Histochemical study of posterior cricoarytenoid muscle reinnervation by a nerve-muscle pedicle in the cat, *Ann Otol Rhinol Laryngol* 96:479, 1987.

39. Feringa ER and others: Cell death in the adult rat dorsal root ganglion after hind limb amputation, spinal cord transection, or both operations, *Exp Neurol* 87:349, 1985.

40. Fink BR: Folding mechanism of the human larynx, *Acta Otolaryngol* 78:124, 1974.

41. Frazier CH: Anastomosis of the recurrent laryngeal nerve with the descendens noni, *JAMA* 83:1637, 1924.

42. Frazier CH, Mosser WB: Treatment of recurrent laryngeal nerve paralysis by nerve anastomosis, *Surg Gynecol Obstet* 43:134, 1926.

43. Friedman B and others: Regulation of ciliary neurotrophic factor expression in myelin-related Schwann cells in vivo, *Neuron* 9:295, 1992.

44. Frostick SP, Yin Q, Kemp GJ: Schwann cells, neurotrophic factors, and peripheral nerve regeneration, *Microsurgery* 18:397, 1998.

45. Gacek M, Gacek RR: Cricoarytenoid joint mobility after chronic vocal cord paralysis, *Laryngoscope* 106:1528, 1996.

46. Gacek RR: Morphologic correlates for laryngeal reinnervation, *Laryngoscope* 111:1871, 2001.

47. Gacek RR, Malmgren LT, Lyon MJ: Localization of adductor and abductor motor fibers to the larynx, *Ann Otol Rhinol Laryngol* 86:770, 1977.

48. Gambino DR, Malmgren LT, Gacek RR: Three-dimensional computer reconstruction of the neuromuscular junction distribution in the human posterior cricoarytenoid muscle, *Laryngoscope* 95:556, 1985.

49. Goding GS, Cummings CW, Bright DA: Extension of neuromuscular pedicles and direct nerve implants in the rabbit, *Arch Otolaryngol* 115:217, 1989.

50. Goding GS Jr., Bierbaum RW: Relationship of the posterior cricoarytenoid muscle to the posterior cricoid lamina, *Otolaryngol Head Neck Surg* 120:493, 1999.

51. Green JG, Neil E: The respiratory function of the laryngeal muscles, *J Physiol (Lond)* 129:134, 1955.

52. Guida HL, Zorzetto NL: Morphometric and histochemical study of the human vocal muscle, *Ann Otol Rhinol Laryngol* 109:67, 2000.

53. Hall SJ, Trachy RE, Cummings CW: Facial muscle reinnervation: a comparison of neuromuscular pedicle with direct nerve implant, *Ann Otol Rhinol Laryngol* 97:229, 1988.

54. Hansson HA and others: Evidence indicating trophic importance of IGF-I in regenerating peripheral nerves, *Acta Physiol Scand* 126:609, 1986.

55. Hast MH: The primate larynx: a comparative physiological study of intrinsic muscles, *Acta Otolaryngol* 67:84, 1969.

56. Hast MH: The respiratory muscles of the larynx, *Ann Otol Rhinol Laryngol* 76:489, 1967.

57. Hast MH: Studies on the extrinsic laryngeal muscles, *Arch Otolaryngol* 88:273, 1968.

58. Hayashi M and others: Loss of large myelinated nerve fibres of the recurrent laryngeal nerve in patients with multiple system atrophy and vocal cord palsy, *J Neurol Neurosurg Psychiatry* 62:234, 1997.

59. Heineke H: Die direkte einpflanzung der nerven in den muskel, *Zentralbl Chir* 41:465, 1914.

60. Henderson CE and others: Neurotrophins promote motor neuron survival and are present in embryonic limb bud, *Nature* 363:266, 1993.

61. Hengerer AS, Tucker HM: Restoration of abduction in the paralyzed canine vocal cord, *Arch Otolaryngol* 97:247, 1973.

62. Hirose H and others: An experimental study of the contraction properties of the laryngeal muscles in the cat, *Ann Otol Rhinol Laryngol* 78:297, 1969.

63. Hiroto I, Hirano M, Tomita H: Electromyographic investigations of human vocal cord paralysis, *Ann Otol Rhinol Laryngol* 77:296, 1968.

64. Hisa Y, Malmgren LT: *Muscle fiber types in the human sternothyroid muscle: a correlated histochemical and ultrastructural morphometric study.* In Baer T, Sasaki C, Harris K, editors: *Laryngeal function in phonation and respiration.* Boston, Mass, 1987, College-Hill, p 29.

65. Hisa Y, Malmgren LT, Lyon MJ: Quantitative histochemical studies on the cat infrahyoid muscles, *Otolaryngol Head Neck Surg* 103:723, 1990.

66. Hoessly H: Uber Nervenimplantation bei recurrenslahmungen eine experimentelle studie, *Beitr Klin Chir* 99:186, 1916.

67. Horsley JA: Suture of the recurrent laryngeal nerve with report of a case, *Trans South Surg Gynecol Assoc* 22:161, 1909.

68. Iwaurma S: Functioning remobilization of the paralyzed vocal cord in dogs, *Arch Otolaryngol* 100:122, 1974.

69. Jacobs IN and others: Reinnervation of the canine posterior cricoarytenoid muscle with sympathetic preganglinic neurons, *Ann Otol Rhinol Laryngol* 99:167, 1990.

70. Kelly JD: Surgical treatment of bilateral paralysis of the abductor muscles, *Arch Otolaryngol* 33:293, 1941.

71. Kernell D, Wang LC: Simple methods for quantifying the spatial distribution of different categories of motoneuronal nerve endings, using measurements of muscle regionalization, *J Neurosci Methods* 100:79, 2000.

72. Kuffler DP: Regeneration of muscle axons in the frog is directed by diffusible factors from denervated muscle and nerve tubes, *J Comp Neurol* 281:416, 1989.

73. Kugelberg E, Edstrom L, Abbruzzese M: Mapping of motor units in experimentally reinnervated rat muscle: interpretation of histochemical and atrophic fibre patterns in neurogenic lesions, *J Neurol Neurosurg Psychiatry* 33:319, 1970.

74. Lahey FH: Successful suture of recurrent laryngeal nerve for bilateral abductor paralysis, with restoration of function, *Ann Surg* 87:481, 1928.

75. Lundborg G and others: Trophism, tropism, and specificity in nerve regeneration, *J Reconstr Microsurg* 10:345, 1994.

76. Lyons RM, Tucker HM: Delayed restoration of abduction in the paralyzed canine larynx, *Arch Otolaryngol* 100:176, 1974.

77. Malmgren LT, Gacek RR: Histochemical characteristics of muscle fiber types in the posterior cricoarytenoid muscle, *Ann Otol Rhinol Laryngol* 90:423, 1981.

78. Manthorpe M and others: Laminin promotes neuritic regeneration from cultured peripheral and central neurons, *J Cell Biol* 97:1882, 1983.

79. May M, Beery Q: Muscle-nerve pedicle laryngeal reinnervation, *Laryngoscope* 96:1196, 1986.

80. May M, Lavorato AS, Bleyaert AL: Rehabilitation of the crippled larynx: application of the Tucker technique for muscle-nerve reinnervation, *Laryngoscope* 90:1, 1980.

81. Meikle D, Trachy RE, Cummings CW: Reinnervation of skeletal muscle: a comparison of nerve implantation with neuromuscular pedicle transfer in an animal model, *Ann Otol Rhinol Laryngol* 96:152, 1987.

82. Meyer M and others: Enhanced synthesis of brain-derived neurotrophic factor in the lesioned peripheral nerve: different mechanisms are responsible for the regulation of BDNF and NGF mRNA, *J Cell Biol* 119:45, 1992.

83. Miyauchi A and others: Ansa-recurrent nerve anastomosis for vocal cord paralysis due to mediastinal lesions, *Ann Thorac Surg* 57:1020, 1994.

84. Miyauchi A and others: Opposite ansa cervicalis to recurrent laryngeal nerve anastomosis to restore phonation in patients with advanced thyroid cancer, *Eur J Surg* 167:540, 2001.

85. Miyauchi A and others: The role of ansa-to-recurrent-laryngeal nerve anastomosis in operations for thyroid cancer, *Eur J Surg* 164:927, 1998.

86. Nathan CF: Secretory products of macrophages, *J Clin Invest* 79:319, 1987.

87. Neal GD, Cummings CW, Sutton D: Delayed reinnervation of unilateral vocal cord paralysis in dogs, *Otolaryngol Head Neck Surg* 89:608, 1981.

88. Nikolajew NA: Zur frage de implantation von nerven in muskeln (nervenuberpflanzung auf kehlkopfmuskeln), *Monatsschr Ohrenheilkd* 61:1005, 1927.

89. Nomoto M and others: Misdirected reinnervation in the feline intrinsic laryngeal muscles after long-term denervation, *Acta Otolaryngol Suppl* 506:71, 1993.

90. Ochs S: *Sensation and neuromuscular transmission.* In Selkurt EE, editor: *Physiology.* Boston, Mass, 1984, Little, Brown & Co., p 46.

91. Olson DE, Goding GS, Michael DD: Acoustic and perceptual evaluation of laryngeal reinnervation by ansa cervicalis transfer, *Laryngoscope* 108:1767-1772, 1998.

92. Paniello RC, Lee P, Dahm JD: Hypoglossal nerve transfer for laryngeal reinnervation: a preliminary study, *Ann Otol Rhinol Laryngol* 108:239, 1999.

93. Paniello RC, West SE: Laryngeal adductory pressure as a measure of post-reinnervation synkinesis, *Ann Otol Rhinol Laryngol* 109:447, 2000.

94. Park DM, Shon SK, Kim YJ: Direct muscle neurotization in rat soleus muscle, *J Reconstr Microsurg* 16:135, 2000.

95. Purves D, Nja A: Effect of nerve growth factor on synaptic depression following axotomy, *Nature* 260:535, 1976.

96. Rende M and others: Immunolocalization of ciliary neuronotrophic factor in adult rat sciatic nerve, *Glia* 5:25, 1992.

97. Rice DH and others: The nerve-muscle pedicle, *Arch Otolaryngol* 109:233, 1983.

98. Rochel S, Robbins N: Effect of partial denervation and terminal field expansion on neuromuscular transmitter release and nerve terminal structure, *J Neurosci* 8:332, 1988.

99. Romanul FC, Van der Meulen JP: Reversal of the enzyme profiles of muscle fibres in fast and slow muscles by cross-innervation, *Nature* 212:1369, 1966.

100. Rosen M, Malmgren LT, Gacek RR: Three-dimensional computer reconstruction of the distribution of neuromuscular junctions in the thyroarytenoid muscle, *Ann Otol Rhinol Laryngol* 92:424, 1983.

101. Sahgal V, Hast MH: Effect of denervation on primate laryngeal muscles: a morphologic and morphometric study, *J Laryngol Otol* 100:553, 1986.

102. Sahgal V, Hast MH: Histochemistry of primate laryngeal muscles, *Acta Otolaryngol* 78:277, 1974.

103. Saika T and others: Effects of nerve crush and transection on mRNA levels for nerve growth factor receptor in the rat facial motoneurons, *Brain Res Mol Brain Res* 9:157, 1991.

104. Saito A, Zacks SI: Fine structure of neuromuscular junction after nerve section and implantation of nerve in denervated muscle, *Exp Mol Pathol* 10:256, 1969.

105. Sanders I and others: The innervation of the human larynx, *Arch Otolaryngol Head Neck Surg* 119:934, 1993.

106. Sanders I and others: The innervation of the human posterior cricoarytenoid muscle: evidence for at least two neuromuscular compartments, *Laryngoscope* 104:880, 1994.

107. Sato F, Ogura JH: Functional restoration for recurrent laryngeal paralysis: an experimental study, *Laryngoscope* 88:855, 1978.

108. Schlaepfer WW, Hasler MB: Characterization of the calcium-induced disruption of neurofilaments in rat peripheral nerve, *Brain Res* 168:299, 1979.

109. Sciote JJ and others: Unloaded shortening velocity and myosin heavy chain variations in human laryngeal muscle fibers, *Ann Otol Rhinol Laryngol* 111:120, 2002.

110. Sercarz JA and others: Physiologic motion after laryngeal nerve reinnervation: a new method, *Otolaryngol Head Neck Surg* 116:466, 1997.

111. Shiotani A, Flint PW: Myosin heavy chain composition in rat laryngeal muscles after denervation, *Laryngoscope* 108:1225, 1998.

112. Shiotani A, Westra WH, Flint PW: Myosin heavy chain composition in human laryngeal muscles, *Laryngoscope* 109:1521, 1999.

113. Siribodhi C, Sundmaker W, Atkins JP: Electromyographic studies of laryngeal paralysis and regeneration of laryngeal motor nerve in dogs, *Laryngoscope* 73:148, 1963.

114. Slack JR, G HW: Neuromuscular transmission at terminals of sprouted mammalian motor neurons, *Brain Res* 237:121, 1982.

115. Staron RS: Human skeletal muscle fiber types: delineation, development, and distribution, *Can J Appl Physiol* 22:307, 1997.

116. Steindler A: Direct neurotization of paralyzed muscles: further studies of the question of direct implantation, *Am J Orthop Surg* 14:707, 1916.

117. Talmadge RJ: Myosin heavy chain isoform expression following reduced neuromuscular activity: potential regulatory mechanisms, *Muscle Nerve* 23:661, 2000.

118. Thomas CK and others: Patterns of reinnervation and motor unit recruitment in human hand muscles after complete ulnar and median nerve section and resuture, *J Neurol Neurosurg Psychiatry* 50:259, 1987.

119. Tucker HM: Combined laryngeal framework medialization and reinnervation for unilateral vocal fold paralysis, *Ann Otol Rhinol Laryngol* 99:778, 1990.

120. Tucker HM: Human laryngeal reinnervation, *Laryngoscope* 86:769, 1976.

121. Tucker HM: Human laryngeal reinnervation: long-term experience with the nerve-muscle pedicle technique, *Laryngoscope* 88:598, 1978.

122. Tucker HM: Long-term results of nerve-muscle pedicle reinnervation for laryngeal paralysis, *Ann Otol Rhinol Laryngol* 98:674, 1989.

123. Tucker HM: Nerve-muscle pedicle reinnervation of the larynx: avoiding pitfalls and complications, *Ann Otol Rhinol Laryngol* 91:440, 1982.

124. Tucker HM: Reinnervation of the paralyzed larynx: a review, *Head Neck Surg* 1:235, 1979.

125. Tucker HM: Reinnervation of the unilaterally paralyzed larynx, *Ann Otol Rhinol Laryngol* 86:789, 1977.

126. Tucker HM, Harvey J, Ogura JH: Vocal cord remobilization in the canine larynx, *Arch Otolaryngol* 92:530, 1970.

127. Tucker HM, Ogura JH: Vocal cord remobilization in the canine larynx: an histologic evaluation, *Laryngoscope* 81:1602, 1971.

128. Tucker HM, Rusnov M: Laryngeal reinnervation for unilateral vocal cord paralysis: long-term results, *Ann Otol Rhinol Laryngol* 90:457, 1981.

129. van Lith-Bijl JT, Mahieu HF: Reinnervation aspects of laryngeal transplantation, *Eur Arch Otorhinolaryngol* 255:515, 1998.

130. van Lith-Bijl JT and others: Laryngeal abductor reinnervation with a phrenic nerve transfer after a 9-month delay, *Arch Otolaryngol Head Neck Surg* 124:393, 1998.

131. van Lith-Bijl JT and others: Selective laryngeal reinnervation with separate phrenic and ansa cervicalis nerve transfers, *Arch Otolaryngol Head Neck Surg* 123:406, 1997.

132. Wang L and others: Regional distribution of slow-twitch muscle fibers after reinnervation in adult rat hindlimb muscles, *Muscle Nerve* 25:805, 2002.

133. Wu YZ and others: New perspectives about human laryngeal muscle: single-fiber analyses and interspecies comparisons, *Arch Otolaryngol Head Neck Surg* 126:857, 2000.

134. Yan Q, Elliott J, Snider WD: Brain-derived neurotrophic factor rescues spinal motor neurons from axotomy-induced cell death, *Nature* 360:753, 1992.

135. Yin Q, Kemp GJ, Frostick SP: Neurotrophins, neurones and peripheral nerve regeneration, *J Hand Surg [Br]* 23:433, 1998.

136. Zheng H and others: Update: laryngeal reinnervation for unilateral vocal cord paralysis with the ansa cervicalis, *Laryngoscope* 106:1522, 1996.

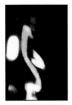

CHAPTER NINETY NINE

MALIGNANT TUMORS OF THE LARYNX AND HYPOPHARYNX

George L. Adams
Robert H. Maisel

INTRODUCTION

There are many similarities between malignant tumors of the larynx and hypopharynx in relationship to etiology, clinical presentation, and surgical treatment, which permits a discussion in a single chapter. In particular, the adverse effects of the surgery on speech and swallowing and reconstructive techniques require an understanding of the close relationship of these tumors. With time, tumors of the larynx can extend to the hypopharynx and vice versa. At the same time, there are distinct differences in the ultimate behavior of these two areas of malignancy. Laryngeal carcinomas are more prevalent in heavy smokers, present earlier, and are less likely with the exception of supraglottic malignancies to metastasize early to the adjacent lymph nodes. On the other hand, hypopharyngeal carcinomas present late, have a high association with alcoholism and other disorders, and commonly present with cervical metastatic disease. Most importantly, because of the early presentation and lack of rich lymphatic drainage of the larynx, tumors confined to the laryngeal framework have a substantially better prognosis. Their early detection, the effectiveness of the American Cancer Society in warning patients of the need for evaluation of persistent hoarseness, and an easier in-office endoscopic examination allows for the earlier detection and treatment. In addition, studies reported in this chapter will show that conservative treatment when not effective still permits reasonable salvage by more radical surgery. On the other hand, hypopharyngeal malignancies do not cause symptoms until the late stage of the disease, and most of the patients have palpable adenopathy in the neck when initially seen. Surgical salvage for recurrent disease is less likely to be successful. History of dysphagia or persistent sore throat, even on office examination, may not reveal an early malignancy, especially on the posterior pharyngeal wall or even in the postcricoid area. Referred otalgia (pain referred to the ipsilateral ear) may be the only initial complaint and can mislead the practitioner.

In the past 10 years, a substantially more conservative approach to the management of advanced malignancies of the larynx and hypopharynx has become evident. Prospective randomized studies have demonstrated that laryngeal preservation with radiation as initial treatment with laryngectomy reserved for recurrent or persistent disease has become accepted. At the same time, there has to be an acceptance of a high incidence of late recurrent disease that will still necessitate laryngectomy, increased surgical morbidity from salvage surgery, and the potential of poor voice and difficulty swallowing when organ preservation is accomplished. Still, quality-of-life studies suggest that preservation of the larynx is a worthwhile goal and objective. The extension of this treatment to tumors of the hypopharynx has been less extensively explored, possibly because of the late presentation of so many of these tumors, difficulty in following these patients, and the overall greater mortality from the primary, locoregional disease, distant disease, and comorbidity factors of patients with hypopharyngeal cancer. With such a multiplicity of management schemas for these patients, an effort will be made to provide the rationale both from an anatomic and pathologic basis, as well as from prospective randomized studies to allow a treatment plan to be made for a given patient. The diversity of protocols and institutional treatment recommendations, particularly in carcinomas of the hypopharynx, results from the fact that no specific treatment has received overwhelming acceptance. Individualization of each patient, including evaluation of their general health, pulmonary status, and ability to accept radical surgery particularly for residual or recurrent disease, has to be included in the assessment. Particularly in more advanced cases, pretreatment assessment by the team of individuals including radiation therapists, oncologists, internists, and others who at some point will become involved in the treatment of the patient has become necessary for these patients.

INCIDENCE

The American Cancer Society predicts that 10,270 new cases of laryngeal cancer will be diagnosed in 2004.[114] This figure is basically consistent with the data provided in 1994 and may actually show a slight decrease. It is interesting to note that this incidence persists, despite continual efforts to make the public more aware of the adverse effects of smoking. The demographics and epidemiology of the disease have changed during the past 40 years. The male/female incidence has dropped from 15:1 to now less than 5:1 in 2004.[114] This statistical change in the United States has been hypothesized to be a result of women obtaining an equal place in the toxic work environment and participating in what has become a more socially acceptable act of public cigarette smoking. The time between these behavioral changes (i.e., since World War II) and the recently altered gender statistics on cancer of the larynx may represent the duration of exposure needed to cause cancer of the larynx.

In the United States, the incidence of hypopharyngeal tumors has consistently been about one-third of that of laryngeal cancers. The incidence of esophageal and laryngeal cancers among blacks is twice that among white Americans.[292] In addition, blacks are often diagnosed at a later stage of disease. Factors that correlate with the development of cancers of the larynx and hypopharynx include tobacco use, alcohol abuse, or a sibling with head and neck cancer. In addition, there is an association among presence of human papillomavirus (HPV), previous radiotherapy, and previous head and neck cancer.[37]

Tobacco is a major risk factor for the development of larynx cancer. Many studies show that risk increases with increasing tobacco use.[228] People who smoked 40 or more cigarettes daily had an age-adjusted death rate of 15/100,000 compared with 0.6/100,000 person-years among nonsmokers. The death rate for pipe and cigar smoking was 5/100,000 person-years. European studies on filtered cigarettes and light (air-cured) tobacco compared with flue-cured or black tobacco showed the former two categories to be somewhat protective (50% lower risk) against cancer of the larynx and hypopharynx.[276] Rolled cigarettes are also more dangerous than commercially packaged cigarettes. La Vecchia and others[144] suggested that smokers of cigarettes with >22 mg of tar had double the incidence of laryngeal cancer compared with smokers of low-tar cigarettes. International studies have confirmed that the risk of laryngeal cancer developing decreases with time after the cessation of smoking. This accumulation of evidence indicates that tobacco acts as a promoter and an initiator in carcinogenesis.

A recent French study showed a 13-fold increase in laryngeal cancer for smokers, and those consuming more than 1.5 L/day of wine had a 34-fold increased risk.[7,95] This model suggests the high risk is multiplicative and without interaction. Additional risk is attributed to early onset and long duration of smoking.

A form of tea known as *mate* in Latin America and *chimarra* in Brazil has been a recognized risk factor for cancer in other aerodigestive sites. DeStefani and others[58,59] calculated a relative risk of 4.9 for laryngeal cancer in those who drink more than 1.5 L/day of this beverage compared with those who consume none. The phenols in the drink may be cancer promoters or may act as a carcinogen solvent.

Chemical carcinogens in the workplace that relate to laryngeal cancer include asbestos, nickel compounds, and certain mineral oils. Glass-wool has been associated with an increased mortality for laryngeal cancer in an Italian study.[24] The consensus of participants in the 1991 International Works on Perspectives on Secondary Prevention of Laryngeal Cancer was that smoking cessation and reduced alcohol drinking are the most effective means of preventing the development and recurrence of laryngeal cancer. A toxin-free work environment and a healthy diet are also important.

Genetics and susceptibility to cancer are hard to separate from lifestyle and the environment. Patients should be educated that cigarettes and, to a lesser degree, pipe and tobacco smoke are associated closely with laryngeal cancer. Beer and hard liquor are suggested to be more at fault than wine, although, as recognized previously, this may reflect only the mores of a country.

High incidence of second primary malignancies in head and neck squamous cell carcinoma has previously been demonstrated. A study in Fukuoka reported in 1998 showed an increased risk of multiple upper aerodigestive tract cancers in individuals with a positive family history for malignancy.[177] In their study, there was a higher incidence of hypopharyngeal esophageal cancer, as well as the disease occurring in younger individuals. They suggest that the same chromosomal change may be responsible for both the increased familial incidence of hypopharyngeal carcinoma and the increased overall incidence of second primary malignancies in patients with upper aerodigestive tract cancer. The extension of this argument is the need for panendoscopic assessment of patients with hypopharyngeal malignancies who have a potential for a second malignancy.

A study in Manchester, England, showed that only 5% of patients with hypopharyngeal cancer had it develop before the age of 45.[11] A clinical impression existed that younger patients did worse and may have presented with later stage disease. This study comparing those younger than age 45 with those older than age 60 showed no difference in prognosis.

Wahlberg[286] conducted a similar study in Sweden comparing the age of both men and women at the time of presentation for hypopharyngeal carcinoma. This study was important because of the decreased incidence of the Plummer-Vinson syndrome in Sweden during this period of time. Men were diagnosed twice as frequently as women, and in the women reported there was no change in survival related to age younger or older than age 60. However, men diagnosed before the age of 60 had a poorer prognosis than those diagnosed after the age of 60.

There have been many recent advances in understanding the genetics of head and neck cancer. There have been investigations into circulating immune complexes.[284] Aneuploidy has been recognized to accompany the progression from dysplasia to head and neck cancer.[313] Knudson's proposal of the two-hit hypothesis, whereby both copies of the retinoblastoma gene, when deleted, lead to clinical disease in retinoblastoma, represents an important modern cancer place theory and has been suggested to occur in head and neck cancer as well.[130]

Vogelstein's theory of inactivation of tumor suppressive genes or activation of proto-oncogene, another pillar of oncologic theory, has been evaluated in laryngeal cancer as well. Genetic alterations of chromosomal region 9p21 seem to occur frequently and early in the progression of preneoplastic abnormal mucosa to invasive cancer.[86,120] This loss affects the p16 gene that acts in cell cycle regulation.[244,319] Failure to have programmed cell death and apoptosis may be the step that immortalizes tumor cells.

Gene locus 17p13 has been implicated to create mutant p53, which, when present, seems to result in progression to invasion by carcinoma and risks further genetic changes.[87,178] Clinically this p53 mutation has been noted in many squamous cell carcinomas[33,201] and when the wild p53 suppressive gene is lost, it is presumed this fits Vogelstein's theory of inactivation of tumor-suppressive gene (TSG) by the mutant copy.

Similarly, activation of a proto-oncogene (11q13) amplifies the oncogene cyclin D1. This oncogene activates cell wall progression (noted in one-third of tumor specimens studied) and is associated with tumor invasion.[78,199]

It is hoped that learning more about these suppressive genes and oncogenes will guide patient therapy once their molecular pathways become better understood.[96] Although the present intense interest in genetics and the molecular biology of laryngeal cancer offers no clinically relevant treatment, studies have

suggested that mutagen-induced chromosome breaks may be an independent risk factor for head and neck cancer. They also seem to correlate with the incidence of second tumors.

HPV has been detected in many lesions of the head and neck, including squamous cell carcinoma. HPV types 16 and 18 have been identified as a major risk for the development of cancer in the cervix. This is presumed because of the E6 and E7 viral protein-mediated degradation of p53. This enzyme is involved in genomic integrity, proliferation, and apoptosis, which are considered important in immortalizing cancer cells. The ability to use this information about HPV is not clear in laryngeal cancer, because many studies have used different techniques, and the results vary in sensitivity and specificity. Although a recent study suggests that oropharyngeal cancer is 14.4 times more likely, with previous HPV exposure, measured by serologic markers,[178] the studies limited to laryngeal cancer are not so clear. Almadori and others[3] suggested one-third of laryngeal tumors had evidence of HPV DNA, but Ha and Califano[96] suggest from their review of the literature that HPV has a reasonable mechanism to promote tumor progression, but its role may be site specific, with a minority of laryngeal cancers influenced by HPV. Clayman and others[44] found 24 of 57 specimens from laryngeal cancer were HPV positive. Their studies suggest detectable HPV may represent a biologically distinct subset of tumors with poor prognosis. In contrast to Clayman's results, Sisk and others[246] suggest the presence of HPV confers a survival advantage among cancer patients, particularly when p53 is wild type.

Koufman[131] reported 31 patients with carcinoma of the larynx, with reflux documented in 84%. In contrast to most series, only 58% were smokers. Although the relationship is not proven, gastroesophageal reflux is regarded as a risk factor for laryngeal carcinoma.[81,131,291]

RISK FACTORS FOR HYPOPHARYNGEAL CANCER

With the exception of postcricoid carcinoma, which was formerly more common in women, all forms of hypopharyngeal malignancy are more common in men, usually aged 55 to 70. A history of heavy alcohol ingestion, cirrhosis of the liver, and heavy smoking is usual.[123] In women, the reverse ratio for postcricoid carcinoma has been related to Plummer-Vinson syndrome. The postcricoid/piriform ratio is also reversed in patients seen and managed in Egypt in whom the postcricoid area was the site for 50% of identifiable malignancies in the hypopharynx.[231] The piriform sinus was the site in only 26%. The disease occurs primarily in men by a ratio of 7:1. In England and the

United States, a postcricoid carcinoma is considered the least common site. One possible explanation for this is nutritional deficiencies in upper Egypt and the presence of schistosomiasis. Similar to Plummer-Vinson syndrome, this combination leads to chronic sideropenic anemia. It may also be associated with vitamin C deficiency.

Plummer-Vinson or Paterson-Brown-Kelly Syndrome

The combination of dysphagia, hypopharyngeal and esophageal webs, weight loss, and iron deficiency anemia in women aged 30 to 50 years of age was first reported in the United States by Plummer in 1914.[93] Vinson[283] elaborated on it further in 1922. Simultaneously in Europe in 1919, Paterson-Brown[124,208] described a similar entity. In 1939, Waldenström referred to this syndrome as *sideropenic dysphagia*.[288] It soon became apparent that this entity was present in most of Europe and North and South America, and it is still most common in the United States, Sweden, and Wales. Of patients, 85% are women.

Initially, the dysphagia is intermittent, but it later becomes constant. Patients accept this and continue to modify their diet to softer food. However, when the disorder is recognized early, management with bougienage, iron replacement, and vitamin therapy can reverse the disease process. When fibrosis develops secondary to chronic inflammation, webs and irreversible long strictures develop. Additional findings include early loss of teeth, development of cheilosis, and glossitis with an atrophic appearing mucosa of the tongue and pharynx. There may be associated splenomegaly, hepatomegaly, and achlorhydria.

Radiologic examination with a barium swallow shows a hypopharyngeal web, most commonly in the low hypopharynx or the area between the postcricoid region and the thoracic esophagus. The web is initially anterior but later becomes circumferential.

The association of the benign syndrome with postcricoid carcinoma was made because of the reverse in the usual 4:1 ratio of male/female prevalence of cancer in other areas of the head and neck. In a series of 322 women who had postcricoid carcinoma develop, one-third to two-thirds had a history of Paterson-Brown syndrome. Malignancies were more common in patients who never sought management. The malignancy began just proximal to the web, possibly because of chronic irritation. In the same study, 76 patients with Paterson-Brown syndrome were followed prospectively, and postcricoid carcinoma developed in only one.[172] In this circumstance, however, most patients had undergone management with iron replacement, vitamin B replacement, and dilation. Currently, in the United States, because of the

reduced incidence of this syndrome, postcricoid carcinoma is more common in men.

Prognosis has not changed significantly in the past 20 years for patients with advanced hypopharyngeal cancer. This relates to the tendency for submucosal extension into the esophageal introitus; metastatic spread to the mediastinal, tracheoesophageal, and jugular nodes; and a higher incidence of distant metastases for hypopharyngeal cancer than for most other head and neck malignancies.

Second Primary Malignancies

Patients with malignancies of the hypopharynx have a significant risk of a second primary malignancy developing or have a second malignancy diagnosed at the time of presentation (metachronous malignancy).[222] Coexisting second primary malignancies are found in 4% to 8% of patients who have one head and neck primary malignancy.[118] Thus, preoperative assessment includes chest radiography, endoscopy, and careful evaluation of any other findings or symptoms the patient might have (e.g., blood in urine, gastrointestinal symptoms, positive stool guaiac finding). The probability of finding a second primary cancer in the lung is low if the chest x-ray is clear. The likelihood of a second primary tumor developing for head and neck cancer is 12.8%.[104] The head and neck and the lung are the most common sites. The likelihood of a second primary tumor developing increases with time and is 23% at 8 years.[47] In a study of 875 patients with epidermoid carcinoma of the head and neck,[143] 207 had second primary malignancies develop within 5 years of their primary or index tumor. Of these patients, 64 (30.9%) had a third primary malignancy develop, and 21 (10%) had a fourth primary malignancy develop. Virtually all patients (203 of 207) had a history of >50 pack-years of smoking. Of the remaining four patients, three had a history of alcohol abuse.

The hypopharyngeal area was the third most common site for patients with floor of mouth cancers to have a second primary malignancy. The mean time between development of first and second primary malignancies was 1.5 years; tumors tended to occur sooner in the hypopharyngeal area than in other sites.

Diagnosis

Early recognition of malignancies of the larynx and hypopharynx is crucial if the cure rate is to be affected. Most patients with hypopharyngeal cancers (70%) manifest stage III disease. However, laryngeal cancers are detected at an earlier stage. Because >95% of malignancies are squamous cell or epidermal carcinoma, malignancy of the larynx and hypopharynx has often been considered synonymous with squamous cell carcinoma. Other malignant tumors in the area are rare; however, because of the similarly presenting symptoms, biopsy confirmation of squamous cell carcinoma is essential before proceeding to definitive management. Hypopharyngeal tumors can cause a chronic sore throat, dysphagia, or referred otalgia and are thus managed with antibiotics, because the process is mistakenly attributed to infectious disease. The rich lymphatic network in the submucosal tissue surrounding the hypopharynx allows early spread to regional lymph nodes and direct extension into adjacent soft tissues. This accounts for the fact that 78% of patients with hypopharyngeal carcinoma have palpable cervical metastases when initially seen.

ANATOMY AND EMBRYOLOGY

The embryologic development of the larynx has been studied by anatomists and laryngologists and relates to the biologic spread of cancer. The development begins from the hypopharynx with the fusion of lateral structures derived from the tracheobronchial primordium (arch 4 or 5) in the midline. This lateral development and the scarcity of lymphatics in the true vocal cord have led to management theories in cancer of the larynx. A surgical division into supraglottis, glottis, and subglottis has embryologic and anatomic correlates and historically has had value in predicting the patterns of tumor invasion and tumor behavior (Figure 99-1). Frazer[79] in 1909 showed that the supraglottis came from the buccopharyngeal primordium (arch 3 or 4) without a midline merger, suggesting the risk of bilateral neck disease, because no midline barrier occurred, whereas glottic tumors usually metastasized ipsilaterally. Current surgical management is undertaken on the basis of the theory of compartmentalization of the larynx, which evolved

from Frazer,[79] Pressman and others,[220] and Tucker and Smith.[274] The supraglottis includes the superior laryngeal nerve as the nerve of the third arch and the superior thyroid artery as its vascular supply. In contrast, arches 4 and 6 create the glottis and subglottis. Pressman and others[220] addressed the theory that this separate derivation explains why supraglottic tumors of substantial bulk do not spread across the laryngeal ventricle to the vocal cord. This region was confirmed as a barrier to tumor spread in experiments that used submucosal vital dyes and radioisotopes. Pressman and others[220] noted that the inferior extent of supraglottic injection was the inferior false vocal cord, with the ventricle defining an anatomic barrier and halting further inferior flow of the dye. Tucker and Smith,[274] using animals and cadavers and whole organ serial sections of human tumor specimens, provided a rational anatomically based confirmation that elastic tissue barriers within the larynx explained the dye studies. These studies form the science underlying partial laryngeal surgery, predict the biologic progress of laryngeal cancer, and enable the surgeon to predict and anticipate metastasis to the neck.

The intrinsic ligaments of the larynx create a preepiglottic and a paraglottic compartment. The former space is bounded by the hyoid bone and the hyoepiglottic ligament superiorly and by the thyrohyoid membrane anteriorly and the epiglottis posteriorly. The adhesion of the anterior fascia to the thyroid cartilage defines the limit of this space, which is filled with fat and connective tissue and may restrict tumor projection externally. However, this space is frequently involved with tumor, probably because the elastic epiglottis cartilage has anatomic perforation and is easily penetrated below the hyoid bone, which

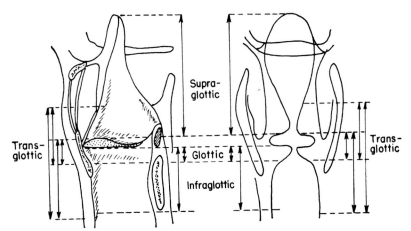

Figure 99-1. Classification of laryngeal lesions by the anatomic area involved. (From Ogura JH, Biller HF: *Partial and total laryngectomy and radical neck dissection.* In *Otolaryngology,* vol 4, New York, 1971, Harper & Row Publishers.)

allows direct extension of infrahyoid supraglottic cancer into this fascia-bound space (Figure 99-2). When neck metastases occur in conjunction with preepiglottic space involvement, bilateral involvement may occur. Therefore, many surgeons believe all supraglottic laryngeal carcinomas need attention directed equally to both sides of the neck. Although the embryologic compartmentalization hypothesized 40 years ago may explain the tendency of supraglottic tumors to not cross the laryngeal ventricle and involve the true vocal cord, studies[297] have challenged this long-held tenet in noting that paraglottic space invasion may produce transglottic carcinoma independent of ventricular invasion (Figure 99-3). However, the ventricular barrier because of separate embryologic growth has been a good predictor of behavior because most tumors, despite considerable bulk, remain supraglottic and extend up and out from their prescribed epicenter while preserving vocal cord integrity free of cancer.

Transglottic tumors cross the ventricle and may initiate as supraglottic or glottic cancers. As they enlarge, these tumors fail the compartmentalization thesis by direct mucosal extension or through the paraglottic space.

Almost 50% of infrahyoid supraglottic carcinomas seem to have preepiglottic space involvement, which upstages these tumors, because radiography and pathologic staging of preepiglottic space involvement designate a T_3 tumor. Computed tomography (CT) and magnetic resonance imaging (MRI) can recognize preepiglottic space involvement that is not apparent clinically.

The paraglottic spaces are lateral and are contained within the piriform sinus mucosa by the quadrangular membrane inferiorly, by the conus elasticus anteriorly and medially, and by the thyroid cartilage laterally. In theory, this space connects to the preepiglottic space, but growth and invasion along this potential path are unusual (Figure 99-4). Muscular invasion and lateral ventricular invasion by supraglottic or glottic cancer may fix the ipsilateral vocal cord and clearly inhibit consideration of partial surgery. Such fixation also suggests invasion of the paraglottic (potential) space, which no longer accepts the bounds of dividing the larynx between a supraglottis and glottis alone. Because the paraglottic space transcends the ventricle without restriction, surgical attention to such a cancer would require a wide-field laryngectomy. Even in the presence of such evidence of extensive local disease, wide-field laryngectomy offers a high likelihood of cure and a local control rate >90%.

Although paraglottic space invasion upstages the cancer, radiation still has a reasonable cure rate in cases of paraglottic space invasion; although local control rates are lower than those with surgery, such

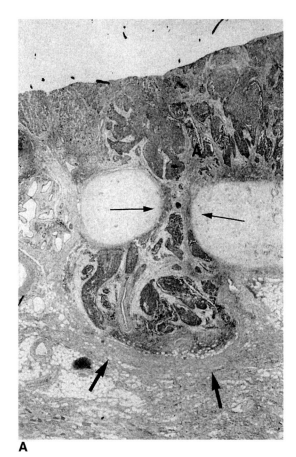

A

Figure 99-2. Histologic sections. **A,** Carcinoma on the laryngeal surface of the epiglottis growing through natural epiglottic fenestration *(light arrows)* into the preepiglottic space. A typical fibroelastic pseudocapsule has formed *(heavy arrows)* around advancing cancer. (Hematoxylin-eosin; original magnification ×40.)

a recommendation for management is acceptable to some patients.

Glottic anatomy, as it affects carcinoma, suggests natural barriers for tumor spread as a result of the scarcity of lymphatics in the body of the vocal cord, which creates a more prolonged course of local and, therefore, more highly curable disease. The conus elasticus, which attaches between the vocalis muscles and the cricoid cartilage, does not bind the cancer, because 20% of deeply invasive glottic tumors have subglottic extension.[238] The ossified portion of the cricoid or thyroid cartilages has been reported to be more likely invaded by cancer, possibly because of the increased vascularity of this portion compared with cartilage. The cartilage itself may resist invasion by presenting a smooth histologic barrier to neoplasia without an active metabolic substrate or blood vessels, except where the anterior commissure tendon attaches and allows penetration beyond the larynx.[314]

Glottic and subglottic tumors have a 2% to 5% risk of neck disease unless the subglottic extension

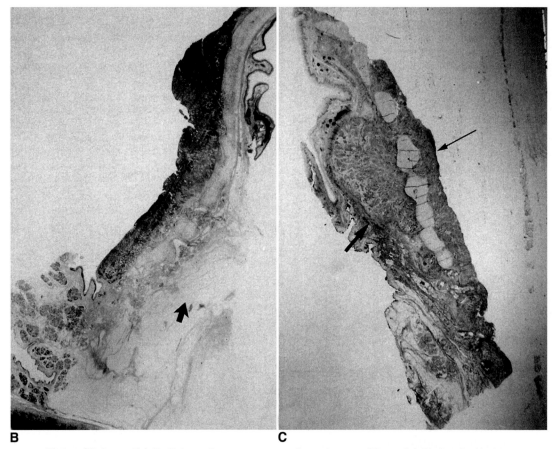

B   **C**

Figure 99-2, cont'd B, Sole routine squamous cell carcinoma of the epiglottis located below
the hyoepiglottic ligament did not grow through the epiglottic foramina into the preepiglottic
space *(arrow).* (Hematoxylin-eosin; original magnification ×10.) **C,** Squamous cell carcinoma
arising on the laryngeal surface of the epiglottis *(light arrow)* and invading the preepiglottic
space *(heavy arrow).* (Hematoxylin-eosin; original magnification ×1.) (From Zeitels SM,
Vaughan CW: *Ann Otol Rhinol Laryngol* 99:951, 1990.)

exceeds 10 mm. Such subglottic tumors usually
spread to the pretracheal Delphian node or to paratracheal nodes on either side of the trachea at a variable frequency, which with extensive disease may
represent an incidence as high as 50%.

Transglottic and supraglottic cancers spread to the
upper and middle chains of the lateral jugular nodes
and usually involve other nodal groups if the neck has
not been violated by previous surgery or biopsy. This
suggests surgical management to the clinically N_0
neck by removal of the jugular envelope of nodes and
can be an excellent predictor of risk for neck disease,
particularly if done bilaterally with microscopic intraoperative control.[57,182] This consideration anticipates
complete and careful surgical dissection of levels II,
III, and IV, which is achieved by unwrapping the fascia of the carotid sheath from the jugular vein so that
no more tissue remains than would be appropriate to
radical neck dissection except for the preserved
nerves, arteries, and veins.

The hypopharynx (laryngopharynx) is the longest
of the three segments of the pharynx. It is wide superiorly and progressively narrows toward the level of
the cricopharyngeal muscle, where it merges with the
cervical esophagus. Enclosed anterolaterally by the
lateral aspects of the thyroid cartilage are two paired
recesses that extend inferiorly to about the same level
as the laryngeal ventricle. They open posteriorly into
the pharynx and are called the piriform (pear-shaped)
sinuses (Figure 99-5). The hypopharynx does not
function solely as a conduit from the oropharynx to
the esophagus but has important dynamic actions that
allow separation of air and food passage and prevent
aspiration. Food enters the hypopharynx during the
third stage of swallowing, when the tongue propels it
rapidly past the epiglottis. Contraction of the constrictor muscles propels the food toward the cricopharyngeal muscle. The cricopharyngeal muscle relaxes,
and the food enters the esophagus, where peristaltic
action again transmits the bolus toward the stomach.

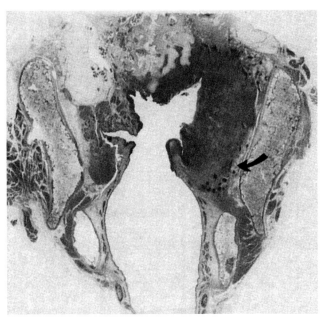

Figure 99-3. T$_3$ supraglottic carcinoma extends to the glottic level through the paraglottic space. Note the extension below the floor of the ventricle *(arrow)* with widening of the paraglottic space. (Hematoxylin-eosin, gross coronal section.) (From Weinstein and others: *Laryngoscope* 105:1131, 1995.)

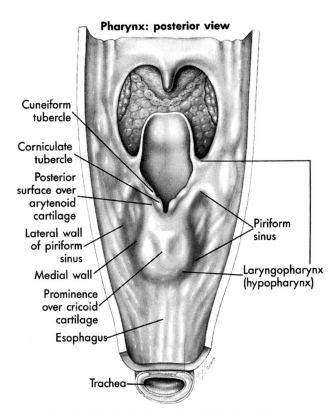

Pharynx: posterior view

Figure 99-5. Anatomic regions of the hypopharynx.

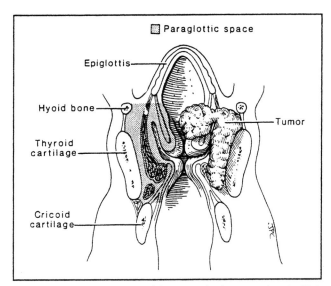

Figure 99-4. Dimensions of the paraglottic space located lateral to the mucosa of the larynx and deep to the cartilaginous framework. (Reprinted with permission from the American Academy of Otolaryngology—Head and Neck Surgery; from Myers EN, Alvi A: *Laryngoscope* 106:561, 1996.)

Innervation of the superior and middle constrictor muscles is through the superior laryngeal nerve and the pharyngeal plexus, which overlies the middle constrictors. It includes the pharyngeal branches of the vagus and glossopharyngeal nerves and contributions from the superior cervical ganglion. The inferior constrictor muscle receives branches from the external and the recurrent laryngeal branches of the vagus nerve. The internal branch of the superior laryngeal nerve passes through the thyroglossal membrane and traverses beneath the mucosa of the anterior piriform sinus. Laryngeal and piriform sinus anesthesia is obtained by topical anesthesia to this area, which is helpful when general anesthesia cannot be used for tumor assessment. This complex muscular coordination is not appreciated until after a major surgical resection in this area. Replacement with an adynamic muscle flap or a tight pharyngeal closure often results in aspiration, even when the laryngeal sphincter mechanism is intact. It may be necessary to resect the cancer-free larynx of patients whose tumor could otherwise be resected without laryngectomy were it not for the concern about chronic aspiration.

The mucosal lining of the hypopharynx is stratified squamous epithelium. It is associated with a rich submucosal lymphatic network that exits through the thyrohyoid membrane and leads to the superior and middle jugular lymph nodes. Inferiorly, the passage is directly through the hypopharynx to the paratracheal lymph nodes and low jugular nodes (Figure 99-6).

Tumor node metastasis (TNM) staging divides the hypopharynx into three distinct regions (Box 99-1). The first is the piriform sinus. This lateral funnel with

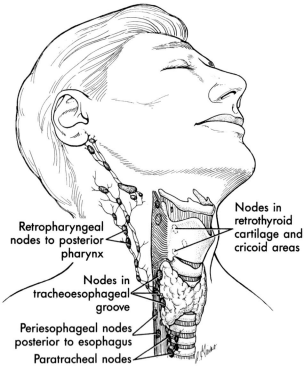

Retropharyngeal nodes to posterior pharynx

Nodes in retrothyroid cartilage and cricoid areas

Nodes in tracheoesophageal groove

Periesophageal nodes posterior to esophagus

Paratracheal nodes

Figure 99-6. Hypopharyngeal carcinomas metastasize primarily to these nodes. The superior jugular and midjugular nodes are the most common sites of the metastases. However, metastasis to the retropharyngeal nodes, paratracheal nodes, paraesophageal nodes, and parapharyngeal space nodes occurs.

its apex at the cricopharyngeal muscle is bound laterally by the medial aspect of the thyroid lamina and posteriorly by the lateral wall of the hypopharynx. It begins superiorly at the glossoepiglottic fold and medially is adjacent to the lateral surface of the arytenoid cartilage.

The second region is the posterior pharyngeal wall, which extends from a plane drawn at the level of the tip of the epiglottis to a plane at the level of the inferior border of the cricoid cartilage. Others describe the superior plane as at the level of the vallecula or hyoid bone. This approximately corresponds to the level of the bodies of the third through sixth cervical vertebrae. The superior and inferior margins of the posterior pharyngeal wall blend with the posterior wall of the oropharynx and the esophagus.

The third area is the postcricoid region, which includes the posterior surface of the aryepiglottic fold and posterior surface of the arytenoid to the inferior border of the cricoid cartilage. This latter area is the most difficult to assess by mirror examination and by direct laryngoscopy, because the tip of the blade of the laryngoscope may obscure an early cancer.

TUMOR NODE METASTASIS STAGING

Tumor Size (T)

T_{is} Carcinoma in situ
T_1 Tumor confined to one site
T_2 Extension of tumor to adjacent region
T_3 Extension of tumor to adjacent region or site with fixation of hemilarynx
T_4 Massive tumor in invading bone or soft tissues of neck

Nodal Involvement (N)

N_x Minimum requirement to assess regional nodes cannot be met
N_0 No clinically positive node
N_1 Single clinically positive homolateral node 3 cm or less in diameter
N_2 Single clinically positive homolateral node >3 cm but not >6 cm in diameter or many clinically positive homolateral nodes, none >6 cm in diameter
N_{2a} Single clinically positive homolateral node >3 cm but not >6 cm in diameter
N_{2b} Multiple clinically positive homolateral nodes, none >6 cm in diameter
N_3 Massive homolateral node(s), bilateral nodes, or contralateral node(s)
N_{3a} Clinically positive homolateral node(s), one >6 cm in diameter
N_{3b} Bilateral clinically positive nodes (in this situation, each side of the neck should be staged separately; i.e., N_{3b}; right, N_{2a}; left, N_1)
N_{3c} Contralateral clinically positive node(s) only

Distant Metastasis (M)

M_x Minimum requirements to assess presence of distant metastasis cannot be met
M_0 No known metastasis
M_1 Distant metastasis present

DIAGNOSIS
Diagnosis of Laryngeal Cancer

Physicians and cancer societies have educated the public to seek evaluation for hoarseness persisting longer than 4 weeks. A small lesion of the vocal fold will cause voice changes by affecting the vocal wave or restricting the direct opposition between the two vocal cords. Patients with reflux laryngitis, heavy smokers, and alcohol consumers often have an edematous, irritated larynx and may not appreciate a voice change from usual chronic hoarseness. Every patient with hoarseness should be examined, and if indicated, the larynx is biopsied. The examination should be satisfactory; although mirror examination gives the best color and depth perception, it may be supplemented by evaluation with a telescope or flexible laryngoscope. A difficult patient, or one with an intense gag reflex, requires supplemental examination, as do patients whose local anatomy prohibits complete examination of the entire intrinsic larynx, epiglottis, false and true vocal cords, and anterior commissure. Both piriform sinuses should be clearly seen with all saliva and secretions swallowed so that the mucosa can be recognized. Vocal cord mobility is assessed and recorded, because it has major implications in staging and management. Photo or video documentation allowing observation of dynamic laryngeal function can be performed in the office with care not to affect the airway when using the flexible scope. When possible, the laryngeal examination can be videotaped during indirect examination with a 70-degree or 90-degree telescope or a nasal flexible scope in questionable cases. This video documentation serves as a clear record as the plan for management is formulated. In selected cases, a small biopsy can be taken through a large channel flexible laryngoscope, allowing cancer to be diagnosed without the need for general anesthesia and endoscopy. Although indirect laryngoscopy can be helpful, the operator should appreciate potential complications. Any suggestions of trouble should abort the attempt, and endoscopy should be reserved for controlled examination in the operating room with an anesthesiologist available and, if necessary, a nurse in the room ready to help perform an emergency tracheostomy.

Dysphagia is usually a symptom of supraglottic or hypopharyngeal lesions, but laryngeal lesions can occasionally present with no change in voice because they start insidiously, with only symptoms of dysphagia or hemoptysis. Often, these symptoms are managed medically before referral for endoscopy. Airway obstruction with no apparent voice change may represent the presenting signs of a large supraglottic or subglottic lesion. The latter can present as refractory asthma without voice change, and referral may be indicated by a flow volume loop showing upper airway obstruction patterns in a patient with known asthma.

It is helpful in a stable patient to image the neck and airway before biopsy and operative endoscopy to recognize the loss of cross-sectional airway and to predict the need for urgent or emergent tracheostomy. In these circumstances, care in endoscopy should be exercised, because a more complete obstruction can be created by manipulation in the operating room. A debulking biopsy with the patient carefully controlled may prevent the need for tracheostomy and allow relief of the airway. The carbon dioxide laser has been used for this purpose. When the patient recovers, the biopsy is interpreted, and careful consultation and education of the patient are possible before

proceeding to definitive management. Any cartilage removed at tracheostomy in a suspected cancer patient should undergo pathologic review.

Laryngeal cancer staging has been useful for studies of cancer management and as a dynamic and modified grade of lesion size and location (Box 99-2). It allows institutional series to be compared, allowing recognition of the differences among different management groups. The two series are matched for tumor size and location. TNM staging is useful for discussing individual tumors in a patient and is required by institutions managing cancer patients and maintaining a tumor registry (Joint Commission on Accreditation of Healthcare Organizations [JCAHO] requirement). The staging was originally clinical but has been amended to allow supplementation with

---

BOX 99-2

CLASSIFICATION OF THE PRIMARY TUMOR FOR LARYNX (UICC AND AJCC)

T_x Primary tumor cannot be assessed
T_0 No evidence of primary tumor
T_{is} Carcinoma in situ

Supraglottis

T_1 Tumor limited to one subsite of supraglottis or glottis with normal vocal cord mobility
T_2 Tumor invades more than one subsite of supraglottis with normal vocal cord mobility
T_3 Tumor limited to larynx with vocal cord fixation or invades postcricoid area, medial wall of piriform sinus, or preepiglottic tissues
T_4 Tumor invades through thyroid cartilage or extends to other tissues beyond the larynx (e.g., to oropharynx, soft tissues of neck)

Glottis

T_1 Tumor limited to vocal cord(s) (may involve anterior or posterior commissures) with normal mobility
T_2 Tumor extends to supraglottis or subglottis, or with impaired vocal cord mobility
T_3 Tumor limited to the larynx with vocal cord fixation
T_4 Tumor invades through thyroid cartilage or extends to other tissues beyond the larynx, (e.g., to oropharynx, soft tissues of neck)

Subglottis

T_1 Tumor limited to the subglottis
T_2 Tumor extends to vocal cord(s) with normal or impaired mobility
T_3 Tumor limited to the larynx with vocal cord fixation
T_4 Tumor invades through cricoid or thyroid cartilage or extends to other tissues beyond the larynx (e.g., to oropharynx, soft tissues of neck)

AJCC, American Joint Committee on Cancer; UICC, Union Internationale Contre le Cancer.

diagnostic radiography, including CT or MRI. Nodes >1 cm or nodes with central necrosis are considered N-positive on radiography. The correlation of the clinically noted categories of presumptive nodal abnormality with pathologic study has been 60% to 70% for a clinical examination (palpation) and varies between approximately 65% and 80% for imaging studies. MRI and CT seem equal in discriminating abnormal nodes. Neither imaging study (unless central necrosis is seen) nor physical examination recognizes nodes 1 cm, which may contain microscopic tumor and extracapsular spread. These clinically N_0 pathologically N-positive nodes represent a management dilemma for the physician.

Diagnosis of Hypopharyngeal Cancer

Hypopharyngeal malignancy is suspected in a patient with an appropriate history of heavy alcohol ingestion; heavy smoking; and persistent dysphagia, persistent sore throat, or a foreign body sensation in the throat. The average duration of symptoms before presentation is 2 to 4 months. A later symptom is pain referred to the ear by Arnold's nerve, a division of the tenth nerve. Referred otalgia suggests a malignancy in the region of the hypopharynx, base of tongue, or supraglottic larynx.

Of patients, 20% have an asymptomatic mass in the neck, usually ipsilateral, a jugulodigastric or midjugular lymph node. Associated symptoms include weight loss and, in most advanced stage disease, hemoptysis and hoarseness when the vocal cord becomes fixed by direct extension into the arytenoid cartilage or muscles.

Indirect laryngoscopy examination includes observation of vocal cord function. An ipsilateral fixed cord suggests a more advanced hypopharyngeal lesion. There may be pooling of secretions on one side of the piriform sinus obstructing adequate visualization of an area. There may be asymmetry of the laryngeal structure and edema in the region of the arytenoid. Lesions in the superior portion of the posterior hypopharynx show ulceration. The edges may be raised, or an ulceration may be identified. Flexible fiberoptic laryngoscopy may be necessary for assessment when mirror examination is not adequate.

Radiologic Assessment of the Larynx and Hypopharynx

Preoperative assessment of advanced malignancies is further clarified with CT. It may show extension of tumor beyond what is detected clinically by endoscopy and will show preepiglottic space and paraglottic space involvement and cartilage erosion.

CT and MRI show the substitution of high-density tumor for fat in the preepiglottic space. MRI using T2-weighted images may be superior to highlight submucosal tumor extension into the preepiglottic and paraglottic spaces.[88] Thyroid cartilage destruction is best assessed by CT.[267] This is reliable when clear destruction has occurred. This finding, when definite, mandates a total laryngectomy (T_4 stage). Munoz and others[179] found only a 46% positive predictive value of CT for detecting cartilage invasion. Nakayama and Brandenburg[185] found that in tumors clinically and radiographically staged as T_3, 50% had microinvasion of the thyroid cartilage, usually at the thyroid notch.

When a malignancy of the hypopharynx is suspected, CT or MRI is preferred before direct laryngoscopy with biopsy. Thus, CT findings of edema are more likely to represent submucosal infiltration than be attributed to edema associated with the biopsy. In addition, CT may draw attention to additional areas that may need to be assessed and require biopsy at the time of endoscopy. CT may show more extensive disease than is appreciated by indirect or direct endoscopy (Figure 99-7).

Chest radiography is performed to evaluate the possibility of metastatic disease and a second primary malignancy in the lung. Bronchoscopy is not routinely indicated when chest radiography is completely normal. Whole-lung CT is required if chest radiography suggests any abnormality.[161]

Endoscopic Evaluation of the Larynx and Hypopharynx

Office endoscopic assessment of the larynx is more useful than evaluation for the extent of disease in the hypopharynx. Most patients, however, even after thorough office examination, including video photography to evaluate vocal cord function (Figure 99-8) and a schematic drawing, require general anesthesia for endoscopic assessment of the extent of disease and biopsy. It is preferable to concentrate on the laryngeal extent of the lesion after assessment of the hypopharynx (including both piriform sinuses and the postcricoid area) using a full esophagoscopy if indicated. The larynx is brought into complete view, and a photograph or drawing is made of the extent of the lesion (Figure 99-9). Cord mobility is best assessed preoperatively. In the operating room, fixation of the cord is differentiated from arytenoid fixation by palpation of the vocal process and can help stage the disease. The laryngeal probe permits assessment of the extension into the ventricle. Telescopes can be passed through the laryngoscope to assess the subglottic extent and better visualize the anterior commissure. The operating microscope also allows better visualization of the larynx. It is important to obtain biopsy specimens from the obvious tumor and any additional suspicious areas, particularly on the contralateral cord. This is

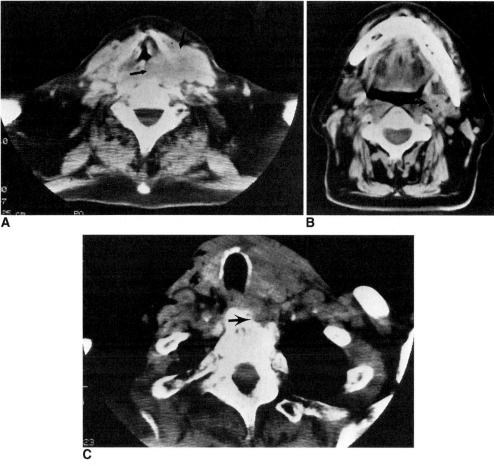

Figure 99-7. Computed tomography shows extension into the soft tissues and bilateral nodal disease. **A,** The tumor is clinically evident only on the left. **B,** There is circumferential tumor involvement of the carotid artery. **C,** Invasion of the prevertebral fascia.

especially needed if a conservation laryngeal procedure is planned.

Endoscopic assessment of the hypopharynx permits biopsy of the tumor and determination of extent. Rigid endoscopic assessment was shown by Fenton and others[68] to be superior to flexible esophagogastrostomy, because flexible endoscopy missed 10 of 12 tumors. Likewise, barium swallow is not as effective in the detection of early hypopharyngeal malignancy as it is in esophageal malignancies. It is particularly important to determine whether the cord is mobile or fixed, whether tumor is on the medial or lateral aspect of the piriform sinus (number of walls involved), whether there is extension into the apex of the piriform sinus or into the esophageal inlet, or whether the tumor extends across the midline when it involves the posterior pharyngeal wall. Endoscopy is also required to rule out the existence of a second or concurrent malignancy and is thus performed to determine the inferior extent of the tumor and to ensure that no skip lesions exist. To be considered resectable, a tumor of

the posterior hypopharyngeal wall cannot invade the prevertebral fascia. Clinically, this is determined by palpation. The tumor should be mobile (back and forth) when slid against the cervical vertebrae.

Topical cocainization of the cords before biopsy limits bleeding and may prevent postoperative laryngeal spasm.

Assessment of Precancerous Laryngeal Lesions

Biopsy is always needed to confirm the diagnosis, because the gross appearance of fungal laryngitis, sarcoidosis, tuberculosis, or Wegener's granulomatosis can be mistaken for advanced carcinoma. Biopsy should be deep and reach necrotic tumor and viable tumor and stroma or muscle to prove the presence of an invasive squamous cell carcinoma.

Squamous cell carcinoma accounts for >95% of primary laryngeal cancers. Biopsy sampling should be simultaneously prudent and aggressive. Small suspicious lesions should be completely excised with a border of healthy laryngeal submucosa so the depth of

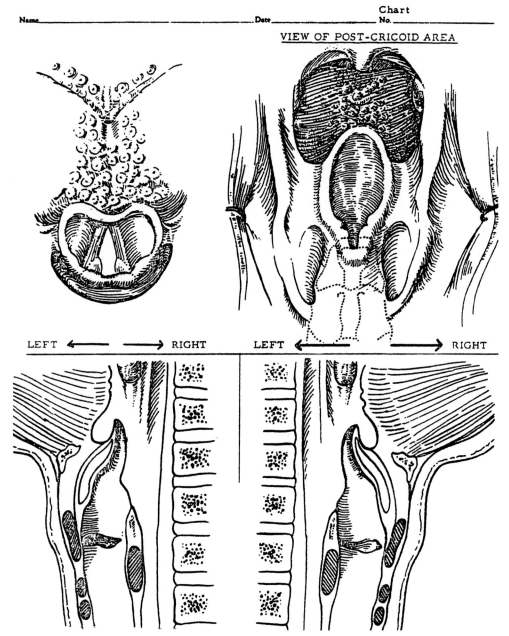

Figure 99-8. Indirect laryngoscopy or fibroscopy findings are mapped and compared with Figure 99-9.

invasion can be measured. Similarly, large lesions should be adequately sampled with the laryngeal biopsy forceps to measure invasion below the basement membrane. Histologic aggressiveness suggested by a lesion that is poorly differentiated has not usually been predictive of biologic behavior; better predictions are deep and extensive invasion by T staging, microvascular invasion, and extracapsular spread in the nodes. In general, endolaryngeal lesions are well to moderately differentiated. Hypopharyngeal lesions are more likely poorly differentiated.

Patients with glottic tumors are seen early because of hoarseness. Clear diagnosis of invasion is difficult with a small biopsy sample of an early lesion. Repeat endoscopy is necessary if an adequate specimen is not obtained. Unless the endoscopist is experienced and confident, a frozen section to confirm invasive squamous cell carcinoma in lesions with generous biopsy material may be useful. When the gross lesion can be safely removed without anticipating undue complications (e.g., notching of the vocal cord), complete excision should be performed to create a satisfactory

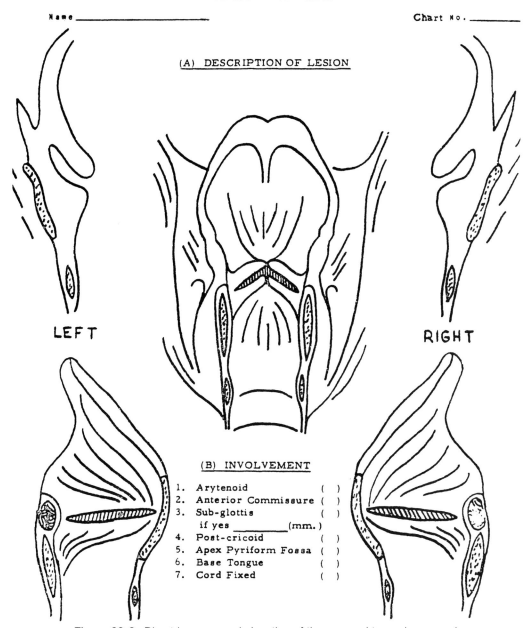

Figure 99-9. Direct laryngoscopic location of the mucosal tumor is mapped.

specimen. Pseudoepitheliomatous hyperplasia (granular cell myoblastoma) of the supraglottic larynx may be misdiagnosed as carcinoma and is a clear example of a situation requiring an adequate biopsy sample. Failure to act in this manner will result in undue management of a benign disease.

MANAGEMENT OF PREMALIGNANT LESIONS AND CARCINOMA IN SITU

Pathologists are usually as comfortable categorizing laryngeal biopsy specimens as uterine cervix biopsy specimens. Although the written report may not be perfectly clear, sitting with the pathologists who reviewed the studies is encouraged. The five categories of laryngeal squamous abnormality run from benign to clearly malignant. They begin with hyperkeratosis, hyperkeratosis with atypia, carcinoma in situ (CIS), superficially invasive carcinoma, and invasive carcinoma (Figure 99-10).

When lesions clearly show hyperkeratosis with atypia and often CIS, management can be conservative if a satisfactory strip of cord is removed. The gross lesion should be microscopically removed. Follow-up and rebiopsy 6 to 12 weeks later is necessary. To apply

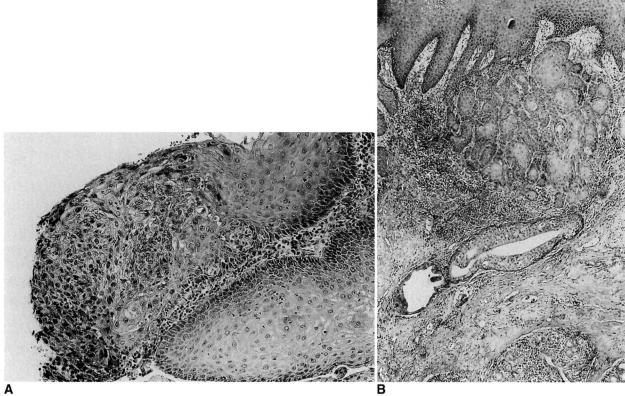

Figure 99-10. A, Carcinoma in situ. **B,** Microinvasive carcinoma. In the early phase of invasion, irregular nests of well-differentiated squamous cells infiltrate the lamina propria and evoke an inflammatory response. A gland with squamous metaplasia is present near deeper carcinomatous cells. (From Ferlito A and others: *Ann Otolaryngol* 105:245, 1996.)

this diagnosis, there should be no carcinoma deep to the basement membrane. Differentiation between severe hyperkeratosis with atypia and CIS is often difficult. Hyperkeratosis with atypia requires review by several pathologists, and the biopsy may show mitoses, poor maturation, cells retaining nuclear material as they rise toward the surface in the epithelial layer, and excess keratin. These lesions frequently are described histologically to reflect poikilocytosis, dyskeratosis, and acanthosis. Although replacement of the epithelium with malignant cells, which do not penetrate the basement membrane, defines CIS, debate among pathologists about these diagnoses is less important to the clinician, because both are harbingers of invasive cancer and are associated (5%–30%) with future invasive cancer (Figure 99-11).

Occasionally, the biopsy represents a poor sample with invasive cancer evident in adjacent mucosa. Laryngeal mucosa may be abnormal at some distance from the area of gross disease and may be positive on biopsy for invasive carcinoma below an intact mucosa without ulcer. The opposite true vocal cord can show hyperkeratosis with atypia and even CIS, as will the epiglottis and false vocal cord if biopsied or reviewed

from sections of laryngectomy. This reflects the at-risk nature of the region to presumed toxic exposure and confirms Slaughter's hypothesis of field cancerization described originally for the oral cavity.[248]

Superficial invasive carcinoma shows foci of invasion deep to the basement membrane. Again, sampling error and pathologist bias can make superficial invasive cancer and CIS difficult to distinguish. These lesions are usually recognized on the central third of the true vocal cord, which is the only site where early symptoms of voice change with a small flat lesion are likely. In other sites, the early lesion will be asymptomatic, may not merit mirror examination, and may progress to invasive cancer with symptoms appropriate to invasion and increased bulk.

Rothfield and others[227] showed only 2 of 20 patients with carcinoma in situ had subsequent invasive carcinoma after microlaryngoscopy and stripping with or without laser ablation (using one to five endoscopies to clear the lesion). Myssiorek and others[184] also noted 83% success in endoscopic management of this intraepithelial malignancy, except for lesions at the anterior commissure. Small and others[249] noted good success with radiotherapy in 19 of 20 patients without

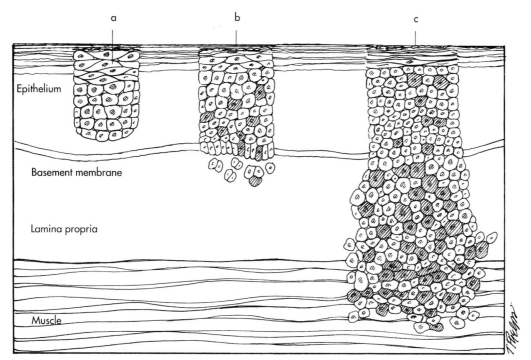

Figure 99-11. Depth of abnormal mucosa in microinvasive and invasive carcinoma in situ.

extension to invasive carcinoma. Nguyen and others[188] had similar success with radiotherapy and surgery and noted that 50% of those managed endoscopically required restripping. Blackwell and others[29] concluded that there is a high rate of progression from intraepithelial dysplasia to invasive carcinoma. This report suggested endoscopy can have similar outcomes to those after partial laryngectomy and after radiotherapy administered before invasive disease develops. Stenerson and others[260] reported a 46% risk of progression of superficial invasive cancer and CIS to invasive carcinoma.

Management of precancerous lesions is conservative surgery. At present, the recommendation for surgery is based on the concern that radiotherapy may fail (10%), eliminating the future option to manage a T_1 or T_2 invasive cancer. Surgery requires obtaining a satisfactory strip of vocal cord mucosa, which includes the entire gross lesion. The patient is informed of the need to rebiopsy for recurrence, and follow-up is planned for many years. Supravital staining with toluidine blue has been used intraoperatively to identify clinically inapparent lesions, which can be excised or lasered. Rapid or frequent recurrence with the same histology (not true for hyperkeratosis without atypia) or progression to histologically proven invasive carcinoma requires cordectomy, hemilaryngectomy, or full-course narrow-field radiation. Many surgeons believe that unless the patient is unreliable, is a significant risk for repeat general anesthesia, or

lives far away, radiation is a second choice for this disease. Recurrence is frequent and can produce invasive carcinoma. A behavioral or medicated smoking cessation program should be part of management.

MANAGEMENT OF LARYNGEAL CANCER
Glottic Cancer

Invasive glottic carcinoma is generally less biologically aggressive than supraglottic or hypopharyngeal squamous cell carcinoma. The histology is usually well to moderately differentiated, and early disease $(T_1–T_2)$ remains localized to the glottic compartment longer without neck or distant metastases. This is presumably because of the sparse submucosal lymphatics in the vocal cord and may reflect a biologic behavior of the well-differentiated carcinoma.

Symptoms present early, because most tumors originate on the free surface of the true vocal fold in its anterior two-thirds where hoarseness invites medical evaluation. Early-stage disease has been successfully managed with radiotherapy or conservation surgery without the need for elective neck management.[183] In general, surgery offers 90% to 95% cure rates for T_1 lesions at select institutions using carefully planned radiotherapy, whereas most community hospitals report cure rates of 75% to 90%. Surgical salvage, often by total laryngectomy, offers equal long-term cure but with different morbidities and financial costs.

Several small series have noted excellent results after surgery. Johnson and others[116] reported a 98%

local control rate by surgery for T_1 tumors, and 24 of 31 T_2 tumors were cured by initial partial surgery with 4 more salvaged by total laryngectomy to result in a 94% cure rate. Thomas and others,[271] reviewing 159 cases, noted a 93% local control rate for T_1 lesions (8 of 11 recurrences eventually had distal disease) and a 3-year survival of 91%.

Important tumor anatomy, which influences the choice of management, includes in decreasing importance vocal cord mobility, subglottic extension, anterior commissure invasion, and arytenoid cartilage involvement. These have been well addressed by partial surgery and, when radiation series are analyzed, represent the sites of most frequent failure. Vocal mobility is impaired because of thyroarytenoid muscle invasion or cricothyroid joint invasion, which can lead to paraglottic space involvement.

The middle third of vocal fold lesions are easiest to cure and respond well to radiotherapy, endoscopic, laser resection, or open cordectomy. Cure rates approach 100% for such lesions excised with good margins and can represent a 95% cure rate for radiotherapy. Radiation failures may be caused by unrecognized deep invasion. If the mucosal lesion is excised by endoscopy, observation is acceptable with radiotherapy used for return of disease. Although radiation alone offers excellent cures, management for a second tumor cannot be offered, and the new tumor may not be amenable to conservation surgery. The patient should be informed of this, particularly patients with increased risk factors for second primary tumors.

The anterior commissure is always of concern regarding radiotherapy. Earlier reports suggested a poor cure rate, but Dickens and others[61] reported radiotherapy for T_1 lesions offered a single modality cure of 92%. Rothfield and others[227] noted that 50% of radiotherapy failures for T_1 glottic cancer failed at the anterior commissure. Of 14 patients managed by hemilaryngectomy, 13 were ultimately cured after radiotherapy failure, whereas 77 radiotherapy failure patients required a total laryngectomy after initially being seen with stage I glottic cancer.

These reports suggest the hemilaryngectomy tenets of Biller and others[26] (Box 99-3) often allow surgical salvage of radiotherapy failures for T_1 and T_2 laryngeal cancer. The cure rate is less than that for primary radiotherapy or for primary surgery and may reflect the aggressive biologic transformation or selection of recurrent tumor and the difficult task of measuring margins after radiotherapy.

Endoscopic surgery for early vocal fold tumor is most often accomplished through the linkage of the operating microscope and the carbon dioxide laser. In 1978, Ossoff and others[204] described 17 successful laser excisions. Others described continued excellent,

---

BOX 99-3

CRITERIA FOR HEMILARYNGECTOMY FOR RECURRENT CANCER AFTER RADIOTHERAPY

Lesion limited to one cord (may involve the anterior commissure)
Body of arytenoid free of tumor
Subglottic extension no >5 mm
Mobile cord
No cartilage invasion
Recurrence correlating with initial tumor

From Biller HF and others: *Laryngoscope* 80:249, 1970.

---

economic management and cure (Table 99-1) with prudent and appropriate care selection.[242] Voice preservation was excellent.[49] Laser cordotomy or cordectomy has been used to offer oncologic relief in T_1 and even selected T_2 lesions.[221]

A specimen to prove negative surgical margins should be obtained and oriented for the pathologist. Understood techniques should include the correct spot size of the laser beam, wattage, premedication, and preparation of the airway.

Hypomobility of the vocal fold reduces the cure rates and emphasizes the advantage of surgery over radiotherapy. This is often related to tumor bulk. Dickens and others[61] noted 4% of tumors <15 mm recurred after radiotherapy, whereas more sizable, similarly staged lesions recurred 26% of the time, even when only one vocal cord was involved.[67] T_2 tumors managed by primary radiotherapy showed a 30% local failure rate, which, when surgically salvaged, improved to 94%.[112] Harwood and De Boer[103] noted that impaired cord mobility resulted in lower control rates in T_2 lesions, and they suggested the classification be divided into T_{2a} and T_{2b} on the basis of mobility. In this analysis, a 70% local control rate was noted for the former category vs 51% in the latter. In 1996, McLaughlin and others[171] noted an 11% recurrence rate for T_{2a} with a 26% recurrent rate for T_{2b}. Surgery

---

TABLE 99-1

LASER MANAGEMENT OF T_1 GLOTTIC CARCINOMA

	DISEASE-FREE PATIENTS (%)	
Primary Therapy	Local Control Rate	Overall Control Rate After Further Excision, Surgery, or Radiotherapy
Laser Therapy	87.3	98.6
Radiotherapy	85.7	94.9

Data from Cragle SP, Brandenburg JH: *Otolaryngol Head Neck Surg* 108:648, 1993.

salvaged six of nine T_{2b} radiation failures. Ogura and others[197] reported an 82% tumor-free survival of 3 years for hemilaryngectomy as a single modality. Of 18 T_3 vocal cord tumors managed by Lesinski and others,[149] 15 obtained local control despite the fact that 8 reportedly had positive margins; and 14 had immobility caused by bulky tumor invading the arytenoid and approaching the medial perichondrial border, but they did not have cricoarytenoid joint invasion.

Positive margins on a hemilaryngectomy specimen were shown to increase the risk of local recurrence by threefold according to Bauer and others[20] and sevenfold according to Wenig and Berry.[302] Despite this increased local recurrence, the 2-year and 3-year cure rate was equal between patients with positive and those with negative surgical margins. There still is debate about whether the positive margins suggested by Bauer and others[20] were close margins, because a second sample from the patient, after the specimen was removed, was not submitted. A positive margin is clearly less dangerous for the pushing slow-growing glottic tumor than for hypopharyngeal or tongue tumors.[320]

Biller and Lawson[27] achieved a 73% 2-year local control by extended partial surgery for such cases. When there is arytenoid invasion, the cricoid arch can be sacrificed, but subsequent swallowing is impaired if >10 mm of the subglottis anteriorly or 4 mm posteriorly is resected. Subsequent dysphagia is preventable with a thyroid cartilage or hyoid bone transplant to replace the missing cricoid. T_2 and early T_3 lesions of the glottis have more recently been managed by supracricoid laryngectomy with cricohyoidoepiglottopexy. This operation was championed in Europe in the late 1970s. Reports of this surgery performed in the United States began to enter the American literature in the early 1990s. The operation requires resection of the entire thyroid cartilage and paraglottic space. The cricoid cartilage, the hyoid bone, much of the epiglottis and at least one arytenoid cartilage must be conserved. A series of 36 patients were reported to have satisfactory deglutition, phonation, and 100% decannulation with a 5% local recurrence rate. Sixty-one percent of the patients had been pretreated with chemotherapy.[139] A current series of 17 patients noted 53% obtained a normal diet and 6 additional patients had moderate oral dietary restriction. Voice quality was limited in range and intensity but was not equal to that after supraglottic laryngectomy.[36] A total laryngectomy with primary tracheoesophageal puncture is another reasonable choice for T_3 glottic cancer. T_3 glottic cancer has a statistically similar survival rate with different treatment protocols. The overall disease-free survival is 67% at 5 years.

The cause of death from cancer included 37 of 200 deaths (18%) because of uncontrollable local or neck disease with 26 (13%) because of metastatic disease and 9% because of a second cancer.[237] The cure rate after total laryngectomy is excellent, and the regional and distant metastasis risk is small.[121]

Local cure by radiotherapy for glottic tumors, which almost always matches tumor-free survival, has not changed since 1974, when Fletcher and Jesse[73] noted 85% control rate, until 1996 when McLaughlin and others[171] noted 89%. Surgical management of radiation failures resulted in a 60% salvage rate, with a 70% salvage rate reported by Biller and Lawson[27] and a 95% salvage rate reported by Rothfield and others.[159,226] The latter result is achieved when partial surgery can be performed despite radiation failure.

No clear advantage of surgery vs radiotherapy is noted in the literature for early glottic tumor, and local mores and abilities should prevail. Surgery is more successful for lesions with subglottic extension and impaired vocal mobility. Postradiation edema for longer than 6 months has a 45% association with deeply invasive recurrence and requires follow-up by endoscopy and imaging.[82,290]

Subglottic Cancer

Subglottic cancer is unusual, with only 1% of 2180 larynx cancers located 1 cm below the vocal cord according to Shaha and Shah.[240] The clinical presentation is usually by airway obstruction; many cases are regarded as symptomatic lower airway problems without response to management for chronic obstructive lung disease.

Patients may have airway insufficiency and obtain immediate relief when intubated. True subglottic lesions arise below the conus elasticus (1 cm below the free edge of the true vocal cord) and spread locally to invade the cricoid cartilage and thyroid gland with lymphatic spread to lower deep jugular nodes, the Delphian node (prelaryngeal), and the paratracheal nodes (Figure 99-12).[99] Welsh[299,300] reported that 96% of the colloidal gold injected into subglottic tissue was initially noted in the paratracheal nodes.

Management requires total laryngectomy, because laryngeal framework invasion is frequent. Ipsilateral thyroidectomy and paratracheal node dissection is necessary. For cases showing positive nodes or deep invasion, postoperative radiotherapy to include the superior mediastinum is needed to prevent stomal recurrence.

Extensive glottic carcinoma of stage T_4 or T_3 requires total laryngectomy in most cases and attention to the ipsilateral nodes, because a 20% risk of lateral metastasis occurs. Tumors larger than 1.5 cm, subglottic extension, and lymph node metastasis

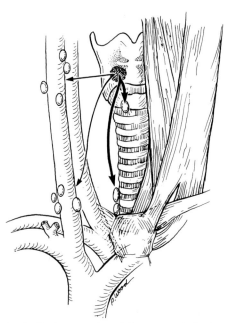

Figure 99-12. Pathways of nodal metastasis from subglottic tumors. Spread occurs along submucosal lymphatics to paratracheal nodes and along lower and midjugular chains.

laterally or to paratracheal or anterior pretracheal nodes predict failure above the clavicle.[75,201]

Kirchner and Som[129] noted that 31 of 52 total laryngectomy specimens of transglottic cancer had cartilage invasion and usually had clinical true vocal cord palsy. The cartilage invaded was usually ossified.

Local control rates approach only 40% for radiotherapy alone; although attempts to avoid total laryngectomy are worthwhile, significant local destruction and persistent edema frequently create a preserved but severely compromised organ with restricted airway and poor voice. Total laryngectomy and appropriate neck dissection with primary tracheoesophageal puncture and postoperative radiotherapy is the preferred management for T_4 laryngeal cancer. T_3 tumors are more amenable to laryngectomy alone, because experience with radiotherapy for the immobile true vocal cord has been poor. The literature reflects this high risk of recurrence (almost 40% after radiotherapy).[132]

Late-Stage Disease

The general neglect that precipitates late presentation is often characterized by other social and medical diseases, including chronic alcoholism with liver and heart disease and severe chronic obstructive pulmonary disease. The tumor creates dysphagia, and significant weight loss should be evaluated and reversed.[123] Gastrostomy to manage caloric and protein intake should be part of the management planning and can be achieved during anesthesia for biopsy

and tumor mapping. A premanagement barium swallow is often helpful, and CT may show extensive neck disease, suggesting the need to occlude the carotid artery electively before neck surgery. More usually for hypopharyngeal than laryngeal tumors, deep posterior invasion may make surgery with clear margins impossible.

Obstructive laryngeal lesions have been managed with premanagement tracheostomy, which has been reported with increased local or stomal recurrence. Often, at endoscopy, significant debulking with laser or directly with surgical forceps can temporarily relieve the airway to allow a full workup and discussion before definitive management. If a tracheostomy is necessary, the literature continues to suggest surgery within 48 hours and removal of the tracheostomy site and bilateral paratracheal node dissection with postoperative mantle radiotherapy. This management seems to reduce local stomal recurrence after glottic cancer to <3%. A high tracheostomy is indicated, so subsequent resection allows preservation of as much tracheal anatomy as oncologically appropriate.

Postoperative radiation is recommended for cartilage destruction, subglottic extension, thyroid gland involvement, or positive paratracheal nodes.

Recurrence at the stoma after laryngectomy is grave. Such diffuse infiltration where amputated trachea and the skin of the neck meet is insidious and rarely discovered before deep, extensive penetration has occurred. The pattern of recurrence has been explained as caused by paratracheal node involvement, thyroid gland infiltration, or an implanted tumor on a fresh stoma, such as that seen with a preoperative tracheostomy. Several authors believe that emergency laryngectomy is needed if a tracheostomy is necessary before surgical resection is initiated.[94] Other authors disagree with this thesis, but large series have shown subglottic cancer is most associated with stomal recurrence because the Delphian and paratracheal drainage ports are presumed to be the pathway to recurrence.[298]

Because even aggressive management of stomal recurrence is morbid and often unsuccessful, prevention of recurrence is paramount. When the risk of infiltration is high, the thyroid gland, at least ipsilateral, is removed and bilateral paratracheal node dissections are accomplished and postsurgical radiation used. The radiation is directed to a lower than usual port that includes the upper mediastinum and paratracheal beds. Of 15 stomal recurrence cases in a large series of laryngectomies by Rubin and others,[230] 12 were subglottic in the primary site. The risk of recurrence was 24% among those without a tracheostomy before management and 30% when tracheostomy was needed. A surgeon presented with a newly diagnosed carcinoma obstructing the glottic or subglottic airway should await final pathologic examination confirming squamous cell carcinoma before embarking on laryngectomy. Although rare, frozen section can be incorrect in its interpretation, and the patient should be left intubated or have tracheostomy at the time of biopsy with plans to complete the microscopic evaluation of the biopsy sample within 48 hours, and laryngectomy should be accomplished if the patient is agreeable.

Sisson[247] pioneered mediastinal dissection and wide local resection for stomal recurrence and proposed four categories of this disease. Better precision and upstaging of the lesion has occurred with advanced soft-tissue imaging with CT and MRI. The Sisson system of staging suggests that stage I and stage II stomal recurrence have, in selected cases, produced a 45% 2-year survival. The significant morbidity and mortality caused by exposure of the great vessels in the chest, severe hypocalcemia, and enteral fistula all result in prolonged hospitalization, risk vascular blowout, and mediastinitis.[298] This high-risk surgery in patients who have already undergone surgery and radiation and are usually in negative nutritional balance has made aggressive management of stage III and stage IV stomal recurrence less certain.[90] Sisson[247] concluded that mediastinal failure was an important factor in survival for advanced head and neck cancer and should be considered for prophylaxis in T_4N_{1-3} glottic and subglottic tumors in which mediastinoscopy was positive for nodes. For some surgeons, a planned mediastinal dissection can be considered for cervical esophageal and high tracheal cancers in view of the good success with rotation and free flap replacement of the dissected and resected soft tissue (Figure 99-13).

Hemithyroidectomy or subtotal thyroidectomy is recommended for cases of palpable abnormality, subglottic tumors, or glottic tumors with >1 cm of subglottic extension, T_4 glottic tumors, and T_4 piriform sinus tumors.[25] Of these thyroid specimens, 3% to 8% will have cancer. The endocrine gland invasion is predicted with positive Delphian nodes or cartilage destruction.

Thyroid function is reduced after larynx cancer management that includes radiotherapy or extensive laryngeal and thyroid surgery. The patient who seems depressed and lethargic months after management may be hypothyroid; this can manifest late.[34,265] Follow-up laboratory studies are suggested at 6 months, 1 year, and when clinically indicated thereafter. The risk of hypothyroidism is 20% after radiotherapy, 50% after laryngectomy and ipsilateral thyroid lobectomy, and >65% if both radiation and surgery are used (Table 99-2).[152]

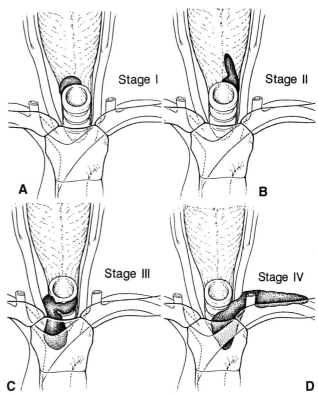

Figure 99-13. Stomal recurrence. **A,** Stage I. **B,** Stage II. **C,** Stage III. **D,** Stage IV. (From Sisson: *Laryngoscope* 99:1264, 1989.)

Supraglottic Cancer

Management of the supraglottic lesion is reasonably clear but should always consider the neck disease. Early supraglottic (epiglottic) tumors, which are suprahyoid, can be grossly excised endoscopically. This can be accomplished by electrocautery or by carbon dioxide laser. The safety of this technique is best for suprahyoid lesions, because no invasion of the preepiglottic space is likely. This space, bound inferiorly by the attachment of the petiole to the thyroid cartilage and posteriorly by the elastic cartilage of the epiglottis and anteriorly by the thyroid cartilage and thyrohyoid membrane, is the first conduit for infrahyoid tumors to extend beyond the cartilaginous confines of the supraglottis. This migration of cancer occurs through the foramina of the elastic epiglottic cartilage. European studies have noted excellent results with endoscopic laser treatment of selected supraglottic carcinoma, but infrahyoid tumors do not fare so well with only laser resection.[5,64] The procedure of endoscopic laser partial laryngectomy requires a bivalved laryngoscope designed for the task and in contrast to the usual cancer surgery tenets is accomplished by sagittal splitting and resection of the suprahyoid epiglottis followed by a split of the infrahyoid supraglottis with evaluation of the extent of

TABLE 99-2

INCIDENCE OF HYPOTHYROIDISM AFTER MANAGEMENT FOR CARCINOMA OF THE LARYNX

Study	Radiotherapy	Laryngectomy and Thyroid Surgery	Larynx and Neck Surgery
Vrabec[206a]	14%	66%	21%
Tami and others[265]	29%	69%	0%
Liening and others[152]	6%	65%	28%
Biel and Maisel[25]	38%	70%	20%

invasion of the tumor at this point. The specimen is removed and subjected to frozen section control. The preepiglottic space is included in the specimen and is often (50%) infiltrated either grossly or microscopically. The resection may require removal of all tissue to the inner perichondrium of the thyroid cartilage and thyrohyoid membrane. False cords are also resected when indicated. Authors report a return to the operating room to evaluate and rebiopsy a presumed positive resection margin may be necessary (12.5%) in the 4 weeks after surgery. For full evaluation and success of the technique, it must be noted that frequent postoperative x-ray therapy is used for indications at the primary site vs a rare need for this accompanying N_0 supraglottic laryngectomy. The neck can be addressed at a subsequent occasion, because the soft tissues are not violated in entering the larynx. This separation of treatment to the neck from the larynx seems to offer better swallowing results and usually eliminates the need for a temporary tracheostomy. Good local control of 89% has been reported when radiation is included in the treatment. Functional results include resumption of an oral diet in 1 to 2 weeks in most patients and is explained by lack of interruption of the tongue base and function of the arytenoids, which are considered important measures of laryngeal protection and recovery of swallowing after supraglottic laryngectomy.[154] Complications of the procedure include failure to eradicate the cancer and early postoperative bleeding, which can be fatal in an unprotected airway.

Reporting in 1994, Zeitels and others[315] used postoperative x-ray therapy in 55% of their 42 cases and considered this treatment as neoadjuvant therapy with histopathologic controlled results. The American experience with laser supraglottic laryngectomy has been increasing,[182,315,317] and this technique requires more evaluation and larger series to determine whether the early advantage of rapid return to an oral diet, absence of a tracheostomy tube, and the opportunity for separate attention to neck disease and the opportunity for postoperative small port x-ray therapy represents better rehabilitation, equal cure rates, and

better economy compared with supraglottic laryngectomy and neck dissection as described later.

Marks and others[162] suggested that more central supraglottic lesions have less metastatic potential than aryepiglottic fold or lateral epiglottic sites. The preepiglottic space may contain the tumor, although epiglottic and anterior false cord tumors can spread across the midline in a horseshoe pattern.[158] The preepiglottic space has been invaded in up to 50% of cases of infrahyoid carcinoma, which cannot be predicted even if CT and physical examination are used.[168] The direct relationship between this invasion and lateral neck metastases is unclear but has been reported to be up to 50% even for early tumors.[317] In 1974, the Centennial Conference on Laryngeal Cancer concluded that preepiglottic space invasion worsened prognosis,[198] and this has been confirmed many times since.[316]

Metastases to either side of the neck can occur, because the preepiglottic space feeds lymphatics to both sides.

Local extension beyond the supraglottis is protected above by the hyoepiglottic ligament, which roofs the preepiglottic space (Figure 99-14). Yeager and Archer[312] suggest that the penetration between the laryngeal compartments occurs where the connective tissue attaches to cartilage. The cancer cells are presumed to separate collagen bundles and form a pathway through the perichondrium at the sites of strongest membrane attachment. Extralaryngeal spread at the anterior commissure and at the cricothyroid membrane fits this theory.

Mucosal extension seems to be resisted at the ventricle of the larynx, but occasionally deep extension through the submucosa of the ventricle to penetrates the paraglottic space occurs without mucosal disease. This can be recognized by imaging, which is best done before manipulation of the laryngeal tumor. Several authors, on the basis of their experience with invasion of the paraglottic space, warn that vocal cord paralysis without mucosal disease may herald this invasion. Evidence of such paraglottic invasion mitigates against partial laryngeal surgery and also suggests against radiotherapy alone.

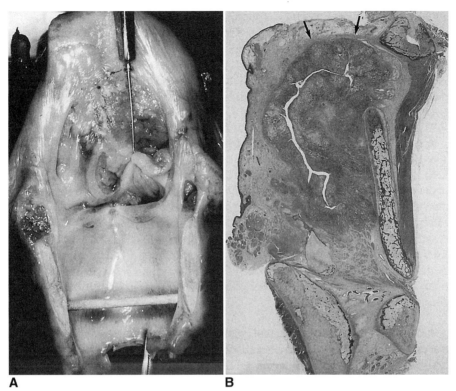

A   **B**

Figure 99-14. A, A gross laryngectomy specimen with deeply invading false vocal cord cancer. **B,** Sagittal section shows cancer filling the paraglottic space without penetrating the hyoepiglottic ligament *(arrows)*. (From Zeitels SM, Kirchner JA: *Ann Otol Rhinol Laryngol* 104:770, 1995.)

Limited supraglottic tumors, which are defined as T_1 to T_3 (because preepiglottic space invasion does not change surgical resection but upstages the lesion), are often managed with supraglottic laryngectomy if the vocal cord is mobile. Alonso[4] used a two-stage procedure, which was modified to a one-stage procedure by Ogura.[191] Som[253] suggested that suturing of the base of the tongue muscle to the perichondrium of the thyroid cartilage is sufficient for primary closure without a fistula. Som[253] insisted that the entire oncologic boundary of the preepiglottic space should be included in resections (Figure 99-15).

Arytenoid involvement allowed partial surgery,[193] as did lateral extension to the medial piriform sinus.[196] However, complications with swallowing are magnified, and the likelihood of single modality therapy is reduced. Extended resections that allow preservation of voice and airway can include removal of the vallecula and base of the tongue up to the level of the circumvallate papilla. Despite reconstruction, this impedes swallowing and, when combined with radiotherapy, reduces the success of rehabilitation.[30,196] Tongue base involvement, no further anterior than the circumvallate papilla, represents the limit of anterior resection and often requires flap reconstruction to rebulk the missing tongue muscle while preserving swallowing.

Patient selection for supraglottic laryngectomy is important. Younger, more vigorous patients with strong motivation and good pulmonary reserve to prevent recurrent pneumonia and regain satisfactory oral diet fare best. Patients should be able to tolerate the mild-to-moderate aspiration that occurs in the early postoperative period and will occur, to some degree, for the rest of the patient's life. Patients with chronic pulmonary disease and reduced pulmonary ciliary clearance are at greater risk for pneumonia, which can complicate postoperative recovery and contribute to long-term mortality from the operation. Even with gastrostomy to circumvent the risk of oral intake aspiration, the remaining salivary aspiration may be overwhelming. Pulmonary insufficiency may even make conversion to a laryngectomy unsatisfactory. Although Beckhard and others[23] studied 46 patients and found a forced expiratory volume (FEV) of 1 and a forced expiratory capacity (FEC) of <50% predictive of aspiration, most surgeons believe these pulmonary tests are too imprecise. A careful history reviewing the patient's overall functions of daily life and motivation for rehabilitation and simple clinical tests such as walking up a flight of stairs are more predictive.

Patients who failed full-course radiation for supraglottic lesions are at increased risk because of unrec-

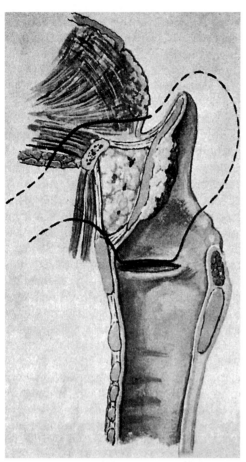

Figure 99-15. A line of extirpation of supraglottic structures as a unit in continuity with the entire preepiglottic space. (From Som ML, Max L: *J Laryngol Otol* 84:657, 1970.)

ognized submucosal tumor spread. Occasionally, when the original tumor configuration is completely understood and the workup for recurrent lesion is especially diligent, including careful and well performed imaging, partial laryngeal surgery is possible. Morbidity secondary to wound healing and persistent edema and pharyngeal dysfunction from radiation fibrosis are much higher than in primary supraglottic laryngectomy.[190,256]

Limitations to supraglottic laryngectomy include thyroid cartilage invasion or anterior commissure involvement, which both imply tumor has broken the anterior inner perichondrial sheath, and a barrier to tumor spread has been broached. Standard cartilage cuts for partial surgery are, therefore, at a high risk. The anterior commissure is a frequent point of spread to the thyroid cartilage, and involvement is generally considered a contraindication to partial surgery, unless it is the surgeon's judgment that tumor invasion is superficial and is not associated with cartilage invasion. Imaging studies may make this decision easier.

Involvement of the glottis and vocal cord fixation by causes other than paraglottic space invasion are

relative contraindications to partial surgery, and the source for cord paralysis should be recognized before leaving a laryngeal remnant. Cricoid cartilage involvement clearly mandates against a supraglottic laryngectomy, because swallowing is severely impaired with laryngeal preservation and cricoid cartilage resection. Bilateral arytenoid cartilage involvement is an absolute contraindication to supraglottic laryngectomy.

Radiotherapy seems to offer less local control than supraglottic laryngectomy and reduces the number of useful, preserved functioning larynges. Most large institutions recommend surgery for supraglottic tumors if partial surgery is planned, and for many, even total laryngectomy is logical for extension of the supraglottic lesion.[56,182]

This understanding of the correct precept for management has led to surgical series reporting 73% 5-year survival after supraglottic surgery.[32] Marks and others[164] noted actuarial 4-year survival is 50%, and cancer-free survival is 74% (Figure 99-16). The risk of local recurrence after supraglottic laryngectomy is 2% to 5%, and the indications for classic supraglottic laryngectomy remain true, with the same expectation for local control if the tumor has not crossed a

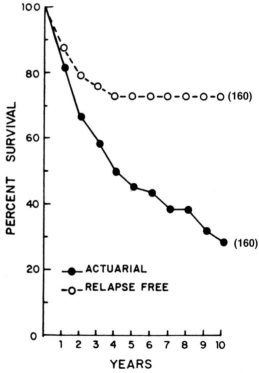

Figure 99-16. Relapse-free and actuarial survival for 160 patients with carcinoma of supraglottic larynx. Patients who were lost or died of causes other than cancer were withdrawn; the relapse-free curve depicts only deaths from cancer. Note that cancer survival is flat at 4 years and after. Of primary and neck recurrences, 85% occurred within 2 years. (From Marks JE and others: *Am J Roentgenol* 132:257, 1979.)

ventricle, gone below the petiole, or caused vocal cord paralysis.

EXTENSION OF SUPRAGLOTTIC LARYNGECTOMY

A three-quarter laryngectomy or foldover has been used successfully in patients with extension to the mobile vocal cord, as has cricohyoidopexy. Subtotal laryngectomy[211,212] preserves voice and swallowing with a retained tracheostomy tube if one mobile arytenoid is left in place. The value of this procedure, which has good local tumor control but does not approach the success rate of supraglottic laryngectomy, was confirmed by other series.[264] A few patients fulfill the criteria for this procedure.

Subtotal laryngectomy with cricohyoidopexy represents a functional laryngectomy that can be offered to appropriate patients with extensive supraglottic carcinoma. It is of value for the surgical treatment of carcinoma extended to the true vocal cord, the ventricle, involving the thyroid cartilage and the paraglottic space. The resection includes the entire thyroid cartilage, the paraglottic space, the epiglottis and the entire preepiglottic space. To be successful, the cricoid cartilage, hyoid bone, and at least one arytenoid cartilage must be spared.[43,138] It must be recognized that this operation has been supported by induction chemotherapy in the European literature and that many of the patients had indications not far different than those making the patient eligible for a supraglottic laryngectomy. The paraglottic space is removed in a supracricoid laryngectomy, and this is integral to success in local control of the cancer.[126]

Local failure after supracricoid partial laryngectomy seems to mimic that after supraglottic laryngectomy. A report of 15 local recurrences suggest a 5% rate with eventual local control of 80% of the failed patients by total laryngectomy or salvage chemotherapy with a 5-year survival of 50%. The series of 322, from which this is derived, may offer a better hint of success in this operation, but whether adjunct therapy including chemoradiation was part of the therapy is not described.[140]

Radiotherapy is a reasonable second choice for patients intolerant to or refusing major surgery. It has been reported to be effective for properly selected lesions of the supraglottic larynx.[174] Several institutions have reported fine results, with careful attention to planning and managing radiotherapy, and have reserved surgical salvage for radiation failure.[207]

For suprahyoid and lateral lesions on the aryepiglottic fold, where the depth of penetration of the tumor is clear, radiotherapy should be appropriate. Infrahyoid tumors involving the epiglottis and false cord may have unrecognized deep invasion of the preepiglottic

and paraglottic space. In centers in which significant expertise exists, hyperfractionation has been used for bulkier lesions or for those with significant depth of invasion. Recurrence of supraglottic lesions, which occurs in 10% to 20% of early T-stage tumors after radiotherapy, results in delayed diagnosis and the need for total laryngectomy.

Control of the neck is the most important aspect of managing supraglottic tumors, because local control is excellent. Although classic radical neck dissection ipsilateral to the largest bulk of tumor was used for many years, Bocca and others[32] began to recognize the opportunity to control the neck disease with bilateral modified neck dissections. The incidence of nodes in the neck dissection has varied widely at different institutions, from 32% palpable and 12% occult[164] to 25% positive as reported by Bocca and others.[32] In general, the range of cervical metastases is 25% to 50% (Figure 99-17).

Shah[239] and Byers[38] suggested that in previously unmanaged necks, nodal involvement in clinical N_0 or N_1 necks is at levels II, III, and IV. Level I disease is very unusual, with no involvement of these other areas. There is a slight incidence of level I involvement, and the surgeon should assess the relative risk of surgical complications by including level I in modified neck management vs leaving disease, particularly when single-modality therapy is planned. Hicks and others[105] noted a significant likelihood of level I pathology but only when level II had disease. Dissecting level I nodes and the submandibular gland eliminates postradiation decision about a firm or

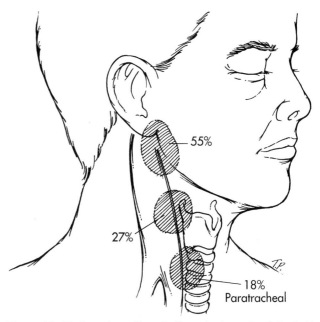

Figure 99-17. Location of lymphatic metastases in clinically N neck for the supraglottic larynx.

enlarged submandibular gland. Such a delayed presentation often requires a subsequent operation to remove a gland with chronic sialadenitis. Shah[239] noted no level I involvement without other levels of positive disease. This has also been true for level V and is the basis of the recommendation by Byers and others,[38] Shah,[239] and Wenig and Applebaum[301] that supraglottic laryngectomy requires only a modified radical neck dissection to include levels II through IV unless the clinical disease is N_2 or N_3. In the latter patients, a comprehensive or classical radical neck dissection may be required. These authors believe that T_4 lesions of the supraglottic larynx deserve more comprehensive neck dissection. In 1972, Lindberg[153] noted frequent bilateral nodes in only 3 of 147 patients with positive nodes having level I involvement and only 13 showing posterior neck (level V) involvement at presentation. A follow-up study from the same institution noted no level I or level V disease.[39]

Spiro and others[259] noted N_0 neck disease with cancer of the larynx and pharynx resulted in a 10% neck failure rate with or without postoperative radiotherapy.

A study of 201 patients with supraglottic tumors[158] showed only four failures in the operated ipsilateral neck and only four failures at the primary site. Surgery with no attention (radiation) to the contralateral neck resulted in 22% recurrence contralaterally, whereas radiotherapy resulted in 17% recurrence contralaterally. In 1994, a series of 76 patients from the same institution[294] had a 9% recurrence rate for surgery after bilateral neck dissections. This, again, occurred regardless of whether surgery alone or surgery plus radiotherapy was the management to the opposite neck. Failure in the neck after radiation and surgery was morbid. An ongoing institutional evaluation was reported in 1996 showing neck failure was more likely after radiotherapy.[182] Only one neck failure after bilateral neck dissection was noted, whereas 27% recurred, usually in the contralateral neck after ipsilateral surgery and radiotherapy. These studies, although retrospective and possibly placing the high-risk patients in radiotherapy categories, support Bocca,[31] who recommends surgery only for N_0 and N_1 necks. Postoperative radiotherapy seems to add little to the control (regional) of low nodal status cases; Ogura and others[196] showed that partial or total surgery with negative surgical margins in T_1 to T_3 cancers allows a 95% to 97% local control rate. Postoperative radiotherapy to the pharynx influences swallowing so severely it should be reserved only for significantly at-risk patients, whom many institutions define as patients with two or more ipsilateral pathologically positive nodes and those with extracapsular spread in the nodes.[252]

VARIANTS OF SQUAMOUS CELL CARCINOMA
Verrucous Carcinoma

Verrucous carcinoma represents an unusual presentation of a well-differentiated squamous cell carcinoma; it was first described as a laryngeal lesion in 1966 by Kraus and Perez-Mesa.[135] The tumor is characterized as slowly growing and locally aggressive, with a gross presentation described as very warty and keratotic. This carcinoma is most common in the oral cavity, and the second most frequent location is the larynx, where it is always endolaryngeal. It has only been reported as a glottic or supraglottic lesion. Verrucous carcinoma accounts for 1% to 2% of laryngeal carcinomas. Diagnosis requires cooperation between the physician and pathologist.

Repeat biopsies are often required before a satisfactory diagnosis is achieved. The lesion is exophytic, fungating, and broadly implanted. Grossly, it looks neoplastic and suggests malignancy. The histologic appearance shows broad, papillomatosis-like, club-shaped, new growth with high rete ridges and typically containing a hyperkeratotic squamous epithelium with minimal cytologic atypia (Figure 99-18).

The tumor margins seem to be pushing rather than infiltrating. Surgeons aware of this expected histologic pattern understand why multiple deep excisions and, on occasion, excision of the lesion should be achieved before diagnosis. There often is significant inflammation adjacent to the tumor, and occasionally, presentation with enlarged inflammatory neck nodes has been seen, which further heightens the suspicion for malignancy. However, no primary presentation with carcinoma in the lymph node has been associated with verrucous carcinoma.[98]

Hybrid verrucous squamous cell carcinoma of the larynx was first reported in 1982 by Batsakis and others[19] and has been noted by others.[157] Orvidas and others[203] reported that these tumors occur in 10% of verrucous cancers and represented the only cancer mortality in their series (all patients died from squamous cell carcinoma). These mixed histology tumors should be managed as squamous cell carcinomas, and if T stage merits it or the nodes are palpable, the neck should be addressed. Once verrucous carcinoma is diagnosed, management is surgery, not radiotherapy, if the patient can tolerate it. Verrucous carcinomas were reported 30 years ago to undergo malignant transformation to undifferentiated carcinoma after radiotherapy and even after cryotherapy. There have been suggestions that even the insult of surgery can dedifferentiate these tumors.

Failure to fully excise the lesion, whose biologic growth is slow, will cause local recurrence, and the tumor can be managed successfully. Several series of patients managed with radiotherapy[98] showed

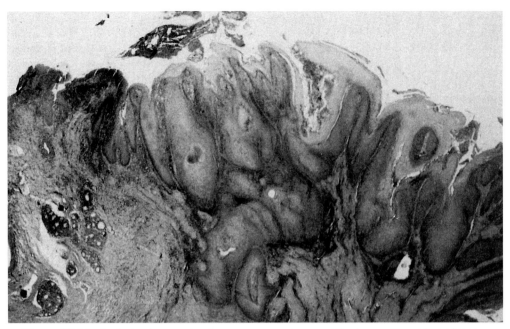

Figure 99-18. A photomicrograph of verrucous carcinoma of the larynx shows hyperkeratosis, papillomatosis, and club-shaped rete ridges. (Hematoxylin-eosin; original magnification ×25.) (From Fliss and others: *Laryngoscope* 104:147, 1994.)

significant recurrence and an 11% risk of anaplastic transformation. On the basis of these reports of dedifferentiation, which have not been well confirmed in more recent literature, and more importantly, in view that local control (<50% cure) is poorly achieved by radiotherapy, this technique is not offered for primary management. Surgery, which has a >85% local control rate, remains the primary modality.[268] When total laryngectomy is required to remove disease, radiotherapy should be considered as primary management, recognizing salvage surgery may be needed.

HPV, particularly HPV 16 and 18, is associated with these tumors, but the relationship between the virus and squamous cell carcinoma is unclear.[74]

Pseudosarcoma

Spindle cell carcinoma has been regarded as epithelial in origin. The pathology literature uses pseudonyms, including pseudosarcoma, carcinosarcoma, and pleomorphic carcinoma. The tumor has been explained in one of three ways in that it may be a collision tumor where two different histologies are present in the same site or it may be a squamous cell carcinoma with a reactive atypical stroma (pseudosarcoma). Another thought is that there may be some dedifferentiation of an epithelial tumor to result in a more spindle cell morphology (sarcomatoid carcinoma).[151]

These tumors generally present as firm, fleshy, polypoid masses noted on the anterior vocal cord. Most are glottic in presentation. The mucosa may be

ulcerated. There has been some suggestion that tumors of polypoid presentation fare better, but Randall and others[223] prove otherwise. Treatment for this unusual tumor is recommended to be surgical when possible, because radiation therapy for small lesions has not been satisfactory.[142] The planned treatment is similar to that for squamous cell carcinoma of similar location and size in that neck dissection is done for hypopharyngeal, supraglottic, advanced glottic, and transglottic tumors.

Basaloid Squamous Cell Carcinoma

Basaloid squamous cell carcinoma is a unique, infrequent variant of squamous cell carcinoma. This tumor occurs most frequently in the piriform sinus, base of tongue, tonsil, or larynx. Case reports have been infrequent; in 1992, a multiinstitutional pathology study found 8 of 40 tumors to occur in the larynx. The original description of Wain and others[287] required four primary microscopic features: (1) solid groups of cells in a lobular configuration; (2) small, crowded cells with scant cytoplasm; (3) dark, hyperchromatic nuclei without prominent nucleoli; and (4) small, cystic spaces containing mucin-like material or pseudoglandular formation. Pathologists should distinguish this tumor from other head and neck cancers with prominent nuclei and scant cytoplasm (e.g., small cell carcinoma, undifferentiated carcinoma, adenoid cystic carcinoma). Basaloid squamous carcinoma has been proposed in the literature to be an aggressive variant of squamous cell carcinoma. Winzenburg and others[306] attempted to match by stage and site this tumor vs those diagnosed as poorly differentiated carcinoma and their opinion and others in the literature is that this aggressive variant of squamous cell carcinoma requires metastatic survey presently to include a CT positron emission tomography (PET) scan at the time of diagnosis to assist in planning therapy. Patients with this diagnosis should not be enrolled in prospective randomized studies in which patients with squamous cell carcinoma are grouped together.[209,306]

SURGICAL PATHOLOGY OF THE HYPOPHARYNX

The characteristics of typical tumor extension and the pathways of spread of hypopharyngeal malignancy are essential in determining the extent of the surgical resection or the irradiation ports.[153] Unrecognized submucosal extension has been a major cause of management failure. Harrison[102] studied whole organ serial section and found recurrent disease after laryngopharyngectomy was primarily caused by submucosal extension inferiorly. Murakami and others[180] found that submucosal extension was superior and inferior. They recommended extending the superior limit of resection to the base of the palatine tonsil.

Kirchner[127] and Harrison[100] found that tumors of the lateral wall extend into the thyroid cartilage and directly into the overlying thyroid gland. Because of these findings, all authors recommended resection of the ipsilateral hemithyroid and isthmus, even if these sites are not clinically involved and there is no clinical evidence of thyroid cartilage invasion. Kirchner[127] confirmed the recommendation by Ogura and others[194] that no patient with involvement of the piriform apex or thyroid cartilage be considered a candidate for partial laryngopharyngectomy. Harrison demonstrated submucosal extension inferiorly into the cervical esophagus, as well as superiorly.

Hiroto believed that submucosal extension was greater superiorly and explained the recurrence rate in the oropharynx.[106] Ho[108] recognized that submucosal extension was greater in patients receiving previous radiation therapy and found tumor extension was greater inferiorly into the cervical esophagus than it was superiorly. Submucosal extension did not correlate with survival, and a "skip" lesion was present in only 1 of the 57 specimens studied.

In no study did the extensiveness of the submucosal disease have a direct effect on survival when negative margins were obtained. It does not necessarily reflect a more aggressive malignancy. These data suggest that the surgeon is obligated to obtain both a superior and inferior negative margin and be prepared to resect up to 3 or more cm in both directions.

Sessions[236] reviewed 195 pathologic specimens from patients with tumors of the hypopharynx. This represented 21% of laryngopharyngeal malignancies. He correlated pathologic findings with 3-year survival. Factors evaluated included location of tumor, margins, differentiation of tumor, and lymph node involvement. Several of these patients managed between 1955 and 1971 underwent preoperative radiotherapy. Of patients with tumors in the inferior hypopharynx who had no tumor in the surgical specimen after preoperative radiotherapy, 38% eventually experienced management failure. When margins were reported as positive in the inferior hypopharynx, only 5% of patients survived. This was in direct contrast to patients with supraglottic tumor, for whom close or involved margins did not always affect survival. The presence of pathologically positive cervical adenopathy was related to tumor size, because patients whose tumors were <4 cm had a 50% incidence of positive cervical adenopathy. Those with tumors >4 cm had an 85% incidence of positive nodes. The incidence of positive cervical metastasis did not correlate with tumor differentiation. However, tumor differentiation at the primary site directly correlated with survival.

Invasion of thyroid cartilage, muscle, or nerve was directly related to cervical adenopathy. There were no survivors among patients who had contralateral cervical metastases. The most common lymph node to be involved was the upper jugular node, even for inferior hypopharyngeal tumors. When positive nodes were present in the posterior inferior cervical triangle, there were no survivors. Martin and others[166] further reviewed pathologic data and correlated it with the TNM system. They found a greater response to preoperative radiotherapy among patients who had nonkeratinizing carcinoma. The response to preoperative radiotherapy did not correlate with the degree of differentiation or whether the tumor had a pushing or infiltrating margin. None of these factors correlated with the development of cervical metastases. Between 10% and 29% of patients had extranodal extension of tumor. Poorest survival was associated with tumor in cervical lymph nodes or at the surgical margins. Patients who had extranodal extension of metastases regardless of T or N staging had an increased incidence of distant metastases.

Histologic differentiation of the tumor correlated with invasion of thyroid cartilage. Tumors of the medial wall of the piriform sinus tended to extend into the region of the supraglottic larynx. Because of these findings, surgical removal of the preepiglottic space is advised when partial pharyngectomy is considered for medial wall tumors. Kirchner[127] and Deleyiannis and others[53] reviewed whole-organ sections to determine suitability of patients for partial pharyngectomy. They showed that piriform sinus malignancies might infiltrate into the posterior cricoarytenoid muscle and thereby affect cord mobility. Cord mobility can also be affected by invasion of the cricoarytenoid joint or direct invasion of the recurrent laryngeal nerve. Tumors spread medially into the larynx and may invade the thyroarytenoid muscle. Tumors extend upward to invade the base of the tongue or inferiorly into the esophagus. A 1-cm submucosal infiltration is invariably present, requiring a surgical margin of at least 2 cm.

Dumich and others[63] studied histopathologic specimens to determine whether piriform apex involvement would permit a near-total laryngopharyngectomy in patients with piriform sinus carcinoma. In a review of 20 total laryngectomy and partial pharyngectomy specimens, they found 17 patients who could have been considered for a near-total laryngectomy. They believed that the anterior larynx could be preserved to establish a sphincteric tracheopharyngeal shunt. Patients should not be considered candidates for this surgery if there was any evidence of involvement of the postcricoid area, bilateral cord fixation, or tumor in the interarytenoid area, because one functioning arytenoid cartilage should be preserved.

MANAGEMENT OF HYPOPHARYNGEAL CANCER

There are a variety of philosophies that are applied to managing hypopharyngeal malignancies. Current management modalities include full-course radiotherapy with surgical salvage, surgery alone, a combination of preoperative or postoperative radiotherapy with surgery, and prospective protocols, including chemotherapy preceding or concomitant with radiotherapy. To understand the current management modalities, it is helpful to examine trends that have developed over the past 30 years.

In the early 1960s, surgery was the primary modality for malignancies of the hypopharynx once it was determined that the patient could undergo an operative procedure. Indications for nonresectability were presence of fixed cervical metastases, involvement of the carotid artery, fixation of the posterior pharyngeal wall (prevertebral fascia invasion), extension into the cervical esophagus, and evidence of distant metastatic disease.

Patients not considered candidates for surgery were offered full-course radiotherapy for palliation. With advances in surgical technique, the limits of resectability were extended. Thus, total laryngopharyngectomy was possible with reconstruction by use of regional flaps[13] and colon interposition rather than local flaps.[181,310] This extended the surgeon's ability to resect recurrent tumors after full-course radiotherapy and to interpose acceptable pharyngeal reconstruc-

tion. Harrison and others[100] pointed out that a cause of surgical failure was tumor extension into the thyroid gland, paratracheal nodes, and upper mediastinal lymph nodes, and, most importantly, submucosal extension inferiorly into the cervical esophagus.

Harrison[101] also recognized the possibility of skip lesions within the esophagus and advised total esophagectomy combined with radical total laryngopharyngectomy for postcricoid carcinoma. His later study of 57 patients with postcricoid carcinoma revealed only one concurrent esophageal carcinoma. Total esophagectomy with gastric pull-up was advised to obtain an adequate resection of the cervical esophagus and limit the number of anastomoses. Partial pharyngectomy was described by Trotter,[273] who used resection and primary closure for limited lesions of the superior lateral hypopharynx and postcricoid area (Figure 99-19). Orton[202] described transhyoid pharyngotomy. Alonso[4] described supraglottic laryngectomy and vertical partial laryngectomy for malignancy of the hypopharynx. In 1960, 1964, and 1979, Ogura and others[194-196] reported on their experiences with partial pharyngectomy, which by 1979 had included 85 patients.

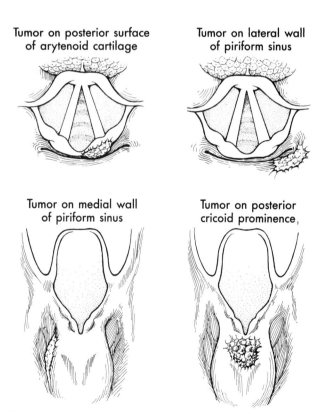

Figure 99-19. Proper endoscopic mapping of tumor is essential in planning therapy. These examples of tumors might be acceptable for partial pharyngectomy. Limited tumor on the posterior cricoid region would be amenable to resection by the laryngeal autograft method.

Extended surgery did not greatly affect overall survival for patients with advanced diseases. Simultaneously, Biller and others,[28] Ogura and others,[194-196] and Goldman and others[92] began to administer low-dose radiotherapy before surgical resection. Dosages were in the range of 2000 to 4500 rad delivered over 1 to 4 weeks. The planned surgical resection was performed 4 weeks later. Initial results, although not randomized, suggested that survival was improved with this combined therapy. Preoperative radiotherapy combined with surgical resection became the most popular management for hypopharyngeal malignancies during the late 1960s and early 1970s.

In the late 1970s, postoperative radiotherapy administered as part of a planned therapy was considered. It was hoped that complications would be lessened if the radiotherapy was administered postoperatively. Doses up to 6000 rad could be administered safely after the wound healed, and pathologic evaluation of the specimen allowed the establishment of criteria to determine who should receive radiotherapy. However, Carpenter and others[42] and Yates and Crumley,[311] in a prospective study, believed that combined therapy was not proved to be better than surgery alone. Still, combined therapy with postoperative radiotherapy for the management of advanced hypopharyngeal malignancies became the trend.

Another advance in surgical management was microvascular surgery, which allowed free jejunal autograft reconstruction. A total laryngopharyngectomy with 6 cm of cervical esophagus could be reconstructed by a single-stage procedure. If total esophagectomy was necessary, gastric pull-up became the preferred method of reconstruction.[101] Reconstruction with colon and local and regional flaps became less popular, because these newer techniques allowed for more rapid reestablishment of healthy swallowing and a shorter hospital stay.

Surgery combined with radiotherapy did not significantly improve overall 5-year survival. What changed was the pattern of recurrence: increased distant metastases and failure in the opposite neck and decreased local and ipsilateral neck recurrences. In an effort to continue to reduce the distant metastases, reduce the extent of surgery required, and improve overall survival statistics, chemotherapy was administered. Prospective studies[187] were initiated and showed that a partial response in the tumor mass could be obtained by administering one to four courses of chemotherapy before definitive surgical resection. In addition, studies were undertaken to administer chemotherapy first followed by, if there was a partial or complete response, full-course radiotherapy rather than surgery. Thus, an effort was made for voice preservation. Persistence of palpable cervical metasta-

tic disease remained an indication for radical neck dissection. In the 1980s, management further changed when it was suggested that a comprehensive or radical neck dissection provided no better survival than modified neck dissection followed by radiotherapy.

Primary Radiotherapy

Radiotherapy (RT) is used for (1) patients who have early malignancies, often confined to the medial wall of the piriform sinus, particularly exophytic tumors without extension into the piriform apex; (2) patients who have primary malignancy of the posterior pharyngeal wall; (3) those who refuse surgical resection or are too ill to undergo resection; and (4) those for whom radiotherapy is used primarily for palliation to reduce the bulk of extensive unresectable malignancies and alleviate pain. Amdur and Mendenhall[6] at the University of Florida summarized their experience in treating 101 T_1 and T_2 hypopharyngeal cancers with RT primarily with planned neck dissection. Local control was achieved in 86% of T_1 and 82% of T_2 cancers with laryngeal preservation. They challenged the need for adjuvant chemotherapy in this group of patients. Surgery was required for cervical metastases.

These results were not obtainable in patients with postcricoid cancer. Axon and others[12] compared their 5-year survival results with radical radiotherapy (23% survival) with surgery and gastric interposition (45%). Results were even better in patients presenting without adenopathy (63% surgery) compared with 25% radiation therapy.

Wang[289] presented the results of 42 patients who had primary malignancy of the posterior pharyngeal wall. This lesion had the poorest prognosis of any area in the hypopharynx. Of patients, 95% were older than 50 years and 70% were older than 60 years. Presenting symptoms, including dysphagia, persistent pharyngeal pain, sensation of foreign body, and referred otalgia, were identical to those of other hypopharyngeal tumors. Most lesions were in the midposterior pharyngeal wall, and some lesions could be seen by simple depression of the posterior tongue. Of patients, 55% had metastatic cervical adenopathy; four had bilateral adenopathy. Thirty-six patients were eligible for 3-year survival assessment. Survival with radiotherapy alone was 25% (9 of 36). However, when patients had T_1, T_2, and T_3 lesions and no adenopathy, the 3-year survival rate was 47%. However, of 17 patients who had clinically evident cervical adenopathy, only 12% were alive at 3 years. Local recurrence along the posterior pharyngeal wall was the primary cause of failure.

In 1996, Garden and others[84] used primary radiotherapy for 84 T_1 and T_2 hypopharyngeal carcinoma patients. Local control was achieved in 89% of T_1 and

77% of T_2 lesions. Neck dissection was used in some node-positive cases. Surgical salvage, however, was only successful in 6 of 19 primary recurrences. Actual 5-year survival rates were 68% for T_1 lesions and 46% for T_2 lesions. Success was attributed to twice-daily hyperfractionation of the radiotherapy and careful selection of patients by premanagement CT.[84]

Some studies suggest that twice-daily radiation has been more effective than conventional radiation.[85,86,119,207] An extensive phase III randomized study was performed by the Radiation Therapy Oncology Group (RTOG) and reported in 2000.[83] This was a four-arm study of more than 1000 patients who had radiation given in four different formats. The first was standard radiation at 2 Gy/fraction/day for 5 days of the week to a total dose of 70 Gy. The second arm included hyperfractionation of 1.2 Gy given twice a day to a total dose of 81.6 Gy. The third arm was an acceleration fractionation, which did require a split with twice daily radiation, but included a 2-week rest period. The fourth arm included both accelerated fractionation and what was referred to as a concomitant boost with a total of 72 Gy given over the 6-week period. The results of the study demonstrated that hyperfractionation, twice daily radiation, or radiation with a concomitant boost had a statistically improved locoregional control rate and a greater disease-free survival. However, the overall survival was the same for all treatments, including the standard radiation therapy arm. Although there was improvement in locoregional control, there was also a greater incidence of significant mucositis; later in this chapter there is discussion of the complexity of salvage surgery in patients having received extensive radiation therapy.

Surgical Options and Results

McGavran and others[169] reported that radiotherapy alone was insufficient management for patients with cervical metastases. The 5-year survival rate was approximately 8% with radiotherapy alone when nodes were present. As in other large series, 84% of patients had pathologically positive cervical adenopathy, primarily in the upper jugular chain. Only 4 of 52 patients had contralateral nodes. When managed by surgery alone, eight patients died of local disease, eight of cervical metastases, and four of distant metastases. No patients who experienced recurrence were salvaged regardless of secondary therapy. In this group, surgery included partial pharyngectomy, total laryngopharyngectomy, and ipsilateral radical neck dissection. Overall 5-year survival rate was 31%. Of patients with T2 lesions, 69% had positive node findings at presentation. They noted that survival decreased by 50% in the presence of positive nodes.

Carpenter and others[42] analyzed management and results in 162 patients. Surgery was the primary, and often only, management modality used; radiotherapy was reserved for palliation. Patients who had mobile cervical metastases underwent surgery with possible combined therapy. Those who had large metastatic cervical nodes were given radiotherapy before attempts at surgical resection. The characteristics of patients managed by Carpenter and others[42] were typical of those in all studies: 84% were men, 85% were in the sixth or seventh decade of life, 96% were active or former smokers, 93% had a history of heavy alcohol ingestion, 67% had cervical adenopathy at the time of presentation, 5% had contralateral disease, and 24% had fixed cervical metastases. Patients with postcricoid carcinoma, the smallest group (six patients), had the best 5-year survival (44%), whereas those with tumors of the posterior pharyngeal wall had only a 22% 5-year survival.

Pingree and others[215] presented data on management modality in 695 patients with carcinoma of the hypopharynx managed between 1973 and 1983. Tumor-free 3-year survival for the group managed by surgery alone was 59%; for radiation alone, 28%; and for surgery plus radiation, 43%. The 5-year survival was 41% for surgery alone, 21% for radiation alone, and 33% for combined surgery and radiation. Five-year survival rates for 156 patients with stages I and II hypopharyngeal cancer showed that the group managed by surgery alone had a survival of 48%; for surgery plus radiation, 40%. A comparison was made, although not randomized, of preoperative vs postoperative radiotherapy. At 5 years, the survival rate for patients who received planned preoperative radiation was 29%; for planned postoperative radiation, it was 32.7%. These findings were similar to those reported by Yates and Crumley[311]; no demonstrable improvement in survival occurred with combined therapy over surgery alone. Because many patients who received radiotherapy may not have been eligible for surgery, it would not be fair to compare management modalities in this series.

In an analysis of 109 patients treated primarily by surgery, Ho[107] confirmed that results are related to stage of the primary and nodal status and not necessarily to the extent of the surgery. The primary cancer was located in the piriform sinus in 83 patients (76%) and postcricoid region in 19 (17%). Initially, all patients underwent laryngopharyngoesophagoscopy, but later the extent of surgery was more conservative, although all patients had a laryngopharyngectomy. The overall 5-year survival was 35% but varied from 74% for stage I to 14% for stage IV. Survival for N_0 neck disease was 57%, but there were no survivors when the neck was staged as N_3. As noted in other studies, 17% of patients had second primary malignancies develop.

Spector and others[257] reported on the 5-year survival rate of 408 patients managed between 1964 and 1991. This study revealed that 69% of patients had positive metastatic disease and 87% of patients had stage III or IV disease when initially seen. Survival was better for patients with one-wall lesions than patients with two walls of the piriform sinus involved (34%). Most patients (302) had combined radiation and surgery. Again, lesions confined to one wall had the most favorable prognosis, and extension to the apex of the piriform sinus or postcricoid carried the most unfavorable prognosis. The overall incidence of distant metastases was 17.7%, and 6.2% of patients had a second primary cancer develop. This improvement in overall survival was attributed to improvements in radiotherapy and surgery. Patients continued to be seen with advanced disease, had distant metastatic disease develop, and had second primary malignancies develop. In addition, patients were generally older than laryngeal cancer patients and had significantly more intercurrent disease. Both the incidence of delayed recurrence and of developing second primary malignancies was three times greater for hypopharyngeal cancer than laryngeal cancer.[258]

Axon and others[12] compared the results of surgery with primary radiation therapy for postcricoid carcinomas. Surgery included pharyngolaryngoesophagoscopy with gastric transport. Excluding patients who had palliative radiation only, the 5-year survival was 45% in the surgical group and 23% in the radiation group. When palpable nodes were present at diagnosis, the 5-year survival fell to 10%. The 5-year survival for salvage surgery after radiation therapy was 25%.

CONSERVATION SURGERY OF THE LARYNGOPHARYNX

Partial laryngopharyngectomy with voice preservation is best understood by studying the chronologic development of the operative procedures used. As in conservation surgery for laryngeal carcinoma, limited surgery for piriform sinus carcinoma is feasible, because the cancer initially remains confined within anatomic boundaries. Early tumor remains ipsilateral with direct extension into the soft tissues and lymph nodes. Extension later is superior and inferior. Wide surgical margins are essential to include the submucosal extension. Select limited lesions, T_1 or T_2, are amenable to conservation surgery. Surgeons who advocate these procedures concur that: (1) the vocal cord should be mobile; (2) there can be no invasion of the thyroid cartilage; (3) the apex of the piriform sinus or cricoid cartilage cannot be involved;

(4) tumors may not extend into the vallecula or involve the epiglottis; (5) there should be no involvement of the preepiglottic fat; (6) there should be no extension into the strap muscles; (7) tumor should be confined to the medial anterior or lateral hypopharyngeal wall; (8) the procedures are not useful for carcinomas of the posterior hypopharyngeal wall or the postcricoid area; (9) there can be no invasion of the paraglottic space on CT or MRI; (10) they should not be applied when bilateral extensive cervical adenopathy is present; (11) they are not useful in patients who have had radiation fail; (12) low-dose preoperative radiotherapy is ineffective in reducing the bulk of tumor mass when combined with conservation surgery; and (13) patients should be selected with comorbidity factors carefully examined.

Because of the silent nature of the initial tumor, few patients fulfill these criteria. Most patients have tumors too extensive to consider conservation surgery and are best served by total or partial pharyngectomy and laryngectomy. At the time of surgery, a tumor believed to be confined to one area may, on frozen section, have submucosal extension to adjacent sites. No boundary exists between the walls of the piriform sinus and posterior hypopharyngeal wall.

Ogura and others[194] reported on an extension of the supraglottic laryngectomy for superior hypopharyngeal cancers. The method requires a midline thyrotomy preceded by a hemithyroidectomy with preservation of the recurrent laryngeal nerve. The inferior strap muscles are transected, allowing exposure of the entire ipsilateral thyroid cartilage. The ipsilateral external perichondrium of the thyroid cartilage is preserved for closure, whereas the actual cartilage is resected. The hypopharynx is entered through the vallecula, and the full extent of the tumor is appreciated. Wide resection is performed, including the preepiglottic space and anterior medial and lateral walls of the piriform sinus. The resection can be extended to remove the false cord and arytenoid if necessary. The defect is closed primarily. Larger lesions require a musculocutaneous flap reconstruction or split-thickness skin graft. Patients are not permitted to swallow for at least 2 weeks. To prevent aspiration, the remaining ipsilateral vocal cord is sutured to the midline of the cricoid.

By 1979, the series by Ogura and others[196] had expanded to include 85 patients who had partial laryngopharyngectomy for piriform sinus carcinomas. Approximately one-half of the patients were eligible for this type of partial pharyngeal surgery. The 3-year actuarial survival rate remained 59% compared with 36% for 57 patients undergoing total laryngopharyngectomy. Recognizably, patients who had total laryngopharyngectomy had more extensive tumors. The most important prognostic factor was the development of palpable cervical disease. The 3-year survival rate for patients without nodal disease was 53% compared with 24% for those with palpable nodal metastases. Overall control of the primary tumor for patients with piriform sinus carcinoma was 47%, with a 66% 3-year survival rate for patients who had conservation surgery. As in patients who had total laryngopharyngectomy, recurrences occurred equally at the primary site, in the neck, and distantly.

More than 50% of patients who had undergone conservation pharyngeal surgery retained their voice. Submucosal spread and extensive lymphatic drainage with cervical adenopathy were more limiting factors in conservation surgery of the piriform sinus than they were for supraglottic malignancies.

Although Ogura and others[191,193,194,198] advocated this method of conservation surgery in the United States, Laccourreye and others[137,141] in Paris developed a technique of supracricoid hemilaryngopharyngectomy (SCHLP). Between 1964 and 1983, they operated on 240 patients with primary lesions of the hypopharynx using SCHLP. Most patients had T_2 tumors, but some limited T_3 tumors were included. Neck dissection was performed at the time of surgery and included ipsilateral thyroidectomy. This approach differs from that advocated by Ogura and others in that the strap muscles are not resected but are rotated medially exposing the posterior border of the thyroid cartilage. A perichondrial incision is made posteriorly, and the perichondrium with the attached strap muscles is rotated medially. Resection of the hyoid bone depends on the location of the primary tumor. The ipsilateral epiglottis is resected midvertically, and the resection includes the preepiglottic space. Access to the site of tumor is performed through a midline thyrotomy and, after resection of the ipsilateral thyroid and preepiglottic space, the incision is carried across the vallecula. The lateral pharyngeal wall and tumor are excised under direct vision. The inferior limit of resection is the cricothyroid membrane. The recurrent laryngeal nerve is not preserved, because the hemilarynx is included in the resection. Closure uses the preserved mucoperichondrial flap, which is sutured to the lateral pharyngeal wall. Laccourreye and others[141] advocate this procedure for T_2 carcinomas of the piriform sinus, reserving the technique described by Ogura and others as an extended supraglottic laryngectomy for T_1 malignancies. To reduce the incidence of functional failures, they advocated no more than 5000 rad postoperatively. The local recurrence rate was low, with most recurrences occurring within 3 years. This has become their preferred technique for limited lesions of the piriform sinus. Laccourreye and others found a 30% incidence of second primary malignancies in these patients within 5 years.

Krespi and Sisson[136] reported their results with voice preservation for piriform sinus carcinoma. They refer to their procedure as hemicricolaryngopharyngectomy. In this technique, the ipsilateral cricoid cartilage ring is not preserved, because it is in an extended supraglottic laryngectomy. The operative procedure begins with a modified or radical neck dissection, depending on whether clinically palpable nodes are present. After separation of the strap muscles, the pharynx is entered through the vallecula. If the ipsilateral strap muscles are included in the surgical resection, the thyroid and cricoid cartilages are divided in the midline, and the larynx is divided posteriorly through the midline to include the ipsilateral cricoid cartilage anteriorly and posteriorly. Residual or contralateral hemilarynx is converted into a tube and the opening maintained with a stent. The large defect after resection of the hemilarynx and hemipharynx is repaired with a pectoralis myocutaneous flap. With this technique, patients retain a permanent tracheostomy. It is a more extensive surgical resection than that proposed by Laccourreye and others,[138] but it preserves a speech tube. The method of resection is oncologically adequate for patients with T_2 and T_3 piriform sinus tumors, because there was no local recurrence of malignancy. Again, patient deaths were reported from second primary malignancies or distant metastatic disease.

Dumich and others[63] evaluated total laryngopharyngectomy specimens in serial sections. They wanted to establish whether piriform sinus carcinoma extended across the midline and a portion of the ipsilateral noninvolved larynx could be preserved in selected cases. Their study showed that in 13 of 20 patients who had undergone total laryngopharyngectomy, a near total laryngopharyngectomy would have been oncologically safe. They showed, however, that involvement of the posterior contralateral larynx would make such preservation of the contralateral larynx unsafe. Any suggestion that the tumor extended across the interarytenoid region would contraindicate any voice preservation or near total laryngopharyngectomy. In the initial 15 cases managed by this technique, with preservation of a mucosal speaking tube similar to near total laryngectomy, there was no evidence of local recurrent disease. Similar to the technique advocated by Sisson,[247] patients have a permanent tracheostomy and a speaking tube consisting of the remaining portion of the contralateral larynx and one functioning vocal cord and arytenoid. Frozen section assessment is essential to establish whether the contralateral larynx is free of tumor.

A prospective study of near total laryngectomy in 40 patients with piriform sinus lesions was reported by Shenoy and others.[243] Their technique adapted the Pearson technique for laryngeal malignancies to piriform cancers. This study emphasizes the issues associated with this procedure in hypopharyngeal cancers. Positive margins were found on permanent section in five patients when the frozen section was negative. Thirty percent of patients had a postoperative fistula develop. Overall complications occurred in 68% of piriform sinus cases. Speech, however, was restored in 76% of these patients. The 5-year disease-free survival was 66% for medial wall lesions and 54% for lateral wall malignancies.

COMBINED RADIATION THERAPY AND SURGERY

The concept of combining radiotherapy with surgical resection in a planned manner began in the early 1960s after initial reports by Goldman and others,[92] Powers,[218] Ogura and Mallen,[195] Martin and others,[166] and others.[128,155] These large series compared patients who had 2000 to 5000 rad of preoperatively administered radiotherapy delivered at 200 rad/day followed by a short waiting period and planned surgical resection with historical control patients from the same institution.

In theory, the primary advantage of preoperative radiotherapy was that well-oxygenated unoperated tissue had a better vascular supply, making delivery more effective than radiotherapy to an operated field. Also, the field and extent of radiotherapy would be more limited, because this modality could be directly applied to the tumor site.[262]

Postoperative radiation gained acceptance in the late 1970s.[9,65,224,279] The advantage of postoperative radiotherapy was the establishment of the pathologic extent of disease, true status of cervical nodes, and status of the surgical margins. To encompass the entire field, radiation had to be delivered to a larger port, requiring 6000 rad over 6 weeks. The disadvantage was that postoperative radiotherapy would be delayed if there were a delay in wound healing (fistula). Vikram[281] pointed out the need to deliver postoperative radiotherapy within 7 weeks of the operative procedure. In 7 of 10 patients to receive postoperative radiotherapy within 7 weeks of surgery, no signs of recurrence developed. In 11 patients in whom the initiation of postoperative radiotherapy was delayed, 3 had regional or local recurrent tumor develop. The need to administer postoperative radiotherapy within 8 weeks of surgery has been a major argument of advocates of preoperative radiotherapy.

In a more recent analysis, a retrospective study reported by Bastit and others[17] in 2001 of 420 patients

with oropharyngeal and hypopharyngeal malignancies could not demonstrate that delay of initiation of postoperative RT was a significant prognostic factor. Their multivariate analysis showed that status of the margins and N stage predicted likelihood of locoregional recurrence. They could not demonstrate RT begun more than 6 weeks postoperatively effected survival and believed that radiation could be delayed in those cases when necessary to allow for adequate wound healing.

El-Badawi and others[65] summarized management results between 1949 and 1976 for piriform sinus carcinomas. Limited to hypopharyngeal cancer only, the study revealed 422 patients with piriform sinus cancer, 91 with posterior pharyngeal wall cancer, and 18 with postcricoid cancer. Postoperative radiotherapy was defined as radiation commencing within 12 weeks after resection of all gross tumor. Radiation fields were enlarged in the 1960s to include parapharyngeal lymphatics and inferiorly to attempt to reduce stoma recurrence by submucosal extension. Survival curves were calculated for surgery vs surgery plus planned postoperative radiotherapy. In the surgery-only group, the survival rate was 25%; in the combined group, it was 40%. The combined group had a slightly higher incidence of pharyngeal stenosis. Significantly fewer recurrences above the clavicle occurred in the group who received postoperative radiotherapy. However, recurrences above the clavicle were related to T stage, with a low incidence (18%) for T_1 and T_2 tumors and a higher incidence (33%) for T_3 and T_4 tumors. Recurrence above the clavicle for all N stages was approximately 30%. Patients with N_2 and N_3 neck disease had a higher incidence of distant metastases (28%) compared with those with N_0 and N_1 stage (16%).

Two major prospective randomized studies were initiated to determine whether preoperative or postoperative radiotherapy was more advantageous. The largest study was performed between 1973 and 1975 under the direction of the RTOG.[133,275] Patients with carcinoma of the oral cavity, oropharynx, supraglottic larynx, and hypopharynx were randomly assigned to receive preoperative radiation of 5000 rad or postoperative radiation in the range of 6000 rad. Of 320 patients, 78 had primary piriform sinus cancers; 35 patients received preoperative radiotherapy, and 38 received postoperative radiotherapy. In the hypopharynx area, the preoperative group had a 50% locoregional control rate, and the postoperative group had a 61% control rate. There was no statistical difference, however, in overall survival.

In a randomized prospective clinical study, Vandenbrouck and others[280] included 260 patients, but the trial was terminated because of a higher incidence of postoperative deaths among patients who had received preoperative radiotherapy. Thus, 49 of 177 patients with hypopharyngeal tumors were randomly assigned. The higher complication rate in the preoperative radiation group was also associated with prolonged healing time (148 hospital days vs 91 days). Overall survival for the preoperative radiation group was 36% and for the postoperative radiation group was 56%.

HYPOPHARYNGEAL RECONSTRUCTION WITH ADJACENT NONINVOLVED TISSUE

Several efforts have been made to develop an operative procedure that would effectively remove the malignancy from the postcricoid area or hypopharynx without the requirement for pectoralis major flap reconstruction or major bowel interposition. In 1956, Som[255] introduced laryngotracheal autograft for postcricoid carcinoma. The procedure was developed primarily to deal with women with postcricoid carcinoma secondary to Paterson-Brown-Kelly syndrome. This limited but often difficult-to-diagnose carcinoma in the postcricoid area comprises only 7% of malignancies of the hypopharynx in the United States. As noted by Som and others,[254] a major cause for failure is not the local disease but the early development of cervical, retropharyngeal, paratracheal, and superior mediastinal node involvement (Figure 99-20). Unlike the procedure described by Asherson[10] in 1954, which preserved the party wall between the hypopharynx and larynx, Som[255] proposed a more limited surgical resection. By preserving the anterior portion of the larynx and trachea and resecting the posterior aspect,

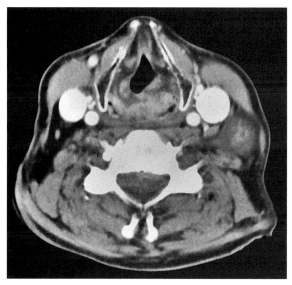

Figure 99-20. Postcricoid carcinoma with metastatic disease in the left neck. The patient's voice was normal, because both vocal cords showed healthy function. The only finding on direct office examination was pooling in the left piriform sinus area.

including the arytenoids and common wall, it was possible to use the anterior larynx as an autograft to reconstruct the pharynx. He analyzed 26 patients with postcricoid carcinoma and found that this method was acceptable in patients with tumor limited to the postcricoid area and not extending caudally into the cervical esophagus. The procedure could not be used in patients who had previously had radiotherapy, and the endolarynx had to be free of tumor.[254] Today this procedure has very limited applicability.

Calcaterra[40] described a procedure using a tongue rotation flap. A horizontal laterally based flap of the posterior tongue is elevated and rotated 90 degrees to augment the closure of the hypopharynx. The tongue flap is sufficient to form three-fourths of the circumference of the newly created hypopharynx. This technique is considered only when a subtotal pharyngectomy has been performed in combination with total laryngectomy.

Lore and others[156] reported a technique for reconstruction of superior hypopharyngeal tumors. To reconstruct the posterior wall, a dermal graft is applied to the prevertebral fascia. The tongue flap forms the anterior three-fourths of the newly reconstructed hypopharynx.

Bocca and Marzaroli (as quoted in and later modified by Barzan and Comoretto) developed another method of reconstruction.[16] This reconstructive method depends on piriform sinus malignancies not extending across the midline. A midline thyrotomy incision is made and extended upward through the hyoid and inferiorly through the cricothyroid membrane, cricoid, and first tracheal ring. Resection is continued through the posterior commissure of the postcricoid region. Thyroid cartilage is removed by subperichondrial dissection on the contralateral or uninvolved side. The arytenoid cartilage on the uninvolved side is not resected for fear of devascularization of the adjacent mucosa. They advise postoperative radiotherapy. Their report again noted the high incidence of local recurrence and second primary malignancies in these patients. A limitation to performing this procedure is involvement of the vallecula, epiglottis, and cervical esophagus. A disadvantage of this procedure is a reported high incidence (29%–50%) of pharyngocutaneous fistulas (Figure 99-21).

HYPOPHARYNGEAL RECONSTRUCTION WITH REGIONAL FLAPS

Reconstruction of the hypopharynx after total laryngectomy and total or near total pharyngectomy requires familiarity with several surgical techniques. Favored reconstruction uses adjacent tissue once the margins are proven to be tumor free. Preoperative assessment by CT or MRI, endoscopic assessment

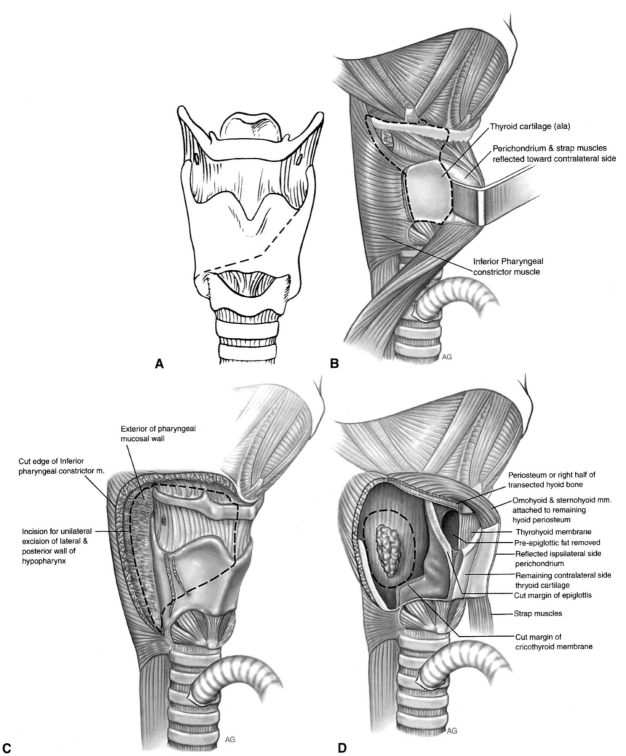

A

B

Thyroid cartilage (ala)

Perichondrium & strap muscles
reflected toward contralateral side

Inferior Pharyngeal
constrictor muscle

AG

Exterior of pharyngeal
mucosal wall

Cut edge of Inferior
pharyngeal constrictor m.

Incision for unilateral
excision of lateral &
posterior wall of
hypopharynx

C

AG

Periosteum or right half of
transected hyoid bone

Omohyoid & sternohyoid mm.
attached to remaining
hyoid periosteum

Thyrohyoid membrane

Pre-epiglottic fat removed

Reflected ispsilateral side
perichondrium

Remaining contralateral side
thryoid cartilage

Cut margin of epiglottis

Strap muscles

Cut margin of
cricothyroid membrane

D

AG

Figure 99-21. A, A lateral pharyngotomy for a limited posterolateral pharyngeal wall lesion.
B, Supracricoid hemilaryngopharyngectomy. The external perichondrium and overlying strap
muscles are rotated medially. A median thyrotomy incision is made, and the piriform sinus
lesion is exposed. The resection includes the lateral portion of the hyoid bone and necessitates transection of the laryngeal pedicle. Closure is obtained by suturing the lateral pharyngeal wall to the preserved perichondrial flap. **C,** A pectoralis major myocutaneous flap serves
best as a patch graft when it can be used for a 360-degree defect, but the swallowing results
are superior when a 3-cm segment of the posterior pharyngeal wall can be preserved.
D, A lateral pharyngotomy incision for a medial piriform sinus lesion. In this technique, the
resection includes the preepiglottic space, but the contralateral laryngeal pedicle and superior
laryngeal nerve are preserved.

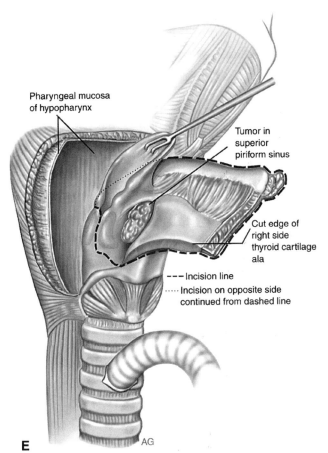

Pharyngeal mucosa
of hypopharynx

Tumor in
superior
piriform sinus

Cut edge of
right side
thyroid cartilage
ala

––– Incision line

····· Incision on opposite side
continued from dashed line

E

AG

Figure 99-21, cont'd E, Cartilage incisions for tumor confined to the superior portion of the piriform sinus. In this technique, the cricoid cartilage and the contralateral laryngeal pedicle are preserved. The cartilage cut preserves the inferior cornu of the ipsilateral cartilage. This procedure is basically an extension of a supraglottic laryngectomy and includes resection of the entire preepiglottic space.

with biopsy and mapping of the tumor, and biopsies of adjacent areas provide information to determine whether transposed tissue such as a pectoralis flap or jejunal interposition will be required. In the United States, more than 75% of tumors of the hypopharynx are in the piriform sinus. When confined to one side, total laryngectomy with partial pharyngectomy is the most common surgical procedure, provides satisfactory margins, and requires the least postoperative care. However, surgical margins cannot always be totally assessed preoperatively. Submucosal extension, particularly inferiorly and across the posterior pharyngeal wall, requires a more complex reconstruction. In most circumstances, primary reconstruction with the preserved contralateral piriform sinus mucosa provides an adequate conduit for swallowing. Too tight a closure, however, invariably leads to stricture or fistula.[167] The neopharyngeal closure should at

least accommodate a No. 14 Salem Sump NG Tube plus the esophageal cardiac lead.

When only a small strip of posterior wall mucosa remains (2.5–3 cm) after resection, a rolled pectoralis major myocutaneous flap can be used (Figure 99-22). Cusumano and others[50] and Schuller[235] recommended the tubed pectoralis major myocutaneous flap to reconstruct pharyngoesophageal defects.[269] This flap has a high success rate. Major problems include fistula formation and stricture at the flap esophageal anastomosis.[225] Swallowing is delayed with this procedure compared with gastric pull-up or jejunal interposition procedures. The major advantage of the technique is that it is possible in elderly or debilitated patients. Such flaps work more effectively when they are not completely circumferential.[263] Even preservation of 2.5 cm of posterior pharyngeal or contralateral piriform mucosa greatly improves swallowing and decreases stenosis. The soft tissue underlying the skin may preclude formation of a pliable tube. The skin paddle should be at least 9 to 10 cm wide to form a tube and usually cannot be longer than 12 cm.

TOTAL HYPOPHARYNGEAL RECONSTRUCTION

Resection of large or circumferential hypopharyngeal malignancies requires total laryngopharyngectomy. As reported by Gluckman and others[89] and Harrison,[101] there is a need for a 5- to 6-cm resection inferiorly or into the cervical esophagus. Options for reconstruction include local regional flaps, colon interposition, free jejunal interposition, and gastric pull-up (Figure 99-23).

Two techniques are preferred for total hypopharyngeal reconstruction. The first method is jejunal interposition, which allows excellent reconstruction if there is no cervical esophageal extension. It can be performed in patients who have recurrence or persistence after radiotherapy. It has the shortest period of rehabilitation, and swallowing is possible in 10 to 18 days (Figure 99-24). The second favored procedure is the gastric pull-up. It is required when there is more extensive disease or when total esophagectomy is indicated (e.g., in postcricoid carcinoma where there may be skip lesions; (<6% of postcricoid carcinomas).

The stomach is mobilized with care to maintain the right gastroepiploic artery. The short gastric vessels are ligated, the lesser curvature of the stomach freed, and the left gastric vessel ligated. A pyloromyotomy is performed. The entire esophagus is carefully dissected away from the trachea bluntly from the abdominal and cervical approach. The distal esophagus is separated from the stomach, and the gastroesophageal junction is closed with staples. With care, the stomach

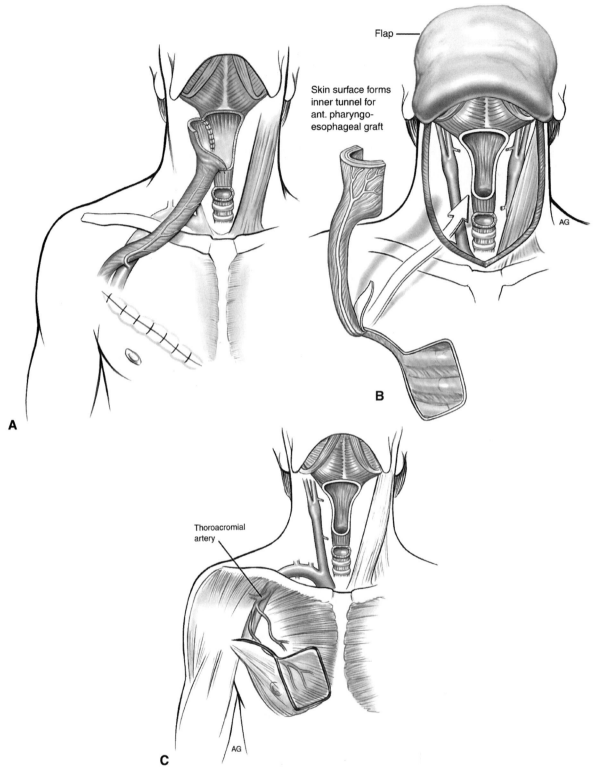

Figure 99-22. A, Rolling of the pectoralis major myocutaneous flap to reconstruct the hypopharynx. The lower anastomoses should be carefully designed to reduce the likelihood of stricture. **B,** In a pectoralis major myocutaneous flap, an 8- × 10-cm skin paddle is outlined and raised on the long axis of the pectoral branch of the thoracoacromial artery. **C,** Outline of the skin paddle over the pectoralis muscle for hypopharyngeal reconstruction. When soft tissue is excessive, a split-thickness skin graft can be applied directly to the muscle to reduce the bulk of the paddle.

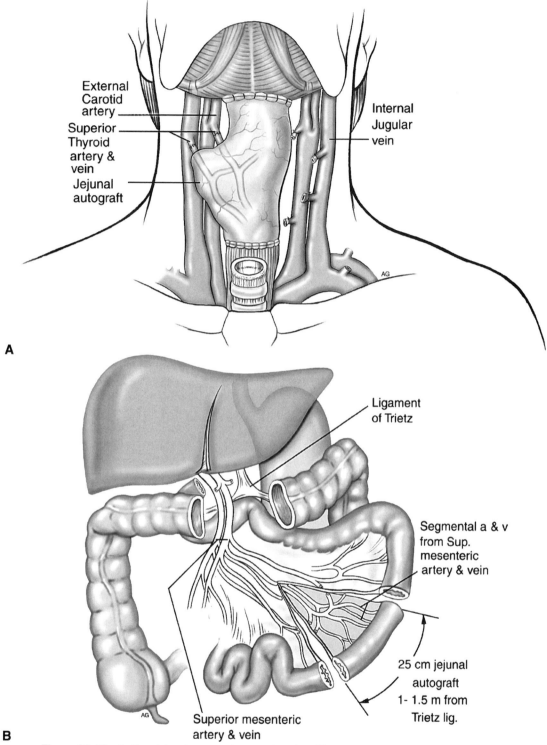

Figure 99-23. A, Free jejunal segment reconstruction. The mesenteric artery is anastomosed to the superior thyroid or external carotid artery. Vein anastomosis to the facial thyroid or end-to-side to the jugular vein is another option. Preservation of a jugular vein is required. Vein is anastomosed to the superior thyroid (facial). **B,** A segment of jejunum is isolated with a complete arcade and an adequate length of the mesenteric artery and vein.

Continued

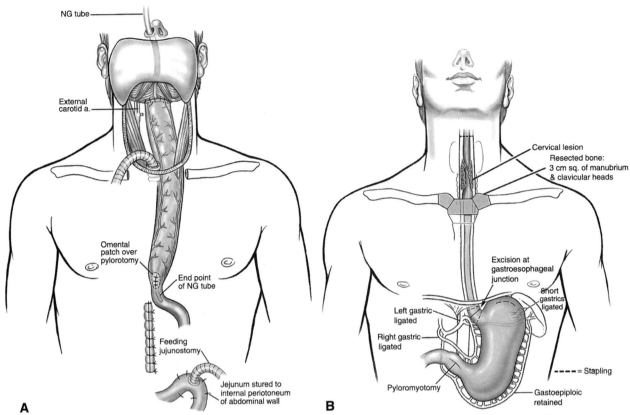

Figure 99-24. A, Gastric transposition. The stomach is passed through the posterior mediastinum. Pyloromyotomy enhances food passage. A jejunostomy will be used for decompression and for temporary feeding. Jejunostomy may be retained when postoperative radiation is planned. **B,** The advantage of the gastric pull-up procedure is no anastomosis within the abdomen or mediastinum. The single anastomosis occurs near the thoracic inlet. Ligation of the short gastric vessels and left gastric artery permits rotation of the greater curvature of the stomach upward through the tunnel created at the time of resection of the esophagus. The stomach is placed in a plastic bag, which allows gentle passage through the posterior mediastinum to the neck.

is passed through the previous esophageal bed into the neck. If necessary so that there is absolutely no compression, a segment of the manubrium and clavicle is resected. Swallowing is permitted in 10 days. Rehabilitation seems to be equal to that for the jejunal technique. The advantage of this method is no intraabdominal anastomosis is required (Figure 99-25 and Table 99-3).

As institutions have acquired greater experience with the gastric pull-up procedure, it has become the most widely accepted reconstruction procedure after total laryngopharyngectomy for postcricoid carcinoma and for any hypopharyngeal carcinoma extending into the cervical esophagus. The advantages of no anastomosis in the abdomen and a single anastomosis in the neck have been the reason for this preference. An endoscopic approach to releasing the stomach and passage through the posterior mediastinum has lessened the morbidity. Radiation can be given postoper-

atively and has not adversely affected the healing results. This procedure has an increased risk when applied in those patients who have had radiation fail or when it has been used primarily for palliation.

Increasing experience with laparoscopic surgery has permitted two major advances that have decreased both the time and morbidity of total laryngopharyngoesophagectomy. Laparoscopic harvest of the jejunal segment for hypopharyngeal reconstruction was achieved by Wadsworth and others.[285] A feeding jejunostomy would also be placed laparoscopically, allowing for early enteral feeding.

Additional studies have demonstrated the decreased morbidity of laparoscopic surgery combined with thorascopic surgery for total esophagectomy.[55,72,293,305] By pulling the stomach into the left lower cervical incision, the anastomosis can be completed.

The jejunal interposition remains an excellent reconstructive technique. The disadvantage is the

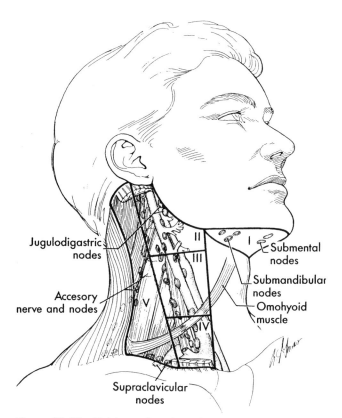

Figure 99-25. Divisions of neck nodes as defined by Sloan-Kettering Memorial Cancer Center. Levels II, III, and IV should be resected at the time of primary resection; even in clinical findings, comprehensive neck dissection including levels I and V is indicated.

(labels on figure: Jugulodigastric nodes; Accesory nerve and nodes; Supraclavicular nodes; II; III; V; IV; I; Submental nodes; Submandibular nodes; Omohyoid muscle)

intraabdominal anastomosis, the increased morbidity, and it may not be able to bridge a large defect. The lower, or jejunal esophagus anastomosis, is the most technically difficult and is not easily performed when it is the low level of the manubrium. The jejunum interposition has an advantage of its higher reach, almost to the skull base if necessary.

The myocutaneous flap reconstruction has the least morbidity and is the preferred technique when a nearly complete laryngopharyngectomy is required and when it is believed safe to retain at least 3 cm of the posterior wall of the hypopharynx. Retaining 3 cm of the contralateral hypopharyngeal wall limits the vascular supply to this tissue and may result in fistula or resultant stricture.

The least effective reconstructive maneuver is the deltopectoral flap. It usually requires a series of operative procedures to control leaks, permit swallowing, and the reconstruction is prone to stricture. It is generally used as a last resort.

The forearm free flap offers an ideal reconstruction in certain circumstances. Notably, posterior wall defects as with the myocutaneous flap are most effective when some mucosa can be preserved. Its lack of

bulkiness and pliability make it an excellent choice in certain circumstances.

The morbidity, mortality, and strictures have limited the use of colon interposition. Its only use at this time is when there is a reason one of the other more favored techniques cannot be used.

Patients who would have undergone a total laryngectomy are now evaluated for possible management with combined chemotherapy and radiotherapy. Avoidance of total laryngectomy in patients who show a complete or partial response to chemotherapy has been a recent goal in head and neck cancer management. The goal to reduce distant metastases and preserve a functional physiologic larynx is very attractive. Studies have not shown any survival advantage over standard surgery for T_3 to T_4 cancer of the larynx. However, survival with or without the larynx intact does not decrease with this protocol when surgical salvage is accepted.

MANAGEMENT OF THE NECK IN HYPOPHARYNGEAL CANCER

Simultaneous with the decision on management of the primary hypopharyngeal malignancy, management of the neck should be decided. As noted in the preceding series for hypopharyngeal lesions, particularly of the piriform sinus, the incidence of occult neck disease varies from 30% to 40%. Thus, the neck should be addressed and managed, even if N_0.

Medina[173] classified the nodal zones affected in modified neck dissection. Among the five nodal groups in the neck, regions II, III, and IV are associated with the jugular vein and should be cleared in every neck dissection for hypopharyngeal cancer (Figure 99-26).

Patients who have palpable cervical metastases, N_1, N_2, and N_3 disease are uniformly managed by comprehensive neck dissection. Candela and others[41] reviewed the metastatic patterns of cervical node metastases in patients with hypopharyngeal malignancies. Of 222 cases of hypopharyngeal malignancies, 91 had piriform sinus malignancies, 35 had posterior pharyngeal wall malignancies, and 4 were postcricoid tumors. It was evident that for piriform sinus tumors with N_0 necks, levels II and III were the areas primarily involved. However, in cases of N-positive nodes, levels II, III, and occasionally IV were involved, but levels I and V also showed substantial involvement. These findings were similar for posterior pharyngeal wall lesions and were different from laryngeal lesions. They concluded that a modified or anterior neck dissection could be considered appropriate in patients with N_0 necks but recommended comprehensive neck dissection in any patient who had clinically positive nodes.

TABLE 99-3

METHODS OF HYPOPHARYNGEAL RECONSTRUCTION

Methods	Advantages	Disadvantages	Complications
Hemipharyngectomy/ hemilaryngectomy	Single-stage, uses adjacent tissue, no stenosis, use in limited posterior wall tumors	Tumor limited to one side, no esophageal extension, no involvement of preepiglottic space or vallecula	Fistula in 29% to 50%
Pectoralis major myocutaneous flap	Less-than-total pharyngectomy, single-stage	Thick flap, stenosis, inability to swallow solids, 60% success	Fistula, adverse effect of radiation
Deltopectoral flap	Thin flap	At least two, often four, stages; stricture formation; poor swallowing	Fistula, stenosis, inability to swallow solids
Radial forearm free flap (fasciocutaneous)	Thin malleable tissue, partial or total pharyngectomy, no abdominal procedure	Requires microvascular anastomosis, short distance only	Adynamic flap necrosis
Free jejunal graft	Single-stage, early rehabilitation (10–18 days)	Total pharyngectomy requires microvascular anastomosis, abdominal anastomosis, and temporary gastrostomy	Success rate is 90%, graft necrosis
Gastric pull-up	Best choice for total esophagectomy, no intraabdominal anastomoses	Necrosis of graft	Mortality is 8% to 15%, complication rate is 26% to 50%
Colon transposition	Single-stage, delayed if jejunum fails	Requires dilation of stenosis, poor swallowing results, two intraperitoneal anastomoses	Esophageal stump

When disease is more limited, the standard neck dissection can be modified if radiotherapy is to be delivered postoperatively. At issue is whether postoperative radiotherapy should always be administered in the patient with palpable nodes who has undergone a complete neck dissection. In the early 1970s, a series of reports suggested that cervical metastatic disease is preferably managed by surgery followed by radiotherapy. This provided better regional control but did not necessarily extend survival.

Ogura and others[192] reported their experience with 98 cases of piriform sinus cancer. Palpable cervical nodes were present in 52% of patients, and occult nodes found during surgery occurred in 38%. No patient who had negative nodes result at presentation or occult nodes found to be positive at the time of surgery experienced recurrence in the neck. However, in 21% of patients who had palpable nodes, neck recurrence developed despite radical neck dissection. Assuming that patients who had recurrence in the neck after radical neck dissection almost uniformly die of disease, Ogura and others[192] thought that radical neck dissection was indicated.

There are still some unresolved issues regarding the contralateral neck. If postoperative radiation therapy is planned, it is always included in this field. Johnson and others[117] retrospectively reviewed 169 patients with hypopharyngeal carcinoma. They found a significant incidence of failure rate in the contralateral neck in medial wall piriform sinus cancer compared with lateral wall lesions. They attribute this to involvement of the marginal zone as is often the case in supraglottic malignancies.

Like Johnson, Murakami[180] is also an advocate for bilateral neck dissections in all but T_2 lesions of the hypopharynx. They found the presence of contralateral metastases in 30% of the hypopharyngeal specimens studied and in 70% of ipsilateral neck specimens. Tumors that extend superiorly toward the inferior tonsil pole may have retropharyngeal space lymph node involvement. At present, the issue is not resolved, but the need to address the contralateral neck by either surgery or radiation is required. Preoperative radiologic evaluation is required to evaluate for retropharyngeal node involvement and contralateral neck metastases.

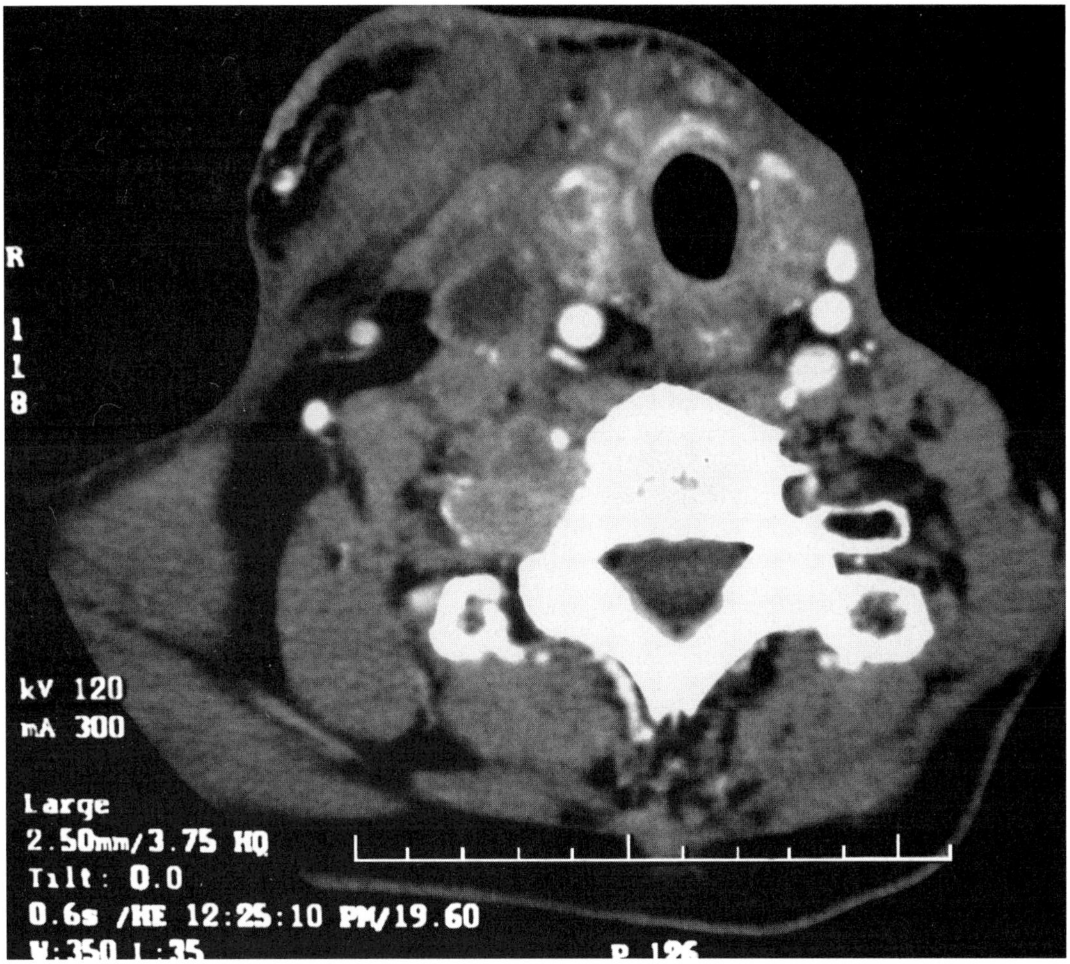

Figure 99-26. Metastatic carcinoma of the piriform sinus presenting with retropharyngeal node involvement. Prevertebral space involvement with early involvement of the cervical spine.

Barkley and others[15] compared 596 patients with neck disease with a control group whose primary tumor was controlled but had recurrence in the neck. The goal was to determine whether postoperative radiotherapy was of value when given electively after modified or radical neck dissection. Postoperative radiotherapy was administered if there were positive margin findings, CIS at the margins, extension of tumor outside the larynx, positive nodes at many levels, or evidence of extracapsular extension. There were no delayed failures in the neck in patients with N_1 and N_2 disease managed by surgery followed by radiation, whereas cervical recurrence developed in 12 of 38 patients managed by surgery alone. They concluded that combined surgery and radiotherapy was the preferred management for patients with N_1 and N_2 disease.

Leemans and others[147] recommend that the indications for postoperative radiotherapy include positive nodes at many levels, extranodal extension, and the presence of more than one positive node. Patients in this study had a comprehensive or standard radical neck dissection. They found a direct correlation between the number of positive nodes in the surgical specimen and the incidence of recurrent disease. The rate of recurrence was 2.6% in N_1, 9.1% in N_2, and 11.3% in N_3 necks. They concluded that patients with one or two positive nodes, regardless of extranodal extension, had the same rate of recurrence as did those who had more extensive neck disease; overall recurrence rate in a surgically managed neck was 7.2%.

Most studies support the use of postoperative radiation for local control,[78] although increased survival has not been shown for patients with N_1 and N_2 cervical disease.[9,35] The issue that then arises in the management of the clinically N_0 neck is whether surgery alone, radiation alone, or a combination is preferred.

Often, the decision is based on the management of the primary tumor.[115,192] For example, if radiation alone is used for the primary tumor, it can be extended to manage the clinically N_0 neck. To control the N_0 neck, a minimum dosage of 5000 rad is required. If radiation is intended to control an N_1 neck, then a minimum dosage of 6500 rad is required. Higher dosages of radiotherapy do not increase control of metastatic disease but have a higher incidence of complications.

In 1992, Marks and others[163] elaborated on the likelihood of contralateral lymphatic metastases for hypopharyngeal carcinoma. They noted that midline cancers of the glossoepiglottic fold and marginal supraglottic cancers had the highest incidence of contralateral metastatic disease. Importantly, the development of contralateral metastatic disease was not related to the size of the primary tumor. The likelihood of the presence of contralateral positive cervical adenopathy was four times greater in patients who were initially seen with palpable ipsilateral cervical adenopathy.

Most studies, however, suggest that when postoperative radiotherapy is to be administered, control of the contralateral neck can be obtained with approximately 6000 rad. In contrast to supraglottic malignancies, contralateral neck dissection is reserved for patients who have palpable nodal disease. If the tumor extends across the midline, contralateral neck dissection, usually modified, is performed.

SELECTION OF TREATMENT FOR PATIENTS WITH HYPOPHARYNGEAL CARCINOMA

Selection of treatment for a particular patient must take into consideration a large number of variables. First, and most importantly, is the general health and status of the patient. Patients with hypopharyngeal carcinoma almost always have some underlying respiratory disease, chronic obstructive lung disease, or emphysema. They may have coronary artery arteriosclerosis or carotid artery disease. There is often a history of alcoholism with associated cirrhosis. Because this disease occurs most often in older individuals, diabetes must also be considered. Although the extent and size of a tumor might determine a preferred treatment, these underlying factors may exclude that recommendation. For example, a patient with chronic lung disease will not be a candidate for an operative procedure that might result in some degree of chronic aspiration. Similarly, radical radiation to the larynx may also compromise this important laryngeal function. The full extent of the disease must first be established. Unlike laryngeal malignancies, which can often be fully assessed and photographed in an endoscopy suite, hypopharyngeal carcinomas may extend into

the cervical esophagus, extend to the posterior wall and cannot be fully assessed in the office setting. General anesthetic is often required to fully determine the extent of the lesion and particularly to see if the lesion is mobile on the posterior wall. CT radiologic assessment cannot determine whether there is prevertebral space invasion unless it is extending into the underlying cervical spine (Figure 99-27). Surgery with curative intent will be excluded when there is apparent prevertebral space involvement, retropharyngeal lymph node involvement, fixation to the carotid artery, or extension into the superior mediastinum or into more than the immediately adjacent cervical esophagus.

It is apparent that a multidisciplinary team is essential from the time of diagnosis for planning the most effective treatment for the patient. For example, a percutaneous endoscopic gastrostomy (PEG) will not be placed when a gastric pull-up is planned. Selection of the reconstruction modality should be made at the time of this initial intervention. Another example of a multidisciplinary issue is that if combined modality therapy or regional flap reconstruction is considered, it is worthwhile to place a PEG at this time and perform necessary dental extractions.

Review of the literature demonstrates that T_1 and selective T_2 lesions can be adequately treated with radiation therapy, although there are many advocates for hyperfractionation in this group of patients. Still, management of the neck will require surgical intervention, because radiation therapy seems to be less effective in managing cervical disease compared with the primary site. Patients with select early lesions may also be candidates for limited surgical intervention as described by Weinstein.[297]

More advanced lesions, T_3 or greater, which is the bulk of patients initially seen with piriform sinus cancer will require at least radiation therapy and surgery, with many advocating now a role for chemotherapy. The standard of treatment for such patients has been laryngopharyngectomy with neck dissection followed by postoperative radiation therapy to be initiated within 6 weeks of resection. Because of data from randomized prospective studies demonstrating that the larynx can be preserved in 40% to 50% of patients even with advanced disease, a role for multimodality therapy has arisen. There are two primary reasons for chemotherapy to be considered. First, in the organ preservation studies, chemotherapy may be given initially to assess the patient for response. Patients not responding are considered a particularly high-risk group and proceed to standard surgery with postoperative radiation. Individuals who respond to induction chemotherapy fall into a more favorable group. In this group, radiation therapy with concomitant

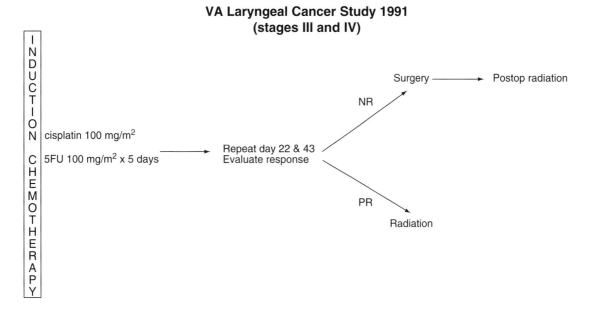

Figure 99-27. Schematic of VA Laryngeal Preservation Study.

chemotherapy may provide the same overall results with preservation of the larynx. However, as noted earlier in this chapter, the need for early detection and recognizing an incomplete response require immediate surgery, including neck dissection. Even when there is a complete response at the primary site, any suggestion of residual disease in the neck should be addressed with surgical intervention. Surgical salvage when performed for late recurrence carries a poor prognosis and a higher morbidity.

Second, in the initial assessment of a large number of patients, up to 30% might be found to be surgically inoperable on initial evaluation. The presence of metastatic disease in the mediastinum or metastatic disease in the lung or fixation to the surrounding structures may determine whether the patient is not operable. These patients can be treated with full-course radiation therapy, with evidence that the survival may be enhanced by combining chemotherapy with radiation therapy.[2]

Even in the best circumstances there remains a high likelihood of recurrent disease in all patients seen with hypopharyngeal carcinoma, thus necessitating the need for all members of the head and neck oncology team to see and assess the patient initially. Simply put, 30% of patients with early T_1 lesions will have recurrence, and the survival rate for patients with advanced disease is 30%. These figures have been unchanged with the advent of the numerous additional modalities. These modalities have length-ened survival and have allowed selected patients to preserve their larynx. Overall survival, however, has not been greatly affected by the combination of therapies that are now available for these patients, especially those with advanced disease. This relates not only to the high incidence of regional failure in the cervical nodes but also the high incidence of distant metastases and second primary malignancies that occur in this group of patients, as well as comorbidity factors.

ORGAN PRESERVATION OF THE LARYNX AND HYPOPHARYNX

In the early 1980s, a series of studies suggested that the addition of chemotherapy preoperatively or before radiation may enhance the survival rate for patients with advanced head and neck malignancies. A second goal was to, if not change survival, allow for less surgery and potentially even reduce the bulkiness of a malignancy before initiation of treatment with either radiation or surgery.

In 1983, Ensley and others[66] demonstrated a correlation between the response to a cisplatinum-based chemotherapy regimen followed by radiation therapy in patients not previously treated for head and neck squamous cell carcinoma. Their initial study included 77 patients treated with cisplatinum, vincristine, and bleomycin infusions, and they were able to obtain a 29% complete response (CR) rate and a 51% partial response (PR) rate. They had even better results with a combination of cisplatinum and a 5-day infusion of 5-fluorouracil (5-FU). Ultimate survival of this group of patients was not altered by the preoperative administration of chemotherapy. Further analysis of the patients did demonstrate a correlation between those who responded to the cisplatinum regimen and the later response to radiation therapy. Interestingly, the size and stage of the disease did not always correlate with the response achieved. Large metastatic tumors exhibiting central necrosis are believed to be poorly oxygenated, and this could account for the poorer response to chemotherapy and radiation. But, some smaller tumors without these characteristics also failed to respond, suggesting that there are additional mechanisms to explain the response rate to chemotherapy.

A series of studies reported in the mid-1980s demonstrated the feasibility of the use of induction chemotherapy to select patients who might avoid surgery and proceed directly to radiation or radiation/chemotherapy. Patients who achieved a CR or PR, and especially a pathologic CR, were reported by Jacobs and others and Demard and others.[54,113]

Jacobs and others[113] in 1987 thought that patients who had a complete response to the induction chemotherapy would not require surgery but could proceed to radiation therapy. Again, a combination of cisplatinum and 5-FU was used for the chemotherapy, and 12 of 30 patients achieved a complete pathologic response. Nonresponders proceeded to surgery. An especially good response was achieved, because 60% of the patients had a complete clinical response and 30% a PR with a 43% overall CR in both the primary and neck. Repeat biopsy, however, demonstrated that 16 of 18 thought to be complete responders still had residual disease. The oropharynx was noted to have the highest incidence of complete clinical response. Although this study suggested that patients having a complete pathologic response to induction chemotherapy might not require surgery, it also showed the need for confirmation of complete clinical response with pathologic response and the need to re-biopsy of the primary site.

Demard and others[54] in France reported on an evaluation of 81 patients with pharyngolaryngeal cancer. In this group, 51% of the laryngeal and 54% of the hypopharyngeal cancers showed a complete response to the regimen of cisplatinum plus 5-FU. That group went on to definitive radiation therapy and avoided surgery. Although overall survival remained poor, this study again showed in those patients who achieved a CR had a more favorable outcome and could avoid laryngectomy. They also caution that patients who have only a partial response or no response must undergo surgical resection.

Urba and Wolf[277] reviewed the application of neoadjuvant chemotherapy from the 1970s for organ preservation. They recognized that with current therapy, 50% of patients would have a local recurrence, there was a high incidence of secondary malignancy, and 30% of patients had distant metastatic disease develop. It was their initial hope that the advent of the addition of chemotherapy might affect these results. They also recognized that the chemotherapy might not necessarily be effective in changing survival but more effective in selecting out a group of patients who would have a more favorable prognosis regardless of additional treatment. Recognition of this finding led to the development of prospective studies that used cisplatinum and 5-FU with the intent not of changing survival but of maintaining the same survival and avoiding laryngectomy or laryngopharyngectomy. As in other studies, the regimen Wolf and others selected was three cycles of cisplatinum (100 mg/m^2) and 5-FU continuous infusion for 5 days given at 15-day intervals. Those who had a CR went on to radiation therapy, whereas those having a PR would have standard surgery followed by postoperative radiation therapy. Patients with primary laryngeal cancer fared better than those with hypopharyngeal carcinoma. Again, in a response rate of 86%, CR and PR was achieved with this regimen, and 51% of patients did not require laryngectomy.

Two phase II laryngeal preservation studies were undertaken between 1986 and 1991 at the MD Anderson Cancer Center.[45,245] A three-cycle regimen of cisplatinum, bleomycin, and 5-FU was used in an effort to preserve the larynx in 55 patients with advanced disease who responded to this induction chemotherapy regimen. They were able to achieve a combined PR and CR rate of 75% in laryngeal cancers and 78% in hypopharyngeal cancers. These individuals went on to definitive radiation therapy, whereas nonresponders underwent surgery. A twice-daily hyperfractionation regimen was used at the primary site of 76.6 Gy. There was no difference in survival between the responders who received chemotherapy and definitive radiation therapy vs the nonresponders who went on to laryngectomy. However, as far as the site of recurrence, those patients in the laryngeal preservation arm had a higher incidence of local recurrence. There was no reduction in the incidence of distant metastatic disease.

It was these and other studies that provided the rationale for the large Veterans Affair (VA) laryngeal cancer study in 1991. This was the first large prospective randomized study to demonstrate the effectiveness of the use of chemotherapy to define the more favorable patients and avoid laryngectomy in responders.

This multiinstitutional VA study reported on 332 patients who, if they responded, were given two to three cycles of 5-FU and cisplatin chemotherapy followed by radiotherapy; nonresponders underwent surgery.[307] Survival with laryngeal anatomic preservation was compared with that for standard surgery and postoperative radiotherapy. A radiotherapy-only arm was not part of this study. The first report suggested 66% of patients randomly assigned to receive chemotherapy and radiation had laryngeal preservation, although only 39% had a fully functioning larynx. In a follow-up evaluation of this landmark group of patients at 60 months, a further 10% drop in the number of those with a functioning larynx was noted.[110]

There was criticism that the VA study did not contain a radiation-therapy-only arm (Figure 99-28). Radiation therapists had advocated that radiation alone could result in retention of the larynx in 50% of patients with T_3 disease and that the effect of chemotherapy was limited. The National Cancer Institute Intergroup then conducted an extensive prospective randomized study that included 517 patients randomly assigned to three arms (Figure 99-29).[76,295] Limited T_4 malignancies were included, that is, question of early cartilage invasion or early invasion into the tongue base. The results showed that concomitant chemotherapy with radiation therapy had a longer time until need for laryngectomy, but both groups ultimately did not show a statistical difference between the chemotherapy/radiation therapy group and radiation therapy for ultimate laryngeal preservation.

HYPOPHARYNGEAL ORGAN PRESERVATION PROTOCOLS

Head and neck surgeons, radiation therapists, and oncologists recognize that organ preservation has become an acceptable treatment concept for the management of advanced laryngeal, hypopharyngeal, and tongue-based malignancies and offers an alternative to the standard treatment of surgery followed by postoperative radiation therapy.

In 1996, the European Organization for Research and Treatment of Cancer (EORTC) reported 3- and 5-year preliminary results for patients given conventional surgery and postoperative radiotherapy vs chemotherapy followed by definitive radiotherapy (Figure 99-30).[148] All patients would have required a total laryngectomy and partial pharyngectomy. Chemotherapy consisted of cisplatin (100 mg/m²) and a 5-day infusion of 5-FU (1000 mg/m²/day). Patients who did not show a CR or PR after two cycles underwent standard surgery. Responders received a third cycle of chemotherapy followed by

EORTC Head & Neck Cancer Cooperative Group

Larynx & Piriform Sinus Preservation Study

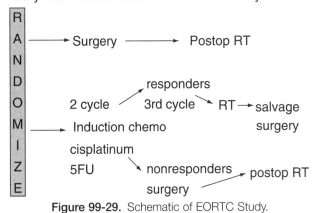

Figure 99-29. Schematic of EORTC Study.

LARYNGEAL PRESERVATION STUDY

Schema

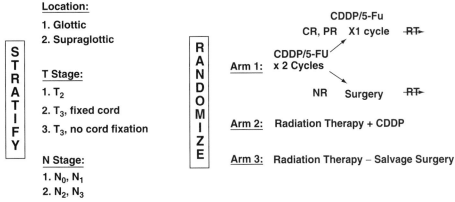

Figure 99-28. Schematic of NCI Intergroup Study.

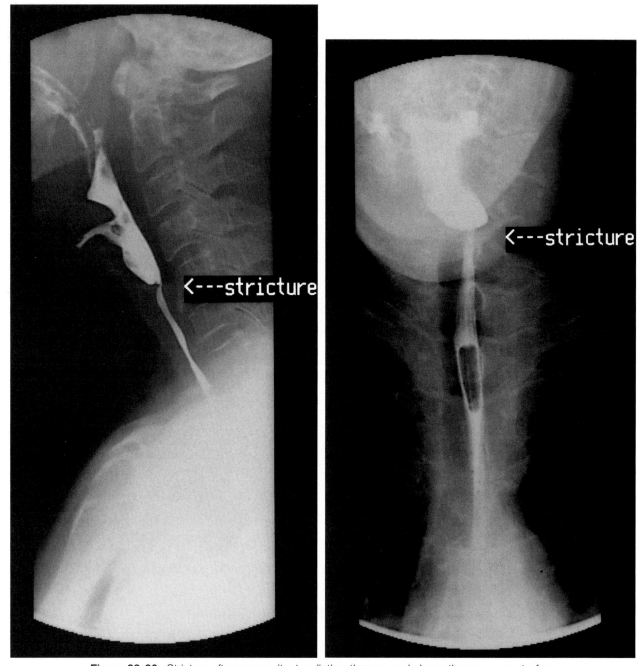

Figure 99-30. Stricture after concomitant radiation therapy and chemotherapy as part of an organ preservation protocol.

definitive radiotherapy. Both arms had equivalent survival results, but 42% of patients retained a functional larynx. The study suggested that the laryngeal preservation study could be applied to select patients with hypopharyngeal malignancy. There was a higher incidence (36%) of distant metastases in the surgery-only arm than in the chemotherapy arm (25%). This was not thought to be a statistical difference, and more distant metastases could potentially occur with further follow-up. Locoregional failure

was the reason for death in most cases, although a high number in both groups had distal disease or second primary malignancies. This study specifically excluded patients who would require complicated reconstruction for hypopharyngeal malignancy, that is, patients requiring myocutaneous flaps or gastric or jejunal interposition.

Kraus and others[134] studied 110 patients prospectively enrolled in a laryngeal preservation cisplatin and radiation protocol. The sites included hypopharynx, oropharynx, and larynx and required generally healthier patients for enrollment. Thirteen nonresponders and 18 management failures received laryngectomy. Complications of surgery included a 42% fistula rate. When laryngectomy was required, a neck dissection was necessary. Recurrent disease was difficult to detect.

In a prospective study of organ preservation in patients with stages III and IV hypopharyngeal carcinoma, Clayman and others[45] administered induction chemotherapy. Twenty-nine patients received at least two cycles of cisplatin and 5-FU. Responders received an additional course of chemotherapy followed by radiotherapy. Nonresponders underwent laryngectomy. Persistent neck disease was managed surgically. Nine patients required laryngectomy, and 13 were disease free with the larynx preserved. All four patients with T_4 cancer died.

These results are not supported by Marks and others,[165] who reported an overall survival rate for 93 patients of 34.6% for surgery alone vs 7.1% for resectable patients receiving radiotherapy with or without chemotherapy. Surgical salvage occurred when radiation was not successful. They cautioned against considering organ preservation protocols for patients with hypopharyngeal cancer.

Likewise, Poulsen and others[217] found disappointing survival results in 314 patients with oral cavity, oropharyngeal, and hypopharyngeal cancer undergoing induction chemotherapy. The 130 responders to the chemotherapy regimen were divided into 57 patients who received surgery and postoperative radiotherapy and 73 patients who received radiotherapy alone. Patients who had a CR to chemotherapy or were managed with surgery and radiotherapy had a 90% 5-year survival rate vs 56% for responders managed with radiotherapy. There was no significant difference in the partial responders, whereas the 5-year survival was 59% for the surgery/radiation group and 53% for the radiation-only group. They believe there is a role for surgery even in patients achieving a CR.

Zelefsky and others[318] administered cisplatin-based induction chemotherapy before radiotherapy in 26 nonrandomized patients with advanced but resectable carcinoma of the hypopharynx. They compared the results with those of 30 patients managed with standard surgery and postoperative radiotherapy. A CR to chemotherapy was achieved in 12 patients (46%), and a partial overall response was achieved in 6 patients (23%). The 5-year local control rate for T_3 to T_4 tumors was essentially identical in both groups (52%), and neck recurrence occurred in approximately one-third of patients. Distant metastases developed in 23% of the chemotherapy group and 40% of the surgery group. The 5-year absolute survival rate for the

chemotherapy/radiation group was 15%, 22% for the surgery group, and approximately 25% of each group died from intercurrent disease. Although this study is not definitive because of the lack of randomization, it suggests that protocols for organ preservation applied to laryngeal cancer may be applied to hypopharyngeal cancer in select situations.

Samant and others[232] assessed 25 patients with advanced piriform sinus squamous cell carcinoma and studied the effect of intraarterial cisplatinum with concomitant radiation therapy in an effort to achieve organ preservation in a small group of patients with more advanced disease. They reported a 92% complete response rate at the primary site, with a 76% response in the neck with this intensive regimen. These results were reported as significantly better than previous reported studies for advanced hypopharyngeal cancer including the EORTC study. In this study only one patient had a recurrence at the primary site, and 78% of the patients were able to swallow adequately at 1 year.

With the general acceptance of the role of chemoradiation as a potential for laryngeal preservation, studies have turned to assess different chemotherapy combinations[14] and modifications in daily vs twice-daily radiation therapy. Such a study was performed by Prades in France in which he combined chemoradiation first using carboplatinum only with bifractionated radiation therapy and compared it with carboplatinum 5-FU and once-daily radiation therapy.[219] In both arms, 60% of the patients were able to retain a functional larynx. Although there was a slight advantage to the twice-daily radiation therapy arm, the overall survival at 2 years was 58% in the twice-daily radiation arm and 50% in the once-daily arm. The overall disease-free survival at 2 years was not significant, with 39% survival in the twice-daily radiation/chemotherapy arm and 41% in the once-daily radiation/chemotherapy arm.

To assess the effectiveness of new treatments, especially the size reduction of these solid tumors in response to nonsurgical treatments, guidelines have been published by the NCI.[270] The longest diameter of the tumor must be decreased by 30% to be recognized as a PR. This is easier to evaluate in cervical metastases and oropharyngeal tumors but more difficult in laryngeal and hypopharyngeal primary sites. CT or MRI may permit evaluation of response in those sites.

An intensive regimen of paclitaxel and 5-FU, as well as hydroxyurea and hyperfractionated radiation therapy, was reported by Kies and others.[125] This regimen consisted of a 5-day infusion of paclitaxel with 20 mg/m² per day plus 5-FU 600 mg/m² per day plus hydroxyurea 500 mg every day combined with twice-daily radiation therapy for a total of five cycles. The performance status of this group of patients who had multiple head and neck sites was 0 or 1 Eastern Cooperative Oncology Group (ECOG). There was an overall 92% locoregional control at 3 years in this advanced group of patients. This intensive regimen made it difficult with patients with PR having negative biopsies and those with CR clinically having a positive biopsy. This confirms the complexity of assessing response to these intensive regimens.

Beauvillain and others[22] reported on 92 patients with advanced T_3 or T_4 hypopharyngeal carcinomas who received preoperative neoadjuvant chemotherapy. Again, the combination of cisplatinum and 5-FU was selected. Patients were randomly assigned to receive either total laryngopharyngectomy and postoperative radiation therapy or radiation therapy alone. In this study, randomization was performed before determining the effect of the chemotherapy. In contrast to some of the other reported studies, patients receiving surgery and postoperative radiation therapy did have statistically better overall 5-year survival of 37%, whereas those going on to radiation therapy only had a 5-year survival of 19%. This was attributed to the overall better locoregional control rate in the patients undergoing surgery. Because response to chemotherapy was not considered in the selection of radiation or surgery, this study adds to the evidence already compiled that response to chemotherapy may select patients who will have a better overall survival.

Karp and others[122] presented their data on combining cisplatinum and 5-FU for hypopharyngeal malignancies. Their study was interesting in that the patients with hypopharyngeal malignancy who initially had the same rate of response to the chemotherapy/radiation therapy had only a 33% 2-year local control rate compared with 77% control for patients with primary laryngeal cancer.

Pignon and others[214] reviewed the literature on the use of chemotherapy as part of the treatment regimen in advanced head and neck cancer. Their meta-analysis of six trials, which included 851 patients, demonstrated only a 4% absolute benefit at 2 and 5 years. They thought that the addition of chemotherapy had a minimal effect on survival. As in other studies, the most significant effects were seen with concomitant radiation/chemotherapy. In assessing laryngeal preservation trials, they believed that there might be an advantage in laryngeal cancer, but this was not apparent in hypopharyngeal malignancies. They caution against accepting neoadjuvant or adjuvant chemotherapy as part of locoregional control as accepted therapy.

In general, however, the concept of organ preservation whether by radiation therapy alone or with con-

comitant chemotherapy has become acceptable,[77] perhaps because of the high patient acceptance of this concept. The particular regimen that would have the least morbidity and be most patient acceptable is still being assessed.[278] There is criticism that these studies did not show the effect on voice quality or particularly on swallowing with potential for stricture development (Figure 99-30). Current studies have a closely associated swallowing assessment pretreatment and posttreatment. Besides a thorough swallowing assessment, there is a quality-of-life instrument being used to assess the ultimate patient experience. Dependence or not on gastrostomy feedings is not an acceptable method to quantitate the adverse effects on swallowing and voice. A more sophisticated evaluation of these areas is required. The barium swallow alone, although helpful, does not always predict the patient's capability to swallow.[270] Some specific issues still need to be addressed: proper patient selection, the frequent need for a pretreatment-placed gastrostomy, the need to maintain this gastrostomy for several months after completion of therapy, and the effectiveness of the preserved larynx for speech and swallowing.

Detection of Recurrent Disease

From the surgical oncologist's view, detection of recurrent disease and its management is difficult. Recall that in all studies, at least 40% of the patients on these protocols will eventually require surgery. Patients will have had not only a full course of radiation therapy but will have received chemotherapy as well. Fortunately, the effects on wound healing with platinum-based regimens has not been as severe as that reported by Corey and others[48] when methotrexate-based regimens were used. Still, there are prolonged wound healing and increased incidence of all wound complications. The incidence of fistula is higher in patients receiving salvage therapy.[52,134,146,234,295]

Early detection of neck recurrence in the firm radiated neck is always difficult. Some advocate frequent use of the CT scan to supplement clinical impression. The advent of the PET scan may ultimately be useful in detecting early recurrence. In the posttreated neck, recurrence may be extracapsular or into the muscles or soft tissue rather than the lymph nodes. These recurrences are difficult to assess even at the surgical neck dissection let alone preoperatively. Because recurrence may be extracapsular, the role of a modified neck vs a radical neck dissection has to be assessed. Is a neck dissection required for an N_2 neck that has had a complete clinical response? There seems to be uniform agreement that the need for surgery in an N_3 neck regardless of the response is required.[233] N_0 and N_1 necks generally do not require surgery if both CT and clinical examination demonstrate a CR.[233] Many authors favor surgery for the N_2 neck as well when the patient was staged with an N_2 neck at the initial diagnosis regardless of the response.[145,229,261,308] If at the completion of therapy, residual disease is detected at the primary malignancy or in the neck either by CT or clinical examination, there is a need for surgery, which should be performed at the earliest possible time.[308] There are advocates of waiting at least 3 months to assess the response before advocating surgical intervention; however, after 8 weeks, the effects on the soft tissues within the neck make surgical resection more difficult.

Early recognition of recurrent disease in the larynx or hypopharynx is also difficult in this situation. In almost all cases, there is mucositis lasting for up to 6 weeks after this combined therapy, with edema of the supraglottic laryngeal structures. Paralyzed or fixed vocal ligament pretreatment may not regain function. Biopsy has been reported to increase the likelihood of chondritis. Posttreatment CT has been more accurate than clinical examination.

McGuirt and others[170] have researched this problem extensively. The PET scan in their study was the most accurate and effective means of demonstrating recurrent or residual disease. Even biopsies may miss a recurrence deeper in the soft tissues, and a negative biopsy can be misleading. In both the hypopharynx and laryngeal prospective organ preservation studies, patients require a planned laryngectomy shortly after completion of radiation when residual disease is suspected. This group did as well as those in the previous combined surgery/postoperative radiation therapy protocols. Those undergoing surgery for later recurrence did poorly. This further accentuates the need to recognize early recurrent disease.

MANAGEMENT OF THE NECK IN ORGAN PRESERVATION STUDIES

In all organ preservation protocols, management of the neck and of the primary site must be considered both individually and together. There is no uniform agreement on the management of the neck in patients when there has been a CR to treatment in both the primary malignancy and in the neck. There is agreement that if any residual disease remains within the neck after completion of radiation and chemotherapy, either by CT scan or by clinic examination, neck dissection is indicated.

In the initial VA study by Wolf,[307] of the 106 patients who underwent combined chemotherapy and radiation therapy, 46 had N_2 or N_3 neck disease. A CR to treatment was obtained in 18 of the 46 patients (39%) with advanced neck disease and a PR in 16 of the 46 patients (35%). There was no response in 12 patients (26%). Fifty percent of the complete responders had N_2 disease, and 33% had N_3 disease. These data demonstrate that there is not a direct correlation between initial node size and response. In fact, in 24% of the patients, response in the neck was better than that obtained at the primary site. Among the 18 patients who obtained a CR in the neck, 5 eventually required a neck dissection. Among the 28 patients who had less than a CR, 19 underwent neck dissection. When there was a delayed recurrence in the neck, survival was poor, less than 30%. When a poor response was obtained in the neck to the combined therapy treatment, salvage by surgery still gave a poor outcome. Wolf, like others, reports the difficulty in detecting early cervical recurrence and recommends early neck dissection in those patients with any question of residual disease as soon as feasible after completion of radiation therapy.

In an organ preservation study, Lavertu[145] examined the presence of residual tumor in patients with N_2 and N_3 nodal disease on completion of treatment. In this group, 67% of patients with a persistent mass had residual positive adenopathy in neck dissection. Even 33% of the complete responders still had positive cervical disease at surgery. Only in patients with N0 and N_1 disease in which a CR was obtained did it seem to be reasonable not to undertake a neck dissection. Of those 53 patients with N_2 and N_3 disease, 23 had a PR and 30 had a CR. Thirty-five patients underwent neck dissection, but 4 of 18 of the complete responders still had residual malignancy in the specimen, and 8 of 17 patients with PRs remained with positive disease.

These authors also concluded that neck dissection was useful when advanced cervical disease was present at the initiation of organ preservation treatment. In an evaluation of oropharyngeal malignancy with metastatic disease in organ preservation studies, Strasser[261] demonstrated that patients with N_2 or N_3 disease had a significant incidence of residual disease after treatment in the neck. Eight of 12 partial responders still had positive findings at surgery, as did two of three complete responders. They, too, advocated the postradiation therapy neck dissection.

In an organ preservation study by Roy and others[229] of 37 patients with N_2, N_3 disease with oropharyngeal cancer, 3 of 9 patients with CR both by clinical examination and CT had residual positive adenopathy at the time of neck dissection. Notably, two-thirds of patients with clinical or CT residual disease in the neck had pathologically confirmed positive nodes. In contrast, a study by Peters and others[213] that used definitive radiation therapy for an oropharyngeal malignancy with nodal disease <3 cm, found no positive histologic findings at neck dissection. They concluded that the size of the node at the initiation of treatment did not correlate with response.

Although most of the studies were for oropharyngeal cancer (tonsil, base of tongue), they provide the only data in the literature demonstrating the relationship of initial nodal disease to response in organ preservation protocols. Current recommendations include neck dissection in all patients with residual disease, either clinically or on CT scan on completion of organ preservation therapy.[8] This surgery is technically easier to perform within 6 to 8 weeks on completion of treatment. There are data to support routine neck dissection in such individuals when the initial adenopathy was >3 cm. Large series data are not available to make a definitive recommendation for the management of the neck when there has been a complete clinical and CT scan response. The decision to perform a neck dissection in such cases is easier if residual disease remains at the primary site as well. Regardless of treatment, when neck disease recurs late, salvage surgery is recommended, but with poor data to substantiate a change in overall survival.

SURGICAL SALVAGE AFTER RADIATION THERAPY

There is an increasing trend toward radiation therapy with concomitant chemotherapy as the first line of treatment for laryngeal and hypopharyngeal carcinoma.[272] Patients who fail to respond to the initial chemotherapy proceed directly to surgery and postoperative radiation. Surgery is also reserved for those patients who recur later whether at the primary site or in the neck. Surgery is occasionally required for chondronecrosis, where the larynx is rendered ineffective to protect the airway during swallowing. The importance and difficulty of early detection of residual or recurrent disease has been discussed.

Radiation therapy has adverse effects on soft tissue, particularly cartilage, by causing increasing fibrosis.[109] There are suggestions that combined radiation and chemotherapy, although more effective in the management of the cancer, may also adversely increase these unwanted effects, particularly the effects on small vessels with intimal proliferation leading to fibrosis and decreased tissue vascularity, which is important in the area of surgical healing.[111] Although this process begins after completion of the radiation therapy, it is progressive for the next year. Surgery, then, during this period is not only technically more difficult but also has an increased risk of postoperative complications.

J. Davidson and others[52] recorded their experience with 88 patients undergoing salvage surgery after radi-

ation therapy without chemotherapy. Five-year survival for recurrent disease was 35%. The survival rate did not correlate with the TNM stage of the original tumor or the time until recurrence was apparent. As expected, the highest rate of surgical complications occurred in patients undergoing pharyngectomy (48%), with pharyngocutaneous fistula occurring in 27% of patients. A pretreatment tracheostomy did not correlate with survival in their study.

Sassler's[234] retrospective study of patients undergoing surgery after organ preservation protocols revealed an overall complication rate of 61%. His study showed that the rate of complications was 77% when surgery was performed within 1 year of treatment and only 20% when performed after 1 year. This was in direct contrast to the Davidson study. In this study and in all others, the risk of complications was associated with entrance into the pharynx. Neck dissection only had a much more acceptable complication rate. Sassler reported a fistula rate of 50% with a mean time until closure of 7.7 months. The use of regional or revascularized flaps improved the results in obtaining a closure.

Panje and others[206] also reported their experience in recurrent cases after multidrug chemotherapy and radiation therapy. They also noted not only the increased incidence of wound complications but there was a delay in the onset of these complications, with the median time to presentation of 22 days. He suggested that the combined treatment had an effect on stem cell depletion with resultant adverse effect on cell repair. This effect was not seen in those patients receiving induction chemotherapy only.

Wound healing and fistula formation in patients undergoing surgical salvage in the NCI Intergroup study was reported by Weber and others.[295] The fistula rate was 30%, which was considered equivalent to the rates reported for radiation therapy alone. This study also did not find a correlation with the timing of the surgery.

Both Lavertu[146] and B. Davidson[51] in their separate studies showed a higher rate of complications (20% and 22%, respectively) when neck dissection only was used with no difference between a modified and a radical neck dissection.

In selection of patients for laryngeal preservation studies, it must be recognized that 40% of these patients will eventually require surgery. The overall survival at 5 years for the recurrent group of patients is generally in the range of 35%. Surgery in such patients when laryngopharyngectomy is required will result in the fistula rate reported from 30% to 60%. The addition of the neck dissection at the time of surgery does not necessarily increase the risk of wound complications. Importantly, though, in most studies, the time to recovery for such fistulas is substantially longer than that reported when patients undergo a laryngectomy as primary initial treatment. Wound infection rate and delay in healing may be related to other metabolic and general health factors of the patient and cannot be attributed to the radiation/ chemotherapy only. When this group of patients requires surgery, their general nutritional status, thyroid status, and general health should be maximized before undertaking surgical intervention.

RARE LARYNGEAL MALIGNANCIES
Sarcomas

Cancers can arise from the structural elements of the larynx; these tumors are usually sarcomas. Although rare, they have a reportable incidence. Chondrosarcoma is the most frequent sarcoma, followed by fibrosarcoma. Other tissue types generally have been reported in single cases, and any management consideration is difficult based on the lack of information.

Chondrosarcomas that arise from hyaline cartilage have been reported by Lewis and others[150] and Nicolai and others.[189] Lewis and others[150] reported on 47 laryngeal cartilage tumors and suggested 44 were low-grade malignancies, whereas three were classified as benign. Similar to previous studies,[189] 70% were based on the cricoid cartilage, whereas 20% were related to the thyroid cartilage, 10% originated on an arytenoid, and only one was epiglottic. Growths originating from the elastic cartilage are not clearly low-grade sarcoma, because some authors regard them as metaplastic cartilage.[60,176] The cytology of the tumor has made the distinction between chondroma and low-grade malignancy difficult in past reports, but Lewis and others[150] thought there was a clear histologic pattern consistent with low-grade malignancy.

Management of this lesion has always been surgical. Because the histologic patterns suggest very slow growth, cases regarded as chondromas can be managed by local enucleation, whereas low-grade chondrosarcoma is usually managed by external laryngeal surgery with partial laryngectomy or by endoscopic resection. Total laryngectomy is reserved for histologically or clinically aggressive lesions, whereas recurrence may require complete laryngectomy. Metastases have been reported; however, most deaths are caused by advanced local disease. This conservative approach resulted in a death rate similar to an age-matched population without tumor and, therefore, conservative management is recommended with neck dissection only for clinical or radiographic metastases.

Nakayama and others[186] reported a differentiated aggressive form with histologic characteristics of fibrosarcoma or osteosarcoma. This aggressive, rare (5%–10%) pattern had a mean survival of 6 months. It is unclear whether the literature reflects a reporting bias to aggressive and lethal disease, because single case reports suggest more active disease than a longitudinal report based on a single institution's experience.

Kaposi's sarcoma is the most frequent malignancy in acquired immunodeficiency syndrome (AIDS). The lesion is often purple or violaceous and polypoid and may involve the glottis, supraglottis, or the aryepiglottic folds. The lesion may appear cystic and is usually not ulcerated. The gross appearance is easily differentiated from squamous cell carcinoma in most cases. Occasionally, a superinfection with fungus makes clinical diagnosis difficult until the infection has cleared.

The lesion differs from that seen in elderly men of Mediterranean or Jewish ancestry and that in Africans who are human immunodeficiency virus (HIV) negative. It has been hypothesized that Kaposi's sarcoma is a reactive phenomenon and would regress if the underlying immunodeficiency were fully reversed as seen in renal transplant patients.

Management with radiotherapy is reported to show a response in 90% of cases, with complete lesion disappearance only in 20%. AIDS patients are very radiosensitive with respect to mucositis edema and radiation-induced dysphagia. Therefore, the dose needs to be moderated in managing this disease. One report suggested a dose per fraction of 2 Gy to a total management dose of 20 Gy with management possible for regrowth of the lesion. Cytoprotective chemicals such as amifostine may allow higher dosing in the future.

Intralesional vinblastine injection for previously unmanaged Kaposi's sarcoma using 0.1 mm/cm^2 of lesion surface has been suggested with monthly management until the lesion was completely flat,[80] whereas Tami and Sharma[266] reported complete resolution of a large lesion with 3 mL of the same solution. Surgery is usually not indicated for these lesions, although laser excision has been used to control the airway obstruction with repeat management as indicated. Controlling the vapor, which may contain viable HIV particles, is most important.

Lymphoma

Laryngeal lymphomas are seen as a mucosa-covered mass in the supraglottic larynx. Workup for staging is required to establish whether the disease is limited to the larynx. In those cases confined to the larynx, radiation therapy is an effective treatment. Only 86 reported cases were noted by 1986.[62] Most laryngeal lymphomas have been B-cell lymphomas in AIDS patients and in nonimmunocompromised hosts. They seem to be arising from the mucosal associated lymphoid tissue. Several cases have been reported in association with AIDS, and a recent T-cell lymphoma was reported in 1995.[250] Management with 3000 Gy is indicated for lymphoma and controls the laryngeal lesion satisfactorily with no recurrence. Long-term follow-up is difficult in AIDS patients, because their primary infectious disease and its complications have not allowed long survival in the past.

Adenocarcinoma

Salivary gland carcinoma is very unusual in the larynx; only 1 of 281 laryngeal cancers were noted by Adams and Duvall[1] to be glandular, as were 18 of 2967 reviewed by Cohen and others.[46] It is suggested that these occur where glandular tissue is seen histologically; in one study, 14 tumors presented supraglottic and four presented subglottic. The literature reports two adenoid cystic carcinomas for each adenocarcinoma, and more than 300 cases have been reported to date. The lesions generally present as submucosal masses without ulceration and present with symptoms typical of the region. Therefore, subglottic tumors have more opportunity to invade deeply, because symptoms are only noted late. Reporting in 1985, the recommendation was for an elective neck dissection for adenocarcinoma, whereas the histologic presentation of adenoid cystic carcinoma does not merit elective neck surgery. Distant extension has frequently been through perineural and hematologic spread, and distant metastasis is present, often without regional disease. As is true of adenoid cystic carcinoma elsewhere, this distant disease is occasionally very stable with slow growth, and therefore, aggressive local management is suggested even in the presence of pulmonary nodules.[97,251]

Salvage after regional recurrence has been successful but has always been associated with distant disease. Radiotherapy generally has been reserved for recurrent disease. In view of a significant risk of metastasis from these tumors, the 5-year survival of 12% to 17% is not surprising.[97]

Mucoepidermoid carcinoma has been reported at about the same frequency as adenocarcinoma. Again, it is primarily supraglottic.[251] The histologic presentation among those reported is similar to that of the major salivary glands, and management should be tendered on the same basis, with conservation surgery without neck dissection for low-grade tumors and elective management of at least the ipsilateral neck and combined surgery and radiation for high-grade malignancies.

Neuroendocrine Carcinoma

Neuroendocrine tumors in the larynx are rare lesions presumed to arise from the amine precursor uptake and decarboxylase (APUD) cells; theoretically, the tumor arises from neuroendocrine cells originating in the neurocrest, which are disbursed throughout body organs, including the larynx. Wenig and others[303] favor endoderm as the site of origin rather than the neurocrest. Small cell cancer involving the larynx was first noted in 1972[200] and has been described with some frequency. The World Health Organization[241] categorizes malignant neuroendocrine tumors of the larynx as carcinoid, atypical carcinoid, and small cell carcinoma. Moisa,[175] Porto and others,[216] and Batsakis and others[18] thought only 13 true carcinoids had been reported as of 1991. The reported carcinoids have been noted to be supraglottic tumors often on the arytenoids or the aryepiglottic fold; treatment based on the scant literature suggests that wide local resection is sufficient treatment, and neck dissection should be performed only if there is obvious clinical disease.

Atypical carcinoids are the most frequent neuroendocrine tumor of the larynx. There is a male preponderance in these tumors, which usually occur in the sixth and seventh decade. Woodruff and Senie[309] noted 127 cases of atypical carcinoid in a literature review and recognized frequent cervical metastases (43%) and distant metastases (44%). Their review suggested 5-year survival of 48% and 30% at 10 years. Lesions seem to be primarily supraglottic, and many patients have had increased calcitonin levels. Total laryngectomy is the primary modality of treatment recommended with elective neck dissection performed because of the high rate of cervical metastases. Chemotherapy and radiation treatment have not been shown to be effective.[71] Symptoms at presentation are similar to squamous cell carcinoma, although the physical examination may show a variable appearance of a tumor that may be polypoid, pedunculated, nodular, or ulcerated but is usually submucosal. The tissue is almost always positive for cytokeratin, carcinoembryonic antigen, and epithelial membrane antigen. The tumors usually stain positive for calcitonin and occasionally for S100 protein. Electromicroscopy usually reveals neurosecretory granules 70 to 420 mm in diameter.[70,160] Ferlito and Friedman[69] found local control to be good, with nodal and distal disease causing death in these patients.

Small cell carcinoma is a disease that carries a very poor prognosis, with 5% survival. It is regarded as a systemic disease even with single site presentation, but usually when present in the larynx is recognized with both nodal and distal metastases on diagnosis.[70] Laryngeal cases often show submucosal lesions with ulceration and can present as glottic, subglottic, or supraglottic tumors. Because virtually all patients are dead within 2 years, management should not include aggressive or disabling surgery as priority treatment. Most cases of small cell carcinoma have widespread disease; the longer survival in cases presenting in the larynx compared with those primary in the lung may result from earlier symptom presentation in the former situation. This would allow a longer natural history being measured from the time of diagnosis. Local lesions may be cleared by chemotherapy with local radiation to the neck considered as the least disabling form of therapy.[91]

Immunocytochemical studies have been similar to those in other small cell carcinoma series, with cytokeratin, neuron-specific enolase, and chromogranin all showing positive staining.[205] It is important to recognize the systemic nature of this diagnosis even if the only presentation is in the larynx. Management should begin with chemotherapy and not surgery, reserving the latter for laryngeal lesions that do not resolve. This seems to be the least disabling management and offers an equal tumor-free interval before death from the disease.[21] There is little in the surgical or pathologic literature suggesting electromicroscopy is important in helping to distinguish among the three neuroendocrine cancers and their benign counterpart; paraganglioma. It is suggested that the immune histochemical battery replaces ultrastructure by electromicroscopy to make a correct diagnosis. There is an overlap in the size of neurosecretory granules recognized on electromicroscopy that limits the use of granule size in categorizing the tumors.

Wick has recently tabulated the three malignant neuroendocrine carcinomas into group I tumors (epithelial) and grades them on the basis of their virulence: grade I (carcinoid), grade II (atypical carcinoid), and grade III (small cell neuroendocrine carcinoma). Laryngeal paragangliomas (benign) are group listed under group II tumors (neuro).[304]

Extramedullary Plasmacytoma

This rare malignancy can present in the region of the supraglottic larynx, subglottic area, or upper trachea. It may present as a smooth-covered pedunculated mass causing airway obstruction, and there can be more than one mass in the region. When biopsy confirms the presence of extramedullary plasmacytoma, it is necessary to make certain that this is not a manifestation of multiple myeloma. An appropriate systemic assessment is necessary. The patient needs to be followed indefinitely for the possible later development of multiple myeloma as well. This malignancy can be treated by surgical resection, which is sufficient if margins are adequate, or by radiation therapy. Most are treated with radiation therapy. Surgery is used when the mass can be resected without substantial morbidity or functional loss. If that would be required, radiation therapy becomes the preferred modality.[296]

SUMMARY

Carcinoma of the larynx remains one of the most common head and neck malignancies. Early recognition by the patient and physician and limited metastatic potential of early glottic lesions has given it one of the highest cure rates. Early malignancies are managed by limited surgery or limited radiotherapy. If the tumor is in the supraglottic area or subglottic region, however, more extensive surgery is indicated, and the neck should undergo radiotherapy or surgery. Recent studies showed that supraglottic malignancy has a high potential of metastases to both sides of the neck, and, therefore, even lateral supraglottic lesions require bilateral supraomohyoid neck dissection. Surgery and radiotherapy provide equal cure rates for early lesions. Choice of management may depend on other factors (e.g., age, patient request, need to retain a healthy voice). Recently, a great deal of attention has been paid to laryngeal preservation studies and protocols. A prospective randomized study showing 39% of patients who ordinarily would have required total laryngectomy can undergo radiotherapy and retain a functional larynx has made a major impact on the management of moderately advanced laryngeal cancer. The final conclusions of the prospective studies in this area have not been established, but in properly selected cases, less aggressive surgery can be offered. Management of the neck for laryngeal cancer still requires a modified neck dissection.

Despite this progress, carcinoma of the hypopharynx continues to have one of the poorest prognoses of all head and neck malignancies. Most patients have metastatic disease or tumors too large for voice-saving operative procedures or primary radiation.

These patients have a high incidence of second primary malignancies and synchronous tumors. Thus, thorough preoperative assessment includes endoscopic evaluation of the entire upper aerodigestive tract to make certain that a synchronous tumor is not present. CT of the head and neck permits evaluation of the extent of the tumor and nodal disease and is of particular value in determining direct extension of the tumor mass into the soft tissues.

In the rare situation in which an early tumor is encountered, patients may be suitable candidates for full-course radiotherapy or voice-conserving limited resection. Even in these cases, the neck should be addressed. In these patients, tumors that are suitable for primary radiation could also be considered for conservation surgery. The status of the cervical nodes, CT evaluation, and institutional preference may determine which mode of therapy is used for these early lesions.

Most studies have shown improved locoregional control when surgery with radiation is used. These results have not necessarily translated into improved survival.[282] Overall survival relates primarily to stage of disease at presentation, particularly to the status of the cervical lymph nodes. Prospective evaluation of the role of chemotherapy is under way. It is hoped that chemotherapy may reduce the incidence of distant metastatic disease and allow for less radical surgical resection (organ preservation). Current chemotherapy trials have not changed the recommendation for surgery and postoperative radiation as standard management.

REFERENCES

1. Adams GL, Duvall AJ: Adenocarcinoma of the head and neck, *Arch Otolaryngol Head Neck Surg* 93:261, 1971.
2. Adelstein DJ and others: An intergroup phase III comparison of standard radiation therapy and two schedules of concurrent chemoradiotherapy in patients with unresectable squamous cell head and neck cancer, *J Clin Oncol* 21:92, 2003.
3. Almadori G and others: Human papillomavirus infection and epidermal growth factor receptor expression in primary laryngeal squamous cell carcinoma, *Clin Cancer Res* 7:3988, 2001.
4. Alonso JM: Conservative surgery of cancer of the larynx, *Trans Am Acad Ophthalmol Otolaryngol* June-July:633, 1947.
5. Ambrosch P, Kron M, Steiner W: Carbon dioxide laser microsurgery for early supraglottic carcinoma, *Ann Otol Rhin Laryngol* 107:680, 1998.
6. Amdur RJ and others: Organ preservation with radiotherapy for T1-T2 carcinoma of the piriform sinus, *Head Neck* 23:353, 2001.
7. Andrew K and others: Role of alcohol and tobacco in the etiology of head and neck cancer: a case-control study in the Doubs region of France, *Eur J Cancer* 31:301, 1995.
8. Armstrong J and others: The management of the clinically positive neck as part of a larynx preservation approach, *Int J Radiat Oncol Biol Phys* 26:759, 1993.
9. Arriagada R and others: The value of combining radiotherapy with surgery in the treatment of hypopharyngeal and laryngeal cancers, *Cancer* 51:1819, 1983.
10. Asherson N: Pharyngectomy for postcricoid carcinoma: one stage operation with reconstruction of the pharynx using the larynx as an autograft, *J Laryngol Otol* 68:550, 1954.
11. Axon PR and others: Carcinoma of the hypopharynx and cervical esophagus in young adults, *Ann Otol Rhin Laryngol* 109:590, 2000.
12. Axon PR and others: A comparison of surgery and radiotherapy in the management of post-cricoid carcinoma, *Clin Otolaryngol* 22:370, 1997.
13. Bakamjian VY: Total reconstruction of pharynx with medially based deltopectoral skin flap, *N Y State J Med* 68:2771, 1968.
14. Bardini R, Ruol A, Peracchia A: Therapeutic options for cancer of the hypopharynx and cervical oesophagus, *Ann Chir Gynaecol* 84:202, 1995.
15. Barkley HT Jr. and others: Management of cervical lymph node metastases in squamous cell carcinoma of the tonsillar fossa, base of tongue, supraglottic larynx, and hypopharynx, *Am J Surg* 124:462, 1972.
16. Barzan L, Comoretto R: Hemipharyngectomy and hemilaryngectomy for piriform sinus cancer: reconstruction with remaining larynx and hypopharynx and with tracheostomy, *Laryngoscope* 103:82, 1993.
17. Bastit L and others: Influence of the delay of adjuvant postoperative radiation therapy on relapse and survival in oropharyngeal and hypopharyngeal cancers, *Int J Radiat Oncol Biol Phys* 49:139, 2001.
18. Batsakis JG, El Naggar AK, Luna MA: Neuroendocrine tumors of larynx, *Ann Otol Rhinol Laryngol* 101:710, 1992.
19. Batsakis JG and others: The pathology of head and neck tumors: verrucous carcinoma. Part 15, *Head Neck Surg* 5:29, 1982.
20. Bauer WC, Lesinski SG, Ogura JH: The significance of positive margins in hemilaryngectomy specimens, *Laryngoscope* 85:1, 1975.
21. Baugh RF and others: Small cell carcinoma of the larynx: results of therapy, *Laryngoscope* 96:1283, 1986.
22. Beauvillain C and others: Final results of a randomized trial comparing chemotherapy plus radiotherapy with chemotherapy plus surgery plus radiotherapy in locally advanced resectable hypopharyngeal carcinomas, *Laryngoscope* 107:648, 1997.
23. Beckhard RN and others: Factors influencing functional outcome in supraglottic laryngectomy, *Head Neck* 16:232, 1994.
24. Bertazzi PA and others: Cancer mortality of an Italian cohort of workers in man-made glass-fiber production, *Scand J Work Environ Health* 12:65, 1986.
25. Biel AM, Maisel RH: Indications for performing hemithyroidectomy for tumors requiring total laryngectomy, *Am J Surg* 150:435, 1985.
26. Biller HF and others: Hemilaryngectomy following radiation failure for carcinoma of the vocal folds, *Laryngoscope* 80:249, 1970.
27. Biller HF, Lawson W: Partial laryngectomy for vocal cord cancer with marked limitation or fixation of the vocal cord, *Laryngoscope* 96:61, 1986.
28. Biller HF and others: Planned pre-operative irradiation for carcinoma of the larynx and laryngopharynx treated by total and partial laryngectomy, *Laryngoscope* 79:1387, 1969.
29. Blackwell KE, Calcaterra TC, Fu Y: Laryngeal dysplasia: epidemiology and treatment outcome, *Ann Otol Rhinol Laryngol* 104:596, 1996.
30. Bocca E: Supraglottic cancer, *Laryngoscope* 85:1318, 1975.
31. Bocca E: Surgical management of supraglottic cancer and its lymph node metastasis: a conservative perspective, *Ann Otol Rhinol Laryngol* 100:261, 1991.
32. Bocca E, Pignataro O, Mosciaro O: Supraglottic surgery of the larynx, *Ann Otol Rhinol Laryngol* 77:1005, 1968.
33. Boyle JO and others: Gene mutations in saliva as molecular markers for head and neck squamous cell carcinomas, *Am J Surg* 168:421, 1994.
34. Brennan JA, Myers AD, Amsjakek BW: The intra-operative management of the thyroid gland during laryngectomy, *Laryngoscope* 101:929, 1991.
35. Briant TDR, Bryce DP, Smith TJ: Carcinoma of the hypopharynx: a five year follow-up, *J Otolaryngol* 6:353, 1978.
36. Bron L and others: Functional analysis after supracricoid partial laryngectomy with cricohyoidoepiglottopexy, *Laryngoscope* 112:1289, 2002.
37. Burch JD and others: Tobacco, alcohol asbestos and nickel in the etiology of cancer of the larynx: a case-control study, *J Natl Cancer Inst* 67:1219, 1981.
38. Byers RM: Modified neck dissection: a story of 967 cases from 1970-1980, *Am J Surg* 150:414, 1985.
39. Byers RM, Wolf PR, Ballantine AJ: Rationale for elective modified neck dissection, *Head Neck Surg* 10:160, 1988.

40. Calcaterra TC: Tongue flap reconstruction of the hypopharynx, *Arch Otolaryngol Head Neck Surg* 109:750, 1983.
41. Candela FC, Kothari K, Shah JP: Patterns of cervical node metastases from squamous carcinoma of the oropharynx and hypopharynx, *Head Neck Surg* 12:197, 1990.
42. Carpenter RJ III and others: Cancer of the hypopharynx: analysis of treatment and results in 162 patients, *Arch Otolaryngol Head Neck Surg* 102:716, 1976.
43. Chevalier D, Piquet JJ: Subtotal laryngectomy with cricoidhyoidopexy for supraglottic carcinoma: review of 61 cases, *Am J Surg* 168:472, 1994.
44. Clayman GL and others: Human papillomavirus in laryngeal and hypopharyngeal carcinomas: relationship to survival, *Arch Otolaryngol Head Neck Surg* 120:743, 1994.
45. Clayman GL and others: Laryngeal preservation for advanced laryngeal and hypopharyngeal cancers, *Arch Otolaryngol Head Neck Surg* 121:219, 1995.
46. Cohen J and others: Cancer of the minor salivary glands of the larynx, *Am J Surg* 150:513, 1985.
47. Cooper JS and others: Second malignancies in patients who have head and neck cancer: incidence, effect on survival and implications based on the RTOG experience, *Int J Radiat Oncol Biol Phys* 17:449, 1989.
48. Corey JP and others: Surgical complications in patients with head and neck cancer receiving chemotherapy, *Arch Otolaryngol Head Neck Surg* 112:437, 1986.
49. Cragle SP, Brandenburg JH: Laser cordectomy or radiotherapy: cure rates, communications and cost, *Otolaryngol Head Neck Surg* 108:648, 1993.
50. Cusumano RJ and others: Pectoralis myocutaneous flap for replacement of cervical esophagus, *Head Neck Surg* 11:450, 1989.
51. Davidson BJ and others: Complications from planned, posttreatment neck dissections, *Arch Otolaryngol Head Neck Surg* 125:401, 1999.
52. Davidson J and others: The role of surgery following radiotherapy failure for advanced laryngopharyngeal cancer, *Arch Otolaryngol Head Neck Surg* 120:269, 1994.
53. Deleyiannis FWB, Piccirillo JF, Kirchner JA: Relative prognostic importance of histologic invasion of the laryngeal framework by hypopharyngeal cancer, *Ann Otol Rhinol Laryngol* 105:101, 1996.
54. Demard F and others: Response to chemotherapy as justification for modification of the therapeutic strategy for pharyngolaryngeal carcinoma, *Head Neck Surg* 12:225, 1990.
55. DePaula AL and others: *Transhiatal approach for esophagectomy*. In Toouli J, Gossot D, Hunter JG, editors: *Endosurgery*, New York, Churchill Livingstone, 1999, p 293.
56. DeSanto LW: Cancer of the supraglottic larynx: a review of 260 patients, *Otolaryngol Head Neck Surg* 93:705, 1985.
57. DeSanto LW: Early supraglottic cancer, *Ann Otol Rhinol Laryngol* 99:593, 1990.
58. DeStefani E and others: Hand-rolled cigarette smoking and risk of cancer of the mouth, pharynx and larynx, *Cancer* 70:679, 1992.
59. DeStefani E and others: Risk factors for laryngeal cancer, *Cancer* 60:308, 1987.
60. Devaney KO and others: Cartilaginous tumors of the larynx, *Ann Otol Rhinol Laryngol* 104:251, 1995.
61. Dickens WJ and others: Treatment of early vocal carcinoma: a comparison of apples and apples, *Laryngoscope* 93:216, 1993.
62. Diebold J and others: Primary lymphoplasmacytic lymphoma of the larynx: a rare localization of malt-type lymphoma, *Ann Otol Rhinol Laryngol* 99:577, 1990.
63. Dumich PS and others: Suitability of near-total laryngopharyngectomy in piriform carcinoma, *Arch Otolaryngol Head Neck Surg* 110:664, 1984.
64. Eckel HE, Thumfart WF: Laser surgery for the treatment of larynx carcinomas: indications, techniques, and preliminary results, *Ann Otol Rhinol Laryngol* 101:113, 1992.
65. El-Badawi SA and others: Squamous cell carcinoma of the piriform sinus, *Laryngoscope* 92:357, 1982.
66. Ensley JF and others: Correlation between response to cisplatinum-combination chemotherapy and subsequent radiotherapy in previously untreated patients with advanced squamous cell cancers of the head and neck, *Cancer* 54:811, 1984.
67. Fein DA and others: T_1-T_2 squamous cell carcinoma of the glottic larynx treated with radiotherapy: a multivariate analysis of variables potentially influencing local control, *Int J Radiat Oncol Biol Phys* 25:605, 1993.
68. Fenton JE and others: Hypopharyngeal tumours may be missed on flexible oesophagogastroscopy, *BMJ* 311:623, 1995.
69. Ferlito A, Friedmann I: Review of neuroendocrine carcinomas of the larynx, *Ann Otol Rhinol Laryngol* 98:780, 1989.
70. Ferlito A, and others: A review of neuroendocrine neoplasms of the larynx: update on diagnosis and treatment, *J Laryngol Otol* 12:827, 1998.
71. Ferlito A, Shaha AR, Rinaldo A: Neuroendocrine neoplasms of the larynx: diagnosis, treatment and prognosis, *ORL* 64:108, 2002.
72. Fernando HC, Christie NA, Luketich JD: Thoracoscopic and laparoscopic esophagectomy, *Semin Thorac Cardiovasc Surg* 12(3):195, 2000.
73. Fletcher GH, Jessee RH: The place of irradiation in the management of the primary lesion in head and neck cancers, *Cancer* 39:862, 1977.
74. Fliss DM and others: Laryngeal verrucous carcinoma: a clinical pathologic study and detection of human papilloma virus using polymerase chain reaction, *Laryngoscope* 104:146, 1994.
75. Foote RW and others: Patterns of failure after total laryngectomy for glottic carcinoma, *Cancer* 64:143, 1989.
76. Forastiere AA , and others: Phase III trial to preserve the larynx: induction chemotherapy and radiotherapy versus concomitant chemoradiotherapy versus radiotherapy alone, Intergroup trial R91-11, *Proc Am Soc Clin Oncol* 20:2A, 2001.
77. Forastiere A and others: Head and neck cancer, *N Engl J Med* 345:1890, 2001.
78. Forastiere AA, Trotti A: Radiotherapy and concurrent chemotherapy: a strategy that improves locoregional control and survival in oropharyngeal cancer, *J Natl Cancer Inst* 91:2065, 1999.
79. Frazer EJ: The development of the larynx, *J Anat Physiol* 44:156, 1909.
80. Friedman M and others: Intralesional vinblastine for treating AIDS-associated Kaposi's sarcoma of the oropharynx and larynx, *Ann Otol Rhinol Laryngol* 105:272, 1996.
81. Fretjie JE and others: Carcinoma of the larynx in patients with gastroesophageal reflux, *Am J Otol* 6:388, 1996.
82. Fu KK and others: The significance of laryngeal edema following radiotherapy of carcinoma of the vocal cord, *Cancer* 49:655, 1982.
83. Fu KK and others: A Radiation Therapy Oncology Group (RTOG) phase III randomized study to compare hyperfractionation and two variants of accelerated fractionation to standard fractionation radiotherapy for head

and neck squamous cell carcinomas: first report of RTOG 9003, *Int J Radiat Oncol Biol Phys* 48(1):7, 2000.

84. Garden AS and others: Early squamous cell carcinoma of the hypopharynx: outcomes of treatment with radiation alone to the primary disease, *Head Neck* 18:317, 1996.

85. Garden AS and others: Hyperfractionated radiation in the treatment of squamous cell carcinomas of the head and neck: a comparison of two fractionation schedules, *Int J Radiat Oncol Biol Phys* 31:493, 1995.

86. Geisler SA, Olshan AF: GSTM1, GSTT1, and the risk of squamous cell carcinoma of the head and neck: a mini-HUGS review, *Am J Epidemiol* 154:95, 2001.

87. Gillison ML and others: Evidence for a casual association between human papillomavirus and a subset of head and neck cancers, *J Natl Cancer Inst* 92:709, 2000.

88. Giron J and others: CT and MR evaluation of laryngeal carcinomas, *J Otolaryngol* 22:284, 1993.

89. Gluckman JF and others: Surgical salvage for stomal recurrence: a multi-institutional experience, *Laryngoscope* 97:1025, 1987.

90. Gluckman JL and others: Partial vs total esophagectomy for advanced carcinoma of the hypopharynx, *Arch Otolaryngol Head Neck Surg* 113:69, 1987.

91. Gnepp DR: Small cell neuroendocrine carcinoma of the larynx. A critical review of the literature, *ORL Otorhinol Rel Spec* 53:210, 1999.

92. Goldman JL and others: Combined therapy for cancer of the laryngopharynx, *Arch Otolaryngol Head Neck Surg* 92:221, 1970.

93. Goldstein F: *Dysphagia with iron deficiency (Plummer-Vinson syndrome, Paterson-Brown syndrome, sideropenic dysphagia)*. In Bockus HL, editor: *Gastroenterology*, ed 3, vol 1, Philadelphia, WB Saunders, 1974.

94. Griebie MS, Adams GL: "Emergency" laryngectomy and stomal recurrence, *Laryngoscope* 97:1020, 1987.

95. Guenel P and others: A study of the interaction of alcohol drinking and tobacco smoking among French cases of laryngeal cancer, *J Epidemiol Commun Health* 42:350, 1988.

96. Ha PK, Califano III JA: Molecular biology of laryngeal cancer, *Otolaryngol Clin North Am* 35:993, 2002.

97. Haberman PJ, Haberman RS: Laryngeal adenocarcinoma, otherwise specified, treated with carbon dioxide laser excision and postoperative radiotherapy, *Ann Otol Rhinol Laryngol* 101:920, 1992.

98. Hagen P, Lyons DG, Haindel C: Verrucous carcinoma of the larynx: role of human papillomavirus, radiation, and surgery, *Laryngoscope* 103:253, 1993.

99. Harrison DF: The pathology and management of subglottic cancer, *Ann Otol Rhinol Laryngol* 80:6, 1971.

100. Harrison DFN: Pathology of hypopharyngeal cancer in relation to surgical management, *J Laryngol Otol* 84:349, 1970.

101. Harrison DFN: Surgical management of hypopharyngeal cancer: particular reference to the gastric "pull-up" operation, *Arch Otolaryngol Head Neck Surg* 105:149, 1979.

102. Harrison DFN: Thyroid gland in the management of laryngopharyngeal cancer, *Arch Otolaryngol Head Neck Surg* 97:301, 1973.

103. Harwood AR, De Boer G: Prognostic factors in T_2 glottic cancer, *Cancer* 45:991, 1980.

104. Haughey BH and others: Meta-analysis of second malignant tumors in head and neck cancer: the case for an endoscopic screening protocol, *Ann Otol Rhinol Laryngol* 101:105, 1992.

105. Hicks WL and others: Patterns of nodal metastasis and surgical management of the neck in supraglottic laryngeal carcinoma, *Otol Head Neck Surg* 121:59, 1999.

106. Hiroto I and others: Pathological studies relating to neoplasms of the hypopharynx and the cervical esophagus, *Kurume Med J* 16:127, 1969.

107. Ho CM and others: Squamous cell carcinoma of the hypopharynx–analysis of treatment results, *Head Neck* 15:405, 1993.

108. Ho CM and others: Submucosal tumor extension in hypopharyngeal cancer, *Arch Otol Head Neck Surg* 123:959, 1997.

109. Hom DB, Adams GL, Monyak D: *Irradiated soft tissue and its management*. In Hom DB, Szachowicz EH, editors: *The otolaryngologic clinics of North America*, vol 28, *Wound healing for the otolaryngologist*, Philadelphia, WB Saunders, 1995.

110. Hong WK and others: Recent advances in head and neck cancer: larynx preservation and cancer chemoprevention: the seventeenth annual Richard and Hinda Rosenthal foundation award lecture, *Cancer Res* 53:5113, 1993.

111. Hopewell JW and others: Vascular irradiation damage: its cellular basis and likely consequences, *Br J Cancer* 53:181, 1986.

112. Howell-Burke D and others: T_2 glottic cancer, *Arch Otolaryngol Head Neck Surg* 116:830, 1990.

113. Jacobs C and others: Chemotherapy as a substitute for surgery in the treatment of advanced resectable head and neck cancer: a report from the Northern California Oncology Group, *Cancer* 60:1178, 1987.

114. Jemal A and others: Cancer statistics, 2004, *CA Cancer J Clin* 54:8, 2004.

115. Jesse RH, Lindberg RD: The efficacy of combining radiation therapy with a surgical procedure in patients with cervical metastasis from squamous cancer of the oropharynx and hypopharynx, *Cancer* 35:1163, 1975.

116. Johnson JT and others: Outcome of open surgical therapy for glottic carcinoma, *Ann Otol Rhinol Laryngol* 102:752, 1993.

117. Johnson JT and others: Medial vs lateral wall piriform sinus carcinoma: implications for management of regional lymphatics, *Head Neck* 16:401, 1994.

118. Jones AS and others: Second primary tumors in patients with head and neck squamous cell carcinoma, *Cancer* 75:1343, 1995.

119. Jortay A and others: A randomized EORTC study on the effect of preoperative polychemotherapy in piriform sinus carcinoma treated by pharyngolaryngectomy and irradiation: results from 5 to 10 years, *Acta Chir Belg* 90:115, 1990.

120. Jourenkova-Miranova N and others: High-activity microsomal epoxide hydrolase genotypes and the risk of oral, pharynx and larynx cancers, *Cancer Res* 60:534, 2000.

121. Karlen RG, Maisel RH: Does primary tracheoesophageal puncture reduce complications after laryngectomy and improve patient communication? *Am J Otolaryngol* 22:324, 2001.

122. Karp DD and others: Larynx preservation using induction chemotherapy plus radiation therapy as an alternative to laryngectomy in advanced head and neck cancer, *Am J Clin Oncol* 14:273, 1991.

123. Keller AZ: Cirrhosis of the liver, alcoholism and heavy smoking associated with cancer of the mouth and pharynx, *Cancer* 20:1015, 1967.

124. Kelly AB: Spasm at entrance to esophagus, *J Laryngol Rhinol Otol* 34:285, 1991.

125. Kies MS and others: Concomitant infusional paclitaxel and fluorouracil, oral hydroxyurea, and hyperfractionated radiation for locally advanced squamous head and neck cancer, *J Clin Oncol* 19:1961, 2001.

126. Kim M-S and others: Paraglottic space and supracricoid laryngectomy, *Arch Otolaryngol Head Neck Surg* 128:304, 2002.

127. Kirchner JA: Piriform sinus cancer: a clinical and laboratory study, *Ann Otol Rhinol Laryngol* 84:793, 1975.

128. Kirchner JA, Owen JR: Five hundred cancers of the larynx and piriform sinus: results of treatment by radiation and surgery, *Laryngoscope* 87:1288, 1977.

129. Kirchner J, Som M: Clinical and histological observations and supraglottic cancer, *Ann Otol Rhinol Laryngol* 80:638, 1971.

130. Knudson Jr AG: Mutation and cancer: statistical study of retinoblastoma. *Proc Natl Acad Sci USA* 68:820, 1971.

131. Koufman JA: The otolaryngologic manifestations of gastroesophageal reflux disease (GERD), *Laryngoscope* 101:1, 1991.

132. Kowalski LP and others: Prognostic factors in T_3 N_{0-1} glottic and transglottic carcinoma, *Arch Otolaryngol Head Neck Surg* 122:77, 1996.

133. Kramer S and others: Combined radiation therapy and surgery in the management of advanced head and neck cancer: a final report of study 73-03 of the Radiation Therapy Oncology Group, *Head Neck Surg* 10:19, 1987.

134. Kraus DH and others: Salvage laryngectomy for unsuccessful larynx preservation therapy, *Ann Otol Rhinol Laryngol* 164:936, 1995.

135. Kraus FT, Perez-Mesa C: Verrucous carcinoma-clinical and pathologic study of 105 cases involving oral cavity, larynx and genitalia, *Cancer* 19:26, 1966.

136. Krespi YP, Sisson GA: Voice preservation in piriform sinus carcinoma by hemicricolaryngopharyngectomy, *Ann Otol Rhinol Laryngol* 93:306, 1984.

137. Laccourreye H and others: Supracricoid hemilaryngopharyngectomy: analysis of 240 cases, *Ann Otol Rhinol Laryngol* 96:217, 1987.

138. Laccourreye H and others: Supracricoid laryngectomy with cricohyoidopexy: a partial laryngeal procedure for selected supraglottic and transglottic carcinomas, *Laryngoscope* 100:735, 1990.

139. Laccourreye H and others: Supracricoid laryngectomy with cricohyoidoepiglottopexy: a partial laryngeal procedure for glottic carcinoma, *Ann Otol Rhinol Laryngol* 99:421, 1990.

140. Laccourreye O and others: Local failure after supracricoid partial laryngectomy: symptoms, management, and outcome, *Laryngoscope* 108:339, 1998.

141. Laccourreye O and others: Supracricoid hemilaryngopharyngectomy in selected piriform sinus carcinoma staged as T_2, *Laryngoscope* 103:1373, 1993.

142. Lambert PR, Ward PH, Burke G: Pseudosarcoma larynx, *Arch Otol* 106:700, 1980.

143. Larson J, Adams G, Fattah HA: Survival statistics for multiple primaries in head and neck cancer, *Otolaryngol Head Neck Surg* 103:14, 1990.

144. La Vecchia C and others: Types of cigarettes and cancers of the upper digestive and respiratory tract, *Cancer Causes Control* 1:69, 1990.

145. Lavertu P and others: Management of the neck in a randomized trial comparing concurrent chemotherapy and radiotherapy with radiotherapy alone in respectable stage III and IV squamous cell head and neck cancer, *Head Neck* 19:559, 1997.

146. Lavertu P and others: Comparison of surgical complications after organ-preservation therapy in patients with stage III or IV squamous cell head and neck cancer, *Arch Otolaryngol Head Neck Surg* 124:401, 1998.

147. Leemans CR and others: The efficacy of comprehensive neck dissection with or without postoperative radiotherapy in nodal metastases of squamous cell carcinoma of the upper respiratory and digestive tracts, *Laryngoscope* 100:1194, 1990.

148. Lefebvre JL and others: Larynx preservation in piriform sinus cancer: preliminary results of a European organization for research and treatment of cancer phase III trial, *J Natl Cancer Inst* 88:890, 1996.

149. Lesinski SG, Bauer WC, Ogura JH: Hemilaryngectomy for T_3 (fixed cord) epidermoid carcinoma of larynx, *Laryngoscope* 86:1563, 1976.

150. Lewis JE, Olsen KD, Inwards CY: Cartilaginous tumors of the larynx: clinical pathologic review of 47 cases, *Ann Otol Rhinol Laryngol* 106:374, 1997.

151. Lewis JE, Olson KD, Sebo TJ: Spindle cell carcinoma of the larynx: a review of 26 cases including DNA content and immunohistochemistry, *Otol Head Neck Surg* 116:47, 1997.

152. Liening DA and others: Hypothyroidism following radiotherapy for head and neck cancer, *Otol Head Neck Surg* 103:10, 1990.

153. Lindberg R: Distribution of cervical lymph node metastases from squamous cell carcinoma of the upper respiratory and digestive tracts, *Cancer* 29:1446, 1972.

154. Logemann JA and others: Mechanisms of recovery of swallow after supraglottic laryngectomy, *J Speech Hear Res* 37:965, 1994.

155. Lord IJ and others: A comparison of pre-operative and primary radiation therapy in treatment of carcinoma of the hypopharynx, *Br J Radiol* 46:175, 1973.

156. Lore JM, Klotch DW, Lee KY: One-stage reconstruction of the hypopharynx using myomucosal tongue flap and dermal graft, *Am J Surg* 144:473, 1982.

157. Luna MA, Tortoledo ME: Verrucous carcinoma, *Contemp Issues Surg Pathol* 10:497, 1988.

158. Lutz CK and others: Supraglottic carcinoma: patterns of recurrence, *Ann Otol Rhinol Laryngol* 99:12, 1990.

159. Maipano J and others: Surgical salvage for recurrent "early" glottic cancers, *Surg Oncol* 40:32, 1989.

160. Maisel R, Schmidt D, Pambuccian S: Subglottic laryngeal paraganglioma, *Laryngoscope* 113:401, 2003.

161. Maisel RH, Vermeersch H: Panendoscopy for second primaries in head and neck cancer, *Ann Otol Rhinol Laryngol* 90:460, 1981.

162. Marks JE and others: The need for elective irradiation of occult lymphatic metastases from cancers of the larynx and piriform sinus, *Head Neck* 8:3, 1985.

163. Marks JE and others: The risk of contralateral lymphatic metastases for cancers of the larynx and pharynx, *Am J Otol* 13:34, 1992.

164. Marks JE and others: Carcinoma of the supraglottic larynx, *Am J Roentgenol* 132:255, 1979.

165. Marks SC and others: Outcome of piriform sinus cancer: a retrospective institutional review, *Laryngoscope* 106:27, 1996.

166. Martin SA and others: Carcinoma of the piriform sinus: predictors of TNM relapse and survival, *Cancer* 46:1974, 1980.

167. McConnel FM and others: Hypopharyngeal stenosis, *Laryngoscope* 94:1162, 1984.

168. McDonald TJ, DeSanto LW, Weiland LH: Supraglottic larynx and its pathology as studied by whole organ sections, *Laryngoscope* 86:635, 1976.

169. McGavran MH and others: Carcinoma of the piriform sinus: the results of radical surgery, *Arch Otolaryngol Head Neck Surg* 78:826, 1963.

170. McGuirt WF and others: Laryngeal radionecrosis versus recurrent cancer: a clinical approach, *Ann Otol Rhinol Laryngol* 107:293, 1998.

171. McLaughlin MP and others: Salvage surgery after radiotherapy failure in T_1, T_2 squamous cell carcinoma of the glottic larynx, *Head Neck* 18:229, 1996.

172. McNab Jones RF: The Paterson-Brown Kelly syndrome: its relationship to iron deficiency and postcricoid carcinoma, *J Laryngol Otol* 75:529, 1961.

173. Medina JE: A rational classification of neck dissections, *Otolaryngol Head Neck Surg* 100:169, 1989.

174. Mendenhall WM and others: Carcinoma of the supraglottic larynx: a basis for comparing the results of radiotherapy and surgery, *Head Neck* 12:204, 1990.

175. Moisa H: Neuroendocrine tumors of the larynx, *Head Neck* 13:498, 1991.

176. Moran CA, Suster S, Carter D: Laryngeal chondrosarcomas, *Arch Pathol Lab Med* 117:914, 1993.

177. Morita M and others: Family aggregation of carcinoma of the hypopharynx and cervical esophagus: special reference to multiplicity of cancer in upper aerodigestive tract, *Int J Cancer* 76:468, 1998.

178. Mork J and others: Human papillomavirus infection as a risk factor for squamous cell carcinoma of the head and neck, *N Engl J Med* 344:1125, 2001.

179. Munoz A and others: Laryngeal carcinoma: sclerotic appearance of the cricoid and arytenoid cartilage. CT pathologic correlation, *Radiology* 189:433, 1993.

180. Murakami Y and others: Excision level and indication for contralateral neck dissection in hypopharyngeal cancer surgery, *Auris Nasus Larynx* 12:S36, 1985.

181. Mustard RA: The use of the Wookey operation for carcinoma of the hypopharynx and cervical esophagus, *Surg Gynecol Obstet* 111:577, 1960.

182. Myers EN, Allvi A: Management of carcinoma of the supraglottic larynx: evolution, current concepts and future trends, *Laryngoscope* 106:559, 1996.

183. Myers EN, Wagner RL, Johnson JT: Microlaryngoscopic surgery for T$_1$ glottic lesions: a cost-effective option, *Ann Otol Rhinol Laryngol* 103:28, 1994.

184. Myssiorek D, Vamburas A, Abramson AL: Carcinoma in situ of the glottic larynx, *Laryngoscope* 104:463, 1994.

185. Nakayama M, Brandenburg JH: Clinical underestimation of laryngeal cancer: predictive indicators, *Arch Otolaryngol Head Neck Surg* 119:950, 1993.

186. Nakayama M, Brandenburg JH, Hafez GR: Dedifferentiated chondrosarcoma of the larynx with regional and distant metastases, *Ann Otol Rhinol Laryngol* 102:785, 1993.

187. National Cancer Institute Head and Neck Contracts Program: Adjuvant chemotherapy for advanced head and neck squamous carcinoma: final report of the head and neck contracts program, *Cancer* 60:301, 1987.

188. Nguyen C and others: Carcinoma in situ of the glottic larynx, excision or irradiation, *Head Neck* 25:223, 1996.

189. Nicolai P and others: Laryngeal chondrosarcoma: incidence, pathology, biological behavior, and treatment, *Ann Otol Rhinol Laryngol* 99:515, 1990.

190. Nichols RD, Stive PM, Greenwald KJ: Partial laryngectomy after radiation failure, *Laryngoscope* 90:571, 1980.

191. Ogura JH: Supraglottic subtotal laryngectomy and radical neck dissection for carcinoma of the epiglottis, *Laryngoscope* 68:983, 1958.

192. Ogura JH, Biller HF, Wette R: Elective neck dissection for pharyngeal and laryngeal cancers, *Ann Otol Rhinol Laryngol* 80:646, 1971.

193. Ogura JH, Dedo HH: Glottic reconstruction following subtotal glottic-supraglottic laryngectomy, *Laryngoscope* 75:865, 1965.

194. Ogura JH, Jurema AA, Watson RK: Partial laryngopharyngectomy and neck dissection for piriform sinus cancer, *Laryngoscope* 70:1399, 1960.

195. Ogura JH, Mallen RW: Partial laryngopharyngectomy for supraglottic and pharyngeal carcinoma, *Trans Am Acad Ophthalmol Otolaryngol* 69:832, 1965.

196. Ogura JH, Marks JE, Freeman RB: Results of conservation surgery for cancers of the supraglottis and piriform sinus, *Laryngoscope* 90:591, 1980.

197. Ogura JH, Sessions DG, Spector GJ: Analysis of surgical therapy for epidermoid carcinoma of the laryngeal glottis, *Laryngoscope* 85:22, 1975.

198. Ogura JH, Sessions DG, Spector GJ: Conservation surgery for epidermoid carcinoma of the supraglottic larynx, *Laryngoscope* 85:18, 1975.

199. Okami K and others: Cyclin D1 amplification is independent of p16 inactivation in head and neck squamous cell carcinoma, *Oncogene* 18:3541, 1999.

200. Olofsson J, van Nostrand AWP: Anaplastic small cell carcinoma of larynx, *Ann Otol Rhinol Laryngol* 81:284, 1972.

201. Olsen KD, DeSanto LW, Peterson BW: Positive delphian lymph node: clinical significance in laryngeal cancer, *Laryngoscope* 97:1033, 1987.

202. Orton HB: Lateral transthyroid pharyngotomy: Trotter's operation for malignant conditions of the laryngopharynx, *Arch Otolaryngol Head Neck Surg* 12:320, 1930.

203. Orvidas LJ and others: Verrucous carcinoma of the larynx: a review of 53 patients, *Head Neck Surg* 20:197, 1998.

204. Ossoff RH, Sisson GA, Shapshay SM: Endoscopic management of selected early vocal cord carcinoma, *Ann Otol Rhinol Laryngol* 94:56, 1985.

205. Overholt SM and others: Neuroendocrine neoplasms of the larynx, *Laryngoscope* 105:789, 1995.

206. Panje WR and others: Surgical management of the head and neck cancer patient following concomitant multimodality therapy, *Laryngoscope* 105:97, 1995.

207. Parsons JT and others: Twice-a-day radiotherapy for squamous cell carcinoma of the head and neck: the University of Florida experience, *Head Neck* 15:87, 1993.

208. Paterson DR: A clinical type of dysphagia, *J Laryngol Otol* 34:289, 1919.

209. Paulino AAF and others: Basaloid squamous cell carcinoma of the head and neck, *Laryngoscope* 110:1479, 2000.

210. Pavelic ZP, Gluckman JL: The role of p53 tumor suppressor gene in human head and neck tumorigenesis, *Acta Otolaryngol (Stockh)* 527:21, 1997.

211. Pearson BW: Subtotal laryngectomy, *Laryngoscope* 91:1904, 1981.

212. Pearson BW, Wood RD, Hartman DE: Extended hemilaryngectomy for T$_3$ glottic carcinoma with preservation of speech and swallowing, *Laryngoscope* 90:1950, 1980.

213. Peters LJ and others: Neck surgery in patients with primary oropharyngeal cancer treated by radiotherapy, *Head Neck* 18:552, 1996.

214. Pignon JP and others: Chemotherapy added to locoregional treatment for head and neck squamous-cell carcinoma: three meta-analyses of updated individual data, *Lancet* 355:949, 2000.

215. Pingree TF and others: Treatment of hypopharyngeal carcinoma: a 10-year review of 1,362 cases, *Laryngoscope* 97:901, 1987.

216. Porto DP and others: Neuroendocrine carcinoma of the larynx, *Am J Otolaryngol* 9:97, 1987.

217. Poulsen M and others: Is surgery necessary in stage III and stage IV cancer of the head and neck that responds to induction chemotherapy? *Arch Otolaryngol Head Neck Surg* 122:467, 1996.

218. Powers WE: Radiation biologic considerations and practical investigations in preoperative radiation therapy, *J Can Assoc Radiol* 16:217, 1965.

219. Prades JM and others: Concomitant chemoradiotherapy in piriform sinus carcinoma, *Arch Otolaryngol Head Neck Surg* 128:384, 2002.

220. Pressman JJ and others: Further studies upon the submucosal compartments and lymphatics of the larynx by the injection of dyes and radioisotopes, *Ann Otol Rhinol Laryngol* 65:963, 1956.

221. Puxeddu R and others: Surgical therapy of T1 and selected cases of T2 glottic carcinoma: cordectomy, horizontal glottectomy and CO_2 laser endoscopic resection, *Tumori* 86:277, 2000.

222. Raghavan U, Quraishi S, Bradley PJ: Multiple primary tumors in patients diagnosed with hypopharyngeal cancer, *Otolaryngol Head Neck Surg* 128:419, 2003.

223. Randall G, Alonso WA, Ogura JH: Spindle cell carcinoma (pseudosarcoma) of the larynx, *Arch Otolaryngol Head Neck Surg* 101:63, 1975.

224. Razack MS, Sako K, Kalnins I: Squamous cell carcinoma of the piriform sinus, *Head Neck Surg* 1:31, 1978.

225. Rees RS and others: Pectoralis major musculocutaneous flaps: long-term follow-up of hypopharyngeal reconstruction, *Plast Reconstr Surg* 77:586, 1986.

226. Rothfield RE, Johnson JT, Myers EN: Hemilaryngectomy for salvage of radiation therapy failures, *Otolaryngol Head Neck Surg* 103:792, 1990.

227. Rothfield RE, Myers EN, Johnson JT: Carcinoma in situ and microinvasive squamous cell carcinoma of the vocal cords, *Ann Otol Rhinol Laryngol* 100:793, 1991.

228. Rothman KJ and others: Epidemiology of laryngeal cancer, *Epidemiol Rev* 2:195, 1980.

229. Roy S and others: Role of planned neck dissection for advanced metastatic disease in tongue base or tonsil squamous cell carcinoma treated with radiotherapy. *Head Neck* 24:474, 2002.

230. Rubin J, Johnson JT, Myers EN: Stomal recurrence after laryngectomy: interrelated risk factor study, *Otolaryngol Head Neck Surg* 103:305, 1990.

231. Saleh EM, Abdullwahab AA, Kammal MM: Age and sex incidence of hypopharyngeal tumours in Upper Egypt: Assuit University experience, *J Laryngol Otol* 109:737, 1995.

232. Samant S and others: Concomitant radiation therapy and targeted cisplatin chemotherapy for the treatment of advanced piriform sinus carcinoma: disease control and preservation of organ function, *Head Neck* 21:595, 1999.

233. Sanguineti G and others: Management of the neck after alternating chemoradiotherapy for advanced head and neck cancer, *Head Neck* 21:223, 1999.

234. Sassler AM, Esclamado RM, Wolf GT: Surgery after organ preservation therapy. Analysis of wound complications, *Arch Otolaryngol Head Neck Surg* 121:162, 1995.

235. Schuller DE: Reconstructive options for pharyngeal and/or cervical esophageal defects, *Arch Otolaryngol Head Neck Surg* 111:193, 1985.

236. Sessions D: Surgical pathology of cancer of the larynx and hypopharynx, *Laryngoscope* 86:814, 1976.

237. Sessions D and others: Management of T3N0M0 glottic carcinoma: therapeutic outcomes, *Laryngoscope* 112:1281, 2002.

238. Sessions DG, Ogura JH, Fried MP: Carcinoma of the subglottic area, *Laryngoscope* 85:1417, 1975.

239. Shah JP: Patterns of cervical lymph node metastasis from squamous carcinomas of the upper aerodigestive tract, *Am J Surg* 160:405, 1990.

240. Shaha AR, Shah JP: Carcinoma of the subglottic larynx, *Am J Surg* 144:456, 1982.

241. Shanmugaratnam K, Sobin LH: The World Health Organization histologic classification of tumours of the upper respiratory tract and ear: a commentary on the second edition, *Cancer* 71:2689, 1993.

242. Shapiro J, Zeitels SM, Fried MP: Laser surgery for laryngeal cancer, operative techniques, *Otolaryngol Head Neck Surg* 3:84, 1994.

243. Shenoy AM and others: Near-total laryngectomy in advanced cancers of the larynx and piriform sinus: a comparative study of morbidity and functional and oncological outcomes, *Ann Otol Rhinol Laryngol* 111:50, 2002.

244. Shiga H and others: Prognostic value of p53 glutathione S-transferase pi and thymidylate synthase for neoadjuvant cisplatin-based chemotherapy in head and neck cancer, *Clin Cancer Res* 5:4097, 1999.

245. Shirinian MH and others: Laryngeal preservation by induction chemotherapy plus radiotherapy in locally advanced head and neck cancer: the M.D. Anderson Cancer Center experience, *Head Neck* 16:39, 1994.

246. Sisk EA and others: Human papillomavirus and p53 mutational status as prognostic factors in head and neck carcinoma, *Head Neck* 24:841, 2002.

247. Sisson GA: 1989 Ogura memorial lecture: mediastinal dissection, *Laryngoscope* 99:1262, 1989.

248. Slaughter JT: Multicentric origin of intra-oral carcinoma, *Surgery* 20:133, 1946.

249. Small W Jr and others: Role of radiation therapy in the management of carcinoma in situ of the larynx, *Laryngoscope* 103:663, 1993.

250. Smith MS, Browne JD, Teot LA: A case of primary laryngeal T-cell lymphoma in a patient with acquired immunodeficiency syndrome, *Am J Otol* 17:332, 1996.

251. Snow RT, Fox AR: Mucoepidermoid carcinoma of the larynx, *J Am Osteopath Assoc* 91:182, 1991.

252. Snyderman NL and others: Extracapsular spread of carcinoma in cervical lymph nodes, *Cancer* 56:1597, 1985.

253. Som ML: Conservation surgery for carcinoma of the supraglottis, *J Laryngol Otol* 84:665, 1970.

254. Som ML: Laryngotracheal autograft for postcricoid carcinoma: a reevaluation, *Ann Otol Rhinol Laryngol* 83:481, 1974.

255. Som ML: Surgical treatment of carcinoma of postcricoid region, *N Y State J Med* 61:2567, 1961.

256. Sorenson H, Munsen M, Thomsen K: Partial laryngectomy following radiation, *Laryngoscope* 90:1344, 1980.

257. Spector JG and others: Squamous cell carcinoma of the piriform sinus: a nonrandomized comparison of therapeutic modalities and long-term results, *Laryngoscope* 105:397, 1995.

258. Spector JG and others: Delayed regional metastases, distant metastases, and second primary malignancies in squamous cell carcinomas of the larynx and hypopharynx, *Laryngoscope* 111:1079, 2001.

259. Spiro RH, Gallo O, Shah J: Selective jugular node dissection in patients with squamous carcinoma of the larynx or pharynx, *Am J Surg* 166:399, 1993.

260. Stenerson TC, Hoel PS, Boysen M: Carcinoma in situ of the larynx: an evaluation of its natural clinical course, *Clin Otolaryngol* 16:358, 1991.

261. Strasser MD and others: Management implications of evaluating the N2 and N3 neck after organ preservation therapy, *Laryngoscope* 109:1776, 1999.

262. Strong MS and others: A randomized trial of preoperative radiotherapy in cancer of the oropharynx and hypopharynx, *Am J Surg* 136:494, 1978.

263. Su CY and others: Near-total laryngopharyngectomy with pectoralis major myocutaneous flap in advanced piriform carcinoma, *J Laryngol Otol* 107:817, 1993.

264. Suits GW, Cohen JI, Everts EC: Near total laryngectomy, *Arch Otolaryngol Head Neck Surg* 122:473, 1996.

265. Tami TA and others: Thyroid dysfunction after radiation therapy in head and neck cancer patients, *Ann J Otol* 13:357, 1992.

266. Tami TA, Sharma PK: Intralesional therapy for Kaposi's sarcoma of the epiglottis, *Otolaryngol Head Neck Surg* 113:283, 1995.

267. Thabat HM and others: Comparison of clinical evaluation and CT accuracy for tumors of the larynx and hypopharynx, *Laryngoscope* 106:589, 1996.

268. Tharp ME, Shidnia H: Radiotherapy in the treatment of verrucous carcinoma of the head and neck, *Laryngoscope* 105:391, 1995.

269. Theogaraj SD and others: The pectoralis major musculocutaneous island flap in single-stage reconstruction of the pharyngoesophageal region, *Plast Reconstr Surg* 65:267, 1980.

270. Therasse P and others: New guidelines to evaluate the response to treatment in solid tumors, *J Natl Cancer Inst* 92:205, 2000.

271. Thomas JV and others: Early glottic carcinoma treated with open laryngeal procedures, *Arch Otolaryngol Head Neck Surg* 120:264, 1994.

272. Tishler RB and others: An initial experience using concurrent paclitaxel and radiation in the treatment of head and neck malignancies, *Int J Radiat Oncol Biol Phys* 43:1001, 1999.

273. Trotter W: Malignant disease of the hypopharynx and its treatment by excision, *BMJ* 19:510, March, 1932.

274. Tucker GF, Smith HR: A histological demonstration of the development of laryngeal connective tissue compartments, *Trans Am Acad Ophthalmol Otolaryngol* 66:308, 1982.

275. Tupchong L and others: Randomized study of preoperative versus postoperative radiation therapy in advanced head and neck carcinoma: long-term follow-up of RTOG study 73-03, *Int J Radiat Oncol Biol Phys* 20:21, 1991.

276. Tuyns AJ and others: Cancer of the larynx/hypopharynx, tobacco and alcohol, *Int J Cancer* 41:483, 1988.

277. Urba S, Wolf GT: Organ Preservation in multimodality therapy of head and neck cancer, *Hematol Oncol Clin North Am* 5:713, 1991.

278. Urba SG and others: Neoadjuvant therapy for organ preservation in head and neck cancer, *Laryngoscope* 110:2074, 2000.

279. Van den Bogaert W, Ostyn F, van der Schueren E: Hypopharyngeal cancer: results of treatment with radiotherapy alone and combinations of surgery and radiotherapy, *Radiother Oncol* 3:311, 1985.

280. Vandenbrouck C and others: Results of a randomized clinical trial of preoperative irradiation versus postoperative in treatment of tumors of the hypopharynx, *Cancer* 39:1445, 1977.

281. Vikram B: Importance of the time interval between surgery and postoperative radiation therapy in the combined management of head and neck cancer, *Int J Radiat Oncol Biol Phys* 5:1837, 1979.

282. Vikram B and others: Failure at distant sites following multimodality treatment for advanced head and neck cancer, *Head Neck Surg* 6:730, 1984.

283. Vinson PP: Hysterical dysphagia, *Minn Med* 5:107, 1922.

284. Vlock DR and others: Clinical correlates of circulating immune complexes and antibody reactivity in squamous cell carcinoma of the head and neck, *J Clin Oncol* 11:2427, 1993.

285. Wadsworth JT, Futran N, Eubanks TR: Laparoscopic harvest of the jejunal free flap fro reconstruction of hypopharyngeal and cervical esophageal defects, *Arch Otolaryngol Head Neck Surg* 128:1384, 2002.

286. Wahlberg PCG and others: Carcinoma of the hypopharynx: analysis of incidence and survival in Sweden over a 30-year period, *Head Neck* 20:714, 1998.

287. Wain SL, Kier R, Vollmer RT: Basaloid-squamous carcinoma of the tongue, hypopharynx and larynx, *Hum Pathol* 17:1158, 1986.

288. Waldenström J, Kjellberg SR: The roentgenological diagnosis of sideropenic dysphagia, *Acta Radiol* 20:618, 1939.

289. Wang CC: Radiotherapeutic management of carcinoma of the posterior pharyngeal wall, *Cancer* 27:894, 1971.

290. Ward PH, Calcaterra TC, Kagan AR: The enigma of postradiation edema and recurrent or residual carcinoma of the larynx, *Laryngoscope* 85:522, 1975.

291. Ward PH, Hanson DG: Reflux as an epidemiologic factor in carcinoma of the laryngopharynx, *Laryngoscope* 99:666, 1989.

292. Wasfie T, Newman R: Laryngeal carcinoma in black patients, *Cancer* 61:167, 1988.

293. Watson DI, Jamieson GG, Devitt PG: Endoscopic cervico-thoraco-abdominal esophagectomy, *J Am Coll Surg* 190(3):372, 2000.

294. Weber PC, Johnson JT, Myers EN: The impact of bilateral neck dissection on pattern of recurrence and survival in supraglottic carcinoma, *Arch Otolaryngol Head Neck Surg* 120:703, 1994.

295. Weber RS and others: Outcome of salvage total laryngectomy following organ preservation therapy, the Radiation Therapy Oncology Group Trial 91-11, *Arch Otolaryngol Head Neck Surg* 129:44, 2003.

296. Wein RO, Topf P, Sham RL: Subglottic plasmacytoma: a case report and review of the literature, *Amer J Otol* 23:112, 2002.

297. Weinstein GS and others: Reconsidering a paradigm: the spread of supraglottic carcinoma of the glottis, *Laryngoscope* 105:1129, 1995.

298. Weisman RA, Coleman M, Ward PH: Stomal recurrence following laryngectomy, *Ann Otol Rhinol Laryngol* 88:885, 1979.

299. Welsh LW: The normal human laryngeal lymphatics, *Ann Otol Rhinol Laryngol* 73:569, 1964.

300. Welsh LW, Welsh JJ, Rizzo TA: Laryngeal lymphatics: current anatomic concepts, *Ann Otol Rhinol Laryngol* 93:19, 1984.

301. Wenig BL, Applebaum EL: The submandibular triangle in squamous cell carcinoma of the larynx and hypopharynx, *Laryngoscope* 101:516, 1991.

302. Wenig BL, Berry BW: Management of patients with positive surgical margins after vertical hemilaryngectomy, *Arch Otolaryngol Head Neck Surg* 121:172, 1995.

303. Wenig BM, Hyams VJ, Heffner DK: Moderately differentiated neuroendocrine carcinoma of the larynx: a clinicopathologic study of 54 cases, *Cancer* 62:2658, 1988.

304. Wick MR: Immunohistochemistry of neuroendocrine and neuroectodermal tumors, *Semin Diagn Pathol* 17:194, 2000.

305. Willson P and others: Laparoscopically-assisted total pharyngolaryngo-oesophagectomy, *Br J Surg* 84:870, 1997.

306. Winzenburg SM and others: Basaloid squamous carcinoma: a clinical comparison of two histologic types with poorly differentiated squamous cell carcinoma, *Otolaryngol Head Neck Surg* 119:471, 1998.

307. Wolf GT and others: Induction chemotherapy plus radiation compared with surgery plus radiation in patients with advanced laryngeal cancer: the Department of Veterans

Affairs Laryngeal Cancer Study Group, *N Engl J Med* 324:1685, 1991.

308. Wolf GT, Fisher SG: Effectiveness of salvage neck dissection for advanced regional metastases when induction chemotherapy and radiation are used for organ preservation, *Laryngoscope* 102:934, 1992.

309. Woodruff JM, Senie RT: Atypical carcinoid tumor of the larynx: a critical review of the literature, *ORL J Otorhinolaryngol Relat Spec* 53:194, 1991.

310. Wookey H: The surgical treatment of carcinoma of the hypopharynx and the esophagus, *Br J Surg* 35:249, 1948.

311. Yates A, Crumley RL: Surgical treatment of piriform sinus cancer: a retrospective study, *Laryngoscope* 94:1586, 1984.

312. Yeager VL, Archer CR: Anatomical routes for cancer invasions of laryngeal cartilages, *Laryngoscope* 92:449, 1982.

313. Zatterstrom UK and others: Prognostic factors in head and neck cancer: histologic grading, DNA ploidy, and nodal status, *Head Neck* 13:477, 1991.

314. Zeitels SM, Kirchner JA: Hyoepiglottic ligament in supraglottic cancer, *Ann Otol Rhinol Laryngol* 104:770, 1995.

315. Zeitels SM and others: Endoscopic treatment of supraglottic and hypopharynx cancer, *Laryngoscope* 104:71, 1994.

316. Zeitels SM, Vaughn CW: Pre-epiglottic space invasion in "early" epiglottic cancer, *Ann Otol Rhinol Laryngol* 100:789, 1991.

317. Zeitels SMK and others: Endoscopic management of early supraglottic cancer, *Ann Otol Rhinol Laryngol* 99:951, 1990.

318. Zelefsky MF and others: Combined chemotherapy and radiotherapy versus surgery and postoperative radiotherapy for advanced hypopharyngeal cancer, *Head Neck* 18:405, 1996.

319. Zheng Z and others: Tobacco carcinogen-detoxifying enzyme UGTIA7 and its association with otolaryngeal cancer risk, *J Natl Cancer Inst* 93:1411, 2001.

320. Zieske LA and others: Squamous cell carcinoma with positive margins, *Arch Otolaryngol Head Neck Surg* 112:863, 1986.

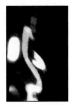

CHAPTER ONE HUNDRED

MANAGEMENT OF EARLY GLOTTIC CANCER

Henry T. Hoffman
Lucy H. Karnell
Timothy M. McCulloch
John Buatti
Gerry Funk

. . . at the start of the 21st century, the oncologist and patient are presented with a bewildering array of choices for laryngeal cancer therapy.

Ferlito and others[51]

BACKGROUND
Demographics

The American Cancer Society estimates that 8900 new cases of laryngeal cancer occurred in the United States in 2002, representing 0.7% of the 1,284,900 new cancers that were diagnosed overall (excluding the most common skin cancers and carcinoma in situ).[4] Although the number of new cancer cases in the United States has overall remained stable (between 1,220,100 and 1,284,900) from 1999 to 2002, the number of new cases of laryngeal cancer have decreased (Figure 100-1). These incidence estimates of new cancer cases (Figure 100-1) are extrapolated from Surveillance, Epidemiology, and End Results Program (SEER) data and are not considered to be as accurate as survival data. Further indirect support for the diminishing incidence in laryngeal cancer is provided from the American Cancer Society, with more accurate mortality data identifying a parallel decrease in the number of deaths from laryngeal cancer during the same time period (Figure 100-2). The decrease in both incidence and mortality from 1999 to 2002 appears to reflect changes primarily among males and parallels the decrease noted in their tobacco use.[30]

Statistics from the National Cancer Database (NCDB) provide insight into contemporary demographics and management of laryngeal cancer in the United States.[33] Analysis of this dataset demonstrated that squamous cell carcinoma is the dominant histologic type of laryngeal cancer in the United

States, representing approximately 95% of cases (Figure 100-3). Unless indicated otherwise, the remainder of the discussion in this chapter focuses on squamous cell carcinoma.[48,134]

Etiology

Squamous cell carcinoma of the larynx is strongly associated with the use of tobacco and alcohol. An increase in the prevalence of cigarette use among females in the past has been linked to a proportionate increase in the number of female patients with laryngeal cancer. Other factors implicated in the development of laryngeal cancer include passive smoking, chronic laryngeal irritation from gastroesophageal reflux, and viral infection.[22,66,74,124,167]

Since 1979 gastric acid reflux has been identified as a risk factor for laryngeal and pharyngeal cancer.[44,114] Alkaline reflux has more recently been identified as a laryngeal carcinogen by Galli and others.[56] These investigators identified a higher than expected number of patients with pharyngolaryngeal cancer associated with achlorhydria and presumed alkaline reflux after gastric resection. They concluded that periodic endoscopy of the upper aerodigestive tract should be performed on gastrectomized patients because of their higher risk for pharyngolaryngeal disorders in general and cancer in particular. These investigators also identified that, among patients with laryngeal squamous cell carcinoma with an intact gastric acid secreting mechanism, 81% showed abnormal acid reflux on 24-hour pH testing.

Human papillomavirus (most notably the oncogenic type 16) has been shown be associated with head and neck cancer.[61,109,144] The role for human papillomavirus (HPV) infection in laryngeal oncogenesis has been supported by previous study but does

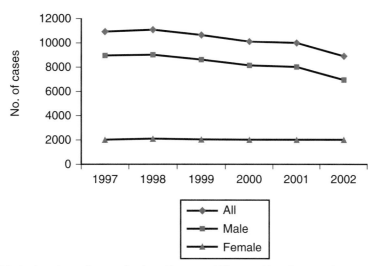

Figure 100-1. American Cancer Society Facts and Figures: New laryngeal cancer cases by year.

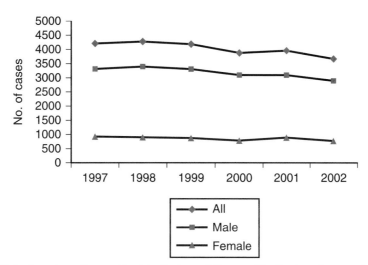

Figure 100-2. American Cancer Society Facts and Figures: Deaths from laryngeal cancer by year.

not have as strong an association as has been identified with cancer of the oropharynx and oral cavity.[2,145] Initial study suggests that a difference exists in behavior between HPV and non-HPV–related squamous cell carcinoma of the upper aerodigestive tract, with a better prognosis afforded the HPV-positive cases.[12]

Differences in exposure to carcinogens or genetic susceptibility may explain the differences in the pre-

dominant types of laryngeal cancer throughout the world. Glottic cancers predominate over supraglottic cancers in the United States at a ratio of 2:1. In France the opposite occurs, where the number of supraglottic cancers exceeds that of glottic cancers at a ratio of 2:1.[169] In Finland the incidence of supraglottic cancer decreased and the incidence of glottic cancers increased between the decades 1976 to 1985 and

HISTOLOGY OF LARYNGEAL CANCER CASES
DIAGNOSED IN 2000 NATIONAL CANCER DATABASE

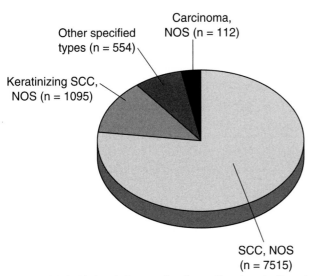

Figure 100-3. National Cancer Database Benchmark Report: Histology of Laryngeal Cancer in the U.S. in 2000. © *Commission on Cancer, American college of Surgeons. NCDB Benchmark Reports, v1.1. Chicago, IL, 2002. (The content reproduced from the applications remains the full and exclusive copyrighted property of the American college of Surgeons. The American College of Surgeons is not responsible for any ancillary or derivative works based on the original Text, Tables, or Figures.)*

1986 to 1995.[156] Supraglottic cancers were more common than glottic cancers in the earlier decade (ratio of 1.4:1). Glottic cancers predominated in the later decade at a ratio of 2:1. The reason for this change in distribution of laryngeal cancers in Finland is not clear. A low exposure to alcohol and a high availability of medical services were factors Brenner and others identified as important determinants to the characteristics of laryngeal cancer in Israel.[23] These investigators linked these factors to the high proportion of laryngeal cancers treated at early stage with an overall better outcome when compared with other countries.[23]

Staging

The most widely accepted system for classifying cancer in the United States, as is currently promoted by the American Joint Committee on Cancer (AJCC), had its beginning in 1959 with the organization of the American Joint Committee for Cancer Staging and End-Results Reporting (AJC).[100] This staging system was first published in 1977 in the *Manual for Staging of Cancer*.[5] The staging system has evolved to its current form as it is codified in the *AJCC Staging Manual, Sixth Edition* published in May of 2002 and

implemented as of January 1, 2003.[64] Major revisions were made to the fifth edition in the head and neck section that were directed primarily to the advanced-stage cases. Although the definitions for stages 0, I, and II laryngeal cancers remained unchanged, alterations to the T_3 definitions in the sixth edition have impacted on the interpretation of T_1 and T_2 classification.

The anatomic definitions and boundaries between sites, as published in the *AJCC Staging Manual*, have remained constant across the multiple editions. The glottis has been defined as the true vocal cords, including the anterior and posterior commissures. Unfortunately, the definition of the posterior commissure remains vague. It is difficult to discriminate between the glottis, the adjacent supraglottis (arytenoids), and the hypopharynx (post-cricoid region) in the region of the posterior commissure.[73] The superior border of the glottis is more clearly defined by a horizontal plane passing through the apex of the ventricle. The inferior limit of the glottis is defined by a line parallel to and 1 cm inferior to this plane.

Glottic cancers are staged primarily by clinical assessment of degree of vocal cord mobility (Table 100-1).[63] Cancers confined to the glottis with normal mobility are staged T_1. Subdivision of T_1 vocal cord

---

TABLE 100-1

PRIMARY TUMOR (T) CLASSIFICATION OF GLOTTIC CANCER*

T_x	Primary tumor cannot be assessed
T_0	No evidence of primary tumor
T_{is}	Carcinoma in situ
T_1	Tumor limited to the vocal cord(s) (may involve anterior or posterior commissure) with normal mobility
	T_{1a} Tumor limited to one vocal cord
	T_{1b} Tumor involves both vocal cords
T_2	Tumor extends to supraglottis or subglottis, or with impaired vocal cord mobility
T_3	Tumor limited to the larynx with vocal cord fixation or invades paraglottic space, or minor thyroid cartilage erosion (e.g., inner cortex)
T_{4a}	Tumor invades through the thyroid cartilage or invades tissues beyond the larynx (e.g., trachea, soft tissues of neck including deep extrinsic muscle of the tongue, strap muscles, thyroid, or esophagus)
T_{4b}	Tumor invades prevertebral space, encases carotid artery, or invades mediastinal structures

*From Greene F, Page D, Fleming I and others: *AJCC cancer staging manual,* ed 6, New York, 2002, Springer Verlag.

cancers is based on extension to involve the opposite cord. A tumor limited to one vocal cord is T_{1a}. A horseshoe lesion that extends around the anterior commissure to involve both vocal cords without impairing mobility is T_{1b}. Despite consistency across all previous editions of AJCC staging manuals indicating that T_4 status is based on "tumor invasion through the thyroid cartilage . . . ," it has been common clinical practice to consider any extent of thyroid cartilage invasion from a glottic cancer to be cause for T_4 classification. Clinically apparent stage I glottic cancers ($T_1N_0M_0$) were reassigned stage IV status ($T_4N_0M_0$) when "microscopic invasion of adjacent cartilage" was identified.[49] Revision to the sixth edition AJCC staging manual identifies that minor cartilage erosion (e.g., inner cortex) should be classified as T_3 rather than T_4.

Glottic cancers continue to be classified T_2 based on two separate criteria: impaired vocal cord motion or transglottic spread beyond the glottis to involve either the supraglottis or subglottis. Although the AJCC does not discriminate between these two criteria, some investigators distinguish T_{2a} from T_{2b} cancers. T_{2a} vocal cord cancers do not impair mobility but are a higher stage than T_1 cancers by virtue of transglottic spread to involve the supraglottis or subglottis. T_{2b} cancers are sufficiently invasive to impair vocal cord mobility without causing complete fixation. Revision to the sixth edition identifies that T_3 classification results from vocal cord fixation or invasion of the paraglottic space. This clarification is helpful to resolve controversy in the interpretation of subtle differences between impaired vocal cord motion and fixation. If the arytenoid remains mobile but the membranous vocal cord is tethered by deep infiltration to the paraglottic space, the cancer is considered a T_3.

Still further clarification is needed to address inconsistencies that persist among publications describing the paraglottic space.[12,84,101,161] Berman defined the borders of the paraglottic space as they have been commonly reported by others:

- Anterolateral: the thyroid cartilage.
- Inferomedial: the conus elasticus.
- Medial: the ventricle and the quadrangular membrane.
- Posterior: the pyriform sinus.[12]

This definition fails to address the controversy as to whether all, part, or none of the thyroarytenoid muscle is part of the paraglottic space.[141] An assessment by Weinstein and others[171] defines the medial border of the paraglottic space as the tissue lateral to the conus elasticus at the glottic level and lateral to the qua-

drangular membrane at the supraglottic level. By this convention, the thyroarytenoid muscle is considered part of the paraglottic space. Others define the glottic portion of the paraglottic space as the fat deep to the intrinsic laryngeal musculature. For the purposes of T classification according to the revised AJCC criteria, it is reasonable to consider that paraglottic space invasion (T_3) occurs when the fat compartment deep to the intrinsic laryngeal musculature is involved with tumor. Impaired vocal cord mobility (T_2) (without paraglottic space involvement) may be considered when the thyroarytenoid or lateral cricoarytenoid muscles are infiltrated but not fully transgressed.

Carcinoma in situ is classified as T_{is}. Accuracy in classifying premalignant changes affecting the laryngeal epithelium is compromised by the subjective nature of the assessment and by a lack of uniformity in terminology. Some pathologists discriminate between severe dysplasia and carcinoma in situ, whereas others group them together as type III intraepithelial neoplasia.[34,52,108] The grading of laryngeal dysplasia as mild, moderate, and severe or as carcinoma in situ originated from a similar classification of preneoplastic diseases of the uterine cervix. Keratinizing dysplastic lesions of the upper airway are more common than in the cervix and are also more difficult to categorize. The differences that exist in the behavior of carcinoma in situ originating at these two distinctly different anatomic sites has also undermined the transfer of concepts governing uterine cervical carcinoma in situ to laryngeal carcinoma in situ.[21] Despite the clearly stated pathologic principle that high grade dysplasia and carcinoma in situ are equivalent terms in describing abnormal laryngeal squamous epithelium, clinical management is generally less aggressive for high grade dysplasia than for carcinoma in situ.

The stage grouping of primary tumor, regional lymph nodes, distant metastatic (TNM) classifications for laryngeal cancer is the same as for other head and neck mucosal sites (Table 100-2). Although the stage groupings have been revised—with the sixth edition introducing the division of stage IV into IV a, IV b, and IV c—the staging of early glottic cancer has remained constant (stages 0, I, and II).

Definitions: Early Glottic Cancer

The appropriate definition of the term *early* as it applies to laryngeal cancer has been debated. Some investigators have loosely used the term to describe laryngeal cancer in the context of management options. By this convention, a laryngeal cancer is considered early if it can be treated by partial laryngeal (conservative) surgery without a neck dissection, by endoscopic excision, or by radiotherapy alone.[50] Others apply the term *early* to stage 0, I, or II tumors

TABLE 100-2

STAGE GROUPING OF LARYNGEAL CANCER*

Stage 0	T_{is}	N_0	M_0
Stage I	T_1	N_0	M_0
Stage II	T_2	N_0	M_0
Stage III	T_3	N_0	M_0
	$T_1, T_2,$ or T_3	N_1	M_0
Stage IV a	T_{4a}	N_0, N_1, N_2	M_0
	$T_1, T_2, T_3,$ or T_{4a}	N_2	M_0
Stage IV b	T_{4b}	Any N	M_0
	Any T	N_3	M_0
Stage IV c	Any T	Any N	M_0

*From Greene F, Page D, Fleming I and others: *AJCC cancer staging manual*, ed 6, New York, 2002, Springer Verlag.

and *late* to stage III or IV tumors. This definition of *early* may be inappropriate. Because the extent of disease—not the rate of growth—determines staging, the term *localized* is more accurate than the term *early*.[46] Similarly, the term *advanced* may be more appropriate than the term *late*.[126] The most accurate grouping uses the terms *localized* for any-TN_0M_0 disease, *regionally spread* or *vicinally spread* for any-$TN+M_0$ disease, and *widely disseminated* for any-T-any-NM_1 disease.[47] Convention and tradition dictate that this chapter continue to use the terms *early* to refer to lower stage (0, I, and II) and *late* to refer to higher stage (III and IV).

National Data

Information regarding the demographics, management, and outcome for laryngeal cancers in the United States is available from past reviews of data accumulated by the NCDB.[63,71] A review of the NCDB published in 1995 included data from 9101 laryngeal cancer cases managed during 1986 to 1989 and 8139 cases from 1992. These data represent approximately 39% and 65% of all laryngeal cancers evaluated in the United States during 1986 to 1989 and 1992, respec-

tively. As with all other NCDB reports, these data were obtained as a convenience sample through voluntary submission by participating hospitals and central registries and may therefore not be representative of the United States.[78] The reviews were limited to squamous cell carcinoma.

Among the 8139 laryngeal cancers identified in 1992, glottic cancers (62%) were more common than supraglottic (37%) and subglottic (2%) cancers (Table 100-3). Accurate staging was available for 87% of these cases and was presented as combined stage, also termed *best stage*. The more precise pathologic staging is used in cases in which surgical resection permits detailed evaluation of a resected specimen. Pathologic staging is not available when definitive management is nonsurgical. Combined stage or best stage reflects the pathologic stage when available or the clinical stage when treatment is nonsurgical.

Most glottic cancers are identified in the early stages (Table 100-3) because hoarseness, a readily identified symptom, generally occurs early in the course of a cancer that is located on the vibrating surface of the vocal cords. Additionally, metastases rarely develop from small glottic cancers because the lymphatics are sparse in this region of the larynx.[132] Supraglottic and subglottic cancers frequently present at more advanced stages because small tumors are often asymptomatic and because the abundant lymphatic drainage in this region of the larynx permits metastases to develop early in the course of disease.

A comparison of treatment modalities for laryngeal cancer at all stages and sites identified that nonsurgical treatment increased from 43.8% during 1986 to 1987 to 47.4% in 1992 (Table 100-4). Across these two periods, an increase in the use of endoscopic resection coincided with a decline in the practice of open partial laryngectomy.

Survival related to stage and management is presented in Table 100-5. These data reflect survival (relative) adjusted for age, race, and gender and should be interpreted with the understanding that, in this retrospective analysis, no control of selection bias influenced choice of treatment. The slightly worse survival

TABLE 100-3

STAGING CHARACTERISTICS OF LARYNGEAL SQUAMOUS CELL CANCER CASES FROM 1992

Anatomic Subsite	STAGE (%)					Early-stage (0, I, II) to Late-stage (III, IV) Ratio	(Cases) (*n*)
	0	I	II	III	IV		
Glottis	7.8	56.8	16.5	11.1	7.8	4.3	3566
Supraglottis	1.0	16.5	21.0	23.9	37.6	0.6	2130
Subglottis	2.1	14.9	28.7	22.3	32.0	0.8	94

TABLE 100-4

SURGICAL MANAGEMENT OF LARYNGEAL SQUAMOUS CELL CANCER CASES

Diagnosis Year	None (%)	Laser Surgery/ Local Excision/ Stripping (%)	Partial Laryngectomy (%)	MANAGEMENT		Laryngectomy Unspecified (%)	Regional Distant (%)	Unknown (%)	Cases (n)
				Total Laryngectomy Without Lymph Node Dissection (%)	Total Laryngectomy with Lymph Node Dissection (%)				
1986–1987	43.8	15.2	6.6	7.2	13.6	2.1	0.5	11.0	8701
1992	47.4	19.9	5.5	7.5	15.8	0.7	0.7	2.5	7692

TABLE 100-5

RELATIVE SURVIVAL FOR EARLY GLOTTIC SQUAMOUS CELL CANCER

		YEARS OF SURVIVAL					
Stage	Management*	1 (%)	2 (%)	3 (%)	4 (%)	5 (%)	Cases (n)
I	Surgery	97	93	89	86	81	193
	Radiation	95	90	84	78	73	678
	Surgery and radiation	97	92	86	81	75	309
	Other	93	88	83	72	68	81
	All	96	91	85	80	74	1261
II	Surgery	89	82	73	69	57	70
	Radiation	92	83	74	69	69	220
	Surgery and radiation	95	87	79	73	70	75
	Other	85	78	65	58	54	31
	All	92	83	74	69	64	396

*Survival data on management are presented to provide a record of outcome experience. Because patients were not randomly assigned to management groups, differences should be interpreted with caution.

for stage I lesions treated with radiotherapy rather than surgery therefore may not represent a greater treatment failure rate. It is possible that only the healthiest patients were selected for surgical treatment. The differences in 5-year survival could reflect the effect of a greater prevalence of death from concurrent illness among those treated with irradiation.

The high percentage of stages I and II cases receiving combined modality therapy appears contrary to the principle that supports the use of a single modality for highly curable early cancers as a means to limit morbidity and cost.[38] This high incidence of combined modality treatment may be an artifact induced by recording the surgical biopsy as cancer-directed therapy. Most patients with stage I or II cancers receiving surgery and irradiation likely underwent a biopsy then received definitive irradiation. Through this interpretation, the use of radiotherapy as initial definitive treatment for early glottic cancers appears to be an even more pervasive practice.

Most stage I glottic cancers (54%) received initial definitive treatment with radiotherapy (Table 100-5). The relative survival for stage I cancer overall was similar whether surgery, radiotherapy, or a combination was used. The 2-year survival rate was in the 90% to 92% range. Among those treated with irradiation, the 5-year survival rate was 73%. Among those treated surgically, the 5-year survival rate was 81%.

For stage II glottic cancers, 2-year survival ranged from 82% to 87% (Table 100-5). For cases initially treated with surgery alone, the 5-year survival was 57%, compared with 69% of those treated with irradiation alone, and 70% of those treated with both surgery and irradiation. The lower survival rate identified among surgically treated stage II cancers may also reflect a selection bias. Cancers stage T_{2b}, based on

impaired vocal cord mobility, are preferentially treated surgically at many centers.[67] The surgery alone group may have contained a disproportionate number of T_{2b} cases, which have a poorer prognosis than T_{2a} glottic cancers.

Data addressing practice in the United States in the late 1990s and early in the millennium are now available from the Benchmark Reports distributed by the American College of Surgeons to certified hospitals.[72] Future analysis of this data will ultimately permit more specific review. At this point, analysis is available only for broad groupings that lump the supraglottic, glottic, and subglottic sites together (Figure 100-4). These data identify the remarkable increase in utilization of chemotherapy combined with radiotherapy for advanced stage laryngeal cancer. Chemoradiation (29%) was the most common treatment of stage III laryngeal cancer and the second most common (25%) for stage IV cancer (Figure 100-4).

In contrast, chemotherapy combined with radiotherapy is not commonly used for early laryngeal cancer (Figure 100-5). Radiotherapy alone is the most common initial management for laryngeal cancer in the United States. The role that salvage surgery played in the treatment of radiation failures is not addressed in this analysis.

Detail addressing treatment-specific survival is not included in the survival analysis from the NCDB, which is published in the sixth edition of the AJCC staging manual. However, stage- and site-specific survival statistics are available as they were analyzed from a data set of patients whose cancer was diagnosed between 1985 and 1991.[64]

The analysis of observed survival (Figure 100-6) employs the end point of death from any cause. Relative survival (Figure 100-7) adjusts these observed

ADVANCED STAGE LARYNGEAL CANCER (ALL SITES)
INITIAL TREATMENT
CASES DIAGNOSED IN 2000
NCDB (1184 REPORTING HOSPITALS)

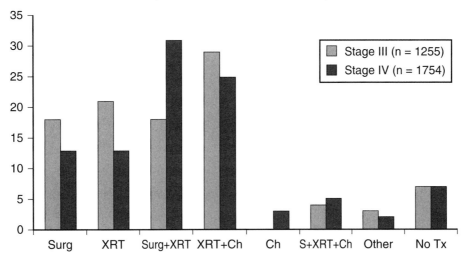

Figure 100-4. Radiotherapy combined with chemotherapy is currently the most common initial treatment modality for stage III laryngeal squamous cell carcinoma in an analysis grouping all sites (supraglottis, glottis, and subglottis) together. © *Commission on Cancer, American college of Surgeons. NCDB Benchmark Reports, v1.1. Chicago, IL, 2002. (The content reproduced from the applications remains the full and exclusive copyrighted property of the American college of Surgeons. The American College of Surgeons is not responsible for any ancillary or derivative works based on the original Text, Tables, or Figures.)*

EARLY STAGE LARYNGEAL CANCER (ALL SITES)
INITIAL TREATMENT
HISTOLOGY = SCC, NOS
CASES DIAGNOSED IN 2000
NCDB (1184 REPORTING HOSPITALS)

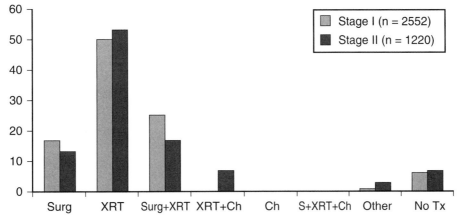

Figure 100-5. Radiotherapy alone is the most common initial treatment modality for early (stage I and II) laryngeal squamous cell carcinoma in an analysis grouping all sites (supraglottis, glottis, and subglottis) together. © *Commission on Cancer, American college of Surgeons. NCDB Benchmark Reports, v1.1. Chicago, IL, 2002. (The content reproduced from the applications remains the full and exclusive copyrighted property of the American college of Surgeons. The American College of Surgeons is not responsible for any ancillary or derivative works based on the original Text, Tables, or Figures.)*

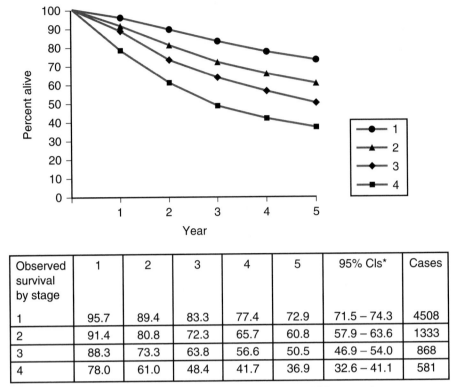

Observed survival by stage	1	2	3	4	5	95% CIs*	Cases
1	95.7	89.4	83.3	77.4	72.9	71.5 – 74.3	4508
2	91.4	80.8	72.3	65.7	60.8	57.9 – 63.6	1333
3	88.3	73.3	63.8	56.6	50.5	46.9 – 54.0	868
4	78.0	61.0	48.4	41.7	36.9	32.6 – 41.1	581

Figure 100-6. Five-year observed survival by "combined" AJCC stage for squamous cell carcinoma of the glottis.

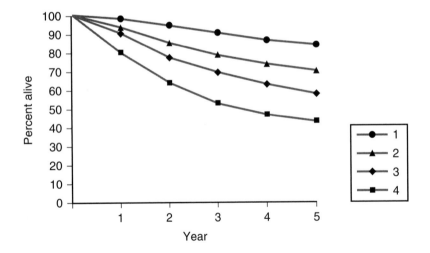

Relative survival	1	2	3	4	5	95% CIs*	Cases
1	97.8	94.1	90.1	86.1	83.4	81.8 – 85.0	4528
2	93.4	84.7	78.3	73.3	69.5	66.3 – 72.7	1340
3	89.9	77.0	69.1	62.6	57.4	53.3 – 61.5	872
4	79.6	63.6	52.5	46.4	42.6	37.7 – 47.4	587

Figure 100-7. Five-year, relative survival by "combined" AJCC stage for squamous cell carcinoma of the glottis, 1985–1991. (*Confidence intervals of 95% correspond to year 5-year survival rates.)

survival rates by the expected age- and gender-matched general population. Although these adjusted relative survival rates are intended to isolate the impact of laryngeal cancer on survival, they do not account for other related causes of death (e.g., comorbidity, tobacco use). Disease-specific survival that uses death as a result of the cancer as the end point would theoretically be the most accurate. Unfortunately information about whether death results from the cancer or other causes is difficult to assign accurately, even through comprehensive retrospective chart review. Therefore, relative survival is a more reasonable approach to analyzing survival in large data sets such as the NCDB.

DIAGNOSIS
Endoscopic Imaging

The initial evaluation of a patient with an early glottic lesion requires inspection of the larynx. The common use of flexible fiberoptic laryngoscopy to supplement indirect mirror examination now permits visualization of the majority of laryngeal cancers in a clinic setting. Videoendoscopy and videostroboscopy offer further refinement in assessing glottic lesions. It has become standard practice in many institutions to permanently record the appearance of all laryngeal cancers through video recording, using rigid or fiberoptic endoscopy. The capacity to refer to these permanent records documenting the extent of the original lesion often improves long-term patient care.

The development of flexible fiberoptic endoscopes designed for transnasal esophagoscopes has also permitted use of these instruments to evaluate the larynx and trachea.[11,14,15,119] The improved optics of these instruments—coupled with the presence of a side port that permits the use of suction, placement of biopsy instruments, and instillation of topical anesthetics—has expanded the capacity to perform in-office laryngeal evaluations (Figure 100-8, *A*). Although direct laryngoscopy remains the most appropriate approach to evaluate and biopsy the majority of lesions suspected of being malignant, in selected cases biopsy can be effected in the clinic (Figures 100-8, *B* and 100-8, *C*).

When videostroboscopy was introduced as a common clinical tool, enthusiasm was high for its potential to help discriminate invasive cancer from epithelial atypia based on the stroboscopic appearance of the vocal fold epithelial pliability.[133,183] Subsequent experience of Colden and others has identified that laryngeal stroboscopy is neither reliable in distinguishing vocal fold atypia from invasive cancer nor useful in determining the depth of invasion of vocal fold cancer.[29] These investigators did suggest that the stroboscopic appearance of a relatively normal mucosal wave indicates that a lesion is superficial and does not extensively involve the underlying vocal ligament.

Advances in technology, coupling physical and biologic analysis to endoscopy, have identified several adjuncts to complement standard imaging of the larynx at the time of direct laryngoscopy. Lugol's solution, as well as toluidine blue, have been used to stain laryngeal tissue in an effort to discriminate normal tissue from tumor.[81,88] These approaches have not met with uniform success and therefore have not been widely adopted. Fluorescent tumor markers such as tetracyclines and hematoporphyrin derivatives are preferentially absorbed by tumor cells and can be used to discriminate tumor from adjacent normal tissue by the red fluorescence they emit when exposed

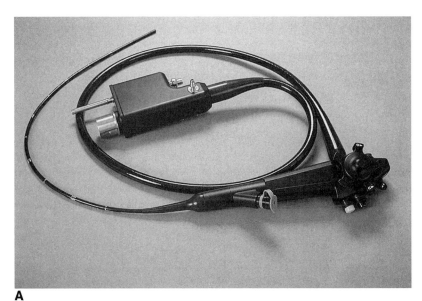

A

Figure 100-8. A, Transnasal esophagoscope (TNE) (Pentax®).

Continued

B   **C**

Figure 100-8, cont'd B, View of oropharynx and hypopharynx through TNE. **C,** Biopsy forceps prepared to remove posterior pharyngeal wall lesion. To view this image in color, please go to *www.ototext.com* or the Electronic Image Collection CD, bound into your copy of *Cummings Otolaryngology—Head and Neck Surgery,* 4th edition.

to ultraviolet light.[98] Additional cost and operating time, as well as problems with skin photosensitivity, have limited the usefulness of this technique. A more promising approach employing autofluorescence laryngoscopy has been reported. Zargi and others have employed the lung imaging fluorescence endoscope (LIFE) system to evaluate laryngeal lesions.[180] Their preliminary work identified differences in the intensity of autofluorescence between normal and tumor tissue when exposed to blue or violet light. They also identified shortcomings in the use of the LIFE system for this purpose, noting that further technical advances are needed to make this endeavor a useful clinical tool.

Stone and others reported that the fluorescence of biologic tissue actually may impede the use of Raman spectroscopic analysis to discriminate normal from malignant laryngeal lesions.[153] These investigators have developed strategies that negates the impact of the natural biologic fluorescence to permit evaluation of the distinctive spectral signatures of tissues elicited when exposed to monochromatic laser excitation. This strategy may develop into a noninvasive tool in the early detection of cancerous and precancerous lesions.

Similarities in the accessibility to and histopathology of the epithelial lining of the uterine cervix and the vocal folds have resulted in the transfer of technology from the field of gynecology to laryngology on many levels. In the past, this has even extended to the use of gynecologic speculums used as direct laryngoscopes.[166] In 1995 Andrea, Dias, and Santos reported laryngeal use of the gynecologic microcolpohysteroscope.[7] This instrument is most commonly used for in vivo and in situ microscopic study of epithelial cells of the uterine cervix. It employs a magnifying telescope that that makes direct contact with the epithelium. Laryngeal epithelium may be evaluated in a similar fashion with the rigid telescope placed through a direct laryngoscope to evaluate the vocal fold epithelium after is has been stained by methylene blue. Further work by Arens and others amplified this concept to include analysis of autofluorescence at the time of contact endoscopy, entitled "Compact Endoscopy."[9] Compact endoscopy (a combination of autofluorescence and contact endoscopy) stimulates autofluorescence of the laryngeal tissue with blue filtered light. This adjunct to standard laryngoscopy is still under development but promises to enable the laryngologist to accurately assess laryngeal cancer and precancerous lesions during microlaryngoscopy without need for a biopsy.

Radiology
Chest X-Ray

A chest radiograph is necessary in the evaluation of patients with glottic cancers to assess for concurrent pulmonary disease and to screen for second primary lung cancers. The incidence of distant metastatic spread of an early glottic cancer to the lung is sufficiently rare that a preoperative chest radiograph is not generally intended to survey for that specific purpose. Annual chest x-rays should be obtained in the course of clinic follow-up examinations primarily because of the high incidence of second primary lung cancers in patients managed for laryngeal cancer.[120]

Magnetic Resonance Imaging and Computed Tomography

The appropriate role for magnetic resonance imaging (MRI) and computed tomography (CT) in early glottic cancers is still being defined.[170] These advanced imaging studies are of questionable value in the assessment of most superficial T_1 lesions of the vocal cords. Selected T_1 lesions with anterior commissure involvement may benefit from MRI or CT imaging if extension of the tumor superiorly into the preepiglottic space or anteriorly into the thyroid cartilage is detected. The more routine use of MRI or CT is advocated in the evaluation of T_2 lesions is not only to help determine tumor extent (and hence T classification), but also tumor volume. Some authors have suggested that CT or MRI of T_2 lesions may help determine radiocurability by assessing tumor volume. Other investigators have not found the size of the tumor to be useful for predicting radiocurability.[111]

Wenig and others[176] contend that surgical treatment of laryngeal cancer with less than a total laryngectomy mandates preoperative MRI in almost all cases. These investigators identify that tumor involvement of the entire vocal cord or the anterior commissure, as well as the presence of vocal fold paresis, are considered indications for the use of MRI. They relate that only the most superficial T_1 lesions of the mobile portion of the vocal cord need not be imaged because MRI will not detect the extent of these lesions. This philosophy is in distinctly opposite from that of Steiner and others, who relate that advanced imaging of laryngeal cancer is fraught with artifact.[150] Steiner and Ambrosch find little value in preoperative imaging of laryngeal cancers and relate that the most accurate assessment of tumor extent comes at the time of endoscopic laser microsurgical resection.

Debate continues as to whether CT or MRI offers the most useful information when imaging the larynx.[172] Advances in the speed with which CTs can now be done offers an advantage to this technique. In 2002 Stadler and others[148] reported that use of rapid imaging spiral CTs of the larynx permits complete evaluation during the course of a single maneuver. This rapid imaging of the larynx may be accomplished as the patient performs either a modified Valsalva maneuver or phonation of the utterance "E." This functional imaging (done during the maneuver) was compared with nonfunctional imaging (done with quiet breathing) and correlated with postsurgical pathology assessments and findings at microlaryngoscopy. Although the numbers in their study were small, Stadler and others conclude that functional CT imaging appears to be more accurate in determining tumor extent than nonfunctional imaging.

Positron Emission Tomography

The role for positron emission tomography (PET) is continuing to expand. Unfortunately, despite the presence of a governing body to accredit nuclear medicine laboratories, significant variability exists in the quality of clinical PET imaging. Current accreditation standards set by the American College of Radiology require that the interpreting radiologists have 20 hours of continuing medical education in PET and that they have interpreted 80 oncologic cases in the preceding 3 years.[106] There was an insufficient number of fellowship-trained nuclear medicine physicians to staff the approximately 250,000 PET cases that were performed in the United States in 2002. The favorable results reported from institutions with substantial experience and the most sophisticated equipment are not necessarily obtained from institutions with limited experience and with less refined equipment. The challenges in performing and interpreting PET images are likely to be more of a problem in the head and neck region than elsewhere. The complex anatomy of the head and neck, coupled with its complex physiology (including areas with normal high glucose metabolism), adds to the variability in the quality of PET imaging in this region.

F-18-fluoro-deoxy-glucose (FDG) PET scanning has been reported as useful in detecting subclinical recurrent or persistent cancer at a stage when it is highly curable.[10] Terhaard and others propose an algorithm for the follow-up of patients treated for laryngeal or hypopharyngeal cancers that emphasizes the use of PET imaging.[157] Through a prospective study of 109 PET scans done on 75 patients with either laryngeal or hypopharyngeal cancer, these investigators concluded that an FDG PET scan should be the first diagnostic step when a recurrence is suspected after treatment with irradiation. As a result of this study, in which the majority of cases were glottic and classified as either T_1 or T_2, these investigators suggested that no biopsy is needed if the scan is negative. In the face of a positive scan and a negative biopsy, a follow-up scan showing decreased FDG uptake would indicate that a recurrence is unlikely. Caution should be exercised in following these guidelines if other clinical indicators support the need for a biopsy. At this point in our experience, endoscopy with a biopsy to sample tissue suspicious in appearance for cancer remains the most critical means by which recurrence is evaluated.

Shortcomings of PET imaging have been noted. Most investigators suggest waiting at least 3 months after treatment to perform PET imaging because false positive results are common if the imaging is done soon after radiotherapy is completed.[104] False positives may also result from infection, radionecrosis, or accumulation of saliva in the vallecula.[77,162] Some of these shortcomings of PET imaging are being addressed by use of pharmaceuticals other than FDG. The presence of viable tumor has been identified through PET imaging with 1-[1-^{11}C]-tyrosine (TYR).

TYR PET imaging analyzes protein synthesis activity and has been reported to be successful in detecting recurrent squamous cell carcinoma of the larynx.[36] Further progress with PET imaging is anticipated with the introduction of other pharmaceuticals.

TREATMENT

The ideal initial management of an early glottic cancer is the one that is most likely to result in cure and to preserve a normal voice without impaired swallowing or breathing. It is not often possible to meet all of these goals. A compromise is generally required, wherein the choice of therapy is based on the desires of an informed patient who understands the shortcomings of the alternatives. The surgeon should be aware of the options to make an informed recommendation to the patient. Ideally the patient will meet with both the surgeon and a radiation oncologist to permit identification of the full spectrum of treatment options from differing perspectives.

The following discussion focuses on specific surgical and radiotherapy techniques and concludes with a review of general management principles, focusing on the impact of management on the voice.

Surgery

Physicians' views vary on the indications for use of a specific procedure or radiotherapy technique. General guidelines for selection of an approach based on the extent of a lesion are listed in Table 100-6 and depicted in Figure 100-9. The choice of therapeutic approach for a patient requires consideration of many other variables in addition to the anatomic extent of the cancer. Overall cure rates and laryngeal preservation figures are high for the surgical management of early glottic squamous cell carcinoma (Table 100-7).

Endoscopic Excision

The histopathologic correlate of a superficial T_1 primary cancer may reveal a lesion without deep extension beyond the superficial layer of the lamina propria.[86] Endoscopic surgical excision of such a lesion may allow for resection with a clear margin without damaging the underlying vocal ligament or vocalis muscle (Figure 100-9).[165] However, not all T_1 glottic cancers are amenable to superficial conservative resection. Up to 20% of T_1 cancers will show normal mobility despite invasion of the vocal ligament.[38] Carcinoma in situ, which by definition does not invade past the basement membrane, is most amenable to complete excision without disruption of the underlying vocal ligament.

Biopsy

In general, discrete lesions of the vocal cords are better sampled through excisional biopsy than through

---

TABLE 100-6

SELECTED SURGICAL PROCEDURES FOR GLOTTIC CANCER

Procedure	Indications	Study
Microlaryngoscopy partial cordectomy with or without carbon dioxide laser (excisional biopsy)	T_1 midcord leukoplakia, T_{is}/microinvasion	Strong and Jako (1972) Kleinsasser (1990) Shapshay, Hybels, and Bohigian (1990)
Cordectomy complete with or without carbon dioxide laser (endoscopy)	T_1 midcord	Strong (1975) Annyas and others (1990) Shapsay, Hybels, and Bohigian (1990) Eckel and Thumfart (1992)
Cordectomy (laryngofissure)	T_1 midcord	DeSanto and others (1977) Bailey (1985)
Frontolateral partial laryngectomy	T_1 with extension to anterior commissure	Leroux-Robert (1975)
Hemilaryngectomy and extended hemilaryngectomy	T_1/T_2 with extension to arytenoid, without anterior commissure fixation (minimal)	Norris (1958) Som (1975) Mohr and others (1983)
Anterior partial laryngectomy with epiglottoplasty or with keel	T_1/T_2 with extension to anterior commissure (without arytenoid)	Tucker and others (1979) Som and Silver (1968)
Subtotal laryngectomy with cricohyoidoepiglottopexy	T_{1b}/T_2 bilateral anterior involvement, may include removal of one arytenoid	Laccourreye and others (1990) Charlin and others (1988)

TABLE 100-7

RESULTS OF SURGICAL MANAGEMENT OF EARLY GLOTTIC CANCER*

Study	Patients (n)	Stage	Type of Management	LESIONS CONTROLLED (%)		After Laryngeal Preservation	SURVIVAL (%)	
				Initially	Ultimately		2-year	5-year
Ton-Van and others[62]	170	T_{1a}		94				
	36	T_{1b}	Cordectomy	78	*98*	*92*	*87*	*84*
	24	T_2		75				
Johnson (1991)	54	T_1	Hemilaryngectomy	98	98	98	98	—
	31	T_2	Hemilaryngectomy	67	90	67	84	—
Laccourreye (1991)	308	T_1	Cordectomy	87	—	—	—	—
	107	T_2	Vertical hemilaryngectomy	78				
Daniilidis (1991)	94	T_1	Cordectomy	90	93	84	—	93
Rothfield (1991)	20	T_{is}–T_{mi}	Microscopic direct laryngoscopy	95	80	95	100	100
Casiano and others[6]	37	T_1	Carbon dioxide laser	62	97	91	—	97
	16	T_1[†]		51	100	69	—	100
Steiner (1993)	29	T_{is}	Carbon dioxide laser		100		97	
	96	T_1		98	100	99	—	87
	34	T_2[‡]		100			78	
Myers (1994)	50	T_1	Carbon dioxide laser	92	100	100	100	
Thomas (1994)	159	T_1	Laryngofissure approach	92	100	94	91	84

*Italicized numbers are mean figures for entire patient group.
†Radiation failure patients.
‡T_2 with mobile cords.

small, piecemeal, random biopsies. The opportunity to effect a cure exists through excisional biopsy if the pathologic assessment shows carcinoma in situ or a minimally invasive cancer. Excisional biopsies also avoid any sampling error wherein small areas of invasive cancer may be missed within a larger field of dysplastic epithelium. Judgment should be exercised in determining the extent of dissection in performing a biopsy on patients who are candidates for irradiation. Smaller biopsies that are sufficient to confirm the diagnosis of invasive cancer impair the posttreatment voice to a lesser degree than larger excisions if irradiation is used as definitive treatment. It is useful to discuss the decision making with the patient in weighing the benefits and risks to approaching the biopsy conservatively or aggressively.

Microflap Technique

The degree of invasion may be assessed clinically at the time of biopsy by using the microflap technique. This approach stresses attention to dissection along the natural tissue plane of the superficial layer of the lamina propria, which separates the epithelium from the vocal ligament. Dissection in this plane creates a microflap of overlying diseased epithelium, which, once the plane is developed, can be removed without damage to the underlying vocal ligament during excisional biopsy. This approach may result in a defect similar to that created with traditional vocal cord stripping but is done in a more controlled manner that has less chance of injuring adjacent healthy tissue. The deep extent of the tumor through the superficial layer of the lamina propria can be evaluated while developing the plane between the epithelium and vocal ligament. Good exposure through an adequate-sized laryngoscope; suspension of the laryngoscope, permitting instrumentation with both hands; improved dissecting instruments; and use of the operating microscope to provide magnification with binocular vision facilitate the assessment of superficial lesions of the vocal cords. Removal of carcinoma in situ or a minimally invasive cancer on the surface of the vocal cord by this approach may be curative. It is not necessary to use a laser in resecting superficial vocal cord lesions. Although the incisions in the epithelium can be made with carbon dioxide lasers without a large amount of adjacent thermal damage, the extra preparation and expense needed to use the

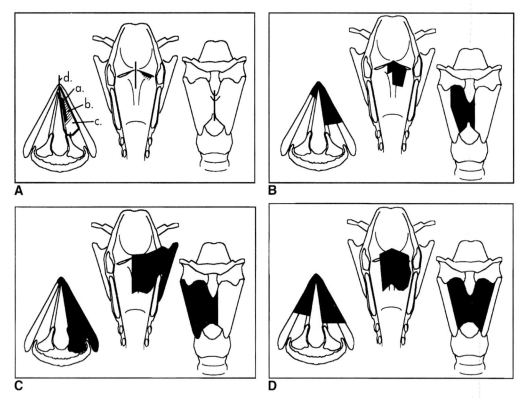

Figure 100-9. Diagrams of vertical partial laryngectomy.

laser to dissect in the relatively avascular glottic larynx do not support its general use. The laser is more useful in the endoscopic management of more invasive glottic cancers and in the resection of adjacent well-vascularized supraglottic structures.

Laser Excision

Principles. The carbon dioxide laser was introduced for resecting laryngeal cancer in 1972 by Strong and Jako.[154] Through the following years, results with laser resection were generally inferior to those with conventional open techniques. These poor results likely reflected the novelty of the technology and the need to establish clinically useful guidelines for selection of this management modality. Recent reports have focused on the successful use of the carbon dioxide laser to manage early glottic lesions[35] (Table 100-8). This technique has been reported with cure rates equivalent to those of laryngofissure with cordectomy, classic hemilaryngectomy, and radiotherapy for selected early lesions.[35,43]

The extent to which laser resection is practiced in the management of glottic cancers varies considerably. The general consensus is that endoscopic resection (with or without the laser) is most appropriate for small cancers involving the free edge of a mobile vocal cord.[38] Controversy persists regarding the use of

endoscopic resection in the management of T_2 lesions of the glottis.[37,43,135,137,182] Although some investigators have reported poor outcome from endoscopic laser treatment of T_{2b} glottic cancers with impaired cord mobility associated with muscular invasion,[43,136] Thumfart and others[158] identified that radical and effective management of transglottic T_2 cancers (T_{2a}) can be effected through endoscopic removal with clear margins ensured by removal of the inner perichondrium of the thyroid and cricoid cartilages and the cricothyroid membrane. They reported that use of fibrin glue to seal the exposed cartilage at the time of the resection helps decrease granulation tissue formation and minimizes postoperative bleeding.

A reassessment of the underlying oncologic principle of en bloc resection has lead some investigators to extend the approach by which glottic cancers are removed endoscopically. Halstead's principle of en bloc resection to avoid tumor spill is reasonable but has not been supported by experience from clinical practice. As Pearson identified, "Halstead did not have a laser."[117] Pearson observed that viable tumor cell implantation is prevented by use of laser as a cutting instrument to sear the cut surfaces.

Steiner and Ambrosch from Germany have condensed years of work into a valuable reference entitled *Endoscopic Laser Surgery of the Upper Aerodigestive*

TABLE 100-8

EARLY MANAGEMENT RESULTS USING THE CARBON DIOXIDE LASER PUBLISHED CURE RATES FOR T_1 GLOTTIC TUMORS MANAGED WITH LASER CORDECTOMY

Study	Patients (n)	Local Control Achieved (n)	Failures (n)	Laser Salvage Management (n)	Total Laryngectomy (n)	X-ray Radiation Management (n)
Koufman (1986)	23	22	1	1	0	0
Wetmore and others (1986)	21	17	4	1	0	3
Blakeslee and others (1984)	35	31	4	0	2*	2
Hirano and others (1985)	8	7	1	0	0	1
Elner and Fex (1988)	31	25	6	3	0	3
Annyas and others (1984)	10	9	1	1	0	0
Cragle and Brandenburg[9]	14	13	1	0	1	0
TOTAL	142 (100%)	124 (87.3%)	18 (12.7%)	6 (4.2%)	3 (2.1%)	9 (6.3%)

From Cragle S, Brandenburg J: Laser cordectomy or radiotherapy: cure rates, communication, and cost, *Otolaryngol Head Neck Surg* 108:648, 1993.
*Both laryngectomies resulted in recurrent tumor and death.

Tract.[150] In this work they relate that adherence to the en bloc resection principle advocated by Halstead may actually impair the capacity to obtain a tumor-free margin in the process of resection. As a result, endoscopic resection of larger tumors is often done with the initial laser cuts made directly through the tumor both to debulk it and to identify (through microscopic dissection) the interface between the tumor and the normal tissue (Figures 100-10, *A* and 100-10, *B*). This approach to endoscopic cancer surgery has permitted more aggressive resections to be done in a controlled fashion as the depth of the tumor

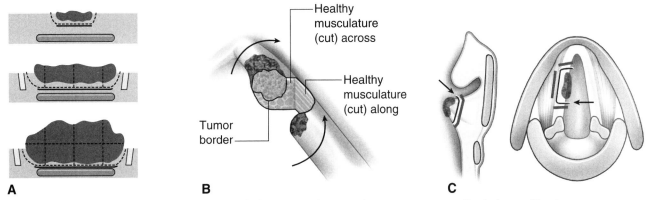

Figure 100-10. A, Endoscopic laser resection may be encompass smaller lesions without transgressing tumor. Larger tumors are best managed with controlled resection in several pieces. **B,** Microscopic evaluation of the cut surface of tumor permits accurate removal with the plane between tumor and normal tissue clearly defined. **C,** Small vocal fold lesions can be resected as a single specimen with care to keep a 1- to 3-mm distance about the lesion and to mark it appropriately to confirm clear margins histologically (Steiner W, Ambrosch P: Endoscopic laser surgery of the upper aerodigestive tract. New York, 2000, Thieme International, pp 43 (A), 54 (B), and 56(C).)

extent is more readily determined. It is not always necessary to cut through tumors to ensure their complete removal. Steiner and Ambrosch identify that smaller tumors may be removed en bloc with a traditional approach to excision (Figure 100-10, *C*). "Cold steel" removal with or without laser assistance can also be used effectively for these smaller lesions (Figure 100-11). Eckel, from analysis of a series of 252 T_1 and T_2 glottic cancers treated with transoral laser surgery (TLS) between 1987 and 1996 concluded that TLS offered local control rates comparable to radiotherapy for T_1 lesions and better than radiotherapy for T_2 lesions.[42] Eckel identified that recurrence rates after TLS were higher than for open conventional partial laryngectomy, but identified that these recurrences are more amenable to retreatment in the absence of previous radiation or open surgery.

Some investigators advocate limiting use of endoscopic laser resection to those patients with good exposure of the glottic region and tumors staged T_{is} or T_1 without deep involvement of the anterior commissure, vocal process, ventricle, or subglottic region.[58] Others have addressed extension to the anterior commissure by combining laser endoscopic resection with a mini-open procedure by a "window" laryngoplasty to remove the cartilage segment at risk.[121,138] The capacity to use the laser to extend a resection to cartilage has been employed by Steiner and Ambrosch[150] to address the more deeply invasive cancers endoscopically without the need for an external incision (Figure 100-12). These investigators report results

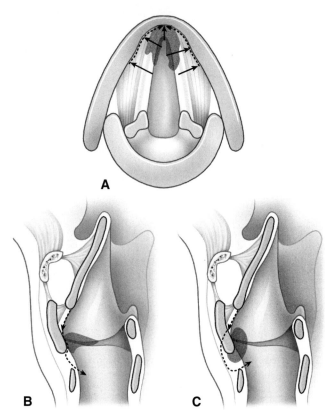

Figure 100-12. Endoscopic laser resection of cancer involving the anterior commissure and subglottis requires sequential resection of tissue in several pieces. This approach permits removal of the inferior aspect of the thyroid cartilage. (Steiner W, Ambrosch P: Endoscopic laser surgery of the upper aerodigestive tract, New York, 2000, Thieme International, p 58).

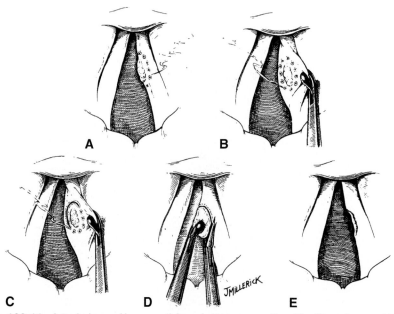

Figure 100-11. A technique of laser partial cordectomy as outlined by Shapshay and Rebeiz.

from endoscopic laser surgery for early and advanced upper airway cancers that are similar to those obtained with more traditional approaches.[3,149,151]

Classification of endoscopic resections. The extent of an endoscopic laryngeal cancer resection is determined by the location and extent of the tumor at the time of microdirect laser laryngoscopy. It is therefore difficult to apply a rigid classification scheme to accurately describe all the options possible through endoscopic laser resection. For research purposes and to provide some broad guidelines for treatment, it is reasonable to group surgical resections along standardized guidelines with these limitations in mind. The European Laryngological Society has developed a classification scheme addressing endoscopic resection of glottic cancer (Table 100-9).[122]

Gallo and others have employed this classification scheme in their analysis of 156 cases of early stage glottic cancer and have generalized the type of resection with regard to T classification (Table 100-10).[58]

Laser vestibulectomy. The false vocal cords may be resected with the carbon dioxide laser at the time of microlaryngoscopy to improve exposure of the true vocal cords. Kashima, Lee, and Zinreich[82] have termed this approach *laser vestibulectomy.* Kerrebijn, deBoer, and Knegt support the use of the laser vestibulectomy in staging and treating glottic tumors.[83] In 20 consecutive patients undergoing evaluation for early-stage vocal cord cancer, these authors identified that laser resection of the false vocal cords improved management without inducing additional morbidity. Laser vestibulectomy improved exposure of the entire upper surface of the vocal folds at the time of microlaryngoscopy, provided access to detect subclinical tumor invasion into the paraglottic space, and improved accuracy of follow-up examinations. Others have argued that routine resection of the false cords may not be advisable. Steiner and Ambrosch suggest that it

TABLE 100-9

ENDOSCOPIC CORDECTOMY: CLASSIFICATION BY EUROPEAN LARYNGOLOGICAL SOCIETY

Subepithelial cordectomy	Type I
Subligmental cordectomy	Type II
Transmuscular cordectomy	Type III
Total or complete cordectomy	Type IV
Extended cordectomy encompassing	
contralateral fold	Type IV a
arytenoids	Type IV b
ventricular fold	Type IV c
subglottis	Type IV d

TABLE 100-10

INDICATION BY STAGE FOR LASER RESECTION

T Stage	Type of Cordectomy	Indication
T_{is}	Type I	Depending on the extension of the involved area and the results of preoperative investigation (e.g., videostroboscopy)
	Type II	
	Type III	
T_{1a}	Type III	Small (0.5–0.7 mm), superficial tumor involving the middle-third of the true vocal fold
T_{1a}	Type IV	Tumor size >0.7 mm or deep infiltrative pattern and/or extension to the anterior commissure
T_{1b}	Type Va	Involvement of the anterior commissure or horseshoe lesion
	Bilateral cordectomy	Multifocal cancer

is important to preserve these structures to permit the compensatory supraglottic phonation as a useful adaptation if glottic incompetence results from glottic resection.[150]

Open Partial Laryngectomy
Laryngofissure

The basic external (open) approach to resection of vocal cord cancer is a laryngofissure (or thyrotomy). After separation of the strap muscles in the midline, an incision is made through the cricothyroid membrane to permit inspection of the subglottic and undersurface of the vocal cord. As with intranasal surgery, injection of the vascular laryngeal structures with a vasoconstrictor before making incisions helps to diminish bleeding and improve exposure. Direct inspection through a cricothyrotomy permits placement of the tips of a hemostat between the vocal cords immediately posterior to the anterior commissure. The vocal cords are then separated by opening the hemostat. This exposure permits safe division of the thyroid cartilage and underlying anterior commissure without transecting the vocal cords. Wide exposure of the endolarynx results from lateral traction on each of the separated thyroid alae. In younger patients, the thyroid cartilage is not ossified and may be transected with a scalpel. The ossified cartilage of older patients generally requires a rotating drill or saw to cut the cartilage. This approach disrupts the laryngeal architecture only at the site of the anterior incisions. Laryngofissure has also been used to describe the procedure whereby the larynx is exposed by dividing the cricoid cartilage in addition to the thyroid cartilage.[25]

Laryngofissure with Cordectomy

Laryngofissure with cordectomy refers to the use of a thyrotomy to permit excision of the vocal cord (see Figure 100-9, A). This procedure is appropriate for T_1 glottic cancers that are not amenable to resection endoscopically because of anatomic constraints preventing adequate laryngoscopic exposure (e.g., limited mouth opening, retrognathia, prominent dentition, or poor neck extension). The open approach via laryngofissure offers the advantage of excellent exposure, which permits precise tumor removal and accurate sampling of adjacent tissue for frozen section analysis. Additionally, the procedure can be extended to include resection of adjacent structures (e.g., underlying thyroid cartilage). Disadvantages of this approach include the usual need for a tracheotomy and potential problems with healing that may compromise the airway, voice, and swallowing. Laryngofissure with cordectomy without glottic reconstruction relies on secondary intention healing to create a neocord. Despite efforts to restore glottic competence through creating a neocord, efforts are commonly unsuccessful and a breathy voice commonly results.

Vertical Partial Laryngectomy

Vertical partial laryngectomy is a more extensive resection that begins with a laryngofissure. Removal of the vocal cord and a segment of the underlying thyroid cartilage is termed *vertical partial laryngectomy* or *hemilaryngectomy*. It may be modified in one of several ways. The ipsilateral thyroid alae and arytenoid may be removed as required for more extensive lesions (see Figure 100-9, B and C). Alternatively, the ipsilateral arytenoid and a posterior strip of thyroid cartilage may be left intact. Unless tumor involves the arytenoid, this structure should be retained to diminish the risk of aspiration.

Further extension of the vertical partial laryngectomy may include resection of the anterior commissure (Figure 100-9, D). Excision of part of the contralateral vocal cord along with the anterior commissure may require that the laryngofissure be done off the midline through the thyroid alae and underlying vocal cord. Direct laryngoscopy immediately before the procedure, coupled with inspection of the undersurface of the glottis after the initial cricothyrotomy, helps direct the cartilage and vocal cord incisions appropriately. Resection of the anterior commissure shortens the anterior-posterior dimensions of the glottis. Placement of an umbrella keel at the time of closure may effectively lengthen the vocal cords to diminish the potential for glottic stenosis. The keel is generally removed 3 to 6 weeks later under a brief anesthetic.

An extended vertical partial laryngectomy may permit resection of tumors with involvement of both vocal cords, the anterior commissure, and the paraglottic space. Giovanni and others identified that this extensive resection is readily reconstructed with an epiglottic flap and offers an alternative to supracricoid laryngectomy (Figures 100-13, A).[62] Giovanni and others reported similar speech and swallowing outcomes for this type of vertical partial laryngectomy when compared with supracricoid laryngectomy. These investigators also identified similar local control rates for T_1 and T_2 disease in comparing these two procedures.

Supracricoid Laryngectomy

Supracricoid partial laryngectomy (SPL) involves removal of both membranous vocal folds and the contents of the adjacent paraglottic spaces in continuity with the entire thyroid cartilage. The resection also includes the base of the epiglottis and can be extended to remove one (but not both) arytenoids, as well as the false cords, the entire epiglottis, and the pre-epiglottic space. This procedure is based on the novel concept that the extent of tumor does not impact on the amount of thyroid cartilage removed. In all cases the entire thyroid cartilage is removed both for oncologic reasons and, more consistently, for reconstructive purposes in order to remove tissue intervening between the cricoid cartilage and hyoid bone.[92] Resection of the entire thyroid cartilage permits reconstruction of a functional larynx by approximating the cricoid cartilage to the hyoid bone with stout sutures to adhere these structures together. A detailed description of the technique is available in the book *Organ Preservation Surgery for Laryngeal Cancer* by Weinstein and others, which includes videos of the technique on four separate CD-ROMs.[175] Modifications of this approach have been described. Adamopoulos and others report that preservation of the posterior segment of the vocal cord on the less involved side is useful in selected cases where surgical margins are not compromised.[1] These investigators identify that their preliminary data support this technique to improve voice quality and decrease swallowing impairment by preserving a larger portion of the valvular structure of the larynx.

The nomenclature most commonly employed to discriminate between the types of supracricoid laryngectomy focuses on the reconstruction. When the epiglottis above the petiole is preserved, the reconstruction is termed a *cricohyoidoepiglottopexy*

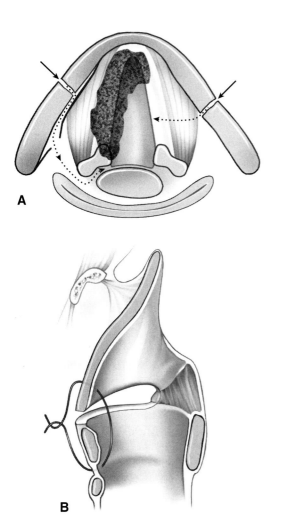

Figure 100-13. A, Extended vertical partial laryngectomy. **B,** Reconstruction with epiglottic flap after extended vertical partial laryngectomy. As described in Giovanni A, Guelfucci B, Gras R and others: Partial frontolateral laryngectomy with epiglottic reconstruction for management of early-stage glottic carcinoma, *Laryngoscope* 111:663–668, 2001.

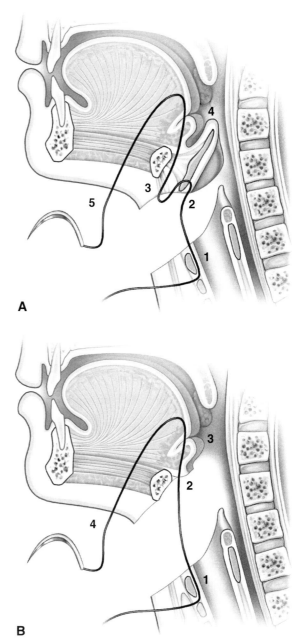

Figure 100-14. A, Lateral view of defect remaining after supracricoid laryngectomy with suture placement for crico-hyoidoepiglottopexy. **B,** Lateral view of defect remaining after supracricoid laryngectomy with suture placement for cricohyoidopexy. From Weinstein GS, Laccourreye O, Brasnu D and others, editors: *Organ preservation surgery for laryngeal cancer,* San Diego, 2000, Singular Thomson Learning, pp 84, 134.]

(Figure 100-14, *A*). When the entire epiglottis is removed, usually along with the contents of the pre-epiglottic space, the reconstruction is via cricohyoidopexy (Figure 100-14, *B*). Supracricoid laryngectomy extends the option of conservation surgery to patients with more extensive glottic cancers than can be encompassed with the more common vertical partial laryngectomy and its extensions. Weinstein and Laccourreye suggest limiting the use of vertical partial laryngectomy to cases in which the mid membranous vocal cord is involved and when a surgical reconstruction (imbrication laryngoplasty) is planned to improve the chance for glottic phonation. They identify that the standardized supracricoid laryngectomy offers predictable results without the need to "invent" a new modification of vertical partial laryngectomy for each case that then requires further innovation in choosing from a large number of reconstructive options.[174]

The wide resection of the anterior glottis is demonstrated through a cadaver dissection specimen identifying the standard resection of an SPL-CHEP (Figure 100-15, *A*). Weinstein and others propose that supracricoid laryngectomy (CHEP) is most useful for early glottic cancer to increase local control rates relative to standard vertical partial laryngectomy or radiotherapy.[172] They identify that it is useful in cases of advanced glottic cancers to avoid total or near-total (Pearson) laryngectomy. More specifically, CHEP is useful for selected glottic carcinoma invading the anterior commissure, the ventricle, and the thyroid cartilage. Weinstein and others also report that supracricoid laryngectomy is appropriate treatment for glottic cancer with impaired motion or, in selected cases, fixation of the true vocal cord. Contraindications of SPL include fixation of an arytenoid cartilage, subglottic extension invading the cricoid cartilage, posterior commissure involvement, and extralaryngeal spread (including outside the outer perichondrium of the thyroid cartilage).

Extensive cancers of the anterior commissure or ventricle should be considered for supracricoid laryngectomy with removal of the epiglottis and preepiglottic space (CHP) to address the high propensity for preepiglottic space invasion. An extensive cancer involving the anterior commissure with extensive involvement of the lower epiglottis with extension to the preepiglottic space was successfully removed by supracricoid laryngectomy and reconstructed with CHP (Figure 100-15, *B*). The same contraindications listed for supracricoid laryngectomy with CHEP pertain for supracricoid laryngectomy with CHP. Superior extension of tumor with major preepiglottic space invasion—with extension under vallecular mucosa, through the thyrohyoid membrane, or abutting the hyoid bone—is considered a contraindication for CHP.

Stepwise progress through a supracricoid laryngectomy is demonstrated for removal of a supraglottic cancer with inferior extension to the anterior commissure (Figure 100-16, *A*). The resulting defect shows forceps on the left vocal process (Figure 100-16, *B*) with subsequent placement of 3-0 Vicryl sutures from the arytenoids to the cricoid cartilage (Figure 100-16, *C*). Placement of three separate 0-vicryl sutures around the cricoid cartilage inferiorly and the hyoid bone superiorly prepares the wound for closure (Figure 100-16, *D*). Tension on the sutures permits assessment of the appropriate level for placement of the tracheotomy, which is performed before closure. Cadaver dissection demonstrates the cricohyoid impaction as the 0-vicryl sutures are approximated with final closure of the strap muscles as an outer layer (Figure 100-17).

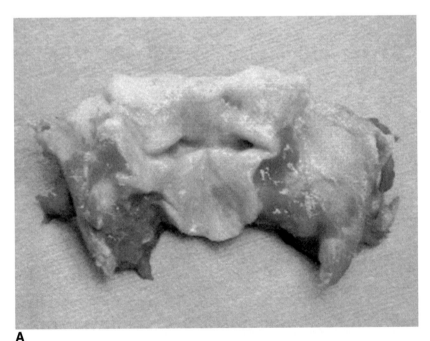

A

Figure 100-15. A, Cadaver demonstrations of resected specimen that includes to lower aspect of the epiglottis and preepiglottic space. Preservation of the upper two-thirds of the epiglottis permits reconstruction with CHEP. To view this image in color, please go to *www.oto-text.com* or the Electronic Image Collection CD, bound into your copy of Cummings Otolaryngology—Head and Neck Surgery, 4th edition.

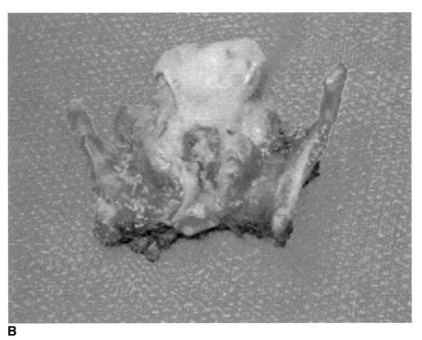

B

Figure 100-15, cont'd B, Resected specimen via supracricoid laryngectomy reconstructed with CHP. Resection of a recurrent (after irradiation) anterior commissure cancer with extension superiorly into the preepiglottic space was successfully reconstructed with CHP. To view this image in color, please go to *www.ototext.com* or the Electronic Image Collection CD, bound into your copy of Cummings Otolaryngology—Head and Neck Surgery, 4th edition.

Bron and others determined that supracricoid laryngectomy with CHEP results in a rough voice that is unstable because of a major loss of air during phonation.[24] These investigators concluded that the strained breathy voice resulting from CHEP is more like the post-total-laryngectomy-voice produced from the upper esophageal sphincter than a voice produced by vocal folds.

Zacharek and others carefully evaluated speech and swallowing in a group of 10 patients treated with supracricoid laryngectomy (four CHPs, six CHEPs). Blindfolded expert listeners identified each as having a breathy hoarse voice but still rated them as highly intelligible.[179] The swallowing evaluation included either a modified barium swallow study in three patients or a fiberoptic endoscopic evaluation of swallowing in the other seven. All three patients who underwent the modified barium swallow study demonstrated substantial degrees of aspiration. All seven evaluated with a fiberoptic endoscopic evaluation exhibited laryngeal penetration with the need for multiple swallows to clear food boluses. Despite the findings, each patient produced a strong cough reflex that cleared the laryngeal inlet. All 10 patients were tolerating a normal oral diet without feeding tubes by the thirtieth postoperative day, with no hospitalization required for pneumonia recorded.

Other complications after supracricoid laryngectomy have been reported to include rupture of the pexis, laryngocele, and laryngeal stenosis. Among 376 consecutive supracricoid laryngectomies evaluated by Diaz and others, only 14 (3.7%) resulted in symptomatic laryngotracheal stenosis.[41] The authors conclude from their retrospective review that in most cases stenosis results from avoidable technical error.

Despite these potential shortcomings, it appears that quality of life, as assessed through questionnaires completed by the patients, is high after supracricoid laryngectomy. Weinstein and others performed a detailed study comparing the quality of life in patients treated with supracricoid laryngectomy to normative data and to patients treated with total laryngectomy with tracheo-esophageal punction speech.[172] The outcome measures of physical functioning, general health, vitality, and physical limitations were significantly better among the 16 patients treated with supracricoid laryngectomy than among 15 matched patients treated with total laryngectomy and tracheo-esophageal punction speech. The group treated with supracricoid laryngectomy actually scored higher than the U.S. norms (55–64 years of age) in every domain within the SF-36 general health status measure. Weinstein and others interpreted this finding as "frame-shifting," wherein a very positive perspective resulted from the outcome of "saving their voice box" in the context of the fear of losing it. Weinstein and others caution that the indications and contraindications for supracricoid laryngectomy must be strictly observed to obtain such favorable results.

An important study offering additional support for an expanded use of supracricoid laryngectomy comes from a retrospective analysis of 204 patients with T_2N_0 glottic cancer who were consecutively managed at Laennec Hospital in France during the years 1962 to 1995.[93] Statistically significant differences favored the 119 supracricoid laryngectomy (with CHEP) over the 85 vertical partial laryngectomy with respect to 10-year survival (66.4% vs 46.2%), local control (94.1% vs 69.3%), and laryngeal preservation rate (94.9% vs 78.1%). Similar low complication rates were identified between those treated with supracricoid laryngectomy (with CHEP) and vertical partial laryngectomy with respect to permanent gastrostomy (2.4% vs 0%),

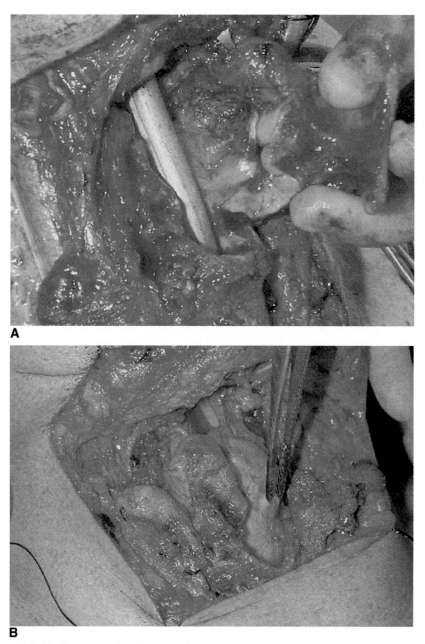

Figure 100-16. Intraoperative photographs of a supracricoid laryngectomy in progress for a supraglottic cancer extending to the anterior commissure. An endoscopic laser approach with debulking (note the epiglottis is gone) was converted to an open procedure to permit adequate removal. To view this image in color, please go to *www.ototext.com* or the Electronic Image Collection CD, bound into your copy of Cummings Otolaryngology—Head and Neck Surgery, 4th edition.

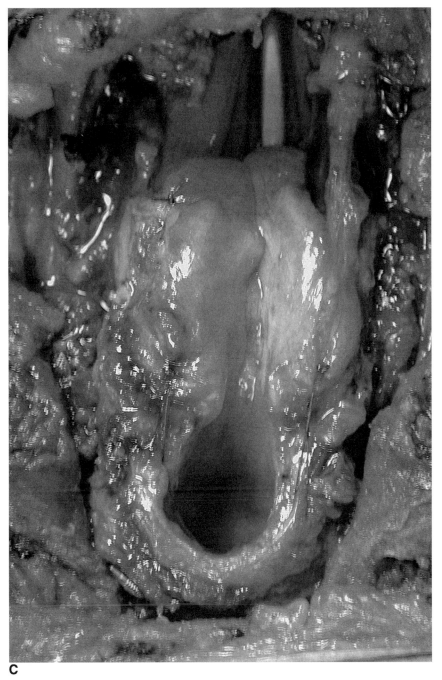

C

Figure 100-16, cont'd.

Continued

completion laryngectomy for functional non-oncologic problems (0.8% vs 1.2%), and permanent tracheostomy (1.2% vs 2.4%). Although the risk of developing aspiration pneumonia was higher after supracricoid laryngectomy (CHEP) than with vertical partial laryngectomy, aggressive treatment with chest therapy, speech therapy, and antibiotic treatment yielded a very small number (1.2%) of cases requiring total laryngectomy to deal with swallowing problems. These investi-

gators concluded that the better local control rate with supracricoid laryngectomy was responsible for preventing the cascade of oncologic events (regional and distant metastases) that are associated with tumor recurrence. These investigators linked a higher local recurrence after treatment with vertical partial laryngectomy to the poorer survival in this group. The investigators offer the opinion that the better local control associated with supracricoid laryngectomy

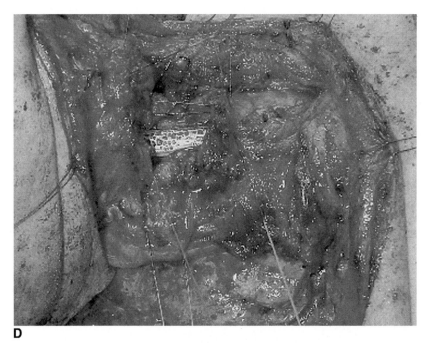

D

Figure 100-16, cont'd.

resulted from technical differences that provide wider exposure, as well as the wider mucosal and paraglottic space resection.

Voice Considerations

Cragle and Brandenburg reported that surgical treatment of early glottic cancers may produce a vocal result that is equivalent to that following irradiation.[35] These investigators evaluated voice profiles in 11 patients treated with laser cordectomy and 20 patients treated with irradiation. Both groups had similar voice profiles, characterized by decreased maximum phonation times and increased jitter, shimmer, and signal-to-noise ratios.

Most investigators contend that, in cases of early glottic cancers, a better voice more reliably follows treatment with radiotherapy rather than with surgery.[26,45,76,128,146] Unlike surgery, radiotherapy does not require removal of adjacent healthy tissue to provide a clear margin around a cancer. However, vocal deterioration may result from radiotherapy and may be significant if loss of vocal cord bulk results from tumor necrosis or if fibrosis develops.

Ton-Van and others[160] evaluated 356 patients with early glottic cancer and determined that the quality of voice after treatment with radiotherapy is "indisputably superior to that after conservation surgery." However, these investigators pointed out that a functional larynx was preserved in 92% of patients treated surgically compared with 81% initially treated with radiotherapy. The investigators acknowledged that these results could have been biased by management, which generally used total laryngectomy for surgical salvage. As a result of these findings, Ton-Van and others[140] advocate the use of surgery as a primary mode of therapy in patients capable of safely undergoing an anesthetic. Exceptions include patients who are willing to accept a greater risk of total loss of the larynx in the effort to preserve the highest quality voice.

For most patients with laryngeal cancer, the absolute quality of their voice may not be as important a consideration in selecting treatment as is their general ability to communicate. For these patients, speech intelligibility may be more meaningful as a criterion to assess results rather than acoustic and aerodynamic measurements. Schuller and others[130] used interviews and questionnaires to evaluate 75 patients treated surgically for early laryngeal cancers. They found that 88% of the respondents were content with the postoperative voice.

The vocal behaviors of most patients after partial laryngectomy are similar to those of patients with glottic incompetence caused by vocal cord paralysis. Leeper, Heeneman, and Reynolds[97] evaluated six patients who had undergone vertical hemilaryngectomy operations. They found that, whereas large variability was noted, the general tendencies for patients after hemilaryngectomy were (1) incomplete glottic closure; (2) vibratory action of the supraglottic structures (ventricular folds, arytenoids); and (3) high average trans glottal airflow with reduced maximum phonation time.

The ability of the vocal tract to regain normal appearance and function is determined by the extent of tumor damage and by the extent of surgical resection. Benninger and others[16] evaluated factors associated with recurrence and voice quality after radiotherapy for early glottic carcinomas. They identified that large excisional biopsies before irradiation increased the risk of poor voice quality.

Glottic Reconstruction
Primary Reconstruction at the Time of Tumor Resection

Multiple approaches support the use of various tissue flaps to reconstruct the glottic larynx after partial laryngectomy.[8] The reconstruction may be done at the time of tumor resection or delayed as a second procedure.[6]

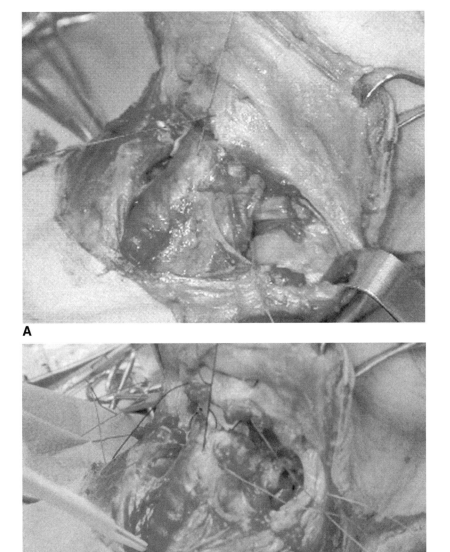

A

B

Figure 100-17. Cadaver demonstration of the cricohyoidopexy secured with three 0-vicryl sutures and final closure of strap muscles after CHP. (Thanks to L. Ollivier Laccourreye for preparation and performance of the cadaver prosection.) To view this image in color, please go to *www.ototext.com* or the Electronic Image Collection CD, bound into your copy of Cummings Otolaryngology—Head and Neck Surgery, 4th edition.

Continued

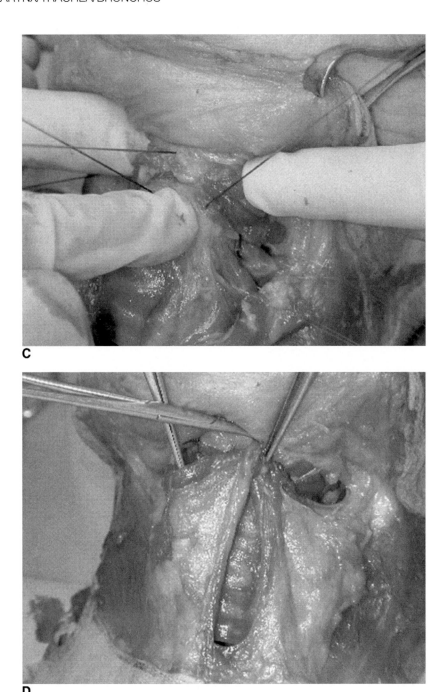

Figure 100-17, cont'd.

Imbrication laryngoplasty. Minimal tumor involvement of a vocal cord permits resection by a laryngofissure and cordectomy with preservation of the false vocal cord and its underlying cartilage. By removing the cartilage underlying the true vocal cord, the upper remnant of the thyroid cartilage can be displaced inferiorly to imbricate the false cord and its underlying cartilage to the level of the normal opposing true vocal cord (Figure 100-18).[118] This imbrication laryngoplasty may offer a greater chance of restoring true glottic phonation by creating a cartilage-supported neocord. Other publications have offered support for use of imbrication laryngoplasty as an effective reconstructive technique.[55] Biacabe and others performed a study randomizing patients either to no reconstruction or to reconstruction with imbrication laryngoplasty (with a false vocal fold myomucosal flap) at the time of vertical partial

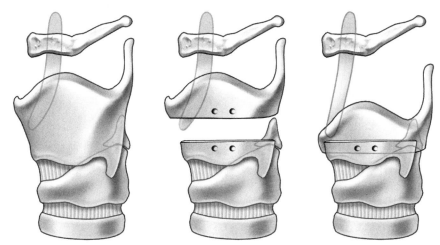

Figure 100-18. Diagram demonstrating removal of a horizontal strip of thyroid cartilage permitting imbrication of the ipsilateral false cord to the glottic level to restore glottic competence.

laryngectomy.[18] These investigators identified that the supraglottic structures participated in voice production in 80% of the cases without glottic reconstruction. The success in restoring glottic phonation was much better after neocord formation with the false vocal fold flap participating in voice production in 54% of those treated with the imbrication procedure.

Free tissue transfer. The shortcomings to reconstruction of the glottis after partial laryngectomy with rotation (or imbrication) of tissue pedicled adjacent to the defect have been addressed by introducing tissue obtained from a distant source. Microvascular free tissue transfer has been used to reconstruct the glottic larynx in the attempt to address the atrophy and stiffening of region tissue (e.g., strap muscles) that commonly occurs.

Initial work to reconstruct the hemilarynx with free flaps was developed for hypopharyngeal cancer cases involving the hemilarynx in which the standard surgical approach would be total laryngectomy.[163] Work has been done utilizing a temporoparietal free flap or forearm fascial flap with an endolaryngeal buccal mucosal graft to reconstruct smaller defects. This technique appears to recreate a mobile neocord with the introduction of supple mucosally covered tissue on the reconstructed side. Optimal results require that the arytenoid on the operated side be mobile. If the arytenoid is involved or fixed after the procedure, the benefit of mobility is lost, and more conventional strap muscle techniques would likely provide a similar result. The procedure has been used in both primary and recurrent cases.[60] The additional time, cost, and morbidity of this procedure needs to be weighed in the context of the standard locoregional recurrence assessment with and emphasis on study of voice and quality of life. A patient treated for a T_1N_0 glottic cancer with free tissue transfer via temporoparietal flap with buccal mucosal free graft is demonstrated in Figure 100-19.

Secondary Reconstruction

Despite efforts to reconstruct a functional neocord from positioning strap muscles, perichondrium, or supraglottic structures at the glottic level, vertical partial laryngectomy often results in glottic incompetence.[103] Inadequate bulk in this neocord commonly causes failure of true glottic phonation. A breathy voice results, with compensatory phonation frequently arising from vibration of the supraglottic structures.

When the resection is limited to disruption of only one vocal cord, it seems reasonable to assume that injection laryngoplasty or medialization laryngoplasty will restore glottic competence and improve voicing by advancing the deficient cord medially.[181] Jiang and Titze identified in an excised canine model that phonation can be restored to near normal when glottic competence is maintained by replacing one vocal cord with a plexiglas plate.[79] A clear voice, that differs from normal only by a 6-dB decrease in sound pressure level, results from this intervention. It follows that application of this principle to medialization of a scarred vocal cord should result in near-normal voicing with restoration of glottic competence.

Unfortunately, the scarring that accompanies the healing after glottic cancer resection often precludes successful medialization through standard injection laryngoplasty or thyroplasty. As a result, special techniques have been developed to address glottic insufficiency in this subgroup of patients.[6] Some question persists as to the overall success of these interventions in preserving or restoring normal glottic function.[17]

Adaptation of an approach designed by Tucker to treat laryngeal paralysis has been used by Sittel and others to restore glottic competence following hemilaryngectomy.[142] These investigators introduced autologous cartilage into a pocket created in the paraglottic space adjacent the scarred vocal fold (Figure 100-20). This procedure may be performed either under local or general anesthesia without a tracheotomy. Sittle and others suggest a waiting period of at least 1 year after the cancer resection before performing the reconstruction to ensure that the risk of recurrence is minimal. As with other surgical procedures, it seems that appropriate patient selection is critical to obtaining

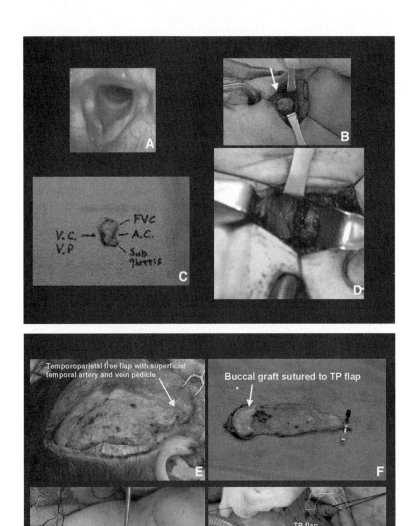

Figure 100-19. Reconstruction of hemilaryngectomy defect using temporoparietal flap, buccal mucosa, and cartilage strut. Procedure developed by Ralph Gilber, M.D. (personal communication). **A,** Appearance of T$_1$ SCCA of left true vocal cord. **B,** Exposure of larynx. **C,** Resected specimen. **D,** Hemilaryngectomy defect. **E,** Elevated temporoparietal flap. **F,** Buccal mucosal graft sutured to distal flap. **G,** Initial flap inset. **H,** Cartilage strut at vocal cord level.

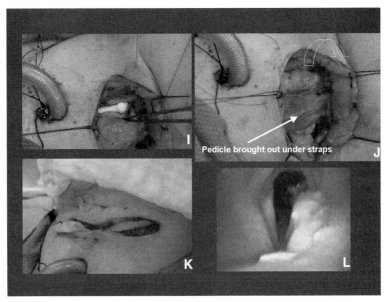

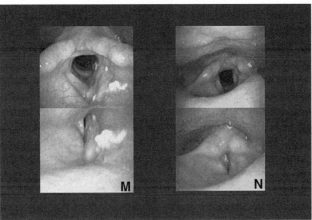

Figure 100-19, cont'd I, Placement of Montgomery stent. **J,** Temporoparietal flap brought out laterally under strap muscles. **K,** Closure over Penrose drain. **L,** Montgomery stent removed 10 to 12 days postoperatively. **M,** Appearance of larynx at 3 months. **N,** Appearance of larynx at 1 year. To view this image in color, please go to *www.ototext.com* or the Electronic Image Collection CD, bound into your copy of Cummings Otolaryngology—Head and Neck Surgery, 4th edition.

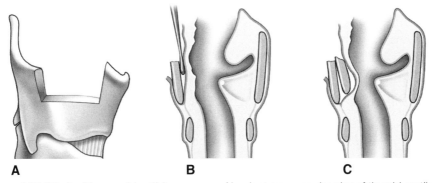

Figure 100-20. A, Diagram identifying source of implant on upper border of thyroid cartilage. **B,** With a pocket created in the paraglottic space lateral to the neo-cord. **C,** With resultant medialization of reconstructed vocal cord. From Sittel C, Friedrich G, Zorowka P: Surgical voice rehabilitation after laser surgery for glottic carcinoma, *Ann Otol Rhinol Laryngol* 111:494, 2002.

good results with this procedure. Extensive scarring or removal of the cartilage underlying the deficient vocal cord would appear to preclude successful use of this technique.

It is generally recognized that resections involving the anterior commissure create greater challenges in restoring glottic phonation than do resections of the mid-membranous vocal folds. Zeitels and others have developed an innovative approach that employs unilateral subluxation of the anterior aspect of the involved thyroid ala via an "anterior commissure laryngoplasty" to address deficiencies following anterior commissure glottic cancer surgery (Figure 100-21).[181] These investigators have successfully employed this approach following previous medialization procedures with fat injection or paraglottic placement of Gore-tex®.

Problems with medializing the posterior glottic has been addressed through modifications of the cricoid collapse procedure reported by Biller and Urken in 1985.[20] Amin and Koufman reported improved voicing by restoring posterior glottic closure through resection of a portion of the cricoid.[6] They were able to collapse the glottic aperture with maintenance of a lumen by temporarily obturating it with a modified Montgomery stent (Figures 100-22 and 100-23). Reconstruction includes rotation of an adjacent vascularized strap muscle as a flap to restore glottic competence. Concern about diminishing the airway is recognized as a potential problem by these investigators. They stress that their results are preliminary, but, that among the six patients treated by this method, they reported no problems with decannulation.

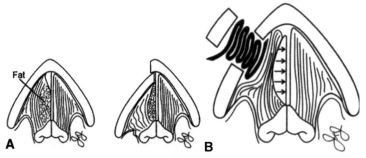

Figure 100-21. A, Limited scarring of the glottis will permit restoration of glottic competence in selected cases by standard thyroplasty technique. **B,** Scarring and deficiency in tissue may prevent true glottic phonation despite efforts such as this anterior commissure laryngoplasty. need permission. From Zeitels SM, Jarboe J, Franco RA: Phonosurgical reconstruction of early glottic cancer, *Laryngoscope* 111:1863, 2001.

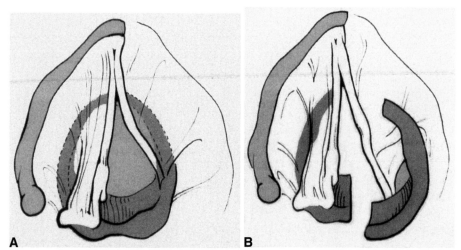

Figure 100-22. Complex procedures have been devised to improve posterior glottic closure. From Amin MR, Koufman JA: Hemicricoidectomy for voice rehabilitation following hemilaryngectomy with ipsilateral arytenoid removal, *Ann Otol Rhinol Laryngol* 110:514–515, 2001.

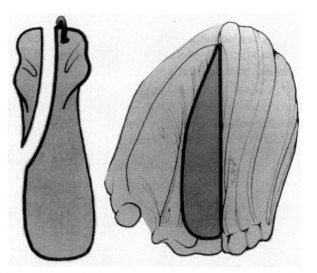

Figure 100-23. Preliminary reports employing a combination of cricoid collapse with introduction of strap musculature temporarily obturated by a modified Montgomery stent has been used successfully in a limited number of patients. (From Amin MR, Koufman JA: Hemicricoidectomy for voice rehabilitation following hemilaryngectomy with ipsilateral arytenoid removal, *Ann Otol Rhinol Laryngol* 110:515, 2001.)

Radiotherapy

Radiotherapy is considered effective treatment for early glottic cancer (Table 100-11). Broad comparisons between outcomes after initial treatment with either irradiation or surgery are often made without addressing the differences in the various approaches to the administration of radiotherapy or different techniques in performing the surgery.[18] Variables in the application of radiotherapy that affect tumor control include fraction size, total dose of radiation delivered, treatment duration, field size, energy of the x-rays, and method of delivery.[85,127,143,152] Rudoltz, Benammar, and Mohiuddin[127] identified duration of treatment as a significant variable in predicting local control and survival in the management of early glottic cancer. Patients completing treatment within 46 days had better local control than those treated over a longer period (Figure 100-24). Treatment applied through fractions of at least 200 cGy for the standard once-a-day, 5-day-a-week dosing also improved control rates relative to treatment with less than 200 cGy per day.[85,107] Ricciardelli and others[123] also supported

TABLE 100-11

RESULTS OF RADIOTHERAPY FOR EARLY GLOTTIC CANCER*

Study	Patients (n)	Stage	Dose Mean (Range)	LESIONS CONTROLLED (%) Initially	LESIONS CONTROLLED (%) Ultimately	After Laryngeal Preservation	SURVIVAL (%) 2-year	SURVIVAL (%) 5-year
Howell-Burke (1990)	114	T_2	70 Gy[†] (65–78 Gy)	68	96	74	—	92[‡] 70
Kersh (1990)	95	T_1	60 Gy	94	100	*91*	100	—
	53	T_2		76	86		86	
Johansen (1990)	295	T_{1a}	—	81	94	—	—	94
	63	T_{1b}						—
Ton-Van and others[62]	68	T_{1a}	60 Gy (50–65 Gy)	70	94	79	—	67
	39	T_{1b}						
	19	T_2						
Pellitteri (1991)	113	T_1	60 Gy	93	98	95	—	87
	48	T_2	64–70 Gy	78	92	79		79
Terhaard (1991)	194	T_1	66 Gy (58–68 Gy)	91	97	92	97	—
Small and others[57]	103	T_1	64 Gy (54–70 Gy)	89	97	89	—	97
Rudoltz, Benammar, and Mohiuddin[45]	91	T_1	64 Gy (59–70 Gy)	80	95	84	—	92
Fein (1993)	19	T_{is}	56 Gy[§] (56–60 Gy)	93	100	93	100	—
Smitt and Goffinet[58]	29	T_{is}	62 Gy (53–66.5 Gy)	92	96	96	—	82

*Italicized numbers are mean figures for entire patient group.
†Ten patients managed twice daily with 1.2 Gy.
‡Disease specific.
§Median dose.

CARCINOMA OF THE LARYNX: T_1 GLOTTIS
LOCAL CONTROL vs ELAPSED DAYS

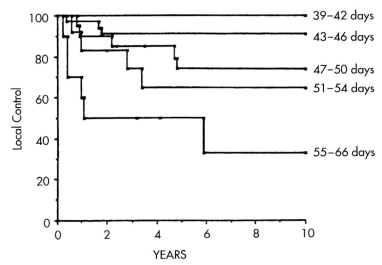

Figure 100-24. T_1 glottic carcinoma of the larynx: local control vs radiotherapy elapsed time. Local control is a function of elapsed days for patients managed with radiotherapy for T_1 squamous cell carcinoma of the glottis. (From Rufdoltz MS, Benammar A, Mohiuddin M: *J Radiat Oncol Biol Phys* 26:768, 1993.)

the use of higher per-dose fractions through a clinical study and in an in vivo tumor model. In 1993 Rudoltz, Benammar, and Mohiuddin[127] reported that accelerated regimens employing higher dose fractions were of value primarily because they allowed for shorter treatment duration.

The benefit derived from accelerated fractionation needs to be balanced against the additional morbidity induced. In a phase III study Hliniak and others compared an accelerated regimen (AF) of 66 Gy given in 33 fractions during 38 days (2 fractions every Thursday) with conventional regimen (CF) of 66 Gy given in 33 fractions during 45 days.[70] A total of 395 patients with $T_{1-3}N_0$ glottic and supraglottic cancer treated between 1995 and 1998 were evaluated. More acute morbidity (acute mucositis with pain and dysphagia) was seen in the AF arm at 1 and 2 months. At 4 months after treatment all types of toxicity except skin telangiectasia were similar in both arms. Although there was no difference in the disease-free survival between the two arms, these investigators calculated that shortening of the overall treatment time by 1 week resulted in a 3% to 5% therapeutic gain ($P = .37$). They suggest that further shortening of the treatment time could be done within the limits of acceptable morbidity, especially if the volume of the irradiated tissue was small (as for T_1 and T_2 tumors).

Another important consideration in the radiotherapeutic management of early glottic cancer is the technique used for planning and delivery. The treatment target for an early cancer is the lesions itself without the need to address the very rare occult metastasis. Conventional techniques initially depended on the physical examination with the placement of a square open field that generally ranged from 44 cm up to 66 cm for larger T_2 lesions. Most of the published experience is based on utilization of either cobalt −60 or linear accelerators of 4 meV or less. The treatment field was traditionally defined by positioning a light field to cover the mid thyroid notch superiorly to the inferior cricoid inferiorly. The posterior border of the treatment field was defined by the physician's estimate of the posterior border of the tumor. Anteriorly, the field was extended to completely cover over the anterior skin with additional margin. Attention to the daily replacing the field carefully based on external anatomic landmarks was a key to accurate targeting. Treatment simulation employed plain radiographs with confirmation of appropriate targeting of the field based on portal films to check the position of the cartilaginous anatomy that is well visualized on lateral radiographs.

Despite this simple and common sense approach to treatment setup, dosimetric misses occurring because of field misplacement, as well as dose calculation considerations in the small air-filled and irregular cavity of the larynx, were problematic. Reports using higher (6 meV) energy beams (which today are more commonly available than lower energy beams) were initially associated with higher failure rates because of a lack of adequate dosimetric considerations.[39,168] With the advent of virtual simulation it has become possible to better account for the 3D anatomic considerations within the glottis. More sophisticated corrections for the air interfaces can also now be made. These advances permit better estimation of the optimal wedge used to shape the beam profile. Multiple field techniques can now be employed to assure homogenous and accurate doses. These new techniques improve success but still depend on verification for accurate daily reproducibility and dosimetry.[53,115]

Most radiation failures of early glottic cancer represent local recurrences rather than regional or distant metastasis.[27] The ability to salvage radiation failures with partial laryngectomy or endoscopic laser resection contributes to the overall success of radiotherapy for initial treatment modality (Table 100-12).[83,91,125,135,136] The extent to which conservation laryngeal surgery (partial laryngectomy) rather than total laryngectomy is used to salvage irradiation failures of T_1 and T_2 glottic squamous cell carcinoma depends on multiple

factors: the intensity of follow-up (designed to identify persistent tumor at an early stage), the desires of the patient, the presence of comorbidity, and the management philosophy of the treating physicians. Differing philosophies likely contribute to the variable success reported with salvage partial laryngectomy.

Toma and others[159] expanded on their initial criteria to permit partial laryngectomy salvage of early glottic irradiation failures unless the tumor invaded:

1. The arytenoid cartilage (except the vocal process).
2. Beyond the anterior half of the contralateral vocal cord.
3. Subglottically more than 10 mm in the anterior half or 5 mm in the posterior half of the larynx.
4. Into the thyroid or cricoid cartilage.

Application of these criteria to 19 recurrent T_1 and T_2 glottic cancers treated with primary radiotherapy at their institution between 1989 and 1998 yielded three failures (recurrences), which were each successfully salvaged with total laryngectomy. These criteria may be considered as general guidelines but should not be applied to all cases for several reasons. Consideration as to anatomic differences in laryngeal size should allow a more subjective assessment of resectability than afforded by the absolute measurement of 10 mm of anterior subglottic extension as a contraindication. A large male larynx will differ from a small female larynx in applying these criteria.

Additionally, Toma and others did not address the role that supracricoid laryngectomy may play in salvaging irradiation failures. Laccourreye and others reported successful use of supracricoid laryngectomy as a salvage procedure with a laryngeal preservation rate among 12 patients who had failed radiotherapy.[96] The major contraindications they pointed to in use of supracricoid laryngectomy were fixation of the ipsilateral arytenoid cartilage, cricoid cartilage invasion, extralaryngeal spread of tumor, and infraglottic spread to the cricoid cartilage.

Successful salvage with voice preservation using partial laryngectomy has been reported to range from 11% to 85%.[89,105] It remains unclear as to whether the successful use of surgical salvage after failure of irradiation provides an overall laryngeal preservation rate comparable with that when the primary treatment is with conservation laryngeal surgery.

Photodynamic Therapy

Preferential uptake of photochemicals by malignant cells has been successfully exploited to treat superficial cancers of the larynx. Photofrin (dihematoporphyrin ether or DHE) is the most extensively studied

---

TABLE 100-12

RECURRENCE RATES OF EARLY STAGE LARYNGEAL CANCER FOLLOWING INITIAL TREATMENT WITH IRRADIATION*

Study	T1 Recurrence	T2 Recurrence
	(%)	(%)
Jose and others, J Surg Oncol, 1984 (summarized 8 reports before 1984)	$T_{1,18}$	T_2, 18
	T_1, 15	T_2, 31
Fisher and others, Arch laryngol Head Neck Surg, 1986	T_1, 8	T_2, 36
Strauss, Laryngoscope, 1988	T_1, 11	T_2, 23
Maipang and others, J Surg Oncol, 1989	T_1, 20	T_2, 36
Foote and others, Mayo Clin Proc, 1992	$T_{1,16}$	T_2, 16
Suzuki and others, Acta Otolaryngol, 1994	T_1, 7	T_2, 82
Parsons and others, Int J Radiat Oncol Biol Phys, 1995	T_1, 4	T_2, 15
McLaughlin and others, Head Neck, 1996	T_1, 6	T_2, 16
Nibu and others, Head Neck, 1997	—	T_2, 11–73

*T_1 approximately 10%; T_2 approximately 30%.

photosensitizer and is postulated to exert its tumoricidal effect after intravenous administration by two modes:

1. Light activation of the photo concentrated DHE in malignant tissue to produce singlet oxygen resulting in mitochondrial insult and apoptosis.
2. Vascular endothelial damage with erythrocyte leakage and ischemic tumor necrosis.[129] Photophrin-mediated photodynamic therapy (PDT) has been given U.S. Food and Drug Administration approval for the treatment of obstructing esophageal and endobronchial tumors, as well as for the treatment of minimally invasive endobronchial non-small cell carcinoma. This promising treatment modality currently has been promoted most vigorously for use in the treatment of superficial laryngeal cancers that are recurrent after irradiation, with expanded applications anticipated with improved technology.[19,129] Broad acceptance of PDT in the treatment of glottic cancer has not occurred at many centers because of the success of other conventional therapies, the difficulties in introducing new technology with new equipment, and the side effects of treatment with PDT, which include generalized skin photosensitization.

Chemotherapy

Because early glottic cancers are highly curable with conventional surgery or radiotherapy, the addition of chemotherapy to most treatment algorithms has not been strongly supported. In addition, past dogma has dictated that invasive squamous cell carcinoma of the upper aerodigestive tract is not curable with chemotherapy alone.[95] Laccourreye and others reported that some of the patients with early glottic squamous carcinoma that they treated with an induction chemotherapy regimen (platinum based) had a complete response clinically and chose to forgo the further treatment that was suggested.[94] Although local recurrence was noted in almost one-third of these patients, none of the patients who had local recurrence ultimately died from their disease or lost their larynx. This finding has prompted further interest in the use of chemotherapy for early laryngeal cancer to the point that prospective trials evaluating this modality are now underway.

CHOSING A TREATMENT MODALITY
Carcinoma in situ

Close interaction between the clinician and pathologist are needed to manage optimally carcinoma in situ ($T_{is}N_0M_0$). Depending on the bias among several pathologists evaluating a biopsy, the same lesion may be reported as grade III intraepithelial neoplasia, high-grade dysplasia, or $T_{is}N_0M_0$.[57] Despite the often stated pathologic principle that high-grade dysplasia and $T_{is}N_0M_0$ are equivalent terms in describing abnormal squamous epithelium, the clinical management is generally less aggressive for high-grade dysplasia than for $T_{is}N_0M_0$. Whereas radiotherapy has commonly been supported as a reasonable treatment alternative for $T_{is}N_0M_0$, it is not recommended in the management of high-grade dysplasia.

Difficulty in discriminating between reactive processes and carcinoma in situ is underscored by a study evaluating imprecision in histopathologic diagnoses. Westra, Kronz, and Eisele reported three cases of laryngeal $T_{is}N_0M_0$ submitted from outside hospitals that were, on review with a second opinion at their hospital, considered to be reactive atypia.[177]

Controversy persists regarding the role for radiotherapy in the management of $T_{is}N_0M_0$. A common management approach has been to address laryngeal $T_{is}N_0M_0$ surgically when conservative endoscopic removal is possible.[131] Persistence after multiple resections or the presence of extensive involvement of multiple sites have been used as indications for irradiating $T_{is}N_0M_0$.[147] Factors such as the anticipated need for multiple endoscopic resections, cost of treatment, voice considerations, reliability of the patient for follow-up, patient's age, and presence of comorbidities are all factors that may influence initial definitive treatment with irradiation.[59]

Issues regarding the appropriate management of $T_{is}N_0M_0$ are unresolved. Local excision and radiotherapy are effective management options.[112] Either approach requires close follow-up.

Invasive Squamous Cell Carcinoma

Selection of an appropriate treatment modality for early glottic cancers ($T_1N_0M_0$, $T_2N_0M_0$) is made difficult by the many opinions that support conflicting approaches. The simplest conceptual approach is offered by Hinerman and others who identified that, in the past at the University of Florida, "Radiation therapy has been the treatment of choice for all previously untreated T_1 and T_2 vocal cord cancers."[68] These investigators later amended this practice to prefer transoral laser excision over radiotherapy for the small subset of patients with limited T1 mid-third vocal cord lesions for whom surgical excision is expected to preserve voice quality.

Although the NCDB survey of laryngeal cancer indicates that in the United States radiotherapy is used most commonly in the management of T_1 and T_2 cancers, there are well-considered arguments for a more liberal use of surgery as the initial management.[71]

Morris, Canonico, and Blank,[110] through an intensive literature review, identified an overall 8.6% failure rate at the primary site for T_1 glottic cancers managed surgically (cordectomy) compared with a 16.7% failure rate among similarly staged cancers managed with radiotherapy.[37] Stronger support comes for use of surgery as the primary treatment for T_2 glottic cancers. In 1990 Howell-Burke and others reported from MD Anderson that, among patients treated with primary irradiation for T_2 glottic cancers, only 74% maintained a functional larynx.[75] Some investigators contend that T_2 glottic cancers initially treated with irradiation have a higher risk that laryngeal function will be lost than when conservation surgery is the initial treatment.[173]

Further support for this concept comes from review of published recurrence rates following initial treatment of early stage laryngeal cancer (see Tables 100-12 and 100-13). A review of these same rates (supplemented by a series of rates from 2000) identifies that the great majority of early laryngeal cancers that recur are ultimately treated with total laryngectomy. A problem leading to this need for total laryngectomy may be identified as difficulty in surveillance permitting early detection. Suzuki and others reported in 1994 that 60% of patients initially identified with an early laryngeal cancer are identified with an increased stage at the time of recurrence.[155]

Barthel and Esclamado reviewed management of 45 patients with early glottic cancer who were treated with primary irradiation at the Cleveland Clinic between 1986 and 1994.[13] These investigators reported that their local control rates of 87.5% for T_1 and 75% for T_2 lesions were consistent with prior published series. Among the nine recurrences that developed, six had tumors that were (retrospectively) considered to be amenable to treatment with a partial laryngec-

TABLE 100-13

PERCENTAGE OF T_1/T_2 LARYNGEAL CANCERS WITH RECURRENCE REQUIRING TOTAL LARYNGECTOMY

Study	Recurrence (%)
Jose and others, J Surg Oncol, 1984	95
Fisher and others, Arch Otolaryngol Head Neck Surg, 1986	100
Maipang and others, J Surg Oncol, 1989	100
Nichols and others, Ann Otol, 1991	>30
Suzuki and others, Acta Otolaryngol, 1994	91
Parsons and others, Int J Radiat Oncol Biol Phys, 1995	>40
McLaughlin and others, Head Neck, 1996	83
Stoeckli and others, Arch Otolaryngol Head Neck Surg, 2000	92

tomy. Among these six cases (all treated with irradiation), only one was successfully salvaged with conservation laryngeal surgery. These investigators concluded that patients with T_2 glottic tumors may be better treated primarily with surgery because T_2 glottic cancers have a high recurrence rate after irradiation and surgical salvage with less than a total laryngectomy was unlikely to be successful.

Valuable insight is provided by a report by Jorgenson and others that addresses 1005 Danish patients treated at a single referral center between 1965 and 1998.[80] The philosophy of treating all but those who had previous treatment with irradiation resulted in remarkably little selection bias regarding treatment choice, with 99% of patients receiving initial management with radiotherapy. Jorgenson and others identify that the presence of a stable patient base within a cachement area of 1.33 million people, coupled with excellent follow-up (only three patients were lost to follow-up), lend further credibility to this study. Among 312 T_1 glottic cancers treated with irradiation, 5-year locoregional control was 88%, which, coupled with surgical salvage, resulted in a 99% 5-year disease-specific survival. Among 233 T_2 glottic cancers treated with irradiation, 5-year locoregional control was 67.4%, which, when coupled with surgical salvage, resulted in an 88.4% 5-year disease-specific survival. These investigators identify that this high recurrence rate (one out of three) for T_2 glottic cancers resulted in an overall laryngeal preservation of 80%, which is substantially lower than the 95% organ preservation reported by Chevalier and others when supracricoid laryngectomy was used as the initial treatment.[28] Based on these data, Jorgensen and others raised the logical question: Why not introduce supracricoid partial laryngectomy as primary standard treatment of T_2 glottic cancer? Jorgenson and others argued that part of the excellent results reported by Chevalier and others reflected a selection bias that favoring surgical results by reserving supracricoid laryngectomy for the more favorable cases. Jorgensen and others additionally pointed out that the voice quality is better after irradiation than after supracricoid laryngectomy. For these reasons, they have not altered their standard approach to managing T_2 glottic cancers with irradiation. They also observed that improved radiotherapy techniques, as well as the capacity to salvage irradiation failures with supracricoid laryngectomy, will likely decrease the ultimate need for total laryngectomy further.[96]

The preceding studies have focused on AJCC (or the International Union Against Cancer) TNM classification as the factor determining treatment. Others have identified specific features of early glottic cancers separate from this classification system that may be helpful in assessing the likelihood of cure with radiotherapy.[54] It is useful to individually evaluate these characteristics that are either not included in the TNM staging (anterior commissure extension and large tumor bulk) or are used to discriminate T_2 from T_1 lesions (impaired vocal cord mobility and subglottic extension). Many investigators support surgery as the preferred initial treatment for patients who have such characteristics.[31]

The anterior commissure has been, in a contradictory fashion, either considered as a barrier to tumor spread or as an early pathway for cancer extension into the laryngeal framework.[87] Shvero and others[139] related that surgical treatment is preferred for cancers arising in this region because of a higher local recurrence rate after radiotherapy with an increased risk for distant metastasis. They contend that the behavior of small cancers in this location is much different from that of other early glottic cancers.[140] Other investigators have attributed the higher rates of failure after radiotherapy for anterior commissure lesions to problems with adequate dosing.[90,184] The distance from the anterior commissure to the skin varies greatly among patients. This variability and the thick overlying thyroid cartilage have been cited as impediments to consistent dosing of radiation to this region.

Insight into poor outcomes after irradiation of cancer affecting the anterior commissure is offered through a retrospective review by Maheshwar and Gaffney of 53 patients with T_1 glottic cancer treated between 1989 and 1996 with a minimum dose of 63 Gy in 30 fractions during 6 weeks with parallel opposed fields.[102] These investigators reported an overall 20.8% locoregional recurrence rate. The recurrence rate (57.1%) with anterior commissure involvement was much higher than the recurrence rate (15.8%) when the anterior vocal cord was involved but did not include the anterior commissure. They hypothesized that a lack of pretreatment CT imaging may have contributed to their poor results. Without this advanced imaging, they may have under staged the group of anterior commissure cancers, which have a high chance of cartilage involvement and hidden tumor bulk. Although some investigators relate that modern radiotherapy techniques with improved dosimetry have adequately addressed these concerns, Maheshwar and Gaffney[102] report in their study that they had addressed the potential to under dose the anterior commissure by adding wax bolus to the region during treatment.

T_{2b} cancers and those with subglottic extension generally have a larger tumor volume that may contribute to the lower cure rates with radiotherapy.[164,178] Many contend that surgery as a single modality is more effective than radiotherapy for managing these larger "early" glottic lesions. Questions persist about the capacity of a management plan that uses definitive radiotherapy coupled with salvage by partial laryngectomy to provide equivalent rates of laryngeal preservation.[38]

A systematic review of the world's literature (including the Cochrane Controlled Trials Register, as well as MEDLINE, EMBASE, CINAHL, and Cancer Lit, up to October 2000) identified three randomized clinical trials (RCTs) comparing treatment of patients with stages I and II glottic cancer with either irradiation or surgery.[40] One trial was excluded because of insufficient numbers of patients[99] and another because of the combination of suboptimal radiotherapy dosimetry, small numbers of patients with glottic cancer, and improper randomization.[69]

The most relevant RCT was an Eastern European multicenter trial to which 234 patients with early laryngeal cancer were randomly assigned, starting in 1979. They were treated with open surgery, radiotherapy, or a combination of radiotherapy and chemotherapy (prospodine) after stratification by anatomical site (glottis or supraglottis) and by tumor stage (T_1 or T_2).[113] The published results (which did not report the number of events or patients at risk in each treatment arm) identified 5-year survival rates of 100% after surgery and 91.7% after radiotherapy for T_1 tumors. For T_2 tumors the 5-year survival rates were 97.4% after surgery and 88.8% after radiotherapy. Although these higher survival rates for patients receiving surgery were not statistically significant, the 5-year disease-free survival rates of 78.7% for surgery and 60.1% for radiotherapy were significant (P = .036). In subsequent review, Dey and others[40] questioned the validity of these results because they believed the patients in the study were inadequately staged before being randomly assigned, that the radiotherapy may have been suboptimal, and that the follow-up was poor. Dey and others concluded from their systematic review that uncertainty remains as to the comparative benefits and societal costs of these different treatment modalities.

A large survey employing Canadian and American data sets to assess outcome as a function of differing management philosophies acknowledged that "current practice is based on reports from individual institutions recommending differing treatment policies."[65] These investigators opine that a clear advantage to one approach will be difficult to identify because randomized trials comparing surgical and non-surgical treatment of glottic cancer will never be conducted because of entrenched beliefs. Although it is clear from the review by Dey and others that RCTs have been done addressing early laryngeal cancer, none has yet compared the effectiveness of endolaryngeal resection with either radiotherapy or open surgery.[40] We hope the completion of an ongoing randomized prospective multicenter study directed by William Coman of Brisbane, Australia, will provide useful data to permit analysis of the comparative value of these two treatment modalities.[32] Coman's study randomly assigns patients with early glottic cancer to treatment with either radiotherapy or endoscopic laser resection and evaluates multiple endpoints but directs its most detailed analysis to voice and quality-of-life outcomes. At the time of this writing, another large study addressing endoscopic laser resection of upper aerodigestive tract cancer by a multicenter coalition in the United States is nearing completion and is also prospective, but without an arm randomized to nonsurgical treatment.[116] It is our hope that studies such as these will offer insight to reduce the unknowns that now dominate the counseling and decision making regarding management of early glottic cancer

SUMMARY

Selection of a treatment modality for early glottic cancers may be simplified by acknowledging that treatment initiated with radiotherapy and careful follow-up employing surgical salvage likely offers a similar chance for a cure as treatment with surgery as the initial approach. The major shortcomings of treatment with radiotherapy include the need for prolonged treatment and the higher risk of requiring a second treatment modality (salvage surgery). Evidence from retrospective studies with unknown selection bias identifies that overall laryngeal preservation for early glottic cancers with anterior commissure involvement, large tumor bulk, or the features defining classification as T2 (transglottic spread or impaired vocal fold mobility) is better with initial surgical treatment rather than with irradiation. The major shortcomings of surgery include exposure to a general anesthetic and the high probability of developing a breathy voice. Potential swallowing impairment, as well as other comorbidities, should be considered when recommending an approach. The patient should be an active and informed participant in the decision-making process. Close follow-up is an important component to any management plan.

REFERENCES

1. Adamopoulos G, Yiotakis J, Stavroulaki P and others: Modified supracricoid partial laryngectomy with cricohyoidopexy: series report and analysis of results, *Otolaryngol Head Neck Surg* 123:288–293, 2000.
2. Almadoria G, Galli J, Cadoni G and others: Human papilloma virus infection and cyclin D1 gene amplification in laryngeal squamous cell carcinoma: biologic function and clinical significance, *Head Neck* 24: 597–604, 2002.
3. Ambrosch P, Kron M, Steiner W: Carbon dioxide laser microsurgery for early supraglottic carcinoma, *Ann Otol Rhinol Laryngol* 107(8):680–689, 1998.
4. American Cancer Society: Facts and figures 2003, *http:www.cancer.org/docroot/STT/stt_0.asp.*
5. American Joint Committee on Cancer Staging: Manual for staging of cancer. Philadelphia, J.B. Lippincott, 1977.
6. Amin M, Koufman J: Hemicricoidectomy for voice rehabilitation following hemilaryngectomy with ipsilateral arytenoid removal, *Ann Otol Rhinol Laryngol* 11:514–518, 2001.
7. Andrea M, Dias O, Santos A: Contact endoscopy during microlaryngeal surgery: a new technique for endoscopic examination of the larynx, *Ann Otol Rhinol Laryngol* 104:333–339, 1995.
8. Apostolopoulos K, Samaan R, Labropoulou E: Experience with vertical partial laryngectomy with special reference to laryngeal reconstruction with cervical fascia, *J Laryngol Otol* 116:19–23, 2002.
9. Arens C, Glanz H, Dreyer T and others: Compact endoscopy of the larynx, *Ann Otol Rhinol Laryngol* 112:113–119, 2003.
10. Austin JR, Wong FC, Kim EE: Positron emission tomograph in the detection of residual laryngeal carcinoma, *Otolaryngol Head Neck Surg* 113:404, 1995.
11. Aviv JE, Takoudes TG, Ma G and others: Office-based esophagoscopy: a preliminary report, *Otolaryngol Head Neck Surg* 125:170–175, 2001.
12. Bailey BJ, Biller JF: *Surgical anatomy of the larynx.* In *Surgery of the Larynx.* Philadelphia, 1985, WB Saunders, p 23.
13. Barthel S, Esclamado R: Primary radiation therapy for early glottic cancer, *Otolaryngol Head Neck Surg* 124:35–39, 2001.
14. Belafsky PC, Postma GN, Daniel E and others: Transnasal esophagoscopy, *Otolaryngol Head Neck Surg* 125:588–589, 2001.
15. Belafsky PC, Postma GN, Koufman JA: Normal transnasal esophagoscopy (comment), *Ear Nose Throat J* 80:438, 2001.
16. Benninger MS, Bellomo A, Ferrero FE and others: Factors associated with recurrence and voice quality following radiation therapy for T_1 and T_2 glottic carcinomas, *Laryngoscope* 104:294, 1994.
17. Bertineo G, Bellomo A, Ferror F and others: Acoustic analysis of voice quality with or without false vocal fold displacement after cordectomy, *J Voice* 15:131–140, 2001.
18. Biacabe B, Crevier-Buchman L, Laccourreye O and others: Phonatory mechanisms after vertical partial laryngectomy with glottic reconstruction by false vocal fold flap, *Ann Otol Rhinol Laryngol* 110:935–940, 2001.
19. Biel M: Photodynamic therapy and the treatment of head and neck neoplasia, *Laryngoscope* 108:1259–1268, 1998.
20. Biller HF, Urken M: Cricoid collapse. A new technique for management of glottic incompetence, *Arch Otolaryngol* 111:740–741, 1985.
21. Bouquot JE, Gnepp DR: *Pathology of the head and neck.* In *Epidemiology,* New York, 1988, pp 263–314.
22. Bradford CR and others: Squamous carcinoma of the head and neck in organ transplant recipients: possible role of oncogenic viruses, *Laryngoscope* 100:190, 1990.
23. Brenner B, Marshak G, Rakowsky E and others: Laryngeal carcinoma—Epidemiological and clinical features: experience of the Rabin Medical Center in Israel, *Oncol Rep* 8:141–144, 2001.
24. Bron L, Pasche P, Brossard E and others: Functional analysis after supracricoid partial laryngectomy with cricohyoidoepiglottopexy, *Laryngoscope* 112:1289–1293, 2002.
25. Burgess LPA: Laryngeal reconstruction following vertical partial laryngectomy, *Laryngoscope* 103:109, 1993.
26. Casiano RR, Cooper JD, Lundy DS and others: Laser cordectomy for T_1 glottic cancer: a 10-year experience and videostroboscopic findings, *Otolaryngol Head Neck Surg* 104:831, 1991.

27. Cellai E, Chiavacci A, Olmi P: Causes of failure of curative radiation therapy in 205 early glottic cancers, *Int J Radiat Oncol Biol Phys* 19:1139, 1990.

28. Chevalier D, Laccourreye O, Brasnu D and others: Cricohyoidoepiglottopexy for glottic carcinoma with fixation or impaired motion of the true vocal cord: 5-year oncology results with 112 patients, *Ann Otol Rhinol Laryngol* 106:364–369, 1997.

29. Colden D, Zeitels SM, Hillman RE and others: Stroboscopic assessment of vocal fold keratosis and glottic cancer, *Ann Otol Rhinol Laryngol* 110:293–298, 2001.

30. Coleman MP, Esteve J, Damiecki P and others: *Trends in cancer incidence and mortality, international agency for research on cancer scientific publications, no. 121..* New York, Oxford University Press, 1993.

31. Coman W, Grigg R, Tomkinson A and others: Supracricoid laryngectomy: a significant advance in the management of laryngeal cancer, *Aust N Z Surg* 68:630–634, 1998.

32. Coman W: Personal communication, August 2003.

33. Commission on Cancer, American College of Surgeons: *NCDB benchmark reports,* vol 1, Chicago, 2002.

34. Crissman JD, Zarbo RJ, Drozdowicz S and others: Carcinoma in situ and microinvasive squamous cell carcinoma of the laryngeal glottis, *Arch Otolaryngol Head Neck Surg* 114:299, 1988.

35. Cragle S, Brandenburg J: Laser cordectomy or radiotherapy: cure rates, communication and cost, *Otolaryngol Head Neck Surg* 108:648, 1993.

36. de Boer JR, Pruim J, Burlage F and others: Therapy evaluation of laryngeal carcinomas by tyrosine-pet, *Head Neck* 25:634–644, 2003.

37. DeSanto LW: Early supraglottic cancer, *Ann Otol Rhinol Laryngol* 99:593, 1990.

38. DeSanto LW, Olsen KD: Early glottic cancer, *Am J Otolaryngol* 15:242, 1994.

39. Deviveni VR, King K, Perez C and others: Early glottic carcinoma treated with radiotherapy: impact of treatment energy on success rate, *Int J Radiat Oncol Biol Phys* 24:106, 1992.

40. Dey P, Arnold D, Wight R and others: Radiotherapy versus open surgery versus endolaryngeal surgery (with or without laser) for early laryngeal squamous cell cancer *Cochrane Database Syst Rev,* 2:2003.

41. Diaz E, Laccourreye L, Veivers D, and others: Laryngeal stenosis after supracricoid partial laryngectomy, *Ann Otol Rhinol Laryngol* 109:1077–1081, 2000.

42. Eckel HE: Local recurrences following transoral laser surgery for early glottic carcinoma: frequency, management and outcome, *Ann Otol Rhinol Laryngol* 110:7–15, 2001.

43. Eckel HE, Thumfart WF: Laser surgery for the treatment of larynx carcinomas: indications, techniques, and preliminary results, *Ann Otol Rhinol Laryngol* 101:49, 1992.

44. El-Serag HB, Hepworth EJ, Lee P and others: Gastroesophageal reflux disease is a risk factor for laryngeal and pharyngeal cancer, *Am J Gastroenterology* 96:2013–2018, 2001.

45. Epstein BE and others: Stage T_1 glottic carcinoma: results of radiation therapy or laser excision, *Radiology* 101:49, 1992.

46. Feinstein AR: A new staging system for cancer and reappraisal of "early" treatment and "cure" by radical surgery, *N Engl J Med* 279:747, 1968.

47. Feinstein AR, Wells CK: A clinical-severity staging system for patients with lung cancer, *Medicine (Baltimore)* 69:1, 1990.

48. Ferlito A: Histological classification of larynx and hypopharynx cancers and their clinical implications: pathologic aspects of 2052 malignant neoplasms diagnosed at the ORL department of Padua University from 1966 to 1976, *Acta Otolaryngol (Stockh)* 1(Suppl 342): 1976.

49. Ferlito A, Carbone A, DeSanto L and others: Early cancer of the larynx: the concept as defined by clinicians, pathologists, and biologists, *Ann Otol Rhinol Laryngol* 105:245–250, 1996.

50. Ferlito A, Rinaldo A: A comment on misuse of the term 'early' laryngeal cancer, *Eur Arch Otorhinolaryngol* 257:347–348, 2002.

51. Ferlito A, Silver C, Howard D and others: The role of partial laryngeal resection in current management of laryngeal cancer: a collective review, *Acta Otolaryngol* 120:456–46, 2000.

52. Flint PW: Minimally invasive techniques for management of early glottic cancer, *Otolaryngol Clin N Am* 35:1055–1066, 2002.

53. Foote RL, Grado GL, Buskirk SJ and others: Radiation therapy for glottic cancer using 6 MV photons, *Cancer* 77:381–386, 1996.

54. Franchin S, Boiocchi M: Brief report: prognostic importance of cellular DNA content in T_1-$2N_0$ laryngeal squamous cell carcinomas treated with radiotherapy, *Laryngoscope* 105:649, 1995.

55. Fukuda H, Tsuiji D, Kawasaki Y and others: Displacement of the ventricular fold following cordectomy, *Auris Nasus Larynx* 17:221–228, 1990.

56. Galli J, Cammarota G, Calo L and others: The role of acid and alkaline reflux in laryngeal squamous cell carcinoma, *Laryngoscope* 112:1861–1865, 2002.

57. Gallo A, de Vincentiis M, Della Rocca C and others: Evolution of precancerous laryngeal lesions: a clinicopathologic study with long-term follow-up on 259 patients, *Head Neck* 23:42–47, 2001.

58. Gallo A, de Vincentiis M, Manciooco V, and others: CO_2 laser cordectomy for early-stage glottic carcinoma: a long-term follow-up of 156 cases, *Laryngoscope* 12:370–374, 2002.

59. Garcia-Serra A, Hinerman RW, Amdur RJ and others: Radiotherapy for carcinoma in situ of the true vocal cords, *Head Neck* 24:390–394, 2002.

60. Gilbert R: Personal communication, 2002.

61. Gillison ML, Koch WM, Capone RB and others: Evidence for casual association between human papillomavirus and a subset of head and neck cancers, *J Natl Cancer Inst* 92:709–720, 2000.

62. Giovanni A, Guelfucci B, Gras R and others: Partial frontolateral laryngectomy with epiglottic reconstruction for management of early-stage glottic carcinoma, *Laryngoscope* 111:663–668, 2001.

63. Greene F, Page D, Fleming I and others: *AJCC cancer staging manual,* ed 6, New York, Springer Verlag, 2002.

64. Greene F, Page D, Fleming I, and others: *AJCC cancer staging manual: part II head and neck sites,* ed 6, New York, Springer Verlag, 2002, pp 17–88.

65. Groome P, O'Sullivan G, Irish J and others: Glottic cancer in Ontario, Canada and the SEER areas of the United States: Do different management philosophies produce different outcome profiles? A detailed analysis of glottic cancer management, *J Clin Epidemiology* 54:301–315, 2001.

66. Harrison DFN: Laryngeal cancer: a preventable disease, In Ferlito A, editors: *Laryngeal cancer: a preventable disease, neoplasms of the larynx,* Edinburgh, 1993, Churchill Livingstone.

67. Harwood AR, DeBoer G: Prognostic factors in T_2 glottic cancer, *Cancer* 45:991, 1980.

68. Hinerman R, Mendenhall W, Amdur R and others: Early laryngeal cancer, *Curr Treat Options Oncol* 3:3–9, 2002.

69. Hintz B, Charyula K, Chandler JR and others: Randomized study of local control and survival following radical surgery or radiation therapy in oral and laryngeal carcinoma, *J Surg Oncology* 12:61–74, 1979.

70. Hliniak A, Gwiazdowska B, Szutkowski Z and others: A multicenter randomized/controlled trial of conventional versus modestly accelerated radiotherapy in the laryngeal cancer: influence of a 1 week shortening overall time, *Radiother Oncol* 62:1–10, 2002.

71. Hoffman HT, Karnell LK: *Laryngeal cancer.* In Steele GD and others, editors: *National cancer data base annual review of patient care 1995,* Atlanta, American Cancer Society, pp 84–99, 1995.

72. Hoffman H, Karnell L and others: National cancer database benchmark reports: a valuable resource for head and neck oncologists.

73. Hoffman HT, Overholt EM, Karnell MP and others: *The larynx.* In Steele GD, Jessup JM, Winchester DP and others, editors: *Granuloma contact ulcers and other posterior lesions,* Philadelphia, 2003, Lippincott Williams & Wilkins, pp 203–224.

74. Hoshikawa T and others: Detection of human papillomavirus DNA in laryngeal squamous cell carcinomas by polymerase chain reaction, *Laryngoscope* 100:647–650, 1990.

75. Howell-Burke D, Peters LJ, Goepfert H and others: T2 glottic cancer: recurrence, salvage, and survival after definitive radiotherapy, *Arch Otolaryngol Head Neck Surg* 116:830–835, 1990.

76. Hoyt DJ and others: The effect of head and neck radiation therapy on voice quality, *Laryngoscope* 102:477–480, 1992.

77. Jabour BA, Choi Y, Hoh CK, and others: Extracranial head and neck: PET imaging with 2-[f-18]-fluoro-2-deoxy-D-glucose and MR imaging correlation, *Radiology* 186:27–35, 1993.

78. Jessup JM, Steele GD, Winchester DP: *Introduction.* In Steele GD, Jessup JM, Winchester DP and others, editors: *National cancer data base annual review of patient care 1995,* American Cancer Society, Atlanta, 1995.

79. Jiang JJ, Titze IR: A methodological study of hemilaryngeal phonation, *Laryngoscope* 103:872–882, 1993.

80. Jorgensen K, Godballe C, Hansen O and others: Cancer of the larynx treatment results after primary radiotherapy with salvage surgery in a series of 1005 patients, *Acta Oncologica* 41:69–76, 2002.

81. Kambic V, Gale N: *Epithelial hyperplastic lesions of the larynx.* Amsterdam, Elsevier, 1995, p 108.

82. Kashima HK, Lee DJ, Zinreich SJ: *Early cancer of the larynx: vestibulectomy in early vocal fold carcinoma.* In Johnson JT, Didolkar MS, editors: *Head and neck cancer: proceedings of the Third International Conference on Head and Neck Cancer, San Francisco, July 26–30, 1992,* vol 3, Amsterdam, 1993, Elsevier Science Publishing.

83. Kerrebijn JD, deBoer MF, Knegt PP: CO_2-laser treatment of recurrent glottic carcinoma, *Clin Otolaryngol* 17:430, 1992.

84. Kim M, Sun D, Park K and others: Paraglottic space in supracricoid laryngectomy, *Arch Otolaryngol Head Neck Surg* 128:304–307, 2002.

85. Kim RY, Marks ME, Salter MM: Early-stage glottic cancer: importance of dose fractionation in radiation therapy, *Radiology* 182:273, 1992.

86. Kirchner JA: One hundred laryngeal cancers studied by serial section, *Ann Otol Rhinol Laryngol* 78:689, 1969.

87. Kirchner JA: What have whole organ sections contributed to the treatment of laryngeal cancer? *Ann Otol Rhinol Laryngol* 98:661, 1989.

88. Kleinsasser O: *Tumors of the larynx and hypopharynx.* Stuttgart, Thieme International, 1988, pp 128–130.

89. Kooper DP, van den Broek P, Manni JJ and others, editors: Partial vertical laryngectomy for recurrent glottic cancer, *Clin Otolaryngol* 20:167, 1995.

90. Krespi YP, Meltzer CJ: Laser surgery for vocal cord carcinoma involving the anterior commissure, *Ann Otol Rhinol Laryngol* 98:105, 1989.

91. Lavey RS, Calcaterra TC: Partial laryngectomy for glottic cancer after high-dose radiotherapy, *Am J Surg* 162:341, 1991.

92. Laccourreye O, Laccourreye H, El-Sawy M, and others: *Supracricoid partial laryngectomy with cricohyoidoepiglottopexy.* In Weinstein G, Laccourreye O, Brasnu D and others, editors: *Organ preservation surgery for laryngeal cancer.* San Diego, 2000, Singular Thomson Learning.

93. Laccourreye O, Laccourreye L, Garcia D and others: Vertical partial laryngectomy versus supracricoid partial laryngectomy for selected carcinomas of the true vocal cord classified as T2N0, *Ann Otol Rhinol Laryngol* 109:965–971, 2000.

94. Laccourreye O, Veivers D, Bassot V and others: Analysis of local recurrence in patients with selected T1-3N0M0 squamous cell carcinoma of the true vocal cord managed with a platinum-based chemotherapy-alone regimen for cure (comment), *Ann Otol Rhinol Laryngol* 111:315–322, 2002.

95. Laccourreye O, Veivers D, Hans S and others: Chemotherapy alone with curative intent in patients with invasive squamous cell carcinoma of the pharyngolarynx classified as T1-T4N0M0 complete clinical responders, *Cancer* 92:1504–1511, 2001.

96. Laccourreye O, Weinstein G, Nauda P and others: Supracricoid partial laryngectomy after failed laryngeal radiation therapy, *Laryngoscope,* 106:495–498, 1996.

97. Leeper HA, Heeneman H, Reynolds C: Vocal function following vertical hemilaryngectomy: a preliminary investigation, *J Otolaryngol* 19:62, 1990.

98. Leonard JR, Beck WL: Hematoporphyrin fluorescence: an aid in diagnosis of malignant neoplasm, *Laryngoscope* 81:365–372, 1971.

99. Li GZ: A comparison of the therapeutic effect between preoperative radiotherapy plus operation and operation alone for laryngocarcinoma: a prospective study of 260 cases, *Chung Hua Erh Pi Yen Hou Ko Tsa Chih—Chinese J Otorhinol,* 28:170–173, 1993.

100. Lydiatt WM, Shah JP, Hoffman HT: AJCC stage groupings for head and neck cancer: should we look at alternatives? A report of the Head and Neck Sites Task Force, *Head Neck* 23:607–612, 2001.

101. Maguire A, Dayal VS: Supraglottic anatomy: the pre- or the periepiglottic space? *Can J Otolaryngol* 3:432–445, 1974.

102. Maheshwar A, Gaffney C: Radiotherapy for T1 glottic carcinoma: impact of anterior commissure involvement, *J Laryngol Otol* 115:298–301, 2001.

103. Mandell DL, Woo P, Behin DS and others: Videolaryngostroboscopy following vertical partial laryngectomy, *Ann Otol Rhinol Laryngol* 108:1061–1067, 1999.

104. McGuirt WF, Keyes JW, Geising KR and others: Positron emission tomography in the evaluation of laryngeal carcinoma, *Ann Otol Rhinol Laryngol* 104:274–278, 1995.

105. McLaughlin MP and others: Salvage surgery after radiotherapy failure in T_1-T_2 squamous cell carcinoma of the glottic larynx, *Head Neck* 18:229–235, 1996.

106. Menda Y: Personal communication, August 2003.

107. Mendenhall WM and others: T_1-T_2 squamous cell carcinoma of the glottic larynx treated with radiation therapy: relationship of dose-fractionation factors to local control and complications, *Int J Radiat Oncol Biol Phys* 15:1267–1273, 1988.

108. Miller AH: Premalignant laryngeal lesions, carcinoma in situ, superficial carcinoma: Definition and management, *Can J Otolaryngol* 3:573, 1974.

109. Mork J, Lie KA, Glattre E and others: Human papilloma virus infection as a risk factor for squamous-cell carcinoma of the head and neck, *N Engl J Med* 344:1125–1131, 2001.

110. Morris MR, Canonico D, Blank C: A critical review of radiotherapy in the management of T_1 glottic carcinoma, *Am J Otolaryngol* 15:276, 1994.

111. Mukherji SK and others: Can pretreatment CT predict local control of T_2 glottic carcinomas treated with radiation therapy alone? *Am J Neuroradiol* 16:655–622, 1995.

112. Nguyen C and others: Carcinoma in situ of the glottic larynx: excision or irradiation, *Head Neck* 8(3):225–228, 1996.

113. Ogoltsova ES, Paches AI, Matyakin EG and others: Comparative evaluation of the efficacy of radiotherapy, surgery and combine treatment of stage I-II laryngeal cancer (T1-2N0M0) on the basis of co-operative studies, *J Otorhinolaryngol* (Moscow) 3:3–7, 1990.

114. Olson N: Effects of stomach acid on the larynx, *Proc Am Laryngol Assoc* 104:108–112, 1983

115. Parson JT, Greene BD, Speer TW and others: Treatment of early and moderately advanced vocal cord carcinoma with 6 MV x-rays, *J Radiat Oncol Biol Phys* 50: 953–959, 2001.

116. Pearson B, Davis K: Personal Communications, August 2003.

117. Pearson B: *Foreword 9*. In Steiner W, Abrosch P: *Endoscopic laser surgery of the upper aerodigestive tract*, New York, 2000, Thieme International, p viii.

118. Pleet L and others: Partial laryngectomy with imbrication reconstruction, *Trans Am Acad Ophthalmol Otolaryngol* 84(5):882–889, 1977.

119. Postma GN, Bch KK, Belafsky PC and others: The role of transnasal esophagoscopy in head and neck oncology, *Laryngoscope* 112:2242–2243, 2002.

120. Rachmat Luci and others: The value of twice yearly bronchoscopy in the workup and follow-up of patients with laryngeal cancer, *Eur J Cancer* 29A:1096–1099, 1993.

121. Rebeiz EE, Wang Z, Annino DJ and others: Preliminary clinical results of window partial laryngectomy: a combined endoscopic and open technique, *Ann Otol Rhinol Laryngol* 109:124–127, 2000.

122. Remacle M, Eckel HE, Anteonelli A and others: Endoscopic cordectomy: a proposal for a classification by the working committee: European Laryngological Society, *Eur Arch Otohinolaryngol* 257:227–231, 2000.

123. Ricciardelli EJ and others: Effect of radiation fraction size on local control rates for early glottic carcinoma, *Arch Otolaryngol Head Neck Surg* 120:737–742, 1994.

124. Ritchie JM, Smith EM, Summergill KF and others: Human papillomavirus infection as a prognostic factor in carcinomas of the oral cavity and oropharynx, *Int J Cancer* 104:336–344, 2003.

125. Rothfield RE and others: Hemilaryngectomy for salvage of radiation therapy failures, *Otolaryngol Head Neck Surg* 103:792–794, 1990.

126. Rubright WC and others: Delay in the diagnosis of oral cavity cancer: an assessment of factors influencing tumor stage at the time of treatment, *Arch Otolaryngol Head Neck Surg* 1996 (in press).

127. Rudoltz MS, Benammar A, Mohiuddin M: Prognostic factors for local control and survival in T_1 squamous cell carcinoma of the glottis, *Int J Radiat Oncol Biol Phys* 26:767, 1993.

128. Rydell R and others: Voice evaluation before and after laser excision vs. radiotherapy of T1A glottic carcinoma, *Acta Otolaryngol* (Stockh) 115:560–565, 1995.

129. Schewitzer VG: Photofrin-mediated photodynamic therapy for treatment of early stage oral cavity and laryngeal malignancies, *Lasers Surg Med* 29:305–313, 2001.

130. Schuller DE and others: Evaluation of voice by patients and close relatives following different laryngeal cancer treatments, *J Surg Oncol* 44:10–14, 1990.

131. Schweinfurth JM, Powitzky E, Ossoff RH: Regression of laryngeal dysplasia after serial microflap excision, *Ann Otol Rhinol Laryngol* 110:811–814, 2001.

132. Sessions RB, Johnson JT, Didolkar MS, editors: *Minimal glottic cancer: head and neck cancer*, vol 3, Amsterdam, Elsevier Science Publishing, 1993.

133. Sessions RB, Miller SD, Martin GF and others: Videolaryngostroboscopic analysis of minimal glottic cancer, *Trans Am Laryngol Assoc* 110:56–59, 1989.

134. Shah and others: Conservation surgery for radiation failure in carcinoma of the glottic larynx, *Clin Otolaryngol* 19:105–108, 1994.

135. Shah JP and others: Conservation surgery for radiation-failure carcinoma of the glottic larynx, *Head Neck* 12:326, 1990.

136. Shapshay SM: Laser technology in the diagnosis and treatment of head and neck carcinoma of the glottic larynx, *Head Neck* 12:326, 1990.

137. Shapshay SM, Rebeiz EE, Silver CE, editors: *Laser management of laryngeal cancer: laryngeal cancer*. New York, Thieme, 1991.

138. Shapshay SM, Wang Z, Rebeiz EE and others: Window laryngoplasty: a new combine laser endoscopic and open technique for conservative surgery, *Ann Otol Rhinol Laryngol* 103:679–685, 1994.

139. Shvero J and others: Early glottic carcinoma involving the anterior commissure, *Clin Otolaryngol* 19:105–108, 1994.

140. Shvero J and others: T_1 Glottic carcinoma involving the anterior commissure, *Eur J Surg Oncol* 20:557–560, 1994.

141. Silver C, Silver CE, Ferlito A, editors: Chapter 2 *Surgical anatomy in surgery for cancer of the larynx and related structures*, ed 2. Philadelphia, 1996, WB Saunders Co, p 25.

142. Sittel C, Friedrich G, Zorowka P and others: Surgical voice rehabilitation after laser surgery for glottic carcinoma, *Ann Otol Rhinol Laryngol* 111:493–498, 2002.

143. Small W Jr and others: Results of radiation therapy in early glottic carcinoma: Multivariate analysis of prognostic and radiation therapy variables, *Radiology* 183:789–794, 1992.

144. Smith EM, Hoffman HT, Summersgill KS and others: Human papillomavirus and risk of oral cancer, *Laryngoscope* 108:1098–1103, 1998.

145. Smith EM, Summersgill KF, Allen J and others: Human papillomavirus and risk of laryngeal cancer, *Ann Otol Rhinol Laryngol* 109:1069–1076, 2000.

146. Smitt MC, Goffinet DR: Radiotherapy for carcinoma-in situ of the glottic larynx, *Int J Radiat Oncol Biol Phys* 28:251, 1994.

147. Spayne JA, Warde P, O'Sullivan and others: Carcinoma-in situ of the glottic larynx: results of treatment with radiation therapy, *Int J Radiation Oncology Biol Phys* 49:1235–1238, 2001.

148. Stadler A, Dontrus M, Kornfehl J and others: Tumor staging of laryngeal and hypopharyngeal carcinomas with functional spiral CT: comparison with nonfunctional CT, histopathology, and microlaryngoscopy, *J Comput Assist Tomogr* 26: 279–284.

149. Steiner W, Ambrosch P, Hess CF and others: Organ preservation by transoral laser microsurgery in piriform sinus carcinoma, *Otolaryngol Head Neck Surg* 124:58–67, 2001.

150. Steiner W, Ambrosch P: *The role of the phoniatrician in laser surgery of the larynx.* In Steiner W, Ambrosch P, editors: *Endoscopic laser surgery of the upper aerodigestive tract,* New York, 2000, Thieme, pp 124–129.

151. Steiner W, Fiereck O, Ambrosch P and others: Transoral laser microsurgery for squamous cell carcinoma of the base of the tongue, *Archives Otolaryngol Head Neck Surg* 129:36–43, 2003.

152. Stevenson JM, Juillard GJ, Selch MT: Stages 1 and 2 epidermoid carcinoma of the glottic larynx: involvement of the anterior commissure, *Radiology* 182:797, 1992.

153. Stone N, Stavroulaki P, Kendall C and others: Raman: spectroscopy for early detection of laryngeal malignancy: preliminary results, *Laryngoscope* 110:(10 Pt 1):1756–1763, 2000.

154. Strong MS, Jako GJ: Laser surgery in the larynx: early clinical experience with continuous CO_2 laser, *Ann Otol Rhinol Laryngol* 81:791, 1972.

155. Suzuki and others: *Acta Otolaryngol* 1994.

156. Teppo H, Koivunen P, Sipila S and others: Decreasing incidence and improved survival of laryngeal cancer in Finland, *Acta Oncological* 40:791–795, 2001.

157. Terhaard C, Bongers V, Van Rijk P and others: F-18-Fluoro-Deoxy-Glucose Positron-Emission tomography scanning in detection of local recurrence after radiotherapy for laryngeal/pharyngeal cancer, *Head Neck* 23(11):933–941, 2001.

158. Thumfart WF: *Early cancer of the larynx: laser-surgery of larynx-carcinomas: indications, techniques and follow-up.* In Johnson JT, Didolkar MS, editors: *Head and neck cancer: proceedings of the Third International Conference on Head and Neck Cancer, San Francisco, July 26-30, 1992,* vol 3, Amsterdam, 1993, Elsevier Science Publishing.

159. Toma M, Kenichi N, Nakao K, and others: Partial laryngectomy to treat early glottic cancer after failure of radiation therapy, *Arch Otolaryngol Head Neck Surg* 128:909–912, 2002.

160. Ton-Van J and others: Comparison of surgery and radiotherapy in T_1 and T_2 glottic carcinomas, *Am J Surg* 162:337–340, 1991.

161. Tucker GF, Smith HR: A histological demonstration of the development of laryngeal connective tissue compartments, *Trans Am Acad Ophthalmol Otolaryngol* 66:308–318, 1962.

162. Uematsu H, Sadato N, Yonekura Y and others: Coregistration of FDB, PET and MRI of the head and neck using normal distribution of FDG, *J Nucl Med* 39:2121–2127, 1998.

163. Urken ML, Blackwell K, Biller HF: Reconstruction of the laryngopharynx after hemicricoid/hemithyroid cartilage resection. Preliminary functional results, *Arch Otolaryngol Head Neck Surg* 123:1213–22, 1997.

164. van den Bogaert W: *What is the treatment of choice in early glottic cancer.* In Johnson JT, Didolkar MS, editors: *Head and neck cancer: proceedings of the Third International Conference on Head and Neck Cancer, San Francisco, July 26-30, 1992,* vol 3, Amsterdam, 1993, Elsevier Science Publishing.

165. Vaughon CW, Gates GA, editors: *Glottic cancer: current therapy in otolaryngology head and neck surgery, ed 5.* St Louis, Mosby, 1993.

166. von Leden H: *The history of phonosurgery.* In Ford CN, Bless DM, editors: *Phonosurgery: assessment and surgical management of voice disorders,* New York, 1991, Raven Press, Ltd., pp 3–24.

167. Ward PH, Hanson DG: Reflux as an etiological factor of carcinoma of the laryngopharynx, *Laryngoscope* 98:1195, 1988.

168. Warde PR, O'Sullivan B, Panzarella T and others: T1/T2 glottic cancer managed by external beam radiotherapy—the influence of beam energy on local control, *Int J Radiat Oncol Biol Phys* 42:2202, 1998.

169. Waterhouse JAH: *Epidemiology.* In Ferlito A, editor: *Neoplasms of the larynx.* Edinburgh, Churchill Livingstone, 1993.

170. Weber RS and others: CT vs MRI for staging carcinoma of the larynx (L) and hypopharynx (HP), American Laryngological Association, Orlando, Florida, May 4, 1996 (abstract).

171. Weinstein GS, Laccourreye O, Brasnu D, and others: *Laryngeal anatomy: surgical and clinical implications.* In Weinstein GS, Brasnu D, Laccourreye H, editors: *Organ preservation surgery for laryngeal cancer.* San Diego, Singular, 2000, pp 18–21.

172. Weinstein GS, El-Sawy MM, Ruiz C and others: Laryngeal preservation with supracricoid partial laryngectomy results in improved quality of life when compared with total laryngectomy, *Laryngoscope* 111:191–199, 2001.

173. Weinstein GS: Surgical approach to organ preservation in the treatment of cancer of the larynx, Oncology, Huntington.

174. Weinstein GS, Laccourreye O: *Vertical partial laryngectomies.* In Weinstein GS, Brasnu D, Laccourreye H, editors: *Organ preservation surgery for laryngeal cancer.* San Diego, Singular, 2000, pp 59–71.

175. Weinstein GS, Laccourreye O, Brasnu D and others: *Organ preservation surgery for laryngeal cancer,* San Diego, Singular Thomson Learning.

176. Wenig BL and others: MR imaging of squamous cell carcinoma of the larynx and hypopharynx, *Otolaryngol Clin North Am* 28:609, 1995.

177. Westra WH, Kronz JD, Eisele DW: The impact of second opinion surgical pathology on the practice of head and neck surgery: a decade experience at a large referral hospital, *Head Neck* 24:684–693, 2002.

178. Yamamoto M, Hada Y, Shirane M and others: The results of radiation therapy for glottic carcinoma: prognostic significance of tumor size in laryngoscopic findings, *Oncol Rep* 7:1275–1277, 2000.

179. Zacharek MA, Pasha R, Meleca RJ and others: Functional outcomes after supracricoid laryngectomy, *Laryngoscope* 111:1558–1564, 2001.

180. Zargi M, Smid L, Fajdiga I and others: Detection and localization of early laryngeal cancer with laser-induced fluorescence: preliminary report, *Eur Arch Otorhinolarynngol* 254:S113–S116, 1997.

181. Zeitels S, Jarboe J, Franco R: Phonsurgical reconstruction of early glottic cancer, *Laryngoscope* 111:1862–1865, 2001.

182. Zeitels SM, Vaughan CW, Domanowski GF: Endoscopic management of early supraglottic cancer, *Ann Otol Rhinol Laryngol* 99:951, 1990.

183. Zhao R, Hirano M, Tanaka S and others: Vocal fold epithelial hyperplasia: vibratory behavior versus extent of lesion, *Arch Otolaryngol Head Neck Surg* 117:1015–1018, 1991.

184. Zohar Y and others: The controversial treatment of anterior commissure carcinoma of the larynx, *Laryngoscope* 102:69–72, 1992.

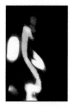

CHAPTER ONE HUNDRED AND ONE

TRANSORAL LASER MICRO RESECTION OF ADVANCED LARYNGEAL TUMORS

Bruce W. Pearson
John R. Salassa
Michael L. Hinnir

TERMS AND DEFINITIONS

Transoral laser microsurgery (TLM) is a surgical treatment strategy for primary cancers of the mouth, pharynx, and larynx. The instrument of excision is a carbon dioxide (CO_2) laser beam. An operating microscope imparts the perspective. The natural passageways of the upper aerodigestive system provide the access.

Two features distinguish TLM from open surgery. (1) Healing is allowed to occur by secondary intention. (2) The tumor block can be subdivided into manageable units by the laser (in situ).

TLM is clearly a conservation strategy, but it is not a reconstructive one. "Piecemeal" removal is a distinguishing feature of TLM—and a key source of controversy. Tumor transection endows important diagnostic dimensions to TLM. Magnification exploits the difference in visual appearance between normal tissue and cancer.

Safe TLM requires two conditions: (1) Adequate exposure through the mouth; (2) a tangible specimen.

TLM is an excision, not a vaporization. A specimen is the basis of meaningful frozen section margins. Individual specimens may be small. But in aggregate, the resected tissue volume parallels that of an open operation.

TLM is a misleading name. Transoral laser microsurgery is *not* totally transoral. Open surgery is still required for nodes in the neck. TLM is not entirely laser either. It depends on endoscopic cautery, vascular clipping, and occasionally blunt and sharp dissection. Finally, TLM is not exclusively surgical. Radiotherapy may be offered (for neck indications, but never to finesse margins).

TLM aims to improve cure *and* function through patient selection and technical excellence. The goal is the cure rate of open surgery and the functional promise of a tissue-conserving treatment like radiotherapy, all of this with less morbidity, at lower cost.

Advanced (as in "advanced laryngeal tumors") is a confusing term. In the context of laser surgery, it once meant any tumor larger than T1a glottic. In traditional discussions, it used to mean cancer with a fixed cord. The staging system suggests a different connotation—positive neck nodes. What is clear is that laryngeal cancer is not one disease. It is many different diseases. And unless we digress and clarify the descriptors of the different laryngeal cancers, all discussions of treatment are ambiguous. The answer to the question "Does an advanced case qualify for TLM?" is "It depends. What do you mean by advanced?" Let's look at the classifications.

Is it cancer? Laser surgery manages everything along the histologic spectrum, but this chapter only relates to the worst actor, invasive squamous cell carcinoma. The Ljubljana taxonomy[16] is probably the closest thing we have to an internationally accepted classification of epithelial hyperplastic laryngeal lesions (EHLL). For the most benign, "simple hyperplasia," acanthosis predominates. "Abnormal hyperplasia" is next, and basal proliferation is the hallmark. "Atypical hyperplasia" features dysplasia and atypia. Fourth is carcinoma in situ (CIS), cytologic neoplasia on an intact basement membrane. All these can be laser resected but TLM is a higher strategy, for a higher challenge, group five, neoplasia with subepithelial penetration (i.e., invasive squamous cell cancer).

Is it TLM? An excellent classification for laser cordectomies has been developed by the European Laryngological Society.[54] It names five types: subepithelial, subligamental, transmuscular, total, and extended cordectomy. The first three are elegant one-piece excisional biopsies, and a laser may be used on them. TLM (and the strategy of depth determination) comes into play for the last two.

What site? Before "multidisciplinary" committees imposed a theoretic anatomical classification (glottic, supraglottic, and subglottic) on laryngeal cancer, surgeons included clinical behavior in the sorting system. For 50 years, laryngeal cancer was "intrinsic" or "extrinsic."[25] Intrinsic was "interior region" cancer, primarily glottic in origin, slow growing, and nodes were late. TLM treats most of these, but not all. Extrinsic cancer was more supraglottic and more malignant. Originating around the laryngeal opening or its pharyngeal surface, extrinsic cancer was more lethal, more metastatic. TLM treats the local disease, but not the metastases.

Now the fashionable categories are glottic, supraglottic, subglottic, and in some quarters, "transglottic" (spanning the ventricle). However, in the anterior larynx, glottic and subglottic act as one).[56] Subglottic cancer often turns out to be glottic, with descent. The height of the glottis is argued (5 mm high, 10 mm high), or excluded posteriorly (sparing the posterior commissure). None of the sites is off limits to TLM.

In discussing local extent, clinicians often reduce their spoken references to "early" and "advanced" laryngeal cancer, the traditional dividing line being vocal cord motion. By this denomination, TLM is primarily an "early" cancer treatment, exceptional in the "advanced" group.

The tumor, node, metastasis (TNM) staging system[4] uses T_X, T_{is}, T_1 (a and b in the glottis), T_2, T_3, T_{4a}, and T_{4b} to define a local tumor, expanding 3 regions to 18 "extents." And this is just for the local disease (T). Nodes multiply the possibilities by 7. Metastases multiply the possibilities by 3, for more than 300 possibilities. Some are suitable for TLM. Some are not. No one knows where we should place the dividing line, or where "advanced" should start (or end). The staging system does encourage a summary format, Stage 1, Stage 2, Stage 3, and Stage 4. But the neck dominates this classification. If the neck is positive, everything is Stage 3 or 4 (advanced), even if the primary is miniscule.

None of the "approved" classifications for laryngeal cancer links stage to therapy. The TNM staging system has, for example, nothing to say about treatment. Staging leaves out all the patient factors (e.g., age, life expectancy, previous treatment, habits, expectations, work, literacy, medical illness, religious beliefs, distance from the treatment facility, etc.). The TNM staging system leaves out the history entirely (e.g., duration, otalgia, odynophagia, hemoptysis, exercise intolerance, etc.). It discards much of the physical exam (e.g., exophytic vs endophytic, keratinized vs ulcerated, stridor, obesity, cachexia, etc.). The labs

are ignored (e.g., hemoglobin, creatinine, blood sugar, liver function tests, human immunodeficiency virus antibodies, bleeding time). No account is taken of the imaging—magnetic resonance imaging (MRI), computed tomography (CT), positron emission tomography (PET) or the special tests (forced expiratory volume, electrocardiogram, cardiac ejection fraction). Staging was developed to facilitate comparisons of outcomes between different treatment centers and different treatment regimens. It is a standardized way to reduce the chance that reported differences do not arise from innate differences in tumor prognosis. Staging was never a prescription for therapy.

This leaves the doctor with the problem of how to interpret the term *advanced* in the context of TLM. It makes little sense to link advanced to a higher TNM stage (3 or 4) if patients with T_1 and T_2 local cancers will be included. (All that is required to make a T2 cancer "Stage 3" is for someone to feel a node in the neck). For example, the 2002 American Joint Committee on Cancer (AJCC) TNM staging of larynx cancer states that Stage III includes T_1, T_2, or $T_3 N_1$ (or $T_3 N_0$), where N_1 is a single node smaller than 3 cm. The AJCC also lists Stage IVA to include T_1, T_2, T_3, or $T_{4a} N_2$ (or $T_{4a} N_1$ or N_2), where N_{2a} is a node between 3 and 6 cm in size, on the same side; N_{2b} is multiple nodes smaller than 6cm, on the same side; and N_{2c} is bilateral or contralateral nodes smaller than 6 cm in size.

This chapter is primarily about the treatment of the local disease (by TLM). Therefore, we need to classify local disease and to help distinguish those for whom TLM is an option and those for whom it is not.

FIVE TYPES OF LOCAL LARYNGEAL CANCER

From the surgeon's standpoint, local laryngeal cancer comes in five different "flavors," each one more damaging (to function) to cure. Severity relates to what stock local excision would be required for complete removal. What would that impose on the patient, in terms of voice, swallow, and nasal breathing? This does not indicate the treatment is surgery. It just ensures that the appropriate local option for surgery is identified, especially to the patient, when the selection amongst various modalities is made. Each flavor can thus be defined by one of five classic excisions. These ascend in severity from laryngoscopic biopsy to total laryngectomy. Each excision removes a customary block, from one nodule to the whole larynx and its coverings. Each has a formal technique. For each we have a published record of local control rates from 98% to 80%. The expected functional outcome ranges from normal voice, swallow, and breathing down to tracheoesophageal puncture (TEP) voice and stomal breathing. Each of these five categories can be named as follows: very early, early, intermediate, advanced, and very advanced.

1. **Very Early**
   Exophytic mid cordal T_{1a} carcinoma. Encompassed by transoral excisional biopsy removal. Includes one-piece subepithelial cordectomy (stripping), subligamental[54] partial cordectomy, and mid-cordal transmuscular cordectomy
2. **Early**
   Two subtypes, glottic and supraglottic.
   a. **Early Glottic**
      T_{1a}, T_{1b}, and T_{2a} true cord carcinoma whose formal external excision would be a vertical partial laryngectomy,[35,66] or hemilaryngectomy.[5,67] The European Laryngological Society's total cordectomy and extended cordectomy[54] concepts probably fit here.
   b. **Early Supraglottic**
      T1 supraglottic carcinoma fitting within a supraglottic laryngectomy block.[1,6,41]
3. **Intermediate**
   Intermediate is laryngeal cancer that fits within a supracricoid partial laryngectomy block.[26,52] Thus, T_2 glottic carcinoma (T_2 by spread to the supraglottis), T_3 glottic (T_3 by thyroid cartilage erosion from the anterior commissure—mobility is preserved), T_2 supraglottic (T_2 by descent to involve the vocal cords), or T_3 supraglottic cancer (if T_3 by involvement of the preepiglottic space PES).[13,29,88]
4. **Advanced**
   T_3 glottic carcinoma (T_3 by unilateral cord fixation and invasion of the paraglottic space or the thyroid ala) is the prototype, because it is lateralized and fits within a near-total laryngectomy.[51] Lateralized invasive T_{2b} glottic carcinoma qualifies if the T_{2b} is by impaired mobility of one vocal cord. Also, advanced glottic carcinoma includes T_2 supraglottic carcinoma, where T_2 means involvement of the vallecula or the medial pyriform wall, and T_3 supraglottic carcinoma, where T_3 means unilateral cord fixation with invasion of the paraglottic space or the thyroid ala.
5. **Very Advanced**
   Bilateral anterior T_3 glottic carcinoma invading both ventricles, bilateral posterior T_3 supraglottic cancer invading the postcricoid region, or T_{4a} glottic or supraglottic carcinoma, which means the cancer has invaded into adjacent structures outside the larynx—the strap muscles, the thyroid gland, the tongue beyond the immediate base, the trachea, or the esophagus. The minimum excision these cancers would require is at least a wide field total laryngec-

tomy (T_{4b} is incurable by surgery). T_{4b} means gross distant extension. But this is virtually unheard of in cancers with no prior treatment. Examples include direct extension into the prevertebral space or the mediastinal structures or encasing the carotid.

Now we can examine TLM in the context of the clinical severity of the local disease. Others can judge the use and validity of the approximate term *locally advanced*.

ACRONYMS

CHEP	Cricohyoidoepiglottopexy.[27] Reconstruction for SCPL.
CHP	Cricohyoidopexy.[14,28] Reconstruction for SCPL.
HSL	Horizontal supraglottic laryngectomy.
NTL	Near-total laryngectomy.[32,48] Frontoanterior VPL with epiglottoplasty, SCPL, and NTL have at various times all been called *subtotal* laryngectomies.[10,34,49,62]
PES	Preepiglottic space.
SCPL	Supracricoid partial laryngectomy. Frontoanterior VPL with epiglottoplasty, SCPL and NTL have at various times all been called *subtotal* laryngectomies.[10,34,49,62]
TLM	Transoral laser microsurgery.
TEP	Tracheoesophageal puncture, tracheoesophageal prosthesis.[18,64]
VPL	Vertical partial laryngectomy. Includes the vertical frontoanterior and frontolateral[22,35,40,66] partial laryngectomies, and hemilaryngectomy.

LASER SURGERY AND TLM IN THE TREATMENT OF EARLY, INTERMEDIATE, AND ADVANCED CANCERS

Laser surgery is not new in larynx cancer. Davis and others[12]; Jako and others[20]; Strong[79]; and Vaughan, Strong, and Jako[83] all treated selected tumors during the 1970s and early 1980s.

Through the 1980s and 1990s, Motta and others[37] and Steiner[72,77] pioneered a new concept: tumor transection in situ. Consider the implications. If infiltrative cancer could be safely resected in pieces, tumor depth could be determined in situ. Incremental resection would become possible—as in Mohs's chemosurgery.[36] (Mohs treated cancer successfully in more sites than just the skin.) One could "follow the tumor," custom tailor the excision to each individual patient. If tumors could be subdivided into manageable subunits, early, intermediate, and even some advanced laryngeal cancers might be candidates.

Of course, transoral cordectomy provided outstanding results long before the laser was added.

Suspension[23,31,33,39] and the microscope were the key, not a laser. What the laser added was questionable—costs for new equipment, time to set up, regulations in the operating room, thermal injury hazards, maintenance issues, anesthesia issues, more suction, filters, retraining requirements, and new credentialing. And what the laser gave up was considerable—the tactile feedback of cold steel micro-instruments, the ability to cut around corners, the plume-free operating site, the char-free pathology specimen, operating room space, an unencumbered microscope, the precision of a cut path vs a vaporization path.

But in the 1980s and 1990s, a sustained experience of endoscopic laser surgery for *larger than T_{1a}* glottic cancers was growing in Germany.[58,72,75,77] This raised additional questions amongst traditionalists. They had concerns about exposure, hemostasis, reconstruction, margins, and wound healing. The greatest concern, however, was tumor transection. Steiner cut right through laryngeal cancer—in situ—through a laryngoscope! The claimed advantage was visualization and confirmation of tumor depth. How did the skeptics respond? First, we were asked to compromise access and work through smoke and an endoscope with no convincing evidence this was meaningful. Then we were asked to give up orientation and violate the principle of en bloc resection—with no laboratory evidence this was safe!

Other concerns fueled the discussion. After a laser supraglottic resection, there was no reconstruction! Open supraglottic laryngectomy always led to aspiration if one failed to repair the gap between the glottic unit and the tongue base.[41,53,80] After laser SCPL, there was no cricohyoidopexy. Yet this was essential in open SCPL.[28,29] And there were so many additional issues a laser did not address—bleeders over 2 mm, ossified cartilage, neck nodes.

Furthermore, the obvious problems of access were troubling. Big tongues, small mandibles, capped teeth, mild trismus, and other challenges all lay in wait, even for the most resourceful of operators. Very early mid-cordal T_{1a} carcinomas may have been okay. But early cancers would require greater exposure, intermediates more, and so on. Some would be too big to extract through an endoscope. A growing plethora of "laser laryngoscopes" raised suspicion that the problem of access remained unsolved.

Another challenge would be quality control from the pathology department. In cancer operations, negative margins are compulsory. If laser specimens were vaporized, the pathologist would have no margins to read. If they were laser-excised, margins would at best be charred. If they were excised in several pieces, positive margins would be meaningless!

In North American practices, these considerations delayed TLM. This, despite much of the pioneering work originating in North America—the entire organ serial section studies from New Haven,[24] Philadelphia,[81] and Toronto[43,82]; the development of the CO_2 laser itself at American Optical Corporation by Polanyi[78] and associates in 1965; the pioneering clinical laryngology of Strong[79]; Jako and others[20]; Vaughan, Strong, and Jako[83]; Davis and others[12]; Ossoff, Sisson, and Shapshay[45]; and Shapshay.[63] But the German centers were leaders in the collaborative development of all the ancillary laryngologic instrumentation needed to capitalize on the technique. They pushed their experience well beyond the concerns recited above, tracked their results, and continue to report on their experience.[*]

In 1996, the authors of this chapter began to study this body of work more closely, and subsequently we took numerous steps to incorporate TLM into our practices. This effort provided new perspectives on laryngeal cancer management and the initial selection of therapy. Now we seek to share what we have learned.

THEORETIC BASIS OF TLM

TLM does violate a time-honored dictum of surgical oncology—en bloc resection. A typical glottic or supraglottic cancer (above T_1) is likely to be extracted in three to six separate pieces!

En bloc has always been a prudent tactic to avoid unseen physical dispersion of viable malignant cells in a wound. When a scalpel penetrates cancer, the cells exposed will be alive. Viable cancer cells may adhere to the blade. Nothing prevents the surgeon from inadvertently transferring unseen cancer to an adjacent site in the wound. If unseen cell transplantation does occur during open surgery, and then we close the wound, how could tumor not recur? In open traditional surgery, this is why we isolate cancer in an unbroken package of normal surrounding tissue—to prevent contact between cancer and a scalpel or a scissor. This way, maybe we can avoid transplanting living malignant cells from the cancer back into the patient.

Rethinking this chain of events in laser micro resections raises a new question. What would be the apparatus of physical transplantation? Cancer cells do not adhere to a beam of light. There *is* no physical carrier to transplant tumor. Then again, grasping forceps and the suction cautery tips are used in TLM. They could do it. But assuming no tearing of the specimen, how would exposed cancer cells be viable? Cells revealed by laser energy are thermocoagulated, not

---

*References 3, 57, 60, 61, 70, 74, 76.

viable. Finally, in the TLM paradigm, we do not close the wound. An unseen cancer cell falls on a thin layer of coagulum, not a healthy tissue surface. This layer is gradually sloughed, not incubated.

These are theoretic reasons we postulate that laser surgery permits local cancer ablation without en bloc resection. Is there any laboratory or clinical data? Werner and others showed (for CO_2 laser incisions) that the lymphatic vessels of the wound margin are sealed immediately, and lymphatic vessels remain sealed for about 10 days after laser surgery.[85] And we also have 20 years of European clinical data.[19,59,69] Steiner and others have been performing TLM since the early 1980s. He and his colleagues have observed a low local recurrence rate (2%–10%), a high survival rate, and a low rate of complications.[71,74] They have not seen an increase in late neck or distant metastases during follow-up of more than 10 years. In other words, the incidence of cure by TLM is the same as the best results reported for open conservation surgery. Put another way, open surgery follows the principle of block resection, but produces no more local cures than TLM! TLM allows laser tumor subdivision, but local failure occurs with the same low incidence as in traditional open conservation surgery.

If tumor transection can be safely accomplished (it's not automatic, care is still important), we have an attractive new technique to determine the depth of cancer invasion before we commit to the plane of excision. If we misjudge and cleave too close to the tumor, this is just another form of tumor transection. We can extend the excision, incrementally. All we have lost is some time.

If tumors can be divided in situ, the tumor itself ceases to be a factor in obstructing our vision. Complete removal always requires that we expose the entire mucosal margin of the tumor. Now we can achieve that goal in a mosaic of views, unrestricted by the bulk of the disease.

If tumors can be extracted in pieces, the internal diameter of the laryngoscope does not set the limit on how large a tumor we can resect. The limit becomes the exposure for each step and our disciplined attention to specimen orientation. Mohs[36] transected cancers in situ successfully—and his attention to orientation was uncompromising.

Later in this chapter we summarize the TLM results reported by Steiner and others.[74] They document a very low incidence of failure at the primary site and also report the ultimate causes of death. Their conclusion: ultraradical treatment of the primary is not justifiable in a disease for which the main causes of death are advanced neck recurrences, distant metastases, second primaries, and serious general diseases. In modern times, quality of life is increasingly salient. In related diseases like hypopharyngeal cancer (TLM treats pyriform cancer too[73]), 5-year survival rates have stood between 15% and 30% for decades. Aggressive combined therapy (chemotherapy, radiotherapy and radical surgery) have not improved the poor prognosis. Again, if we can effect local control with conservation laser surgery, the argument in favor of radical ablation clearly declines.

TLM COMPARED WITH OPEN CONSERVATION SURGERY

Open operations approach intralaryngeal carcinoma from its "blind side." The surgeon cannot see the primary cancer until he or she has opened the neck, divided the fascia, separated the strap muscles, opened the framework, and penetrated the lumen at a critical point, determined by the local anatomy. Once exposed, field margins are oozy, not laser cut. Structures within the field relocate with the surgery, instead of maintaining a fixed position. The tumor margins are diminutive, not magnified; headlight illuminated, not microscope super-illuminated. For safety and reproducibility, open operations closely replicate a named excision block, chosen without the benefit of intraoperative depth information. For example, supraglottic laryngectomy removes the superstructures above the cords, which produces a predictable wound, requires a characteristic reconstruction, and can be repeated for numerous supraglottic cancer patients, despite the fact each has unique anatomy, distinctive preoperative findings, and slightly different tumor characteristics. Since the neck will be opened, the timing of a node dissection is determined. Since the neck dissection is continuous with the primary wound, steps must be taken to prevent a fistula. Since the framework is elevated to the tongue base and both swell, airway safety demands a temporary tracheotomy. Supraglottic laryngectomy supports the principle of en bloc resection, but this was necessitated by the scalpel, not the cancer. It facilitates teaching, but for gross anatomy, not for the microanatomy and micropathology. Open supraglottic laryngectomy provides the access needed for reconstruction, but the open surgery necessitated the reconstruction.

By approaching laryngeal carcinoma through the mouth, TLM requires no disassembly for access. The laryngeal framework continues to support the airway. A tracheotomy is usually superfluous in a supraglottic TLM. The strap muscles retain their swallowing contribution. Through the endoscope, the operator confronts the authentic primary right from the beginning of the resection—no preparatory dissection. The laryngoscope stabilizes the field. The magnification and brilliant illumination unveil important subtleties, dysplasia at a margin for example. With no disturbance of the neck, and no connection of a neck wound with a laryngeal wound, pharyngocutaneous fistulae disappear from the list of potential complications.

During TLM, diagnosis continues.[91] Wherever the local tumor extends, the microscope and the laser try to follow. Magnified tissue appearances acquire new significance. Some tumors change the vascular patterns in the mucosa. Deeper in, invasive cancer tends to appear pale and dysmorphic. Tissues give up subtle information about their consistency as they are retracted. Cancer is stiff or soft (soft can progress to friability and bleeding). Beyond the tumor, the expected microarchitecture is striated muscle, fat, seromucinous glands, fibrous perichondrium, (ossified) cartilage, or bone. Fat looks yellow and lobulated; mucous glands are pale and lobulated but more noticeably vascular. Muscle is striated. Fibrous tissue is white and dry. Ossified cartilage and bone carbonize to a dominoes-like appearance. The undersurface of the strap muscles is loose and areolar.

TLM is a natural ally of combined treatment. Once the tumor is out, the locoregional microvasculature is still undisturbed—the best milieu for post operative radiotherapy. And complete 3D resection under the microscope has minimized the chances of a positive margin.

During the weeks after TLM, the endolaryngeal wound heals by secondary intention (in many ways similar to a tonsil bed). The framework resists stenosis because it remains intact. The thermal damage from laser resection is superficial (after electrocautery, it is deeper). No local flaps are mobilized or transposed—no chance to bury residual tumor. "Second look" endoscopies become a meaningful way to revisit the primary site.

Months later, persistent granulation may signal the need for endoscopic removal, to improve voice. Follow-up laryngoscopy also allows the removal of small, ossified cartilage sequestra, which sometimes develop after a laser resection has been carried down to the framework. Re-epithelialization seems to forecast recovery but does not completely eliminate all risk of recurrence. Not even a negative second look excludes later recurrence. An overhanging anterior glottic scar may hide an unsuspected nubbin of residual tumor—still a salvageable circumstance, by simple laser resection, if discovered in time by this tactic. Before recommending TLM, discuss the willingness of the patient to return for a "second look."

INSTRUMENTAION AND TECNIQUES OF TLM
Instruments

We use a floor-model CO_2 laser console (Laserscope Paragon 50™), which generates an output beam of 1 to 50 W. Two modes, pulsed and continuous, are possible. Pulsed mode produces the fastest vaporization, the least adjacent thermal injury—the least char, hence the best clear recognition of the texture at the cut surface. But any vessel larger than an arteriole will bleed, and the bleeding must be arrested with electrocautery. Pulsed mode at low power (2–3 W) is ideal for glottic mucosa. One can maintain control over the cut (working slowly), avoid collateral heat (especially unintended thermal injury to the anterior commissure), and also avoid a "hole" of unintended depth (by pausing). For most normal laryngeal incisions, we use continuous mode at around 6 W of power. This setting provides excellent hemostasis but not enough char to upset the pathologists. Most mucosa bleeds too much in pulsed mode. Continuous mode results in a little more coagulation (about 50–100 µm).

The overall spectrum of power in laryngeal work is wide—1 W (focused, pulsed mode, for fine cutting of cordal mucosa), to 15 W (defocused, continuous mode, to vaporize friable semi necrotic centers inside bulky cancer (one of the few justifications for vaporization).

Besides mode and power, four more variables influence the effect:

- Speed: How quickly one moves the beam. Thermal transmission takes some time.
- Focus: Defocus the beam to create a superficial cautery effect but turn up the power, especially for broad forward advancement. Defocusing reduces the density of the power.
- Target tissue: Normal tissue (moist, not running wet) cuts best. Wet tissue (fluid is visible) cuts slowly, with a lot of thermal artifact from the boiling that has to take place first.
- Bleeding: Flowing blood stops laser surgery cold. It has to be ended (with electrocautery) before the excision can continue. Bleeding tissue just takes refuge under an expanding black char ball. Paradoxically, a beam set for the least char may impose the greatest char, by requiring the use of electrocautery.

An articulated arm brings the laser beam to the microscope body. From here we direct it with the joystick on a Sharplan Acuspot 712™ micromanipulator. The frame of the micromanipulator bears a gimbaled half-silvered mirror through which we see the target and with which we manipulate the laser beam. The narrowness of the micromanipulator frame is very important. Anything wider than the microscope body will conflict with the introduction of instruments (22–23 cm long). Unimpeded maneuvering and hemostasis at the primary site demand a clear path alongside the microscope for the grasping forceps and suction cautery tubes.

The CO_2 cutting beam is invisible, at 10,600 nm (far infra-red). The wavelength of visible light is 400 nm (violet) to 700 nm (red). The surgeon observes a red spot on the target produced by an integral red Helium Neon (HeNe) beam at 632.8 nm (visible red). A video camera is mounted on the microscope as in otologic microsurgery. A monitor displays the operative field, so the operating room nurses can anticipate and assist.

More than anything else, laser micro resection requires sophisticated skills in direct laryngoscopy. Much of this is experience, but part of it is an understanding of the laryngoscopes. Narrow tubular endoscopes (i.e., narrow side-to-side) overcome difficult exposure best. The tongue is incompressible (a fluid) and confined by the arch of the mandible. It can only be distorted. Wherever the scope contacts the tongue, it employs strong pressure, and deforms it such that a straight path to the anterior commissure results. The narrower an endoscope, the more it can sink into the tongue, and the more the tongue can squeeze around the sides.

A narrow vertically oval instrument like the Hollinger anterior commissure laryngoscope is the optimal tool to overcome difficult anterior visualization. But a narrow monocular laryngoscope is too narrow to accommodate the side-by-side dual optical pathways of an operating microscope. A Dedo anterior commissure laryngoscope overcomes this limitation. It provides just barely enough width to accommodate a microscope. Zeitels Endocraft™ laryngoscope[90] maintains this advantage and adds a useful tip enhancement for glottic work—less bevel. A blunt tip is better for holding aside the false cords. Regular tips actually cover the anterior commissure by the time the rest of the barrel reaches distal enough to lateralize the false cords. Zeitels's scope also features proximal slots along the sides to improve access for the instruments. Special modifications load both the Dedo and the Zeitels instruments with extra light and needed extra suctions carriers. Laser plume is the most troublesome limitation to clear vision during TLM, so the optimum allocation of suctions is important.

Storz™ and others have developed a specific assortment of laryngoscopes for TLM. Their standard adult laser laryngoscope (8661 CN) has a dome-shaped cross-section, a lip at the tip (anterior commissure), and an unobtrusive suction channel incorporated into the upper wall of the blade and the handle. For larger tumors, distending laryngoscopes are the best. Two we have considered indispensable are the Weerda distending operating laryngoscope (8588 L) and the Weerda/Rudert distending supraglottiscope (8588 E). These instruments are wider, independently adjustable, and fitted with great suction tubes. The upper blade features flares at the side to help hold the tongue out of the way. The lower blade mounts on a strong left proximal C arch (8588 L), or a strong ring (8588 E) to provide minimal encroachment on instrument access.

The best vallecular laryngoscope is probably the Lindholm instrument (8587 A). The essential laser laryngoscopes for difficult access and subglottic access are the Steiner models. These are long and thin. The "half dome" subglottiscope (8661 DN) sinks into a large tongue the best and the suction channel is incorporated into the handle. The flat-bodied subglottiscope (8661 E) gets past prominent incisor teeth the best, and a separate suction can be clipped.

We protect the incisors by fashioning a custom splint of heated Aquaplast™ (PS-1685), a thermoplastic substance that sets to a hard stable cap and diffuses the pressure over five or six teeth (WFR/Aquaplast Corp., Wyckoff, NJ). Sometimes we compress the cricothyroid with a band of tape across the table to help tip the larynx.

You can never have too much suction for plume evacuation—suction tubes on the laryngoscopes, suction tubes on the grasping instruments, suction in the insulated cautery, and plain dedicated suction tubes. Support each one with a separate suction line. Then add special suction tubes for blood. We prefer plain suction tubes for cleanup and gentle tissue manipulation and insulated suction-cautery tubes for flowing blood (two of each). Insulated (model 8606) suction cauteries come in various diameters—the insulation is necessary to prevent them sparking out to the endoscope. Prevent suction trauma (and worse, sticking to a friable specimen and tearing it) with a small relief hole in the tubing or at the sucker tip.

Larger vessels sometimes require something more targeted than suction cautery. Insulated model 8663 alligator forceps will pick up a small bleeder around a corner for electrocoagulation. Control the lateral vascular pedicles coming into the supraglottis with insulated MicroFrance™ CE 0459 bipolar cautery-forceps (specify 22.5-cm length). Place titanium clips on named arteries, like the superior laryngeal and the anterior cricothyroid arteries. Delayed secondary hemorrhage would be a formidable complication in a patient with no tracheotomy. Stop this problem before it arises by using laryngeal vascular clip applicators (model 8665 works well).

Bouchayer fenestrated forceps (8662 R or L) are excellent grasping instruments for small cordal specimens. But to secure the grip we need on the larger specimens we manipulate in TLM, normal laryngeal micro instruments are too delicate. Saw-tooth grasping forceps meet the need. Use one (model 8662 EL, FL, GL, or HL) to maintain a stable grip on tumor subunits. Use two to advance by double grasping. The L denotes a suction channel.

Controlled resection is only as certain as the stability we create for the micromanipulator. A rock-steady microscope stand, like a Universal S3, serves our Zeiss OPMI 111™ very well. Reduce the wrist and finger movements you transmit to the system with adjustable armrest stabilizers on a pneumatic chair (like the Möller-Wedel™ Combisit E). Adjust the microscope and the patient to a comfortable position for you (as in otologic microsurgery) instead of the other way around.

During TLM, operating laryngoscopes require frequent redirection. This is why a rack-and-pinion chest table (like the Storz Göttingen™ model) is worthwhile. It permits efficient breakdown and redirection of the suspension system, which affords the operator the opportunity to quickly reestablish a different stable vantage point several times per case. Coupled with table-height and tilt adjustment (controlled from the head end of the table too), the operator can repeatedly reestablish the optimal line of sight.

Techniques

To enhance endoscopic exposure of the anterior commissure, one can laser-transect the ventricular bands (i.e., the inferior free margin of the false cord or upper lip of the ventricle) from their anterior anchorage on the framework of the larynx. But this diminishes the contribution undisturbed false cord tissues might have made to voice. (Exposure of the anterior commissure for lasering presupposes that the anterior glottic contribution to voice will be lost.)

Do not rely completely on the pathologist. Study the mucosal margin around the tumor yourself. The operator enjoys the advantage over the pathologist when it comes to dodging a falsely negative margin reading. The pathologist will only see some of the margin, a rolled edge, its telltale vascular network empty and collapsed. The surgeon gets to view the living margin under brilliant illumination, extended by traction, and further described by its vascular patterning.

Once beneath the mucosa, follow the cancer in an orderly way. Use your knowledge of cross-sectional anatomy. Use the telescopes—inspect beyond the tumor. Use the power of laser surgery to resect one piece at a time and maintain constant orientation. Replace finger palpation with instrument palpation. Pull tumor into the field with grasping forceps. Finish an area before changing the tension and exposure in favor of another.

For laryngeal cancers that we choose to remove in sections, the plan of TLM is to complete each sub resection a block (or view) at a time. Use transection at the edge of the field to find the healthy tissue plane and deliver all the cancer that will be taken in that established view. Tumor transection defines the plane of separation from the rest of the cancer. Consider marking it with ink. This surface will be the plane we need to place within the next view we "capture," to maintain a continuous resection. Like a Rubik's cube, as each new tumor subcomponent is delivered, an adjacent component becomes more accessible.

As each subunit is resected, three obligations are paramount:

1. Maintain continuous orientation to the cancer. Recognize what has been completed and what next to expose. Know what remains to be done.
2. Orient the resected specimen for the pathologist. The deep margin is the margin of interest, not the margin released from the rest of the tumor, which is known to be cancerous. It usually remains unmarked, or bears the specific color we use to designate tumor transection surfaces.
3. Ink the deep surface margins, the surgical margins, which are expected to be negative, with the previously agreed on study color—black usually.

Anytime TLM is applied to intermediate or advanced cancer, some patients will present with significant disease in the *subglottic* larynx. This can be a challenging location for exposure. Among the most helpful ploys: a small endotracheal tube, proper choice of the endoscopes, top-to-bottom sequencing of the resection, and special positioning of the larynx. Tip the larynx up by elevating the thyroid cartilage with the laryngoscope blade and depress the cricoid with tape. Most patients with subglottic cancer have glottic cancer. Excise the glottic component first and exposure is automatically improved for the subglottic disease. When cancer descends to the inferior margin of the thyroid cartilage, include the cartilage margin itself in the resection. It is possible to encounter (and recognize) the Delphian node when laser resections extend forward through the lower margin of the thyroid cartilage. Resection with the cricothyroid soft tissues provides an opportune method to identify an important mode of extralaryngeal nodal spread, a finding that usually calls for further treatment of the nodes in the neck.[44] Laser resection and histopathologic study of the Delphian node should probably be a routine part of any significant subglottic resection.

TLM is not just a simple combination of already familiar techniques. It forces us to reconsider the detailed anatomy of the larynx—to learn it "inside out." Otolaryngologists introducing TLM into their practice should watch someone do it. Take a course. Be prepared to train an assistant and a scrub nurse too. If facilities permit, fresh frozen cadaver dissection has merit. Some of the goals would be to distinguish the greater horn of the hyoid vs the upper edge and cornu of thyroid cartilage, the preepiglottic fat vs the glands around the ventricle, the distribution of the superior laryngeal artery and its main branches,[50] the form and attachments of the conus elasticus, as well as other parts of the neck.

If you biopsy a cancer at a separate sitting, use this opportunity to evaluate your preparedness and equipment for TLM. Determine whether your exposure will be adequate. When it comes to making the transition from study and observation to practice and application, start with small cancers and edentulous patients, the easiest to expose. Then work your way up.

PATHOLOGY ISSUES

TLM tends to be a "one-surgeon" operation. But it is by no means a one-doctor operation. An interested, enthusiastic, and involved frozen-section pathologist is an essential partner. Multiple specimen blocks require mutual understanding and clear communication. The step-section technique works nicely for a single block (like a T1a glottic specimen). It is not appropriate for the usual multi block TLM case.[2]

When a tumor has been subdivided in situ, as already noted in this chapter, not all raw borders are margins. We have outlined one way to ink the margin in question on the specimen (Davidson Marking System™). Another is to cut separate margin specimens from the wound. You may be surprised at how easily a specimen becomes disoriented. Orientation is often lost by the time the specimen reaches the lips! If you want the pathologist to work from the primary specimen itself, ink the margin in situ, *before* the specimen is detached. In complex resections, ink the site of detachment too, so the subsequent readings will be easier to track. If you prefer, cut specific separate margin specimens *from the wound*. Then all the pathologist has to do is evaluate the entire submitted specimen. Is it yes or no? Is tumor is present or not? The surgeon's responsibility is to avoid three errors—errors of sampling, errors of communication, and errors of identification. Sampling is the art of providing a dead specimen and getting the pathologist to tell you what will happen with the adjacent living tissue still present in the patient. Communication means providing the pathologist with key information, like whether the patient was irradiated before. Identification means

keeping track of the sites of the sources of the biopsies. Use hemo clips, maps, lists, ink of different colors. Number the specimens and link them to a map or a color. Make sure you and the cytopathologist share the same site names.

TLM IN RELATION TO EACH OF THE FIVE CLINICAL CATEGORIES OF LARYNGEAL CANCER
Very Early Laryngeal Cancer

Very early laryngeal cancers provide a good initiation to laser laryngology, but the laser is just a "stand in" for microforceps and cautery with little tangible advantage. Expert laryngologists commonly cure mid-cordal T1a glottic lesions by transoral laser excision. But all they perform is a simple excisional biopsy. Suspension microlaryngoscopy is a key asset. But the secret to the high cure rate in "very early" cancer is patient selection, skillful laryngoscopic exposure, careful en bloc excision, and negative margins. The advantage lies not with a laser, but with the nature of the disease. Very early glottic cancers are an exceptional neoplasm, small, localized, and off the anterior commissure. No new principles were really required and no old principles were really challenged.

Early Laryngeal Cancer

"Early" laryngeal cancer comprises two groups, loosely similar to previously untreated T1B and T2A glottic cancer and previously untreated T1 supraglottic cancer. These are: (1) glottic cases falling within the purview of an open vertical partial laryngectomy; (2) supraglottic cases falling within the boundaries of a supraglottic laryngectomy.

Transoral laser microresection clearly meets or exceeds expectations in early laryngeal cancer:

- The cure rate matches the open operations (vertical partials and supraglottics) while the morbidity and functional losses decline.[74]
- TLM does not require a temporary tracheotomy to treat early cancer. Hospital time contracts to 3 days[46] and costs fall.[8]
- Radiotherapy may outperform open VPL for *voice* in early glottic cancer, but only if cure is obtained. TLM provides the same high cure rate of VPL, but a better voice than VPL.[55] The major advantages of TLM relate to the efficiency of cure (obtained with only one treatment), and speed of completion (treatment is finished at the same direct laryngoscopy and biopsy the patient would *require* to start radiation treatment).
- Radiotherapy may surpass open supraglottic laryngectomy (HSL) in resisting aspiration (but it loses on cure and efficiency). TLM preserves

better swallowing[21] than HSL and, unlike radiotherapy, requires no diminution of lubrication or taste.

- Over a lifetime, up to 25% of laryngeal cancer patients develop a second cancer.[68] Half involve the upper aerodigestive system. Patients who opted for TLM retain every possible option for the second cancer (including radiotherapy and laser surgery). Patients who accepted radiotherapy—and even prevailed—have narrowed their de facto future options to surgery in an irradiated field.

The conduct of TLM in early laryngeal cancer proceeds as follows. Intubate for general anesthesia with a small laser-approved endotracheal tube. (To minimize trauma, consider doing it yourself). Our tubes have two balloons filled with water. Set up the laser for parfocal operation, for the smallest microspot (0.25 mm), and for continuous mode. Ask for 3 W power if you are a beginning laser surgeon, more as you learn to work faster. Establish the initial laryngoscopic exposure and the video image. Protect the face with a wet towel.

For early glottic cancer, using the laser, retracting with the suction, outline the tumor margins. Then subdivide the lesion into a "middle plus anterior" and a "posterior" subunit.[71] Identify the depth of infiltration into the thyroarytenoid muscle and the extent onto the arytenoid. Laser-resect the posterior block. Resuspend the laryngoscope and transect the remaining tumor between the "middle" and "anterior" block. Laser-resect the middle block, so all that remains is the front. Reconfirm the depth by frozen section. Finally, reposition the laryngoscope and resect the anterior block. Traction with Bouchayer forceps works well to clarify the resection line at the anterior commissure.

In anterior commissure cancer, the voice is usually bad due to the disease. Voice after TLM for anterior commissure cancer is usually no worse.[46] However, the mechanism is different. Extensive resection of *anterior commissure/anterior glottic* cancers changes the glottis to a keyhole shape. It also bares the inner aspect of the thyroid cartilage. Healing on the inner aspect of cartilage will produce thin mucosa on a solid base, cartilage or fibrous scar with tethered restriction points. Thus we obtain stiffness. And stiffness produces hoarseness. Also, the intact thyroid cartilage will brace open the defect to produce an anterior glottic gap. And a gap produces breathiness.

In some cases, breathiness can be reduced with phonosurgery (e.g., cartilage implantation[65]) to reduce the anterior glottic gap. The correction of hoarseness due to stiffness awaits future advances. The principal strategy now is the intelligent preser-

vation of uninvolved tissues and the avoidance of unnecessary desiccation of the normal tissues left behind. (TLM preserves glandular elements better than radiotherapy.)

For early supraglottic cancer (confined to the supraglottis—the glottis and both arytenoids are free), split the suprahyoid epiglottis[60] vertically in the midline (even if this transects cancer crossing the midline). Identify the hyoid bone. Cut the vallecula and expose more hyoid to each side. Pass down the thyrohyoid membrane and clearly identify the upper margin of the thyroid cartilage. Plan to capture the bilateral supraglottic vascular pedicles with insulated grasping forceps or the bipolar cautery forceps. Resect suprahyoid tissues before infrahyoid tissues, in planned subsections, proximal to distal. Above the plane of the thyroid alar margin, you will not harm the glottis. Below this plane, improve your access and vision by having resected all of the suprahyoid tissues on both sides. When resecting the false cords, take advantage of the angled suction protectors (model 8596) to shield the vocal cords. Insert the "baffle" into the ventricle or above the anterior commissure. In every supraglottic case, the surgeon should work to resect *all* of the preepiglottic space.

Intermediate Laryngeal Cancer

Earlier we defined "intermediate" laryngeal cancer to be one that would require SCPL to be encompassed by an open operation. Most "intermediate" glottic or supraglottic cancers can be treated by laser micro resection, open SCPL, or radiation with surgical salvage. The problem with radiation and salvage is intermediate cancers that fail radiotherapy are not cured by conservation operations. SCPL has a better record of local control,[9,28] but patient selection and surgical execution require tremendous sophistication. SCPL pushes function to the limit—it is probably the most extensive open resection one can do and still restore swallowing and an internalized airway (i.e., the tracheotomy is temporary).

Experience refutes the allegation that TLM cannot encompass intermediate cancers. When an anterior commissure lesion too big for a vertical partial (but too mobile for a near total or total laryngectomy),[46] TLM provides a very logical resection. TLM clearly rivals open SCPL for functional results. The morbidity is more than we see after TLM for *early* cancer, but clearly less than we expect after open SCPL for *intermediate* cancer.[38] Case selection may be more forgiving than it is for open SCPL because of the intraoperative diagnostic advantage of TLM.

Full exposure of intermediate cancer is only slightly more difficult than for early cancer. The larger challenge is continuity and orientation. Start with early cases to master exposure. Then progress to intermediate cases and the greater manipulative and directional tests they offer. Intermediate anterior glottic cancers typically involve the thyroid cartilage, but spare the arytenoids. Of course, anterior laryngeal resections can include large pieces of the thyroid cartilage and the subglottis. Ossified framework can be devitalized with heat and outlined for endoscopic resection with Jackson laryngeal scissors (Pilling™).

If motion on one side of the anterior glottis is at all impaired (T2b), look for extraconal cancer during TLM. And bear in mind that once external to the conus, tumor descends to escape outside the larynx (through the cricothyroid triangle).[50] Borders of the cricothyroid triangle are the inferior margin of the thyroid cartilage, the lateral edge of the cricothyroid ligament, and the medial border of the cricothyroid muscle. An "intermediate" cancer found to extend outside the larynx should probably be converted. It might well be better to open the neck and to permit the formal resection of, say, a near-total laryngectomy, which includes strap muscles and the thyroid isthmus and lobe.[47] The price is the permanent stoma that accompanies NTL, but this is better than recurrent cancer.

TLM can also treat T_2 supraglottic cancers if the reason for "T_2" is invasion of the glottis or the medial pyriform wall. Once, a total laryngectomy was rationalized in these cases (by the notion that the tumor exceeded the limits of a supraglottic laryngectomy). That was why SCPL was a real advance. When TLM is feasible for T_2 supraglottic cancer, TLM becomes the next advance. Note that the patient undergoing TLM for intermediate cancer reaps the additional benefit of continuing diagnosis. Under brilliant magnification and stable exposure, little extensions of unexpected cancer[11] are likely to be recognized and removed. So are erythroplasia and keratosis, future sites of origin of the next cancer. When TLM cannot be done for intermediate cancer, the attempt to perform a laser excision may demonstrate why transoral laser or open SCPL are both unsafe (in that patient).

Intermediate TLM risks glottic stenosis. The maximum safe preservation of intralaryngeal mucosa and cricoid cartilage resist it. Preemptive suppression of reflux with antacid medical regimens also makes sense. If you anticipate losing an arytenoid at TLM, do a tracheotomy at the time of the laser surgery. Take advantage of the view (no endotracheal tube), and protect the patient against initial aspiration with a cuff.

TLM may generate the most logical resection for intermediate cancer, but the wound is still left to granulate and contract by itself. Open SCPL calls for a strong cricohyoidopexy.[30] The return of swallowing after TLM implies cricoarytenoid elevation is accomplished by other means. Perhaps this is preservation of the strap muscles—no suprahyoid dissection, no circum-hyoid suturing.

The risk of a fistula after TLM for intermediate laryngeal cancer is nil—the neck dissection never connects to the primary site.

Advanced Laryngeal Cancer

"Advanced" laryngeal cancers are glottic, supraglottic, transglottic, aryepiglottic, or even medial pyriform cancers distinguished by two fundamental features: (1) Permeation of the paraglottic space. (Therefore advanced cancers impair the motion on one side.) (2) A clearly lateralized disposition. (Advanced cancers seem to permeate the "hemilarynx.")

The block to encompass such a cancer corresponds to a near-total laryngectomy.[47] NTL is a complete supraglottic laryngectomy plus an extended hemilaryngectomy—combined to include all of one paraglottic space and all of its contiguous neighbors. (Neighbors are the thyroid lobe and isthmus, the hemi cricoid, the arytenoids, the pyriform, the anterior commissure and subglottis, and however much contralateral anterior glottis is necessary to encompass the cancer. Patients undergoing NTL retain a lung-powered voice—a prosthesis-free tracheopharyngeal fistula voice—but their stoma is permanent.

What saves these patients from being classified "*very* advanced" are the following characteristics.

1. Most of the subglottic mucosa within the cricoid, certainly all of it on the "good" side, is free of cancer.
2. The contralateral ventricle is clear of cancer
3. The contralateral vocal cord is only involved in the superficial mucosa and the most anterior glottic musculature.
4. The posterior commissure and post-cricoid regions are completely clear.

To recognize patients with "advanced" laryngeal cancer, we have to be able to identify and exclude the "very advanced" cancers, for which near-total laryngectomy would not be not safe. "Very advanced" means the only dependable ablative option is total laryngectomy and the preferred voice strategy is TEP. Typical "very advanced" laryngeal cancers are midline and bilateral, not lateralized. For example:

1. Massive "horseshoe" glottic/subglottic cancers (both ventricles and both muscular vocal cords are cancerous).
2. Significant subglottic cancers (generally involve the cricoid bilaterally and often present with airway obstruction).

3. Posterior commissure/postcricoid cancers (both arytenoid complexes are involved).

Near-total laryngectomy is the most logical open "block" for advanced cancers. But NTL requires a very specialized lateral laryngotomy. The challenge is to enter the lumen *without* encountering cancer and *without* compromising the future speaking shunt. In many candidates, it would be easier to outline the block from within the lumen of the larynx. And the laser would be the ideal tool. More subglottic mucosa could be saved (which improves the tapered capacity of the inferior shunt—the tracheocricoid entry into the speaking shunt). More interarytenoid soft tissue could be saved (which contributes to the shunt's voicing and valving capacities). Occasionally, it might be recognized that both arytenoids were actually clear. That is, the cancer was "intermediate" not "advanced," and a very logical laser *supracricoid* operation could be performed. This would confer an important advantage for the patient—no permanent tracheotomy.

Generally, we find "advanced" cases *cannot* be treated by TLM, because *reconstruction* is required. The value of TLM lies not in complete excision, but in prereleasing the crucial tissue that really *needs* to be excised—this can define whether the cancer actually rises to the level of a near-total laryngectomy. Prerelease occurs with visible direction from familiar endolaryngeal landmarks and it avoids the cancer itself. Then the surgeon can perform open delivery through the neck. No concerns about the site of entry, where the true margins lie, or where unseen submucosal cancer might extend. Perhaps the pharyngeal augmentation flap (to be turned down from the ipsilateral side to participate in the shunt[47]) can be precut with the laser as well. Voice shunt reconstruction would then be a simplified assembly with precut margins, no mucosal bleeding, and the least chance of cautery damage to the nerve supply or the muscular components of the shunt.

Very Advanced Laryngeal Cancer

A laser might be *capable* of total laryngectomy in a well-defined previously untreated very advanced cancer, but not the restoration required. The pharyngotomy must be repaired. A stoma must be fashioned. Sometimes the hypopharynx needs reconstruction. The neck must be opened. Not much justification for a prerelease. Total laryngectomy is an anatomical excision.

Most patients present with very advanced laryngeal cancers that are in a sea of inflammation. Many have failed earlier radiotherapy. Many are treacherous for their submucosal extent. Keeping tiny remnants of the larynx in cases like these is oncologic brinksman-

ship, and it never supports meaningful function. So TLM has no apparent application in the "very advanced" category of laryngeal cancer. The exception might be the emergency treatment of neglected cancer with airway obstruction.[7]

TLM AND NECK DISSECTION

The neck nodes are treated as they always have been—by open surgery or post-operative radiotherapy. We *can* carry out a neck dissection at the same sitting as TLM on the primary, but laser endoscopic surgery cancels the argument to perform a node dissection *now* because "the neck is already violated" (to access the primary). A better time might be weeks afterwards. One unproven hypothesis suggests later is better, because the micrometastases "in transit" at the time of the TLM will have had time to lodge in the nodes. A more practical reason would be to wait until a patient with serious comorbidities has recovered from the primary resection, or until after an elderly patient has regained swallowing after a laser supraglottic laryngectomy, or until after we know exactly what the pathologist has to say about the invasive nature of the primary cancer. Since a "second look" is possible after TLM, this might be a suitable time to operate on the deferred neck. With respect to the patient with a very low tolerance for complications, we have already mentioned that staging the primary and the neck surgery at separate sittings reduces the chance of a pharyngocutaneous fistula to zero.

TLM AND RADIOTHERAPY

TLM undoubtedly works best as a primary treatment. But surgeons who can offer TLM are not always consulted when the initial therapy is being selected. About half our anterior commissure patients had already received previous treatment by the time we were called on to consider laser surgery.[46] Therefore, surgeons *will* be confronted with patients who seek TLM for radio recurrent disease.

Prior radiotherapy complicates the planning of TLM and increases the morbidity attributable to delayed wound healing. It diminishes the accuracy of clinical judgment and the specificity of preoperative imaging. Radio recurrent cancer is often submucosal and sometimes discontinuous.[17] These factors complicate the decision to even attempt TLM. If TLM is undertaken, magnification does help disclose atypical patterns of spread. But magnification comes with its own danger—the temptation to cut normal-looking margins too close.

In our anterior commissure series,[46] 5 of 16 patients with intermediate laryngeal cancers received *postoperative* radiotherapy. The indication was suspected disease in the neck, never a positive margin at the primary site. A positive margin at the laser site is an indication for further surgery, not radiotherapy.

TLM gives us a way to remove the primary without first disturbing the neck. After TLM, postoperative radiation faces the novel circumstance that no one has first disturbed the microcirculation with an open operation. Maybe the obligation to include the primary site in the radiotherapy fields is more questionable after TLM, when margins were clear and radiotherapy is being given for neck indications. TLM patients tend to heal as quickly as patients with open surgery. But more importantly, the risk of a complication (necrosis, a fistula, an infection in the neck) is diminished. Therefore, TLM may be a more logical choice for the excisional component of combined therapy. Indicated radiotherapy will not likely be delayed by the prior performance of a TLM.

COMPLICATIONS OF TLM

The complications of stray laser light include unwanted burns. Tiny pinpoint burns to normal laryngeal or pharyngeal mucosa are not rare. The beam can easily pop the endotracheal cuff. Important burns or to facial skin or worse, to the eyes or the airway are extremely rare but potentially devastating. We use small wet precut toweling strips to cover fields beyond the target site. Angled suction protectors shield the cords. Cover the face and eyes of the patient with wet toweling after you position the laryngoscope. The microscope itself will save the operator's eyes from harm. All other personnel need protective eyewear in the operating suite. Give the laser pedal to the surgeon (only), and the cautery pedal to the assistant (only). Control the concentration of oxygen in the airway, and use a double-cuffed laser endotracheal tube with saline in each cuff to maintain the seal confining the oxygen to the distal trachea.

Prolonged endoscopic displacement of the tongue causes obvious, sometimes severe, lingual contusion, swelling, and subsequent dysphagia, with or without long-term lingual dysesthesia. Chipped or loosened teeth follow difficult intubations or forceful endoscopic suspension in the dentulous patient. Sponges used to protect mucosa easily drift out of sight to be left behind when an endoscope is repositioned. Arteries can bleed voluminously into the wound in the larynx, particularly in the patient recently taking platelet inhibitors. All of these complications threaten the airway—with swelling, foreign bodies, or blood.

Many patients undergoing TLM require no tracheotomy. However, every consideration should be given to one in the intermediate and advanced cases where the role of a tracheotomy may be different. Here are some potential indications:

- To bypass expected edema from prolonged pressure on the tongue base in a lengthy case with difficult exposure.
- To bypass the specter of serious hemorrhage in the supraglottic region in the absence of airway protection.
- To avoid the impediment to exposure an endotracheal tube can pose, especially in the subglottis.
- To allow cuffed resistance to laryngotracheal aspiration in a patient with susceptible lungs.

Sudden secondary bleeding—without a tracheotomy—is probably the most dangerous risk.[84] The best treatment is avoidance. Never trust the cautery to provide sustained control of a named artery (like the superior laryngeal). Clip named arteries. And never trust the standard mouth guards to protect the teeth. Cover the upper incisors with thermosetting plastic and cool it with ice water. We mentioned the small square of double-folded Aquaplast™ we use, the same material used to fashion rhinoplasty splints. As much as possible, the surgeon should pick up the tempo of the TLM to avoid prolonged tongue pressure. Do not be slowed down by inadequate plume suction, a weak laser beam, or a medium power beam weakened by defocusing. Learn to adjust the power and focus to the optimal settings for pace. Lengthy surgery risks tissue stasis and deep vein thromboembolism. Consider timed repositioning and apply antiembolism devices to all but the "very early" cases.

TLM imposes obvious limitations on reconstruction, but, in practice, the fact that the wound must heal by secondary intention is usually an advantage. The surface we will eventually be following in the office will be recovered by indigenous mucosa, not by a skin graft, not by a regional flap, not by irradiated mucosa. This should improve our ability to monitor for local recurrence. Secondary intention healing involves contraction and granulation tissue of course. But the preserved laryngeal framework does a surprisingly good job resisting contraction and stenosis is not very common. Beware the patient with reflux. Reflux slows healing, which encourages fibrous stenosis. Be prepared to give proton-pump inhibiting medications on minimal evidence. Leaving the wound unreconstructed may yield two additional benefits. Free cancer cells (if any) will fall on a slightly more inhospitable surface than the one we "bury" by reconstruction in open operations. Also, at a future date, not having buried that surface, we preserve the possibility of a second chance through the discovery of persistent cancer at a "second look."

Whenever the inner surface of the cartilage is exposed by TLM, a sizeable granuloma is almost inevitable. Small osseocartilaginous sequestrae will perpetuate a granuloma until they are removed. At the anterior commissure, extensive resection leads to a rounded open anterior glottic defect. The opening produces breathiness. The walls consist of thin new mucosa, directly applied to the cartilage. The stiffness begets hoarseness. Prevention involves the optimal preservation of laryngeal mucosa,[89] plus the recognition and removal of any cartilage that undergoes laser thermal devitalization. Treatment of the breathiness draws upon one's phonosurgical experience.[65] The stiffness is so far resistant to intervention.

TLM incurs new expenses. The institution incurs new costs, for training and equipment, and increased demands are made on the cytotechnicians and frozen-section pathologists. Some patients require a "second look" laryngoscopy (a few patients require more than one "second look"). Other patients will seek phono surgical procedures. Some patients will receive post-operative radiotherapy (but their indications will be the same as in open surgery, so this cannot be considered an extra cost). TLM requires more travel for some patients, because of its limited availability in the United States (although travel for radiotherapy is also common, and the time required away is considerably longer). Despite these extra costs, TLM reduces costs considerably.[8,46] Unfortunately, in practice, many patients do not receive TLM until after they have already incurred the expense of a previous therapy (that has failed). If TLM gains broader acceptance as an initial option, the potential for expense reduction may further improve.

TLM is a more difficult skill to transfer to the residents than is open surgery. The subtleties of orientation defer the assignment of part to the resident, part to the consultant. TLM tends to be a one-person start-to-finish operation. There is not the usual sharing of duties possible with open surgery, or the formal laboratory experience familiar to ear surgeons who prepared themselves on the temporal bone. TLM requires new judgment from laryngeal surgeons with respect to case selection and more advanced skills in laryngeal endoscopy because of the challenges of proper exposure. There are additional procedures to master, including second-look direct laryngoscopies, new phono-surgical procedures, and the artful management of the complications noted earlier.

CONTRAINDICATIONS TO TLM

Extensive tumor spread to the neck (e.g., great vessels, the esophagus, the thyroid gland) is an absolute contraindication to TLM. So is inability to expose (with caveats if the upper teeth are the only impediment). The patient might consider the extraction of (carious) teeth, especially if it might save an open approach and a separate dental charge. Radiotherapists advise patients who have cancer to have pretreatment extractions. Preparation would include receiving patient consent and the taking of a dental impression.

TLM should not be advised for unresectable cancer, advanced cancer needing reconstruction, patients with functional disorders after extensive partial resections (like severe persistent aspiration or secondary stenosis), or the patient with overwhelming comorbidities. TLM is not very successful in any palliative role. It will usually prove unhelpful at the primary site in a patient with an N_3 neck or distant metastasis. A fixed (not impaired) cord is probably a contraindication to TLM. Recurrent cancer in an irradiated "bed" is a relative contraindication.

TLM has the potential to attract more patients with unrealistic expectations, those for example with advanced or very advanced laryngeal cancer after chemoradiation failure, or patients with major systemic comorbidities hoping to avoid a needed open operation for cancers that are advanced or very advanced. Sometimes a patient seeking TLM has built up too much faith in "the laser myth," while denying the realities of his or her predicament. TLM cannot repair tissues or functions already lost to cancer, radiotherapy, or previous surgery. It cannot restore tissues currently compromised by cancer. TLM cannot bring back lubrication, it will not reverse soft tissue or chondro-osseous necrosis, and it does not improve edema or painful soft tissue induration after radiotherapy.

RESULTS OF TLM

After an open operation or radiotherapy, laryngeal cancer reappearing at the original site is properly designated as "local persistence" or "recurrence." Local recurrence is disease that reappears after the initial treatment program has been completed. In TLM, a "second look" is often a planned second phase of treatment. The discovery of residual cancer amenable to cure by laser resection at the time of the second look should *not* be listed as "local persistence" or "recurrence." These are diagnoses one would logically withhold until *after* a second look strategy has been completed (or after one has been refused). This convention would be similar to the standard for chemotherapy, where persistent cancer at the primary site is not considered a failure if only the first cycle has been given.

GOTTINGEN GROUP RESULTS

After first observing TLM by Wolfgang Steiner and Petra Ambrosch in 1996, and later by Heinrich Rudert in Kiel, Germany, the authors attempted to emulate these techniques in their own practices. Around that time, a comprehensive report on the results of TLM was given by Steiner and his colleagues at the European Federation of Oto-Rhino-Laryngological Societies (EUFOS) in Budapest. Because many North American laryngologists remain unfamiliar with this important presentation and, because our own combined experience in more than 400 TLM patients seems congruent with this original work, we have tried to summarize Steiner's data here.

His reports were based on 606 patients treated from 1979 to 1986 in Erlangen-Nurnberg or 1986 to 1993 in Göttingen. The last Erlangen entry was in January 1994, and the last Göttingen entry was in December 1995. The only exclusions were patients with simultaneous second primary cancers, thus not treatable for cure. Of the patients, 360 had early glottic cancer, 43 had early supraglottic disease, 147 had late glottic carcinoma, and 56 had late supraglottic cancer. The T distributions were pT_{is}; 45 patients, pT_1; 228 patients, pT_2; 231 patients, $pT3$; 69 patients and $pT4$; 33. As might be expected, the T_{is} and T_{1a} cases did extremely well and will receive no further comment.

Attempting to reclassify all of Steiner's glottic cases as "very early" (pT_{is} or pT_{1a} for 236 patients) and "early" (pT_{1b} pT_{2a} for 124 patients), there were 18 recurrences (15%) in the 124 "early" cases. Among the 26 pT_{1b} glottic cancer patients, 5 local tumors recurred. Of the 98 patients with pT_{2a} glottic cancers, 13 experienced recurrences. Combining the very early and early patients, there were 35 recurrent cancers amongst 360 TLMs. Of these 35 recurrences, 5 occurred more than 5 years after initial treatment (thus possibly were second primaries).

Of the 35 patients, 27 were salvaged by functional surgery, mainly by transoral laser micro-re-resection. Eight patients proceeded to laryngectomy. Of the 360 (0.5%), 2 died from the glottic cancer. Six developed neck metastases, 3 with their primary controlled and 3 with recurrent cancer at the primary site. During the course of their follow-up, 23 patients (6.4%) developed second primaries, and 16 (5%) died of their second primary. The commonest cause of death in the whole group was intercurrent disease—64 patients (17.5%). The 5-year Kaplan-Meier survivals were 87% for the "very early" glottic group and 83% for the "early" cases. TLM preserved voice in 352 of the 360 patients (98%), and was judged to be of satisfactory quality in 90%. One patient bled. No one needed a tracheotomy.

Steiner reported 43 previously untreated patients with supraglottic cancers. Of these, 18 (42%) underwent TLM to the primary only. Of the 43 patients, 23 (53%) also had open surgery on their neck. Two (5%) received postoperative radiotherapy. Again, trying to apply our clinical definitions to Steiner's supraglottic cases, we judged none to be "very early," 10 to be "early," and 33 to be "intermediate." Only 4 (9.5%) developed a local recurrence (or second primary) within 5 years, and 3 of these were salvaged by functional operations (1 open supraglottic laryngectomy and 2 transoral laser re-resections). No one lost their larynx. Five (12%) died from their supraglottic cancer—1 who refused treatment of a local recurrence, 1 who was never controlled in the neck, and 3 with distant metastases. In addition, 5 (11.3%) developed second primaries, 2 (5%) ultimately fatal. Six supraglottic patients (14%) died of intercurrent disease, while in 1 patient the cause of death was unknown. As in the glottic cancer patients, intercurrent disease placed ahead of laryngeal cancer as a cause of death. The 5-year Kaplan-Meier overall survival was 73%.

Of the 43 patients undergoing laser supraglottic resection, 36 (84%) required a feeding tube. One received a tracheotomy at the time of the laser surgery, and 1 needed a tracheotomy postoperatively. Two patients with dyspnea (5%) required assistance, including one of the temporary tracheotomies. The other was managed by lasering. Two with aspiration required treatment, 1 by tracheotomy to allow a cuffed tube, the other by conservative means. Two patients (5%) had bleeding, and 1 of these had to be returned to surgery for cautery under general anesthesia.

TLM was used for glottic cancer staged T_{2b} and above in 147 patients in Steiner's report. There were 93 pT_{2b} glottic cancers, 40 pT_3, and 14 pT_4. Using our clinical classification, this was about 93 early or intermediate and 54 intermediate or advanced. Ninety (61%) were TNM stage 2, 38 (26%) stage 3, and 19 (13%) stage 4. Ninety-five (65%) of the 147 glottic patients received laser treatment of the primary (only). Thirty-two (22%) were treated with TLM at the primary site plus open surgery in the neck. Four more (3%) underwent TLM and radiotherapy. Eight (5%) had laser micro resection, neck surgery, and postoperative radiotherapy. All in all, 40 patients (27% of the "T_{2b} and above" glottic cancer patients) underwent neck dissections, mainly selective dissections of levels 2 and 3. Twenty patients (14%) received radiotherapy after surgery.

Amongst the 147 patients treated by TLM for early/intermediate/advanced glottic cancer, there were 45 local recurrences (including possible second primaries). The 5-year Kaplan-Meier survival overall was 59%. During 40 months, the recurrence rates broken out by clinical stage ran as follows: 28 of the 93 patients with early and intermediate glottic cancer and 17 of the 54 intermediate to advanced. Seven patients developed neck metastases in addition to their recurrence at the primary site. One grew nodal disease without a primary recurrence. Three (2%) patients acquired distant metastases.

In the entire 147 patients undergoing TLM for T_{1b} early or T_2 intermediate or T_3 advanced glottic cancer, 45 developed local recurrences. In 21, this lead to a total laryngectomy, 8 of whom also received postoperative radiotherapy. Four patients received open vertical partial laryngectomies. Ten were salvaged by TLM, and 6 more were salvaged by TLM and radiotherapy. Four of the patients who developed local recurrences received palliative care only. Thirteen of the 93 early/intermediate cases and 12 of the 54 patients with intermediate/advanced cancer died from their glottic disease. Thus 25 (17%) of the 147 patients with larger tumors died. Only 11 of the 25 died of local/locoregional recurrence. One died from regional recurrence alone, and 13 died from distant metastases. The number of second primaries was 14 (9.5%), with only 1 in the head and neck. Ten patients (7%) died of a second primary and 29 (20%) died of intercurrent disease. Once again, intercurrent disease beat glottic cancer treated by TLM as the cause of death in these patients.

Steiner's report to EUFOS included 56 patients with higher TNM stage supraglottic cancer. One had pT_1 local disease, 7 had pT_2, 29 had pT_3, and 19 had pT_4. Therefore, 48 of 56 patients had pT_3 or pT_4 supraglottic cancer. Eight (14%) underwent only TLM. One (2%) had TLM and radiotherapy. Of the 56 supraglottic TLM patients, 47 (84%) also received neck surgery, mainly of selective dissection of levels II and III. Twenty six (46%) had neck surgery only; 21 (37.5%) had postoperative radiotherapy as well. In the whole group of 56 patients with higher stage supraglottic cancer, 22 (39%) had radiotherapy after surgery. Of the 56, 11 (19.5%) developed local recurrences (or second primaries). Eleven patients developed neck metastases, 5 with their primary controlled, 6 with recurrence at the primary site (locoregional recurrence). Of these, 3 also developed distant metastases.

No local recurrence was salvaged with an open partial laryngectomy. Three were salvaged with radiotherapy and 6 patients required a total laryngectomy, 2 also receiving postoperative radiotherapy. Two patients with recurrence received palliative treatment only. The overall 5-year Kaplan-Meier survival for these patients with higher stage supraglottic cancer (where the primary was treated by TLM) was 50%.

In Steiner's 1996 series, 48 patients had pT_3 or pT_4 supraglottic cancers. Complications in this group included 3 patients with early stenosis. One was lasered. Two required a permanent tracheostomy. Five patients suffered significant aspiration, leading to total laryngectomy in 3. One responded to a temporary cuffed tracheotomy, and 1 accepted a gastrostomy tube. Four patients experienced bleeding that required endoscopic coagulation under general anesthesia.

In the pT_3/pT_4 supraglottic cancer group, 11 recurrences (or second primaries) (23%) appeared. Six patients with recurrence (12.5%) were laryngectomized (2 with postoperative radiotherapy). Nine second primaries (16%) arose, 4 in the head and neck. Of these patients, 7 (12.5%) died from their second primary. Six patients (11%) died of intercurrent disease. Of the patients, 13 (23%) died from supraglottic cancer; 4 from local/locoregional recurrence, 5 of regional recurrence, 4 from distant metastasis, and 1 of causes unknown. Notice that, if TLM failed locally in pT_3 or pT_4 supraglottic cancer, half the patients required a laryngectomy (6 of 11 or 55%). And again, intercurrent disease and second primary cancers combined to cause death as often as locally advanced supraglottic cancer treated primarily with TLM.

For interested readers, Steiner also reported his TLM results for pyriform cancer to EUFOS.[73] Of 103 previously untreated patients with hypopharyngeal cancer, mainly pyriform, 63 patients had pT_2 cancers and 14 had pT_3. Sixty percent had proven neck disease. Steiner excluded patients with simultaneous second primaries, very advanced neck disease (N3), or distant metastases (i.e., not treatable for cure). All patients underwent TLM, but 75% also had neck surgery and 50% had postoperative radiotherapy. Of these 103 patients, 93 were controlled locally—there were only 10 local recurrences during a 44-month mean follow-up period. The 5-year Kaplan-Meier survivals mirrored supraglottic cancer (69.2 % for combined stage I and II, 52.5 % for stage III and IV), validating Krishaber's classic differentiation of "intrinsic" vs "extrinsic" disease. More laser surgery, open surgery, and radiotherapy were used to address failure. Eighteen patients (17%) died from pyriform cancer. Nearly as common (as causes of death) were intercurrent disease (16, or 15%) and second primaries (13 deaths amongst 16 second primaries or 13% of the total group).

CONCLUSIONS

TLM is not cancer surgery through a keyhole. In fact, it has oncologic advantages. The diagnostic component supports accurate verification of the tumor extent. The patient receives not the largest resection, but the most logical resection. The strategy of "follow the tumor" reduces the risk of undertreatment. Tissues adjacent to the resection site do not require dissection, which ensures preservation of the local microcirculation—the optimum precondition for adjuvant radiotherapy. And TLM leaves behind an open resection site—no chance to bury residual cancer cells, and all the better in follow-up.

TLM offers meaningful functional advantages—fewer tracheotomies, no fistulae, less disfigurement, less pain (nurse's observations), earlier swallowing, and a lower risk of over treatment. It also carries certain socioeconomic advantages—reduced treatment costs from the shorter length of stay and the low rate of retreatment (for local control). TLM is a repeatable treatment (radiotherapy is not). And TLM anticipates the real problem of second primaries. After TLM, all treatment options remain.

Some things have changed with the introduction of TLM and others have not. Time spent in the operating room for example—it takes us just as long to perform a transoral resection as an open one. More time is spent on the resection and the frozen sections. Less time is spent on open approaches and closures. The indications for and performance of neck dissection remain the same. The only variation is the greater opportunity to stage the neck. The indications for adjunctive radiotherapy remain the same. And of course, so does the need for expert anesthesia, and skilled postoperative care.

In the United States, opinions once held that TLM should never be done, because it contravened oncologic principles—transected cancer, burned specimen margins, and replaced brilliant reconstructive techniques with healing by secondary intention. Now TLM is receiving more and more attention. Block excision can be seen as just a tactic to spill no viable cancer in the wound, and TLM as a strategy that supports this goal, but with a different tactic. It turns out that pathologists can read laser micro resection specimens well. There are more specimens to study, and the surface coagulation is only several cells deep—less than what electrocoagulation will sometimes produce in an open surgery specimen. Secondary intention healing is no longer seen as a disadvantage, as TLM selects patients for whom secondary intention healing provides excellent results.

Of course, not all change is progress. Predictions that laser surgery would (or should) produce miracles, because laser technology was new, easier, faster, and bloodless, were clearly exaggerations. TLM is a demanding endoscopic intervention and a complex resection, with no savings in time and its own special set of challenges. Bleeding does occur. It can stop the laser in its tracks. Cautery and hemo clips remain entirely necessary. Laser surgery does require us to invest in new equipment and accept new safety regulations. Laboratory evidence of oncologic efficacy still lags, but it may be a bit late for animal evidence, given the excellent cure rates reported in actual human application.[60,71,74] Detailed documentation of quality-of-life outcomes is starting to come. The TNM system retains its due respect as a reporting system, but we feel we have better concepts to guide initial treatment selection. Some will claim long-term multiinstitutional cooperative trials have supported other modalities in the United States[15,86] and not TLM. But chemoradiation is for very advanced cancers by protocol, properly not the patients transoral laser surgery generally treats. TLM does not rule out chemotherapy or radiation whenever they can add to the outcome. Radiotherapy cannot be used until a direct laryngoscopy and biopsy have been done, and this is usually a perfect opportunity for laser micro resection.

Cartilage involvement and subglottic extension were once thought to constitute contraindications to TLM, but this turns out not to be so. Margins are not unobtainable just because the thyroid cartilage is involved. Laser micro resection of the arytenoid was predicted to cause inevitable intolerable aspiration, but again, this proves to be a strong overstatement. Subglottic resection is challenging but now special techniques and special endoscopes[87,90] are available to overcome the limits on exposure.

TLM is eminently suited to the treatment of laryngeal cancer because squamous carcinoma starts in the epithelium and the epithelium is accessible through the mouth. The tumor needs to be accessible to endoscopy, but it does not need to be completely exposed in a single field of view. The cancer will need to be completely resected, with negative margins, but it will not need to be removed in one single piece. The resection site will need to have the time and conditions to heal by secondary intention, and the support to resist stenosis—but it will not require primary closure. T stage *in and of itself* does not rule out TLM as worthy of consideration. In a series of laryngeal cancers involving the anterior commissure,[46] transoral laser excision was valid in selected carcinomas staged pT_2b, and a small number of pT_3 and pT_4 anterior commissure cancers were also treated successfully.

In patients with very early laryngeal cancer, suspension micro laryngoscopies and laser excisional biopsies might best be considered "beginners TLM." When possible, it avoids 6 weeks of radiotherapy.

In early glottic cancer, TLM virtually replaces conventional VPL and hemilaryngectomy in our practice. We have experienced the same for early supraglottic cancer. TLM basically puts conventional HSL out of business. (The minimum prerequisite is at least one mobile arytenoid cartilage.)

TLM challenges supracricoid laryngectomy, and it replaces partial laryngeo-pharyngectomy (Ogura's "PLP"[42]). Laryngeal cancer extension outside the framework contraindicates TLM but in cases of doubt, this decision can be made during treatment, because endoscopic surgery can always be converted to open surgery. The need for reconstruction is considered a relative contraindication to TLM. But the vertical closures familiar in HSL and SCPL have not proven necessary in patients treated by TLM.

TLM probably has a role to play in some (few) advanced laryngeal cancers, but the arytenoid complex must be preserved bilaterally to resist aspiration. It otherwise has only a subsidiary role—to prepare for open NTL—by "pre-release"edge selection, and the clarification of where the laryngeal lumen can be entered with safety.

TLM has no role in very advanced laryngeal cancer, except possible palliative relief of airway obstruction until definitive open laryngectomy.

Transoral laser microsurgery is clearly one of the important treatment options for squamous cell cancer of the larynx. Advantage is taken of the operating microscope, laser micromanipulators, and advanced laryngoscopic instrumentation to provide the most logical tumor resection, the least loss of normal tissue, and the best opportunity to follow tumor extension beyond what was visible in the office and to the scanners. With fewer tracheotomies, shorter hospitalizations, and no limitation on additional treatment, laser resection seems to combine the promise of the "light scalpel" with endoscopic advances and the realities of laryngeal cancer. For many patients, transoral laser micro resection can provide the optimum combination of cure and quality of life.

APPENDIX ON THE CLINICAL CLASSIFICATION USED IN THIS CHAPTER

"Early" and "advanced" were ancient designations intended to differentiate whether the cord was fixed. Fixation meant advanced, which meant total laryngectomy. Early glottic cancer had two operations: resection via direct laryngoscopy or laryngofissure and cordectomy. Early meant a low volume of cancer and a reasonable prospect of cure by radiotherapy. Advanced meant radiation usually failed, and surgery would usually be required. But sometimes radiotherapy worked and avoided a total laryngectomy.

Some early cancers were so favorable they could be cured by a biopsy. This could falsely inflate treatment results—irradiation after an excisional biopsy would invariably produce a "cure." Therefore this subgroup was given its own category, namely "very early."

Conservation surgeons recognized that some cases with a fixed cord could have less than a total laryngectomy. These types of cancers kept the name advanced, but those cancers that everyone agreed had

no chance with anything less than a total laryngetomy came to be called "very advanced."

A clinical classification of local laryngeal cancer thus evolved. There were four categories, very early, early, advanced, and very advanced. Early could be handled by classical conservation operations like the vertical and horizontal partials. Advanced was defined as lateralized cancer pervading one paraglottic space and sparing enough mobile innervated glottic tissue on the contralateral side to make a voicing shunt. The cord was fixed but advanced could be controlled by a near-total laryngectomy.

Naturally, some laryngeal cancers fell in between a supraglottic laryngectomy and a near-total laryngectomy. We called them "intermediate" (between early and advanced). As it happens, these cancers fit the supracricoid partial laryngectomy block quite nicely.

REFERENCES

1. Alonso J: Conservative surgery of cancer of the larynx, *Trans Am Acad Ophthalmol Otolaryngol* 51:633–642, 1947.
2. Ambrosch P, Brinck U, Fischer G and others: Spezielle Aspekte der histopathologischen Diagnostik bei der Lasermikrochirurgie von Karzinomen des oberen Aerodigestivtraktes [Special aspects of histopathologic diagnosis in laser microsurgery of cancers of the upper aerodigestive tract], *Laryngorhinootologie* 73:78–83, 1994.
3. Ambrosch P, Kron M, Steiner W: Carbon dioxide laser microsurgery for early supraglottic carcinoma, *Ann Otol Rhinol Laryngol* 107:680–688, 1998.
4. American Joint Committee on Cancer: *AJCC cancer staging handbook.* In Greene FL, Page DL, Fleming ID and others, editors: *AJCC cancer staging manual,* ed 6, New York, 2002, Springer-Verlag, p 469.
5. Biller H, Ogura J, Pratt L: Hemilaryngectomy for T2 glottic cancers, *Arch Otolaryngol* 93:238–243, 1971.
6. Bocca E: *Supraglottic laryngectomy and functional neck dissection.* London, Royal Society of Medicine, Section of Laryngology, 1966.
7. Bradley PJ: Treatment of the patient with upper airway obstruction caused by cancer of the larynx, *Otolaryngol Head Neck Surg* 120:737–741, 1999.
8. Brandenburg J: Laser cordotomy vs. radiation therapy: an objective cost analysis, *Ann Otol Rhinol Laryngol* 110: 312–318, 2001.
9. Bron L, Brossard E, Monnier P and others: Supracricoid partial laryngectomy with cricohyoidoepiglottopexy and cricohyoidopexy for glottic and supraglottic carcinomas, *Laryngoscope* 110:627–634, 2000.
10. Chevalier D, Piquet JJ: Subtotal laryngectomy with cricohyoidopexy for supraglottic carcinoma: review of 61 cases, *Am J Surg* 168:472–473, 1994.
11. Davidson T, Haghighi P, Astarita R and others: Microscopically oriented histologic surgery for head and neck mucosal cancer, *Cancer* 60:1856–1861, 1987.
12. Davis RK, Shapshay SM, Strong MS and others: Transoral partial supraglottic resection using the CO_2 laser, *Laryngoscope* 93:429–432, 1983.
13. Dayal V, Bahri H, Stone P: The preepiglottic space. An anatomic study, *Arch Otolaryngol* 95:130, 1972.
14. de Vincentiis M, Minni A, Gallo A: Supracricoid laryngectomy with cricohyoidopexy (CHP) in the treatment of laryngeal

cancer: a functional and oncologic experience, *Laryngoscope* 106:1108–1114, 1996.

15. Forastiere AA, Goepfert H, Maor M and others: Concurrent chemotherapy and radiotherapy for organ preservation in advanced laryngeal cancer, *New Engl J Med* 349:2091–2098, 2003.

16. Gale N, Kambic V, Michaels L and others: The Ljubljana classification: a practical strategy for the diagnosis of laryngeal precancerous lesions, *Adv Anat Pathol* 7:240–251, 2000.

17. Gilbert RW, Lundgren JA, van Nostrand AW and others: T3N0M0 glottic carcinoma—a pathologic analysis of 41 patients treated surgically following radiotherapy, *Clin Otolaryngol* 3:467–479, 1988.

18. Hilgers F, Schouwenburg P: A new low-resistance, self-retaining prosthesis (Provox) for voice rehabilitation after total laryngectomy, *Laryngoscope* 100: 1202–1207, 1990.

19. Iro H, Waldfahrer F, Altendorf-Hofmann A and others: Transoral laser surgery of supraglottic cancer: follow-up of 141 patients, *Arch Otolaryngol Head Neck Surg* 124:1245–1250, 1998.

20. Jako GJ, Vaughan CW, Strong MS and others: Surgical management of malignant tumors of the aerodigestive tract with carbon dioxide laser microsurgery, *Int Adv Surg Oncol* 1:265–284, 1978.

21. Jepsen MC, Gurushanthaiah D, Roy N and others: Voice, speech, and swallowing outcomes in laser-treated laryngeal cancer, *Laryngoscope* 113:923–928, 2003.

22. Kambic V, Radsel Z, Smid L: Laryngeal reconstruction with epiglottis after vertical hemilaryngectomy, *J Laryngol Otol* 90:467–473, 1976.

23. Killian G: *Suspension laryngoscopy.* In Jackson C, editor: *Peroral endoscopy and laryngeal surgery,* St Louis, 1915, Laryngoscope Co, pp 133–154.

24. Kirchner J: One hundred laryngeal cancers studied by serial section, *Ann Otol Rhinol Laryngol* 78:678–709, 1969.

25. Krishaber M: Contribution a l'etude du cancer du larynx, *Gaz Bebd Med Chir* 16:518, 1879.

26. Labayle J, Bismuth R: La laryngectomie totale avec reconstitution, *Ann Otolaryngol Chir Cervicofac* 88:219–228, 1971.

27. Laccourreye H, Laccourreye O, Weinstein G and others: Supracricoid laryngectomy with cricohyoidoepiglottopexy: a partial laryngeal procedure for glottic carcinoma, *Ann Otol Rhinol Laryngol* 99:421–426, 1990.

28. Laccourreye H, Laccourreye O, Weinstein G and others: Supracricoid laryngectomy with cricohyoidopexy: a partial laryngeal procedure for selected supraglottic and transglottic carcinomas, *Laryngoscope* 100:735–741, 1990.

29. Laccourreye O, Brasnu D, Merite-Drancy A and others: Cricohyoidopexy in selected infrahyoid epiglottic carcinomas presenting with pathological preepiglottic space invasion, *Arch Otolaryngol Head Neck Surg* 119:881–886, 1993.

30. Laccourreye O, Brasnu D, Laccourreye L, and others: Ruptured pexis after supracricoid partial laryngectomy, *Ann Otol Rhinol Laryngol* 106:159–162, 1997.

31. Lillie J, DeSanto L: Transoral surgery of early cordal carcinoma, *Trans Am Acad Ophthalmol Otolaryngol* 77:ORL92–96, 1973.

32. Lima RA, Freitas EQ, Kligerman J and others: Near-total laryngectomy for treatment of advanced laryngeal cancer, *Am J Surg* 174:490–491, 1997.

33. Lynch R: Intrinsic carcinoma of the larynx, with a second report of cases operated on by suspension and dissection, *Trans Am Laryngol Assoc* 42:119–124, 1920.

34. Maurice N, Crampette L, Mondain M and others: Subtotal laryngectomy with cricohyoidopexy. Carcinologic results and early functional follow-up. Apropos of 49 cases, *Ann Otolaryngol Chir Cervicofac* 111:435, 1994.

35. Mohr RM, Quenelle DJ, Shumrick DA: Vertico-frontolateral laryngectomy (hemilaryngectomy). Indications, technique, and results, *Arch Otolaryngol* 109:384–395, 1983.

36. Mohs F: Chemosurgery. A microscopically controlled method of cancer excision, *Arch Surg* 42:279–295, 1941.

37. Motta G, Villari G, Motta G Jr., and others: The CO_2 laser in laryngeal microsurgery, *Acta Otolaryngol Suppl* 433:1–30, 1986.

38. Naudo P, Laccourreye O, Weinstein G and others: Complications and functional outcome after supracricoid partial laryngectomy with cricohyoidoepiglottopexy, *Otolaryngol Head Neck Surg* 118:124–129, 1998.

39. New GB, Dorton HE: Suspension laryngoscopy in the treatment of malignant disease of the hypopharynx and larynx, *Mayo Clin Proc* 16:411–416, 1941.

40. Norris C: Technique of extended fronto-lateral partial laryngectomy, *Laryngoscope* 68:1240–1250, 1958.

41. Ogura J and H Dedo: Glottic reconstruction following subtotal glotticsupraglottic laryngectomy, Laryngoscope 75: 865–878, 1965.

42. Ogura JH, Jurema AA, Watson RK: Partial laryngopharyngectomy and neck dissection for pyriform sinus cancer, *Laryngoscope* 70:1399–1417, 1960.

43. Olofsson J, Van Nostrand A: Growth and spread of laryngeal and hypopharyngeal carcinoma with reflections on the effect of preoperative irradiation, *Acta Otolaryngol Suppl* 308:1–84, 1973.

44. Olsen KD, DeSanto LW, Pearson BW: Positive Delphian lymph node: clinical significance in laryngeal cancer, *Laryngoscope* 97:1033–1037, 1987.

45. Ossoff RH, Sisson GA, Shapshay SM: Endoscopic management of selected early vocal cord carcinoma, *Ann Otol Rhinol Laryngol* 94:560–564, 1985.

46. Pearson BW, Salassa J: Transoral laser microresection for cancer of the larynx involving the anterior commissure, *Laryngoscope* 113:1104–1112, 2003.

47. Pearson BW, DeSanto L: Near-total laryngectomy, *Oper Tech Otolaryngol Head Neck Surg* 1:28–41, 1990.

48. Pearson BW, DeSanto LW, Olsen KD and others: The results of near-total laryngectomy, *Ann Otol Rhinol Laryngol* 107:820–825, 1998.

49. Pearson BW: Subtotal laryngectomy, *Laryngoscope* 91: 1904–1912, 1981.

50. Pearson BW: Laryngeal microcirculation and pathways of cancer spread, *Laryngoscope* 85:700–713, 1975.

51. Pearson BW, Woods II RD, Hartman DE: Extended hemilaryngectomy for T_3 glottic carcinoma with preservation of speech and swallowing, *Laryngoscope* 90:1950–1961, 1980.

52. Piquet JJ, Desauty A, offmann Y and others: La chirurgie sub-totale et reconstructive dans le traitement des cancers de larynx, *Ann Otolaryngol Chir Cervicofac* 91:311–320, 1974.

53. Rademaker AW, Logemann JA, Pauloski BR and others: Recovery of postoperative swallowing in patients undergoing partial laryngectomy, *Head Neck Surg* 15:325–334, 1993.

54. Remacle M, Eckel HE, Antonelli A and others: Endoscopic cordectomy. A proposal for a classification by the Working Committee, European Laryngological Society, *Eur Arch Oto-Rhino-Laryngol* 257:227–231, 2000.

55. Rosier JF, Gregoire V, Counoy H and others: Comparison of external radiotherapy, laser microsurgery and partial laryngectomy for the treatment of $T_1N_0M_0$ glottic carcinomas: a retrospective evaluation, *Radiother Oncol* 48:175–183, 1998.

56. Rucci L, Gammarota L, Borghi Cirri MB: Carcinoma of the anterior commissure of the larynx: I. Embryological and anatomic considerations, *Ann Otol Rhinol Laryngol* 105:303–308, 1996.

57. Rudert HH, Werner JA: Endoscopic resections of glottic and supraglottic carcinomas with the CO_2 laser, *Eur Arch Oto-Rhino-Laryngol* 252:146–148, 1995.

58. Rudert HH: CO_2 laser treatment of carcinoma of the larynx, *Laryngol Rhinol Otol* 67:261–268, 1988.

59. Rudert HH: *Laser surgery for carcinomas of the larynx and hypopharynx*. In Panje, WR, Herberhold C, editors: *Neck,* New York, 1998, Thieme Medical Publishers, pp 355–370.

60. Rudert HH, Werner JA, Hoft S: Transoral carbon dioxide laser resection of supraglottic carcinoma, *Ann Otol Rhinol Laryngol* 108:819–827, 1999.

61. Rudert HH: *Transoral CO_2-laser surgery in advanced supraglottic cancer*. In Smee R, Bridger GP, eds: *Laryngeal cancer*, Amsterdam, 1994, Elsevier Science B.V., pp 457–461.

62. Schechter G: Epiglottic reconstruction and subtotal laryngectomy, *Laryngoscope* 93:723–734, 1983.

63. Shapshay SM: *Newer methods of cancer treatment: laser therapy for the cancer patient*. In DeVita VT Jr., Hellman S, Rosenberg SA, editors: *Cancer principles and practice of oncology,* ed 2, Philadelphia, 1985, Lippincott.

64. Singer MI, Hamaker RC, Blom ED and others Applications of the voice prosthesis during laryngectomy, *Ann Otol Rhinol Laryngol* 98:921–925, 1989.

65. Sittel C, Friedrich G, Zorowka P and others: Surgical voice rehabilitation after laser surgery for glottic carcinoma, *Ann Otol Rhinol Laryngol* 111:493–499, 2002.

66. Som M, Silver C: The anterior commissure technique of partial laryngectomy, *Arch Otolaryngol* 87:42, 1968.

67. Som M: Hemilaryngectomy: a modified technique for cordal carcinoma with extension posteriorly, *Arch Otolaryngol* 54:524–533, 1951.

68. Spayne JA, Warde P, O'Sullivan B and others: Carcinoma-in situ of the glottic larynx: results of treatment with radiation therapy, *Int J Radiat Oncol Biol Phys* 49:1235–1238, 2001.

69. Steiner W, Ambrosch P: *Endoscopic laser surgery of the upper aerodigestive tract,* New York, 2000, Georg Thieme Verlag, p 147.

70. Steiner W, Ambrosch P: Laser Microsurgery for cancer of the larynx. Minimally invasive therapy and allied technology 5:159–164, 1996.

71. Steiner W, Ambrosch P: *Laser Microsurgery for laryngeal carcinoma*. In Steiner W, Ambrosch P, editors: *Endoscopic laser surgery of the upper aerodigestive tract*, New York, 2000, Georg Thieme Verlag, p 47–82.

72. Steiner W: *Endoscopic therapy of early laryngeal cancer. Indications and results*. In Wigand ME, Steiner W, Stell PM, eds: *Functional partial laryngectomy*, New York, 1984, Springer-Verlag, pp 163–170.

73. Steiner W, Ambrosch P, Uhlig P and others: CO_2 laser microsurgery for hypopharyngeal carcinoma. In 3rd European Congress of the European Federation of Oto-Rhino-Laryngological Societies "EUFOS," 1996, Budapest (Hungary): Monduzzi Editore S.p.A. Bologna.

74. Steiner W, Ambrosch P, Martin A and others: *Results of transoral laser microsurgery of laryngeal cancer. In 3rd European Congress of the European Federation of Oto-Rhino-Laryngological Societies "EUFOS,"* Budapest, 1996, Bologna Monduzzi Editore S.p.A.

75. Steiner W: Experience in endoscopic laser surgery of malignant tumours of the upper aero-digestive tract, *Adv Otorhinolaryngol* 39:135–144, 1988.

76. Steiner W: Results of curative laser microsurgery of laryngeal carcinomas, *Am J Otolaryngol* 14:116–121, 1993.

77. Steiner W: *Transoral microsurgical CO_2-laser resection of laryngeal carcinoma*. In Wigand ME, Steiner W, Stell PM, eds: *Functional partial laryngectomy*, New York, 1984, Springer-Verlag, pp 121–125.

78. Strong MS, Jako GJ, Polanyi T and others: Laser surgery in the aerodigestive tract, *Am J Surg* 126:529–533, 1973.

79. Strong MS: Laser excision of carcinoma of the larynx, *Laryngoscope* 85:1286–1289, 1975.

80. Sylva N, Lore J: Partial horizontal supraglottic laryngectomy: a method of reconstruction, *Laryngoscope* 87:1164–1168, 1977.

81. Tucker G: Some clinical inferences from the study of serial laryngeal sections, *Laryngoscope* 73:728–748, 1963.

82. van Nostrand A, Brodaree I: Laryngeal carcinoma—modifications in surgical technique based on our understanding of tumor growth characteristics, *J Otolaryngol* 11:186–190, 1982.

83. Vaughan C, Strong M, Jako G: Laryngeal carcinoma: transoral treatment utilizing the CO_2 laser, *Am J Surg* 136:490–493, 1978.

84. Vilaseca-Gonzalez I, Bernal-Sprekelsen M, Blanch-Alejandro JL and others: Complications in transoral CO_2 laser surgery for carcinoma of the larynx and hypopharynx, *Head Neck* 25:382–388, 2003.

85. Werner JA, Lippert BM, Schunke M and others: Tierexperimentelle Untersuchungen zur Laserwirkung auf Lymphgefasse. Ein Beitrag zur Diskussion um die laserchirurgische Resektion von Karzinomen in mehreren Teilen. [Animal experiment studies of laser effects on lymphatic vessels. A contribution to the discussion of laser surgery segmental resection of carcinomas], *Laryngo Rhino Otologie* 74:748–755, 1995.

86. Wolf G, Urba S, Hazuka M: Induction chemotherapy for organ preservation in advanced squamous cell carcinoma of the oral cavity and oropharynx, *Recent Results Cancer Res* 134:133–143, 1994.

87. Zeitels S, Vaughan C: "External counterpressure" and "internal distention" for optimal laryngoscopic exposure of the anterior glottal commissure, *Ann Otol Rhinol Laryngol* 103:669–675, 1994.

88. Zeitels S, Vaughan C: Preepiglottic space invasion in "early" epiglottic cancer, *Ann Otol Rhinol Laryngol* 100:789–792, 1991.

89. Zeitels SM, Hillman RE, Franco RA and others: Voice and treatment outcome from phonosurgical management of early glottic cancer, *Ann Otol Rhinol Laryngol* 190:3–20, 2002.

90. Zeitels S: Universal modular glottiscope system: the evolution of a century of design and technique for direct laryngoscopy, *Ann Otol Rhinol Laryngol Suppl* 179:2–24, 1999.

91. Zeitels SM, Vaughan CW, Domanowski GF: Endoscopic management of early supraglottic cancer, *Ann Otol Rhinol Laryngol* 99:951–956, 1990.

CONSERVATION LARYNGEAL SURGERY

Ralph P. Tufano
Gregory S. Weinstein
Ollivier Laccourreye

INTRODUCTION

There are a variety of open surgical approaches available that, when applied for the appropriate indications, have an excellent ability to control laryngeal cancer while conserving laryngeal function. Conservation laryngeal procedures are historically the original "organ preservation" techniques; the first hemilaryngectomy for malignancy was performed by Billroth in 1874.[159] Long before nonsurgical approaches were available to attempt to preserve the entire structure of the larynx, innovative surgical techniques were being used to remove enough of the larynx to allow for local control of the malignancy while preserving adequate structure to allow the larynx to function.[154] There exists a spectrum of laryngeal malignancies for which there is a complementary spectrum of conservation laryngeal procedures available. This chapter will review the open conservation laryngeal procedures in the organ preservation surgical paradigm available for managing the spectrum of selected glottic, transglottic, and supraglottic carcinomas. These techniques allow for the maintenance of physiologic speech and swallowing without the need for a permanent tracheostoma. The modern head and neck surgeon must have a comprehensive understanding of both surgical and nonsurgical organ preservation strategies to allow for the most comprehensive care in the treatment of the patient with laryngeal cancer.

Although the origins of conservation surgery of the larynx are more than a century old, during the second half of the last century, the conservative options were limited to vertical hemilaryngectomy and supraglottic laryngectomy. The inherent limitations of these procedures in terms of indications led to these procedures losing favor among many physicians with experimental approaches, with chemotherapy and radiation dominating the management of advanced laryngeal cancer. Then, in the last decade of the 20th century in the United States, the introduction of supracricoid partial laryngectomies as well as the introduction of endoscopic laser resections created a renaissance in surgical organ preservation for laryngeal cancer. At present, this surgical renaissance in organ preservation surgery for laryngeal cancer has evolved into the standard of care for the 21st century.

The common thread in the history of conservation laryngeal surgery is that these procedures were first developed outside the United States and then imported to its shores. Improvements in antibiotics and anesthetic techniques fostered the development of conservation laryngeal surgery.[109] Vertical hemilaryngectomy, which was first described by Billroth[159] in Germany and popularized in Europe by Leroux-Robert and Portmann,[127] was refined in the United States by Som,[147] Norris,[117] and Conley.[32] A French surgeon named Huet described a procedure in which a portion of the supraglottis was excised without the upper portion of the thyroid cartilage in 1938.[53] Later, a Uruguayan surgeon named Alonso extended this procedure to resect the upper portion of the thyroid cartilage together with the supraglottic structures, thereby defining the supraglottic laryngectomy.[2,3] The supraglottic laryngectomy was popularized in Europe by Bocca[17] and in the United States by Ogura,[118] Som,[147] and Kirchner.[69] The supracricoid laryngectomies originally were described in 1959 by the Austrian surgeons Majer and Reider[98] approximately one decade after Alonso had described the supraglottic laryngectomy.[2] The supracricoid laryngectomies were later promoted in Europe by Labayle[72] and Piquet[129] and were imported to numerous institutions in the United States during the 1990s.[82]

The first of two major classes of techniques that developed was the *vertical partial laryngectomy*, in which entry into the endolarynx is through a vertical thyrotomy, the most notable example of which is the vertical hemilaryngectomy. The second major class of techniques is the *horizontal partial laryngectomy,* in which endolaryngeal entry is made through a transverse or horizontal thyrotomy (i.e., supraglottic partial laryngectomy). During the 1960s through the 1980s, innovative surgeons* reported numerous small series of patients in which the indications and extent of resection of these basic techniques were extended in an attempt to manage larger lesions. The commonalities among these series were: (1) the relatively small numbers of patients; (2) variable local control rates compared with the strict previous indications for the procedure that was being extended; and (3) complex reconstructions requiring cartilage and mucosa rotation flaps with variable functional results.† These variable results made it difficult for other surgeons to use these extended procedures in the treatment of larynx cancer. Despite these innovations of the pioneers of conservation laryngeal surgery, the techniques that most surgeons became facile with, as reflected by the large numbers of series in the literature, were the standard vertical hemilaryngectomy and standard supraglottic laryngectomy. A common surgical solution in the United States for lesions considered too large for these standard conservation laryngeal procedures was total laryngectomy, with the innovations being in the area of alaryngeal speech and speech shunt development.[125,143]

In many European countries, laryngectomy, with its concomitant permanent stoma, was considered an anathema to be avoided when possible, and a different approach evolved. In 1959 in Austria, Majer and Reider[98] reported on a new horizontal partial laryngectomy technique in which the entire thyroid cartilage, true cords, false cords, and all or a portion of the epiglottis and preepiglottic space were resected. The reconstruction was with a pexy either between the cricoid and hyoid (cricohyoidopexy) or between the cricoid and the remaining epiglottis and hyoid (cricohyoidoepiglottopexy). This procedure, known as the *supracricoid partial laryngectomy*, allowed for a complete resection of the preepiglottic and paraglottic spaces and of the surrounding cartilage and soft tissue, resulting in higher local control in glottic, supraglottic, and transglottic cancers that equaled total laryngectomy, resulting in speech and swallowing without a permanent tracheostomy. Unlike the plethora of extensions of the vertical partial laryngectomy and the supraglottic laryngectomy, the supracricoid laryngectomies were repeated in many patients by numerous European centers during the 1970s through the 1990s with consistently excellent local control and functional results.‡

CONSERVATION LARYNGEAL SURGERY TODAY

Although conservation surgery of the larynx had its origins in the 19th century, the standard of care in the 21st century dictates that when vertical partial laryngectomy, supraglottic laryngectomy, or supracricoid laryngectomy are alternatives for a given patient, these options should be discussed with the patient. In most cases, it is the general otolaryngologist–head and neck surgeon who makes the diagnosis of laryngeal cancer, and therefore these are frequently the physicians who first counsel the patients concerning their treatment options. Standard of care dictates that a discussion based on the literature be given to the patient concerning both surgical and nonsurgical approaches to organ preservation. A physician will sometimes argue that since "I don't do these procedures," he or she will send the patient to the radiation therapist—but this may not be in the best interest of the patient.

An analogy can be made with free tissue reconstruction surgery. If a patient has a large jaw carcinoma and the superior option from the oncologic and functional perspective is a free flap, we would not offer him or her a lesser surgical procedure or chemotherapy and radiation. The patient would be sent to a surgeon with a special expertise in free flap surgery. This is possible because, in the last 20 years, a cadre of head and neck subspecialists have cropped up that have a particular interest and expertise in performing free flap surgery. In fact, over the last decade we have witnessed a similar phenomenon in the United States in the area of organ preservation surgery for laryngeal cancer. A subspecialty niche has developed within the field of head and neck surgery in which the surgeon has a special expertise in open and endoscopic approaches for laryngeal organ preservation in the face of laryngeal cancer.

The focus of this chapter is to provide the general otolaryngologist–head and neck surgeon with an introduction to these techniques. This information is important because it is the responsibility of the general otolaryngologist–head and neck surgeon to understand the indications for the full spectrum of open and endoscopic organ preservation surgical approaches and either gain the expertise to perform these procedures or refer the patient to surgeons who have this subspecialty interest.[174]

During the 1970s and 1980s, the functional and oncologic results after supraglottic laryngectomy were reported in numerous series in the United States, defining the role of this technique among the plethora of surgical and nonsurgical options available for supraglottic carcinoma.[39,91,146] During the same period and into the 1990s, the role of vertical partial laryngectomy for glottic carcinoma has been reexamined

---

*References 13, 15, 26, 28, 44, 120.
†References 13, 15, 26, 28, 44, 110, 120, 140.
‡References 20, 46, 56, 73, 99, 100, 126, 129, 130, 133, 165.

because of advances in nonsurgical and laser endoscopic approaches to similarly staged disease.[57,109] In the 1990s, the supracricoid laryngectomies were imported to numerous institutions in the United States, and the European functional results have been reproduced.[82,168,172] The supracricoid laryngectomies have broadened the spectrum of reliable techniques available to the conservation laryngeal surgeon.[109]

At present, a renaissance is occurring in the United States in the area of conservation laryngeal surgery. Many factors have fostered the rekindled interest in conservation laryngeal surgery, including: (1) a clearer understanding of the three-dimensional extent of laryngeal carcinoma, which has stemmed from numerous clinicopathologic studies and from advances in radiologic techniques; (2) numerous long-term studies of outcome after the application of a broad spectrum of techniques; and (3) the introduction of new techniques during the past two decades. Today, there are a variety of techniques available for selected laryngeal malignancies, with predictable functional and oncologic outcome based on analyses in the literature of many patients. The full spectrum of surgical techniques allows the surgeon to consistently offer patients, with selected lesions, excellent local control that will result in speech and swallowing without the need for a permanent tracheostoma. This may provide the patient with an alternative to nonsurgical organ preservation modalities. There are organ preservation principles to which the surgeon must adhere to maximize both oncologic and functional outcome. Conservation laryngeal surgery is precision surgery,[34] and to achieve successful oncologic and functional results, the conservation laryngeal surgeon should have a firm grasp on the clinical assessment of laryngeal cancer and a complete understanding of the surgical techniques. The art of correctly staging the lesion as one appropriate for a conservation laryngeal procedure requires an in-depth knowledge of both the static and dynamic anatomy of the larynx and how the tumor relates to it.

ANATOMY, PHYSIOLOGY, AND TUMOR SPREAD

In 1966, Bocca elegantly stated that, "often cancer seems to have limits, while the surgeon seems to have none. We should make efforts to force upon our knife the same limits as those which surrounding tissues or structures force upon cancer and its spread."[17] Bocca's eloquent statement underscores that successful outcome in conservation laryngeal surgery is predicated on a thorough knowledge of the pertinent surgical anatomy and on an understanding of the behavior of the malignancy in a particular anatomic site. Much of what is known concerning the three-dimensional spread of malignancy through the larynx

has been derived from clinicopathologic studies in which the entire larynx was sectioned. These whole organ section studies are the basic science foundation for clinicians performing conservation laryngeal surgery.

The surgical anatomy of the larynx can be understood in terms of the skeleton and connective tissue barriers, the spaces delineated by these structures, and the soft-tissue structures, which include the fat, musculature, vessels, nerves, and adnexa that fill these spaces. The skeleton of the larynx (Figure 102-1) is dominated by the thyroid cartilage, which articulates posteriorly and inferiorly through the inferior cornua with synovial joints on the posterolateral aspects of the cricoid cartilage. A thick tendon originates from the superior cornua and attaches to the lateralmost aspect of the "crown" of the larynx, the hyoid bone. Anteriorly there is a notch, and the lateral aspect of the laminae is traversed by the oblique line, which is the point of attachment of the strap musculature. The extension of cancer into the thyroid cartilage tends to occur in areas of ossification of the cartilage.[47] The mode of invasion into the ossified bone has been attributed to osteoclast formation,[128] extension along collagen bundles,[178] or through areas of high vascularity.[122] The most common site of invasion of the thyroid cartilage was at the angle,[88] although other sites of predilection for carcinoma invasion are the points of attachment of the cricothyroid membrane and the anterior origin of the thyroarytenoid musculature.[178] The perichondrium provides an excellent barrier to invasion, and once the carcinoma is within the cartilage, the cancer can extend throughout the

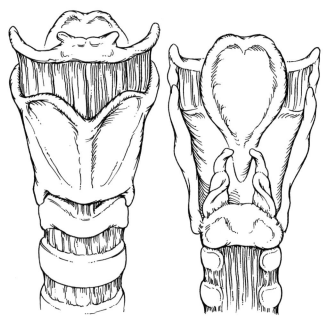

Figure 102-1. Skeletal structure of the larynx.

cartilage behind an intact perichondrium, precluding surgical cuts through the cartilage, as is done in some partial laryngectomies.[65] Nakayama and others[111] noted that a large proportion of patients staged clinically as T_3 actually had thyroid cartilage invasion when the specimens were analyzed by whole organ sectioning, and they noted that in these patients with T_3 glottic cancers, any combination of two factors including significant degree of calcification of the cartilage, tumor length >2 cm, and anterior commissure involvement resulted in a higher incidence of cartilage invasion (71%–92%).

The cricoid cartilage is the only circumferential ring in the airway, and preservation or reconstruction of its ring-shaped structure allows for decannulation after conservation laryngeal surgery. The arytenoid cartilages sit atop the cricoid, to which they are attached by a synovial joint. The two muscular processes of the arytenoid cartilages are oriented posteriorly and laterally, and the vocal cord tendon originates from the tip of the vocal process and spans anteriorly to the thyroid cartilage. The most common site of cricoid cartilage invasion by carcinoma is at its posterior superior border, and the most common site of arytenoid invasion is at the points of attachment of the joint capsule.[177]

The epiglottis, with its numerous fenestrations, originates from the tendinous attachment on the thyroid cartilage, fanning out from its most inferior point known as the *petiole* to a widened superior aspect above the hyoid. The carcinoma on the infrahyoid surface of the epiglottis readily extends through the fenestrations of the epiglottic cartilage through blood vessels[122] and the ducts of the seromucinous glands.[24] The hyoid bone is almost never involved by supraglottic carcinoma. Kirchner[62] noted no cases of hyoid bone invasion in 55 supraglottic carcinomas evaluated by whole organ section, although in Kirchner's series,[62] two patients had cancer up to the periosteum, one of which could be palpated at the level of the thyrohyoid membrane and one which had vallecula mucosa involvement. Among 172 patients with supraglottic carcinoma reported by Timon and others,[155] only four patients had hyoid bone invasion, and a common feature of all of these patients was vallecula mucosal involvement. Preservation of the hyoid bone helps with swallowing postoperatively. Understanding this concept is essential and makes it possible to perform supracricoid laryngectomy with cricohyoidopexy in selected transglottic tumors. These authors concluded that it is sound to preserve the hyoid bone in cases without palpable submucosal vallecula carcinoma or vallecula mucosal involvement.[62,155]

There are numerous condensations of fibrous tissue that traverse the three-dimensional anatomy of the larynx. Some of the modern knowledge of these structures comes from the pioneering work of Tucker and Kirchner, both of whom studied whole organ sections of larynges and analyzed this anatomy.[64,157,158] The conus elasticus (Figure 102-2) spans from each vocal cord down laterally to the cricoid cartilage. The conus elasticus provides a temporary barrier for the spread of early glottic carcinoma, but ultimately, for larger cancers, it serves as the gateway to the subglottic and extralaryngeal spread of carcinoma.[67] Posteriorly, it also is attached to the arytenoid, providing stability to the arytenoid and the vocal tendon. The vocal tendon, which essentially is a medial condensation of the conus elasticus, attaches anteriorly to the thyroid cartilage at the Broyles ligament or the anterior commissure tendon.[25] Although the anterior commissure tendon is devoid of perichondrium, the ligament constitutes a dense fibrous attachment to the cartilage and sends slips of fibrous tissue superiorly to the thyroepiglottic ligament. Kirchner and Carter[67] have noted that the anterior commissure tendon is a point of dense adhesion of fibrous tissue, and it is rare for an early glottic cancer with anterior commissure involvement to erode into the thyroid cartilage here. However, the anterior commissure tendon provides access to cartilage invasion for larger cancers, which spread superiorly or inferiorly.[67] Anteriorly, there is a superior inferior condensation of the conus elasticus called the *cricothyroid ligament*, which is a central structure and does not spread out laterally to provide a connective tissue barrier along the circumference of the cricoid.[88] This is different than its superior counterpart, the thyrohyoid membrane. The thyrohyoid membrane drapes along the entire circumference of the thyroid cartilage superiorly and spreads upward to the hyoid bone (Figure 102-3).

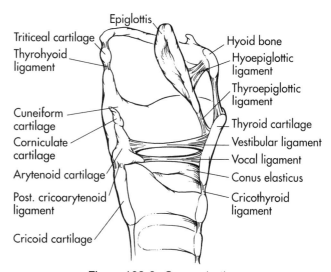

Figure 102-2. Conus elasticus.

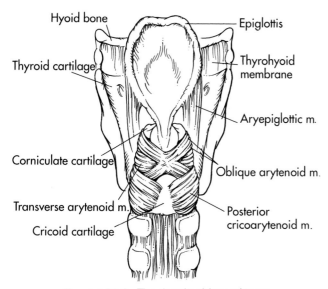

Figure 102-3. The thyrohyoid membrane.

Extension out of the larynx through the thyrohyoid membrane alone is rare and typically is seen when cancer exits the larynx through the upper portion of the thyroid cartilage.[88] The quadrangular membrane (Figure 102-4) originates from the top of the arytenoid posteriorly and from the lateral aspect of the epiglottis anteriorly and then extends inferiorly like a curtain to an inferior condensation of fibrous tissue, which spans between the inferior aspect of the arytenoid posteriorly and the petiole of the epiglottis anteriorly. The hyoepiglottic ligament recently was elegantly described by Zeitels and Kirchner,[181] who

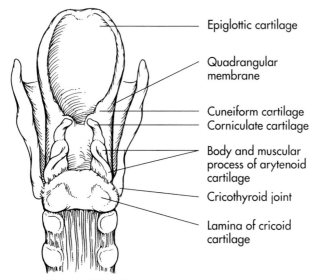

Figure 102-4. The quadrangular membrane.

showed this structure to be a resilient barrier to malignant spread from the supraglottis to the tongue base when the cancer is confined to the laryngeal membranes and does not clinically invade the suprahyoid epiglottis.

The skeleton and fibrous tissue barriers demarcate a number of spaces within the larynx. The superiormost space is the preepiglottic space (Figure 102-5), which is filled with fat and traversed by blood and lymphatic vessels.[37] Kirchner and Carter[67] noted that carcinoma tends to invade within the preepiglottic space with a "pushing edge," which is almost "encapsulated" after it reaches the elastic tissue membranes in the preepiglottic space, contributing to the oncologic safety in saving the hyoid bone during supraglottic surgery. The boundaries of this space are the vallecula mucosa and the hyoid superiorly, the thyrohyoid membrane and the thyroid cartilage anteriorly, and the epiglottis posteriorly. Posterolaterally, on either side, the preepiglottic space is bounded by the superior portions of the paraglottic space.[89]

There is a paraglottic space on either side of the larynx (Figure 102-6). Superiorly, the medial boundary is the quadrangular membrane, whereas inferiorly, the medial margin is the conus elasticus. It originates superiorly within the aryepiglottic fold, where it fades to a peak. The paraglottic space makes up the substance of the true and false cords and within it are the thyroarytenoid musculature and the mucosa-lined, air-filled space known as the *ventricle* and its superior extension, the *saccule*. Inferiorly, it follows the conus elasticus down to the top of the cricoid cartilage. Anteriorly, it abuts the preepiglottic space and the anterior third of the thyroid cartilage, and the posterolateral boundary is the mucosa of the medial aspect of the pyriform sinus. The paraglottic space traverses the supraglottis, glottis, and subglottis laterally within the larynx. Rather than having a distinct barrier to superior–inferior spread, cancer seems to be impeded in its course through the paraglottic space to varying degrees by the hourglass shape of the space, which is made by the indentation of the ventricle and saccule.[175] One additional space is Reinke's space, which actually is a potential space under the true vocal cord mucosa and provides no barrier to invasion.

The behavior of carcinoma in the supraglottis is modified by the soft tissue, connective tissue barriers, and the skeleton of the larynx (Figure 102-7). Kirchner[64] showed, in an analysis of whole organ sections, that supraglottic carcinomas that overlie the epiglottic cartilage have a tendency (9 of 10 cases) to extend into the preepiglottic space, at least microscopically, through the fenestrations in the epiglottic cartilage. In addition, Bridger,[24] working with the

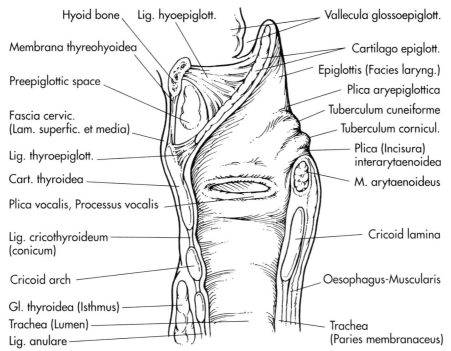

Figure 102-5. The preepiglottic space.

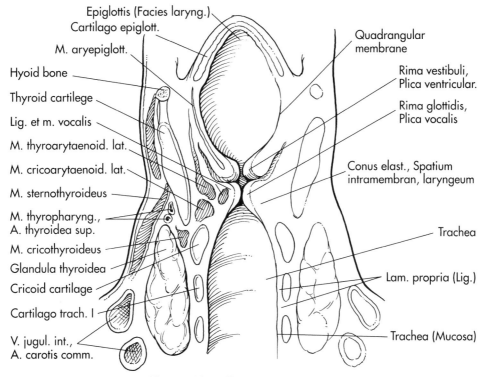

Figure 102-6. The paraglottic space.

whole organ section collection at Johns Hopkins, showed that seromucinous tubuloalveolar glands extend through the fenestrations and provide a route of spread of cancer into the preepiglottic space. Although it had been suggested in the past that embryologic fusion planes somehow provide protection against inferior spread of carcinoma from the supraglottis to the glottis, a recent study that evaluated all of the series of whole organ sections in the literature revealed that the incidence of spread of

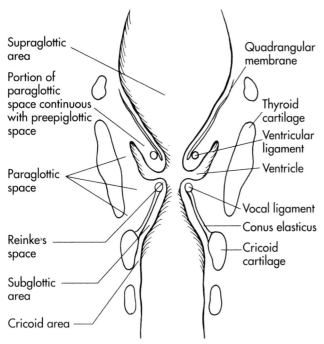

Figure 102-7. Connective tissue barriers within the larynx.

supraglottic carcinoma to the glottic level is between 20% to 54%.[175] This study indicated that there was a statistically significant relationship between the presence of abnormal cord mobility or involvement of carcinoma below the false cord and glottic level extension, most commonly through the paraglottic space.[175]

Carcinomas at the glottic level tend to begin at the junction of the anterior one-third and posterior two-thirds of the vocal cord. They readily pass through Reinke's space to the tissues below. Early studies by Pressman,[134] with submucosally injected dyes and radioisotopes, indicated that barriers existed between the two sides of the glottis and the supraglottis. Welsh and others[177] demonstrated that as dye concentration increases, these barriers become less effective. For early lesions, the conus elasticus provides a barrier to extension; as the lesion enlarges, this barrier becomes less pertinent.[66]

The sensation to the supraglottis is supplied by the superior laryngeal nerves, whereas the glottis and subglottis are innervated by the recurrent laryngeal nerve. The neural structures play an important role in timely postoperative functional rehabilitation.[124] Whenever possible, the main trunks of the superior and recurrent laryngeal nerves and the hypoglossal nerves, bilaterally, should be preserved during conservation laryngeal surgery.

Certain aspects of physiology of the larynx are pertinent to successful application of conservation laryngeal surgery. Hirano and others,[51] in a whole organ

analysis of the normal larynx, noted that 50% to 65% of the entire adult airway is located posterior to the tips of the vocal processes and concluded that the posterior larynx is the respiratory airway and the anterior portion is the phonatory airway. This is because all of the musculature that opens and closes the glottic chink, the lateral cricoarytenoid musculature, changes the position of the vocal processes during speech and swallowing. The arytenoids are responsible for opening the airway for breathing and for closing during swallowing and speaking. The vocal cords provide vocal quality during phonation; therefore, loss of one or both vocal cords results in hoarseness, but preservation of at least one arytenoid and an intact circumferential ring at the level of the cricoid is sufficient for speech and swallowing without a tracheostomy.[12,74–76,162,167]

PRINCIPLES OF ORGAN PRESERVATION SURGERY

The otolaryngologist–head and neck surgeon must adhere to certain key principles to determine a patient's eligibility for a conservation laryngeal surgery. The advent of the supracricoid laryngectomy makes us direct our focus away from the vocal fold and concentrate on the cricoarytenoid unit as the essential functional unit of the larynx. The organ preservation principles are formulated to help provide consistent oncologic and functional outcomes.[173] These can then be compared with current nonsurgical organ preservation options to allow the patient and physician to make educated decisions regarding treatment. Adopting these principles will enable the surgeon to maximize oncologic and functional outcomes for a number of glottic, supraglottic, and transglottic malignancies.

First Principle: Local Control

Local control is the most important principle. Survival from the index cancer is compromised if there is a local failure after radiation therapy or surgery to the supraglottis and glottis.[164] Early detection of the primary site recurrence may be difficult for a number of reasons. Medical and surgical organ preservation modalities alter the topography of the larynx and make definitive evaluation of recurrent cancer difficult. Symptoms may be attributed to the treatment intervention or recurrent tumor, although increasing pain, persistent ear pain, and dysphagia are ominous signs. Repeat endoscopy and biopsy of the original primary site is warranted. Computed tomography (CT), magnetic resonance imaging (MRI), and positron emission tomography (PET) may also be helpful in explaining recurrent or persistent cancer. Organ preservation laryngeal procedures should be used only when resection of the tumor can be accomplished comfortably with local control rates approximating those of total laryngectomy.

Second Principle: Accurate Assessment of the Three-Dimensional Extent of Tumor

The second principle of organ preservation surgery is to be able to confidently predict the extent of tumor. A comprehensive appreciation of laryngeal anatomy and function is necessary. The inability to accurately predict the extent of tumor in a conservation laryngeal procedure may lead to total laryngectomy when another organ-sparing approach may have been possible.

Third Principle: Cricoarytenoid Unit is the Basic Functional Unit of the Larynx

The cricoarytenoid unit is the basic functional unit of the larynx. The cricoarytenoid unit consists of an arytenoid cartilage, the cricoid cartilage, the associated musculature, and the superior and recurrent laryngeal nerves for that unit. Preservation of at least one functional cricoarytenoid unit makes it possible to consider an organ preservation procedure. This is a foreign concept to most surgeons who perform vertical partial laryngectomy and supraglottic laryngectomy. The surgeons, along with the T-staging system for laryngeal cancer, focus on the vocal fold rather than on the cricoarytenoid unit. The paradigm shift form the vocal fold to the cricoarytenoid unit is essential for the head and neck surgeon to be able to use the full spectrum of organ preservation surgeries. It is the cricoarytenoid unit, not the vocal folds, that allows for physiologic speech and swallowing without the permanent need for a tracheostoma after supracricoid laryngectomy.

Fourth Principle: Resection of Normal Tissue to Achieve an Expected Functional Outcome

This principle may seem counterintuitive because we are talking about "conservation laryngeal surgery." What we are conserving is the function of the larynx, not necessarily all the regions of the larynx that are uninvolved with cancer. This resection of normal tissue is necessary to achieve consistent functional outcomes in terms of speech and swallowing. A reliable reconstruction for each organ preservation surgical choice that is proven with regard to speech and swallowing outcome should make the surgeon feel more at ease when comparing nonsurgical and surgical organ preservation results for a patient. Reconstructions based on the extent of tumor resection for clear margins alone often result in novel reconstructions and the surgeon's trepidation regarding functional outcome. A better approach is to perform a standard resection where a consistent functional outcome is known.

PREOPERATIVE EVALUATION

The preoperative evaluation includes an oncologic assessment of the primary site, regional nodes, and distant sites. In addition, it includes an assessment of the patient's ability to medically undergo the surgery and postoperative treatment. Finally, patient and family insight, emotional state, and ability and willingness to undergo the postoperative rehabilitation should be considered.

Clinical Evaluation of the Primary Site

Before examining the larynx, the physician should listen to the patient speak and breathe. The degree of airway impairment and the voice quality should be assessed. Glottic carcinomas that affect the phonatory structures tend to cause hoarseness; supraglottic cancers frequently are above the cords and cause a muffled "hot potato" voice as they enlarge. Hoarseness from a supraglottic carcinoma may indicate impairment of cord mobility as a result of arytenoid involvement or glottic level involvement. Next, both sides of the neck should be palpated for nodal disease. The thyroid cartilage itself should be palpated for irregularities, as should the areas directly above and below the thyroid cartilage. A bulge or mass at the level of the thyrohyoid membrane may indicate massive preepiglottic space invasion. A mass at the level of the cricothyroid ligament may indicate a delphian lymph node, which indicates subglottic extension of the malignancy.[152] Indirect mirror or fiberoptic laryngoscopy is used to assess the larynx and surrounding structures. The important gross pathologic characteristics that need to be evaluated are airway impairment, endophytic vs exophytic, superficial spread vs deep invasion, mucosal structures involved, arytenoid and vocal cord mobility, and extensions out of the endolarynx.

The clinical assessment of laryngeal mobilities provides excellent insight into the three-dimensional extension of carcinoma within the larynx. Mobility of the vocal cord itself, without attention to arytenoid mobility, is adequate when planning for management that is directed to the entire organ, such as total laryngectomy or radiotherapy. Biller and Lawson[14] and Ogura's team[92] have noted that assessment of arytenoid mobility and cord mobility is important in the preoperative planning for conservation laryngeal surgery, particularly when the vocal cord itself is fixed. Assessment of vocal cord mobility is best clinically assessed during indirect laryngoscopy by having the patient speak or breathe deeply, whereas arytenoid mobility is best assessed by having the patient cough gently.

Cancers involving the glottis and supraglottis have different effects on vocal cord mobility and arytenoid mobility. Impaired mobility from glottic carcinoma may be a result of superficial thyroarytenoid invasion or bulk on the surface of the cord in an exophytic lesion.[66] Hirano and others[52] assessed the degree of thyroarytenoid muscle invasion in glottic carcinoma and found fixed cords had deeper invasion into the musculature than impaired cords. Numerous studies have demonstrated that glottic carcinoma associated with a fixed vocal cord most commonly results from extensive invasion of the thyroarytenoid muscle.[52,70,121] In some patients, subglottic extension with fixation to the cricoid cartilage and lateral extension with adherence to the thyroid cartilage resulted in fixation of the cord[70] and invasion of the lateral cricoarytenoid musculature and the cricoarytenoid joint.[121] At the supraglottic level, cancer invasion into the thyroarytenoid musculature at the glottic level is less likely, and the most common cause of cord fixation, noted by Hirano and others,[52] was deep arytenoid cartilage invasion superiorly. Montgomery[108] and Ogura[54] assessed vocal cord and arytenoid mobility, independently, in preparation for conservation laryngeal surgery of the supraglottis. Brasnu and others,[23] in a whole organ section series, noted two types of impairment in arytenoid mobility—namely the "weight impact" of the tumor—in which the arytenoid motion seems impaired superiorly causing "pseudofixation" vs actual fixation from the malignant involvement of the intrinsic laryngeal musculature, the cricoarytenoid joint, or both (Figure 102-8). They are distinguished by careful evaluation of the vocal fold; if any motion of the cord is noted in the presence of what seems to be arytenoid fixation from a supraglottic cancer, this is "pseudofixation."[23] This information is valuable to the conservation laryngeal surgeon, because it is unlikely that a larynx with a "pseudo-fixed" arytenoid has cricoarytenoid joint and musculature involved, whereas these areas are involved in more than two-thirds of patients when "true fixation" of the arytenoid is present. The authors have found that the fiberoptic scope has use in the assessment of vocal cord mobility in the presence of exophytic supraglottic carcinomas, because the tip of the scope can be manipulated past the lesion to look at the structures below. The clinical implication is that careful assessment of the vocal cord and arytenoid mobilities is essential when planning for conservation laryngeal surgery to attempt to understand which deep structures are invaded and which in turn may improve the likelihood of applying the appropriate surgical technique.

The final aspect of the physical examination of the primary site is performed during direct laryngoscopy during general anesthesia. The direct laryngoscopy allows for biopsy of the lesion to be performed and for a thorough visual evaluation of the larynx and surrounding structures with the routine use of the operating microscope or rigid endoscopes. Palpation of the lesion and surrounding structures with endoscopic instrumentation can yield valuable information concerning submucosal extent of disease. Palpation of the vallecula with a finger and of the posterior floor of mouth provides a critical assessment of submucosal extent of disease in these areas from supraglottic carcinoma.

After this clinical assessment, the conservation laryngeal surgeon should have a clear understanding of the extent of the lesion and have in mind which surgical or nonsurgical options are optimal for the patient.

Radiologic Evaluation of the Primary Site

Although imaging studies frequently are available before the clinical evaluation of the primary site, the best role of these studies is to corroborate the clinical findings noted on indirect and direct laryngoscopy and to corroborate clinical evidence of deep growth of lesions. This is because although there are specific findings that are particularly useful to assess with imaging studies, there are limitations to the value of these studies, and they may either overpredict or underpredict tumor in certain situations. One caveat is that when evaluating particularly small lesions or the superficial extension of a large lesion, CT[4] or MRI may demonstrate little abnormality. This is because these modalities are insensitive to superficial mucosal masses. Another pitfall is seen in those with large exophytic lesions. When lesions have large extensions into the airway, they may sit up against adjacent mucosal sites, such as the pyriform sinus, tongue base, floor of mouth, the lateral pharyngeal wall, or

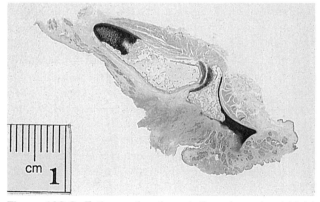

Figure 102-8. Entire section through the cricoarytenoid joint with fixation of the true cord and the arytenoid revealing cricoarytenoid joint invasion.

the ventricle or saccule. Although the point of the attachment of the cancer may be small and discrete, the scan may deceptively indicate that all mucosal surfaces are involved. In these patients, the endoscopist has a better view of the lesion, and the clinical examination takes precedence over the radiologic evaluation. Valsalva maneuver performed during the CT scan may be useful if these issues cannot be resolved at endoscopy.[176] Occasionally, tumors may be isodense (CT) or isointense (MRI) with the surrounding tissues, which at times may overestimate or underestimate the size of the lesion noted on the clinical examination.[5] In these patients, the radiologist and surgeon should work together to find the true extent of tumor.

There are a number of areas in which laryngeal imaging studies have been useful. Occasionally, the bulk of the lesion extends submucosally into the subglottis. In these patients, MRI more so than CT can be useful to demonstrate the direct invasion or secondary thickening or asymmetry caused by the lesion in this area. Coronal T1-weighted MRI scans are particularly elegant in demonstrating submucosal transglottic spread. The cricoarytenoid area is best evaluated with axial scans, and sclerotic changes on CT are indications of perichondrial or direct arytenoid cartilage involvement.[7,176] Sagittal MRI has been shown to be a sensitive and specific test for varying degrees of preepiglottic space invasion.[96] Because the cartilages of the larynx calcify starting in the second decade in an inhomogeneous fashion, loss of calcification of the cartilage on CT is an unreliable indicator of tumor extension.[59] MRI has been shown to be highly sensitive to cartilage invasion, particularly if fat-suppressed and post-gadolinium scans are performed. Enhancement into cartilage on post-gadolinium fat-suppressed scans is highly sensitive to invasion, but it suffers from reduced specificity because inflammation and chondronecrosis will show similar findings. Kirchner[63] noted that the most common site of thyroid ala invasion from glottic carcinoma is the lower edge, and questionable isolated involvement of the superior aspect of the thyroid cartilage may represent random calcification patterns within the cartilage. The authors agree with Kikinis and others[61] that MRI has been more useful for evaluating tumor extension into or through laryngeal cartilages. Fluorodeoxyglucose (FDG) PET has gained popularity among physicians in the staging and surveillance of head and neck cancer.[182] Its most promising role in larynx cancer appears to be in the delineation of posttreatment effect (medical organ preservation strategies) from recurrent tumor. The role of FDG PET in organ preservation for the larynx paradigm is currently being assessed in a prospective study.

T Stage

The larynx by convention is divided into three discrete parts for the purpose of T staging. The supraglottis begins inferiorly at the lateral angle of the ventricle. Although the supraglottis extends superiorly up to the tip of the epiglottis, the vallecula mucosa is part of the oropharynx. The glottis begins at the lateral angle of the ventricle, and it extends 1 cm inferiorly at the midcord level. The subglottis begins at the inferior aspect of the glottic level and extends to the inferior aspect of the cricoid cartilage. Although this partitioning of the larynx is somewhat artificial, it allows for a staging system that, despite its shortcomings, allows for comparison of treatment modalities and prognostication.[29] Although the T-staging system is useful when comparing modalities that encompass the entire larynx, such as radiotherapy or total laryngectomy, it lacks the precision necessary to determine whether conservation laryngeal surgery may be performed at all and, if so, which particular procedure is indicated. Within each of the four T stages, at each site there is a spectrum of lesions for which a variety of conservation laryngeal procedures may be used with successful outcome. When planning for conservation laryngeal surgery, numerous factors that go beyond the level of detail required in the T-staging system should be evaluated. The factors that are clinically important include the precise extent of mucosal involvement, the depth of invasion of the malignancy, and the vocal cord and arytenoid mobilities. Although it has frequently been stated that millimeter margins are adequate for conservation laryngeal surgery, the caveat to this axiom is that for any given conservation laryngeal technique, millimeters of tumor extension within the larynx may preclude performing that technique and may result in intraoperative conversion to total laryngectomy. The conservation laryngeal surgeon should describe the lesion in more detail than the T-staging system to allow for application of the appropriate conservative laryngeal technique.

Overall Clinical Assessment

The primary medical issues important to the conservation laryngeal surgeon are the patient's ability to successfully tolerate the general anesthesia required to perform the procedure, the patient's lack of severe systemic medical problems that may dramatically impair wound healing, and the patient's pulmonary reserve to tolerate the postoperative course. The standard criteria are available for assessing anesthesia-related risks before surgery and should be used. Systemic illnesses that may predispose to poor wound healing include severe nutritional depletion, medications associated with organ transplantation, diabetes mellitus, and gastroesophageal reflux.

The degree to which the severity of pulmonary disease is used in the decision to proceed with conservation laryngeal surgery remains controversial in the literature. The real question is how well the patient will tolerate some degree of aspiration during the early postoperative period.[97] The amount of postoperative aspiration varies with the type of surgery contemplated. Vertical hemilaryngectomy sparing arytenoid typically causes little impact on swallowing function, whereas extensions of standard or extended supraglottic laryngectomy may result in increased dysphagia and aspiration risk.[135] Some authors advocate pulmonary function tests routinely for all patients,[8] whereas others use clinical evaluation such as walking up two flights of stairs without getting short of breath.[97,159] The percutaneous gastrostomy tube has been useful for patients who require long periods of no nutrition by mouth.[42] The literature actually leaves a fair amount of leeway for the clinician in terms of the pulmonary workup and in terms of how to use this information in clinical decision making. The authors rarely use pulmonary function testing preoperatively, unless requested by a medical consultant or anesthesiologist in preparation for a general anesthetic. If the patient has chronic obstructive lung disease but can walk up two flights of stairs without being winded and is active in his or her daily life, then the risks, benefits, and alternatives of conservation laryngeal surgery are discussed with the patient. If the pulmonary status indicates severe impairment of activity and a likelihood of morbidity or mortality after the procedure, then the authors do not recommend conservation laryngeal surgery for that particular patient. In actual practice, each surgeon should know, over time, the limitations of a particular surgical technique in "their hands." Using this approach, there rarely will be patients who need functional laryngectomy for intractable aspiration, although there also will be many patients who have had their larynges spared with conservation laryngeal surgery.

An important factor in patient selection is the patient's insight into the problem and the ability of the patient to play an active role in his or her rehabilitation. The issue of age often has been discussed in the literature. Some authors have strict age criteria for performing partial laryngeal surgery.[1] Others have stated that it is the biologic age and the patient's overall constitution that is more important than the chronologic age.[42,48,159] In addition, conservation laryngeal surgery is a "team endeavor," and if the patient and family prefer to "sit on the sidelines" rather than be actively involved in the rehabilitation process, it is the authors' experience that the patient will likely have a protracted course with increased morbidity. In the authors' institutions, the assessment

of the patient's willingness and ability to be rehabilitated is a joint decision between the speech pathologist, the otolaryngologist, the patient, and the family. Although the authors do not obtain preoperative modified barium swallow, all patients are assessed by a speech pathologist, and the rehabilitation is discussed with the patient. The sine qua non for a cooperative and functional patient postoperatively is extensive preoperative counseling by the surgeon and speech pathologist. The patient and family should understand that much work is required on their part for rehabilitation. Some patients may choose alternative nonsurgical approaches to their problem or even total laryngectomy to avoid the swallowing rehabilitation required for some conservation laryngeal procedures.

The literature is replete with nonsurgical strategies for the preservation of the larynx for all stages of laryngeal carcinoma. All surgical and nonsurgical therapies have expected sequelae, risks, and complications, which are balanced by the ability of a given technique to control the malignancy. The two central issues of great importance to the patient, his or her family, and the physician are: (1) the quality of life; and (2) cancer control. The clinician weighs each of these factors carefully in advising a patient on which modality is preferred in a particular case. It is tempting for clinicians to apply their value system to what is good for a patient, although when making recommendations, it is clinicians' ethical and legal responsibility to offer patients the risks, benefits, and alternatives to the variety of treatment options that are available for their cancer.

SURGICAL TECHNIQUES

The next section will review the various conservation laryngeal techniques available for the management of the spectrum of laryngeal carcinomas. The discussion will be limited to open surgical approaches in which the functional goal is speech and swallowing without a permanent tracheostomy. The main category of surgical technique will be introduced with a review of the literature analyzing the oncologic results, basic surgical technique, key surgical points, extensions of the procedure, expected functional outcome, and complications.

Indications and Contraindications

The indications for particular surgical techniques, presented in the literature, have varied over time. Indications frequently vary, depending on the stage of development of the technique. When a technique is first introduced, most surgeons advocate conservatism in its application.[2,154] Later, pioneering surgeons attempt to cautiously extend the use of techniques, frequently on the basis of applications of their surgical skills combined with their knowledge of surgical anatomy and by necessity without the benefit of long-term oncologic follow-up evaluation.[18,116] The final stage in the development of a technique, according to Daly,[35] is reevaluation followed by acceptance of the technique on the basis of reported results. Before the last stage of development, the indications for a particular technique usually are parochial and based on the anecdotal experiences at a particular institution or the pronouncement of a pundit in the field. Reliance on the literature for indications and contraindications is, therefore, frequently not helpful, because surgeons usually have attempted to use techniques for a large spectrum of tumor stages. To address this problem, the authors have provided, for each technique, a thorough literature review in terms of oncologic results, functional outcome, and complications. The surgeon can use this information when advising patients concerning the risks, benefits, and alternatives for a particular surgical procedure.

Conservation Laryngeal Surgery for the Lesions Originating in the Glottic Level
Vertical Partial Laryngectomies

All vertical partial laryngectomies share a common approach, which includes a vertical transection through the thyroid cartilage and paraglottic space. The extent of resection is decided on the basis of the preoperative and intraoperative assessment of the tumor extent. Although this vertical approach provides useful and expeditious access to the endolarynx, they all share a common characteristic, which is "blind" entry into the larynx through a narrow exposure.[87] Depending on the extent of the primary lesion, the initial vertical cut may be close to or distant from the cancer. This point should be considered when these procedures are used.

Vertical Hemilaryngectomy

Oncologic results. Among the series in the English language literature in which local control has been reported in terms of the T stage, the local recurrence rates for T_1 lesions ranged from 0% to 11%, with five of six series having a local control of >90% (Table 102-1). In one large series of 248 patients, the local control was 93% (104 of 112) for patients with malignancy confined to the true cords without anterior commissure involvement.[87] In that same series, patients with anterior commissure involvement without impaired mobility or extension beyond the glottis had local failure rate of 25% (8 of 32). When the anterior commissure is involved, the most common site of recurrence is the subglottis, as demonstrated in a series in which 14% (8 of 58) of patients with anterior commissure involvement had vertical hemilaryngectomy failure;

in 7 of 8 of these patients, the recurrence was in the subglottis.[68] When the anterior commissure is involved by cancer, a wide surgical margin is indicated in the subglottis. Another factor that portends poor local control is extension beyond the confines of the glottis or impaired mobility.

Mohr and others[107] reported the highest local control in the literature for T_2 glottic carcinoma after extended vertical hemilaryngectomy, but the authors included only T_2 lesions with impaired mobility and excluded lesions that extended beyond the midventricle (only five patients) or beyond 5 mm into the subglottis because of the known high local failure rate for these lesions.[107] Subglottic extension has been associated with cricoid cartilage invasion, which is not resected in the standard vertical hemilaryngectomy.[45] Extension into the supraglottis through the ventricle should alert one to the possibility of thyroid cartilage invasion, which may account for the higher local recurrence in this patient group.[107] The difficulty in managing T_2 glottic carcinoma with vertical hemilaryngectomy was noted in a number of series

TABLE 102-1
LOCAL RECURRENCE AFTER VERTICAL HEMILARYNGECTOMY FOR T_1 GLOTTIC CARCINOMA

Author	Year	T_1	LR	LR (%)
Thomas and others[144]	1994	94	8	9
Lui, Ward, and Pleet[88]	1986	24	1	4
Bailey and Calcaterra[6]	1971	9	0	0
Mohr, Quenelle, and Shumrick[100]	1983	25	2	8
Laccourreye and others[74]	1991	146	16	11
Rothfield and others[130]	1989	54	2	4

LR, Local recurrence.

TABLE 102-2
RECURRENCE AFTER VERTICAL HEMILARYNGECTOMY FOR T_2 GLOTTIC CARCINOMA

Author	Year	T_2	LR	LR (%)
Lui, Ward, and Pleet[88]	1986	14	2	14
Bailey and Calcaterra[6]	1971	18	3	17
Mohr, Quenelle, and Shumrick[100]	1983	27	1	4
Kirchner and Som[58]	1975	58	8	14
Som[138]	1975	104	25	24
Biller, Ogura, and Pratt[10]	1971	58	3	5
Laccourreye and others[74]	1991	102	26	26
Johnson and others[51]	1993	31	7	23

LR, Local recurrence.

that had local failure >20%,[55,87,146] and six of the eight series in the English language literature that correlated local recurrence with T stage reported a local recurrence rate of >14% (Table 102-2). One cause for impaired cord mobility is varying degrees of thyroarytenoid muscle invasion within the paraglottic space, which, in the authors' opinion, may account for the higher local failure rates in vertical hemilaryngectomy in which the paraglottic space is routinely transected.[66]

The local control after the management of T_3 glottic carcinoma with vertical partial laryngectomy has yielded variable local failure rates ranging from 0% to 46%, with four of the eight series reporting local failure rates of >36% (Table 102-3). This finding may be related to the fact that many cases may be understaged[111] and may have thyroid cartilage invasion, which routinely is partially resected during vertical hemilaryngectomy.

The authors' analysis reveals that consistently excellent oncologic results can be expected for T_1 glottic carcinomas involving the mobile membranous vocal cord, although once the anterior commissure is involved or if there is extension beyond the glottis or impaired cord mobility, vertical hemilaryngectomy should be used cautiously. On the basis of the authors' review of the oncologic results in the literature, they do not recommend vertical hemilaryngectomy for those with advanced T_2 lesions or any T_3 or T_4 glottic carcinomas.

Surgical technique. A tracheostomy routinely is performed. A horizontal skin incision is used that is separate from the tracheostomy site. The midline raphe between the strap muscles is dissected from the cricoid cartilage to just above the superior aspect of the thyroid cartilage. When feasible, the authors prefer to resect the window of thyroid cartilage adjacent to the vocal cord, allowing reconstruction through imbrication laryngoplasty.[132] The external thyroid perichondrium is scored in the midline with a blade, and the perichondrium is elevated as a single flap in continuity with the strap musculature. This is done with an elevator such as a Freer and by cutting the perichondrium sharply with a knife at its superior and inferior attachments to the thyroid cartilage. A variety of techniques have been described in which varying amounts of ipsilateral thyroid cartilage is excised, ranging from no cartilage[6] to the entire ipsilateral ala.[146] The authors use the technique described by Pleet and others,[132] in which a window of cartilage is outlined with a marker lateral to the level of the true vocal cord. The inferior aspect of the resected cartilage begins approximately 5 mm above the inferior aspect of the thyroid cartilage, and the resected portion is approximately 1.5 cm in height.[95] It extends from the midline to the posterior aspect of the thyroid cartilage. At this point, the midline thyrotomy and other cuts are made with a knife, drill, or a saw, depending on the degree of calcification of the thyroid cartilage and the preference of the surgeon. A No. 15 blade is used to make a midline vertical cricothyrotomy.

At this point, the patient is paralyzed, the cords are held apart from below with a mosquito clamp, and a No. 12 blade is used to gently transect the anterior commissure, as in laryngofissure and cordectomy. The true and false cords are separated sharply up to the level of the petiole of the epiglottis. The cancer is visualized. The soft-tissue resection is accomplished with a No. 15 blade for the anterior and posterior cuts. A right-angled Beaver blade or small right-angled scissors are useful for the posterior cut.

TABLE 102-3				
Local Recurrence After Vertical Hemilaryngectomy for T_3 Glottic Carcinoma				
Author	**Year**	**T_3**	**LR**	**LR (%)**
Lesinski, Bauer, and Ogura[87]	1976	18	3	17
Bailey and Calcaterra[6]	1971	4	0	0
Biller and Lawson[14]	1986	11	4	36
Mohr and others[100]	1983	5	0	0
Som[138]	1975	26	11	42
Kessler and others[56]	1987	27	3	11
Mendenhall and others[97]	1984	13	6	46
Kirchner and Som[60]	1971	22	9	41

LR, Local recurrence.

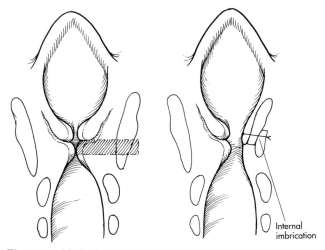

Figure 102-9. Imbrication laryngoplasty—reconstructive technique.

Internal imbrication

A variety of reconstructive options exist, including no replacement of the glottic level allowing healing to occur by secondary intention, strap muscle flap with thyroid cartilage preservation,[6] and skin flaps.[32] In imbrication laryngoplasty,[132] the authors elevate a composite flap that includes the superior portion of the thyroid cartilage and the undermined false cord (Figure 102-9).[95] This flap of vascularized, innervated false vocal cord is stabilized by the imbrication of the cartilage. It allows not only for soft-tissue coverage from the false cord, but also the inset of the superior thyroid cartilage on the inferior remnant ensures medialization of the mucosal surface, which may improve phonation when compared with no reconstruction.[95]

Extended procedures. A number of extensions of the standard procedure have been described.

Frontolateral vertical hemilaryngectomy. Frontolateral vertical hemilaryngectomy has been used for lesions that approach or involve the anterior commissure or opposite true vocal cord anteriorly.[117] In this case, the vertical thyrotomy is made through the thyroid lamina of the less involved side, allowing for removal of the anterior angle of the thyroid cartilage, anterior commissure, and a portion of the contralateral true vocal cord.

Posterolateral vertical hemilaryngectomy. Posterolateral vertical hemilaryngectomy is used for cancers that extend posteriorly to involve the ipsilateral arytenoid mucosa.[147] The thyrotomy approach is the same as the standard operation, and the modification lies in the posterior extension of the resection to encompass part or all of the ipsilateral arytenoid cartilage and mucosa.

Extended vertical hemilaryngectomy. A number of procedures have been described in which extensive resection is accomplished through a vertical approach. Common characteristics include resection of the entire ipsilateral hemilarynx with the option of resecting the superior aspect of the cricoid cartilage. A variety of reconstructions have been proposed for these radical resections, including sparing a posterior strip of the ipsilateral thyroid cartilage and fashioning a new hemilarynx, strap muscle reconstruction,[6] or pyriform sinus mucosal flap advancement into the hemilaryx.[107]

Functional outcome. The functional outcome after the standard vertical hemilaryngectomy is some degree of permanent hoarseness, which varies with the reconstructive technique. A more impaired voice tends to accompany no reconstruction, whereas the best voice was associated with replacement of the glottis with an adjacent false cord flap.[95] Hirano and others[49] com-

pared the vocal function after a variety of reconstructions and noted that poor outcome was least often associated with free mucosal grafts, although this report did not evaluate the imbrication technique. Blaugrund and others[16] noted that the supraglottic structures were responsible for voicing postoperatively predominantly in patients in whom one arytenoid was resected but also in patients in whom both arytenoids were spared. The supraglottic voicing was rougher and associated with a lower fundamental frequency than glottic voicing. Chronic dysphagia is not associated with the standard vertical hemilaryngectomy with or without resection of the vocal process, and 92% (11 of 12) of patients resumed a normal postoperative diet within 1 month.[135] It is not clear from the literature how extended vertical hemilaryngectomy affects function in terms of speech and swallowing.

Key surgical points.

1. As in cordectomy, always tack the petiole of the epiglottis back into position with a 3-0 Vicryl stitch so that the epiglottis will not prolapse posteriorly postoperatively, obscuring the view of the glottis.
2. Also as in cordectomy, suture the anterior commissure on the noninvolved side anteriorly at the external thyroid perichondrium with a 4-0 Vicryl stitch so that the cord will be in normal position and so the vocal tendon will have proper tension.

Complications. Uncommonly, wound complications such as seroma or hematoma might occur. Again, as in cordectomy, fistula is uncommon. In extended procedures, there is a higher incidence of complications, including delay in decannulation, stenosis, and long-term dysphagia.[14] Persistent airway edema can be managed expectantly or with laser laryngoscopy.

Epiglottic Laryngoplasty

Oncologic results. Epiglottic laryngoplasty was first described by the Czechoslovakian surgeon Sedlacek,[139] then reported by Kambic[58] in Yugoslavia, and later popularized in the United States by Tucker.[161] The history of the development of this technique is classic for conservation laryngeal surgery in general; it was first developed in Europe and later imported and popularized in the United States. The term *epiglottic laryngoplasty* refers to the reconstruction, which is done by undermining the epiglottis and advancing it inferiorly and laterally to reconstruct the larynx after vertical hemilaryngectomy or anteroinferiorly to reconstruct after a bilateral vertical partial laryngectomy.

The entrance into the larynx, like in all vertical partial laryngectomies, is through two vertical thyrotomies: one just anterior to the posterior aspect of the thyroid cartilage on the more involved side, and the other can be anywhere from a midline thyrotomy when the reconstruction is applied to the standard vertical hemilaryngectomy or symmetrically placed on the opposite thyroid ala for extensive bilateral lesions. In the most extensive resection, both cords, true cords, and one arytenoid may be resected. Tucker and others[162] reported on a series of patients who underwent the procedure with a minimum follow-up period of 2 years and in which there were no local recurrences among 4 T_{1a}, 8 T_{1b}, and 11 T_3 cancers and one recurrence in 8 (12.5%) T_2 cancers. Tucker[160] noted a 50% local recurrence rate for lesions with >6 mm of subglottic extension anteriorly.

Surgical technique.[161] A tracheostomy is performed. The authors will describe the procedure in which both thyroid ala are resected to manage a bilateral lesion. The midline raphe of the strap muscles is identified. The thyroid perichondrium is incised in the midline. The perichondrium is elevated in continuity with the overlying strap musculature. The vertical thyrotomies are made 3 to 4 mm anterior to the posterior aspect of the thyroid cartilage on the more involved side and placed more anteriorly on the less involved side. A transverse cricothyrotomy is performed. Right-angled scissors are used to transect the soft tissue of the paraglottic space on the less involved side through the previously made thyrotomy. The resection on the involved side can resect the arytenoid, taking care to preserve the posterior arytenoid mucosa. The epiglottis is undermined to the level of the vallecula, which is not transgressed (Figure 102-10). It is advanced inferiorly and sutured to the cricothyroid membrane or cricoid cartilage and laterally to the thyroid cartilage remnants. The external thyroid perichondrial flap and strap muscles then are sewn across the midline.

Key surgical points.

1. At least one functional arytenoid should be saved, and care should be taken not to damage the cricoarytenoid joint during the resection.
2. The preepiglottic space is dissected away from the anterior surface of the epiglottic cartilage, and this dissection should be brought up through the median hyoepiglottic ligament to allow for the epiglottis to be advanced far enough inferiorly.
3. No internal mucosal stitches are necessary, although the inferior suture line should be under no tension to prevent dehiscence.

Extended procedures. One extension of the epiglottic laryngoplasty has combined the procedure of the

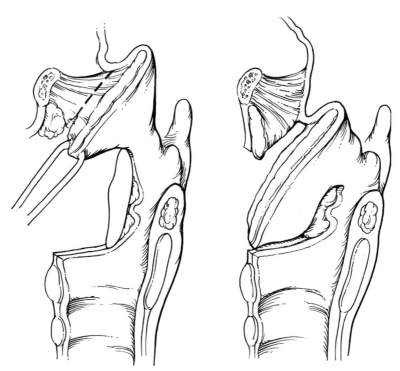

Figure 102-10. Epiglottic laryngoplasty—undermining of the epiglottis in the preepiglottic space before closure.

supracricoid partial laryngectomy with cricohyoi-doepiglottopexy as described by Guerrier and others,[46] in which an epiglottic advancement flap and pexy of the cricoid and the hyoid are performed.

Functional outcome. In Tucker's[161] original description, all patients were taking food by mouth from 1 to 18 days after decannulation, although as in all conservation laryngeal procedures in which one arytenoid is resected, some degree of temporary dysphagia is to be expected. Other authors have encountered increased degrees of postoperative aspiration and an extremely breathy voice, which they attributed to the wide anterior posterior dimension of the airway that prevents appropriate sphincteric function of the posterior glottis.[114] Nong and others[115] have responded to this problem by modifying the procedure by use of a number of endolaryngeal flaps to reconstruct the neolarynx to decrease aspiration and breathiness while preserving respiration.

Complications. Reported complications have included delayed decannulation from postoperative aspiration and mild upper airway obstruction.[161]

Horizontal Partial Laryngectomies

Horizontal partial laryngectomies are so called because the initial entry into the laryngeal lumen is through a transverse or horizontal cut. This incision is distant from the cancer, which allows for safe entry into the endolarynx followed by inspection of the lesion before making additional incisions. Although in the past the term *horizontal partial laryngectomy* has been used by some authors interchangeably with *supraglottic partial laryngectomy*, this is one type of horizontal technique that is used for supraglottic carcinomas. During the past two decades, the supracricoid partial laryngectomy with cricohyoi-doepiglottopexy, another horizontal technique with use for managing selected glottic carcinomas, has been developed.

Supracricoid Partial Laryngectomy with Cricohyoido–Epiglottopexy

Oncologic results. The supracricoid partial laryngectomy with cricohyoidoepiglottopexy allows for resection of both true cords, both false cords, the entire thyroid cartilage, both paraglottic spaces bilaterally, and a maximum of one arytenoid. Speech and swallowing without a permanent tracheostomy are achieved. The technique's main use has been for the management of selected T_2 and T_3 carcinomas of the glottis, although it has been reported that it was used for T_{1b} and selected T_4 glottic carcinomas. There were no local recurrences among nine patients

with T_1 glottic carcinomas (one T_{1a} and eight T_{1b}).[75] The local control for T_2 lesions is 4.5% (3 of 67).[79] The local recurrence for selected T_3 glottic carcinomas was 10% (2 of 20).[84] Piquet and Chevalier[128] reported the local recurrence for a group of 104 (T_1, 12; T_2, 77; T_3, 15) previously untreated patients to be 5%, although local recurrence was not reported by T stage in this series. One of the reasons for the consistently low local recurrence rates may be the complete resection of the entire thyroid cartilage and the bilateral en bloc resection of the paraglottic spaces.

Transglottic lesions have been defined as carcinomas that extend across the laryngeal ventricle, involving the true and false cords.[102] Although the exact origin of these cancers frequently is unclear, the origin is attributed to the site in which the epicenter of the tumor resides. In carcinomas with transglottic extension, the local recurrence after conservation approaches that use extended vertical hemilaryngectomy or extended supraglottic laryngectomy has yielded a local failure rate of 23% (7 of 30).[106] One caveat is that the supracricoid laryngectomy with cricohyoidoepiglottopexy does not result in a complete resection of the supraglottis, and therefore the authors prefer to perform supracricoid laryngectomy with cricohyoidopexy for transglottic extension.

Surgical technique.[75] After the creation of a U-shaped incision in line with the tracheostomy site, which will be placed later in the procedure, the superior flap is elevated to approximately 2 cm above the hyoid bone, exposing the underlying strap muscles. Next, the sternothyroid and the thyrohyoid muscles are transected individually, from medial to lateral, along the superior aspect of the thyroid cartilage. The sternohyoid muscle is elevated inferiorly, allowing for the exposure of the sternothyroid muscle. Typically, there is a blood vessel that pierces the deep strap musculature to the more superficial layer that should be ligated at this point bilaterally. The sternothyroid muscle is then carefully is transected along the inferior edge of the thyroid cartilage. Care is taken at this point not to cut the underlying thyroid gland. The constrictor muscles then are transected along the posterior and superior–lateral aspect of the thyroid cartilage, and the pyriform sinus mucosa is elevated off of the internal surface of the thyroid cartilage bilaterally, as is done in a total laryngectomy. A Freer elevator is used to disarticulate the cricoarytenoid joint bilaterally, taking care to protect the recurrent laryngeal nerves. The recurrent laryngeal nerves never are actually visualized. The isthmus of the thyroid gland is transected and ligated. At this point, a blunt finger dissection of the cervicomediastinal trachea is done to the level of the carina, as is done in a tracheal resection and anastomosis, to close the tracheal defect. A transverse cricothyrotomy is performed just above the cricoid cartilage, and the endotracheal tube is removed from above and placed into the cricothyrotomy. The larynx then is entered through a transverse transepiglottic laryngotomy. The scissors are oriented obliquely and inferiorly to allow transection of the epiglottis at the level of the petiole, if the lesion is amenable to such an approach, and to allow for entry just above the false cords and preservation of as much epiglottis as possible.

The endolaryngeal excision now is performed on the non–tumor-bearing side first, and the incision is brought down in the sagittal plane with a scissors at the junction between the false cord and arytenoid. The transection is carried inferiorly just posterior to the ventricle and then through the vocal process of the arytenoid. Special care is taken to avoid entering the cricoarytenoid joint with the scissors. Just above the cricoid cartilage, the orientation of the scissors changes to allow connection of this incision, through the cricothyroid muscle, to the previously made cricothyrotomy. The larynx is opened up on its anterior spine like a book (Figure 102-11). The cut on the tumor-bearing side may be made through just posterior to the ventricle again or may transect all or part of the arytenoid cartilage. This incision can be done by cutting the subglottic mucosa with a No. 15 blade and following posteriorly and superiorly to the level of the arytenoid. Nonetheless, the posterior arytenoid mucosa should be spared so that it can be used in the endolaryngeal reconstruction to cover the cricoarytenoid joint area on the cricoid. This forms a cushion, postoperatively, against which the remaining arytenoid will abut to allow for closure of the larynx.

The reconstruction is begun by pulling the arytenoid cartilages forward with 3-0 Vicryl suture material by placing a stitch just at or just above the vocal process and sewing them (or the posterior arytenoid mucosa in the case of unilateral arytenoid resection) anterolaterally to the cricoid cartilage. In this way, the arytenoid will not prolapse backward postoperatively. Impaction of the cricoid to the hyoid is performed with three centrally placed 2-0 Vicryl sutures on a 65-mm round needle. The first stitch is placed circumferentially, submucosally around the cricoid cartilage, in the midline. The stitch then is passed through a few millimeters of inferior epiglottic cartilage, submucosally, so that when the stitch is tied down, the epiglottic mucosa will be approximated to the cricoid mucosa. Next, the same first stitch is passed back into the preepiglottic fat and up around the hyoid bone and deep into the tongue base. This large needle allows the suture to be passed deeply into the tongue base, submucosally, while it is carefully palpated with a finger on the tongue base mucosa to pull it back and have a bulge of tongue-base tissue over the airway postoperatively (Figure 102-12).

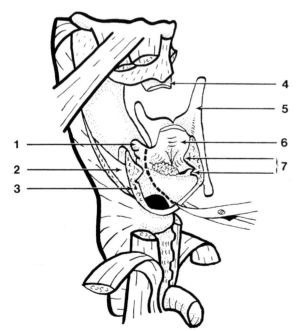

Figure 102-11. Supracricoid partial laryngectomy with cricohyoidoepiglottopexy—exposure of malignancy. *1,* Arytenoid; *2,* internal thyroid perichondrium; *3,* vocal process; *4,* inferior aspect of transected epiglottis; *5,* thyroid cartilage; *6,* petiole of the epiglottis; *7,* false and true vocal cords.

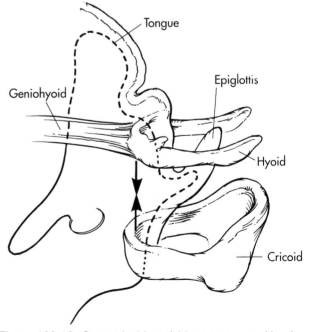

Figure 102-12. Supracricoid partial laryngectomy with cricohyoidoepiglottopexy—laryngoplasty using circumferential cricoid, hyoid, epiglottic, and tongue base sutures.

Before tightening the sutures, the two lateral sutures are pulled taut, which places the trachea in its postoperative position, and the tracheostomy is performed in line with the skin incision. With the two lateral cricohyoidoepiglottopexy sutures under tension, the central pexy stitch is tied, followed by the two lateral stitches. The strap muscles are closed as a second layer closure with 3-0 Vicryl. A cuffed tracheostomy tube is put into place. The skin wound is closed in two layers, taking special care to separate the tracheostomy site from the remainder of the wound with a subcutaneous stitch placed between the skin and the underlying strap muscles above the tracheostomy site.

Key surgical points

1. During the exposure, elevate the skin flaps to approximately 2 cm above the hyoid bone to prevent tethering of the skin in the closure postoperatively.
2. When disarticulating the cricoarytenoid joint, be careful not to injure the recurrent laryngeal nerve.
3. When making the vertical prearytenoid incision just posterior to the ventricle, be careful not to enter the cricoarytenoid joint.
4. Always save the posterior arytenoid mucosa in the case of a transected arytenoid cartilage, and sew this mucosa anteriorly to the cricoid cartilage during the closure.
5. The three tongue base sutures should be placed precisely 1 cm apart and arched up deeply into the tongue base. The authors use a 2-0 Vicryl on a 65-mm needle.
6. Perfect alignment between the cricoid cartilage and the hyoid bone should be created to reduce the risk of dysphagia postoperatively.
7. Submucosal stitches in the inferior aspect of the epiglottic remnant should be performed to avoid posterior rotation of the epiglottis that may cause airway compromise postoperatively.
8. Gentle internal palpation of the upper esophageal sphincter with a finger will allow for assessment of hypertonia, which should prompt the consideration of cricopharyngeal myotomy except in the presence of gastroesophageal reflux.
9. The dissected inner thyroid perichondrium should be gently sewn anteriorly with one 3-0 Vicryl stitch after the creation of the cricohyoidoepiglottopexy to reposition the pyriform sinus in a closer approximation to normal.
10. Always put the tracheostomy in line with the main incision, and always pull up the trachea before placing the tracheostomy so that it will be in line with the incision postoperatively.

Extended procedures. Extensions of the basic technique include resection of one arytenoid. Anterior subglottic extension may be managed with resection of the anterior arch of the cricoid,[83] which is closed with a pexy between the first two tracheal rings and the hyoid or a tracheohyoidoepiglottopexy.

Functional outcome. Temporary dysphagia immediately postoperatively is to be expected, but long-term dysphagia is rare. Review of the functional results in the world literature revealed a range of days to removal of nasogastric tube postoperatively from 9 to 50 days (Table 102-4). The need for removal of the larynx for intractable aspiration was low and ranged from 0% in 4% of seven studies and ranged from 1% to 4% in the remaining three studies (see Table 102-4). These results compare favorably with the functional laryngectomy rate for aspiration noted after supraglottic laryngectomy (Table 102-5). The vocal quality after supracricoid partial laryngectomy has been studied in a prospective fashion, and by the sixth month, speech parameters of phrase grouping and number of words per minute were similar to normal speakers, although the mean fundamental frequency was lower and wider than normal, suggesting some voice instability postoperatively.[33] In addition, the authors found that the degree of voicelessness parameters increased, suggesting difficulties in achieving consistent neoglottic closure during speech.[33]

Complications. In one series, the only complication was progressive hyoid necrosis, resulting from underlying severe vasculitis.[75] Three patients in Piquet's series had neolaryngeal stenosis develop requiring placement of a Montgomery T-tube for 3 months.[128]

Conservation Laryngeal Surgery for Lesion Originating in the Supraglottic Level

The management scheme at most institutions managing supraglottic carcinoma has included surgical and nonsurgical approaches. Table 102-6 categorizes patients with supraglottic carcinoma, from a number of large series, treated in the United States by various approaches including partial laryngectomy, total laryngectomy, or radiotherapy alone.[36,91,97,180] The range of percentages of patients undergoing primary surgical management varied from 47% to 90%. When the authors analyzed the number of patients undergoing total laryngectomy in these series, they noted that the range was from 42% to 66%. Although numerous surgical series have had overall local recurrence rates, including all T stages, of <5%[31,39,40,91,97] in most series (Table 102-7), most patients undergoing primary surgical treatment of the supraglottis underwent total removal of the larynx (see Table 102-6).

TABLE 102-4

FUNCTIONAL OUTCOME AFTER SUPRACRICOID LARYNGECTOMY WITH CRICOHYOIDOEPIGLOTTOPEXY

Author	Patients (n)	Duration NG	Func Laryn	Func Laryn (%)
Guerrier and others[46]	58	9–50	1	1.7
Vigneau and others[165]	52	19*	2	3.8
Traissac and Verhulst[156]	97	10–33	1	1.0
Piquet and Chevalier[129]	104	21–45	0	0
Laccourreye and others[76]	67	11–40	0	0
Piquet and others[127]	46	10–90	0	0
Pech and others[126]	17	10–40	0	0

Func laryn, Functional laryngectomy for aspiration; NG, nasogastric tube.
*Average duration.

TABLE 102-5

ADVERSE RESULTS AFTER SUPRAGLOTTIC LARYNGECTOMY*

Author	Series Includes Extended Procedures	SGL	Permanent Gastrostomy (%)	Death from Pneumonia (%)	Functional Laryngectomy (%)
Herranz-Gonzales and others[48]	N	110	0 (0.00)	0 (0.00)	1 (0.91)
Soo and others[148]		78	0 (0.00)	0 (0.00)	0 (0.00)
Hirano and others[50]	Y	38	0 (0.00)	0 (0.00)	3 (7.89)
Burstein and Calcaterra[27]		40	0 (0.00)	0 (0.00)	1 (2.50)
Flores and others[42]		46	4 (8.70)	2 (4.35)	5 (10.87)
Lee and others[91]		60	1 (1.67)	1 (1.67)	3 (5.00)
Beckhardt and others[8]		49	2 (4.08)	1 (2.04)	4 (8.16)
Spaulding and others[150]		33	0 (0.00)	0 (0.00)	1 (3.03)

This table includes series that reported functional results.
*Includes all laryngectomies done for chronic aspiration.

TABLE 102-6

THE THERAPEUTIC MANAGEMENT OF SUPRAGLOTTIC CARCINOMA

Author	Period	Patients Surgery (n)	Patients Partial (n)	Patients Total (n)	Patients Primary RT (n)	Surgery (%)	Total (%)
Zamora and others[180]	1952–1985	445	258	187	75	0.86	0.42
DeSanto[39]	1971–1980	227	103	124	24	0.90	0.55
Lee and others[91]	1974–1987	190	65	125	211	0.47	0.66
Lutz and others[97]	1975–1986	202	72	130	99	0.67	0.64

TABLE 102-7

LOCAL RECURRENCE AFTER SURGICAL MANAGEMENT OF SUPRAGLOTTIC CARCINOMA

Author	Patients Partial (n)	LR Partial	Patients Total (n)	LR Total	Overall LR
DeSanto[39]	103	3	124	6	0.04
Coates and others[31]	40	1	117	4	0.03
Lee and others[91]	65	0	125	—	0.00
Lutz C and others[97]	72	1	130	3	0.02

LR, local recurrence.

The conservative surgical option among the patients in Table 102-7 (with the exception of five patients in the Mayo series who were treated with transoral epiglottectomy) was standard or extended supraglottic partial laryngectomy. The main use of the standard supraglottic laryngectomy is for those with selected T_1 and T_2 supraglottic carcinomas,[147] whereas its extensions are used for those with highly selected T_3 and T_4 cancer.[19]

Horizontal Partial Laryngectomies

Supraglottic laryngectomy

Oncologic results. When series of supraglottic laryngectomy from the United States were analyzed, it was noted that the local recurrence varied from 0% to 12.8%, with seven of eight of the large series having a local control of 90% or higher.* When local recurrence after supraglottic laryngectomy was analyzed by T stage, one saw consistently high local control for selected T_1 and T_2 lesions but an extremely variable success rate for those with T_3 and T_4 lesions, with local recurrence rates as high as 75% for the former and 66.7% for the latter (Table 102-8). It is not clear from the literature which patients with specific T_3 or T_4 lesions were at highest risk for recurrence; therefore, until this is evaluated further in the literature, supraglottic laryngectomy should be performed with caution for those with highly selected T_3 and T_4 lesions of the supraglottis. Lee and others[91] noted improved local control among intermediate-sized supraglottic carcinomas with the addition of postoperative radiotherapy after supraglottic laryngectomy, although the tradeoff for local control seemed to be decreased functional results after extended supraglottic laryngectomy and radiotherapy in that series. Nonetheless, supraglottic laryngectomy provides consistently excellent oncologic results among patients with selected T_1 and T_2 lesions. The authors' recent analysis of the extension of supraglottic carcinoma to the glottic level revealed a statistically significant increase in glottic involvement for those with lesions with impairment of the vocal cord or involvement of the ventricle.[175] These findings support the contentions that extension below the false cord and impaired cord mobility are contraindications for supraglottic laryngectomy.[108]

Surgical technique. The authors perform an apron incision, in line with the tracheostomy, and routinely perform bilateral modified neck dissection. The main trunk of the superior laryngeal nerve should be spared bilaterally in the nonextended supraglottic laryngectomy. The fascia between the

strap muscles at the level of the superior aspect of the thyroid cartilage is divided. In addition, the fascia between the strap muscles is divided inferiorly, and the thyroid isthmus is transected and ligated routinely. The intervening fascia between the strap muscles is left intact. The sternohyoid and the thyrohyoid muscles at the superior border of the thyroid cartilage are divided, with care taken laterally to avoid damaging the superior laryngeal nerves. The constrictor muscles are sharply cut at the posterior and superior edge of the thyroid cartilage laterally all the way to the top of the superior cornua. The superior edge of the thyroid cartilage is scored with a knife, and a Freer elevator is used to elevate the periosteum off of the thyroid cartilage. The external thyroid cartilage perichondrium is elevated halfway down the cartilage from the superior edge to allow for the transverse thyrotomy to be made at the level just above the anterior commissure. The pyriform sinuses then are freed up bilaterally for endolaryngeal tumors, as is done in total laryngectomy, and unilaterally for tumors that involve the pyriform sinus. A tracheostomy is then performed. The next step in the procedure depends on whether the tumor involves the endolarynx alone or is in the vallecula.

The following is the standard technique for T_1 and T_2 endolaryngeal supraglottic carcinomas. If the tumor has not involved the vallecular mucosa and if it was not palpable beneath the vallecula mucosa in the preepiglottic space, then it is oncologically sound to spare the hyoid bone, and it is skeletonized from below with an electrocautery. The horizontal thyrotomy is made through the thyroid cartilage at the appropriate level with a sagittal saw. The vallecula is entered, and the epiglottis is pulled externally with an Allis clamp. The resection is done close to the epiglottis sparing both arytenoids. The cut is made anterior to the arytenoid cartilage bilaterally in a superior-to-inferior direction with one scissor blade in the laryngeal lumen and one scissor blade between the thyroid cartilage and the previously elevated internal thyroid perichondrium (Figure 102-13). This will allow sparing of the pyriform sinuses bilaterally. The cut is brought down to the level of the ventricle, at which point the transection is made through the ventricle at right angles to the previously made transection in front of the arytenoid. The specimen then is removed for frozen section analysis.

The reconstruction is accomplished by first sewing either the remnant of false cord mucosa or the lateral aspect of the floor of the ventricle to the external perichondrium at the corresponding level of the remaining thyroid cartilage. The stitch should be placed to reposition the anterior commissure into normal position if necessary. There have been numerous reports

---

*References 27, 31, 39, 91, 97, 145, 147, 150.

TABLE 102-8

LOCAL RECURRENCE VS T STAGE AFTER SUPRAGLOTTIC LARYNGECTOMY

Author	T_1	LR T_1	LR T_1 (%)	T_2	LR T_2	LRT$_2$ (%)	T_3	LR T_3	LRT$_3$ (%)	T_4	LR T_4	LRT$_4$ (%)
Bocca and others[19]	59	5	9	296	38	13	46	8	17	28	7	25
Burstein and Calcaterra[27]	3	0	0	20	3	15	16	1	6	1	0	0
Lee and others[91]	3	0	0	32	0	0	21	0	0	4	0	0
Alonso and others[1]	167	16	10				42	19	45	22	13	59
Spaulding and others[150]	4	0	0	16	0	0	4	3	75	9	6	67
Herranz-Gonzales and others[48]	37	3	8	55	2	4	8	0	0	10	1	10

LR, local recurrence.

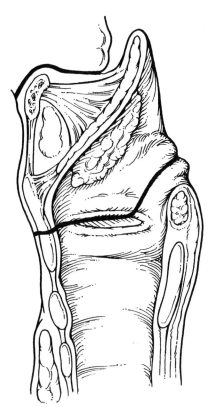

Figure 102-13. Supraglottic laryngectomy—superior to inferior of the false cord, to the level of the ventricle, anterior to the arytenoids.

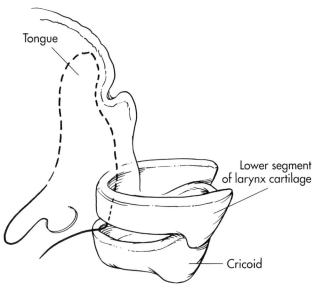

Figure 102-14. Supraglottic laryngectomy—laryngoplasty performed with three closure stitches circumferentially around the inferior half of the thyroid cartilage and submucosally into the tongue base, as is done in the supracricoid partial laryngectomies.

in the literature on various techniques for closure and laryngoplasty after supraglottic laryngectomy.[62,101,119] The technique the authors use is similar to the closure used in supracricoid laryngectomy. The concept is to provide mucosa-to-mucosa closure while creating a prominence of tongue-base tissue right over the central aspect of the larynx and the laryngeal inlet. This is done by passing stitches submucosally deep into the tongue base. Three 1-0 Vicryl stitches are used as in supracricoid laryngectomy (Figure 102-14). The first stitch is place circumferentially around the remnant of the thyroid cartilage, taking care to remain submucosal and to not damage the anterior commissure. The stitch then is arched high up around the hyoid and submucosally deep into the tongue base, using the entire circumference of the needle. Two additional stitches are placed 1 cm lateral; again care is taken to pass the stitches around the entire circumference of the remaining inferior thyroid ala, subperichondrially on the internal surface of the thyroid cartilage, so that the thyroarytenoid musculature is not tethered by the stitch. Each of these stitches is passed around the hyoid bone, if it is present, and submucosally deep into the tongue base. The two lateral stitches are held tight by the assistant while the central stitch is tied down. The two lateral stitches then are tied. The

periosteum with the overlying inferior strap muscle flap is sewn superiorly to the suprahyoid musculature. The skin flaps are closed, with special care to separate the tracheostomy site from the remainder of the neck wound with a semicircular running 3-0 Vicryl stitch placed subcutaneously in the upper flap to the strap muscles above the tracheostomy site.

Key surgical points

1. The authors locate the main trunk of the internal and external branches of the superior laryngeal nerve routinely at the time of bilateral modified neck dissection (Figure 102-15). This is accomplished by dissection of the fat pad, which is anterior to the carotid artery, inferior to the hypoglossal nerve, and lateral to the superior laryngeal nerves. The superior thyroid artery runs through this fat pad and is transected proximally and distally to perform this dissection. This procedure also requires removal of the lymphatics, which travel adjacent to the larynx, allowing the main trunk of the superior laryngeal nerves to be spared bilaterally.

2. The superior aspects of the pyriform sinus are dissected from the inner aspect of thyroid cartilage when they are not involved by the malignancy.

3. The superior aspects of the arytenoid are spared, unless the malignancy is directly involving this area.

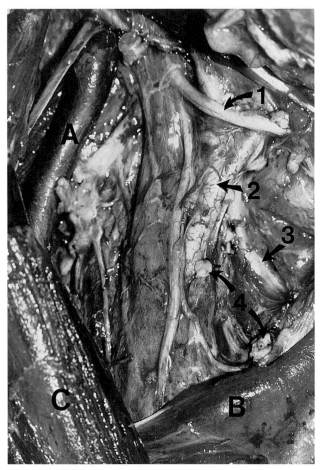

Figure 102-15. Superior laryngeal lymph node dissection—exposure of the superior laryngeal nerve at the time of modified neck dissection. **A,** Internal jugular vein; **B,** omohyoid muscle; **C,** sternocleidomastoid muscle. *1,* hypoglossal nerve; *2,* carotid artery; *3,* superior laryngeal nerve; *4,* transected proximal and distal ends of the superior thyroid artery.

4. The hyoid bone is not spared when the malignancy involves the vallecula or tongue base.
5. The greater cornua of the hyoid is resected in those with marginal lesions.
6. The tongue base sutures are placed in the midline and 1 cm off of the midline, avoiding damaging the hypoglossal nerves and the lingual arteries.

Extended procedures. There are two basic extensions of the supraglottic laryngectomy, including: (1) resection of one arytenoid or the upper part of the pyriform sinus; and (2) resection of a portion of the tongue base.[19] Modifications of the standard procedures can be accomplished systematically by the following two approaches.

Arytenoid, aryepiglottic fold, or superior medial pyriform involvement from supraglottic carcinoma. Skeletonize the hyoid bone, and free up the lateral cor-

nua of the hyoid if it is to be resected. Only free up the internal thyroid perichondrium on the uninvolved side. Enter the endolarynx through the vallecula on the uninvolved side or through the thyrotomy inferiorly if the vallecula is involved. Cut anterior to the uninvolved arytenoid and through the false cord. Bring the resection around the upper pyriform on the involved side, which is transected at the level of the ipsilateral true vocal cord. When the pharyngoepiglottic fold is involved, resect a generous margin of the posterior tonsillar pillar and a portion of the ipsilateral tongue base. If the posterior tonsillar pillar and tongue base have been unilaterally resected, close this portion of the defect separately, taking care to advance the tongue base posteriorly. Close the tongue base with three large stitches.

Base of tongue extension from supraglottic carcinoma. Enter inferiorly through the thyrotomy. Do not skeletonize the hyoid bone. If necessary, free up the twelfth nerves and move them out of the line of resection. Cut above the hyoid bone and do not skeletonize. Make the tongue base resection under direct visualization from below with a 2-cm margin. The resection should leave at least 1 cm of tongue base posterior to the circumvallate papillae to allow for adequate function postoperatively. The closure is with the submucosal tongue base sutures.

Functional outcome. Although there is some variability in vocal quality after supraglottic laryngectomy combined with radiotherapy, among patients who have undergone decannulation within the first three postoperative weeks, microstrobolaryngoscopic findings reveal normal vibration of the cords and normal vibration amplitudes, and results of sonographic evaluations are normal, with some abnormalities related to removal of the resonance space above the cords.[124] One study, which assessed the subjective voice qualities, found that 87% of patients had normal-to-mild breathiness and that 67% had mild or no evidence of hoarseness.[71]

The stages of wound healing and stabilization may take months, although a reasonable measure of progression of swallowing rehabilitation, in the literature, has been the point at which the patient no longer relies on tube feedings for nutrition. Hirano and others[50] noted that 84% (32 of 38) of patients had removal of the nasogastric tube within 30 days postoperatively, whereas some patients required tube feeding for 3 months. Padovan and Oreskovic[124] noted that complete rehabilitation takes at least 3 months, and this may be prolonged in irradiated patients. The factors that Hirano and others[50] found to be significantly related to duration of nasogastric intubation were extent of removal of the arytenoid and asymmetric removal of the false cords, whereas resection of the hyoid and tongue base was not related to swallowing outcome. Flores and others[42] also noted that arytenoid resection was associated with failure to attain swallowing function and that resection of the hyoid and tongue base did not worsen swallowing outcome. Although Flores and others[42] could not find a significant correlation between transection of one vs two superior laryngeal nerves and swallowing outcome, it is interesting to note that all nine patients who failed to swallow had at least one superior laryngeal nerve resected, and there were no patients in this series with the nerves spared bilaterally with which to make a comparison. Although Padovan also agreed that arytenoid preservation is important in swallowing outcome, his group stressed the importance of bilateral preservation of the superior laryngeal nerve to achieve timely swallowing function.[124] This nerve can be visualized after modified neck dissection, and when the pyriform sinus is not involved by the malignancy, the main trunks of the internal and external branches of the superior laryngeal nerve frequently can be spared bilaterally. Staple and Ogura,[151] in a cineradiographic study of 36 patients who had undergone supraglottic laryngectomy, emphasized the association of impaired neuromotor function of the tongue through the hypoglossal nerves and significant degrees of aspiration.

Impaired swallowing function has been associated with extended supraglottic laryngectomy.[42,91,135] The literature was reviewed, and the results from series that assessed the extreme adverse outcomes of permanent gastrostomy, functional laryngectomy, and death resulting from aspiration pneumonia were tabulated in Table 102-5. The series of patients undergoing supraglottic laryngectomy without extended procedures[48,147] seem to be less likely to undergo functional laryngectomy compared with the series that included extended procedures.

Complications. The reported fistula rate after supraglottic laryngectomy has been 0% to 12.5%.[27] Other reported complications, reported in large series, include aspiration pneumonia (0%–10.8%),[8,136] inability to decannulate the tracheostomy (0%–5.5%),[27,48] and tracheocutaneous fistula.[147]

Supracricoid laryngectomy with cricohyoidopexy.

Oncologic results. Supraglottic carcinomas that are not amenable to supraglottic laryngectomy because of glottic level involvement either through the anterior commissure or the ventricle, preepiglottic space invasion, decreased cord mobility, or limited thyroid cartilage invasion frequently will be resectable with supracricoid laryngectomy with cricohyoidopexy.

These lesions are not rare, and in one study, the incidence of spread of supraglottic carcinoma to the glottic level was between 20% and 54% in the literature.[175] Glottic level invasion should be suspected when there is either impaired cord mobility or extension of carcinoma to the ventricle.[175] In a series of selected supraglottic carcinomas, Laccourreye and others[75] found there were no local recurrences in 68 patients (T$_1$, 1; T$_2$, 40; T$_3$, 26; and T$_4$, 1) with a minimum follow-up period of 18 months. Laccourreye and others[78] later reported on 19 patients with gross pathologic invasion of the preepiglottic space, with a minimum of follow-up period of 5 years, and noted a local control of 94.4% (18 of 19). Chevalier and Piquet[30] reported on their series of 61 consecutive cases of supraglottic carcinoma managed with supracricoid laryngectomy with cricohyoidopexy and noted a local recurrence rate of 3.3% (2 of 61). They attributed the oncologic success to the en bloc resection of the bilateral paraglottic spaces, the preepiglottic space, and the entire thyroid cartilage. Contraindications to the procedure include: (1) subglottic extension >10 mm anteriorly and 5 mm posteriorly because of the potential for cricoid cartilage involvement; (2) arytenoid fixation; (3) massive preepiglottic space invasion with involvement of the vallecula; (4) extension to the pharyngeal wall, vallecula, base of tongue, postcricoid region, and interarytenoid region; and (5) cricoid cartilage invasion.[75]

Surgical technique.[75] The approach and many of the steps are the same as in supracricoid laryngectomy with cricohyoidoepiglottopexy, although in this procedure, the entire epiglottis and preepiglottic space is resected. A U-shaped incision is made in line with the tracheostomy site, which will be placed later in the case, and the superior flap is elevated to approximately 2 cm above the hyoid bone, exposing the underlying strap muscles. The incision is made up to the mastoid tip to accommodate the bilateral modified neck dissections that are done in the case of supraglottic carcinoma. The sternothyroid and the thyrohyoid muscles are transected individually from medial to lateral, along the superior aspect of the thyroid cartilage. The thyrohyoid muscle is elevated inferiorly, allowing for the exposure of the thyroid muscle. As in supracricoid laryngectomy with cricohyoidoepiglottopexy, there is a blood vessel that pierces the deep strap musculature to the more superficial layer, which needs to be ligated bilaterally. The sternothyroid muscle then is carefully transected along the inferior edge of the thyroid cartilage. Care is taken not to cut the underlying thyroid gland, which will cause undue bleeding and obscure the surgical field. The constrictor muscles then are transected along the posterior and superior–lateral aspect of the thyroid cartilage, and the pyriform sinus mucosa is elevated off of the internal surface of the thyroid cartilage bilaterally, as is done in total laryngectomy. A Freer elevator is used to disarticulate the cricoarytenoid joint bilaterally, taking care to protect the recurrent laryngeal nerves. The recurrent laryngeal nerves are never actually visualized, although the area posterior and lateral to the inferior cornua of the thyroid cartilage is respected and avoided. The isthmus of the thyroid gland is transected and ligated. A blunt finger dissection of the cervicomediastinal trachea is done to the level of the carina, as is done in a tracheal resection and anastomosis to close the tracheal defect. A transverse cricothyrotomy is performed just above the cricoid cartilage, and the endotracheal tube is removed from above and placed into the cricothyrotomy. Now, rather than entering the larynx through a transverse transepiglottic laryngotomy and transecting the epiglottis as is done in supracricoid laryngectomy with cricohyoidoepiglottopexy, the authors resect the entire epiglottis and preepiglottic space. To do this, the superior aspect of the transected sternothyroid and sternohyoid muscles are elevated off of the thyrohyoid membrane. The upper aspect of the preepiglottic space is dissected off of the inferior aspect of the hyoid bone with an electrocautery unit. The dissection is done medially to create an opening in the vallecula just large enough to allow the epiglottis to be pulled externally and grasped with an Allis clamp. One scissor blade is placed in the endolaryngeal lumen, and one blade is placed externally. The cut is made in a superior-to-inferior direction to allow for resection of the entire preepiglottic space, although the cut is made medial to the main trunk of the internal branch of the superior laryngeal nerve to keep this intact. The scissors are advanced with one blade in the lumen and the other between the elevated internal thyroid perichondrium and the thyroid cartilage. This cut is made anterior to the pyriform sinus, which remains intact posteriorly.

The endolaryngeal excision now is performed on the non–tumor-bearing side first, in the same fashion as in supracricoid laryngectomy with cricohyoidoepiglottopexy. The incision is brought down, in the sagittal plane, with a scissor blade at the junction between the false cord and arytenoid. The transection is carried inferiorly just posterior to the ventricle and then through the vocal process of the arytenoid. Special care is taken to avoid entering the cricoarytenoid joint with the scissors, avoiding cricoarytenoid ankylosis. Just above the cricoid cartilage, the orientation of the scissors changes to allow connection of this incision, through the cricothyroid muscle, to the previously made cricothyrotomy. The larynx is opened up on its anterior spine like a book, which allows for direct visualization of the lesion (Figure 102-16). The cut on the tumor-bearing side may be made just posterior to the ventricle or may transect all or part of the arytenoid cartilage. This can be done by cutting the subglottic mucosa with a No. 15 blade and following posteriorly and superiorly to the level of the arytenoid. The posterior arytenoid mucosa should be spared to be used in the endolaryngeal reconstruction and to cover the cricoarytenoid joint area on the cricoid. This forms a cushion, postoperatively, against which the remaining arytenoid will abut to allow for closure of the larynx. The patient will have severe swallowing impairment postoperatively unless this posterior arytenoid mucosa is spared.

The reconstruction is begun by pulling the arytenoid cartilages forward with 3-0 Vicryl suture material by placing a stitch just at or just above the vocal process and sewing them (or the posterior arytenoid mucosa in unilateral arytenoid resection) anterolaterally to the cricoid cartilage. In this way, the arytenoid will not prolapse backward postoperatively. The impaction of the cricoid to the hyoid is performed with three centrally placed 2-0 Vicryl sutures on a 65-mm round needle. The first stitch is place circumferentially, submucosally around the cricoid cartilage, in the midline. The stitch is placed submucosally in

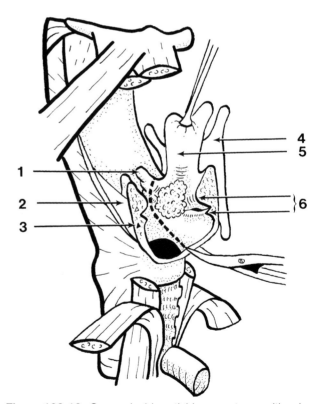

Figure 102-16. Supracricoid partial laryngectomy with cricohyoidopexy—exposure of malignancy. *1,* Arytenoid; *2,* external thyroid perichondrium; *3,* vocal process; *4,* thyroid cartilage; *5,* epiglottis; *6,* false and true cord.

the subglottis. Next, the same first stitch is passed up around the hyoid bone and deep into the tongue base. This large needle allows the suture to be passed deeply into the tongue base, submucosally, while it is carefully palpated with a finger on the tongue base mucosa, to pull it back and have a bulge of tongue base tissue over the airway postoperatively (Figure 102-17). A self-release needle should not be used, because it may become embedded in the tongue base muscula-

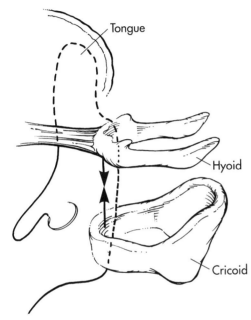

Figure 102-17. Supracricoid partial laryngectomy with cricohyoidopexy—laryngoplasty using three circumferential cricoid, hyoid, and tongue base stitches.

ture. Before tightening the sutures, the two lateral sutures are pulled taut, which places the trachea in its postoperative position, and the tracheostomy is performed in line with the skin incision. With the two lateral cricohyoidoepiglottopexy sutures under tension, the central pexy stitch is tied, followed by the two lateral stitches. The strap muscles are closed as a second layer closure with 3-0 Vicryl. A cuffed tracheostomy tube is put into place. The skin wound is closed in two layers, taking special care to separate the tracheostomy site from the remainder of the wound, with a subcutaneous stitch placed between the skin and the underlying strap muscles above the tracheostomy site.

Key surgical points. The key surgical points are the same as those in supracricoid laryngectomy with cricohyoidoepiglottopexy.

Extended procedures. The extension of the basic technique, as in supracricoid laryngectomy with cricohyoidoepiglottopexy, is the resection of one arytenoid.[75]

Functional outcome. When the world literature is analyzed, variability was noted in the duration of tube feedings with a range from 13 days[78] to 365 days (Table 102-9).[20] The percent of patients undergoing functional laryngectomy for intractable aspiration varied from 0% to 10.8% (see Table 102-9). In the large series, with more than 65 patients analyzed, the need for functional laryngectomy remained <5%, which may indicate that experience is of value in achieving successful functional results.[73,75,130] Dysphagia is more common after supracricoid laryngectomy with cricohyoidopexy when one arytenoid is resected.[30,76] Success in postoperative swallowing results has been

TABLE 102-9				
FUNCTIONAL OUTCOME AFTER SUPRACRICOID LARYNGECTOMY WITH CRICOHYOIDOPEXY				
Author	**Patients**	**Duration NG**	**Func Laryn**	**Func Laryn (%)**
Labayle and Dahan[73]	101	?	3	3.0
Piquet and others[129]	72	?	3	4.2
Alajmo and others[1]	17	?	1	5.9
Botazzi[20]	21	20–365	2	9.5
Pech and others[126]	32	33*	2	6.3
Prades and others[133]	29	30*	1	3.4
Marandas and others[99]	57	34*	4	7.0
Junien-Lavillauroy and others[56]	37	33*	4	10.8
Laccourreye and others[84]	68	13–70	0	0.0
Traissac and Verhulst[156]	25	20–56	3	12.0
Laccourreye and others[80]	19	13–29	0	0.0
Maurice and others[100]	43	17–120	1	2.3

Func laryn, functional laryngectomy for aspiration; *NG,* nasogastric tube.
*Average duration.

attributed to careful attention to preoperative patient selection, intraoperative technique, and postoperative rehabilitation.[80]

The duration and frequency characteristics of normal speakers was compared with 14 patients who had undergone supracricoid laryngectomy with cricohyoidopexy.[81] The findings in that study revealed that although the average F_0 among the supracricoid laryngectomy group was within normal range, the operated group was significantly less efficient in jitter, shimmer, maximum phonation time, and phase grouping.[81] The authors attributed these findings to the instability of the neoglottis, resulting from the wide surgical resection and the fact that the neoglottis allows for air escape during phonation.

Complications. Among the extremely rare complications reported in the literature are rupture of the cricohyoidopexy,[77] pneumonia caused by severe gastroesophageal reflux,[76] chondroradionecrosis,[78] and glottic stenosis.[78]

ORGAN PRESERVATION SURGERY SPECTRUM FOR GLOTTIC AND SUPRAGLOTTIC CANCER

Organ laryngeal preservation surgery is based on three fundamental keys. The surgeon needs to be able make an accurate assessment of the patient as a surgical candidate, be able to accurately assess the origin and extent of the lesion, and have a thorough understanding of the available surgical techniques and preoperative issues. Figures 102-18 and 102-19 are schematic representations of the surgical disease spectrum of glottic and supraglottic carcinomas, respectively.[173] Below the schematics are a number of possible variables that are important clinical factors that have a bearing on the application of organ preservation surgery of the larynx. There are representative examples of carcinomas from the smallest on the left to the largest on the right. Every other schematic is blank, enabling the surgeon to consider placement of a lesion in its appropriate space designating the appropriate organ preservation surgeries available. This schematic allows the surgeon to formulate an organ preservation surgical plan by comparing the tumor to known lesions while accounting for certain key organ preservation variables. It is meant to be used as a helpful teaching aid in learning the concepts of organ preservation surgery for larynx cancer.

Intraoperative Conversion to Total Laryngectomy

Accurate preoperative staging is critical to avoid intraoperative conversion to total laryngectomy, including an accurate prediction of the surface extension and the depth of invasion. In general, the problem occurs when there are close margins intraoperatively that necessitate resection of structures that are needed for the postoperative functional reconstruction. Whole organ section studies reveal that deep and superficial lesions are commonly surrounded by a penumbra of microinvasion carcinoma, carcinoma in situ, and dysplasia.[45] Deep invasion is best appreciated preoperatively during the clinical evaluation, which includes visualization of mobility, palpation during direct laryngoscopy, and radiologic studies. The surface invasion is best evaluated by indirect and direct endoscopy. The penumbra of surface changes surrounding the deeply invasive carcinoma may be particularly difficult to assess clinically because of natural tendency to focus on the obvious cancer during endoscopy and because of the difficulty in assessing subtle mucosal changes on a mucosal surface, which is tangential to direct vision with the naked eye or the microscope. If either subtle granularity or erythema is noted in a critical area on the mucosal surface that would obviate the conservation technique that is contemplated, it should undergo microscopic biopsy at the time of endoscopy. The authors do not perform random microscopic biopsies of normal-appearing mucosa, because the excoriations of these sites may lead to confusion at the time of the definitive resection.

One area that results in conversion to total laryngectomy when dealing with supraglottic laryngectomy is extension to the glottic level. In the past, it has been suggested that supraglottic carcinoma rarely, if ever, extended to the glottic level. A recent analysis of whole organ sections of laryngeal carcinoma and a literature review have revealed that the true incidence of glottic level extension from the supraglottis is between 20% and 54%.[175] The most common route of extension is the paraglottic space. Surgeons relying on the previously held assumption that the carcinoma is unlikely to extend to the glottis, regardless of the proximity of the cancer to the glottis, may need to convert to total laryngectomy in 25% of patients.[69]

The area in glottic carcinoma for which involvement may result in intraoperative conversion to total laryngectomy is invasion of the cricoarytenoid joint. Fixation of the joint is an indication that the joint capsule, the joint itself, or the surrounding musculature is involved by carcinoma.[22] This should be fully assessed, and the joint involvement should be predicted to avoid the necessity of intraoperative conversion to total laryngectomy when performing either vertical partial laryngectomy or supracricoid laryngectomy.

The best approach to avoid intraoperative conversion to total laryngectomy is preoperative planning. The surgeon has a wide spectrum of conservative techniques available with consistent functional and oncologic outcome in the literature. The authors do

GLOTTIC ORGAN PRESERVATION SURGERY SPECTRUM

Patient Name _____ Medical Record Number _____ Date _____ Pathology _____ T__ N__ M__

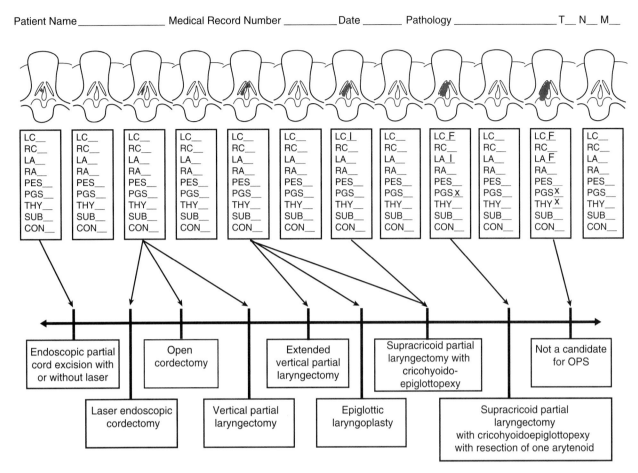

LC, left vocal cord mobility; RC, right vocal cord mobility; LA, left arytenoid mobility; RA, right arytenoid mobility; PES, preepiglottic space involvement; PGS, paraglottic space invasion; THY, early radiologic evidence of thyroid cartilage invasion; SUB, subglottic extension > 1cm at midcord, or > 0.5 cm posterior cord level; CON, tumor and nontumor contraindications. At the top of the form is the series of schematic diagrams of the larynx with additional descriptors in the text box below. At the bottom of the form is the spectrum of organ preservation surgeries that are applicable. Representative cancers are shown in a spectrum from least extensive on the left through most extensive on the right. The mucosal extent is documented on the schematic. Mobility is documented with either a "blank" for normal mobility, "I" for impaired mobility, and "F" for fixation. An "x" documents involvement of the preepiglottic space, paraglottic space, thyroid cartilage, and a tumor- or nontumor-related contraindication. This form may be used in surgical planning by drawing the lesion into a blank laryngeal schematic, in the appropiate place on the spectrum.

Figure 102-18. Glottic organ preservation surgery spectrum (From Weinstein and others: *Organ preservation surgery*).

not advocate conversion from one type of conservation laryngeal surgery intraoperatively to another to avoid total laryngectomy. In their opinion, this conversion will lead to poor oncologic and functional outcome. Rather, to avoid intraoperative conversion to total laryngectomy, the procedure of choice should be decided on preoperatively, and this should be the technique that affords the safest oncologic margins for that particular lesion. Nonetheless, the surgeon always should obtain consent from the patient for the possibility of intraoperative conversion to total laryngectomy, with the understanding that in rare instances,

removal of the entire larynx may be necessary. The patient who cannot accept this option is not a good candidate for conservation laryngeal surgery.

All patients undergoing attempts at conservation laryngeal surgery must give their consent for possible total laryngectomy. Careful preoperative planning can help to reduce the incidence of conversion to total laryngectomy. If the patient can't accept this possibility or if the surgeon feels that there is a distinct possibility for total laryngectomy, the patient should be encouraged to pursue an organ preservation medical strategy if appropriate.

SUPRAGLOTTIC ORGAN PRESERVATION SURGERY SPECTRUM

Patient Name_____ Medical Record Number _____ Date _____ Pathology _____ T__ N__ M__

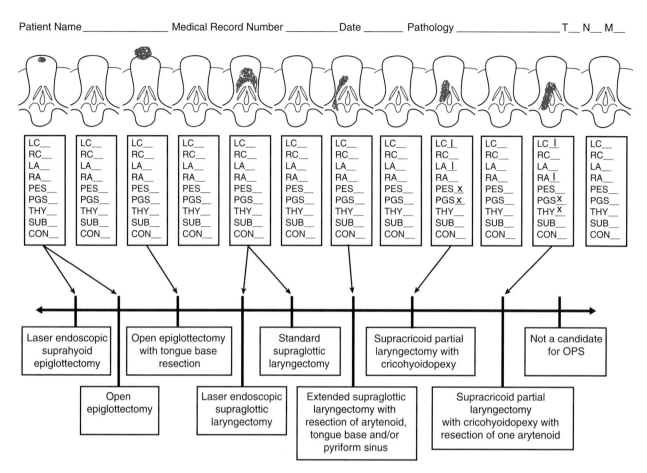

LC, left vocal cord mobility; RC, right vocal cord mobility; LA, left arytenoid mobility; RA, right arytenoid mobility; PES, preepiglottic space involvement; PGS, paraglottic space invasion; THY, early radiologic evidence of thyroid cartilage invasion; SUB, subglottic extension > 1cm at midcord, or > 0.5 cm posterior cord level; CON, tumor and nontumor contraindications. At the top of the form is a series of schematic diagrams of the larynx with additional descriptors in the text box below. At the bottom of the form is the spectrum of organ preservation surgeries that are applicable. Representative cancers are shown in a spectrum from least extensive on the left through most extensive on the right. The mucosal extent is documented on the schematic. Mobility is documented with either a "blank" for normal mobility, "I" for impaired mobility, and "F" for fixation. An "x" documents involvement of the preepiglottic space, paraglottic space, thyroid cartilage, and a tumor- or nontumor-related contraindication. This form may be used in surgical planning by drawing the lesion into a blank laryngeal schematic, in the appropiate place on the spectrum.

Figure 102-19. Supraglottic organ preservation surgery spectrum (From Weinstein et al: *Organ preservation surgery*).

Current Organ Preservation Paradigm for Laryngeal Cancer

The trial conducted by the Department of Veteran's Affairs Laryngeal Cancer Study Group 1991 compared induction chemotherapy (cisplatin plus fluorouracil) followed by radiation vs surgery (total laryngectomy) and radiation for advanced laryngeal cancer.[38] The conclusion from this study was that induction chemotherapy followed by radiation was able to preserve the larynx while not affecting survival. This provided an alternative to total laryngectomy for these patients with advanced laryngeal cancer. Recently, the Radiation Therapy Oncology Group (RTOG) Trial 91-11 was performed to examine the contributions of chemotherapy and radiation therapy to medical larynx-preserving regimens.[43] The conclusion from this study was that concurrent chemotherapy and radiation was superior to both induction chemotherapy followed by radiation and radiation alone for larynx preservation in patients with stage III and stage IV disease (T_2, T_3, or T_4 not extending to tongue base or through cartilage). The study states that radiation with concurrent cisplatin should be the standard of care for the above staged patients.

The study fails to recognize that organ preservation surgical strategies for laryngeal cancer have gained widespread acceptance throughout the last decade.* These strategies offer an alternative to concurrent cisplatin and radiation for similarly staged lesions (T_2, T_3, and selected T_4). The majority of the patients in the RTOG 91-11 trial were staged as T_3 tumors. Previously, the only surgical option available to most of these patients was a total laryngectomy. With the worldwide acceptance of organ preservation surgical approaches (in particular, supracricoid laryngectomy), these patients now have an established surgical alternative to concurrent cisplatin and radiation with defined oncologic and functional outcomes.†

It is incumbent upon all physicians caring for patients with laryngeal cancer to understand all of the available options for treatment. Correct staging is absolutely essential to this and requires an interpretation of dynamic laryngeal function that at present can only be made by direct examination of the larynx. This mandates the need for a head and neck surgeon's examination and interpretation of the larynx. The discussion held before treatment must include all organ-preservation approaches available for that patient's particular tumor. The ability of the patient to choose from these options allows for a tailoring of treatment that best suits the patient's needs and wishes. These options should be to the benefit of the patient with larynx cancer and should not be preferentially excluded.

Conservation Laryngeal Surgery and Radiotherapy

Essential differences exist between nonsurgical organ-sparing modalities vs conservation laryngeal surgery. In nonsurgical approaches, the clinician accepts that when treating those with larger lesions within the spectrum of malignancy that more patients will have local recurrence and rely on surgical salvage when possible, which frequently is total laryngectomy.[164] The advantage to this approach is that for the patients without local recurrence, the entire larynx is spared, and it is inferred that for those patients, the functional outcome is maximized. The approach of the conservation laryngeal surgeon is the opposite. When managing progressively larger lesions within the spectrum of malignancies, the procedure is chosen from the spectrum of conservation laryngeal procedures that then maximize local control while progressively removing more laryngeal tissue. The loss of functional anatomy usually manifests as permanent hoarseness when the glottis is resected

and as temporary dysphagia when the supraglottis is resected. Long-term severe dysphagia for conservation laryngeal surgery is rare (see Tables 102-4, 102-5, and 102-9). The conservation laryngeal approach to organ preservation accepts decreased laryngeal function for the entire population of patients to decrease the morbidity and mortality associated with local recurrence. The nonsurgical approach to organ preservation accepts the sequelae of local recurrence in an effort to preserve anatomic structure for selected patients.

Although functional outcome after conservation laryngeal surgery is well documented in the literature, this has not been the case of the nonsurgical organ-sparing regimens for intermediate-stage to high-stage lesions. Outcomes in terms of vocal quality, long-term dysphagia, reliance on long-term enteral feeding, and need for tracheostomy need to be evaluated in future studies for the nonsurgical approaches to verify that preservation of anatomic structure ensures improved functional outcome.

Surgical salvage with conservation laryngeal surgery has been well documented in the literature. Early diagnosis of failure after radiotherapy for laryngeal carcinoma often is difficult because of posttherapeutic edema, erythema, and changes in laryngeal mobilities.[166] This often leads to late discovery of the recurrence, leaving most patients who are eligible for surgical salvage needing to undergo total laryngectomy.[40,144] Patients with failure at the glottic level who were amenable to vertical hemilaryngectomy in the preradiation period and in whom the tumor has not enlarged may undergo the procedure and expect a local control rate of 83.3% (15 of 18).[9] Although in the DeSanto and others[40] series, 80% (24 of 30) of patients with supraglottic carcinoma who underwent radiotherapy and failed would have been theoretically amenable to supraglottic laryngectomy before radiotherapy, only 30% (9 of 30) underwent conservation laryngeal surgery for postradiation failure. Sorensen and others[149] reported poor oncologic and functional results after supraglottic laryngectomy for radiation failure and advocated total laryngectomy in these patients. Lavey and Calcaterra[90] have stated, after a review of the literature, that vertical hemilaryngectomy should be contraindicated in the radiation failure case if: (1) the tumor involves the arytenoid; (2) there is >10 mm of subglottic extension anteriorly and >5 mm posteriorly; and (3) cartilage invasion into the thyroid or the cricoid is present. Shaw[141] stated that supraglottic laryngectomy is contraindicated in the postradiation failure setting unless: (1) the primary tumor is small; (2) the recurrence is located anteriorly; and (3) the carcinoma has never involved the anterior commissure. One alternative

---

*References 21, 41, 86, 93, 142, 163.
†References 94, 112, 169–171, 174, 179.

for larger lesions is to use either supracricoid laryngectomy with cricohyoidopexy or cricohyoidoepiglottopexy as the salvage procedure, which has a reported local control of 83.3% (10 of 12).[85]

It seems that supracricoid laryngectomy may be ideally suited to treat early (T_1 and T_2) glottic radiation failures. The en bloc resection of the entire thyroid cartilage and its contents along with a significant portion of the anterior subglottic mucosa makes it particularly attractive in those with anterior commissure recurrences. Often, the only salvage modality offered to these patients is total laryngectomy. The role of supracricoid laryngectomy in salvage of glottic radiation failures will be explained as more institutions use the technique.

Management of metachronous primary tumors is an important consideration. Roberts and others[137] reported that the average annual risk for a second malignant neoplasm developing after a glottic carcinoma was 3.1% a year over the ensuing 10 years. Seventy-one percent of these second lesions occurred in the upper aerodigestive tract or in the lungs.[137] The physician also should consider the future management of second primary malignancies when planning treatment for the patient with primary cancer.

POSTOPERATIVE MANAGEMENT ISSUES

Although postsurgical management varies from institution to institution, the central issues generally center on the timing of tracheal decannulation and on the approach to swallowing rehabilitation. The authors will discuss their approach to these management issues. They deflate the tracheotomy tube as early as possible postoperatively. In the absence of contraindications such as ventilator dependence, the authors drop the tracheostomy cuff on day one. Second, they remove the tracheostomy early, and their first attempts at decannulation are between days 3 and 5. The tracheostomy should be kept in for prolonged periods if there is laryngeal edema or salivary stasis. As a rule, patients undergoing vertical partial laryngectomies or supracricoid laryngectomies can be decannulated sooner than those undergoing supraglottic laryngectomies. Swallowing rehabilitation is not begun until the tracheostomy is removed, the stoma is closed, and until the patient is swallowing his or her saliva. The larynx always should be visualized with indirect laryngoscopy before decannulation. If there are any ensuing airway problems, the tracheotomy tube should be immediately replaced. Although stridor is the sentinel sign of laryngeal airway impairment, other signs such as sweating or agitation should be carefully evaluated even in the absence of audible stridor. Finally, the speech pathologist is central to the speech and swallowing rehabilitation and is consulted early postoperatively.

SUMMARY

A spectrum of conservation laryngeal procedures are available that allow for management of the broad spectrum of laryngeal carcinomas. The vertical partial laryngectomy, supraglottic laryngectomy, and supracricoid laryngectomy are accepted worldwide with established oncologic and functional outcomes. No single surgical approach is a panacea, and a conservation laryngeal surgeon may only perform a few of each technique to manage a large number of laryngeal carcinomas. Accurate understanding of the anatomy and physiology of the larynx and the behavior of neoplasm in a particular site is necessary to assess the three-dimensional extent of the malignancy preoperatively. A thorough understanding of the whole organ section literature is paramount for success in conservation laryngeal surgery. The conservation laryngeal surgeon uses a variety of surgical approaches to allow for the preservation of a functional larynx. The functional goals of conservation laryngeal surgery are speech and swallowing without a permanent tracheostomy. The acute functional sequelae vary but typically include temporary dysphagia and a tracheostomy. Among the procedures that have gained acceptance in multiple centers, including vertical hemilaryngectomy, supraglottic laryngectomy, and supracricoid laryngectomy, the rate of severe dysphagia requiring functional laryngectomy for aspiration has been low. The most common long-term functional sequela of conservation laryngeal surgery is hoarseness. If the choice of surgical procedure is based on sound principles gleaned from large series of patients reported in the literature, successful oncologic results in terms of local control are attainable. Open surgical approaches for laryngeal preservation afford the surgeon the opportunity to perform laryngoplasty to maximize functional outcome.

REFERENCES

1. Alajmo E and others: Conservation surgery for cancer of the larynx in the elderly, *Laryngoscope* 95:203, 1985.
2. Alonso JM: Conservative surgery of the larynx, *Trans Am Acad Ophthalmol Otolaryngol* 51:633, 1947.
3. Alonso JM: La chirurgie conservatrice pour le cancer du larynx et de l'hypopharynx, *Ann Otolaryngol Chir Cervicofac* 67:567, 1950.
4. Archer CR and others: Computed tomography of the larynx, *J Comput Assist Tomogr* 2:404, 1978.
5. Archer CR, Yeager VL: Computed tomography of laryngeal cancer with histopathological correlation, *Laryngoscope* 92:1173, 1982.
6. Bailey B, Calcaterra TC: Vertical, subtotal laryngectomy and laryngoplasty, *Arch Otolaryngol* 93:232, 1971.
7. Becker M and others: Neoplastic invasion of the laryngeal cartilage: comparison of MR imaging and CT with histopathologic correlation, *Radiology* 194:661, 1995.

8. Beckhardt RN and others: Factors influencing functional outcome in supraglottic laryngectomy, *Head Neck* 16:232, 1994.

9. Biller HF and others: Hemilaryngectomy following radiation failure for carcinoma of the vocal cords, *Laryngoscope* 80:249, 1970.

10. Biller HF, Ogura JH, Pratt LL: Hemilaryngectomy for T2 glottic cancers, *Arch Otolaryngol* 93:238, 1971.

11. Biller HF and others: Decreasing limitations of partial laryngectomy for vocal cord cancer, *Can J Otolaryngol* 4:432, 1975.

12. Biller HF, Lawson W: Bilateral vertical partial laryngectomy for bilateral vocal cord carcinoma, *Ann Otol Rhinol Laryngol* 90:489, 1981.

13. Biller HF, Lawson W: Partial laryngectomy for transglottic cancers, *Ann Otol Rhinol Laryngol* 93:297, 1984.

14. Biller HF, Lawson W: Partial laryngectomy for vocal cord cancer with marked limitation or fixation of the vocal cord, *Laryngoscope* 96:61, 1986.

15. Biller HF, Som ML: Vertical partial laryngectomy for glottic carcinoma with posterior subglottic extension, *Ann Otol Rhinol Laryngol* 86:715, 1977.

16. Blaugrund SM and others: Voice analysis of the partially ablated larynx. A preliminary report, *Ann Otol Rhinol Laryngol* 93:311, 1984.

17. Bocca E: Supraglottic laryngectomy and functional neck dissection, Section of Laryngology, Royal Society of Medicine, 1966.

18. Bocca E: Limitations of supraglottic laryngectomy and conservative neck dissection, *Can J Otolaryngol* 4:403, 1975.

19. Bocca E and others: Extended supraglottic laryngectomy. Review of 84 cases, *Ann Otol Rhinol Laryngol* 96:384, 1987.

20. Botazzi D: La laryngectomie subtotale reconstructive selon Labayle. Experience clinique sur 21 sujets, *Rev Laryngol* 107:207, 1986.

21. Brasnu DF: Supracricoid laryngectomy with cricohyoidopexy in the management of laryngeal carcinoma, *World J Surg* 27:817, 2003.

22. Brasnu D and others: False vocal cord reconstruction of the glottis following vertical partial laryngectomy: a preliminary analysis, *Laryngoscope* 102:717, 1992.

23. Brasnu D and others: Mobility of the vocal cord and arytenoid in squamous cell carcinoma of the larynx and hypopharynx: an anatomical and clinical comparative study, *Ear Nose Throat J* 69:324, 1990.

24. Bridger GP, Nassar VH: Cancer spread in the larynx, *Arch Otolaryngol* 95:497, 1972.

25. Broyles EN: The anterior commissure tendon, *Laryngoscope* (May):342, 1942.

26. Burgess LP, Yim DW: Thyroid cartilage flap reconstruction of the larynx following vertical partial laryngectomy: an interim report, *Laryngoscope* 98:605, 1988.

27. Burstein FD, Calcaterra TC: Supraglottic laryngectomy: series report and analysis of results, *Laryngoscope* 95:833, 1985.

28. Calcaterra TC: Bilateral omohyoid muscle flap reconstruction for anterior commissure cancer, *Laryngoscope* 97:810, 1987.

29. Cancer AJCO: *Manual for staging of cancer*, Philadelphia, 1988, JB Lippincott.

30. Chevalier D, Piquet JJ: Subtotal laryngectomy with cricohyoidopexy for supraglottic carcinoma: review of 61 cases, *Am J Surg* 168:472, 1994.

31. Coates HL and others: Carcinoma of the supraglottic larynx. A review of 221 cases, *Arch Otolaryngol* 102:686, 1976.

32. Conley JJ: The use of mucosal flaps for wound rehabilitation in partial laryngectomy, *Arch Otolaryngol* 700, 1959.

33. Crevier-Buchman L and others: Evolution of speech and voice following supracricoid partial laryngectomy, *J Laryngol Otol* 109:410, 1995.

34. Cummings C and others: *Atlas of laryngeal surgery*, St Louis, Mosby, 1984.

35. Daly JF: Limitations of cordectomy, *Can J Otolaryngol* 4:420, 1975.

36. Daly JF, Kwok FN: Laryngofissure and cordectomy, *Laryngoscope* 85:1290, 1975.

37. Dayal VS, Bahri H, Stone PC: The preepiglottic space. An anatomic study, *Arch Otolaryngol* 95:130, 1972.

38. The Department of Veteran's Affairs Laryngeal Cancer Study Group: Induction chemotherapy plus radiation compared with surgery plus radiation in patients with advanced laryngeal cancer, *N Engl J Med* 324:1685, 1991.

39. DeSanto LW: Cancer of the supraglottic larynx: a review of 260 patients, *Otolaryngol Head Neck Surg* 93:705, 1985.

40. DeSanto LW and others: Surgical salvage after radiation for laryngeal cancer, *Laryngoscope* 86:649, 1976.

41. de Vincentiis M and others: Supracricoid partial laryngectomies: oncologic and functional results, *Head Neck* 20:504, 1998.

42. Flores TC and others: Factors in successful deglutition following supraglottic laryngeal surgery, *Ann Otol Rhinol Laryngol* 91:579, 1982.

43. Forastiere AA and others: Concurrent chemotherapy and radiotherapy for organ preservation in advanced laryngeal cancer, *N Engl J Med* 349:2091, 2003.

44. Friedman WH and others: Contralateral laryngoplasty after supraglottic laryngectomy with vertical extension, *Arch Otolaryngol* 107:742, 1981.

45. Glanz HK: Carcinoma of the larynx. Growth, p-classification and grading of squamous cell carcinoma of the vocal cords, *Adv Otorhinolaryngol* 32:1, 1984.

46. Guerrier B and others: Our experience in reconstructive surgery in glottic cancers, *Ann Otolaryngol Chir Cervicofac* 104:175, 1987.

47. Harrison DF: Significance and means by which laryngeal cancer invades thyroid cartilage, *Ann Otol Rhinol Laryngol* 93:293, 1984.

48. Herranz-Gonzales J and others: Supraglottic laryngectomy: functional and oncologic results, *Ann Otol Rhinol Laryngol* 105:18, 1996.

49. Hirano M, Kurita S, Matsuoka H: Vocal function following hemilaryngectomy, *Ann Otol Rhinol Laryngol* 96:586, 1987.

50. Hirano M and others: Deglutition following supraglottic horizontal laryngectomy, *Ann Otol Rhinol Laryngol* 96:7, 1987.

51. Hirano M and others: Posterior glottis morphological study in excised human larynges, *Ann Otol Rhinol Laryngol* 95:576, 1986.

52. Hirano M and others: Vocal fold fixation in laryngeal carcinomas, *Acta Otolaryngol (Stockh)* 111:449, 1991.

53. Huet PC: Cancer de l'epiglotte. Hyo-thyro-epiglottectomie, *Ann Otolaryngol Chir Cervicofac* 2:1052, 1938.

54. Iwai H: Limitations of conservation surgery in carcinoma involving the arytenoid, *Can J Otolaryngol* 4:434, 1975.

55. Johnson JT and others: Outcome of open surgical therapy for glottic carcinoma, *Ann Otol Rhinol Laryngol* 102:752, 1993.

56. Junien-Lavillauroy C and others: La crico-hyoido-pexie. Resultants preliminaires et indications therapeutiques (A propos de 41 cas.), *JFORL* 37:3, 1988.

57. Kaiser TN, Sessions DG, Harvey JE: Natural history of treated T1N0 squamous carcinoma of the glottis, *Ann Otol Rhinol Laryngol* 98:217, 1988.

58. Kambic V, Radsel Z, Smid L: Laryngeal reconstruction with epiglottis after vertical hemilaryngectomy, *J Laryngol Otol* 90:467, 1976.

59. Katsantonis GP and others: The degree to which accuracy of preoperative staging of laryngeal carcinoma has been enhanced by computed tomography, *Otolaryngol Head Neck Surg* 95:52, 1986.

60. Kessler DJ and others: The treatment of T$_3$ glottic carcinoma with vertical partial laryngectomy, *Arch Otolaryngol Head Neck Surg* 113:1196, 1987.

61. Kikinis R and others: Larynx: MR imaging at 2.35 T. *Radiology* 171:165, 1989.

62. Kirchner JA: Closure after supraglottic laryngectomy, *Laryngoscope* 89:1343, 1979.

63. Kirchner JA: Invasion of the framework by laryngeal cancer, *Acta Otolaryngol (Stockh)* 97:392, 1984.

64. Kirchner JA: One hundred laryngeal cancers studied by serial section, *Laryngoscope* 78:689, 1969.

65. Kirchner JA: Pathways and pitfalls in partial laryngectomy, *Ann Otol Rhinol Laryngol* 93:301, 1984.

66. Kirchner JA: Two hundred laryngeal cancers: patterns of growth and spread as seen in serial section, *Laryngoscope* 87:474, 1977.

67. Kirchner JA, Carter D: Intralaryngeal barriers to the spread of cancer, *Acta Otolaryngol (Stockh)* 103:503, 1987.

68. Kirchner J, Som ML: The anterior commissure technique of partial laryngectomy: clinical and laboratory observations, *Laryngoscope* 85:1308, 1975.

69. Kirchner JA, Som ML: Clinical and histological observations on supraglottic cancer, *Ann Otol* 80:638, 1971.

70. Kirchner JA, Som ML: Clinical significance of fixed vocal cord, *Laryngoscope* 81:1029, 1971.

71. Klein AD and others: Rehabilitation of partial laryngectomy patients, *Trans Am Acad Ophthalmol Otolaryngol* 84:324, 1977.

72. Labayle J: Laryngectomie totale avec reconstruction, *Ann Otolaryngol Chir Cervicofac* 88:219, 1971.

73. Labayle J, Dahan S: Reconstructive laryngectomy (author's translation), *Ann Otolaryngol Chir Cervicofac* 98:587, 1981.

74. Laccourreye H and others: Supracricoid hemilaryngopharyngectomy: analysis of 240 cases, *Ann Otol Rhinol Laryngol* 96:217, 1987.

75. Laccourreye H and others: Supracricoid laryngectomy with cricohyoidoepiglottopexy: a partial laryngeal procedure for glottic carcinoma, *Ann Otol Rhinol Laryngol* 99:421, 1990.

76. Laccourreye H and others: Supracricoid laryngectomy with cricohyoidopexy: a partial laryngeal procedure for selected supraglottic and transglottic carcinomas, *Laryngoscope* 100:735, 1990.

77. Laccourreye O, Brasnu D, Weinstein G: Ruptured pexy following supracricoid laryngectomy, *Ann Otol Rhinol Laryngol* (in press).

78. Laccourreye O and others: Cricohyoidopexy in selected infrahyoid epiglottic carcinomas presenting with pathological preepiglottic space invasion, *Arch Otolaryngol Head Neck Surg* 119:881, 1993.

79. Laccourreye O and others: A clinical trial of continuous cisplatin-fluorouracil induction chemotherapy and supracricoid partial laryngectomy for glottic carcinoma classified as T$_2$, *Cancer* 74:2781, 1994.

80. Laccourreye O and others: Deglutition and partial supracricoid laryngectomies, *Ann Otolaryngol Chir Cervicofac* 109:73, 1992.

81. Laccourreye O and others: Duration and frequency characteristics of speech and voice following supracricoid partial laryngectomy, *Ann Otol Rhinol Laryngol* 104:516, 1995.

82. Laccourreye O and others: Editorial response, *Cancer* 76:149, 1995.

83. Laccourreye O and others: Extended supracricoid partial laryngectomy with tracheocricohyoidoepiglottopexy, *Acta Otolaryngol (Stockh)* 114:669, 1994.

84. Laccourreye O and others: Glottic carcinoma with a fixed true vocal cord: outcomes after neoadjuvant chemotherapy and supracricoid partial laryngectomy with cricohyoidoepiglottopexy, *Otolaryngol Head Neck Surg* 114:400, 1996.

85. Laccourreye O and others: Supracricoid partial laryngectomy after failed laryngeal radiation therapy, *Laryngoscope* 106:495, 1996.

86. Laccourreye O and others: Supracricoid partial laryngectomy with cricohyoidoepiglottopexy for "early" glottic carcinoma classified as T$_1$-T$_2$N$_0$ invading the anterior commissure, *Am J Otolaryngol* 18:385, 1997.

87. Laccourreye O and others: Vertical partial laryngectomy: a critical analysis of local recurrence, *Ann Otol Rhinol Laryngol* 100:68, 1991.

88. Lam KH: Extralaryngeal spread of cancer of the larynx: a study with whole-organ sections, *Head Neck Surg* 5:410, 1983.

89. Lam KH, Wong J: The preepiglottic and paraglottic spaces in relation to spread of carcinoma of the larynx, *Am J Otolaryngol* 4:81, 1983.

90. Lavey RS, Calcaterra TC: Partial laryngectomy for glottic cancer after high-dose radiotherapy, *Am J Surg* 162:341, 1991.

91. Lee NK and others: Supraglottic laryngectomy for intermediate-stage cancer: U.T. MD Anderson Cancer Center experience with combined therapy, *Laryngoscope* 100:831, 1990.

92. Lesinski SG, Bauer WC, Ogura JH: Hemilaryngectomy for T3 (fixed cord) epidermoid carcinoma of larynx, *Laryngoscope* 86:1563, 1976.

93. Levine PA and others: Management of advanced stage laryngeal cancer, *Otolaryngol Clin North Am* 30:101, 1997.

94. Lima RA and others: Supracricoid laryngectomy with CHEP: functional results and outcome, *Otolaryngol Head and Neck Surg* 124:258, 2001.

95. Liu C, Ward PH, Pleet L: Imbrication reconstruction following partial laryngectomy, *Ann Otol Rhinol Laryngol* 95:567, 1986.

96. Loevner L and others: Can MR accurately predict pre-epiglottic fat invasion, 81st Scientific Assembly and Annual Meeting of the Radiologic Society of North America, Chicago, 1995.

97. Lutz CK and others: Supraglottic carcinoma: patterns of recurrence, *Ann Otol Rhinol Laryngol* 99:12, 1990.

98. Majer H: Technique de laryngecomie permetant de conserver la permeabilite' respiratoire la cricohyoido-pexie, *Ann Otolaryngol Chir Cervicofac* 76:677, 1959.

99. Marandas P and others: Functional surgery in cancer of the laryngeal vestibule. Apropos of 149 cases treated at the Institut Gustave-Roussy, *Ann Otolaryngol Chir Cervicofac* 104:259, 1987.

100. Maurice N and others: Subtotal laryngectomy with cricohyoidopexy. Carcinologic results and early functional follow-up. Apropos of 49 cases, *Ann Otolaryngol Chir Cervicofac* 111:435, 1994.

101. Maves MD, Conley J, Baker DC: Laryngopharyngeal closure following supraglottic laryngectomy, *Laryngoscope* 88:1864, 1978.

102. McGavran MH, Bauer WC, Ogura JH: The incidence of cervical lymph node metastases from epidermoid carcinoma of the larynx and their relationship to certain characteristics of the primary tumor, *Cancer* 14:55, 1961.

103. McGavran MH, Spjut H, Ogura J: Laryngofissure in the treatment of laryngeal carcinoma. A critical analysis of success and failure, *Laryngoscope* 69:44, 1959.

104. Mendenhall WM and others: Stage T3 squamous cell carcinoma of the glottic larynx treated with surgery and/or radiation therapy, *Int J Radiat Oncol Biol Phys* 10:357, 1984.

105. Micheau CLB, Sancho H, Cachin Y: Modes of invasion of cancer of the larynx. A statistical, histological and radioclinical analysis of 120 cases, *Cancer* 38:346, 1976.

106. Mittal B, Marks JE, Ogura JH: Transglottic carcinoma, *Cancer* 53:151, 1984.

107. Mohr RM, Quenelle J, Shumrick DA: Vertico-frontolateral laryngectomy (hemilaryngectomy), *Arch Otolaryngol* 109:384, 1983.

108. Montgomery W: *Surgery of the upper respiratory system*, Philadelphia, 1989, Lea & Febiger.

109. Myers EN, Alvi A: Management of carcinoma of the supraglottic larynx: evolution, current concepts, and future trends, *Laryngoscope* 106:559, 1996.

110. Nagahara K and others: Laryngeal reconstruction by free flap transfer, *Plast Reconstr Surg* 57:604, 1976.

111. Nakayama M, Brandenburg JH: Clinical underestimation of laryngeal cancer, *Arch Otolaryngol Head Neck Surg* 119:950, 1993.

112. Naudo P and others: Complications and functional outcome after supracricoid partial laryngectomy with cricohyoidepiglottopexy, *Otolaryngol Head Neck Surg* 118:124, 1998.

113. Neel B, Devine DD, Desanto LW: Laryngofissure and cordectomy for early cordal carcinoma: outcome in 182 patients, *Otolaryngology Head Neck Surg* 88:79, 1980.

114. Nong HT and others: Epiglottic laryngoplasty after extended hemilaryngectomy for glottic cancer, *Chin Med J (Engl)* 103:925, 1990.

115. Nong HU and others: Epiglottic laryngoplasty after hemilaryngectomy for glottic cancer, *Otolaryngol Head Neck Surg* 104:809, 1991.

116. Norris CM: Role and limitation of vertical hemilaryngectomy, *Otolaryngol* 4:426, 1975.

117. Norris CM: Technique of extended fronto-lateral partial laryngectomy, *Laryngoscope* 68:1240, 1958.

118. Ogura JH: Conservation surgery for cancer of the pharynx and larynx: an evaluation, *Trans Pac Coast Otoophthalmol Soc Annu Meet* 44:215, 1963.

119. Ogura JH: Hyoid muscle flap reconstruction in subtotal supraglottic laryngectomy: a more rapid rehabilitation of deglutition, *Laryngoscope* 89:1522, 1979.

120. Ogura JH and others: Glottic reconstruction following subtotal glottic-supraglottic laryngectomy, *Laryngoscope* 75:865, 1965.

121. Olofsson J, Lord IJ, van Nostrand AWP: Vocal cord fixation in laryngeal carcinoma, *Acta Otolaryngol* 75:496, 1973.

122. Olszewski E: Vascularization of ossified cartilage and the spread of cancer in the larynx, *Arch Otolaryngol* 102:200, 1976.

123. Ossoff RH and others: Endoscopic management of selected early vocal cord carcinoma, *Ann Otol Rhinol Laryngol* 94:560, 1985.

124. Padovan IF, Oreskovic M: Functional evaluation after partial resection in patients with carcinoma of the larynx, *Laryngoscope* 85:626, 1975.

125. Pearson BW: Subtotal laryngectomy, *Laryngoscope* 91:1904, 1981.

126. Pech A and others: Requisite selection of surgical technics in the treatment of cancer of the larynx, *Ann Otolaryngol Chir Cervicofac* 103:565, 1986.

127. Pinel J and others, editors: *Cancers du larynx (indications therapeutiques, resultants)*, Paris, Arnette, 1980.

128. Piquet JJ, Chevalier D: Subtotal laryngectomy with crico-hyoido-epiglotto-pexy for the treatment of extended glottic carcinomas, *Am J Surg* 162:357, 1991.

129. Piquet JJ, Desulty A, Decroix G: Crico-hyoido-pexie. Technique operatoire et results fonctionels, *Ann Otolaryngol Chir Cervicofac* 91:681, 1974.

130. Piquet JJ and others: La chirurgie reconstructive du larynx resultats carcinomlogiques et fonctionele, *JFORL* 33:215, 1984.

131. Pittam MR, Carter RL: Framework invasion by laryngeal carcinomas, *Head Neck* 4:200, 1982.

132. Pleet and others: Partial laryngectomy with imbrication reconstruction, *Trans Am Acad Ophthalmol Otolaryngol* 84:882, 1977.

133. Prades JM and others: Reconstructive laryngectomies. Technical and functional aspects, *Ann Otolaryngol Chir Cervicofac* 104:281, 1987.

134. Pressman JJ: Submucosal compartmentation of the larynx, *Ann Otol Rhinol Laryngol* 65:766, 1956.

135. Rademaker AW and others: Recovery of postoperative swallowing in patients undergoing partial laryngectomy, *Head Neck* 15:325, 1993.

136. Robbins KT and others: Conservation surgery for T2 and T3 carcinomas of the supraglottic larynx, *Arch Otolaryngol Head Neck Surg* 114:421, 1988.

137. Roberts TJ and others: Second neoplasms in patients with carcinomas of the vocal cord: incidence and implications for survival, *Int J Radiat Oncol Biol Phys* 21:583, 1991.

138. Rothfield RE and others: The role of hemilaryngectomy in the management of T1 vocal cord cancer, *Arch Otolaryngol Head Neck Surg* 102:677, 1989.

139. Sedlacek K: Reconstructive anterior and lateral laryngectomy using the epiglottis as a pedunculated graft, *Ceskoslovenka Otolaryngologie* 8:328, 1965.

140. Sessions DG: Extended partial laryngectomy, *Ann Otol Rhinol Laryngol* 89:556, 1980.

141. Shaw HJ: Role of partial laryngectomy after irradiation in the treatment of laryngeal cancer: a view from the United Kingdom, *Ann Otol Rhinol Laryngol* 100:268, 1991.

142. Shenoy AM and others: Supracricoid laryngectomy with cricohyoidopexy: a clinico oncological & functional experience, *Indian J Cancer* 37:67, 2000.

143. Singer MI: Tracheoesophageal speech: vocal rehabilitation after total laryngectomy, *Laryngoscope* 93:1454, 1983.

144. Skolnik EM and others: Radiation failures in cancer of the larynx, *Ann Otol Rhinol Laryngol* 84:804, 1975.

145. Som ML: *Conservation surgery for carcinoma of the supraglottis*, London, 1969, University of London.

146. Som ML: Cordal cancer with extension to the vocal process, *Laryngoscope* 85:1298, 1975.

147. Som ML: Hemilaryngectomy—modified technique for cordal cancer with extension posteriorly, *Arch Otolaryngol* 54:524, 1951.

148. Soo KC and others: Analysis of prognostic variables and results after supraglottic partial laryngectomy, *Am J Surg* 156:301, 1988.

149. Sorensen H and others: Partial laryngectomy following irradiation, *Laryngoscope* 90:1344, 1980.

150. Spaulding CA and others: Partial laryngectomy and radiotherapy for supraglottic cancer: a conservative approach, *Ann Otol Rhinol Laryngol* 98:125, 1988.

151. Staple TW, Ogura JH: Cineradiography of the swallowing mechanism following supraglottic subtotal laryngectomy, *Radiology* 87:226, 1966.

152. Thaler E and others: The clinical significance of the delphian lymph node in laryngeal carcinoma, *Laryngoscope* (Submitted for publication.)

153. Thomas JV and others: Early glottic carcinoma treated with open laryngeal procedures [see comments], *Arch Otolaryngol Head Neck Surg* 120:264, 1994.

154. Thompson S: Intrinsic cancer of the larynx: operation by laryngo-fissure: lasting cure in 80% of cases, *BMJ* 355, 1912.

155. Timon CI and others: Hyoid bone involvement by squamous cell carcinoma: clinical and pathological features, *Laryngoscope* 102:515, 1992.

156. Traissac L, Verhulst J: Indications techniques resultats des laryngectomies reconstructives, *Rev Laryngol* 112:55, 1991.

157. Tucker GA: A histological method for the study of the spread of carcinoma within the larynx, *Ann Otol Rhinol Laryngol* 70:1, 1961.

158. Tucker GF, Smith HR: A histological demonstration of the development of laryngeal connective tissue compartments, *Trans Am Acad Ophthalmol Otolaryngol* May-June:308, 1962.

159. Tucker HM: Conservation laryngeal surgery in the elderly patient, *Laryngoscope* 87:1995, 1977.

160. Tucker HM: *The larynx*, New York, 1993, Theime.

161. Tucker HM and others: Glottic reconstruction after near total laryngectomy, *Laryngoscope* 89:609, 1979.

162. Tucker HM and others: Near-total laryngectomy with epiglottic reconstruction. Long-term results, *Arch Otolaryngol Head Neck Surg* 102:1341, 1989.

163. Tufano RP: Organ preservation surgery for laryngeal cancer, *Otolaryngol Clin North Am* 35:1067, 2002.

164. Viani L and others: Recurrence after radiotherapy for glottic carcinoma, *Cancer* 67:577, 1991.

165. Vigneau D and others: Indications techniques et resultats carcinologique et fonctionnele, *Rev Laryngol* 109:145, 1988.

166. Ward PH and others: The enigma of post-radiation edema and recurrent or residual carcinoma of the larynx, *Laryngoscope* 85:522, 1975.

167. Weinstein GS, Laccourreye O: Supracricoid laryngectomy with cricohyoidoepiglottopexy, *Otolaryngol Head Neck Surg* 111:684, 1994.

168. Weinstein GS and others: *Functional analysis of speech and deglutition following supracricoid laryngectomy,* Annual Meeting of the American Academy of Otolaryngology–Head and Neck Surgery, San Diego, California, 1990.

169. Weinstein GS and others: Laryngeal preservation with supracricoid partial laryngectomy results in improved quality of life when compared with total laryngectomy, *Laryngoscope* 111:191, 2001.

170. Weinstein G and others: Laryngeal organ preservation with supracricoid partial, laryngectomy with cricohyoidoepiglottopexy: correlation of videostroboscopic findings and voice parameters, *Ann Otol Rhinol Laryngol* 111:1 2002.

171. Weinstein GS and others: Larynx preservation with supracricoid partial laryngectomy with cricohyoidoepiglottopexy: correlation of videostroboscopic findings and voice parameters, *Am Otol Rhinol Laryngol* 111:1, 2002.

172. Weinstein GS and others: *Optimizing functional results in supracricoid laryngectomy,* Eastern Sectional Meeting of the Triological Society, Boston, 1992.

173. Weinstein GS and others: *Organ preservation surgery for laryngeal cancer.* San Diego, California, 2000, Singular Publishing Group.

174. Weinstein G and others: Organ preservation surgery for laryngeal cancer: the evolving role of the surgeon in the multidisciplinary head and neck cancer team, *Oper Techn Otolaryngol Head Neck Surg* 14:1, 2003.

175. Weinstein GS and others: Reconsidering a paradigm: the spread of supraglottic carcinoma to the glottis, *Laryngoscope* 105:1129, 1995.

176. Weinstein GS and others: The role of CT and MR in planning conservation laryngeal surgery, *Neuroimag Clin North Am* (in press).

177. Welsh LW, Welsh Louis J, Rizzo TA: Laryngeal spaces and lymphatics: current anatomic concepts, *Ann Otol Rhinol Laryngol* 92(Suppl 105):19, 1983.

178. Yeager VL, Archer CR: Anatomical routes for cancer invasion of laryngeal cartilages, *Laryngoscope* 92:449, 1982.

179. Zacharek MA and others: Functional outcomes after supracricoid laryngectomy, *Laryngoscope* 111:1558, 2001.

180. Zamora RL and others: Clinical staging for primary malignancies of the supraglottic larynx, *Laryngoscope* 103:69, 1993.

181. Zeitels SM, Kirchner JA: Hyoepiglottic ligament in supraglottic cancer, *Ann Otol Rhinol Laryngol* 104:770, 1995.

182. Zinreich SJ: Imaging in laryngeal cancer: computed tomography, magnetic resonance imaging, positron emission tomography, *Otolaryngol Clin North Am* 35:971, 2002.

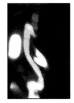

TOTAL LARYNGECTOMY AND LARYNGOPHARYNGECTOMY

Christopher H. Rassekh
Bruce H. Haughey

TOTAL LARYNGECTOMY
Historical Development

Although Patrick Watson of Edinburgh often is credited with performing the first total laryngectomy in 1866, there is no recorded proof that the operation actually was done by him. Research into Watson's own article[64] apparently answers this question; Watson stated he performed only a tracheotomy while the patient was alive and then did a postmortem laryngectomy of the syphilitic larynx. Billroth of Vienna, on December 31, 1873, carried out the first total laryngectomy for a patient with laryngeal cancer. One month earlier, he had performed a vertical cricothyrotomy and local intralaryngeal excision of this patient's lesion. Gross pathologic recurrence necessitated further radical ablation,[63] but the total laryngectomy was punctuated by considerable bleeding, coughing, and arousal from the anesthetic. A large pharyngocutaneous fistula was created, but the patient was fed successfully by mouth and was even fitted with an artificial larynx.[22]

Billroth and Gussenbauer's patient died 7 months after surgery,[1] but Bottini of Turin in 1875 performed a total laryngectomy on a patient who survived for 10 years. Thiersch (also of split-skin graft renown) reported another long-term survivor in 1880, but Gluck in 1880 and others subsequently noted retrospectively that operative or early postoperative mortality rates were approximately 50%. This high mortality rate led Gluck of Germany to develop a two-stage procedure in which the tracheal separation was performed first, such that a healed tracheocutaneous stoma was present when the laryngectomy and pharyngeal closure were performed 2 weeks later. In the 1890s, with his pupil Sorenson, he then developed a successful single-stage operation, similar to contemporary techniques, in which the larynx was removed from above downward.[30] Solis-Cohen, advancing from

partial laryngectomies in the 1860s,[1] reported at the 1892 Philadelphia County Medical Society Meeting carrying out a total laryngectomy by use of similar Gluck-Sorenson techniques, although Frederick Lange of New York apparently reported performing the first total laryngectomy in the United States in 1879.[30] Radiation therapy was popular for treatment of patients with laryngeal cancer during the first half of the twentieth century, although with improvements in surgical and anesthetic technique and a recognition of radiation therapy's limitations, surgery (including total laryngectomy) plays a major contemporary role.

Indications
Malignant Disease

With the spectrum of organ preservation surgery that is now available,[5,48,82] the need for total laryngectomy as the only surgical option for those with laryngeal cancer has decreased. Organ preservation surgery includes specific procedures for supraglottic and glottic cancer. There are two major organ preservation surgical strategies, transoral (endoscopic) and open. Transoral procedures range from the very limited endoscopic resections that most surgeons can accomplish to extensive laser procedures that require greater surgical experience and specialized instrumentation.[32,65] Open procedures include the more conventional vertical partial laryngectomy group of procedures and horizontal (supraglottic) partial laryngectomy group. More recently, a group of operations called the supracricoid partial laryngectomy has become more popular. The supracricoid partial laryngectomy with cricohyoidopexy (SCPL-CHP) for selected supraglottic carcinomas and the supracricoid partial laryngectomy with cricohyoidoepiglottopexy (SCPL-CHEP) for selected glottic carcinoma have extended the spectrum of tumors that can be managed surgically while avoiding total laryngectomy.[37]

Organ preservation surgery can safely be used after radiotherapy but with a higher complication rate.[38] Another operation that avoids total laryngectomy is the "near-total laryngectomy."[51,68] This procedure cannot be viewed as truly an organ preservation operation, because it does not maintain an airway without a tracheostome. Essentially, it can be viewed as a total laryngectomy with an epithelialized voice tract.[52] It has not been very popular in most centers. Nonsurgical treatment for patients with laryngeal malignancy also is established as primary treatment in some centers. Management includes definitive radiation alone with surgery for salvage for patients with primary lesions up to T_3[15,44] or neoadjuvant chemotherapy and radiotherapy, with total laryngectomy reserved for those with unresponsive tumors.[26,33,75,76,81] The frequently cited Veterans Affairs study[12,83] randomly assigned patients with advanced laryngeal cancer to chemotherapy and radiotherapy or total laryngectomy. No differences in survival were identified. Criticisms of the study prompted a head and neck intergroup trial that randomly assigned patients to three groups and compared radiation alone vs concurrent vs sequential chemotherapy with radiotherapy. This study has recently been published and demonstrates that concurrent chemotherapy with radiotherapy is superior to sequential chemotherapy followed by radiotherapy or radiation alone in terms of local control and organ preservation.[18] Other studies have shown that if nonsurgical organ preservation is to be used, concurrent chemotherapy with hyperfractionated radiotherapy is more effective than radiotherapy alone[6] and that hyperfractionated radiotherapy is more effective than standard radiation alone.[19] Newer trials are investigating the impact of induction chemotherapy to assess tumor response. A complete (or near complete) response to chemotherapy then selects the patients for concurrent chemotherapy and radiotherapy.[73] Those who do not respond to chemotherapy are treated surgically. Results of such trials at a national and international level will be very interesting. No biologic marker yet identified can reliably predict which patients are better treated surgically. This is also the topic of investigations in concurrent studies.[73,84] Because the survival of the two treatment strategies is equivalent, quality-of-life issues are of paramount importance. Recently, a study demonstrated that in the intergroup trial, patients who had total laryngectomy after radiotherapy had a high complication rate, including a risk of pharyngocutaneous fistula of up to 30%, highest in the concurrent chemotherapy group.[81] Before that, studies have evaluated the quality of life after nonsurgical management of advanced laryngeal cancer.[15,71] Although the details of such studies are beyond the scope of this chapter, the results indicate that more extensive analysis of the quality of life are important. These studies are difficult to accomplish, because many patients are not available after the study, and the quality of life of the survivors might be significantly different than those of the patients who have died. Total laryngectomy still remains a viable option as the primary surgery for cancer or as salvage surgery after radiotherapy and finally for a group of less common conditions. There is overlap between these indications. For example, a patient with radionecrosis of the larynx may be found to have residual tumor on permanent sections and, as such, the surgery was salvage in hindsight. Similarly, a tumor that fails radiotherapy may also be causing chronic aspiration and may be too large to allow for any sort of organ preservation surgery. This sort of patient has three (or more) of the following indications for a undergoing the procedure.

Indications

1. Advanced tumors with cartilage destruction and anterior extralaryngeal spread; particularly presenting initially with laryngeal dysfunction (including vocal cord paralysis) that includes airway obstruction or severe aspiration (these patients are not good candidates for "organ preservation," because the organ already has been damaged and will not likely function even if preserved anatomically).[62]
2. Posterior commissure or bilateral arytenoid tumor involvement.
3. Circumferential submucosal disease with or without bilateral vocal cord paralysis.
4. Subglottic extension to involve the cricoid cartilage.
5. Completion laryngectomy for failed conservation or extensive endoscopic surgery.
6. Hypopharyngeal tumor originating at or spreading to the postcricoid mucosa.
7. Massive neck metastases or thyroid tumors (usually recurrent) invading both sides of the larynx from outside the laryngeal skeleton.
8. Advanced tumors of certain histologic types that are incurable by endoscopic resection, chemotherapy, or radiotherapy (e.g., adenocarcinoma, spindle cell carcinoma, soft tissue sarcomas, minor salivary gland tumors, and large cell neuroendocrine tumors); chondrosarcomas of the thyroid cartilage.
9. Extensive pharyngeal or tongue base resections in patients who are at high risk for aspiration problems.
10. Radiotherapy or chemoradiation failures; including those who have also had partial laryngectomy fail.

11. Radiation necrosis of the larynx, despite tumor control, unresponsive to adequate antibiotic and hyperbaric oxygen management.

12. Severe irreversible aspiration, with the laryngectomy used for complete separation of the air and food passages. This indication should be rare, considering the variety of other separation or closure procedures available.

Patient Selection and Workup

The following patient requirements should be met before a total laryngectomy is performed.

1. Candidate for general anesthesia; consider severe comorbid conditions as a relative contraindication.

2. Informed consent, including realistic understanding of total laryngectomy state and lifestyle after surgery (including the risk of drowning and the need to avoid swimming and certain risky activities and the lack of sense of smell in the event of fire, smoke, or toxic fume exposure.

3. Sufficient performance status, especially dexterity, to allow basic self-care of stoma. The workup required for a total laryngectomy includes the anesthetic-related assessment of general health (not elaborated here) and specific tests relevant to the larynx. Assuming the patient has a laryngeal carcinoma, the following are required:

    1. History (especially details of any previous radiation) and physical examination.

    2. A comprehensive head and neck examination, especially the neck, for detection of cervical metastasis.

    3. Biopsy proof of malignancy and careful endoscopic assessment of tumor location; use of both microscopic and telescopic endoscopy can help determine the need for total laryngectomy and can also help determine which patients are likely to have extensive subglottic extension or submucosal extension in the hypopharynx.

    4. Synchronous primary tumor screening, including bronchoscopy, esophagoscopy and/or barium swallow, chest radiography, and chest computed tomography (CT) in selected cases.

    5. Metastatic screen, including chest imaging plus bone, brain, and liver studies for high-stage lesions (evidence does not support this very well; some advocate positron emisssion tomography (PET) scan as the best screen for pulmonary metastasis and abdominal CT or

magnetic resonance imaging (MRI) for patients with elevated liver function tests, but the data to support these tests are lacking, so cost-efficacy is dubious.[35] In the laboratory evaluation, diabetes and hypothyroidism should be evaluated and managed appropriately, because they increase the risk of complications.

    6. Neck CT for assessment of cartilage or preparaepiglottic space invasion in those with advanced or radiation-recurrent lesions and for assessment of radiologically detectable neck metastasis.[87] The role of PET scans for detection of tumor in radiated or scarred field still is being evaluated.[55,70]

Surgical Technique
Resection

Proper patient positioning provides access to the anterior part of the neck for the surgeon and the assistant. Positioning is best achieved by placing the patient on a table fitted with a head holder, allowing the head to be cantilevered out but remain well supported. This also facilitates bilateral neck dissection, which is often performed "in-continuity" and allows surgeons to position themselves all the way around the head. The table is turned 180 degrees from the anesthesiology team to further facilitate access to the patient. Before the operation day, airway management is planned with the anesthesiologist, so that an agreement is reached regarding timing of tracheotomy and intubation. In the nonobstructed larynx, the anesthesiologist may pass an orotracheal tube with anesthetic induction, which may be removed at subsequent tracheotomy or left in situ until tracheal transection is performed at the end of the laryngectomy. With an obstructed airway or in a case in which intubation may displace malignant tissue into the lower airway, a preliminary tracheotomy with the patient under local anesthesia is performed. The tracheotomy skin incision is made at the intended site of the final stoma. The stoma can be placed in the line of the incision or 2 to 3 cm inferior to the incision (Figure 103-1, *A* and *B*). The advantage of the former is that creation of the stoma is more reliable and avoids a bipedicled bridge of skin between the flap incision and the tracheostomy incision, which can result in stenosis of the stoma. The advantage of the latter is that in the event of pharyngocutaneous fistula, which requires diversion, the stoma is less likely to be involved in the resulting wound. The latter consideration is perhaps more important in previously irradiated patients, because the risk of fistula in primary total laryngectomy is low. This configuration also avoids the technical nuances of bilateral, three-point closures at the stoma necessitated by

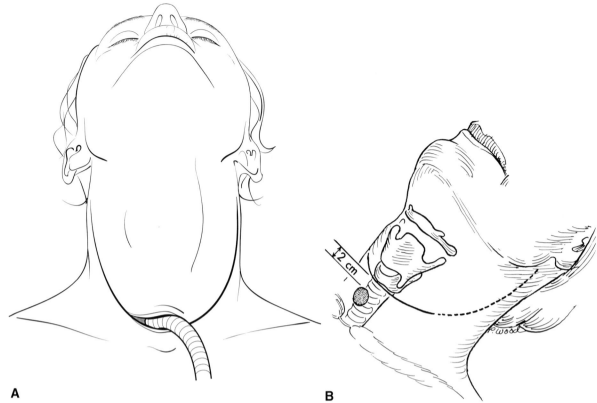

A   **B**

Figure 103-1. Incision options for total laryngectomy and total laryngopharyngectomy. **A,** Long apron flap without separate incision for tracheostomy from mastoid tip to mastoid tip intersecting the midline at approximately the level of the cricoid cartilage, usually about 2 cm above the sternal notch in the midline. **B,** Short apron flap with separate tracheostome incision 2 to 3 cm inferior to the flap incision. A U-shaped incision (not shown) is rarely used, but feasible when neck dissection is not performed.

exteriorizing the lower cut tracheal end through the laryngectomy skin incision. In the long flap approach, the three-point closure is performed after the inferior aspect of the stoma is completed, elongating it with the technique shown in Figure 103-6. This is somewhat more difficult to accomplish with the stoma created 2 to 3 cm into the inferior flap, because the trachea is not anchored to the lateral aspect of the dissection. Ultimately, the comfort level of the surgeon determines the choice of incision.

Every attempt should be made to enter the trachea with a horizontal cut at the ultimate level intended for tracheal transection, but in the event that a tracheotomy already is in place, the tracheal transection will be 2 cm inferior to the existing tracheotomy site (if possible). A precurved or flexible reinforced cuffed tube then is passed into the trachea, and adequate ventilation is confirmed. The cuff of the tube is prepped into the field so that the tube can be removed intermittently for suture placement during creation of the stoma.

For access to the larynx itself, a curved, horizontal neck skin incision is preferred because of its minimal intersection with the pharyngeal closure and its potential for extension laterally into a neck dissection incision. Once the incision is deepened through, but not beyond, the platysma, flaps are elevated superiorly and inferiorly in the subplatysmal plane until there is exposure above to the upper border of the hyoid bone and below to the cervical trachea. The anterior jugular veins and the prelaryngeal Delphian node are left undisturbed on the specimen, as are the strap muscles. The sternocleidomastoid muscle then is identified along its anterior border on each side. The investing layer of cervical fascia is incised longitudinally from the hyoid above to the clavicle below. The omohyoid then is divided, which allows entry to the loose areolar compartment bounded laterally by the sternomastoid muscle and carotid sheath and medially by the pharynx and larynx contained in the visceral compartment of the neck. Appropriate neck dissections are performed. The extent of neck dissection is beyond the scope of this chapter, but a few points merit mention. For supraglottic carcinoma, the minimal neck dissection to be performed is selective neck dissection, stations II, III, and IV bilaterally. It is extended if lymphadenopathy indicates the need. For advanced glottic carcinoma with supraglottic involvement, the same procedure is recommended. Unilateral (ipsilateral) neck dissection can be considered for T3

glottic carcinoma. For patients who have previously been irradiated, evidence still supports selective neck dissection.[79] In general, both neck dissections can be pedicled at the thyrohyoid membrane area, and the resection can easily be done en bloc.

The strap muscles then are divided inferiorly from their sternal origins and elevated to expose the thyroid gland (Figure 103-2, *A*). Controversy exists with

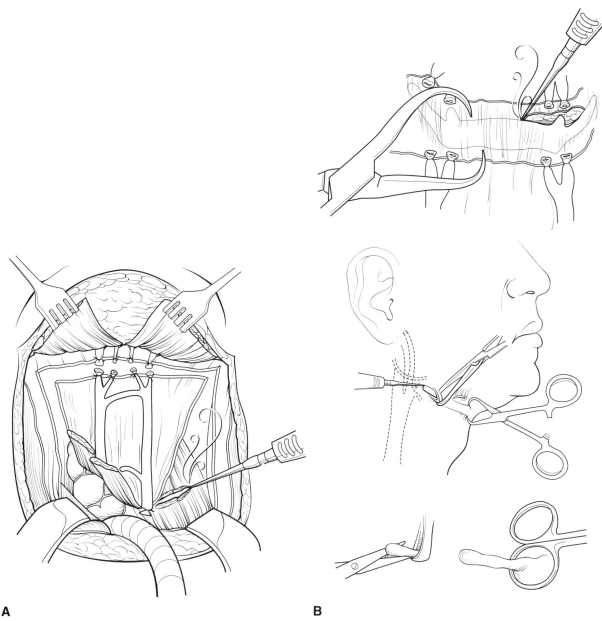

A

B

Figure 103-2. Skeletonization of the larynx. **A,** Division of the strap musculature after elevation of a subplatysmal flap. The omohyoid is divided inferiorly, usually during the neck dissection. The sternothyroid and sternohyoid muscles are divided inferiorly to expose the thyroid gland and trachea. **B,** Division of suprahyoid musculature. This is performed staying close to the superior aspect of the hyoid bone. Cautery is avoided lateral to the lesser cornu to avoid injury to the hypoglossal nerve. In this area, the hyoid is retracted in such a way as to distract the greater cornu inferiorly, and a scissor is used to release the cornu staying right on the bone.

Continued

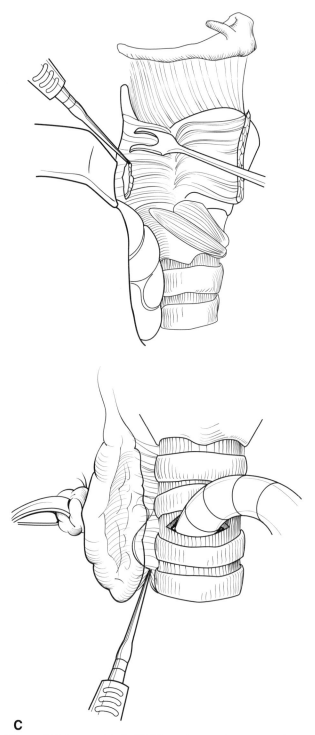

C

Figure 103-2, cont'd C, Division of constrictor musculature along the lateral aspect of the thyroid cartilage and dissection of the thyroid. If the thyroid is to be resected, it is elevated, and the dissection proceeds directly to the tracheoesophageal groove. If the thyroid is to be preserved, the lobe is dissected away from the tracheoesophageal groove after division of the isthmus. Electrocautery dissection is useful to minimize bleeding in this area. The degree of skeletonization depends on tumor extent. Once the thyroid cartilage is skeletonized, the superior laryngeal neurovascular bundle can be divided to decrease bleeding during the resection.

regard to thyroidectomy as part of a total laryngectomy. Studies note that involvement of the thyroid gland is rare.[16] However, when there is nodal disease in the jugular chain from glottic or subglottic cancer, the thyroid is at high risk because of the paratracheal and parapharyngeal lymphatics associated with the thyroid. Also, in patients who have invasion of the thyroid or cricoid cartilage in close proximity to the thyroid gland, the gland may become directly involved by the tumor. The risk to the thyroid is highest with transglottic cancers that extend more than 1 cm subglottic.[9] In some cases, both lobes of the thyroid should be removed because of these risk factors. When the lobe of the thyroid is to be removed, the superior and inferior thyroid vascular pedicles are therefore ligated and divided, as is the middle thyroid vein. The lobe(s) to be preserved then is (are) dissected off the laryngotracheal skeleton from medial to lateral, thereby preserving blood supply to the remaining thyroid and parathyroid parenchyma by way of inferior thyroid vessels (the superior thyroid artery can be preserved also if oncologically sound, but this is not necessary). An effort should be made to preserve the vascularity to the parathyroid glands, but if a parathyroid gland is noted that is poorly vascularized after the procedure, this can be reimplanted into the neck musculature as is done for parathyroidectomy in thyroid cancer. It is neither necessary nor advisable to reimplant parathyroids into the arm in cancer patients. This is only done in parathyroid hyperplasia to avoid confusion between a hyperfunctional graft and residual parathyroid in the neck so that sestamibi scanning can distinguish the two. Hyperfunction of the graft is not an issue in laryngeal cancer (or thyroid cancer, for that matter). Next, after dividing and ligating the upper and lower extent of the anterior jugular veins, the superior aspect of the hyoid bone is skeletonized by detaching the mylohyoid, geniohyoid, digastric sling, and hyoglossus in sequence from medial to lateral (Figure 103-2, *B*). "Cold" knife dissection should be used lateral to the lesser cornu, avoiding excess electrical stimulation or direct damage to the hypoglossal nerve. Caution is advised for supraglottic cancers that involve the aryepiglottic fold, pyriform sinus, or vallecula, because too much skeletonization of the hyoid bone may put the surgeon in close proximity to the deep extent of the tumor, which might seem to be a positive margin histologically. The sternohyoid and thyrohyoid muscle attachments on the lower border of the hyoid bone remain undisturbed. Further laryngeal cartilage skeletonization now is performed if the tumor does not extend outside the pyriform fossa. The posterior border of the thyroid cartilage lamina is rotated anteriorly by upward traction, allowing sharp release of the constrictor muscles from the inferior to the superior cornu (Figure 103-2, *C*). Above the superior cornu, the laryngeal branch of the superior thyroid artery should be identified, ligated, and divided before it penetrates the thyrohyoid membrane.

The pharyngotomy incisions and definitive laryngeal removal now are performed. To avoid contact with the neoplasm or cutting through its submucosal extensions, the pharynx is entered contralateral to the tumor. If superior extension to the tongue base is present, lateral pharyngotomy behind the thyroid cartilage is performed, and by use of a headlight, the extent of tumor is inspected. A safe 2-cm margin of normal-looking mucosa then is preserved with further cuts from below, progressing superiorly behind the thyrohyoid membrane, around the hyoid bone, and then transversely across the vallecula or tongue base. By contrast, if the disease is confined below the level of the hyoid, entry by way of the vallecula is feasible with a direct anteroposterior approach (Figure 103-3) in the horizontal plane of the upper hyoid border. Strict maintenance of this plane, avoiding excessive inferior traction on the hyoid itself, precludes violation of the preepiglottic space. Once the mucosa is breached, the epiglottis' tip is identified, grasped with an Allis forceps if tumor-free, and gently pulled anteriorly out of the pharyngotomy. A view of the endolarynx and pharynx now is possible to assess tumor extent and to plan appropriate mucosal cuts (Figure 103-2, *D*).

With a Mayo scissors, bilateral, inferiorly direct cuts are made, releasing the lateral pharynx from the larynx. The inside scissors blade is on mucosa, and the outside blade is on constrictor musculature. As these vallecula-to-pyriform sinus incisions are made, the larynx is further angled anteriorly out of the wound until it is released to the apices of the pyriform sinuses. The postcricoid mucosa is exposed and is incised sharply in the transverse direction connecting the inferior extent of both lateral incisions across the lower half of the cricoid lamina. A plane of blunt dissection initially behind the posterior cricoarytenoid muscle, but from there down between the trachealis and longitudinal esophageal muscle, then is opened until the desired level of tracheal transection is reached. Optimum exposure of the trachea at this stage is achieved by further lateralization of the preserved thyroid lobe and then followed by knife transection of the trachea itself. This cut is bevelled upward from anterior to posterior (see Figure 103-6, *A*), with special care not to encroach on any subglottic tumor extension. If the latter is present, a 1.5- to 2.0-cm margin of healthy appearing trachea should be resected in continuity with the larynx to avoid stomal recurrence.[56] If a preliminary tra-

cheotomy had not been performed, the oral endotracheal tube is next withdrawn from the tracheal stump, and a new, cuffed, flexible tube is inserted for connection to new anesthesia tubing. As an alternative, the steps can be altered slightly as indicated by the pathology. As long as there is not extensive subglottic spread, preliminary tracheotomy facilitates the resection greatly. This is performed after dissection of the thyroid gland and skeletonization of the thyroid cartilage. The trachea is entered 2 cm below the inferior extent of tumor, and careful inspection is performed on entry. The endotracheal tube is withdrawn, and the trachea is further incised laterally with a beveled cut (Figure 103-6, *A*). A reinforced tube is placed and a sterile connector passed through the drapes to connect to the circuit. The trachea is then transected by making a notched incision in the posterior wall. This is taken down to the esophageal musculature. Once the ligamentous attachments and the recurrent laryngeal nerve are divided, blunt dissection can be performed up to the level of the posterior cricoarytenoid musculature. Then, when the surgeon enters the larynx and completes the mucosal cuts from superiorly along the aryepiglottic folds, the specimen is pedicled on the postcricoid mucosa only, and this facilitates the final transection, which can reduce the blood loss. The surgeon places a pack in the pharynx and neck while inspecting the specimen for orientation and margin assessment (Figure 103-4). After the specimen is passed from the table, it is carefully inspected for adequacy of resection, and a pathologist's frozen section study of all the patient's cut margins, including trachea, tongue, and pharyngeal mucosa, is requested. The tracheal margin is critical, because there are patients in whom submucosal occult microscopic disease spreads down the trachea, despite relatively normal-looking mucosa. Excising all disease helps prevent stomal recurrence. The wound is thoroughly irrigated, all clots are removed, and hemostasis is achieved.

If a primary tracheoesophageal puncture is to be performed, creating the tracheostome before pharyngeal repair may be considered, because it enables definitive positioning of the trachea relative to the esophagus and skin before a puncture site is selected. A pair of right-angled forceps then is passed into the esophagus, with the tip elevating the posterior tracheal wall at the intended puncture site (Figure 103-7). A tracheoesophageal stab incision is made, exposing the forceps tip, and with these, a 14-French gauge feeding tube is grasped, pulled into the pharynx, and then fed down the esophagus until its end is positioned in the stomach. This is secured to the anterior chest wall skin with an op-site and suture.

The previously described resection technique clearly needs to be modified according to the extent of tumor spread. A common variation is the "wide-field" laryngectomy, in which overlying neck skin is resected in continuity with the larynx and thyroid gland (Figure 103-8). This method is recommended for radiation-recurrent tumors that have invaded soft tissue outside the laryngeal skeleton.

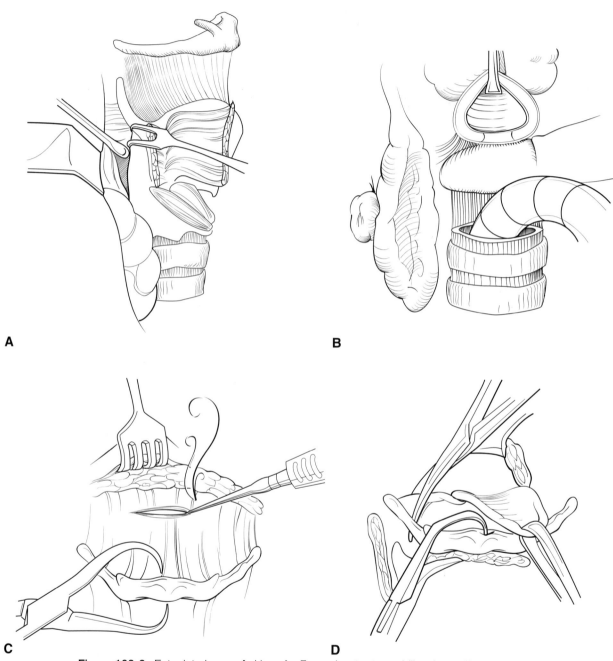

A

B

C

D

Figure 103-3. Entry into larynx. **A,** Use of a Freer elevator to mobilize the pyriform sinus and internal perichondrium from the thyroid cartilage. This should not be performed if the pyriform sinus is likely to be involved by the tumor. **B,** The trachea is transected, and the ligamentous attachments are divided permitting dissection of the trachea away from the upper esophagus up to the level of the posterior cricoarytenoid musculature. This cut is beveled as shown in Figure 103-2. This step is delayed if there is concern about significant subglottic extension. **C,** Dissection follows the hyoepiglottic ligament to the epiglottis and vallecula to avoid entry into the preepiglottic space. **D,** If clinically uninvolved, the vallecula is entered on the nontumor side, and if it is not involved, the tip of the epiglottis is grasped.

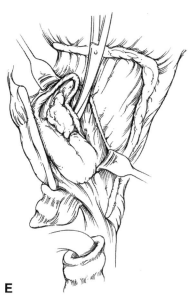

E

Figure 103-3, cont'd E, The pharyngoepiglottic fold cuts are extended. If uninvolved, the previously preserved pyriform sinus mucosa is preserved by transecting the mucosa close to the aryepiglottic fold. This is accomplished by placing one scissor blade in the lumen and the other between the previously released internal perichondrium and the thyroid cartilage. This leaves the larynx pedicled only on the mucosa of the anterior esophageal inlet, which can be transected under direct vision preserving as much mucosa as is oncologically sound. If the trachea was not previously transected, it is done at this time to release the specimen.

Repair and Reconstruction

Pharynx. Pharyngeal reconstruction is currently performed by direct closure or flap augmentation. Configurations for a direct repair are T-shaped or linear (horizontal or longitudinal) (Figure 103-5). Selection of closure type is on the basis of an assessment of the shape and size of the pharyngeal defect, elasticity of remaining tissue, and simulated wound approximation before suturing. The least-tensioned apposition of wound edges is the best and usually is T-shaped and results in minimal or no horizontal pharyngeal shelf formation.[10]

The pharyngeal wall is closed in two layers, the first being mucosal and submucosal and the second being muscle. A running or interrupted closure, according to the surgeon's preference, is used with particular attention to inversion of the mucosal edges into the pharynx. This inversion is achieved with an absorbable stitch that runs horizontally through the submucosa, without penetration of the mucosal surface. A longer retained material, such as polyglycolic acid (3-0), is used and is adequate for irradiated tissue. The muscle layer closure requires advancement of the cut constrictor margins over the mucosal closure for reinforcement. This maneuver always tightens the neopharynx to some extent and should be left undone at points where narrowing may be excessive. One

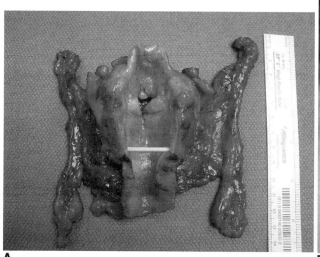

A

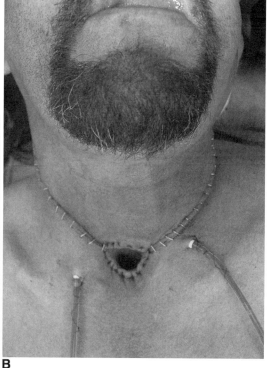

B

Figure 103-4. Specimen and resulting wound. **A,** Total laryngectomy specimen in continuity with bilateral selective neck dissections. **B,** Final closure with stoma in long flap approach. To view this image in color, please go to *www.ototext.com* or the Electronic Image Collection CD, bound into your copy of Cummings Otolaryngology—Head and Neck Surgery, 4th edition.

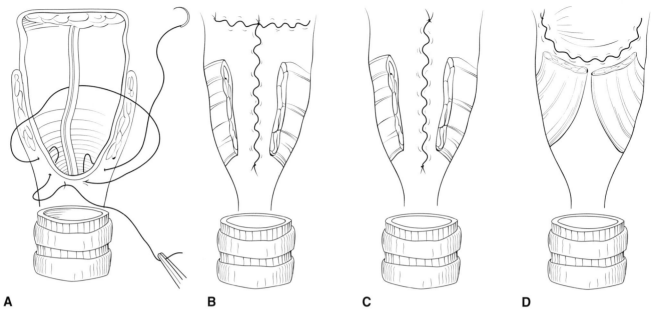

Figure 103-5. A, Closure of pharynx with detail of suturing technique. **B,** T-closure. **C,** Vertical closure. **D,** Horizontal closure.

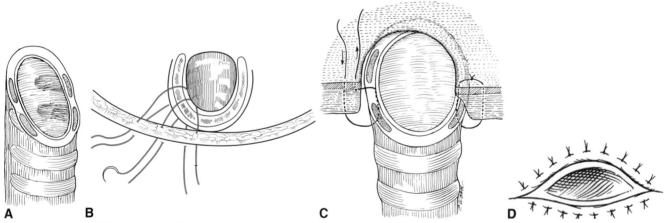

Figure 103-6. Steps to avoid stenosis in creation of tracheostome (long flap incision). **A,** Bevel the tracheal cut such that more posterior wall is preserved. This is done by curving a scissor upward as the anterior tracheostomy is extended laterally. The posterior wall is transected with a **V**-shaped incision in the mucosa to lengthen it and prevent scar contracture. **B,** Elongate the anterior edge of the stoma by placing sutures from midline outward, proceeding farther along the skin than the trachea and by continuing this well onto the lateral portion of the trachea. **C,** Bury the exposed tracheal cartilage with a half-buried vertical mattress suture from far on the skin around the tracheal cartilage and then back through the near edge of the skin tying the suture on the skin. To minimize granulation tissue, an effort should be made to place these sutures submucosally. Absorbable sutures are preferred. 2-0 Vicryl is advisable for the central suture, and 3-0 Vicryl is used for the remainder. **D,** Final closure including appearance of stoma using long-flap approach and the stoma technique described in **A** through **C**. Note the quite ample diameter of the stoma that results from suture placement in the manner described.

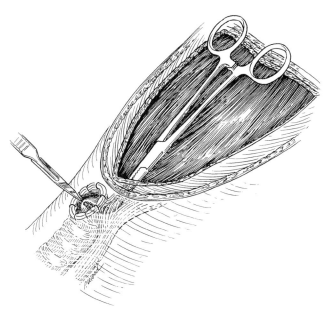

Figure 103-7. Technique of tracheoesophageal puncture. See text for description of technique.

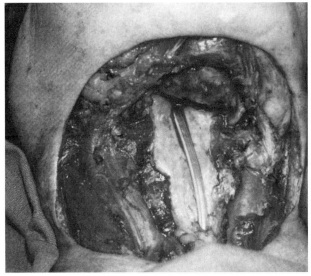

Figure 103-8. Wide-field laryngectomy defect for radiation recurrent tumor, including anterior neck skin, thyroid, sternomastoid, and selective neck node resection.

study[49] has shown that a mucosal closure alone is sufficient for sound healing. Closure of muscle can lead to difficulty with tracheoesophageal speech.[78]

If there is insufficient pharyngeal wall to close over a 36 French dilator, a flap repair should be considered to increase the circumferential dimension of the neopharynx. Hui and others[31] recently addressed the question of the width of the pharyngeal wall remnant relative to postoperative dysphagia and concluded that a remnant as small as 1.5-cm wide was sufficient to avoid dysphagia, although the study included only one patient with a remnant as small as 1.5 cm. Reconstructive

options include a myocutaneous flap, a muscle flap, or a microvascular free flap. Donor tissue for the latter could include the radial forearm free flap,[34] which also has been proposed for patients needing neoglottic reconstruction,[23] and the V-split jejunal patch. Whatever method of closure is used, it sometimes is prudent to fashion a control fistula for prevention of uncontrolled, complicated wound breakdown or infection. Patients with previous radiation therapy or other impediments to rapid wound healing, such as poor nutrition, diabetes, or immunosuppression, are suitable candidates for this procedure. The "mushroom" end of a 16 French or 18 French Malecot catheter is inserted into the neopharynx and secured in position with chromic catgut. The pharyngeal wall closure then is approximated closely to the circumference of the catheter stem, which is led out through the wound away from the carotid arteries and stoma. If a myocutaneous flap has been used for closure, the catheter may pierce the muscle belly for additional security and may be led out through a separate stab incision in the neck skin. Low, continuous wall suction is administered through the catheter for salivary decompression of the pharyngeal repair for 7 to 10 days, after which the catheter is removed. A small amount of discharge sometimes continues from the catheter track for several days, but thereafter it spontaneously heals.

Tracheal stoma. For the long flap approach, the stoma is inserted into the center of the lower flap with a central suture of 2-0 Vicryl excising an ellipse of skin if needed. In the short flap, the permanent end-tracheal stoma is created by excising a shield-shaped skin island from the lower neck flap in the midline, just above the sternal notch. Any excess adipose tissue or bulky sternomastoid muscle or tendon is excised deep to the skin flap to minimize tracheostenosis. The central suture is then secured to the lower aspect of the shield-shaped defect. The circumferential suture line should provide support for the trachea and accurate skin–mucosa apposition without cartilage exposure. These sutures should be placed beginning in the center and each subsequent suture placed lateral to the prior one. For each suture, the surgeon proceeds farther along the skin edge than the mucosal edge, which serves to pull the trachea outward. In addition, the trachea is not sewn in a circular fashion, but by bringing the lateral trachea down to the inferior flap, the inferior aspect of the stoma is elongated producing a more horizontally based trapezoid (shield) shape that avoids the circumferential stenosis or slitlike vertical stomas, which may result in a need for revision. This is best achieved by a modified ("half-buried") vertical mattress suture that traverses (1) skin (peripherally);

(2) cartilaginous tracheal wall (extramucosally); and (3) skin (centrally).

So, to summarize, we have Figure 103-6, *C*, which demonstrates that the three ways to maximize stoma size are (1) "bevel the trachea"; (2) "elongate the base"; and (3) "cover the cartilage." A 2-0 Vicryl is used for the central suture and a 3-0 Vicryl for the remaining inferior sutures. A trifurcating suture can be used (either 3-0 or 4-0 Vicryl where the superior flap comes into contact with the lateral aspect of the stoma bilaterally (in the long flap approach). Absorbable sutures are preferable, because suture removal is undesirable in the stoma region.

Postoperative Management and Complications

Apart from routine postsurgical care, the specific treatment of early postlaryngectomy patients includes the following monitoring: systemic vital signs, fluid balance, oxygenation, wound drain vacuum retention and output, and neck flap viability. Postoperative treatment includes ventilator assistance, as per respiratory status; tracheostomy tube care (cleaning, cuff pressure checks); airway humidification; bronchodilator treatments or chest physical therapy; suture line care three times daily; and nasogastric or tracheoesophageal fistula tube feeding once bowel sounds are present. Drains are removed when output <25 mL/day for 2 consecutive days, and oral feeding normally is begun 7 days after surgery in the nonirradiated patient. Laryngectomees previously radiated are fed 12 to 14 days after surgery to allow a longer healing time for the pharyngeal repair.

Early Complications

Early complications usually occur during the patient's postoperative hospitalization.

Drain failure. Drains unable to hold a vacuum represent a serious threat to the wound. There usually is either a leak in the pharynx or the skin and stoma closure that needs to be promptly detected and sealed.

Hematoma. Although rare, a hematoma requires prompt intervention to avoid pressure separation of the pharyngeal repair and compression of the upper trachea. The patient is returned to the operating room; the clot is evacuated, and any detectable bleeding is controlled. New drains are inserted, because blockage of the original ones with clot is inevitable.

Infection. A subcutaneous infection after total laryngectomy is recognized by increasing erythema and edema of the skin flaps 3 to 5 days after surgery. Associated odor, fever, and elevated leukocyte count occur. If an infected collection is present, the wound

is opened during sterile conditions, and the pus is evacuated and cultured. Dead space between the neopharynx and skin flap is managed with repeated antiseptic gauze packing until healed. Antibiotic coverage is modified according to culture results, and a pharyngocutaneous fistula is suspected if wound discharge continues or increases. A chyle fistula should be ruled out if neck dissection was performed.

Pharyngocutaneous fistula. Patients with poor preoperative nutritional status and positive surgical margins are at high risk for fistula development.[58] Early studies[56,72] did not show a significantly increased fistula rate in patients who have had preoperative radiotherapy, but subsequent studies seem to refute this.[54,77,81] A fistula begins as a major accumulating salivary leak from the pharyngeal closure into the subcutaneous space beneath the skin flaps and may be encouraged by a tight distal hypopharyngeal closure. Its existence often is heralded by increased turbid drain output and by erythema and edema around part of the wound closure, which, on opening, drains purulent material and saliva.

Such fistulas may occur 1 to 6 weeks postoperatively, depending on the presence or absence of previous radiation, and communication from the skin to the pharynx is confirmed by a methylene blue swallowing test. Persistent or recurrent tumor always should be ruled out.

Initial management is by regular, antiseptic gauze fistula-track packing, dressings, antibiotic therapy, and by giving the patient nothing by mouth. An active drain can often be converted to a passive drain to allow diversion of the saliva and prevention of salivary collection. A pressure dressing is sometimes useful. Conservative therapy attempts to allow the fistula to close from the inside toward the skin. A useful adjunct is to "sterilize" the fistula from within by administering 10 mL of 0.25% acetic acid by mouth or an antibiotic or other antiseptic preparation three to four times daily. If the previously described measures are unsuccessful in sealing off the pharynx from the neck within 2 weeks in a nonirradiated patient or 3 weeks in a radiated patient, operative closure should be considered. Although spontaneous closure may occur up to 6 weeks after onset, most patients prefer a more rapid resolution so that oral feeding may begin.

An excellent option for fistula closure before complete epithelialization is a pedicled muscle flap (pectoralis, trapezius, or latissimus dorsi) slipped between the pharyngeal and skin defects. Such flaps endow excellent blood flow and antibacterial benefits to an avascular, infected bed.[21] A control pharyngostome catheter suction system, as described in the discussion of surgical technique, also may be used to direct saliva away from the carotids. Further surgery at this stage also should correct any benign pharyngeal stricture distal to the fistula.

Wound dehiscence. Wound dehiscence may accompany a tensioned skin closure, the postradiation state, wound infection, fistula, or poorly designed ischemic neck flaps. Local wound care should suffice for healing by secondary intention, but if the carotid becomes persistently exposed, vascularized muscle flap coverage is advisable.

Late Complications

Stomal stenosis. Prolonged use (6–12 months) of a laryngectomy tube or stoma button should prevent stenosis, especially if the patient has received or will receive radiotherapy after surgery. Tracheoesophageal fistula speech and prosthesis management are inhibited by this situation; therefore, a stomatoplasty may be more expeditious for rehabilitation. The "fish-mouth" design of stomal revision is usually effective, but it should be delayed until 6 months after radiation is completed to avoid wound-healing problems. With meticulous attention to detail in creation of the stoma as previously described, this complication is rare, so that laryngectomy tubes and stomatoplasty are rarely required.[80]

Pharyngoesophageal stenosis and stricture. Tumor recurrence should be suspected but once excluded by endoscopy and biopsy, outpatient dilation usually is effective. An adequate lumen (36 French) is necessary not only for swallowing and nutrition but also for tracheoesophageal speech production. If dilatation is unsuccessful, flap augmentation, such as a jejunal free flap, may be necessary[6] for successful rehabilitation.

Chronic pharyngocutaneous fistula. Presentation of patients in this state often has been preceded by multiple conservative or operative attempts to close the defect. If the fistula is well matured, with a well-healed, intact skin mucosal junction, recurrent malignancy is less likely, although pharyngoesophageal stenosis at or beyond the distal end of the fistula is likely. The most expeditious and successful method of closure is a bipaddled fasciocutaneous free flap, such as the radial forearm flap. By folding it 180 degrees along its length and deepitheliating the apex of the fold, a secure, two-layered closure is achieved, which brings fresh, well-vascularized tissue to the field. When recipient vessels or comorbid conditions make microvascular surgery too high a risk, a pedicled pectoralis flap works well also.

Hypothyroidism. Preoperative or postoperative radiotherapy plus hemithyroidectomy usually is sufficient to induce a low thyroid state.[60,69] Thyroid function tests every 1 to 2 months after completion of all treatment indicate when supplemental thyroid medication is required.

Rehabilitation
Swallowing

Oral intake usually is commenced 7 days after surgery, although waiting until after 14 days is advisable if the patient has had preoperative radiotherapy. In a Brazilian study, 625 laryngectomees were fed 3 days after surgery and showed no increase in complications. They were able to avoid use of a nasogastric tube altogether.[3] Further study has replicated this finding,[47] but in reality, feeding patients this early is not always feasible because of postoperative edema. Because of this, length of hospital stay was found not to be significantly affected by early oral feeding in one study.[57] In general, once the patient can swallow saliva, it seems reasonable to consider oral feeding. The literature shows that most pharyngocutaneous fistulas occur at or just after postoperative day 7. In uncomplicated cases with minimal edema, it may be possible to be certain there is no fistula sooner than that. Our experience has been that we do tend to feed people who have previously been irradiated later and more carefully. Because of this, the recognition of the fistula has sometimes been delayed well beyond a week. It is our experience that fistula is more common after radiotherapy. Regardless of the timing of oral feeding, the key is recognition of the fistula if it does occur. A higher index of suspicion of pharyngocutaneous fistula should be maintained in patients with edema or prior radiotherapy or in patients with comorbid conditions such as diabetes mellitus, renal insufficiency, or on immunosuppressive agents. Every effort should be undertaken to avoid positive margins not only for cancer control but also because it can result in fistula as well. A gastrostomy may be of benefit in patients who are likely to have a pharyngocutaneous fistula or dysphagia postoperatively. Once a soft diet is tolerated, the patient may advance to normal intake, but edentulous patients should be especially cautious about solid food.

If dysphagia prevents adequate caloric or fluid intake, pharyngeal stricture, tumor recurrence, stenosis, or tongue weakness may be responsible. A modified barium swallow test[41] or manofluorography[45] helps diagnose which component or components of the swallowing tract or mechanism are faulty. Radiation fibrosis of the neck, causing pharyngeal stenosis some months or years after completion of treatment, should be counteracted by regular dilatation. Neuromuscular paralysis or weakness may be either preexisting or iatrogenic from radiotherapy or from surgical damage to the hypoglossal nerve. In these patients, except those with radiation neuritis, time and speech therapy exercises assist recovery.

Occasionally, circumferential spasm of the pharyngoesophageal segment may be sufficient to cause dysphagia, in which case Botox A injections or myotomy may be helpful.[24,29]

Voice

Mechanical devices. Mechanical devices are useful in the early, postoperative phase, before it is safe for the healing pharyngeal wall to be insufflated. Some patients also use them for permanent communication. Their major disadvantages are the monotonous, mechanical sound production, poor intelligibility, and the need for a cumbersome external device.

Esophageal speech. Although esophageal speech is mastered only by a few patients,[20] a good esophageal speaker eventually may undertake public speaking engagements. Air charging is achieved by thrusting the tongue back and forcing a bolus through the cricopharyngeus. The air bolus then is regurgitated through the pharyngoesophageal segment, which vibrates to produce sound. Spasm of the pharyngoesophageal musculature or fixed stricture may prevent acquisition of this technique, as may poor patient motivation. The former may be managed by botulinum toxin injection.[29]

Tracheoesophageal speech. The principle behind tracheoesophageal speech is diversion of exhaled air into the pharynx by way of a permanent, surgically constructed tracheoesophageal fistula. The pharyngoesophageal segment above the fistula vibrates, producing a neovoice. Singer and Blom[61] and Panje[50] have developed prosthetic devices that allow airflow to the pharyngoesophagus and prevent salivary leak into the trachea. Tracheostomal occlusion is either digital or by wearing a valved stoma button that flaps shut with forceful exhalation. The tracheoesophageal puncture may either be done primarily at the time of laryngectomy or as a secondary procedure when wound healing is complete. Most surgeons advise a waiting period of 6 months after completion of radiotherapy before secondary puncture, which allows the acute radiation reaction and thickening in the peristomal tissues and mucosa to regress sufficiently for rapid fistula epithelialization. Also, manipulation of peristomal tissue and vibratory excursion of pharyngoesophageal mucosa ensues once phonation training begins. Both may cause excessive edema, unless thorough tissue recovery from radiation has occurred. A stoma at least 1 cm in diameter is required, so stomatoplasty often is done simultaneously with the puncture procedure. Refer to Chapter 105 for further details of tracheoesophageal speech and prosthesis management. Tracheoesophageal speech is a major factor in improving quality of life in laryngectomy patients[8] and is the preferred method for rehabilitation. Nevertheless, long-term problems with the puncture site do occur. One possible solution to this is a laryngoplasty using radial forearm free flap with cartilage to recreate a voice shunt and neoepiglottis.[23,68]

Ultravoice. A speaking device built into a denture is another option for patients who are unable to acquire tracheoesophageal speech.[42]

TOTAL LARYNGOPHARYNGECTOMY

Total laryngopharyngectomy is a total laryngectomy and associated circumferential pharyngectomy. The vertical extent of the pharyngectomy may be from the nasopharynx above to the cervical esophagus below, depending on tumor location and spread. Advanced squamous carcinoma of the hypopharynx or cervical esophagus with pharyngeal extension is the most common clinical entity requiring this operation.

Historical Development

Total laryngopharyngectomy was a logical extension of total laryngectomy. Thus, after Billroth's landmark total laryngectomy in 1873, von Langenbeck removed a larynx plus much of the pharynx and cervical esophagus in 1875. Czerny, who had assisted Billroth in the first total laryngectomy, performed the first total laryngopharyngectomy in 1877.[59] According to Macbeth,[43] little had been done to reconstitute the pharynx until the 1920s, when Trotter introduced the concept of skin flaps turned in from the neck to form a posterior pharyngeal wall at stage one, followed by circumferential tubing for the second stage. Gluck, operating in the late 19th century, also is credited with discovering this concept,[59] in which bilateral, laterally based neck skin flaps were used.

Once the complications of sepsis and perioperative mortality had been minimized, attention turned to better reconstruction. Wookey[85] in Toronto published a series of total laryngopharyngectomies followed by a unilaterally based skin flap reconstruction. Since then, advances have centered on more sophisticated forms of single-stage reconstruction, with the resectional techniques for the larynx and pharynx remaining standard.

Indications

Assuming surgery is advised, patients with advanced tumors of the hypopharynx with the following features require total laryngopharyngectomy.

Pyriform Sinus Carcinoma

Posterior pharyngeal spread across the postcricoid region beyond the midline posteriorly or extension into the esophageal inlet necessitates circumferential pharyngectomy. The larynx, even if not directly involved, is sometimes sacrificed, because it loses its dynamic pharyngeal support for swallowing or it becomes denervated. An operation also is described in which the uninvolved larynx is splayed open and used for food passage lining.[59] Total pharyngeal resection and reconstruction with laryngeal preservation have been described[7] but require superb patient performance status. A series of patients in whom the larynx was preserved achieved an appreciable level of functional return.[28] This result is the exception rather than the norm in the hypopharyngeal cancer population. Laryngeal spread, especially if it involves the posterior cricoarytenoid muscle to cause abductor paralysis, as indicated previously, nearly always necessitates total laryngectomy.

Again, some patients may be suitable candidates for near-total laryngectomy,[19,52] but these patients also usually require flap reconstruction of the pharynx. Alternatively, supracricoid hemilaryngopharyngectomy[36] has been advocated for select patients with carcinoma of the pyriform sinus. More recently, Steiner's group has reported on a series of endoscopically excised hypopharyngeal tumors with creditable survivorship.[66,67] The goal of treatment of any patient requiring surgery of the laryngopharynx is to achieve cancer control and restore airway, swallowing, and speech. The authors believe this goal is achievable with appropriate reconstruction even in patients undergoing total laryngopharyngectomy.

Larynx preservation without jeopardizing survival seems feasible in patients with cancer of the hypopharynx. On the basis of these observations, the European Organization for Research and Treatment of Cancer has now accepted the use of induction chemotherapy followed by radiation as the new standard treatment in its future phase III larynx preservation trials.[40] Organ preservation rates are lower in hypopharyngeal carcinoma than in laryngeal carcinoma with the chemotherapy and radiation strategy.

Carcinoma of Posterior Hypopharyngeal Wall

When carcinoma of the posterior hypopharyngeal wall extends anteriorly into the pyriform sinuses or inferiorly below the level of the arytenoids, total laryngopharyngectomy is necessary.

Postcricoid Carcinoma

Postcricoid carcinoma usually is seen late, after spread downward into the esophageal inlet has occurred. In these patients, total laryngopharyngec-

tomy is required, especially if there is vocal cord paralysis caused by infiltration of the posterior cricoarytenoid muscles or cricoarytenoid joints.

Patient Selection and Workup

The same general patient considerations apply as outlined for total laryngectomy. Special features of the preoperative workup of patients with hypopharyngeal cancer include nutritional assessment and supplementation, careful scan staging of local and distant disease extent, and endoscopy with mapping biopsies. An assessment of resectability then is made (carotid artery, vertebral column, and extensive neck metastatic involvement is common), followed by complete evaluation of potential donor sites for pharyngoesophageal reconstruction. Preoperative calcium and thyroid hormone levels are assessed as a baseline for postoperative management.

Surgical Technique
Resection

Patient positioning and anesthetic considerations are the same as for those undergoing total laryngectomy with the addition of donor sites, such as the forearm, lateral thigh, or abdomen prepared for flap harvest or, in patients with gastric pull-up, stomach mobilization.

The neck dissection usually is performed first; the specimen is pedicled medially on the pharyngeal wall from the hyoid level down to the cricopharyngeus. Suitable arterial stumps (lingual, facial, superior thyroid, transverse cervical) are preserved, provided no oncologic compromise results, to allow a microvascular free tissue transfer. Similarly, the external jugular, anterior jugular, internal jugular tributaries, or transverse cervical vein may be kept, unless a classic radical neck dissection is necessary. If esophageal resection well inferior to the thoracic inlet is required to obtain clear margins, a total esophagectomy and visceral transposition may be the best reconstruction, obviating the need for recipient vessel preservation and avoiding the potential leakage of saliva or refluxate into a suture line near the great vessels. In such cases, a mediastinal tracheostomy may also be necessary to facilitate tracheal resection.

The initial dissection steps for laryngopharyngectomy are the same as for total laryngectomy, except that mobilization of the larynx, pharynx, and cervical esophagus as a unit is performed by extending the lateral dissection into the retropharyngeal and retroesophageal space. This actually makes this operation much simpler, because the pyriform mucosa is not dissected free. The skeletonization of the larynx is not performed laterally, so the dissection can be done bluntly once the deep cervical fascia is divided medial to the carotid artery along the prevertebral fascia adjacent to the lateral masses of the vertebral bodies. Careful observation is maintained for spread beyond the buccopharyngeal and prevertebral fasciae into the prevertebral muscles or vertebral bodies. The prevertebral fascia itself is a moderately resistant barrier to tumor spread, but it is resected in continuity with the specimen if necessary. Some surgeons would discontinue resection once prevertebral fascia involvement was proven.[53]

Once the pharynx, larynx, and upper cervical esophagus are circumferentially mobilized, the thyroid gland should be dissected free from its vascular pedicles to be removed with the specimen. The parathyroid glands contralateral to the tumor's epicenter often may be preserved but may have to be removed to ensure clearance of the surrounding paratracheal nodes. If there is no oncologic risk, parathyroid

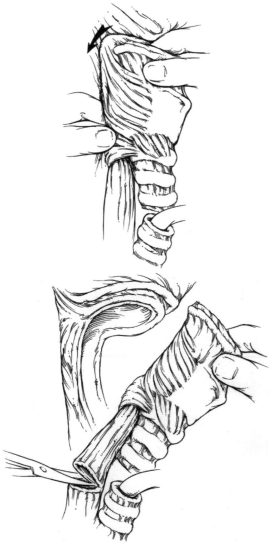

Figure 103-9 Total Laryngopharyngectomy. The retropharyngeal dissection has been performed. Now superior and inferior cuts that are circumferential will complete the resection.

reimplantation into a muscle bed is effective to avoid long-term hypocalcemia.

The pharynx is entered above the hyoid contralateral to the site with the most superior spread. Piriform sinus tumors may extend superiorly into the base of the tongue, thereby requiring a wide margin of resection during direct observation. In such patients, performing a contralateral lateral pharyngotomy improves the view without inhibiting a subsequent total laryngopharyngectomy if deemed necessary. The pharyngeal mucosal cuts then are continued horizontally around and onto the posterior pharyngeal wall at least 2 cm above the highest extent of the lesion, such that the entire upper pharynx and larynx are free. The trachea then is transected, followed by the cervical esophagus at a level appropriate to the tumor extent. The operation can be summarized in three steps: (1) mobilizing a large tube that includes the larynx and pharynx; (2) cutting the superior end of the tube (base of tongue and pharyngeal walls; and (3) cutting the inferior end (esophagus). If total esophagectomy is to be performed, blunt dissection of the esophagus continues from above downward until the inferior esophageal dissection from the abdomen is encountered (Figure 103-10). Superior mediastinal adenopathy is dealt with by use of a manubrial resection approach (Figure 103-11).[25]

Reconstruction

An extensive history and voluminous surgical literature deals with reconstruction of circumferential pharyngeal defects. We prefer to use a tubed skin flap, such as the radial forearm flap[34] (Figures 103-12 and 103-13), but a jejunal free transfer[11,86] is an alternative (see Figure 103-10). If the esophageal resection extends well below the thoracic inlet, a visceral transposition (gastric pull-up) is used, thus avoiding anastomoses in the mediastinum. Quality of life after high pharyngogastric anastomosis is poor in our experience. With adequate access created by sternectomy, a tubed free skin flap reconstruction endows other major advantages such as avoiding thoracoabdominal transgression. Further details of hypopharyngeal reconstruction are given in Chapter 104.

Postoperative Management and Complications
Postoperative Management

The same management applies as that described for total laryngectomy, although one or more neck dissections and abdominal or extremity donor sites frequently are used, and this greater magnitude of surgery necessitates special attention to pulmonary function; fluid nutritional balance; and local wound conditions in the neck, thorax, and donor site. Regular postoperative checks of calcium, magnesium, and phosphorus

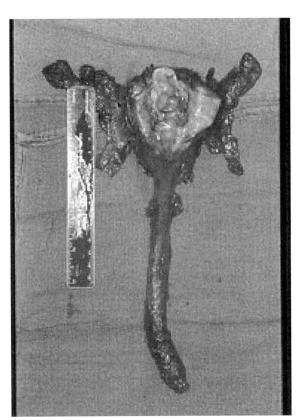

Figure 103-10. Total laryngopharyngoesophagectomy specimen en bloc with bilateral neck dissections and thyroidectomy. This patient had one hypopharyngeal tumor and a second, distal esophageal tumor.

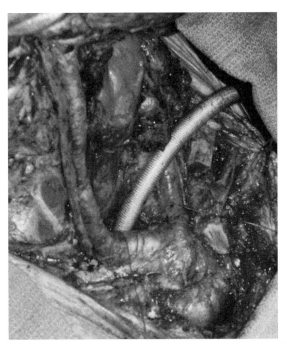

Figure 103-11. Superior mediastinal resection defect, including heads of clavicles and sternal manubrium. All node-bearing tissue is excised, preserving brachiocephalic and common carotid arteries. Ventilation tube enters cut tracheal stump.

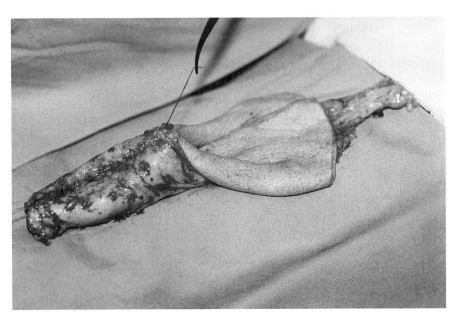

Figure 103-12. Radial forearm flap pretubed on the forearm before transfer to the neck. Note proximal skin paddle to be folded through 180 degrees, separated by a deepithelialized transverse strip and inset in one stage to provide neck coverage.

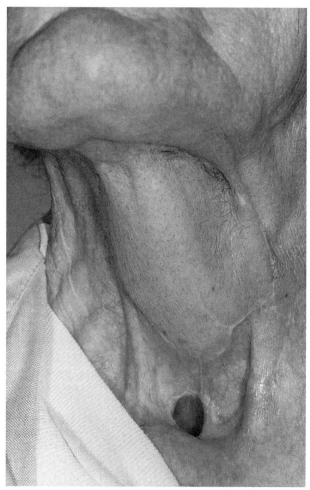

Figure 103-13. Postoperative result at 2 years. Patient maintains normal diet, and skin paddle pliability facilitates neck movement. Contour of tubed neopharyngeal component is visible deep to radial skin paddle.

levels are necessary, and supplementation with calcium, magnesium, and 1,25-dihydroxycholecalciferol usually is required.

Early Complications

Early fistula formation is more common than in patients undergoing total laryngectomy alone and needs especially aggressive management because of the mediastinitis risk. When a fistula or infection in the neck is detected, the wound is opened widely and left open with the track packed and is directed to pass away from the carotids and microvascular pedicle. A tight, distal closure of the pharyngoesophageal reconstruction is a prime cause of early fistula formation. Leaking pharyngeal or esophageal anastomoses, especially if secreting gastric or jejunal tissue has been used for reconstruction, may need to be controlled with pharyngostome formation and, if healing is poor, should be reinforced with fresh, vascularized, nonirradiated flap tissue (e.g., pectoralis or trapezius muscle flaps).

Late Complications

Stricture. Strictures are more common at the inferior, esophageal end of the pharyngeal reconstruction than superiorly, where the recipient lumen of the pharynx is wider. A stricture causing dysphagia may develop some weeks or months after surgery or after radiotherapy is complete.

Whether the reconstruction is skin or viscera, the principles of stricture management are the same as for patients after total laryngectomy alone: repeated, outpatient dilatation once tumor recurrence is excluded by endoscopy and biopsy, progressing to surgical revision if the latter is unsuccessful or poorly tolerated.

Recently, a strategy that uses a salivary bypass tube in combination with a radial forearm free flap has been reported to be encouraging in pharyngoesophageal reconstruction.[74] Another innovation that has been reported is the topical application of mitomycin C just after dilation.[2]

Functional swallowing problems. The jejunal free flap frequently maintains its contractility after transposition to the neck. This has been shown to cause functional dysphagia in some patients if the food bolus is delivered simultaneously with circumferential contractions.[45] Even myotomy of the bowel wall does not completely obliterate jejunal motility, according to a canine model.[27] Regurgitation of food is a recognized complication of the gastric transposition procedure, and it usually is caused by loss of the gastric reservoir or narrowing at the pylorus rather than anastomotic stricture and may be variable in its severity.

Frequent, mechanically blenderized meals eaten slowly usually are sufficient to maintain nutrition. It is possible that a passive segment of a tubed skin flap is superior for swallowing, although no prospective comparison studies have been performed.

Rehabilitation

The considerations in swallowing are the same as those noted previously in the discussion of functional swallowing problems after total laryngectomy.

Voice

Despite the interposition of circumferential visceral, skin, or myocutaneous tissue, voice may be attained with a tracheoneodigestive tract fistula technique. The stomach,[4] the jejunum,[85] and skin or myocutaneous flaps[46] are capable of sufficient vibration to produce intelligible speech.[28] Detailed analysis of voice characteristics after radial forearm flap reconstruction has been documented.[13] A tracheoesophageal puncture procedure may be safely performed as a primary procedure if the fistula tract does not communicate with the main resection site.

SUMMARY

A review of contemporary indications, techniques, and rehabilitation for patients undergoing total laryngectomy or total laryngopharyngectomy is presented. Most patients requiring these operations have head and neck cancer, and the scope of the chapter is limited to the relevant clinical details of operative and perioperative events. Readers are referred elsewhere[17,39] to consider the effectiveness of these operations in cancer control.

REFERENCES

1. Alberti PW: The evolution of laryngology and laryngectomy in the mid-19th century, *Laryngoscope* 85:288, 1975.
2. Annino DJ, Goguen LA: Mitomycin C for the treatment of pharyngoesophageal stricture after total laryngopharyngectomy and microvascular free tissue reconstruction, *Laryngoscope* 113:1499, 2002.
3. Aprigliano F: Use of the nasogastric tube after laryngectomy: is it truly necessary? *Ann Otol Rhinol Laryngol* 99:513, 1990.
4. Bleach N, Perry A, Cheesman A: Surgical voice restoration with the Blom-Singer prosthesis following laryngopharygoesophagectomy and pharyngogastric anastomosis, *Ann Otol Rhinol Laryngol* 100:142, 1991.
5. Bocca E, Pignataro O, Oldini C: Supraglottic laryngectomy: 30 years of experience, *Ann Otol Rhinol Laryngol* 92:14, 1983.
6. Brizel DM and others: Hyperfractionated irradiation with or without concurrent chemotherapy for locally advanced head and neck cancer, *N Engl J Med* 338:1798, 1998.
7. Calteaux N, Hamoir M, deConinck A: Tumor of the hypopharynx: free jejunal transfer with conservation of the larynx: a case report, *J Reconstr Microsurg* 2:153, 1986.
8. Clements KS and others: Communication after laryngectomy. An assessment of patient satisfaction, *Arch Otolaryngol Head Neck Surg* 123:493, 1997.
9. Dadas B and others: Intraoperative management of the thyroid gland in laryngeal cancer surgery, *J Otolaryngol* 30:179, 2001.
10. Davis RK and others: The anatomy and complications of "T" versus vertical closure of the hypopharynx after laryngectomy, *Laryngoscope* 92:16, 1982.
11. deVries EJ and others: Jejunal interposition for repair of stricture or fistula after laryngectomy, *Ann Otol Rhinol Laryngol* 99:496, 1990.
12. Department of Veterans Affairs Laryngeal Cancer Study Group: Induction chemotherapy plus radiation compared with surgery plus radiation in patients with advanced laryngeal cancer, *N Engl J Med* 324:1685, 1991.
13. Deschler DT and others: Tracheoesophageal voice following tubed free radial forearm flap reconstruction of the neopharynx, *Ann Otol Rhinol Laryngol* 103:929, 1994.
14. Dumich PS, Pearson BW, Weiland LH: Suitability of near total laryngopharyngectomy in pyriform carcinoma, *Arch Otolaryngol* 110:664, 1984.
15. Eisenbruch A and others: Objective assessment of swallowing dysfunction and aspiration after radiation concurrent with chemotherapy for head and neck cancer, *Int J Radiat Oncol Biol Phys* 53:23, 2002.
16. Fagan JJ, Kaye PV: Management of the thyroid gland with laryngectomy for cT3 glottic carcinomas, *Clin Otolaryngol* 22:7, 1997.
17. Foote RL and others: Patterns of failure after total laryngectomy for glottic carcinoma, *Cancer* 64:143, 1989.
18. Forastiere AA and others: Concurrent chemotherapy and radiotherapy for organ preservation in advanced laryngeal cancer, *N Engl J Med* 349:2091, 2003.
19. Fu KK and others: A radiation therapy oncology group (RTOG) phase III randomized study to compare hyperfractionation and two variants of accelerated fractionation to standard fractionation radiotherapy for head and neck squamous cell carcinomas: first report of RTOG 9003, *Int J Radiat Oncol Biol Phys* 48:7, 2000.
20. Gates GA and others: Current status of laryngectomy rehabilitation. I. Results of therapy, *Am J Otolaryngol* 3:1, 1982.
21. Gosain A and others: A study of the relationship between blood flow and bacterial inoculation in musculocutaneous and fasciocutaneous flaps, *Plast Reconstr Surg* 86:1152, 1990.
22. Gussenbauer C: Ueber die erste durch Th. Billroth am Menschen ausgefulmte Kehlkopf-Etirpation, *Arch Klin Surg* 17:343, 1876.
23. Hagen R: Laryngoplasty with a radial flap from the forearm: a surgical procedure for voice rehabilitation after total laryngectomy, *Am J Otolaryngol* 7:85, 1990.
24. Hamaker RC, Blom ED: Botulinum neurotoxin for pharyngeal reconstrictor muscle spasm in tracheoesophageal voice restoration, *Laryngoscope* 113:1479, 2003.
25. Harrison DFN: Surgical management of cancer of the hypopharynx and cervical esophagus, *Br J Surg* 56:95, 1969.
26. Harwood AR and others: Management of advanced glottic cancer, *Int J Radiat Oncol Biol Phys* 5:899, 1979.
27. Haughey BH, Forsen JM: The jejunal free graft: effects of longitudinal myotomy, *Ann Otol Rhinol Laryngol* 101:333, 1991.
28. Haughey BH and others: Vibratory segment (VS) function for speech and swallowing after free flap reconstruction of the pharyngoesophagus, *Laryngoscope* 205:487, 1995.
29. Hoffman HT and others: Botulinum neurotoxin injection after total laryngectomy, *Head Neck Surg* 19:92, 1997.
30. Hollinger PH: A century of progress of laryngectomies in the northern hemisphere, *Laryngoscope* 85:322, 1975.
31. Hui Y and others: Primary closure of pharyngeal remnant after total laryngectomy and partial pharyngectomy: how much residual mucosa is sufficient? *Laryngoscope* 106:490, 1996.
32. Iro H, Waldfaherer F, Altendorf-Hofmann A: Transoral laser surgery of supraglottic cancer: follow-up of 141 patients, *Arch Otolaryngol Head Neck Surg* 124:1245, 1998.
33. Kaplan MJ and others: Glottic carcinoma: the roles of surgery and irradiation, *Cancer* 53:2641, 1984.
34. Kato H and others: Primary reconstruction after resection of cancer in the hypopharynx or cervical esophagus: comparison of free forearm skin tube flap, free jejunal transplantation and pull-through esophagectomy, *Jpn J Clin Oncol* 17:255, 1987.
35. Korver KD and others: Liver function studies in the assessment of head and neck cancer patients, *Head Neck* 17:531, 1995.
36. Laccourreye O and others: Supracricoid hemilaryngectomy in selected pyriform sinus carcinoma staged as T2, *Laryngoscope* 103:1373, 1993.
37. Laccourreye H and others: Supracricoid laryngectomy with cricohyoidopexy: a partial laryngeal procedure for selected supraglottic and transglottic carcinomas, *Laryngoscope* 100:735, 1990.
38. Laccourreye O and others: Supracricoid partial laryngectomy after failed laryngeal radiation therapy, *Otolaryngol Head Neck Surg* 113:242, 1995.
39. Lam KH, Lau WF, Wei WI: Tumor clearance at resection margins in total laryngectomy: a clinicopathologic study, *Cancer* 61:2260, 1988.
40. Lefebvre JL and others: Larynx preservation in pyriform sinus cancer: preliminary results of a European Organization for Research and Treatment of Cancer phase III trial. EORTC Head and Neck Cancer Cooperative Group, *J Natl Cancer Inst.* 88:890, 1996.

41. Logemann JA: *Videofluoroscopic procedure*. In Logemann JA, editor: *Evaluation and treatment of swallowing disorders*, San Diego, 1983, College-Hill Press.
42. Lowry LD and others: An intraoral self-contained artificial larynx, *Otolaryngol Head Neck Surg* 90:208, 1982.
43. Macbeth R: The treatment of carcinoma of the hypopharynx: the gutter graft operation, *J Laryngol Otol* 83:119, 1969.
44. McCombe AW, Jones AS: Radiotherapy and complications of Laryngectomy, *J Laryngol Otol* 107:130, 1991.
45. McConnel FMS and others: Manofluorography of deglutition after total laryngopharyngectomy, *Plast Reconstr Surg* 81:346, 1988.
46. Medina JE and others: Voice restoration after total laryngopharyngectomy and cervical esophagectomy using the duckbill prosthesis, *Am J Surg* 154:407, 1987.
47. Medina JE, Kfafif A: Early oral feeding following total laryngectomy, *Laryngoscope* 111:368, 2001.
48. Ogura JH, Thawley SE: *Treatment for early carcinoma including carcinoma in situ of the endolarynx: surgery is the treatment of choice*. In Snow JB, editor: *Controversy in otolaryngology*, Philadelphia, 1980, WB Saunders.
49. Olson HR, Callaway E: Nonclosure of pharyngeal muscle after laryngectomy, *Ann Otol Rhinol Laryngol* 99:507, 1990.
50. Panje WR: Prosthetic vocal rehabilitation following laryngectomy: the voice button, *Ann Otol Rhinol Laryngol* 90:116, 1981.
51. Pearson BW: Subtotal laryngectomy, *Laryngoscope* 91:1904, 1981.
52. Pearson BW and others: Results of near-total laryngectomy, *Ann Otol Rhinol Laryngol* 107:820, 1998.
53. Righi PD and others: Evaluation of prevertebral muscle invasion by squamous cell carcinoma. Can computed tomography replace open neck exploration? *Arch Otolaryngol Head Neck Surg* 122:660, 1996.
54. Grau C, Johansen LV, Hansen HS: Salvage laryngectomy and pharyngocutaneous fistulae after primary radiotherapy for head and neck cancer: a national survey from DAHANCA, *Head Neck* 25:711, 2003.
55. Schwartz DL and others: Staging of head and neck squamous cell cancer with extended-field FDG-PET, *Arch Otolaryngol Head Neck Surg* 129:1173, 2003.
56. Sessions DG, Ogura JH, Fried MP: Carcinoma of the subglottic area, *Laryngoscope* 85:1417, 1975.
57. Seven H, Calis AB, Turgut S: A randomized controlled trial of early oral feeding in laryngectomized patients, *Laryngoscope* 113:1076, 2003.
58. Shemen LJ, Spiro RH: Complications following laryngectomy, *Head Neck Surg* 8:185, 1986.
59. Simpson JF: Some facets of hypopharyngeal surgery, *J Laryngol Otol* 80:1077, 1966.
60. Sinard RJ and others: Hypothyroidism after treatment for nonthyroid head and neck cancer, *Arch Otolaryngol Head Neck Surg* 126:652, 2000.
61. Singer MI, Blom ED: An endoscopic technique for restoration of voice after laryngectomy, *Ann Otol Rhinol Laryngol* 89:529, 1980.
62. Staton J and others: Factors predictive of poor functional outcome after chemoradiation for advanced laryngeal cancer, *Otolaryngol Head and Neck Surg* 127:43, 2002.
63. Stell PM: The first laryngectomy for carcinoma, *Arch Otolaryngol* 98:293, 1973.
64. Stell PM: Total laryngectomy, *Clin Otolaryngol* 6:351, 1981.
65. Steiner W: Personal communication, 1996.
66. Steiner W and others: Therapy of hypopharyngeal cancer. IV. Long term results of transoral laser microsurgery for hypopharyngeal cancer, *HNO* 42:147, 1994.
67. Steiner W and others: Organ preservation by transoral laser microsurgery in piriform sinus carcinoma, *Otolaryngol Head Neck Surg* 124:58, 2001.
68. Tanabe M, Honjo I, Isshiki N: Neoglottic reconstruction following total laryngectomy, *Arch Otolaryngol* 3:39, 1985.
69. Tell R and others: Hypothyroidism after external radiotherapy for head and neck cancer, *Int J Radiat Oncol Biol Ohys* 39:303, 1997.
70. Terhaard CH and others: F-18-flurodeoxy-glucose positron emission tomography scanning in detection of local recurrence after radiotherapy for laryngeal/pharyngeal cancer, *Head Neck* 23:933, 2001.
71. Terrell JE, Fisher SG, Wolf GT: Long-term quality of life after treatment of laryngeal cancer, the Veterans Affairs Laryngeal Cancer Study Group, *Arch Otolaryngol Head Neck Surg* 123:496, 1997.
72. Thawley SE: Complications of combined radiation therapy and surgery for carcinoma of the larynx and inferior hypopharynx, *Laryngoscope* 41:677, 1981.
73. Trask DK and others: Expression of Bcl-2 family proteins in advanced laryngeal squamous cell carcinoma: correlation with response to chemotherapy and organ preservation, *Laryngoscope* 112:638, 2002.
74. Varvares MA and others: Use of the radial forearm fasciocutaneous free flap and Montgomery salivary bypass tube for pharyngoesophageal reconstruction, *Head Neck* 22:463, 2000.
75. Viani L, Stell PM, Dalby JE: Recurrence after radiotherapy for glottic carcinoma, *Cancer* 3:577, 1991.
76. Vikram B and others: New strategies for avoiding total laryngectomy in patients with head and neck cancer, *Natl Cancer Inst Monogr* 5:361, 1988.
77. Virtaniemi JA and others: The incidence and etiology of postlaryngectomy pharyngocutaneous fistulae, *Head Neck* 23:29, 2001.
78. Wang CP and others: The techniques of nonmuscular closure of hypopharyngeal defect following total laryngectomy: the assessment of complication and pharyngoesophageal segment, *J Laryngol Otol* 111:1060, 1997.
79. Wax MK, Touma BJ: Management of the N0 neck during salvage laryngectomy, *Laryngoscope* 109:4, 1999.
80. Wax MK, Touma BJ, Ramadan HH: Tracheostomal stenosis after laryngectomy: incidence and predisposing factors, *Otolaryngol Head Neck Surg* 113:242, 1995.
81. Weber RS and others: Outcome of salvage total laryngectomy following organ preservation therapy: the Radiation Therapy Oncology Group trial 91-11, *J Arch Otolaryngol Head Neck Surg* 129:44, 2003.
82. Weinstein GS, Laccourreye O, Rassekh CH: *Conservation laryngeal surgery*. In Cummings C and others, editors: *Otolaryngology—head and neck surgery*, St Louis, 1998, Mosby p 2200.
83. Wolf GT: A new strategy to preserve the larynx in the treatment of advanced laryngeal cancer: progress report of VA CSP 268. Abstracts of the Second International Conference on Head and Neck Cancer, Boston, July 1988.
84. Wolf GT and others: Immune reactivity does not predict chemotherapy response, organ preservation, or survival in advanced laryngeal cancer, *Laryngoscope* 112:1351, 2002.
85. Wookey H: The surgical treatment of carcinoma of the pharynx and upper esophagus, *Surg Gynecol Obstet* 75:499, 1942.
86. Ziesman M and others: Speaking jejunum after laryngopharyngectomy with neoglottic and neopharyngeal reconstruction, *Am J Surg* 158:321, 1989.
87. Zinreich SJ: Imaging in laryngeal cancer: computed tomography, magnetic resonance imaging, positron emission tomography, *Otolaryngol Clin North Am* 35:971, 2002.

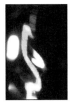

CHAPTER ONE HUNDRED AND FOUR

RADIATION THERAPY FOR THE LARYNX AND HYPOPHARYNX

‖ Parvesh Kumar

EPIDEMIOLOGY AND ETIOLOGY

Tumors of the larynx constitute about 1.5% of all cancers in the United States. The ratio of glottic to supraglottic carcinomas is about 3:1. The American Cancer Society estimates that 9500 cases of laryngeal cancer will be diagnosed and that 3800 patients will die of this disease in the United States in 2003.[2]

Cancers of the larynx and pyriform sinus have been associated with heavy smoking and alcohol intake, whereas those of the lower hypopharynx or postcricoid region have been associated with the nutritional deficiencies of vitamin C and iron.[69,71,72] The risk of the development of cancer of the larynx increases with increasing amounts smoked (Figure 104-1) and decreases with time after cessation of smoking (Figure 104-2).[70] Tuyns and others[64] reported that the carcinogenic effect of alcohol is present even at the lowest levels of tobacco consumption and that alcohol influences the development of epilaryngeal and hypopharyngeal cancers more than it does the development of endolaryngeal cancer. Alcohol presumably bathes the mucosa of the epilarynx and hypopharynx but does not have access to the mucosa of the endolarynx. It seems that tobacco and alcohol act separately and synergistically to increase the risk of cancers of the laryngopharynx.

The molecular basis for laryngeal cancer is beginning to evolve. Mutation of the p53 gene is common, and it is seen in 47% of the patients who are smokers but in only 14% of those who are nonsmokers. Fifty-five percent of tumors among drinkers and 20% among nondrinkers had p53 mutations.[8]

ANATOMY

A fundamental knowledge of laryngeal and hypopharyngeal anatomy is necessary to allow the clinician to understand the following: (1) how a particular cancer affects pharyngeal and laryngeal function to produce signs and symptoms; (2) how patterns of local invasion and lymphatic and distant spread differ for individual cancers of the larynx and hypopharynx; and (3) how the extent of tumor within the larynx and hypopharynx determines management selection.

The larynx is contiguous with the lower portion of the pharynx superiorly and is connected with the trachea inferiorly, separating the functions of respiration and phonation from swallowing. Anatomically the larynx extends from the tip of the epiglottis at the level of the lower border of the C3 vertebra to the lower border of the cricoid cartilage at the level of the C6 vertebra. The laryngeal vestibule is separated from the pyriform sinus laterally by the marginal structures of the larynx (the free margin of the epiglottis, the aryepiglottic fold, and the arytenoid), and the glottic and subglottic regions are separated posteriorly from the hypopharynx by a common partition—the cricoid cartilage (Figure 104-3). Thus food passes laterally into the laryngopharyngeal sulci and then posterior to the cricoid cartilage into the upper cervical esophagus without entering the upper airway. The larynx is subdivided into three anatomic regions: the supraglottis, the glottis, and subglottis regions (Figure 104-4). The anterior limits of the larynx consist of the lingual surface of the suprahyoid epiglottis, the thyrohyoid membrane, the anterior commissure, and the anterior wall of the subglottic region, which is composed of the thyroid cartilage, the cricothyroid membrane, and the anterior arch of the cricoid cartilage. The posterior and lateral limits include the aryepiglottic folds, the arytenoids, the interarytenoid space, and the posterior surface of the subglottic space, which is formed by the mucous membrane that covers the cricoid cartilage. The superolateral limits consist of the tip and the lateral borders of the epiglottis, and the inferior limit is the inferior edge of the cricoid cartilage. These various anatomic structures of the larynx can also be appreciated on computed tomography (CT) scans (Figure 104-5).

The supraglottic region extends from the superior margin of the true vocal cord and includes the

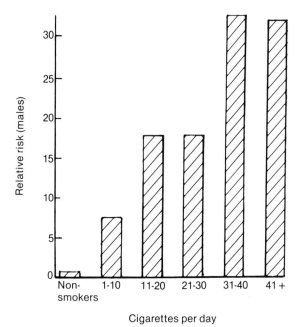

Figure 104-1. The risk of cancer of the larynx as a function of the amount of cigarettes smoked per day. From Wynder EL, Broso IJ, Day E: A study of environmental factors in cancer of the larynx, *Cancer* 9:86, 1956. Copyrighted by the American Cancer Society.

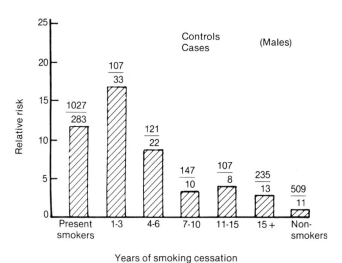

Figure 104-2. The risk of cancer of the larynx as a function of time after cessation of smoking. From Wynder EL, Mushinski MH, Spivak JC: Tobacco and alcohol consumption in relation to development of multiple primary cancers, *Cancer* 40:187, 1977. Copyrighted by the American Cancer Society.

ventricle, the false vocal cords, the epiglottis, the aryepiglottic folds, and the arytenoids. The glottis consists of the true vocal cords and the anterior and posterior commissures. It is important to note that the anterior commissure is usually within 1 cm of the skin surface. The lower boundary of the glottis extends 5 mm below the free margin of the vocal cords. The subglottis extends from the lower boundary of the glottis to the inferior margin of the cricoid cartilage. Cancers that involve the supraglottic region above and the glottic and subglottic regions below are referred to as *transglottic* cancers.

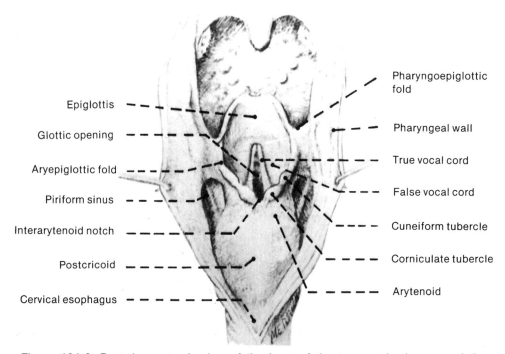

Figure 104-3. Posterior anatomic view of the base of the tongue, the larynx, and the hypopharynx, showing the piriform sinus, the pharyngeal wall, and the postcricoid region.

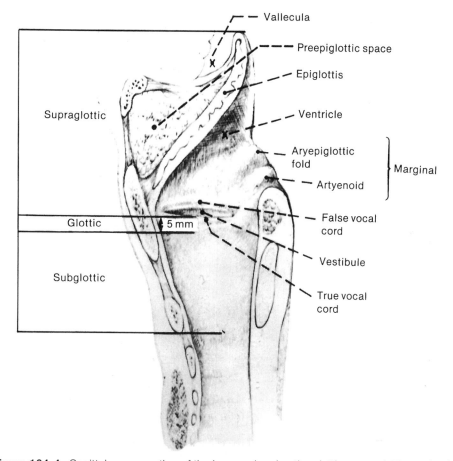

Figure 104-4. Sagittal cross-section of the larynx, showing the glottic, supraglottic, and subglottic regions.

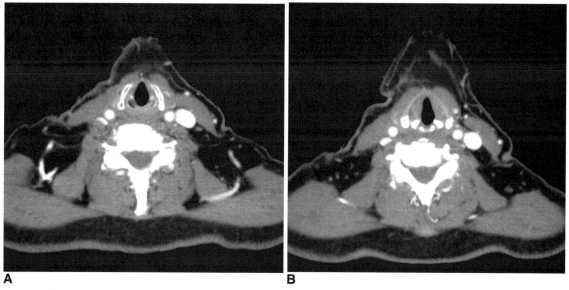

Figure 104-5. Computed tomography scans showing the various anatomic structures of the larynx.

The thyroid, cricoid, and most of the arytenoid cartilages are composed of hyaline cartilage, which begins to ossify when a person is about 20 years old. The epiglottis, corniculate, and cuneiform cartilages and the apex and vocal process of the arytenoids are made up of elastic cartilage, which does not ossify and therefore is not radiopaque.

PATHOLOGY

Squamous cell carcinoma makes up approximately 95% of all malignant neoplasms of the larynx, although many different histologies can originate from the larynx (Table 104-1). Carcinomas arising from the true vocal cords are usually well differentiated or moderately well differentiated; carcinomas of the supraglottis and subglottis are less differentiated than those of the vocal cords. Carcinoma in situ usually occurs in the true vocal cord region.

TABLE 104-1

PRIMARY MALIGNANCIES OF THE LARYNX BY HISTOLOGY

Epithelial cancers
Squamous cell carcinoma
  Carcinoma in situ
  Invasive (well to poorly differentiated)
  Verrucous carcinoma
  Lymphoepithelial carcinoma
  Pseudosarcoma
  Anaplastic carcinoma
  Transitional cell carcinoma
Adenocarcinoma
  Adenocarcinoma (well to poorly differentiated)
  Mucoepidermoid carcinoma
  Adenoid cystic carcinoma
Neuroendocrine tumors
  Small cell carcinoma
  Paraganglioma
  Carcinoid tumor
Oncocytic carcinoma
Melanoma
Carcinoid tumor
Lymphoma
Nonepithelial cancers
Sarcomas
  Chondrosarcoma
  Fibrosarcoma
  Rhabdomyosarcoma
  Osteosarcoma
  Leiomyosarcoma
  Hemangiosarcoma
  Giant cell sarcoma
  Lymphosarcoma

Verrucous carcinoma is a low-grade squamous cell carcinoma that is extremely rare. True verrucous carcinoma does not metastasize, and its anaplastic transformation after radiation therapy (RT) remains controversial.[5]

PATTERN OF SPREAD
Lymphatic Drainage

The low incidence of lymphatic metastases from cancers of the true vocal cord is generally a result of a paucity of lymphatic vessels in the region of the true glottis. The incidence of lymphatic metastases progressively increases as one proceeds above and below the true glottis and from the central supraglottis outward. The supraglottis has a rich lymphatic network. The lymphatic channels from the supraglottis pass through the thyrohyoid membrane and drain into the upper jugular (subdigastric or jugulodigastric), midjugular (jugulocarotid), and lower jugular (juguloomohyoid) nodes of the jugular chain.

The lymphatic network is less developed in the subglottis. Lymphatic channels from the subglottic area unite to form three lymphatic pedicles (one anterior and two posterolateral). The anterior channels pass through the cricothyroid membrane and drain into the mid- and lower jugular nodes or terminate in the prelaryngeal node (Delphian node), from which lymphatics drain into the pretracheal and supraclavicular nodes. The posterolateral lymphatic channels pass through cricotracheal membrane and terminate in the highest paratracheal nodes.

The true vocal codes are devoid of lymphatic capillaries. Lymphatic spread from glottic cancer occurs when there is tumor extension into the supraglottis or the subglottis.

The incidence of lymph node metastasis from carcinoma of the supraglottis increases with the T stage and when there is extension into the base of the tongue and the hypopharynx. The incidence of lymph node metastasis at the time of diagnosis is 55%, with 16% of cases being bilateral.[40] The subdigastric and midjugular nodes are most commonly involved. For carcinoma of the vocal cords, the incidence of lymph node metastasis at diagnosis is low: virtually 0% for T_1 lesions, approximately 5% for T_2 lesions, 15% to 20% for T_3 lesions, and 20% to 30% for T_4 lesions.[33,39,45] The incidence of lymph node metastasis from carcinoma of the subglottis varies from 20% to 50%.[45] The prelaryngeal (Delphian), lower jugular, paratracheal, pretracheal, and upper mediastinal lymph nodes are the most commonly involved nodal stations.

CLINICAL PRESENTATION

The most common presenting symptom of early-stage vocal cord cancer is hoarseness. The symptoms of advanced disease include sore throat, localized pain as a result of cartilage invasion, otalgia, and dyspnea as a result of airway compromise.

The most common presenting symptoms of carcinoma of the supraglottis are sore throat and odynophagia. Quite often a neck mass may be the first sign of carcinoma of the supraglottis as a result of the high incidence of lymph nodal metastases. Unilateral otalgia occurs as referred pain from the involvement of the vagus nerve and the auricular nerve of Arnold. Hoarseness is usually not an initial symptom, and it occurs with invasion of the vocal cords. Weight loss, dyspnea, foul breath, and aspiration occur with advanced disease.

Carcinoma of the subglottis is relatively asymptomatic during the early stage. With advanced-stage disease, dyspnea becomes predominant as a result of narrowing of the airway; other less common symptoms include hoarseness, odynophagia, and hemoptysis.

DIAGNOSTIC EVALUATION

The diagnostic evaluation of a patient who is suspected of having a cancer of the larynx should begin with a mandatory history and physical examination. The mainstay of the physical examination is the flexible fiberoptic endoscope, which allows for excellent visualization of the infrahyoid epiglottis and anterior commissures; these regions may be difficult to see with indirect laryngoscopy. In addition to determining the tumor extent, assessment of the mobility of the vocal cords is absolutely critical. The neck should be carefully palpated to determine the size, number, and location (ipsilateral, bilateral, or contralateral) of lymph node metastasis (Table 104-2).

Routine laboratory tests include a complete blood count and liver function tests. If the liver function tests or serum alkaline phosphatase are abnormal, further studies (e.g., liver and bone scans) may be indicated.

Imaging studies include a chest x-ray and a CT scan with contrast enhancement of the head and neck region. The CT scan should be performed before the biopsy, because postbiopsy edema may overestimate tumor extent. CT slices 3-mm thick should be obtained at 3-mm intervals throughout the larynx. The relative usefulness of CT scanning versus magnetic resonance imaging (MRI) remains controversial. MRI is more useful for delineating the soft-tissue extent of the primary tumor and cartilage invasion, whereas CT scanning is better for evaluating early bone invasion and the remainder of the laryngeal anatomy. The disadvantages of MRI are longer scanning time and motion artifact.

Direct laryngoscopy with biopsy of the tumor is the most important step in the diagnosis of carci-

---

TABLE 104-2

DIAGNOSTIC EVALUATION AND STAGING WORKUP OF PATIENTS WITH SUSPECTED LARYNGEAL CANCER

Clinical examination
History and physical examination: assessment of size, number, and location of affected lymph nodes
Fiberoptic endoscopic examination: mobility of vocal cords, assessment of anterior commissure involvement

Radiographic studies
Chest x-ray
Computed tomography scan of head and neck (3-mm slices)
Magnetic resonance imaging (as indicated)
Computed tomography scan of chest (if CXR is abnormal)

Laboratory studies
Complete blood count with differential and platelets
Comprehensive metabolic panel

Direct Laryngoscopy with Biopsy
Panendoscopy (bronchoscopy and esophagoscopy) for advanced-stage disease

---

noma of the larynx. In advanced-stage disease, a panendoscopy (bronchoscopy and esophagoscopy) should be performed to rule out synchronous tumors.

STAGING

The most recent TNM staging system of the American Joint Committee on Cancer (seventh edition) for carcinoma of the larynx is shown in Table 104-3. Primary tumor (T) staging is based on the extent of involvement within the larynx, extralaryngeal extension, cartilage invasion, and mobility of the vocal cords. Regional lymph node (N) staging is based on size, number, and location (ipsilateral, bilateral, or contralateral) of lymph nodes.

OVERALL MANAGEMENT, RADIOTHERAPY TECHNIQUE AND DOSE, AND OUTCOME

The major goal of the treatment of cancer of the larynx is to maximize the cure rate while preserving speech and swallowing function. Recent advances in surgical techniques, delivery of RT, and different ways of combining chemotherapy with RT have improved cure rates while maintaining organ function. A variety of conservative surgery procedures, such as those outlined below, have led to better preservation of organ function while still maintaining local-regional tumor control rates that are comparable with those achieved with radical surgery:

TABLE 104-3

AMERICAN JOINT COMMITTEE ON CANCER STAGING SYSTEM FOR CANCER OF THE LARYNX
AND THE HYPOPHARYNX (SIXTH EDITION, 2002)

Primary tumor (T)

T_X Primary tumor cannot be assessed
T_0 No evidence of primary tumor
Ti_s Carcinoma in situ

Supraglottis

T_1 Tumor limited to one subsite of the supraglottis, with normal vocal cord mobility
T_2 Tumor invades mucosa of more than one adjacent subsite of the supraglottis or glottis or a region outside of the supraglottis (e.g., mucosa of the base of the tongue, the vallecula, the medial wall of the pyriform sinus), without fixation of the larynx
T_3 Tumor limited to the larynx, with vocal cord fixation and/or invasion of any of the following: postcricoid area, preepiglottic tissues, paraglottic pace, and/or minor thyroid cartilage erosion (e.g., inner cortex)
T_{4a} Tumor invades through the thyroid cartilage and/or invades tissues beyond the larynx (e.g., trachea; soft tissues of the neck, including the deep extrinsic muscle of the tongue, the strap muscles, the thyroid, or the esophagus)
T_{4b} Tumor invades the prevertebral space, encases the carotid artery, or invades mediastinal structures

Glottis

T_1 Tumor limited to the vocal cord(s) (may involve anterior or posterior commissure), with normal mobility
T_{1a} Tumor limited to one vocal cord
T_{1b} Tumor involves both vocal cords
T_2 Tumor extends to the supraglottis and/or the subglottis, with or without impaired vocal cord mobility
T_3 Tumor limited to the larynx, with vocal cord fixation and/or invasion of paraglottic space and/or minor thyroid cartilage erosion (e.g., inner cortex)
T_{4a} Tumor invades through the thyroid cartilage and/or invades tissues beyond the larynx (e.g., trachea; soft tissues of neck, including the deep extrinsic muscle of the tongue, the strap muscles, the thyroid, or the esophagus)
T_{4b} Tumor invades the prevertebral space, encases the carotid artery, or invades mediastinal structures

Subglottis

T_1 Tumor limited to the subglottis
T_2 Tumor extends to the vocal cord(s), with normal or impaired mobility
T_3 Tumor limited to the larynx, with vocal cord fixation
T_{4a} Tumor invades the cricoid or thyroid cartilage and/or invades tissues beyond the larynx (e.g., trachea; soft tissues of neck, including the deep extrinsic muscles of the tongue, the strap muscles, the thyroid, or the esophagus)
T_{4b} Tumor invades the prevertebral space, encases the carotid artery, or invades mediastinal structures

Hypopharynx

T_1 Tumor limited to one subsite of the hypopharynx and is 2 cm or less in its greater dimension
T_2 Tumor involves more than one subsite of the hypopharynx or an adjacent site or measures more than 2 cm but not more than 4 cm in its greatest diameter, without fixation of the hemilarynx
T_3 Tumor measures more than 4 cm in its greatest dimension or involves fixation of the hemilarynx
T_4 Tumor invades adjacent structures (e.g., thyroid/cricoid cartilage, carotid artery, soft tissues of neck, prevertebral fascia/muscles, thyroid and/or esophagus)

Regional lymph nodes (N)

N_X Regional lymph nodes cannot be assessed
N_0 No regional lymph node metastasis
N_1 Metastasis in a single ipsilateral lymph node 3 cm or less in its greatest dimension
N_2 Metastasis in a single ipsilateral lymph node, more than 3 cm but not more than 6 cm in its greatest dimension, or in multiple ipsilateral lymph nodes, none more than 6 cm in its greatest dimension, or in bilateral or contralateral lymph nodes, none more than 6 cm in its greatest dimension

TABLE 104-3

AMERICAN JOINT COMMITTEE ON CANCER STAGING SYSTEM FOR CANCER OF THE LARYNX AND THE HYPOPHARYNX (SIXTH EDITION, 2002)—cont'd

N_{2a} Metastasis in single ipsilateral lymph node more than 3 cm but not more than 6 cm in its greatest dimension

N_{2b} Metastasis in multiple ipsilateral lymph nodes, none more than 6 cm in its greatest dimension

N_{2c} Metastasis in bilateral or contralateral lymph nodes, none more than 6 cm in its greatest dimension

N_3 Metastasis in a lymph node more than 6 cm in its greatest dimension

Distant metastasis (M)

M_X Distant metastasis cannot be assessed

M_0 No distant metastasis

M_1 Distant metastasis

Stage grouping

Stage	T	N	M
Stage 0	T_{is}	N_0	M_0
Stage I	T_1	N_0	M_0
Stage II	T_2	N_0	M_0
Stage III	T_3	N_0	M_0
	T_1	N_1	M_0
	T_2	N_1	M_0
	T_3	N_1	M_0
Stage IVA	T_{4a}	N_0	M_0
	T_{4a}	N_1	M_0
	T_1	N_2	M_0
	T_2	N_2	M_0
	T_3	N_2	M_0
	T_{4a}	N_2	M_0
Stage IVB	T_{4b}	Any N	M_0
	Any T	N_3	M_0
Stage IVC	Any T	Any N	M_1

1. Cordectomy
2. Endoscopic stripping
3. Laser excision
4. Laryngofissure
5. Supracricoid laryngectomy
6. Partial laryngopharyngectomy
7. Hemilaryngectomy
   a. Vertical hemilaryngectomy (lateral or frontal hemilaryngectomy)
   b. Horizontal hemilaryngectomy

Improvements in the delivery of RT include three-dimensional conformal RT (3D CRT) and, more recently, intensity-modulated RT (IMRT). Both of these technologic advances provide a better capability of delineating and localizing the target (tumor) and surrounding normal tissues so that higher doses of radiation dose can be delivered to the tumor while sparing the adjacent critical organs. The recent combined modality and organ preservation therapeutic strategies have focused on adding systemic chemotherapy to RT. There are several ways to do this: sequentially, alternatingly, concurrently, and sequentially followed by concurrently. Each approach has a different therapeutic focus, with its own unique toxicity profile. Three recent metaanalyses looked at the role of systemic therapy in advanced head and neck cancer and have shown that the overall absolute survival benefit of adding chemotherapy to local therapy varies from 4% to 6.5%; neoadjuvant and adjuvant chemotherapy marginally improve survival rates by only 1% to 2%, whereas the concurrent approach provides the greatest survival benefit of 8% to 12%.[14,52,56]

Radiotherapy Technique and Dose

Generally irradiation of laryngeal carcinoma is accomplished with a series of lateral opposed shrinking fields that encompass the primary tumor and the upper cervical lymph nodes with an initial minimum 2- to 3-cm margin. A single anterior low-neck field is used to irradiate the lower neck. Patients are immobilized in the supine position with bite blocks and thermoplastic immobilization masks. Ideally the upper and lower fields should be set up using a "half-beam" technique so that the potential overlap in the spinal cord region can be dosimetrically reduced. Nonetheless, a safety spinal cord block should still be placed either in the inferior-posterior portion of the lateral upper neck fields or the upper mid-center position of the lower neck field so that any areas of gross disease are not blocked. Coverage of nodal areas should follow the basic RT principle of treating the gross disease and the next uninvolved echelon nodal station. For example, if the upper jugulodigastric lymph nodes are involved, then the retropharyngeal nodes (anterior and above C1) should be included in the treatment volume. The lower border of the lateral fields should encompass the larynx, usually at or below the level of C5. When there is extensive subglottic involvement and/or positive lymph nodes in the low neck or supraclavicular fossa, a mediastinal T-field is used for the initial treatment volume up to 45 to 50 Gy. The lateral limits of the T-field should be below the clavicle, and the center portion of the T-field should extend 5 cm below the lower border of the clavicle head to include the upper mediastinum. Another method of treating laryngeal cancers with transglottic spread or extensive nodal disease in the lower neck is with the mini-mantle field technique. In this technique, matching anteroposterior and posteroanterior fields are used, with the patient in the hyperextended position to achieve homogenous dose distribution and to prevent shielding of the upper neck by the jaw (Table 104-4).

Linear accelerators with 4 to 6 MV photons or ^{60}Co machines and 6 to 15 MeV electrons for supplemental boosting to the nodes are commonly used. Treatment distance should be at least 80-cm source-to-skin distance. Because of the skin- and lymph-node–sparing effects of higher-energy photons, bolus material is used with photon energies of 6 MV.

Initially gross disease and areas at risk for subclinical disease should be treated to 45 Gy at standard fractionation (1.8 or 2.0 Gy/fraction [fx] given once daily). Generally, T_1 lesions should be treated to a total dose of 66 Gy, and T_2 lesions should be treated to 70 Gy. For T_3 or T_4 lesions, the dose of the RT depends on whether a single modality or a combined modality approach is used. The doses of RT are much higher (i.e., 74–76 Gy standard fractionation or 76.8–81.6 Gy at 1.2 Gy/fx twice daily with a hyperfractionated approach) if it is the only curative modality being used. When RT is used in conjunction with chemotherapy or surgery, lower doses of radiation are typically used. Preoperative doses are usually in the range of 45 to 50 Gy. Postoperatively, doses in the range of 60 to 70 Gy are used, depending on the histopathologic features (i.e., number of positive lymph nodes, presence of extracapsular extension, and status of surgical margins of the primary tumor). When combined with chemotherapy, standard radiation doses are 70 to 74 Gy. For lymphatic nodal disease measuring 1 to 2 cm, standard radiation doses of 66 to 70 Gy should be used. For nodal disease measuring 3 cm, a minimum standard dose of 70 Gy should be used, although boost doses as high as 74 to 76 Gy may be necessary, depending on the response. Typically, successive doses of radiation are given with a shrinking field technique, with field reductions at 50 Gy and 60 Gy; sometimes an additional reduction may also be necessary, depending on the total dose (Figure 104-6). With each successive field reduction, the margin around the primary tumor and gross nodal disease is reduced from 2 to 3 cm initially to 1.5 cm and then to 1.0 cm. Tissue equivalent compensators or wedges with appropriate angles based on the contours of the neck or CT scan treatment planning should be used to achieve uniform dose distribution within the target volume. The spinal cord should be shielded after 45 Gy, and electrons with appropriate energies should be used for supplemental boosting to the posterior neck lymph nodes.

Recently technical advances in the delivery of irradiation such as 3D CRT and IMRT have allowed for the escalation of radiation dose and/or minimization of late toxicity (e.g., xerostomia) by reducing doses to the salivary glands.[7,13,37,73] At the University of Southern California, we plan all of our curative laryngeal cancer cases using a 3D CRT approach. For those patients with nodal disease who may require significant irradiation to the parotid gland, an IMRT approach is used to spare the salivary glands. Additionally, radioprotectors such as Ethyol are given as supplements with these modern techniques to reduce the risk of permanent xerotsomia.[4,9]

TABLE 104-4

VOLUME- AND DOSE-FRACTIONATION* GUIDELINES FOR TREATMENT OF LARYNGEAL CARCINOMA

Disease	Total Dose*
Subclinical, microscopic	50.0 Gy
T_1	66.0 Gy
T_2	66.0 to 70.0 Gy
T_3/T_4	70.0 to 74.0 Gy†
Nodal disease:	
≤1 cm	60.0 to 66.0 Gy
≥1 to 2≤ cm	66.0 to 70.0 Gy
3 cm	70.0 to 74.0 Gy
>3 cm‡	70.0 to 74.0 Gy or more

*Assuming standard fractionated RT at 1.8 or 2.0 Gy/fx.
†RT should be delivered with shrinking field technique, with 2.0- to 3.0-cm margin to 45 to 50 Gy, then 1.5-cm margin to 60.0 Gy and 1.0-cm margin to ≥70.0 Gy.
‡Neck dissection (dependent on response rate to radiotherapy).

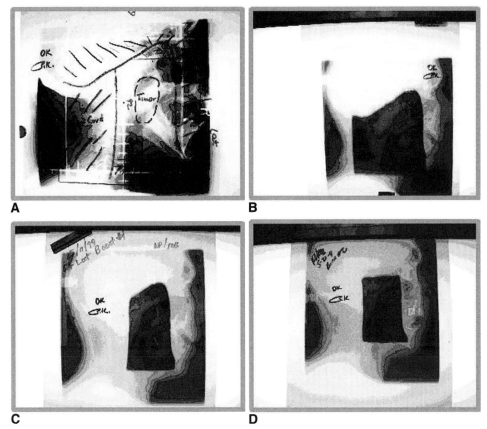

Figure 104-6. Series of scans showing reduced doses of radiation therapy throughout treatment. To view this image in color, please go to *www.ototext.com* or the Electronic Image Collection CD, bound into your copy of Cummings Otolaryngology—Head and Neck Surgery, 4th edition.

Early-Stage Laryngeal Carcinoma
General Management

Early-stage laryngeal disease can often be cured with either RT or surgery. Selection of a treatment modality for an individual patient depends on a number of factors, including the following: vocal cord mobility, size and extent of disease involvement, general medical condition of the patient, occupation, patient compliance for close follow-up examinations, gender of the patient, cost, availability of surgical or radiation oncology expertise, and, of course, patient preference. Because the volume of tissue irradiated for these tumors is relatively small, chronic side effects are minimal. Additionally, RT also addresses subclinical disease, which is another advantage over surgery. Another critical factor in the choice between surgery and RT is the quality of voice after therapy. For example, laser excision of a lesion in the region of the anterior commissure can result in permanent hoarseness as a sequela of surgery. On the other hand, the same laser excision of a mid–vocal-cord lesion often leaves patients with excellent voice quality as compared with voice quality after RT. Harrison and colleagues[25] studied voice quality in irradiated patients and concluded that the resultant voice quality was excellent.

Supraglottic Carcinoma: Management and Outcome

Early (T_1) superficial exophytic lesions can be treated with RT or supraglottic laryngectomy, with excellent local control and preservation of voice (Figure 104-7).

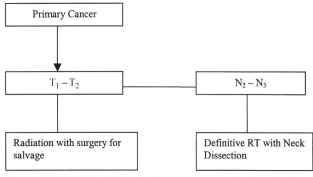

Figure 104-7. Algorithm for the management of early-stage supraglottic cancer.

However, not every patient with early-stage disease is a candidate for supraglottic laryngectomy. From an anatomic standpoint, supraglottic laryngectomy is contraindicated under the following conditions: (1) more than minimal extension into the medial wall of the pyriform sinus; (2) involvement of the post-cricoid region; (3) arytenoid fixation or bilateral arytenoid involvement; (4) impaired vocal cord mobility or fixation; (5) invasion of the thyroid or cricoid cartilage; (6) extension into the infrahyoid epiglottis or into the ventricle within 5 mm of the anterior commissure and/or the true vocal cord(s); and (7) extension into the base of the tongue to involve both lingual arteries and/or extension anterior to the circumvallate papillae. Of course, from a functional standpoint, elderly patients or those with poor lung function who may have difficulty swallowing and consequent complications of aspiration are also not good candidates for conservation surgery.

RT is the preferred initial treatment for superficial exophytic lesions involving the vocal cords (T_2, N_{0-1}), with surgery reserved for RT failures. Moderately advanced supraglottic carcinoma with vocal cord involvement and extensive neck disease (T_2, N_{2-3}) can be treated with RT followed by a radical neck dissection, with preservation of voice. Because of the propensity for lymphatic spread, the treatment volume for carcinoma of the supraglottis should include the primary lesion as well as the regional lymphatics in the neck.

Local control after RT for T_1 supraglottic carcinoma is excellent, ranging from 88% to 100% (Table 104-5).* For T_2 lesions, local control after RT varies from 73% to 89%.* In most series, once-daily RT to total doses of 66 to 74 Gy was used for both T_1 and T_2 lesions. In some series, such as those reported by Wang and Montgomery[66] and Hinerman and colleagues,[28] twice-a-day hyperfractionation approach was used. Hinerman and others[28] used twice-a-day hyperfractional RT to a total dose of 74.4 to 76.8 Gy at 1.2 Gy/fx. A minimum daily interfraction interval of 6 hours is recommended to minimize late normal tissue toxicity. With the split-course accelerated hyperfractional RT schedule used by Wang and Montgomery[66] at the Massachusetts General Hospital, a total dose of 67.2 Gy was delivered at 1.6 Gy/fx, twice a day, 5 days per week, with a 2-week rest after 38.4 Gy.

Glottic Carcinoma: Management and Outcome
Carcinoma in situ

The optimal management of early-stage carcinoma of the glottis is controversial, and this includes that of carcinoma in situ of the true vocal cords. The management of carcinoma in situ ranges from observation to vocal cord stripping, cordectomy, or open partial laryngectomy to primary RT. An incidence of 16% to 63% of the development of invasive carcinoma has

---

*References 17, 24, 28, 53, 59, 65, 66.

TABLE 104-5

LOCAL CONTROL AFTER RADIOTHERAPY FOR EARLY-STAGE SUPRAGLOTTIC CARCINOMA

Series	Stage	Patients (n)	Local Control
Fletcher and others (1974)[17]	T_1	24	88%
	T_2	56	79%
Ghossein and others (1974)[24]	T_1	17	94%
	T_2	64	73%
Wall and others (1985)[65]	T_1	38	89%
	T_2	132	74%
Wang and others (1991)[66]	T_1 } BID	23	89%
	T_2	79	89%
Nakfoor and others (1998)[53]	T_1	24	96%
	T_2	73	86%
Skyes and others (2000)[59]	T_1	65	92%
	T_2	136	81%
Hinerman and others (2002)[28]	T_1	22	100%
	T_2	125	86%

been reported after treatment by conservation surgery.[29,50] Results of conservative surgical approaches, such as microexcision, laser ablation, and vocal cord stripping, are often good, but they are compromised by multiple stripping procedures in the attempt to achieve local control. Maran and colleagues[44] noted that patients, on average, undergo two and up to six stripping procedures. Multiple stripping procedures result in suboptimal voice quality, and they are cost-inefficient. In a literature review of multiple weighted series by Garcia-Serra and others,[22] the local control rate was only 72% at 5 years, with vocal cord stripping alone as the initial mode of treatment; however, an ultimate local control rate of 92% at 5 years was obtained using RT or surgery (laryngofissure and cordectomy, hemilaryngectomy, or total laryngectomy) as salvage therapy. Conversely, a local control rate of 87.4% at 5 years was achieved with RT as the initial mode of therapy, with an ultimate 5-year local control rate of 98.4% with salvage treatment. For the management of carcinoma in situ, we favor a primary

RT approach, which results in excellent local control and the preservation of a high quality of voice (Figure 104-8). The dose-fractionation scheme and the RT technique for carcinoma in situ are similar to those used for early-stage T_1 and T_2 glottic disease, which is discussed next.

Early Stage (T₁ and T₂) Vocal Cord Carcinoma

RT is the treatment of choice for early-stage T_1 and T_2 glottic carcinoma. At the University of Southern California, a 3D CRT approach is used to treat patients with early-stage laryngeal carcinoma. The planning CT scan is done with the patients in a supine treatment position, with the head hyperextended and immobilized with a face mask. For T_1 and very early T_2 lesions, two small opposing lateral fields, usually measuring 5×5 cm² to 6×6 cm², are used. The fields usually extend from the upper thyroid notch superiorly to the lower border of the C6 vertebral body inferiorly. The anterior border should be 1-cm anterior to the skin surface at the level of the vocal cords. The

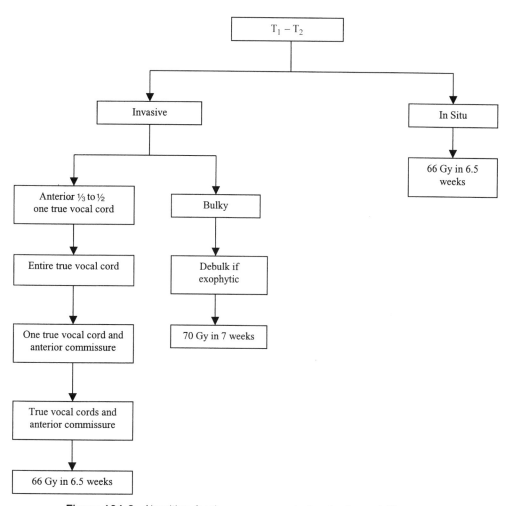

Figure 104-8. Algorithm for the management of early-stage glottic cancer.

posterior border of the field should include the anterior portion of the vertebral bodies (Figure 104-9). The lymph nodes are not treated in patients with T_1 disease because of the virtually nonexistent incidence of lymphatic nodal metastases. However, the need for elective neck irradiation for T_2N_0 vocal cord carcinoma is controversial.[46,68] For nonbulky T_{2a} disease in which the mobility of the vocal cords is not impaired, the treatment of lymphatic nodal disease is not recommended. However, for bulky T_{2b} disease in which the risk of lymph nodal metastases can be as high as 15%, treatment of at least the first-echelon lymph nodes (subdigastric and midjugular) is recommended.

Multiple-dose fractionation schemes have been used to treat patients with T_1 and T_2 glottic carcinoma, with total dose of 66 to 70 Gy at 2 Gy/fx per day, 63 Gy at 2.1 Gy/fx per day, or 60.75 Gy to 65.25 Gy at 2.25 Gy/fx per day, 5 days per week. Lower total doses are used for small tumors, and higher total doses are used for larger tumors. Wedged, open, or mixed fields are used, depending on the shape of the neck. At our institution, we use a total dose of 66 Gy at 2.0 Gy/fx for T_1 and for early, mini-

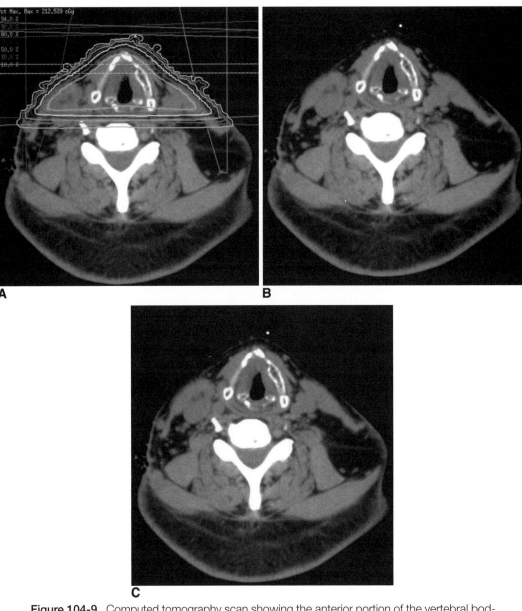

Figure 104-9. Computed tomography scan showing the anterior portion of the vertebral bodies in a patient with early-stage vocal cord carcinoma. To view this image in color, please go to *www.ototext.com* or the Electronic Image Collection CD, bound into your copy of Cummings Otolaryngology—Head and Neck Surgery, 4th edition.

mal T_2 glottic lesions; for bulky T_2 disease, a total dose of 70 Gy at standard fractionation is used.

Local control rates between 83% and 94% at 5 years have been reported with RT alone for T_1 glottic carcinoma (Table 104-6). With surgical salvage, ultimate local control rates between 94% and 99% at 5 years can be achieved after RT. For T_2 glottic lesions, initial local control rates vary between 68% and 88% at 5 years with RT alone (Table 104-7). Failures of RT for T_2 lesions can be salvaged in the majority of patients, so ultimate local control rates between 76% and 96% at 5 years can be achieved with salvage surgery. Although similar cure rates can be achieved with hemilaryngectomy or cordectomy for selected T_1 and T_2 vocal cord carcinomas, voice quality is usually better after RT than after surgery.

Verrucous Carcinoma

Treatment of verrucous carcinoma of the vocal cords remains controversial. Some regard it as a lesion with limited radioresponsiveness, and anaplastic transformation has been reported to occur after RT.[36] However, others have found that RT and surgery are equally effective and that anaplastic transformation rarely occurs.[16,61] Treatment for this rare lesion should be based on the extent of the disease. Small tumors can be treated by excision or partial laryngectomy. RT is recommended for large tumors that would require total laryngectomy if treated surgically.

ADVANCED-STAGE LARYNGEAL CARCINOMA
General Management

Historically, locally advanced carcinoma of the larynx (i.e., T_3 and T_4 and/or N_2 and N_3 disease) has usually been treated with combined surgery and pre- or postoperative RT or RT alone for unresectable disease. The disadvantages of a primary surgical approach include loss of organ function. Locoregional tumor control rates with total laryngectomy and postoperative RT are high (80%–90%), and, with tracheoesophageal

TABLE 104-6

LOCAL CONTROL OF T_1 CARCINOMA OF THE GLOTTIS TREATED WITH DEFINITIVE RADIOTHERAPY AND SURGICAL SALVAGE

Reference	Patients (n)	Initial Local Control	Ultimate Local Control
Elman and others (1979)[15]	T_{1a}, 210	T_{1a}, 94%	T_{1a}, 98%
	T_{1b}, 61	T_{1b}, 93%	T_{1b}, 98%
Fletcher and others (1980)[18]	332	89%	98%
Mittal and others (1983)[51]	177	83%	96%
Amornmarn and others (1985)[3]	86	92%	99%
Wang (1990)[68*]	723	90%	97%
Johansen (1990)[32]	358	83%	94%
Akine and others (1991)[1]	154	89%	94%

TABLE 104-7

T_2 CARCINOMA OF THE GLOTTIS: LOCAL CONTROL WITH RADIOTHERAPY AND SURGICAL SALVAGE

Reference	Patients (n)	Initial Local Control	Ultimate Local Control
Elman and others (1979)[15]	T_{2a}, 146	T_{2a}, 80%	T_{2a}, 96%
	T_{2b}, 82	T_{2b}, 72%	T_{2b}, 96%
Fletcher and others (1980)[18]	175	74%	94%
Mittal and others (1983)[51]	327	69%	—
Howell-Burke and others (1990)[30]	114	68%	76%
Karim and others (1987)[35]	156	81%	95%
Wang (1990)[68*]	173	69%	86%
Amornmarn and others (1985)[3]	34	88%	94%

punctures for voice restoration, patients can regain their verbal communication skills. This treatment is still ideal for patients in whom surveillance would be difficult. The addition of postoperative RT to a primary surgical approach is crucial to reducing the rate of locoregional failures.

Currently, the standard for the management of advanced laryngeal carcinoma is evolving. In the last 10 years, three major randomized trials have evaluated the addition of chemotherapy to local therapies for laryngeal carcinoma (Table 104-8).[12,19,57] Two of these randomized studies investigated induction chemotherapy as an initial treatment vs immediate surgery consisting of total laryngectomy, and they concluded that induction chemotherapy does not compromise survival rates and allows for larynx preservation in the majority of patients. Recently, the RTOG (Protocol 9111) and the Head and Neck Intergroup completed a three-arm phase III trial that randomized patients with stage III and IV laryngeal cancer to standard RT alone (70 Gy in 35 fractions); induction cisplatin (100 mg/m^2 on days 1 and 22); or 5-FU (1000 mg/m^2 daily continuous infusion for 5 days for two cycles); this was followed by the same standard RT or concurrent cisplatin (100 mg/m^2 on days 1, 22, and 43) with the same RT.[19] The two-year survival estimates were not significantly different among the three arms (75% for RT alone, 76% for the induction chemotherapy arm, and 74% for the concurrent chemoradiation arm). However, the 2-year rates of locoregional tumor control were significantly improved with concurrent chemoradiation therapy (78%) as compared with induction chemotherapy (61%, $P = .003$) or RT alone (56%, $P < .001$). In addition, the rates of laryngeal preservation at two years were also significantly better in the concurrent chemoradiation therapy arm (88%) as compared with the induction

chemotherapy arm (75%, $P = .005$) or the RT-alone arm (70%, $P < .001$). Hence, on the basis of the RTOG and the Head and Neck Intergroup Laryngeal Preservation trials, concurrent chemoradiation therapy should be considered a viable alternative to a primary surgical approach for advanced laryngeal carcinoma. However, the cost of achieving better locoregional tumor control and larynx preservation with concurrent chemoradiation therapy comes with a price of increased toxicity; the rate of severe toxicity (acute and late effects) was significantly higher with concurrent chemoradiation therapy (82%) as compared with RT alone (61%).

Radiotherapy Technique and Dose

The general RT techniques used to treat patients with laryngeal patients have been previously discussed. Certain dose-volume nuisances are important to appreciate when treating advanced laryngeal carcinoma. When preoperative RT is given in conjunction with total laryngectomy, a dose of 50 to 54 Gy is delivered at 1.8 Gy/fx per day, 5 days per week. A lower total dose of 45 Gy is given before supraglottic laryngectomy to reduce wound complications, because tissues are under more tension at closure.

For postoperative RT after total laryngectomy, a minimum total dose of 60 Gy at 1.8 to 2.0 Gy/fx per day, 5 days a week, is delivered to the tumor bed and the upper neck using a shrinking field technique. The spinal cord is shielded at 45 Gy when RT is used alone. An additional 5 to 10 Gy is delivered through reduced fields to areas of positive margins or gross residual disease. A dose of 50 Gy is delivered to the supraclavicular fossa. The tracheal stoma is usually included in the anterior low-neck field. It is usually not necessary to bolus the stomal site if ^{60}Co or 4 MV x-rays are used. If higher-energy x-rays are used,

---

TABLE 104-8

Randomized Trials of Advanced Laryngeal Carcinoma

Trial	Primary Tumor Site	Patients (n)	Local Control	2-Year Overall Survival	Larynx Preservation Rate
Department of Veterans Affairs Laryngeal Cancer Study Group[12]	Larynx	332	Surgery, 93% Induction CT, 80%	68% in both arms	Surgery, N/A Induction CT, 64%
GETTEC[57]	Larynx (T3)	68	Surgery, 87.5% Induction CT, 75%	Surgery, 84% Induction CT, 69%	N/A 42%
RTOG[19]	Larynx	547	RT, 56% CT→RT, 61% CT/RT, 78%	RT, 75% CT→RT, 76% CT/RT, 74%	RT, 70% CT→RT, 75% CT/RT, 88%

CT, Chemotherapy; RT, radiation therapy; CT→RT, induction CT followed by RT; CT/RT, concurrent CT and RT.

bolus of the stomal site is recommended. An additional 5 to 10 Gy is delivered through a reduced boost field to the tracheal stoma using 9 to 12 MeV electrons with a 0.5-cm bolus. With preoperative RT, surgery is performed 4 to 6 weeks after completion of the RT. Postoperative RT should be started within 3 to 6 weeks after surgery, when the wound has healed. The RT dose-volume guidelines have been previously discussed (see Table 104-4). When RT is combined with concurrent chemotherapy, the spinal cord dose is generally limited to 40 Gy if standard fractionated irradiation is used.

ADVANCED SUPRAGLOTTIC CARCINOMA: MANAGEMENT AND OUTCOME

For advanced operable carcinoma of the supraglottis, management options include surgery combined with RT, chemotherapy combined with RT, or RT alone. When RT is combined with surgery, it is usually given postoperatively because of the ability to tailor the dose more optimally on the basis of histopathologic information (i.e., the number of positive nodes, the presence of extracapsular extension, and/or the status of the primary surgical margins) and because there are generally lower rates of complications. In a randomized trial by RTOG (Protocol 7303) that compared postoperative (60 Gy) and preoperative (50 Gy) RT for the treatment of stage III and IV carcinoma of the supraglottis and the hypopharynx, local control was significantly better with postoperative RT (70%) as compared with preoperative irradiation (58%, $P = .05$), although there was no significant difference in survival (29% vs 20%, respectively).[63] However, the major complication rate was somewhat lower with postoperative RT (5%) as compared with preoperative RT (9%). Hence, RT should preferentially be given postoperatively, except when it is combined with supraglottic laryngectomy. When combined with a supraglottic laryngectomy, low-dose (45 Gy) preoperative RT is preferable to high-dose (≥60 Gy) because

of increased laryngeal edema and higher rates of complications associated with the higher doses. The contraindications to supraglottic laryngectomy have been previously discussed. In another small randomized trial of 72 patients that was conducted at the Tata Memorial Hospital, radical RT was compared with total laryngectomy and postoperative RT for stage III and IV supraglottic and pyriform sinus cancers.[6] Definitive RT was comparable with surgery for achieving locoregional tumor control (66% in both arms) and for overall survival (77% vs 73%, $P = .79$, respectively).

As discussed previously, randomized trials have shown that combined chemotherapy and RT is comparable with a primary surgical approach for achieving similar survival outcome but with the preservation of organ function. Selected patients with advanced supraglottic carcinoma and patients who are medically unsuitable for surgery and/or chemotherapy can be treated with RT alone. In patients with T3 and T4 disease, local control rates after definitive RT vary from 46% to 76% and 43% to 91%, respectively (Table 104-9).*

ADVANCED GLOTTIC CARCINOMA: MANAGEMENT AND OUTCOME

Fixed vocal cord lesions are indicative of deep muscle or cartilage infiltration. The management options for advanced glottic carcinoma vary between a primary surgical approach, chemotherapy combined with RT (a concurrent approach is favored over a neoadjuvant approach), or RT alone. This decision depends on a number of factors, including performance status, comorbid conditions, suitability for surgery/chemotherapy, and patient preference. The obvious disadvantage of surgery is the loss of voice function, and recent randomized trials have shown that a nonsurgical approach

---

*References 17, 24, 28, 53, 59, 65, 66.

TABLE 104-9

T_3 Carcinoma of the Glottis: Results of Definitive Radiotherapy and Surgical Salvage

Reference	Stage	Patients, n	Initial Local Control	Ultimate Local Control
Lundgren and others (1988)[41]	T_3	141	44%	59%
Harwood and others (1980)[27]	T_3N_0	112	51%	77%
Pameijer and others (1997)[55]	T_3	42	62%	NR
Bryant and others (1995)[10]	T_3	55	55%	NR
Stewart and others (1975)[60]	T_3	67	57%	69%
Lustig and others (1984)[42]	T_3	47	65%	NR
Mendenhall and others (1992)[47]	T_3	47	62%	81%

NR, Not reported.

does not compromise survival but does provide preservation of the larynx.

As discussed previously, locoregional tumor control rates are approximately 80% with concurrent chemoradiation therapy, 60% with induction chemotherapy followed by RT, and 55% with RT alone for stage III and IV disease.[12,19] For selected T3 lesions, local control rates with RT alone vary between 44% and 65%, and approximately two thirds of the failures can be salvaged by surgery (Table 104-10).*

For T_4 lesions, the results from the Veterans Administration and the RTOG/Head & Neck Intergroup Trials suggest that that combination of chemotherapy and RT may be a viable alternative to total laryngectomy.[12,19] Total laryngectomy is the preferred treatment for more advanced lesions with bilateral vocal cord involvement and compromised airway; very few series report results with RT alone for T_4 glottic lesions. Hardwood and others[26] and Karim and others[34] reported local control rates of 56% (39 patients) and 63% (38 patients), respectively, with T_4 disease.

When surgery is used as the primary definitive therapy, postoperative RT is usually added to reduce the risk of locoregional failure. Postoperative RT is indicated when there is tumor at or close to the surgical margins; cartilage invasion; involvement of the soft tissues of the neck; extensive subglottic infiltration; multiple (more than one) lymph node metastasis; extracapsular nodal extension; and perineural, lymphatic, or vascular invasion. A neck dissection is usually performed when there are positive lymph nodes.

SUBGLOTTIC CARCINOMA: MANAGEMENT AND OUTCOME

Primary carcinomas of the subglottis are rare. RT data about the management of subglottic carcinoma is sparse. Recently, Paisley and colleagues[54] reported their retrospective analysis of 43 patients with subglottic cancer who were treated with primary RT alone. Overall, the initial local control was 56% with RT alone, with an ultimate local control rate of 81.4% with surgical salvage. When broken down by T stage, the initial local control rates for T_1, T_2, T_3, and T_4 lesions with primary RT alone were 63.6%, 66.7%, 50%, and 41.7%, respectively. With surgical salvage, the ultimate local control rates for T_1, T_2, T_3, and T_4 lesions were improved to 91%, 100%, 75%, and 58.3%, respectively. Most subglottic lesions are relatively advanced at the time of diagnosis and are managed primarily with surgery followed by postoperative RT. However, definitive RT offers a viable alternative to surgery for the management of subglottic carcinomas.

CARCINOMA OF THE HYPOPHARYNX: MANAGEMENT AND OUTCOME

Early-stage hypopharyngeal carcinoma can be effectively managed with RT alone. Local control rates range from 74% to 90% for T_1 disease and from 59% to 79% for T_2 disease.[23,48,67] Recently, the use of hyperfractionation appears to have improved local control

---

*References 10, 26, 27, 41, 42, 47, 55, 60.

TABLE 104-10

LOCAL CONTROL AFTER RADIOTHERAPY FOR ADVANCED-STAGE SUPRAGLOTTIC CARCINOMA

Series	Stage	Patients, n	Local Control
Fletcher and others (1974)[17]	T_3	29	62%
	T_4	17	47%
Ghossein and others (1974)[24]	T_3	35	46%*
	T_4	87	52%
Wall and others (1985)[65]	T_3	50	70%
	T_4	28	46%
Wang and others (1991)[66]	T_3	95	71%
	T_4	12	91%
Nakfoor and others (1998)[53]	T_3	51	76%
	T_4	16	43%
Skyes and others (2000)[59†]	T_3	83	67%
	T_4	47	73%
Hinerman and others (2002)[28‡]	T_3	99	62%
	T_4	28	62%

*All had vocal cord fixation.
†All were N_0, and some were salvaged with total laryngectomies.
‡1998 American Joint Committee on Cancer staging.

rates for early-stage disease. More recent results have suggested an improvement in control rates with the use of hyperfractionated radiation. Mendenhall and others[48] reported local control in 94% of patients with T_2 pyriform sinus cancer treated with twice-a-day RT. Wang[67] reported a 5-year actuarial local control rate of 76% in patients with T_2 pyriform sinus cancer treated with split-course accelerated RT. Garden and colleagues[23] reported a local control rate of 86% for early-stage hypopharyngeal carcinoma.

The treatment of choice for patients with T_3 and T_4 hypopharyngeal cancer is surgery. Because of the high risk of local failure after surgery, postoperative RT is usually given to most patients. An analysis by Frank and others[20] found that patients with hypopharyngeal cancer who received postoperative irradiation had only a 14% rate of locoregional failure as compared with 57% in those treated with surgery only, despite the fact that patients treated with combined therapy had more advanced disease.

The European Organization for the Research and Treatment of Cancer conducted a voice preservation study of patients with hypopharyngeal carcinomas.[38] In this trial, 202 patients were randomized to either immediate surgery followed by postoperative RT (50-70 Gy) or induction cisplatin (100 mg/m^2 on day 1) and 5-fluorouracil (1000 mg/m^2 daily on days 1 through 5) for three cycles followed by RT (70 Gy). The locoregional failure rates were similar for both the surgery arm (31%) and the induction chemotherapy arm (40%). Survival rates were equivalent in the two treatment groups at 5 years (35% for the surgery arm vs 30% for the induction chemotherapy arm), but patients in the chemotherapy group had a 5-year voice preservation rate of 35). However, only 5% of the patients in the European Organization for the Research and Treatment of Cancer trial had T_4 disease. Another strategy for the treatment of advanced pyriform sinus carcinomas involves the use of high-dose intraarterial cisplatin (100 mg/m^2 on days 1, 8, 15, and 22) with concurrent RT (68-74 Gy).[58] This method is called the "RADPLAT" strategy, and 25 patients with stage III (24%) and stage IV (76%) pyriform sinus carcinoma were treated with this organ-preserving approach. Seventeen patients presented with bulky nodal disease, whereas 10 were diagnosed with T_4 lesions. At a median follow-up interval of 42 months, none of the 25 patients had experienced a local recurrence at the primary site, and only one patient relapsed regionally in the lymph nodes (this patient was subsequently salvaged with surgery). Moreover, the larynx preservation rate was 88%. Hence, combining chemotherapy with RT offers an alternative to patients with advanced-stage disease.

COMPLICATIONS

The acute and late effects of RT are directly dependent on such factors as total dose,[49,60] dose per fraction,[21,43,49] treatment volume,[21,31,43] overall treatment time,[62] and daily interfraction interval with hyperfractionated RT.[11] Other factors that also influence the late complication rate include the stage of disease,[21,49,62] the sequence of RT and surgery (i.e., pre- vs postoperative RT),[63] and chemotherapy.[11] Both acute and late normal tissue effects may be exacerbated in the presence of other medical conditions, such as hypertension, diabetes, immune suppression, and collagen vascular disease.

Acute reactions occurring during fractionated RT for carcinoma of the vocal cords are usually mild. Increases in hoarseness, sore throat, dysphagia, patchy mucositis, erythema, and erythema of the skin in the radiation field may develop, generally beginning during the second to fourth week of RT. These acute reactions may initially increase and then stabilize toward the later part of the treatment course, and they usually subside completely within six to eight weeks after completion of treatment. In the majority of patients, the voice returns to normal within a few months after treatment. In addition to hoarseness and sore throat, change or loss of taste, dry mouth, dysphagia, and weight loss can occur. The severity of these acute reactions increases with treatment volume. The acute reactions of twice-daily hyperfractionated or accelerated fractionated RT are usually more severe than those seen with once-daily conventional fractionated RT.

Laryngeal edema of varying degrees may persist after RT for carcinoma of the glottis or supraglottis. In patients who have been irradiated for carcinoma of the glottis, the incidence of mild to moderate laryngeal edema persisting for more than 3 months after RT is about 15.4% to 25%.[21] The incidence of severe laryngeal edema is about 1.5% to 4.6%,[3,30,31,49] and this increases with greater total dose, field size, dose per fraction, and T stage of the lesion.[31,43,49] In a randomized trial conducted by Inoue and colleagues,[31] 116 patients were treated with a total dose of 60 Gy in 30 fractions over 6 weeks using 4 MV x-rays and wedge filters. Persistent laryngeal edema occurred in 4% of the patients with 5 × 5 cm^2 fields and in 21% of the patients with 6 × 6 cm^2 fields ($P < .02$). However, local control rates were similar at 93% and 95% for field sizes of 5 × 5 cm^2 and 6 × 6 cm^2, respectively. Initially these patients should be managed conservatively with voice rest, abstinence from alcohol and cigarettes, and careful, close follow-up examinations. Antibiotics and steroids may be used when there is suspicion of infection or when the edema is severe enough to significantly compromise the airway. However, if the edema is progressive and unresponsive to conservative measures and recurrent disease is strongly suspected, biopsies are carried out to establish the diagnosis. Salvage surgery is performed if biopsies are positive. Late laryngeal necrosis after RT is rare, with a reported incidence of about 0.5% to 1.8% for glottic cancer.[3,6,51]

REFERENCES

1. Akine Y and others: Radiotherapy of T_1 glottic cancer with 6 MeV x-rays, *Int J Radiat Oncol Biol Phys* 20:1215, 1991.
2. American Cancer Society: *Cancer facts & figures*, 2003, p 5.
3. Amornmarn R and others: A therapeutic approach to early vocal cord carcinoma, *Acta Radiol Onco)* 24:321, 1985.
4. Anne P and others: A phase II trial of subcutaneous amifostine and radiation therapy in patients with head and neck cancer (WR-B060) [abstract], *Int J Radiat Oncol Biol Phys* 51:84 (Abstract 150), 2001.
5. Batsakis JG and others: The pathology of head and neck tumors: verrucous carcinoma, part 15, *Head Neck Surg* 5:29, 1982.
6. Bhalavat RL and others: Radical radiation vs surgery plus post-operative radiation in advanced (resectable) supraglottic larynx and pyriform sinus cancers: a prospective randomized study, *Eur J Surg Oncol* 29:750, 2003.
7. Braaksma MJJ and others: Optimisation of conformal radiation therapy by intensity modulation: cancer of the larynx and salivary gland function, *Radiother Oncol* 66:291, 2003.
8. Brennan JA and others: Association between cigarette smoking and mutation of the p53 gene in squamous cell carcinoma of the head and neck, *N Engl J Med* 332:712, 1995.
9. Brizel DM and others: Phase III randomized trial of amifostine as a radioprotector in head and neck cancer, *J Clin Oncol* 18:3339, 2000.
10. Bryant GP and others: Treatment decision in T3N0M0 glottic carcinoma, *Int J Radiat Oncol Biol Phys* 31:285, 1995.
11. Cox JD, Pajack TF, Marcial VA: ASTRO plenary: interfraction interval is a major determinant of late effects, with hyperfractionated radiation therapy of carcinomas of upper respiratory and digestive tracts: results from Radiation Therapy Oncology Group protocol 8313, *Int J Radiat Oncol Biol Phys* 20:1191, 1991.
12. Department of Veterans Affairs Laryngeal Cancer Study Group: Induction chemotherapy plus radiation compared with surgery plus radiation in patients with advanced laryngeal cancer, *N Engl J Med* 324:1685, 1991.
13. Eisbruch A and others: Dose, volume, and function relationships in parotid salivary glands following conformal and intensity-modulated irradiation of head and neck cancer, *Int J Radiat Oncol Biol Phys* 45:577, 1999.
14. El Sayed S, Nelson N: Adjuvant and adjunctive chemotherapy in the management of squamous cell carcinoma of the head and neck region: a meta-analysis of prospective and randomized trials, *J Clin Oncol* 14:838, 1996.
15. Elman AJ and others: In-situ carcinoma of the vocal cords, *Cancer* 43:2422, 1979.
16. Ferlito A: Diagnosis and treatment of verrucous squamous cell carcinoma of the larynx: a critical review, *Ann Otol Rhinol Laryngol* 94:575, 1985.
17. Fletcher GH, Goepfert H: *Larynx and pyriform sinus*. In Fletcher G, editor: *Textbook of radiotherapy*, ed 3, Philadelphia, 1980, Lea & Febiger, p 330.
18. Fletcher GH, Hamberger AD: Causes of failure in irradiation of squamous-cell carcinoma of the supraglottic larynx, *Radiology* 111:697, 1974.
19. Forastiere AA and others: Concurrent chemotherapy and radiotherapy for organ preservation in advanced laryngeal cancer, *New Engl J Med* 349:2091, 2003.
20. Frank JL and others: Postoperative radiotherapy improves survival in squamous cell carcinoma of the hypopharynx, *Am J Surg* 168:476, 1994.
21. Fu KK and others: The significance of laryngeal edema following radiotherapy of carcinoma of the vocal cord, *Cancer* 49:655, 1982.
22. Garcia-Serra A and others: Radiotherapy for carcinoma-in-situ of the true vocal cords, *Head Neck* 24:390, 2002.
23. Garden AS and others: Early squamous cell carcinoma of the hypopharynx: outcomes of treatment with radiation alone to the primary disease, *Head Neck* 18:317, 1996.
24. Ghossein NA and others: Local control and site of failure in radically irradiated supraglottic laryngeal cancer, *Radiology* 112:187, 1974.
25. Harrison LB and others: Prospective computer-assisted voice analysis for patients with early stage glottic cancer: a preliminary report of the functional result of laryngeal irradiation, *Int J Radiat Oncol Biol Phys* 19:123, 1990.
26. Harwood A and others: $T_4N_0M_0$ glottic cancer: an analysis of dose-time volume factors, *Int J Radiat Oncol Biol Phys* 7:1507, 1981.
27. Harwood AR and others: T_3 glottic cancer: an analysis of dose-time volume factors, *Int J Radiat Oncol Biol Phys* 6:675, 1980.
28. Hinerman RW and others: Carcinoma of the supraglottic larynx: treatment results with radiotherapy alone or with planned neck dissection, *Head Neck* 24:456, 2002.
29. Hints B and others: A "watchful waiting" policy for in-situ-carcinoma of the vocal cords, *Arch Otolaryngol Head Neck Surg* 107:746, 1981.
30. Howell-Burke D and others: T_2 glottic cancer: Recurrence, salvage, and survival after definitive radiotherapy, *Arch Otolaryngol Head Neck Surg* 116:A30, 1990.
31. Inoue T, Chatani M, Teshima T: Irradiated volume and arytenoid edema after radiotherapy for T_1 glottic carcinoma, *Strahlenther Onkol* 168:23, 1992.
32. Johansen LV and others: Primary radiotherapy of T_1 squamous cel carcinoma of the larynx: analysis of 478 patients treated from 1963 to 1985, *Int J Radiat Oncol Biol Phys* 18:1307, 1990.
33. Kaplan MJ and others: Glottic carcinoma: the roles of surgery and irradiation, *Cancer* 53:2641, 1984.
34. Karim A and others: Radiation therapy for advanced (T_3-T_4N_0-N_3M_0) laryngeal carcinoma: the need for a change of strategy. A radiotherapeutic viewpoint, *Int J Radiat Oncol Biol Phys* 13:1625, 1987.
35. Karim AB and others: Heterogeneity of stage II glottic carcinoma and its therapeutic implications, *Int J Radiat Oncol Biol Phys* 13:313, 1987.
36. Kraus FT, Perez-Mesa C: Verrucous carcinoma: clinical and pathologic study of 105 cases involving oral cavity, larynx and genitalia, *Cancer* 19:26, 1966.
37. Lee N and others: Intensity modulated radiation therapy for head-and-neck cancer: the UCSF experience focusing on target volume delineation, *Int J Radiat Oncol Biol Phys* 57:49, 2003.
38. Lefebvre JL and others: Larynx preservation in pyriform sinus cancer: preliminary results of a European Organization for Research and Treatment of Cancer phase III trial. EORTC Head and Neck Cancer Cooperative Group, *J Natl Cancer Inst* 88:890, 1996.
39. Letterman M: Cancer of the larynx: I. Natural history in relation to treatment, *Br J Radiol* 44:569, 1971.

40. Lindberg RD: Distribution of cervical lymph node metastases from squamous cell carcinoma of the upper respiratory and digestive tracts, *Cancer* 29:1446, 1972.

41. Lundgren JAV and others: T3N0M0 glottic carcinoma-a failure analysis, *Clin Otolaryngol* 13:455, 1988.

42. Lustig RA and others: The patterns of care outcome studies: results of the national practice in carcinoma of the larynx, *Int J Radiat Oncol Biol Phys* 10:2357, 1984.

43. Maciejewski B, Taylor JMG, Withers HR: Alpha/beta value and the importance of size of dose per fraction for late complications in the supraglottic larynx, *Radiother Oncol* 7:323, 1986.

44. Maran D, MacKenzie SR: Carcinoma-in-situ of the larynx, *Head Neck Surg* 7:28, 1984.

45. McGavran MH, Bauer WC, Ogura JH: The incidence of cervical lymph node metastasis from epidermoid carcinoma of the larynx and their relationship to certain characteristics of the primary tumor. A study based on the clinical and pathological findings for 96 patients treated by primary en bloc laryngectomy and radical neck dissection, *Cancer* 14:55, 1961.

46. Mendenhall WM, Parsons JT, Brant TA: Is elective neck treatment indicated for T_2N_0 squamous cell carcinoma of the glottic larynx? *Radiother Oncol* 14:199, 1989.

47. Mendenhall WM, Parsons JT, Million RR: T_1-T_2 squamous cell carcinoma of the glottic larynx treated with radiation therapy: relationship of dose-fractionation factors to local control and complications, *Int J Radiat Oncol Biol Phys* 15:1267, 1988.

48. Mendenhall WM and others: Radiotherapy alone or combined with neck dissection for T_1-T_2 carcinoma of the pyriform sinus: an alternative to conservation surgery, *Int J Radiat Oncol Biol Phys* 27:1017, 1993.

49. Mendenhall WM and others: Stage T_3 squamous cell carcinoma of the glottic larynx: A comparison of laryngectomy and irradiation, *Int J Radiat Oncol Biol Phys* 23:725, 1992.

50. Miller A, Fisher HR: Clues to the life history carcinoma-in-situ of the larynx, *Laryngoscope* 1981;81:1475.

51. Mittal B and others: Role of radiation in the management of early vocal cord carcinoma, *Int J Radiat Oncol Biol Phys* 9:997, 1983.

52. Munro AJ: An overview of randomised controlled trials of adjuvant chemotherapy in head and neck cancer, *Br J Cancer* 71:83, 1995.

53. Nakfoor BM and others: Results of accelerated radiotherapy for supraglottic carcinoma: a Massachusetts General Hospital and Massachusetts Eye and Ear Infirmary experience, *Head Neck* 20:379, 1998.

54. Paisley S and others: Results of radiotherapy for primary subglottic carcinoma, *Int J Radiat Oncol Biol Phys* 52:1245, 2002.

55. Pameijer FA and others: Can pretreatment computed tomography predict local control in T_3 squamous cell carcinoma of the glottic larynx treated with definitive radiotherapy? *Int J Radiat Oncol Biol* 37:1011, 1997.

56. Pignon JP and others: Chemotherapy added to locoregional treatment for head and neck squamous-cell carcinoma: three meta-analyses of updated individual data. MACH-NC Collaborative Group. Meta Analysis of Chemotherapy on Head and Neck Cancer, *Lancet* 355:949, 2000.

57. Richard J and others: Randomized trial of induction chemotherapy in larynx carcinoma, *Oral Oncol* 34:224, 1998.

58. Samant S and others: Concomitant radiation therapy and supradose intra-arterial targeted cisplatin chemotherapy for the treatment of advanced pyriform sinus squamous cell carcinoma: disease control and preservation of organ function, *Head Neck* 21:595, 1999.

59. Skyes AJ and others: 331 cases of clinically node-negative supraglottic carcinoma of the larynx: a study of a modest size fixed field radiotherapy approach, *Int J Radiat Oncol Biol Phys* 46:1109, 2000.

60. Stewart JG, Jackson AW: The steepness of the dose response curve both for tumor cure and normal tissue injury, *Laryngoscope* 85:1107, 1975.

61. Sullivan BO and others: Outcome following radiotherapy in verrucous carcinoma of the larynx, *Int J Radiat Oncol Biol Phys* 32:611, 1995.

62. Taylor JMG and others: The influence of dose and time on wound complications following post-radiation neck dissection, *Int J Radiat Oncol Biol Phys* 23:41, 1992.

63. Tupchong L and others: Randomized study of preoperative versus post-operative radiation therapy in advanced head and neck carcinoma: long-term follow-up of RTOG study 73-03, *Int J Radiat Oncol Biol Phys* 20:21, 1991.

64. Tuyns AT and others: Cancer of the larynx/hypopharynx, tobacco and alcohol: IARC international case-control study of Turin and Varese (Italy), Zaragosa and Navarra (Spain), Geneva (Switzerland) and Calvados (France), *Int J Cancer* 41:483, 1988.

65. Wall TJ and others: Relationship between lymph node status and primary tumor control probability in tumors of the supraglottic larynx, *Int J Radiat Oncol Biol Phys* 11:1895, 1985.

66. Wang CC, Montgomery WM: Deciding on optimal management of supraglottic carcinoma, *Oncology* 5:41, 1991.

67. Wang CC: *Radiation therapy for head and neck neoplasms,* New York, 1997, Wiley-Liss, p 205.

68. Wang CC: *Carcinoma of the larynx.* In Wang CC, editor: *Indications, techniques and results,* Chicago, 1990, Yearbook Medical Publishers, p 223.

69. Wynder EL and others: Environmental factors in cancer of the larynx: a second look, *Cancer* 38:1951, 1976.

70. Wynder EL and others: Environmental factors in cancer of the upper alimentary tract, *Cancer* 10:470, 1957.

71. Wynder EL, Broso IJ, Day E: A study of environmental factors in cancer of the larynx, *Cancer* 9:86, 1956.

72. Wynder EL, Mushinski MH, Spivak JC: Tobacco and alcohol consumption in relation to development of multiple primary cancers, *Cancer* 40:1872, 1977.

73. Zhou J, Fei D, Wu Q: Potential of intensity-modulated radiotherapy to escalate doses to head-and-neck cancers: what is the maximal dose? *Int J Radiat Oncol Biol Phys* 57:673, 2003.

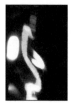

VOCAL REHABILITATION FOLLOWING LARYNGECTOMY

|| Joshua S. Schindler

[Total laryngectomy] affords little prospect of success, and the conditions of existence after its performance are so utterly miserable, the patient being almost cut off with intercourse with his fellow-beings, and having to take food in such a distressing way that suffocation is constantly imminent and that death from starvation not infrequently takes place.

Morrell Mackenzie, 1888[80]

INTRODUCTION

This statement, made by Sir Morrell Mackenzie in his account of *The Fatal Illness of Frederick the Noble*, describes not only the challenges facing the nineteenth century head and neck surgeon, but also underscores the hardships experienced by the first laryngectomy patients. These hardships, including loss of normal phonatory and swallowing function, loss of Valsalva with weakening of cough and upper-body strength, impairment of smell and taste, and inability to control nasal and respiratory secretions, have tremendous physical and social impact on the lives of laryngectomy patients. Although perioperative mortality has declined substantially with advances in surgical technique, antibiotic administration, and enteral nutrition, the challenges faced by recovering laryngectomy patients are little different today than at the turn of the twentieth century. Despite efforts to superannuate this procedure through advances in partial laryngectomy surgery and organ preservation chemoradiation protocols, total laryngectomy is still commonly performed and remains the treatment of choice for many advanced laryngeal malignancies and for patients with poor performance status. Because of the importance of total laryngectomy in the management of head and neck malignancy, active investigation into methods of postoperative rehabilitation continues.

While the larynx has many physiologic functions, loss of phonatory function has historically been considered the most significant deficit facing a laryngectomee. Since the development of laryngectomy procedures, this assumption has driven tremendous surgical and mechanical innovation. Although recent quality-of-life studies suggest that phonation is not the primary concern after laryngectomy,[34] such findings may more accurately reflect our commitment to restore voice after laryngectomy than the weight patients place on communication.

PHYSIOLOGY OF ALARYNGEAL SPEECH

Before discussing the evolution of voice rehabilitation after laryngectomy, it is important to understand the basic physiology of the most common forms of alaryngeal speech. There are three primary methods of speech production following total laryngectomy: esophageal, fistula- (or shunt-) based, and external vibratory voice. Fundamental differences in power supply of the sound wave generator, segment of aerodigestive tract vibrated, and reliance on external prostheses separate these methods. These differences influence not only the quality and intelligibility of voice production, but, in many cases, determine the suitability to individual patients and social acceptance. The three basic methods are described here with further discussion of their acquisition, patient suitability, and complications (later in the chapter).

Esophageal Voice

In many ways, esophageal speech is the simplest form of alaryngeal communication. After the removal of the larynx and primary or augmented closure of the neopharynx, patients commence phonation by passing air into the esophagus. The esophagus may be filled through one of several different methods incorporating closure of the lips, relaxation of the pharyngoesophageal (PE) segment, and retropulsion of the tongue. Once filled, the esophagus acts as a bellows for sustained voice production, containing as much as 80 cc of air for phonation.[27] A vibratory sound wave is produced through controlled regurgitation of air past the undulating mucosa of the PE segment using gentle contraction of the abdominal and chest muscles. As air passes through this segment, the mucosa of the anterior and posterior walls approximates because of a bulge in the posterior pharyngeal wall between the fourth and seventh vertebrae.[40,61,140] This approximated mucosa forms a neoglottis (sometimes called a *pseudoglottis*), which can be tuned to some degree through contraction of the thyropharyngeus, or middle pharyngeal constrictor muscle.[97]

Esophageal speech is simple in that it requires no additional surgery or prostheses. Despite its simplicity, esophageal voicing has significant limitations. The duration of phonation depends on the amount of ingested air and control of its release by the speaker. With only 80 cc of air, the duration of speech can be limited to only a few syllables per injection and result in a choppy, low amplitude phonatory quality. The best esophageal speakers are able to store air in the stomach with greatly improved duration of speech. Although some esophageal speakers can attain exceptional vocal quality, pitch modulation remains difficult because of functional limitations in the ability to change the conformation of the pharyngoesophageal segment. As a result, the fundamental frequency remains low (about 65 Hz), causing difficulty with gender identification and the conveyance of emotion.

Fistula-Based Voice

Restoration of the lungs as the primary energy source for voice production has been a goal of post-laryngectomy rehabilitation since the earliest procedures. Unlike esophageal speech, fistulas from the trachea to the upper digestive tract allow the speaker to use the lungs as the bellows by shunting air from the trachea into the digestive tract. Under controlled release in the PE segment, the entire inspiratory capacity (more than 3000 cc) is at the disposal of the speaker for phonation. Placement of the fistula determines the region of PE segment vibration. Most modern methods direct the prosthesis into the cervical esophagus directly posterior to the membranous wall of the tracheostoma, but procedures for other configurations are of historical interest.

The increased capacity and pressure gained by using the lungs as the bellows substantially affects the quality of speech production. Greater air pressure across the PE segment generates voice with a slightly higher fundamental frequency than that produced by esophageal speakers.[107] In addition, use of the lungs allows much greater range and control of vocal intensity. Consequently, tracheoesophageal (TE) speakers may perform better in noisy environments than esophageal speakers. Finally, greater air capacity allows longer duration of speech production than that

attained by esophageal speakers. In addition, shunted voice production can be acquired by most laryngectomees and is more readily accepted by listeners because the bellows refills naturally during respiration. Despite attempts to create stable biologic fistulas that allow voice production and competent swallowing function, nearly all methods of TE speech require a prosthesis with a finite lifespan and patient-specific acceptability.

External Vibratory Voice

Sound waves can also be created by external mechanical sources. Devices, either electrical or pneumatic, have been designed to vibrate a column of air within the oral cavity and oropharynx, allowing speech production. Pneumatic devices use musical reeds to produce sound waves and are often introduced into the oral cavity with a straw. Electric devices use vibration of a pad to produce monotone sound waves. These devices can be applied to the skin overlying the oral cavity or oropharynx, depending on patient habitus, presence of facial hair, and quality of speech production. Once applied, the vibration is transmitted with variable fidelity to the oral cavity where it is modulated by the tongue, cheeks, palate, and lips into speech. Alternatively, the patient may generate a vibrating column of air in the oral cavity using an electric device fitted with a straw, which is placed in mouth.

Although external vibratory speech may be acquired by nearly all laryngectomees with adequate dexterity to use the devices, this modality remains limited by its monotone sound production. Although the mucosal-wave form of speech may yield limitations in pitch control, external vibratory speech allows only a single pitch based on the vibratory frequency of the reed or electric device. This single pitch results in a monotone sound with a synthetic quality that can draw unwanted attention to the speaker and be distracting to the listener. When compared with other methods of alaryngeal speech, patients generally find external vibratory voicing the least socially acceptable method of post-laryngectomy communication.

HISTORY OF ALARYNGEAL SPEECH

As one might expect, the history of alaryngeal speech parallels the history of total laryngectomy and is as colorful and innovative as any endeavor in medicine. In the early nineteenth century, treatment of laryngeal diseases was at its infancy. Tracheotomy was well understood and used frequently to treat laryngeal phthisis, a term used to describe any "chronic alteration of the larynx which may bring on consumption or death in any way."[4] Direct observations of the larynx may have been made as early as 1743,[79] but were not widely performed until Manuel Garcia's description of indirect laryngoscopy in 1855.[46] Evaluation and treatment were often performed simultaneously as thyrotomy was the procedure of choice for laryngeal disease until the last quarter of the nineteenth century. Voicing was poorly understood, but descriptions of the larynx as the seat of phonation can be found as early as 1791.[77] Ernst Wilhelm von Brucke established the foundations for alaryngeal speech in 1858 when he noted that sounds used in speech production did not all come from the larynx.[23] Using a "sound locator," similar to a stethoscope, Brucke cataloged different sounds and their apparent location within the upper respiratory tract.

Proof of Brucke's observations came the following year with the first demonstration of a prosthetic larynx. In 1859, Johann Nepomuk Czermak used a prosthesis to restore phonation to a young girl with complete laryngeal stenosis. Fashioned by Brucke, the prosthesis directed air from the girl's tracheostomy site to the pharynx by way of a nasotracheal tube.[32] As with most of the early devices, air vibration was produced by a reed. After the procedure, Czermak noted that his patient could produce voice of low volume and that some sounds were absent. Despite these observations, the young girl was able to produce faint, but intelligible speech. Dubbed the "artificial larynx," Czermak's device demonstrated that alaryngeal speech was possible and served as a prototype for prosthetic restoration of voice following total laryngectomy. Interestingly, Czermak noted that his patient's phonation was independent of airflow through the tracheostomy tube and even surmised that the sound was produced by the muscular vibration of air in the oropharynx. One therefore wonders whether the credit for alaryngeal speech restoration belongs to Czermak's device or the young girl for acquiring esophageal speech![77]

In 1873, Theodore Billroth performed the first total laryngectomy for cancer.[52] Although about 8 years earlier Patrick Watson may have performed the first total laryngectomy for syphilis,[3] Billroth's procedure deserves particular distinction as that it was the first time that laryngeal rehabilitation was attempted. His patient was a 36-year-old gentleman with laryngeal carcinoma treated extensively with silver nitrate cautery. Primary closure of the pharynx had not been successful in dog experiments,[33] and, therefore, Billroth removed the larynx, leaving the epiglottis and a persistent oropharyngeal tract for controlled salivary drainage through a common tracheopharyngostome. This tract, which was essential for wound healing, was maintained by a tracheostomy tube designed by Billroth's Viennese assistant, Carl Gussenbauer, and fashioned by the musical instrument maker, Joseph Leiter. The original tube was made of hard rubber and similar to modern T-tubes with both inferior (tracheal) and superior (pharyngeal) limbs. A reed device was in place at the junction of the two limbs for vibrating exhaled air.[98] The literature is confusing in that it contains many different descriptions of Gussenbauer's device. In fact, Billroth's patient actually had three different devices made by different manufacturers. The final device was fashioned by Thuerriegl and was similar to the first device except that it was smaller and made of metal (Figure 105-1). The device could be fitted with an obturator in the pharyngeal limb, which allowed swallowing to resume while maintaining respiration. It could also be fitted for phonation with a one-way valve, allowing inspiration through the tracheostomy and expiration through the pharyngeal segment.

Gussenbauer reported the success of the surgery and device at the Third Congress of the German Company of Surgeons in 1874.[52] In this report, the patient was described as having acceptable vocal function with intelligible speech that could be heard in a large hospital room. As with Czermak's patient, the most significant deficit was pitch control as the neoglottic voicing was noted to be monotone. In addition, Gussenbauer noted that speaking with the artificial larynx required more effort from the patient. Although Billroth's patient died of persistent disease 7 months later, devices similar to the Gussenbauer prosthesis were used for years in the rehabilitation of laryngectomy patients. Many of these devices were very similar to Gussenbauer's original design and their placement became standard for total laryngectomy. In a testimony to the success of the artificial larynx (and that of total laryngectomy for the treatment of glottic cancer), Caselli and Bottini reported on a cancer survivor who used the modified tracheostomy with useful alaryngeal speech for more than 38 years (Figure 105-2).[58]

Advances in total laryngectomy technique created new challenges in alaryngeal speech rehabilitation by the end of the nineteenth century. At this time, total laryngectomy surgery was generally frowned on by the medical community because of the high mortality that accompanied post-operative aspiration pneumonia and wound infection. A number of surgeons sought to improve the outcomes through complete separation of the respiratory and digestive tracts. Jacob Da Silva Solis-Cohen, an American laryngologist practicing at Jefferson Medical College, recognized this necessity and was the first to completely isolate the trachea by sewing it to the skin in 1892.[122,144] This effectively limited the aspiration by isolating the trachea from the pharyngoesophagostome. Gluck

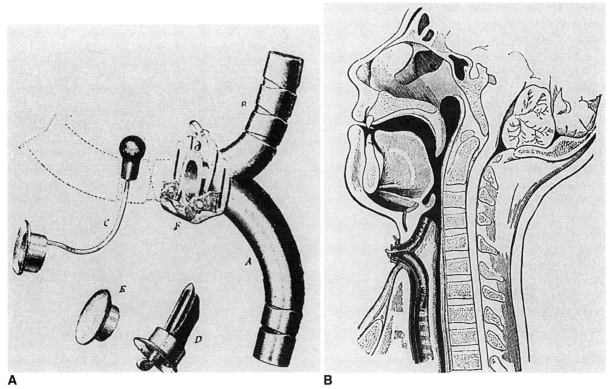

Figure 105-1. A, Gussenbauer's and Thuerriegl's prosthesis. **B,** Gussenbauer's prosthesis in situ.

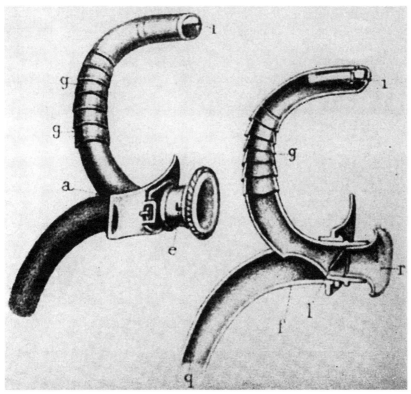

Figure 105-2. Caselli's prosthesis.[58]

described the modern laryngectomy procedure 2 years later, by eliminating the pharyngoesophagostome and closing the pharynx primarily.[49] Although this advance lead to the acceptance of total laryngectomy for glottic carcinoma, it created new challenges for alaryngeal speech rehabilitation.

Interestingly, shortly before Solis-Cohen's and Gluck's modifications of laryngectomy technique, laryngologists began to notice that patients did not require an artificial larynx to acquire speech after total laryngectomy. In 1888, Struebing wrote a review of alaryngeal speech to date and focused on a laryngectomy patient whose tracheopharyngeal opening stenosed completely.[77,125] Despite the absence of a connection between the pharynx and trachea, this patient spoke forcefully and clearly with a rough voice that Struebing deemed superior to the musical and metallic sound obtained with an artificial larynx. Acquisition of esophageal speech was a well-known phenomenon in cases of laryngeal stenosis, but wasn't initially thought possible in laryngectomy patients. Struebing's observations lead him to posit the source of alaryngeal voice in the base of the tongue and he felt that a more natural phonation could be achieved through oropharyngeal muscle exercise. One year after his review, Struebing and Landois presented the development of a "natural" pseudo-voice after total laryngectomy without artificial larynx rehabilitation.[126] Such voicing became known as "whisper voice" and Poppert suggested that patients not receive an artificial larynx immediately in case they develop this pseudo-voice.[104] By 1896, Stoerk presented numerous laryngectomy patients with spontaneous acquisition of speech and declared the use of laryngeal prostheses "antiquated."[124] While the exact nature of voice acquired by these patients cannot be known as it was another 13 years before Gutzmann coined the terms for buccal and esophageal speech in his descriptions of spontaneous alaryngeal voice,[55] it was clear that many patients required no assistive devices to attain speech after laryngectomy.

Despite the observation of spontaneous alaryngeal speech, advances in prosthetic vocal rehabilitation continued throughout the 20th century. With the growing acceptance of laryngectomy technique and marked reduction in post-operative morbidity, the literature became peppered with reports of devices and procedures used to restore vocal function. The designs for assistive speaking devices became increasingly intricate and complex as inventors struggled to overcome limitations of pitch control and social acceptance. Gluck presented a number of devices including an artificial larynx activated intraorally by a denture[50] and an electric device that used a phonograph cylinder to play prerecorded vocals from a

singer and delivered these sounds to the nose or mouth.[51] Most of these devices failed secondary to technical problems, but the concepts spurred the development of modern artificial larynges.

Numerous reports of reed-based devices powered by the patient through tracheostomal exhalation continued through the 1930s as investigators continued to experiment with artificial larynges.[39,86,128] Then, as Louis Lowry notes in a review of artificial larynges, there was a 30-year period almost "devoid" of any reports of mechanical or electrical devices.[77] The beginning of this period coincides with Seeman's studies of esophageal speech published in 1926. Using x-rays, Seeman was the first to describe the vibratory mucosa of the pseudoglottis and outline the mechanism of esophageal speech.[111,112] In his report, Seeman echoed Stoerk's sentiments regarding the artificial larynx and noted that its use "must today be regarded as a backward step which cannot be reconciled to the newest progresses of phoniatry."[112] Seeman's work, along with continued positive reports of spontaneous acquisition of alaryngeal speech by surgeons, allowed esophageal speech to become the unchallenged gold standard of post-laryngectomy rehabilitation until the 1980s.

In spite of the appeal of alaryngeal speech production without a prosthetic device, esophageal speech was noted to have limitations. Acquisition of useful esophageal speech could take as long as a year and, contrary to the opinion held by many surgeons and therapists that esophageal voicing could be acquired by all laryngectomees, some patients failed to generated serviceable speech without assistive devices despite months of rehabilitation. In addition, while the quality of esophageal speech was good, the voice was often soft and difficult to project in a crowd. These limitations continued to drive the development of laryngeal prostheses.

One of the most significant contributions was the electric larynx. The first devices, the Western Electric Models 2A and 2B (Figure 105-3), were introduced in the 1930s, but were not well received because of the emphasis on more "natural" esophageal speech. These devices were reed-based with intraoral straws used to deliver vibrating air. By the 1950s, advances in electric circuitry including the transistor and miniaturization of the components and batteries allowed the production of smaller, more socially acceptable devices.[127] Unlike the original Western Electric devices, the new artificial larynges, produced by Bell Labs, Aurex, and others, were compact, self-contained electric devices that were applied transcervically.[16,77] This placement allowed better speech quality for many patients because the mouth was unobstructed and the vibration was placed more posteriorly in the orophar-

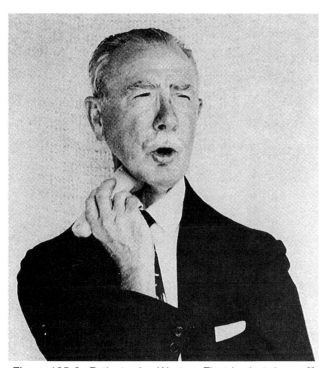

Figure 105-3. Patient using Western Electric electolarynx.[89]

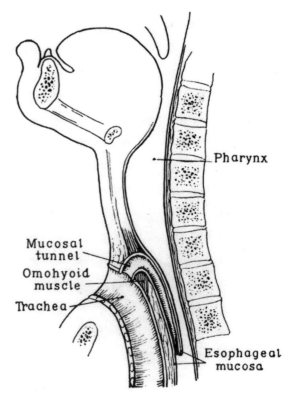

Figure 105-4. Conley's tracheoesophageal shunt.[30]

ynx. In addition, as Barney posited, the "pharynx and nasal cavities do not have the same resonating effect as they would if the sound were introduced at the glottis."[13] In studies performed at Ohio State University in the mid-1950s, speakers using electrical larynges were found not only to have similar speech intelligibility to that of esophageal speakers, but their speech was actually preferred to that of skilled esophageal speakers.[60]

During this same period, head and neck surgeons continued to experiment with ways to reestablish phonation after laryngectomy without relying on cumbersome and inefficient prostheses to maintain separation of the respiratory and digestive tracts. In 1958, John Conley, Felix DeAmesti, and MK Pierce described the creation of a mucosal shunt in laryngectomy patients for just this purpose (Figure 105-4).[30] Following successful work in dogs, they created a 5-cm mucosal shunt using the anterior wall of the cervical esophagus. This shunt was initially brought to the skin as an esophagostome above the tracheostome. In a second stage, the esophagostome was taken down and connected to the superior aspect of the trachea. Thus, Conley's procedure created a mucosal shunt between the trachea to the esophagus with the tracheal inlet approximately 4 cm above that of the esophagus.

Although the initial results were promising, the procedure was technically difficult and problems with salivary leakage, stenosis, and inflammation prevented widespread acceptance.

Over the next 20 years, surgeons continued to experiment with methods of voice restoration using a combination of shunts, prostheses, and surgical innovation. Working at the University of Kobe, Japan, Ryozo Asai experimented with progressively more complicated procedures to restore vocal function. By the mid-1960s, the "Asai Technique" involved a three-stage skin-lined subcutaneous shunt that connected a pharyngostome to the tracheostome.[9,10] Asai's voice results were acknowledged to be outstanding with patients achieving fluent speech, whistling, and even singing. Unfortunately, there were continued problems with aspiration of thin liquids requiring digital occlusion of the subcutaneous shunt during swallowing.[89] Reproducing Asai's voice results proved very difficult and, as with Conley's procedure, shunt stenosis was a frequent problem. These difficulties, as well as the multiple stages required to complete the procedure, caused many to continue looking for alternatives.

During this same period, surgeons working at the University of Padua, Italy, were rethinking the need for a shunt entirely. Following extensive trials in dogs and monkeys, Arslan and Serafini reported a radically new procedure aimed at restoring voice and, potentially, respiration after subtotal laryngectomy.[8,113] Operating on patients with tumors entirely limited to the endolarynx, they performed a laryngectomy from the interspace between the cricothyroid and first tracheal cartilages and extending superiorly to the junction of the body and petiole of the epiglottis (Figure 105-5, *A*). Reconstruction included primary tracheohyoepiglottipexy by mobilizing the distal trachea and anastomosing it to the pharyngeal defect with impaction of the hyoid and suprahyoid epiglottis to the first tracheal ring (Figure 105-5, *B-D*).

The initial success of the Arslan-Serafini procedure was remarkable, with patients achieving soft, but usable speech that improved with time. In addition, normal inspiration was achieved in 14 of 35 patients and confirmed by spirometry after closure of the tracheotomy site in 14 of 35 patients.[8] Of these patients, 90% were able to resume swallowing solid and semi-solid food within 2 weeks after surgery. Although the authors credit elevation and anterior displacement of the larynx with preventing aspiration in their patients, preservation of the epiglottis is likely critical to their success and, as such, their procedure is only appropriate for very limited lesions of the glottis.

Aspiration of thin liquids continued to be problematic, and, unlike the Asai Procedure, patients had no shunt to occlude. As noted, success of the Arslan-Serafini laryngectomy depended on limited laryngeal resection with preservation of the preepiglottic space and therefore, it is not surprising that the rate of tumor persistence was unacceptably high.[119] Despite these limitations, the procedure was a significant step toward successful partial laryngectomy procedures.

Focus turned away from complicated multistage procedures and toward stable fistulae of the posterior tracheal wall into the esophagus. Mutsuo Amatsu, also at the University of Kobe, built on the work of Asai and pioneered a single-stage tracheoesophageal shunt fashioned from posterior tracheal wall mucosa.[5] The procedure was simple to reproduce and allowed complete extirpation of the larynx. Unfortunately, like Asai's procedure, the shunt failed to provide adequate resistance to retrograde flow during swallowing, and patients suffered from leakage of liquids with aspiration. Staffieri tried similar procedures employing pharyngeal muscle to create a dynamic phonatory shunt that acted as a valve around the tracheopharyngeal shunt.[123] Although his results were reproducible and

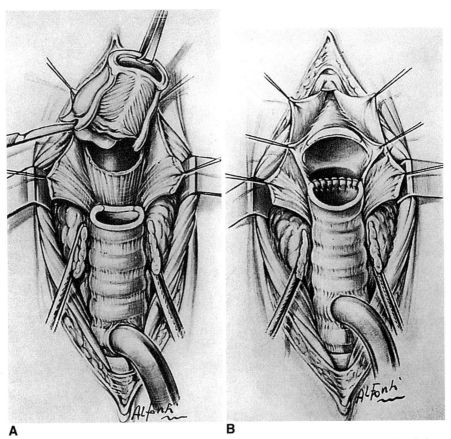

A **B**

Figure 105-5. Serafini laryngectomy. **A,** Limited laryngectomy. **B,** Pharyngo-tracheal closure.

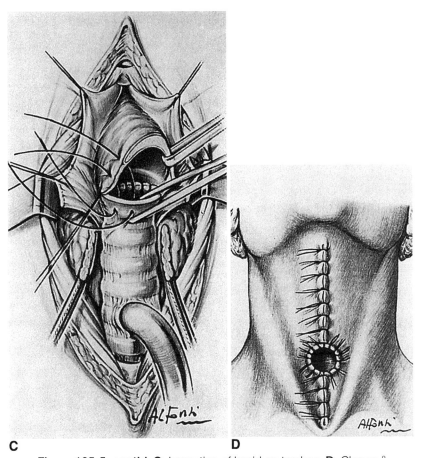

C   D

Figure 105-5, cont'd **C,** Impaction of hyoid on trachea. **D,** Closure.[8]

initially good in 84 of 97 patients, over time, the neoglottis became incompetent and stenotic, leading to aspiration.[85] Other groups, attempting to reproduce Staffieri's procedure found a high rate of aspiration, as well as late speech failure secondary to stenosis of the tract.[134] In comparing the recovery of this procedure to that of matched patients undergoing conventional total laryngectomy, these surgeons found an almost twofold increase in pharyngocutaneous fistula formation and substantially longer hospitalization in those patients undergoing dynamic phonatory shunt procedure.

By the late 1970s the stage was set for a revolution in voice rehabilitation after total laryngectomy. Despite their failures, the work of Amatsu and Staffieri clearly defined the problems of maintaining a dynamic tracheoesophageal fistula that allowed the passage of air and prevented passage of liquids. For the preceding 50 years, the surgical community shunned prosthetic devices for post-laryngectomy speech because of device failure, added nuisance for the patient, and poor biocompatibility. However, in 1980, Mark Singer and Eric Blom set aside this surgical dogma and presented a simple method of estab-

lishing a stable tracheoesophageal fistula using a silastic prosthesis.[114]

The concept of a tracheoesophageal fistula to regain voicing after laryngectomy was not new. Indeed, the procedure was first described in 1931 when Guttman reported the successful acquisition of tracheoesophageal speech by a frustrated patient who created the fistula himself with a heated icepick.[53] With his finger over his stoma to direct airflow through the fistula, Guttman's patient could produce very fluent and speech with near normal timbre. Although he tried to reproduce this result using needle diathermy, Guttman's efforts failed in more than two-thirds of patients, secondary to stenosis and infection.[54] Singer and Blom recreated Guttman's fistula by puncturing the thinnest part of the tracheoesophageal wall in the midline. The puncture site was subsequently dilated with a 14 Fr rubber catheter, which was removed on postoperative day 2 and replaced with a removable prosthesis. In order to prevent leakage from the esophagus, they fashioned a simple valve by making a slit through the long axis of the esophageal lumen of the prosthesis. Ultimately manufactured in silastic, this "duckbill" prosthesis was placed into the tracheoesophageal fistula site and taped into place (Figure 105-6, *A*). The procedure was performed endoscopically with a rigid esophagoscope as early as 4 weeks following laryngectomy (Figure 105-6, *B*).

The initial results with the Blom-Singer prosthesis were outstanding. Of their patients, 90% were able to achieve fluent voices after the procedure and there were no wound complications. Voicing was simple when compared with esophageal speech as patients routinely required only 3 to 5 days to begin speaking after device placement. Aspiration was manifest only as leakage around the prosthesis and only one patient required closure of the site for this problem. Of the five patients who failed to produce satisfactory voice, all had their fistulas closed without difficulty in the office setting. Some difficulties with the prosthesis were noted immediately. The prosthesis caused local irritation over time, necessitating daily removal and cleaning. Accidental extrusion could occur with subsequent aspiration, but this problem was quickly corrected with a retention collar placed on the esophageal end of the prosthesis. Over time, a subpopulation of patients were found to fail with the original prosthesis because they were unable to generate sufficient air pressure to open the valve and produce voice.[117] By 1982, the "duckbill" valve was replaced with a low pressure internal valve that facilitated voicing and decreased the percentage of failures.[20]

Work on tracheoesophageal prostheses continued through the 1980s and early 1990s. As surgical experience with the technique increased, primary tracheoesophageal puncture became commonplace and substantially reduced the postoperative period of voicelessness. Building on the success of the Blom-Singer prosthesis, other devices soon became available.[7,56,101] The State University of Groningen in the Netherlands produced an indwelling device that could be cleaned *in situ*.[7] Although this device dramatically simplified care and safety by eliminating the need for daily prosthesis removal, the internal valve required high opening pressure for use (50–150 mm H_2O), which was difficult for some patients to use. In 1990, Atos Medical of Sweden and Entermed of the Netherlands addressed this problem with introduction of the Provox prosthesis.[56] With its wide low-pressure valve (about 20 Fr) and short length (6–10 mm), the Provox greatly facilitated voicing by decreasing the airflow resistance better than previous prostheses. In addition, with careful cleaning, studies have demonstrated average life spans of nearly 10 months.[72] Simple methods of placement, patient satisfaction, and decreased device complications and failure have all contributed to the growing acceptance of tracheoesophageal puncture technique by both surgeons and patients

MODERN ALAYNGEAL SPEECH
TE Fistula Speech

Since the early 1980s, TE puncture has become the voice rehabilitation method of choice after total laryngectomy, and studies demonstrate that this preference is increasing among head and neck surgeons.[31,76,102,136]

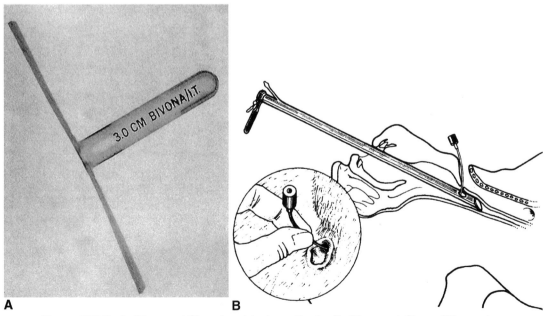

A   **B**

Figure 105-6. A, Blom and Singer's original prosthesis. **B,** Blom and Singer TE puncture technique with fenestrated esophagoscope.[114]

Similar trends can be demonstrated among speech-language pathologists who perform vocal rehabilitation. In a recent study of 151 such therapists, there was a trend noted toward increased application of TE speech, and 69% of those surveyed believed that TE speech was the best method of post-laryngectomy rehabilitation.[31] Interestingly, this study also found that patients are being given more opportunity to participate in their method of speech rehabilitation and believed that "it is reasonable to expect increased use of TEP in the future."

Growing preference for TE speech after laryngectomy is a result of a number of factors. Probably the most significant of these is patient satisfaction with alaryngeal speech acquisition. Since Singer and Blom's first report, many surgeons and centers have reported their success rates with TE speech. Depending on criteria used in the study, the percentage of successful users varies from 37% to 91%,* with most studies reporting rates near 80%. Long-term follow-up of 40 patients who underwent laryngectomy with TE puncture demonstrated that two-thirds of the patients continued to use their prostheses.[48] Other studies have reported even higher rates of continued use.[12,99] Early speech rehabilitation has always been a goal and some studies have noted higher success rates in patients who receive primary tracheoesophageal fistulas.[64,67] Recently, Karlen and Maisel noted that patients will favor the first method of speech presented after laryngectomy, even if it is less comprehensible (e.g., an electrolarynx).[65] Such findings argue in favor of primary TEP placement and reignite controversy that has existed for years over the use of assistive devices before or during esophageal speech training.

The quality of TE speech is another reason for its growing popularity. Although not equivalent to normal speech, most investigators found average intelligibility rates of about 70%, with some greater than 90%.[41,88,103] These numbers are similar when reported by naïve listeners.[121] Other studies compared the intelligibility and quality of TE voice with electro laryngeal and esophageal speech. As expected, in a direct comparison between electrolarynx and TE fistula use in the same patient, Merwin, Goldstein, and Rothman found that both naïve and experienced listeners found TE speech more intelligible and preferable to vibromechanical speech.[88] Similar studies have shown a preference for TE speech over esophageal speech, although the differences are not as marked.[143] The quality of TE voice is often described as low pitched and harsh. While the fundamental frequency of TE speech is lower than that of normal speech, most

experienced users can vary pitch to some degree for intonation and accent. Some women laryngectomees find the low fundamental frequency and limited pitch control stigmatizing, as gender identification can be difficult.[132,137]

Finally, nearly all laryngectomy patients can undergo TE puncture for speech rehabilitation. The ability to create a fistula is independent of the extent of laryngeal resection and, therefore, does not pressure surgeons to "cheat" on their oncologic margins. Not only can TE puncture be performed successfully after extensive hypopharyngeal resection and regional flap reconstruction, but fistulas may be created through gastric and free colonic or jejunal interposition grafts.[25,36,37,66] Limited patient dexterity and mental acuity may preclude or complicate the usage and care of a TE prosthesis as such patients may be unable to digitally occlude their stoma or clean their prosthesis. Although difficult to quantify, patient motivation may be the greatest predictor of successful vocal rehabilitation and should be considered when choosing alaryngeal speech options. While patients develop TE puncture speech much more rapidly than esophageal speech, poorly motivated patients may become discouraged in the teaching period and perform better with artificial larynges.

TEP TECHNIQUE
Secondary TE Puncture

TEP can be performed at any time after the creation of the laryngectomy stoma. If not performed at the time of surgery, most surgeons delay the procedure until 2 to 4 weeks after laryngectomy to allow healing of the tracheostoma. Some surgeons choose to delay creation of the TE fistula until after radiation therapy or if the patient suffers from significant comorbid conditions (e.g., diabetes, immunosuppression for transplant, chronic steroid use). Although radiation therapy is not a specific contraindication to TEP, some investigators have reported that few patients use this modality after therapy and that as many as 50% of those who undergo the procedure are not using the prosthesis after 5 years.[62,87] These failures may be related to pain and swelling around the puncture site, contributing to delayed voicing and decreased motivation.[70] Irradiation can cause stoma stenosis and hypersensitivity, which are relative contraindications to secondary TE puncture as patients require a stoma diameter of at least 1 cm and the ability to tolerate instrumentation. The extent of laryngeal and hypopharyngeal resection is a relative indication for secondary procedure as many surgeons prefer to delay puncture in patients undergoing free flap reconstruction of the pharynx.

One of the most appealing features of TEP for head and neck surgeons is the simplicity of the technique.

*References 2, 48, 56, 64, 67, 71, 99, 117, 143.

Singer's original description was a single-stage endoscopic procedure that can be performed by a single surgeon. A rigid esophagoscope is placed into the patient's neopharynx and gently passed to the cervical esophagus. Singer modified a 7 × 1.3 × 30-cm esophagoscope to include a hole several centimeters proximal to the distal end; however, the procedure can be performed with a standard scope. The surgeon selects a suitable site in the midline of the posterior tracheostomal wall. The site should allow easy access to the prosthesis, but must allow unobstructed closure of the stoma by the patient's finger. This position is usually 5 to 15 mm from the mucocutaneous junction depending on the prosthesis planned and geometry of the stoma. After selecting a suitable site on the posterior stomal wall for the puncture, a needle is passed under direct vision into the hole of the esophagoscope. This puncture site is serially dilated until it accommodates a 14 Fr red rubber catheter. A No. 11 blade may be used to carefully widen the puncture site, if necessary. After insertion, the proximal end of the catheter is secured to the skin and distal end is passed into the esophagus.

Many authors have described modifications of Singer's original technique to surmount patient-specific obstacles. The most common difficulty is exposure of the cervical esophagus because of contraction of the neck after surgery and radiation therapy. Rigid esophagoscopy can be technically demanding in such patients and carries a significant risk of esophageal perforation. Mohr, Paddock, and Boehler have reported a safe method using a flexible endotracheal tube instead of a rigid esophagoscope for patients with poor pharyngeal access.[92] Visualization was achieved using a flexible nasopharyngoscope passed through the endotracheal tube. Noting poor general visibility through a rigid esophagoscope, Koch describes TEP using a flexible esophagoscope and a Russell Percutaneous Gastrostomy Kit (Cook, Inc., Bloomington, In).[69] The procedure is analogous to percutaneous tracheostomy in speed and safety as it involves few steps and is performed under continuous visualization. Office-based creation of TE fistulas has also been described using only local anesthesia in selected patients.[38]

Primary TE Puncture

TE puncture performed at the time of laryngectomy was first reported by Maves and Lingerman in 1982.[84] This procedure was immediately noted to carry several advantages over secondary TEP including elimination of a second operative procedure, elimination of the nasogastric tube for feeding, optimization of the pharyngoesophageal segment and stoma for TE prosthesis placement, and psychological benefit to the patient. Since its introduction, many studies have confirmed the safety of primary TE puncture, as well as the cost savings.[45,93] Although occasionally debated, there is no demonstrable difference between the voices of those who undergo primary or secondary TEP.[22] Finally, the extent of pharyngeal resection and reconstruction does not preclude primary procedures, as TE puncture may be performed at the time of free flap reconstruction without increased complications.[1]

Like secondary fistula creation, primary TE puncture is also a simple procedure. After laryngectomy, but before closure of the pharyngeal defect, the posterior tracheal wall is carefully inspected for a suitable fistula site. Selection of the site can be tricky, as the surgeon must predict where the fistula will lie when the stoma is matured at the conclusion of the procedure. The simplest means to determine this is to grasp the superior edge of the posterior tracheal wall with an atraumatic clamp such as a Babcock. With gentle superior traction, the trachea may be raised from the mediastinum to estimate its final position relative to the skin flaps and sternal notch. Once positioned, a suitable site for puncture may be selected in the midline of the posterior tracheal wall approximately 1 to 1.5 cm from the superior edge. The distance depends on the amount of mucosa required for closure, the anticipated diameter of prosthesis used, and the geometry of the stoma.

Once a site is selected, a right-angle clamp may be placed in the esophagus through the pharyngeal defect and pressed against the tracheoesophageal party wall immediately under the chosen puncture site. Using a No. 11 blade, a small vertical incision is made in the posterior tracheal wall, which allows the right-angle clamp to be passed through. The clamp grasps a 16 Fr red rubber catheter that is drawn through the pharyngeal defect. Smaller catheters may be used, but they may clog in the postoperative period and result in a small TE fistula that must be dilated for prosthesis placement. The catheter is then redirected into the esophagus and the tip is passed into the stomach. The surgeon should straighten any kinks in the catheter with his or her finger and confirm patency of the catheter by gently flushing it with sterile saline after placement. A catheter that does not permit easy flushing may not allow parenteral feeding in the postoperative period. After the pharyngeal defect is closed and the stoma is matured to the skin flaps, a nonabsorbable suture may be used to affix the catheter to the skin close to the puncture site on the superior skin flap. This suture will prevent accidental loss of the catheter during coughing and keep the catheter from occluding the stoma. Antibiotics, ample nutrition, aggressive stoma cleaning ,and humidification in the postoperative period will help maintain a healthy fistula and speed mucosalization.

Prostheses Fitting

Insertion of the prosthesis takes place approximately 7 to 14 days after puncture to allow healing of the fistula tract and stoma. Most of the swelling in the tracheoesophageal party wall has subsided, and the length of the fistula tract can be assessed after removal of the catheter. Gentle dilation of the tract may be performed using a set of puncture dilators. Use of surgical lubricant containing 2% lidocaine can make prosthesis placement more comfortable. The position of the prosthesis may be confirmed using a 2-mm rigid endoscope passed through the valve and into the esophagus.

While several different manufacturers of TE puncture prostheses exist, the devices can be divided into two major categories: indwelling and non-indwelling. Non-indwelling devices are similar to the original Blom-Singer device in that they are designed to be removed daily by the patient for cleaning and maintenance. Examples include the Panje Voice Button (Hood Laboratories, Pembroke, Ma) and the Blom-Singer Duckbill Prosthesis (InHealth Technologies, Carpinteria, Ca). They are easy to place in anterograde fashion because they have only a small retaining collar to hold them in the esophageal lumen. The unfortunate corollary of their easy placement is that they are prone to migrate or extrude if not fitted properly and can be aspirated by the patient. They generally include a flange that is long enough to prevent entry through the stoma or a string to allow easy retrieval if aspirated.

Indwelling prostheses such as the Groningen Voice Button (Hood Laboratories, Pembroke, Ma), Provox and Provox2 (Atos Medical AB, Horby, Sweden), and the Blom-Singer Indwelling Voice Prosthesis (InHealth Technologies, Carpinteria, Ca) were introduced in the mid-1980s in an effort to simplify the care of TE fistula tracts. These prostheses may remain in the TE fistula tract until they fail and are replaced by the therapist or surgeon. Device life varies between the devices and is somewhat patient specific. Most devices function for an average of 2 to 10 months, with a range of 1 to 48 months.[12,56,72,99] Their design differs from that of non-indwelling devices in that they have a larger diameter to accommodate in situ cleaning by the patient with a small brush or saline syringe. The larger diameter of these devices has implications for the position of the TE puncture site and should be considered at the time of fistula creation.

Insertion techniques for placement of indwelling prostheses are product specific and can be more difficult because of their larger diameter and retaining collar size. The Groningen Voice Button and Provox prostheses are designed to be placed in retrograde fashion with topical anesthesia. A semi-rigid catheter is first passed into the tract and brought out the oral cavity. The device is then affixed to the end of the catheter and withdrawn into the fistula through the oropharynx and cervical esophagus. A small hemostat may be used to facilitate passage of the outer collar through the posterior tracheal wall. The Blom-Singer Indwelling and Provox2 prostheses are designed for anterograde placement using proprietary insertion devices. Anterograde insertion is simpler to perform and more comfortable for the patient.

In addition to reduced patient manipulation, indwelling prostheses also have the advantage of immediate placement during primary or secondary TE puncture. When performed at the time of laryngectomy, proponents of this technique argue that the prosthesis will stabilize the tract, preventing separation of the TE party wall and reducing salivary leakage.[22] Although voicing still begins about the postoperative day 10 to allow healing of the pharynx, patients are spared the discomfort of device placement shortly after their procedure. Others disagree with immediate device placement, arguing that it complicates early care of the stoma and mandates a nasogastric tube for feeding. Thinning of the party wall also occurs in the postoperative period, which may lead to poor device fit and early replacement.

In the past, decisions regarding the type of device used were largely determined by the surgeon and voice rehabilitation therapist. With numerous devices now available and tremendous amounts of information readily available on the Internet, patients are becoming increasingly involved in the selection process. While studies have demonstrated a two-fold patient preference for indwelling over non-indwelling devices,[22] comparisons of the low-pressure devices suggest that the vocal quality and ease of use are similar between different brands.[28,35,131] Given these similarities—cost, comfort, ease of replacement, and access to health care services become important patient-specific considerations when selecting TE voice prosthesis.

VOICING

Initiation of voicing can begin immediately after prosthesis placement under the guidance of a voice rehabilitation therapist. Realistic expectations of vocal ability and quality should be discussed and, if possible, patients should become familiar with tracheoesophageal speech preoperatively either through patient interaction or videotape. Instruction in breathing, timing, and complete stoma occlusion should begin after placement. Application of excessive abdominal pressure may make voicing difficult and lead to transient lightheadedness. Patients often acquire usable speech with the first post-operative visit and will continue to improve with practice. On average, patients require 4 to 7 visits to become accomplished and fluent TE speakers.

A small, but growing, number of patients can become successful "hands-free" speakers.[44,74] Two-way valves can be fitted to adhesive peristomal housings (InHealth Technologies, Atos Medical, and others) or intra stomal retaining collars (Barton Button, Bivona Medical Technologies, Gary, In) to allow patients to speak without digital occlusion of the stoma. While not speaking, the tracheostomal valve does not engage, and the device permits free inspiration and expiration. With rapid exhalation, the valve engages and air is directed through the TE prosthesis. Unfortunately, recent studies have shown that only about half of successful TE speakers could use the hands-free valves.[74] Most of the problems with hands-free speech were related to stomal geometry. Prominent clavicular heads and irregular stomas prevent adequate sealing of the peristomal housing or retaining collar. Routine division of prominent clavicular heads, undermining inferior skin flaps around the tracheal closure, and maintenance of a single intact tracheal ring at the skin edge may help increase the success of such devices.

FAILURE TO ACQUIRE TE VOICE

Despite appropriate patient selection and proper TE puncture technique, some patients fail to produce usable voice. The majority of these failures seem to be related to tonicity of the pharyngoesophageal segment.[15] Although hypotonicity of the PE segment has been reported, hypertonicity is more commonly the culprit and such patients will note markedly increased effort required for phonation.[115,116] Clinically, these patients will produce a strong Valsalva maneuver in an effort to voice and produce choppy sounds of short duration (usually less than 6 seconds). Videofluoroscopy with barium sulfate will demonstrate a smooth bulge in the posterior pharyngeal wall during phonation and should be performed in the evaluation of hypertonic PE segment to identify the level of obstruction (Figure 105-7). Although many patients will spontaneously resolve this problem during the next 4 to 6 weeks, as many as 25% of these patients fail to improve despite therapy and become too frustrated to continue voicing.[118]

The physiology and etiology of PE segment hypertonicity is poorly understood. Much of this difficulty comes from the variability of laryngeal resection dictated by tumor extension and the many different closure techniques used to repair the pharyngeal defect. Radiographic studies of patients with hypertonic PE segments demonstrate dynamic obstruction at the level of the upper esophageal sphincter (UES) in

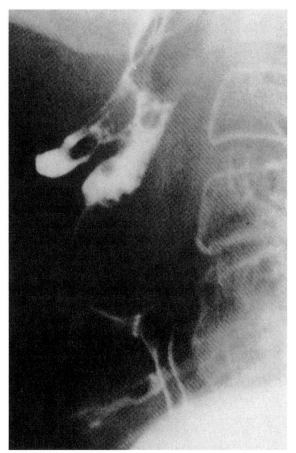

Figure 105-7. Hypertonic PE segment after TE puncture. Note prominent pharyngeal constrictor bulge and reduced barium column preventing airflow.[115]

response to insufflation of the esophagus.[120] While the components of the UES, including the cricopharyngeus, inferior constrictor, and upper esophageal muscles, are transected at the time of laryngectomy, these muscles may be reconstituted during closure of the pharyngeal defect either by postoperative scarring or by multilayer closure to reinforce the mucosal suture line.

PE segment hypertonicity was recognized shortly after the initial descriptions TE puncture technique. Blom, Singer, and Hamaker[21] and Lewin, Baugh, and Baker[73] attempted to identify patients at risk for PE segment problems preoperatively by performing esophageal insufflation through a transnasal catheter. Unfortunately, despite accurate prediction of immediate postoperative voicing in a small cohort of patients, esophageal insufflation testing failed to predict successful TE puncture use 6 months after laryngectomy.[24]

Without reliable methods of predicting success with TE puncture preoperatively, surgeons have advocated various techniques to prevent hypertonicity of the PE segment at the time of laryngectomy.[22] Methods include posterolateral cricopharyngeal and constrictor myotomy, unilateral pharyngeal plexus neurorrhaphy, and non closure of the pharyngeal musculature. The surgeon often palpates the diameter of the upper esophageal segment after removal of the specimen to determine whether myotomy of the proximal esophagus and remaining cricopharyngeus is necessary.[70,100] Before removal of the larynx specimen, the main branch of the pharyngeal plexus can be identified in the hiatus between the inferior and middle constrictor muscles. The surgeon should confirm the identity of the nerve using a handheld nerve stimulator. Once confirmed, the nerve should be ligated and transected before it divides in order to denervate both the middle and inferior constrictor muscles. Incorporating these techniques, one group found postoperative PE segment hypertonicity in only 6% of laryngectomees undergoing primary TE puncture.[100] In addition to these techniques, at least two groups have looked at non-closure of the pharyngeal musculature over the mucosal suture line during repair of the pharyngeal defect as another means of preventing hypertonicity.[29,135] The results, in a total of 50 patients treated between the two studies, demonstrated successful voice acquisition, normal tracheal pressures, and no increase in postoperative fistula development.

Similar procedures for pharyngeal neurorrhaphy and UES myotomy following secondary TE puncture have been described, but these procedures are technically difficult and many patients are reluctant to undergo further surgery.[115,116] Fortunately, less-invasive procedures show great promise in alleviating PE segment hypertonicity. Several investigators have reported the successful use of botulinum toxin under fluoroscopic or EMG guidance.[19,75,105,129] After injection of 45 to 100 units of botulinum toxin A (Botox, Allergan, Inc., Irvine, CA) into the pharyngeal musculature, investigators have noted resolution of PE segment hypertonicity and improvement in vocal quality in 70% to 87% percent of patients. Interestingly, most patients resolve their voicing difficulties with the first procedure and the average duration of effect in 1 study was more than 20 months.[75] Citing variable and unpredictable results with botulinum toxin, Bastian and Muzaffar have reported an endoscopic technique for lysis of the cricopharyngeus muscle.[14] Their technique uses a Weerda diverticuloscope placed into the pharynx to expose the bulge of the cricopharyngeus muscle in the posterior wall. Once properly exposed, the cricopharyngeus muscle may be cut vertically using a CO_2 laser. They report having performed the procedure in two patients with successful voice acquisition postoperatively and no complications.

COMPLICATIONS OF TE PUNCTURE
Major Complications

While a number of adverse events have been reported in association with TE puncture, major complications are extremely rare. Aspiration pneumonia, device aspiration, false passage dissection, mediastinitis, deep neck abscess, esophageal stenosis, vertebral osteomyelitis, necrosis of the TE party wall, and death have all been reported.[6,63,109] Of these problems, dislodgement of the prosthesis is probably the most common serious complication and recent studies suggest an incidence about 10%, depending on the type of prosthesis used and population studied.[63] Although potentially quite dangerous, device aspiration can occur after spontaneous dislodgement, but rarely leads to serious sequelae (Figure 105-8). In most cases, the device does not cause dyspnea and is usually located just above the carina or in the right mainstem bronchus. Izdebski and others noted that the prostheses could often be expelled with a strong cough; however, on occasion, fiberoptic-assisted recovery is necessary. The incidence of aspiration ranges from 0% to 13%[63,99,117] and appears to be decreasing with the newer indwelling prostheses because of larger esophageal flanges. If a dislodged prosthesis is not replaced quickly (usually in fewer than 36 hours), spontaneous closure of the fistula may occur, and the patient may require a repeat operative procedure once healing is complete. For this reason, many surgeons and speech therapists provide their patients with red rubber catheters (about 14 Fr) or dilators to be placed in the fistula should the prosthesis become dislodged and not be easily replaced. Once the fistula is stabilized, the patient may return at their convenience for tract dilation and prosthesis replacement in the office.

Serious infections after prosthesis placement are fortunately very rare. Such problems usually occur if there is disruption of the tracheoesophageal party wall either during primary or secondary procedures or by accidental esophageal perforation during esophagoscopy. Improper technique or prosthesis fit, rough tissue

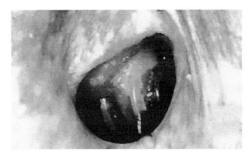

Figure 105-8. Spontaneous extrusion of prosthesis. Courtesy of Atos Medical.

handling, poor patient selection, and irradiation may contribute to salivary leakage into the deep neck spaces or mediastinum. Extension of the infection to involve the vertebral column has been reported.[6,109] Patients may present several weeks after their procedure with fever, lethargy, and dysphagia or odynophagia. CT scans should be performed of the neck and chest in order to identify areas of salivary collection and abscess formation. Videofluoroscopic swallowing studies may confirm the diagnosis and can also be used to follow closure of the esophageal leak. Aggressive drainage of the collections, intravenous antibiotics, and temporary cessation of oral intake or enteral feeding through a nasogastric tube will usually result in spontaneous closure of the fistulas. If a nasogastric tube is used, it should be placed under direct vision at operation or with the assistance of fluoroscopy. Post-duodenal placement of the nasogastric tube may help prevent reflux and speed healing. Large or stubborn esophageal leaks may require repair with healthy tissue.

Prosthesis migration and progressive enlargement of the fistula tract are also serious complications (Figure 105-9). Pressure necrosis from poorly fitted prostheses or unusual angulation of the tract, prior irradiation, poor patient selection, and improper technique have all been cited as contributing factors. Substantial salivary leakage and aspiration can occur as the fistula widens beyond the diameter of the device. Initial management should be directed at systemic problems such as inadequate nutrition, infection, hypothyroidism, and tumor persistence. Once systemic factors are optimized for would healing, careful cleaning and judicious use of chemical cautery agents such as silver nitrate can induce closure of the site. Often the device must be removed in order to obdurate the site with large diameter catheters. These may be serially downsized as healing occurs. Recently,

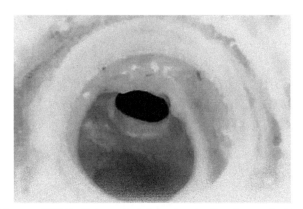

Figure 105-9. Enlarged fistula tract. Courtesy of Atos Medical.

one surgeon has reported successful occlusion of the fistula site using a silicone septal button.[91] Once the TE party wall thins to about 4 mm, spontaneous closure is unlikely and surgical intervention should be considered.[70,108] Several surgical procedures have been used successfully including 2-layer mucosal, 3-layer mucosal including interposed dermis or fascia, and 3-layer mucosal including muscle advancement.[59,108]

Minor Complications

The most common minor complication is premature device failure. While reasonable expectations of device lifespan should be at least 3 months to maintain patient satisfaction, clinicians have noted that tremendous variation in prosthesis longevity exists from patient to patient. Many factors have been blamed for the rapid demise of prostheses in certain patients including prior radiation therapy, volume of salivary tissue radiated, residual salivary flow, presence of dental prostheses, and drug therapy. Shortly after TE prostheses were introduced, fluffy white yeast colonies could be found covering the devices (Figure 105-10). Subsequent studies confirmed that elevated *Candida* species counts were the most common cause of premature device failure and that the use of antifungal medications can prolong device life.[81,82,133] More recent studies have focused on biofilms developing on prostheses and their effect on increasing airflow resistance. Although many species of bacteria and fungi have been recovered from TE prostheses, careful comparisons of the biofilms surrounding short lifespan and extended lifespan devices found significant differences between isolation of *C. albicans*, *C. tropicalis*, and the bacterium *Rothia dentocariosa*.[42] Other studies have implicated *Staphylococcus aureus* in the early failure of TE prostheses. As with denture stomatitis, some have suggested that bacterial colonization is required for subsequent fungal colonization and this has been demonstrated *in vitro*.[90,96] Such findings suggest that topical antibacterials may be as important as antifungal therapy.

In an attempt to decrease leakage and improve device lifespan, at least one group has experimented with a prosthesis containing a *Candida*-resistant fluoro plastic valve and a pair of magnets that allow the valve to close actively.[57] Active valve closure reduces bolus and salivary flow through the device, which minimizes colonization by fungi. In a prospective study of 18 patients with poor device longevity, the group demonstrated a 14-fold increase in device lifespan and no interference with MRI scanning. While such gains do come at a cost of increased valve opening pressure, necessitating the use of lubricant to ease speech, these findings suggest that leakage and device longevity may be less problematic in the future.

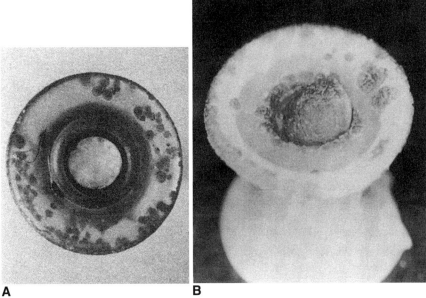

A   **B**

Figure 105-10. A, Yeast harmlessly growing on flange. Courtesy of Atos Medical. **B,** Yeast obstructing device valve.[70]

Signs of *Candida* colonization include fluffy white colonies on the flanges, brittle and stiff retention collars, and rolled appearance of the valve. Patients with previous radiation treatment are at greater risk for colonization, probably because of mucosal changes and decreased salivary flow. Within the laryngectomy community, there are many anecdotal reports of regimens to help promote device longevity. Some of these regimens, including use of dairy products, caffeinated soda, and clearing of the prosthesis with intermittent coughing have been suggested to be helpful when combined with daily cleaning. If fungal colonization continues to be problematic, treatment with oral antifungal medication such as nystatin may help reduce the oropharyngeal yeast counts. Alternatively, nystatin may be used topically to flush or clean the device. Finally, as different devices seem to be more susceptible to different species of bacteria and fungi, it may be appropriate to try a different prosthesis in refractory cases of early failure.

Leakage around the prosthesis is also a common problem. Typically, such leakage occurs after ingestion of thin liquids and can result in near-continuous salivary aspiration. Usually, such drainage is simply inconvenient and not dangerous. While there are several possible causes of leakage around the device, the most common cause is improper device fit. If the device is longer than required by the fistula tract, the fistula may leak through a pistoning movement of the device during swallowing.[99] This problem is easily corrected by replacing the prosthesis with a shorter one and is very common as the tract heals in the postoperative period or during radiation therapy. Temporary removal of the prosthesis (3–6 days) may also allow contraction of the site, sealing leakage when the prosthesis is reinserted. In selected cases, augmentation of the site with collagen or polysaccharide gel can be performed.[78,106] Alternatively, a small purse-string closure of the tracheal mucosa with absorbable suture can be effective and avoids the need for enteral feeding during prosthesis removal.[99]

Other minor complications include mucosal hypertrophy, scarring, granulation tissue formation, and chronic low-grade infection of the site. Mucosal hypertrophy and granulation tissue formation are often patient-specific reactions to foreign material contact (Figure 105-11). Local excision or chemical cauterization of the excess mucosa can all be performed in the office setting. Careful prosthesis sizing (often upsizing to reduce motion) and cleaning can help minimize this problem. Patients with scarring around the site will often complain about tightness or discomfort after prosthesis replacement with the same size device. Such problems often require division of scar bands, either by dilation or incision, and can be performed under local anesthesia. Once the scar has been lysed, temporary upsizing of the prosthesis will permit comfortable use. Chronic local site irritation can be caused by cellulitis and may respond well to antibiotics. Gastroesophageal reflux can also occur in laryngectomees and a trial of therapy may be indicated in refractory cases. Overall, these local site

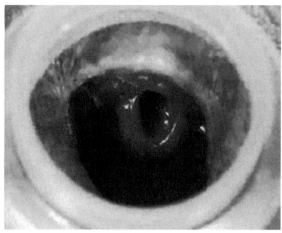

Figure 105-11. Granulation tissue around TE fistula. Courtesy Atos Medical.

problems occur in about one in five of patients who undergo TE puncture, but only rarely lead to fistula closure.[11,83,99]

ESOPHAGEAL SPEECH

For decades the gold standard of speech restoration, esophageal speech remains an excellent option for many patients after total laryngectomy. In motivated patients with contraindications to TE puncture, such as arthritis, tracheostomal stenosis, poor pulmonary function, and previous failed TE fistula, esophageal speech can yield remarkably intelligible and fluent communication. Advantages of this method of rehabilitation include "hands-free" speech of good to excellent quality, freedom from prosthesis maintenance and replacement, and markedly decreased cost in the long term.[68] Both perceptual and voice analysis studies have shown that good esophageal speech compares well with TE speech.[17,95] Unfortunately, successful acquisition of esophageal speech can take months under the guidance of a speech therapist, and many patients seem completely unable to develop this mode of communication. Success rates vary from 14% to 75%,[47] with large studies reporting rates of about 24% before the widespread use of TE puncture.[110] While radiation therapy has been associated with failure to attain esophageal speech, most known factors predictive of patient success are related to an individual's independence and motivation.[47]

Three primary methods exist of producing esophageal speech: consonant injection, glossopharyngeal press, and inhalation method. While the best speakers will use some combination of all three of these methods, consonant injection is the most efficient method for teaching.[18] This method involves injection of air using the base of the tongue while simultaneously producing a consonant (often a plosive consonant such as /p/, /b/,

or /g/). The patient prepares the esophagus by lifting the esophageal sphincter and lowering the base of tongue. The oral cavity is closed, and air is injected from the pharynx into the esophagus.[94] Initially, these injections are performed during intra phrase pauses or rest intervals, but, with practice, patients can learn to inject air with each bilabial, plosive, or fricative consonant. Once patients master the production of a single plosive, they may advance to consonant-vowel combinations and short words.

The glossopharyngeal press method involves pressing the tongue firmly against the hard palate and alveolar ridge. With piston-like pumping action, the patient pushes the tongue posteriorly, forcing air into the esophagus. This method can only be used during pauses or rests, and the patient must be cautioned to avoid swallowing air into the stomach. Like the glossopharyngeal press, the inhalation method can only be used during pauses or rests and is not as effective as consonant injection. It can, however, be used with the other two methods to generate more natural speech. Patients begin by relaxing the PE segment and generate negative intrathoracic pressure by inhaling. This action allows air to enter the esophagus for phonation. Other methods of speech production including buccal and pharyngeal speech may also be incorporated with injection or inhalation methods by some patients, but are not taught as primary modalities.[138]

ARTIFICIAL LARYNGES

While pneumonic larynges are rarely seen, electro larynges are still commonly used artificial speech aides by many laryngectomees. Although generally regarded as unnatural and stigmatizing by many surgeons, therapists, and patients, electro larynges can provide an easy, safe, and effective means of communication for patients. In at least one study, there was no significant difference between the intelligibility of TE fistula, esophageal, or electrolarynx-generated speech among naïve listeners.[142] Though speech from an artificial larynx may be intelligible, proficiency varies widely between speakers, and most patients have difficulty with intonation.[26,139] Certain sounds, such as voiceless fricatives (e.g., /h/) are nearly impossible to express and can cause listeners to become confused. In the same manner, expressions such as laughter remain silent. Despite these shortcomings, electro larynges are easy for patients to begin using and do not interfere with postoperative healing. Before the development of reliable TE speech, many surgeons felt strongly that patients should not be exposed to electro larynges after surgery or they would not develop esophageal speech. Such views are no longer held true and many surgeons or therapists will offer patients devices for temporary use before TE prosthesis fitting.

Two primary modes of electrolarynx are in use. The devices may be applied directly to the lateral neck, just beneath the angle of the mandible, the cheek, or the submental region. Patients and therapists will have to experiment to determine the optimal site for speech production. If the device is used immediately during the postoperative period, swelling, tenderness, over healing incisions, and the extent of surgery may result in some difficulties producing usable speech. In such cases, the device may be used trans orally with a straw adapter. Most long-term users of the electro larynges find the transoral route limiting and more socially unacceptable. Some dexterity is required for both methods, as the device must be inactivated to avoid monotone buzzing during pauses in speech.

ALARYNGEAL SPEECH AND QUALITY OF LIFE

While studies of patient mastery, intelligibility, and continued use of various means of alaryngeal speech are important to guide postoperative planning and care, quality-of-life (QOL) measures are critical to understand the impact of these interventions and tailor future advances in management. As discussed previously in this chapter, patients who undergo laryngectomy quickly note numerous alterations in daily functioning and physiologic processes. Alteration or loss of smell, taste, swallowing, nasal breathing, ability to control secretions, upper body strength, and overall fitness level accompany marked changes in communication, appearance, social interaction, and mood. These and other factors contribute to a laryngectomee's overall sense of well-being after surgery.

Although communication is an important component of post-laryngectomy rehabilitation, recent QOL studies, using validated instruments for evaluating head and neck cancer patients, suggest that speech is not the most important concern after laryngectomy. Activity level, recreation, and swallowing all appeared more important than speech to patients after laryngectomy in a pilot study from the University of Washington.[34] While it is difficult to assess the significance of these findings because the authors did not discuss the methods of voice rehabilitation in their population, it is intriguing that communication is not the most important determinant of well-being after laryngectomy as previously assumed. Most of the QOL studies performed to date compare organ-preservation protocols with total laryngectomy in an effort to determine how best to manage advanced laryngeal cancer. In a long-term follow-up evaluation of patients enrolled in the Veterans Affairs Laryngeal Cancer Study, Terrell, Fisher, and Wolf found no significant difference in the speech and communication abilities between the patients in the organ preservation cohort and those in the total laryngectomy cohort.[130] Terrell, Fisher, and Wolf and the University of Washington groups have posited that, with time, laryngectomees adapt to their communication disabilities and compensate effectively with whatever mode of rehabilitation they choose.[34,130,141] Although comprehensive studies of different methods of alaryngeal speech and QOL have not been performed, at least one study found that patients who use TE fistula speech score higher in most general QOL assessments than those who use an electrolarynx.[43]

REFERENCES

1. Ahmad I and others: Surgical voice restoration following ablative surgery for laryngeal and hypopharyngeal carcinoma, *J Laryngol Otol* 114:522, 2000.
2. Akbas Y, Dursun G: Voice restoration with low pressure Blom-Singer voice prosthesis after total laryngectomy, *Yonsei Med J* 44:615, 2003.
3. Albers JFH: *The history of laryngeal biopsy.* In Jackson C, Jackson CL: *Cancer of the larynx,* Philadelphia, 1939, WB Saunders, p 241.
4. Alberti PW: Panel discussion: the historical development of laryngectomy. II. The evolution of laryngology and laryngectomy in the mid-19th century, *Laryngoscope* 85:288, 1975.
5. Amatsu M: A one stage surgical technique for postlaryngectomy voice rehabilitation, *Laryngoscope* 90:1378, 1980.
6. Andrews JC and others: Major complications following tracheoesophageal puncture for voice rehabilitation, *Laryngoscope* 97:562, 1987.
7. Annyas AA and others: Groningen prosthesis for voice rehabilitation after laryngectomy, *Clin Otolaryngol* 9:51, 1984.
8. Arslan M: Reconstructive laryngectomy: report of the first 35 cases, *Ann Otol Rhinol Laryngol* 81:479, 1972.
9. Asai R: Asai's new voice production method: a substitution for human speech, Eighth International Congress of Otorhinolaryngology, Tokyo, 1965.
10. Asai R: Laryngoplasty after total laryngectomy, *Arch Otolaryngol* 95:114, 1972.
11. Aust MR, McCaffrey TV: Early speech results with the Provox prosthesis after laryngectomy, *Arch Otolaryngol Head Neck Surg,*123:966, 1997.
12. Balle VH, Rindso L, Thomsen JC: Primary speech restoration at laryngectomy by insertion of voice prosthesis—10 years experience, *Acta Otolaryngol Suppl* 543:244, 2000.
13. Barney HL: A discussion of some technical aspects of speech aids for postlaryngectomized patients, *Ann Otol Rhinol Laryngol* 67:558, 1958.
14. Bastian RW, Muzaffar K: Endoscopic laser cricopharyngeal myotomy to salvage tracheoesophageal voice after total laryngectomy, *Arch Otolaryngol Head Neck Surg* 127:691, 2001.
15. Baugh RF, Lewin JS, Baker SR: Vocal rehabilitation of tracheoesophageal speech failures, *Head Neck* 12:69, 1990.
16. Bell Laboratories: New artificial larynx, *Trans Am Acad Opthalmol Otolaryngol,* 63:548, 1959.
17. Bellandese MH, Lerman JW, Gilbert HR: An acoustic analysis of excellent female esophageal, tracheoesophageal, and laryngeal speakers, *J Speech Lang Hear Res,* 44:1315, 2001.

18. Blalock D: Speech rehabilitation after treatment of laryngeal carcinoma, *Otolaryngol Clin North Am* 30:179, 1997.

19. Blitzer A and others: Voice failure after tracheoesophageal puncture: management with botulinum toxin, *Otolaryngol Head Neck Surg* 113:668, 1995.

20. Blom ED, Singer MI, Hamaker RC: Tracheostoma valve for postlaryngectomy voice rehabilitation, *Ann Otol Rhinol Laryngol* 91:576, 1982.

21. Blom ED, Singer MI, Hamaker RC: An improved esophageal insufflation test, *Arch Otolaryngol* 111:211, 1985.

22. Brown DH and others: Postlaryngectomy voice rehabilitation: state of the art at the millennium, *World J Surg* 27:824, 2003.

23. Brucke EW: Nachschrift zu Prof. Joseph Kudelka's adhandlung, betitelt: Ueber herrn Dr. Brucke's lautsystem, nebst einigen beobachtungen ueber die sprache bei mangel des gaumensegels sitzbungsh, *K Akad Wissensch* 28:63, 1858.

24. Callaway E and others: Predictive value of objective esophageal insufflation testing for acquisition of tracheoesophageal speech, *Laryngoscope* 102:704, 1992.

25. Chen HC, Tang YB, Chang MH: Reconstruction of the voice after laryngectomy, *Clin Plast Surg* 28:389, 2001.

26. Choi HS and others: Functional characteristics of a new electrolarynx "Evada" having a force sensing resistor sensor, *J Voice* 15:592, 2001.

27. Christensen JM: Esophageal speaker articulation of /s,z/: a dynamic palatometric assessment, *J Commun Disord* 25:65, 1992.

28. Chung RP and others: In vitro and in vivo comparison of the low-resistance Groningen and the Provox tracheoesophageal voice prostheses, *Rev Laryngol Otol Rhinol (Bord)* 119:301, 1998.

29. Clevens RA and others: Vocal rehabilitation after total laryngectomy and tracheoesophageal puncture using nonmuscle closure, *Ann Otol Rhinol Laryngol* 102:792, 1993.

30. Conley JJ, DeAmesti F, Pierce JK: A new surgical technique for vocal rehabilitation of the laryngectomized patient, *Ann Otol Rhinol Laryngol* 67:655, 1958.

31. Culton GL, Gerwin JM: Current trends in laryngectomy rehabilitation: a survey of speech-language pathologists, *Otolaryngol Head Neck Surg* 118:458, 1998.

32. Czermak JN: Ueber die sprache bei luftdichter verschliessung des kehlkopfes, Sitzungsb *K Akad D Wissensch Math–Naturw Cl* 35:65, 1859.

33. Czerny V: Versuche ueber kehlkopfexstirpation, *Wein Med Wochenschr* 24:557, 1870.

34. Deleyiannis FW and others: Quality of life after laryngectomy: are functional disabilities important? *Head Neck* 21:319, 1999.

35. Delsupehe K and others: Prospective randomized comparative study of tracheoesophageal voice prosthesis: Blom-Singer versus Provox, *Laryngoscope* 108:1561, 1998.

36. Deschler DG and others: Tracheoesophageal voice following tubed free radial forearm flap reconstruction of the neopharynx, *Ann Otol Rhinol Laryngol* 103:929, 1994.

37. Deschler DG and others: Quantitative and qualitative analysis of tracheoesophageal voice after pectoralis major flap reconstruction of the neopharynx, *Otolaryngol Head Neck Surg* 118:771, 1998.

38. Desyatnikova S and others: Tracheoesophageal puncture in the office setting with local anesthesia, *Ann Otol Rhinol Laryngol* 110:613, 2001.

39. Diaz JL: Consideraciones sobre laringectomia y aparato de fonacion en los laringectomizados, *Sem Med* 3:27, 1924.

40. Diedrich WM, Youngstrom AK: *Alaryngeal speech, ed 3,* Springfield, Illinois, 1977, Charles C Thomas.

41. Doyle PC, Swift ER, Haaf RG: Effects of listener sophistication on judgments of tracheoesophageal talker intelligibility, *J Commun Disord* 22:105, 1989.

42. Elving GJ and others.: Comparison of the microbial composition of voice prosthesis biofilms from patients requiring frequent versus infrequent replacement, *Ann Otol Rhinol Laryngol* 111:200, 2002.

43. Finizia C, Bergman B: Health-related quality of life in patients with laryngeal cancer: a post-treatment comparison of different modes of communication, *Laryngoscope* 111:918, 2001.

44. Fujimoto PA, Madison CL, Larrigan LB: The effects of a tracheostoma valve on the intelligibility and quality of tracheoesophageal speech, *Am Speech Hearing Res* 34:33, 1991.

45. Fukutake R, Yamashita R: Speech rehabilitation and complications of primary tracheoesophageal puncture, *Acta Otolaryngol (Stockh)* 500:117, 1993.

46. Garcia M: Physiological observations on the human voice, *Proc Roy Soc* VII:36, 1855.

47. Gates GA, Hearne EM III: Predicting esophageal speech, *Ann Otol Rhinol Laryngol* 91:454, 1982.

48. Geraghty JA and others: Long-term follow-up of tracheoesophageal puncture results, *Ann Otol Rhinol Laryngol* 105:501, 1996.

49. Gluck T: Der gangewaertige stand der chirugie des kehlkopfes pharynx-oesophagus und der trachea, *Monatsechr Ohrenh* 38:89, 1904.

50. Gluck T: Die chirugie im dienste der laryngologie. Vortrag auf dem I. Internat Laryngo-Rhinol Kongr. Wein, pp 66–105, 1908.

51. Gluck T: Patienten mit totalexstirpation de pharynx, larynx und oesophagus, denen eine kuenstliche stimme durch einen automatisch arbeitenden apparat geliefert wird, *Berl Klin Woschenschr* 47: 33, 1910.

52. Gussenbauer C: Ueber die erste durch Th. Billroth am menschen ausgefuehrte kehlkopf-exstripation und die anwendung eines kuenstlichen kehlkopfes, *Arch Klin Chir* 17:343, 1874.

53. Guttman MR: Rehabilitation of the voice of laryngectomized patients, *Arch Otolaryngol* 15:478, 1932.

54. Guttman MR: Tracheo-hypopharyngeal fistulization, *Trans Am Laryngol Rhinol Otol Soc* 41:219, 1935.

55. Gutzmann H: Stimme und sprache ohne kehlkopf, *Z. Laryngol,* 1:221, 1909.

56. Hilgers FJ, Schouwenburg PF: A new low-resistance, self-retaining prosthesis (Provox) for voice rehabilitation after total laryngectomy, *Laryngoscope* 100:1202, 1990.

57. Hilgers FJ and others.: A new problem-solving indwelling voice prosthesis, eliminating the need for frequent *Candida-* and "underpressure"-related replacements: Provox ActiValve, *Acta Otolaryngol* 123:972, 2003.

58. Holinger PH: Panel discussion: the historical development of laryngectomy. V. A century of progress of laryngectomies in the northern hemisphere, *Laryngoscope* 85:322, 1975.

59. Hosal SA, Myers EN: How I do it: closure of tracheoesophageal puncture site, *Head Neck* 23:214, 2001.

60. Hyman M: An experimental study of artificial-larynx and esophageal speech, *J Speech Hear Disorders* 20:291, 1955.

61. Isman KA, O'Brien CJ: Videofluoroscopy of the pharyngoesophageal segment during tracheoesophageal and esophageal speech, *Head Neck* 352, 1992.

62. Izdebski K and others: The effects of irradiation on a laryngeal voice of totally laryngectomized patients, *Int J Radiat Oncol Biol Phys* 14:1281, 1988.

63. Izdebski K and others: Problems with tracheoesophageal fistula voice restoration in totally laryngectomized patients. A review of 95 cases, *Arch Otolaryngol Head Neck Surg* 120:840, 1994.

64. Kao WW and others: The outcome and techniques of primary and secondary tracheoesophageal puncture, *Arch Otolaryngol Head Neck Surg* 120:301, 1994.

65. Karlen RG, Maisel RH: Does primary tracheoesophageal puncture reduce complications after laryngectomy and improve patient communication? *Am J Otolaryngol* 22:324, 2001.

66. Kawahara H A new surgical technique for voice restoration after laryngopharyngoesophagectomy with a free ileocolic graft: preliminary report, *Surgery* 569, 1992.

67. Kerr AI, Shiraishi T, Yasugawa H and others: Blom-Singer prostheses—an 11 year experience of primary and secondary procedures, *Clin Otolaryngol* 18:184, 1993.

68. Kesteloot K and others: Costs and effects of tracheoesophageal speech compared with esophageal speech in laryngectomy patients, *Acta Otorhinolaryngol Belg* 48:387, 1994.

69. Koch WM: A failsafe technique for endoscopic tracheoesophageal puncture, *Laryngoscope* 111:1663, 2001.

70. Koch WM: Total laryngectomy with tracheoesophageal conduit, *Otolaryngol Clin North Am* 35:1081, 2002.

71. Leder SB, Erskine MC: Voice restoration after laryngectomy: experience with the Blom-Singer extended-wear indwelling tracheoesophageal voice prosthesis, *Head Neck* 19:487, 1997.

72. Lequeux T and others: A comparison of survival lifetime of the Provox and the Provox 2 voice prosthesis, *J Laryngol Otol* 117:875, 2003.

73. Lewin JS, Baugh RF, Baker SR: An objective method for prediction of tracheoesophageal speech production, *J Speech Hear Disord* 52:212, 1987.

74. Lewin JS and others: Experience with Barton button and peristomal breathing valve attachments for hands-free tracheoesophageal speech, *Head Neck* 22:142, 2000.

75. Lewin JS and others: Further experience with Botox injection for tracheoesophageal speech failure, *Head Neck* 23:456, 2001.

76. Lopez MJ and others : Voice rehabilitation practices among head and neck surgeons, *Ann Otol Rhinol Laryngol* 96:261, 1987.

77. Lowry LD: Artificial larynges: a review and development of a prototype self-contained intra-oral artificial larynx *Laryngoscope* 91:1332, 1981.

78. Luff DA, Izzat S, Farrington WT: Viscoaugmentation as a treatment for leakage around the Provox 2 voice rehabilitation system, *J Laryngol Otol* 113:847, 1999.

79. Mackenzie M: *The use of the laryngoscope,* ed 2, Philadelphia, 1869, Lindsay and Blakiston, p 11.

80. Mackenzie M: *The fatal illness of Frederick the Noble,* London, 1888, William Clowes & Sons, Ltd., p 244.

81. Mahieu HF and others: Oropharynx decontamination preventing *Candida* vegetation on voice prostheses, *Arch Otolaryngol Head Neck Surg* 112:1090, 1986.

82. Mahieu HF and others: *Candida* vegetations on silicone voice prostheses, *Arch Otolaryngol Head Neck Surg* 112:321, 1986.

83. Manni JJ, Van den Broek P: Surgical and prosthesis-related complications using the Groningen button voice prosthesis, *Clin Otolaryngol* 15:515, 1990.

84. Maves MD, Lingeman RE: Primary vocal rehabilitation using the Blom-Singer and Panje voice prostheses, *Ann Otol Rhinol Laryngol* 91:458, 1982.

85. McConnel FM, Teichgraeber J: Neoglottis reconstruction following total laryngectomy: the Emory experience, *Otolaryngol Head Neck Surg* 90:569, 1982.

86. McKesson EI: A mechanical larynx, *JAMA* 88:645, 1927.

87. Mendenhall WM et al and others: Voice rehabilitation after total laryngectomy and postoperative radiation therapy, *J Clin Oncol* 20:2500, 2002.

88. Merwin GE, Goldstein LP, Rothman HB: A comparison of speech using artificial larynx and tracheoesophageal puncture with valve in the same speaker, *Laryngoscope* 95:730, 1985.

89. Miller AH: *First experiences with the Asai technique for vocal rehabilitation after laryngectomy.* In Snidecor JC, editor: *Speech Rehabilitation of the Laryngectomized,* ed 2, Springfield, Illinois, 1968, Charles C Thomas Publishing.

90. Millsap KW and others: Adhesive interactions between voice prosthetic yeast and bacteria on silicone rubber in the absence and presence of saliva, *Antonie Van Leeuwenhoek* 79:337, 2001.

91. Mirza S, Head M, Robson AK: Silicone septal button in the management of a large tracheo-oesophageal fistula following primary puncture in a laryngectomee, *ORL J Otorhinolaryngol Relat Spec* 65:129, 2003.

92. Mohr RM, Paddock BH, Boehler J: An adaptation of tracheoesophageal puncture, *Laryngoscope* 93:1086, 1983.

93. Morrison MD, Ogrady M: Primary tracheo-esophageal puncture voice restoration with laryngectomy, *J Otolaryngol* 15:69, 1986.

94. Moses PJ: Rehabilitation of the postlaryngectomized patient. The vocal therapist: place and contribution to the rehabilitation program, *Trans Am Laryngol Rhinol Otol Soc* 79:83, 1958.

95. Most T, Tobin Y, Mimran RC: Acoustic and perceptual characteristics of esophageal and tracheoesophageal speech production, *J Commun Disord* 33:165, 2000.

96. Neu TR and others: Microflora on explanted silicone rubber voice prostheses: taxonomy, hydrophobicity and electrophoretic mobility, *J Appl Bacteriol* 76:521, 1994.

97. Omori K, Kojima H, Nonomura M and others: Mechanism of tracheoesophageal shunt phonation, *Arch Otolaryngol Head Neck Surg* 120:648, 1994

98. Onodi A: Ergebnisse der abteilung fuer hoer-, sprach-, stimmstoerungen und tracheotomierte vom kriegsschauplatze mit einem rhino-laryngologischen anhang, *Monatsschr Ohrenh* 52:85, 1918.

99. Op de Coul BM and others: A decade of postlaryngectomy vocal rehabilitation in 318 patients: a single institution's experience with consistent application of Provox indwelling voice prostheses, *Arch Otolaryngol Head Neck Surg* 126:1320, 2000.

100. Op de Coul BM and others: Evaluation of the effects of primary myotomy in total laryngectomy on the neoglottis with the use of quantitative videofluoroscopy, *Arch Otolaryngol Head Neck Surg* 129:1000, 2003.

101. Panje WR: Prosthetic voice rehabilitation following laryngectomy: the voice button, *Ann Otol Rhinol Laryngol* 90:116, 1981.

102. Parker AJ, Yardley M, Lacy P and others: Trends in voice rehabilitation in the United Kingdom, *Folia Phoniatr Logop* 47:286, 1995.

103. Pindzola RH, Moffet B: Comparison of ratings of four artificial larynges, *J Commun Disord* 21:459, 1988.

104. Poppert P: Zur frange der totalen kehkopfexstirpation, *Dtsch Med Wochensch,* 19:833, 1893.

105. Ramachandran K and others: Botulinum toxin injection for failed tracheo-oesophageal voice in laryngectomees: the Sunderland experience, *J Laryngol Otol* 117:544, 2003.

106. Remacle M, Hamoir M, Marbaix E: Gax-collagen injection to correct aspiration problems after subtotal laryngectomy, *Laryngoscope* 100:663, 1990.

107. Robbins JA and others: Selected acoustic features of tracheoesophageal, esophageal, and laryngeal speech, *Arch Otolaryngol* 110:670, 1984.

108. Rosen A, Scher N, Panje WR: Surgical closure of persisting failed tracheoesophageal voice fistula, *Ann Otol Rhinol Laryngol* 106:775, 1997.

109. Ruth H, Davis WE, Renner G: Deep neck abscess after tracheoesophageal puncture and insertion of a voice button prosthesis, *Otolaryngol Head Neck Surg* 93:809, 1985.

110. Schaefer SD, Johns DF: Attaining functional esophageal speech, *Arch Otolaryngol* 108:647, 1982.

111. Seeman M: Speech and voice without larynx, *Cas Lek Ces* 41:369, 1922.

112. Seeman M: Phoniatrische Bemerkungen zur laryngekotomie, *Arch Klin Chir* 140: 285, 1926.

113. Serafini I: Total laryngectomy with maintenance of natural respiration. Report on the first case recently operated on with a personal technique, *Minerva Otorhinolaryngol,* 20:73, 1970.

114. Singer MI, Blom ED: An endoscopic technique for restoration of voice after laryngectomy, *Ann Otol Rhinol Laryngol* 89:529, 1980.

115. Singer MI, Blom ED: Selective myotomy for voice restoration after total laryngectomy, *Arch Otolaryngol* 107:670, 1981.

116. Singer MI, Blom ED, Hamaker RC: Pharyngeal plexus neurectomy for alaryngeal speech rehabilitation, *Laryngoscope* 96:50, 1986.

117. Singer MI: *Voice rehabilitation after laryngectomy.* In Bailey BJ editor: *Head and neck surgery—otolaryngology.* Philadelphia, 1993, JB Lippincott.

118. Singer MI: *Voice rehabilitation.* In Cummings CW, and others: *Otolaryngology—Head and Neck Surgery,* ed 2, St. Louis, 1995, Mosby.

119. Sisson GA, Goldman ME: Pseudoglottis procedure: update and secondary techniques, *Laryngoscope* 90:1120, 1980.

120. Sloane PM, Griffin JM, O'Dwyer TP: Esophageal insufflation and videofluoroscopy for evaluation of esophageal speech in laryngectomy patients: clinical implications, *Radiology* 181:433, 1991.

121. Smith LF, Calhoun KH: Intelligibility of tracheoesophageal speech among naive listeners, *South Med J* 87:333, 1994.

122. Solis-Cohen J: Two cases of laryngectomy for adenocarcinoma of the larynx, *Trans Amer Laryngol Assoc* 14:60, 1892.

123. Staffieri M and others : Surgical rehabilitation of speech after total laryngectomy: the Staffieri techniques, *Laryngol Rhinol Otol (Stuttg)* 57:477, 1978.

124. Stoerk K: Tracheotomie (larynx carcinome. – Die operative behandlung. – Operations – statistik. – Larygoskopische befunde bei larynx. – und Pharynx. – Carcinomen.), *Arch Laryngolo* 5:22, 1896.

125. Struebing P: Pseudostimme nach ausschaltung des kehlkopfs, speciell nach exstirpation desselben, *Dtsch Med Wochenshr* 14:1061, 1888.

126. Struebing P, Landois D: Erzeugung einer (natuerlichen) pseudo-stimme bei einem manne mit totaler exstirpation des kehlkopfes, *Arch Klin Chir* 38:143, 1889.

127. Tait RV: The oral vibrator, *Br Dent J* 107:392, 1959.

128. Tapia AG: Presentacionde un laringuectomizado hablando con un sencillisimo aparato artificial, *Rev Esp Laringol (Madrid)* 4:49, 1914.

129. Terrell JE, Lewin JS, Esclamado R: Botulinum toxin injection for postlaryngectomy tracheoesophageal speech failure, *Otolaryngol Head Neck Surg* 113:788, 1995.

130. Terrell JE, Fisher SG, Wolf GT: Long-term quality of life after treatment of laryngeal cancer. The Veterans Affairs Laryngeal Cancer Study Group, *Arch Otolaryngol Head Neck Surg* 124:964, 1998.

131. van den Hoogen FJA and otherset: The Groningen, Nijdam and Provox Voice Prostheses: a prospective clinical comparison based on 845 replacements, *Acta Otolaryngol (Stockh)* 116:119, 1996.

132. van der Torn M and others: Female-pitched sound-producing voice prostheses—initial experimental and clinical results, *Eur Arch Otorhinolaryngol* 258:397, 2001.

133. van Weissenbruch R and others : Deterioration of the Provox silicone tracheoesophageal voice prosthesis: microbial aspects and structural changes, *Acta Otolaryngol* 117:452, 1997.

134. Vuyk H, Tiwari R, Snow GB: Staffieri's procedure revisited, *Head Neck Surg* 8:21, 1985.

135. Wang CP and others: The techniques of nonmuscular closure of hypopharyngeal defect following total laryngectomy: the assessment of complication and pharyngoesophageal segment, *J Laryngol Otol* 111:1060, 1997.

136. Webster PM, Duguay MJ: Surgeons' reported attitudes and practices regarding alaryngeal speech, *Ann Otol Rhinol Laryngol* 99:197, 1990.

137. Weinberg B, Bennett S: Selected acoustic characteristics of esophageal speech produced by female laryngectomees, *J Speech Hear Res* 15:211, 1972.

138. Weinberg B, Westerhouse J: A study of pharyngeal speech, *J Speech Hear Disord* 38:111, 1973.

139. Weiss MS, Basili AG: Electrolaryngeal speech produced by laryngectomized subjects: perceptual characteristics, *J Speech Hear Res* 28:294, 1985.

140. Wetmore SJ: Location of the vibratory segment in tracheoesophageal speakers *Otolaryngol Head Neck Surg* 93:355, 1985.

141. Weymuller EA and others : Quality of life in head and neck cancer, *Laryngoscope* 110:4, 2000.

142. Williams SE, Watson JB: Differences in speaking proficiencies in three laryngectomee groups, *Arch Otolaryngol* 111:216, 1985.

143. Williams SE, Watson JB: Speaking proficiency variations according to method of alaryngeal voicing, *Laryngoscope* 97:737, 1987.

144. Zeitels SM: Jacob da Silva Solis-Cohen: America's first head and neck surgeon, *Head Neck* 19:342, 1997.

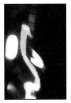

CHAPTER ONE HUNDRED AND SIX

MANAGEMENT OF THE IMPAIRED AIRWAY IN THE ADULT

David Goldenberg
Nasir Bhatti

INTRODUCTION

Acute airway situations should be approached in a systematic manner. The simplest adequate form of control should be selected and the lowest level of airway obstruction should be ascertained. Control should be established by securing an airway below that level. In addition, acute airway problems often evolve in association with other medical problems.

The commonest symptoms of acute airway obstruction are voice change, dyspnea, local pain, and cough. Physical findings may include stridor; hoarseness; restlessness; intercostal, suprasternal, and supraclavicular retraction; drooling; and, if trauma is involved, bleeding, subcutaneous emphysema, and deformation of the normal surgical landmarks.

The severity or completeness of airway obstruction is defined as follows:

- Complete obstruction: No detectable airflow in or out of lungs.
- Partial obstruction: The patient has stridor or respiratory difficulty because of a narrowing of the major airway.
- Potential or impending airway obstruction: The potential or fear for a patient developing airway compromise because of a known anatomical or physical condition if the respiratory physiology or the conscious level was altered.

THE DIFFICULT AIRWAY

Securing a patent airway remains one of the fundamental issues to be addressed in patients undergoing surgery. The most widely used techniques and devices used in clinical practice to secure an airway are orotracheal intubation, nasotracheal intubation, laryngeal mask airway, and fiberoptic intubation. These methods maintain airway patency by way of manipulation of the structures of the upper airway. Success in maintaining a patent airway using any of these techniques involves a detailed understanding of their interaction with the structures of the upper airway.[4] The failure to achieve this goal inevitably results in hypoxic brain injury or death. Benumof and Scheller estimated that up to 30% of deaths attributable to anesthesia are caused by the inability to successfully manage the difficult airway.[6] Caplan and others found that three mechanisms of injury resulted in 75% of adverse respiratory events during surgical anesthesia. These mechanisms included inadequate ventilation, unrecognized esophageal intubation and unanticipated difficult tracheal intubation.[11]

Timely identification of the potentially difficult airway is critical. To do so, the physician should be able to (1) define the nature of a difficult airway; (2) examine the airway for anticipated difficulty; (3) formulate a thorough plan for management of the airway using the American Society of Anesthesiologists (ASA) Difficult Airway Algorithm as a guide (ASA Task Force on Management of the Difficult Airway); and (4) possess the requisite skills to successfully use a variety of airway devices that form the foundation of difficult airway management in a variety of clinical situations such as fiberoptic intubation, laryngeal mask airway, and, if necessary, attaining a surgical airway.

The guidelines for management of the difficult airway developed by the ASA Task Force on Management of the Difficult Airway provide the following definitions:

- Difficult mask ventilation: A situation in which it is impossible for the unassisted.
  Anesthesiologist to prevent or to reverse the signs of inadequate ventilation during positive pressure mask ventilation.
- Difficult rigid laryngoscopy: When it is impossible to visualize any portion of the vocal cords with conventional laryngoscopy.

• Difficult intubation: A situation in which insertion of an endotracheal tube requires more than three attempts or longer than 10 minutes.

The clinical assessment of the airway begins with a rapid comprehensive assessment of the patient's ventilatory and respiratory status. If the airway distress is impending, prevention measures must be instituted to prevent further deterioration. If the patient is found to be ventilating inadequately, the airway must be secured definitively through either medical or surgical means. If the medical techniques to secure an airway fail, an urgent tracheotomy or cricothyrotomy must be performed.

If the situation does not mandate an immediate intervention, the physician may proceed with a diagnostic assessment. This should include a complete history and physical examination of the upper airway. The most valuable assessment in a modern setting is direct flexible fiberoptic nasopharyngolaryngoscopy. This technique affords unparalleled visualization and lends itself to video documentation.

A chest radiograph, arterial blood gas status, and a computed tomography scan may be obtained only if the general status of the patient is stable. If the individual circumstances allow, a review of any systemic disease requiring special attention during airway management must be undertaken.[4]

Mallampati and others originally published three distinct classes: Class I—uvula, faucial pillars, soft palate visible; Class II—faucial pillars and soft palate visible; and Class III—only soft palate visible.[29] Samsoon and Young modified the Mallampati classification to include a fourth class: Class IV—only hard palate visible.[41]

Another widely used method of assessment of the difficult airway is Cormack and Lehane's classification, which defines the difficulty of intubation according to the view of the glottis afforded at the time of direct laryngoscopy.[15,16]

One of the most important concepts in the ASA Difficult Airway Algorithm is to have a strategic plan in place for individual patient situations. This plan requires that the necessary equipment be readily available and that the operator be comfortable with a variety of airway management techniques. These techniques and devices should be practiced electively on patients with "normal" airways.[4]

A well-equipped, organized difficult-airway cart should be readily available. The ideal difficult-airway cart is an easily transportable storage unit that contains a variety of equipment necessary for management of the difficult airway. The cart can be customized to serve the expertise of the group of operators that it serves.

When findings from a thorough physical examination and history of the patient reveal that laryngoscopy, intubation, or mask ventilation is going to be difficult, the life-threatening "cannot intubate, cannot ventilate" situation may arise. This is best handled by placement of an endotracheal tube while the patient is awake.[47] Awake techniques provide rapid and ongoing assessment of the patient's neurologic status. Awake intubation techniques in patients who have been swabbed with appropriate topical anesthesia are easy to perform. Awake techniques preserve the normal position of the larynx. With the induction of anesthesia and paralysis, the larynx moves anteriorly, making conventional intubation more difficult.[42]

Awake nonsurgical intubation techniques can be accomplished by various methods, including awake fiberoptic intubation, awake "look" techniques of direct laryngoscopy, awake placement of a supraglottic airway device (laryngeal mask airway), or retrograde intubation. Awake surgical techniques include the performance of awake tracheostomy and will be discussed later in this chapter (Table 106-1).

Surgical Anatomy

The sternal notch, thyroid, and the cricoid cartilage usually can be easily palpated through the skin. The cricoid, described as a reverse signet ring just inferior to the thyroid cartilage, can be found by using either the sternal notch below or the thyroid cartilage above as reference points. The cricothyroid membrane stretches between the thyroid and cricoid cartilages and can be identified by palpating a slight indentation in the skin inferior to the laryngeal prominence. The

---

TABLE 106-1

INDICATIONS FOR TRACHEOSTOMY

Prolonged intubation
Facilitation of ventilation support
Inability of patient to manage secretions including:
  Aspiration
  Excessive bronchopulmonary secretions
Upper airway obstruction with any of the following:
  Stridor
  Air hunger
  Retractions
  Obstructive sleep apnea with documented arterial
    desaturation
  Bilateral vocal cord paralysis
Inability to intubate
Adjunct to major head and neck surgery
Adjunct to management of major head and neck
  trauma

right and left cricothyroid arteries traverse the superior part and anastomose near the midline.

The cricothyroid muscle arises from the anterior surface of the cricoid and travels superiorly, posteriorly, and laterally to attach laterally to the surface of the thyroid cartilage. This muscle rotates the thyroid anteriorly and lengthens the vocal cords. The vocalis muscles arise from the inner surface of the thyroid cartilage in the midline and pass superiorly and posteriorly to attach to the length of the vocal cords. They shorten the cords and vary the tension on the cords. These two pairs of muscles and the vocal cords themselves are vulnerable to injury during cricothyrotomy.

The innominate or brachiocephalic artery crosses from left to right anterior to the trachea at the superior thoracic inlet and lies just beneath the sternum. Its pulsations can sometimes be palpated during dissection. The trachea is made up of semicircular cartilaginous rings anteriorly and laterally, which can be palpated through the skin in a thin person. The trachea is membranous posteriorly, as are the spaces between the rings.

The thyroid gland lies anteriorly to the trachea with a lobe on either side, with the isthmus crossing the trachea at the level of the second to fourth tracheal rings. This tissue is extremely vascular and must be dealt with gently to prevent bleeding.

The recurrent laryngeal nerves and inferior thyroid veins that travel in the tracheoesophageal groove are paratracheal structures that are vulnerable to injury if dissection strays from the midline. The great vessels too could be damaged should dissection go lateral.

TRACHEOTOMY INTRODUCTION

Tracheotomy is a surgical procedure in which an opening is made in the anterior wall of the trachea to establish an airway. This procedure is often temporary and reversible if the patient is able to breathe through an unobstructed upper airway.

In contrast, tracheostomy is the surgical creation of and opening into the trachea through the neck, with the tracheal mucosa being brought into continuity with the skin. This procedure is most often but not always permanent. The terms are often used interchangeably. Today, because of advancements in intensive care and the widespread use of mechanical ventilation, tracheotomy is one of the most commonly performed surgical procedures.

The 1989 Consensus Conference on Artificial Airways in Patients Receiving Mechanical Ventilation recommended performing a tracheotomy in patients whose need for prolonged artificial airway is anticipated.[15,39] It also recommended that the conversion from translaryngeal intubation to tracheotomy be made as early as possible to minimize the duration of translaryngeal intubation. Evidence suggests that the risk of long-term airway complications significantly increases with translaryngeal intubation beyond the tenth day.[47,50] Prolonged translaryngeal intubation is associated with increased laryngeal injury, glottic and subglottic stenosis, infectious complications, and tracheal injury such as tracheomalacia, and tracheal stenosis. Converting intubation to a tracheotomy also may facilitate suctioning, feeding, and mobility; promote early return of speech; and decrease the work of breathing. In fact, tracheotomy may actually expedite weaning in patients with marginal ventilatory capacity by reducing the airway resistance.[25,9]

Tracheotomy Timing

When a decision has to be made on the appropriate time to perform a tracheotomy, consider the following:

- Emergent (also known as slash trach): Only indicated when emergency airway distress and impending death of a patient exist. This is usually the exact indication for a cricothyrotomy. A slash trach should be considered only when it is impossible to intubate or perform a cricothyrotomy.[21] The complication rate for emergency tracheotomy is as high as 21%.[19]
- Urgent (awake): This is indicated when a patient is in respiratory distress and needs immediate surgical intervention. This is best performed in a controlled environment (the intensive care unit or the operating room) while using local anesthesia on an awake patient. These patients are typically very minimally sedated.
- Elective: Most elective tracheostomies are performed on patients who are already intubated and who are having a tracheostomy for prolonged intubation. Additionally, patients undergoing extensive head and neck procedures may receive a tracheostomy during the operative procedure to facilitate airway control during convalescence.[21]

INDICATIONS FOR TRACHEOTOMY

Current indications for tracheotomy are: prolonged intubation and mechanical ventilation, bypass of an upper airway obstruction, easier management of secretions, as an adjunct to chest or head and neck surgery in which ventilation problems or prolonged intubation are anticipated (Table 106-2).

The earliest indication for the procedure was upper airway obstruction resulting from trauma or infection. As late as the 1950s, the major indication for

TABLE 106-2

RELATIVE CONTRAINDICATIONS TO PERFORM
PERCUTANEOUS DILATIONAL TRACHEOTOMY

Children younger than 12 years of age
Anatomic abnormality of the trachea
Pulsating palpable blood vessel over the tracheotomy
   site
Active infection over the tracheotomy site
Occluding thyroid mass or goiter over the
   tracheotomy site
Short or obese neck
Positive end-expiratory pressure >15 cm H_2O
Platelet count <40,000/mm^3
Bleeding time >10 min
Prothrombin time or partial thromboplastin time
   >1.5 times control
Limited ability to extend the cervical spine
History of difficult intubation

tracheotomy was upper airway obstruction because of infectious disease including diphtheria, polio, Ludwig's angina, tetanus, and laryngotracheobronchitis.[29,41,49]

Other causes of upper airway obstruction necessitating tracheotomy include obstruction due to neoplastic processes, or functional obstruction such as bilateral vocal cord paralysis or edema secondary to smoke inhalation or caustic agent ingestion. In such cases, patients are usually stabilized by tracheal intubation or with a cricothyrotomy and tracheotomy later.

Although facial fractures in and of them selves are not an indication for tracheotomy, in cases of severe maxillo-facial trauma, tracheotomy is sometimes used to secure an airway where intubation would be difficult or damaging.

Today, the most common indication for tracheotomy is prolonged tracheal intubation, usually with mechanical ventilation. A recent review of more than 1000 consecutive tracheotomies found that 76% were performed to facilitate mechanical ventilation.[21]

Surgical Technique

Tracheotomy is optimally performed under general anesthesia in the operating room. If necessary, the procedure may be performed under local anesthesia or in an intensive care setting.[29] In case a tracheotomy is being performed under local anesthesia, the surgeon and the anesthetist have to work in tandem to keep the patient maximally reassured. On most occasions the anesthetist may use minimal sedation to achieve patient comfort without compromising the ability to breathe spontaneously. Another critical precaution to keep in mind is to avoid the use of Bovie

cautery. The surgical field may be getting the oxygen-rich gas mixture from the nasal cannula or the ventilating mask. This simple precautionary measure will avert the risk of igniting fire in the surgical field.

The basic technique consists of either a vertical incision from the cricoid cartilage, 1.5 inches inferiorly or a horizontal incision midway between the sternal notch and the cricoid cartilage (Figure 106-1). The incision is carried down through the skin, subcutaneous tissue, and platysma to reveal the strap muscles. If the patient is obese and the adipose tissue obtrusive, a minimal cervical lipectomy may be performed.[23] At this level, the dissection should be in a vertical plane regardless of the skin incision chosen. The strap muscles are separated by a vertical incision through the bloodless midline raphe (linea Alba) and retracted from one another revealing the thyroid isthmus which typically lies over the third and fourth tracheal ring (Figure 106-2). The isthmus may be dealt with in a number of ways. This decision is based on the position of the isthmus relative to the wound and the surgeon's personal preference. It may be superiorly retracted, transected, and suture-ligated (Figure 106-3), transected slowly using a monopolar cautery (Bovie)[10,28] (Figure 106-4), or inferiorly retracted (least commonly used method).[28] The trachea is revealed and the third and fourth tracheal rings are identified using the cricoid as a landmark. As with the skin incision, there are equally reasonable choices for the entrance into the trachea. An inferiorly based trap door flap (Bjork flap) can be created using a Mayo scissor and sutured to the subcutaneous tissue using 3-0 chromic suture.

Alternatively the anterior section of a single tracheal ring can be resected or a round or vertical oval window spanning two tracheal rings be excised[15,29,47] using a scalpel, curved Mayo scissor, or a tracheotomy punch (Figures 106-5 and 106-6). The endotracheal tube cuff is deflated and the tube slowly withdrawn by the anesthesiologist until the inferior tip of the tube is lined up with the superior border of the newly formed tracheal opening. A tracheotomy tube is then inserted through the tracheotomy into the airway and the patient is ventilated.

Tracheotomy Complications

The complications of tracheotomy may be categorized by the interval from the procedure to the onset of the complication and are thus divided into intraoperative, early, and late postoperative. It should be noted that there may be an overlap in the timeframe in which early, intermediate, and late complications present. It is important to note that specific patient populations, such as the pediatric, post head trauma, obese, burn patient, or seriously debilitated are more susceptible to complications related to tracheotomy.[20]

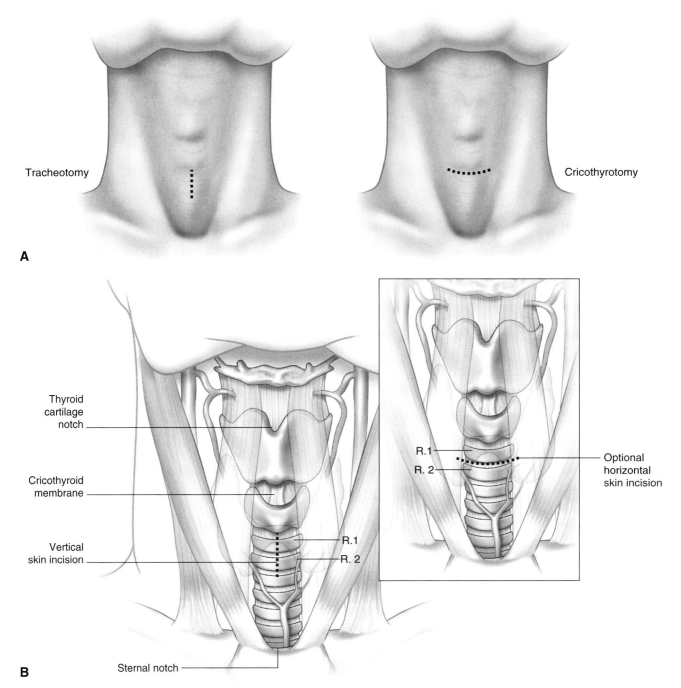

Figure 106-1. **A,** Surface anatomy of the neck with skin incision for the tracheotomy (*left*) and cricothyrotomy (*right*). **B,** A vertical skin incision is made between the cricoid and second tracheal ring as assessed by palpation through the skin.

Tracheotomy holds a complication rate of between 5% to 40% depending on study design, patient follow-up, and the definition of the different complications.[46] In a recent study of 1130 surgical tracheotomies, the major complication rate for surgical tracheotomy was found to be as low as 4.3%, with a mortality rate of 0.7%.[20] Death from tracheotomy is caused most often by hemorrhage or tube displacement. It is important to note that the incidence of complications in emergency tracheotomy is 2 to 5 times that found in an elective procedure.

The most common complication has classically been hemorrhage (3.7%), followed by tube obstruction (2.7%), and tube displacement (1.5%) The incidence

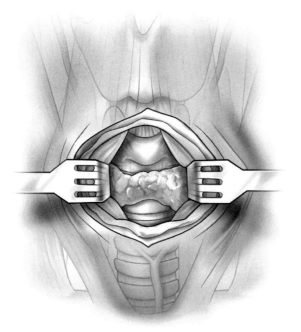

Figure 106-2. The strap muscles are separated through the bloodless midline raphe to reveal the underlying thyroid isthmus.

of pneumothorax, tracheal stenosis, and tracheoesophageal fistula is less than 1%.

Immediate Complications

Immediate complications of tracheotomy include those present during or at the termination of the operation. Although these complications are usually caused during surgery, they may appear hours or days after the tracheotomy is performed.

Bleeding during the performance of a tracheotomy is most commonly the result of errors in surgical technique. Frequent sites of bleeding are the anterior jugular veins, the thyroid isthmus, and vascular variants such as the thyroid ima artery.[36] Other immediate complications include insertion of the tracheotomy tube into a false route, electrocautery-induced intraoperative fire,[1] and surgical injury to adjacent structures.

Intermediate Complications

Intermediate complications develop during the first hours to days after surgery.

Again, hemorrhage may be a frequent postoperative complication of tracheotomy.

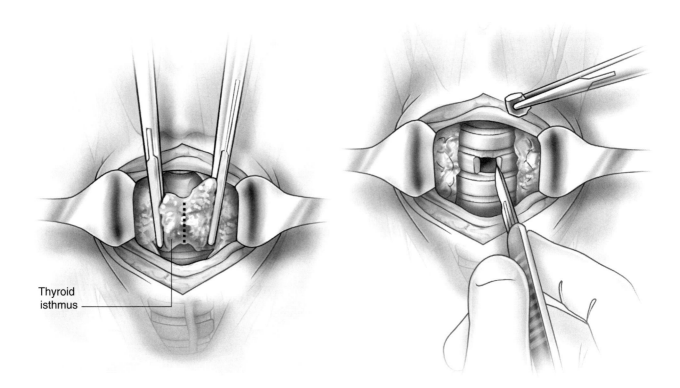

Thyroid isthmus

Figure 106-3. The thyroid isthmus may be retracted or suture ligated.

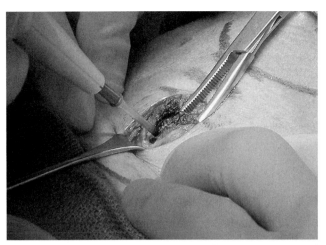

Figure 106-4. The thyroid isthmus may be safely transected slowly using a monopolar cautery (Bovie) when it obscures the proposed entrance site into the trachea.

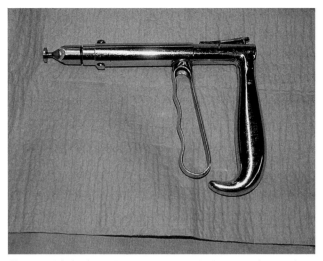

Figure 106-6. A tracheotomy punch is then used to make a circular window in the anterior wall of the trachea.

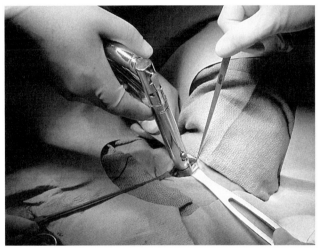

Figure 106-5. A horizontal incision can be made in the intracartilaginous space.

Because many of these patients are hypotensive, bleeding does not occur until arterial blood pressure is restored or venous pressure is increased by coughing associated with canula placement. Minor oozing may be managed by light packing with oxidized cellulose, microfibrillar collagen, or tranexamic acid-soaked gauze packs.[27]

Transient tracheitis and stomal cellulitis may occur, and all fresh tracheotomies should be attended to with strict local hygiene. Severe infection such as mediastinitis, clavicular osteomyelitis, and necrotizing fasciitis are rare, but have been reported after tracheostomy and must be treated aggressively.[48]

Other known early postoperative complications include subcutaneous emphysema, pneumomedi-

astinum, and pneumothorax. All of these may result from excessive dissection of tissue planes at the time of tracheostomy, blockage of the cannula, or assisted ventilation with excessive pressure, causing dissection of air along the pretracheal fascia. The incidence of subcutaneous emphysema is 0% to 9% and the incidence of pneumothorax is 0% to 4% in adults.[43]

Obstruction of the tracheotomy tube on the first few postoperative days is likely to result from blood clot, partial displacement, or tube impingement on the posterior tracheal wall. The incidence of tube obstruction is 2.5%.[43]

Routine postoperative care including observation, humidification, and frequent gentle suctioning prevents tube obstruction.

Dislodgment of the tracheotomy tube may be a fatal complication in the first few days after tracheotomy. Several factors that play a role in tube dislodgment are the length of the tube, thickness of the neck, site of tracheostomy, postoperative swelling, and method of securing the tube. As a general rule, the ties should be secured snugly, yet allow passage one finger between the ties and the neck to prevent neck constriction. We suture the flanges to the skin with monofilament suture in addition to the ties. In an emergent situation of accidental decannulation during the initial 48 hours after the tube placement, one failed attempt at replacement must be followed with orotracheal intubation. This often-neglected intervention can save many unnecessary mishaps.

Late Complications

A late complication such as delayed hemorrhage may be a result of traction on granulation tissue or from innominate artery erosion. Immediate investigation into the cause of bleeding is thus mandatory. Trachea-innominate fistula with massive hemorrhage occurs in 0.4% of tracheotomies.[14] Long-term tracheal intubation and ventilation with a cuffed tracheotomy tube may result in cartilage necrosis of the tracheal wall. Erosion may also occur with a cuffless tube if the tip of the tube is lodged anteriorly, the innominate artery is high in the neck, or the tracheostomy is placed too low.

This complication may be heralded by a "sentinel" bleed that may occur 3 days to 3 weeks before massive hemorrhage and should prompt an immediate fiberoptic tracheal examination.[26] If there is evidence of erosion or necrosis, the patient must be immediately evaluated in the operating room under general anesthesia, with the patient prepared for mediastinal exploration and thoracotomy. In instances of massive hemorrhage, direct digital pressure on the anterior wall of the stoma tract (posterior wall of the vessel) has been effective in controlling bleeding. Tracheal-innominate artery blowout carries a mortality rate of 85% to 90%.[7,8,37]

Tracheoesophageal fistula is rare, with a reported incidence of 0.01% to 1%.[51] Tracheoesophageal fistula is thought to result from incidental damage to the posterior tracheal wall at the time of surgery or to be the product of two factors: an over inflated and improperly fitted cuffed tube, which places pressure on the posterior tracheal wall, together with an indwelling nasogastric tube in the esophagus.

The diagnosis should be suspected clinically by coughing during eating, chronic cough on swallowing saliva, recurrent aspiration, and pneumonia. Barium swallow or methylene blue instilled into the esophagus and flexible fiberoptic evaluation may be diagnostic; however, generally a combination of these studies, with endoscopic evaluation, is often necessary. Once the diagnosis is confirmed, definitive surgical repair is undertaken.[22,40]

Tracheal stenosis and subglottic stenosis are complications predisposed by previous endotracheal tube intubation, high tracheostomy or cricothyroidotomy, and trauma to the airway. Patients at increased risk for tracheal stenosis include children and patients tracheotomized for closed head trauma. Meticulous surgical technique, aggressive treatment of postoperative infections, and the use of the high-volume, low-pressure cuffed tube help minimize the risk of tracheal stenosis.

Tracheocutaneous fistula is a late complication, which is more common as the stomal tract is epithelialized with long-term cannulation. A persistent fistula causes continual tracheal secretions with skin irritation, disturbed phonation, and frequent infections. Infection and granulation tissue may play a role in persistent stomal fistulas. Persistent fistulas require excision of the fistula tract.

Contraindications

No absolute contraindications exist to open surgical tracheostomy.

CRICOTHYROTOMY: CONIOTOMY

Cricothyrotomy is a procedure for establishing an emergency airway where other methods are unsuitable or impossible. Emergency cricothyrotomy is performed in approximately 1% of all emergency airway cases in the emergency room.[3] The access site is the cricothyroid membrane. This procedure is especially suited for gaining control of the airway in cases of severe hemorrhage or massive facial trauma, foreign bodies, or emeses not permitting visualized intubation. Other cases are when teeth are clenched, repeated failed intubation occurs, and a possibility exists of cervical spine injury. In these cases cricothyrotomy becomes the safest and quickest way to obtain an airway.[13] If a patient has sustained respiratory insult associated with burns or smoke inhalation, it may be indicated to perform an elective prophylactic cricothyrotomy early to prevent fatal respiratory obstruction occurring during transport.[35]

Cricothyrotomy Surgical Technique

The cricothyroid membrane is identified by palpating a slight indentation in the skin inferior to the laryngeal prominence. The membrane is immediately subcutaneous in location with no overlying large veins, muscles, or fascial layers, allowing easy access. A vertical skin incision and a horizontal entrance into the cricothyroid membrane is advised. For incision into the cricothyroid membrane itself, a low horizontal stab is made to avoid laterally placed vessels.[33] Either a small tracheotomy tube or a small standard endotracheal tube can be used in cricothyrotomy. Tube size is important in ensuring successful cannulation without excessive trauma. Once the patient is stabilized, the cricothyrotomy should be converted to a formal tracheotomy for adequate ventilation (Figure 106-7).

Contraindications to Cricothyrotomy

Contraindications to cricothyrotomy are patients who have an increased risk of subglottic stenosis, pre-existing laryngeal disease, malignancy, inflammatory processes in near proximity, epiglottitis, severe distortion of normal anatomy, and bleeding diathesis. Also, cricothyrotomy should be avoided in infants and children.

Needle Cricothyrotomy

Needle cricothyrotomy is performed in dire emergencies when either the appropriate equipment or

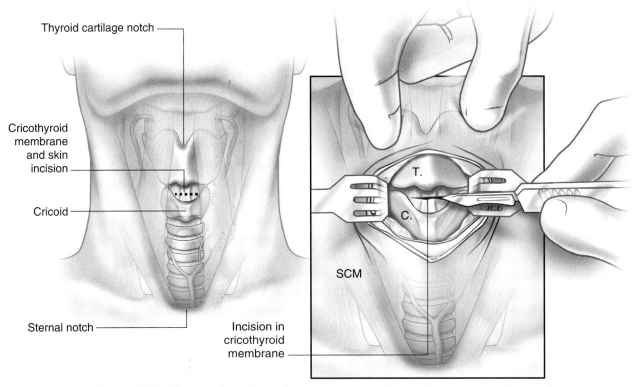

Figure 106-7. The cricothyroid membrane is palpated through the skin using the thyroid notch and cricoid cartilage as reference points.

knowledge to perform a formal emergency cricothyrotomy or intubation is impossible. A large-gauge needle and cannula with a syringe attached is introduced through the cricothyroid membrane until air can be aspirated. The cannula is then advanced off the needle down the airway (Figure 106-8). The cannula is connected to an oxygen supply. The patient can then be oxygenated, but ventilation to remove carbon dioxide is not achieved and respiratory acidosis may ensue rapidly.

A needle cricothyrotomy will ensure a supply of oxygen for a short time only and it must be converted to a surgical cricothyrotomy or tracheotomy in a timely fashion to allow adequate ventilation.

Transtracheal Needle Ventilation

The transtracheal needle ventilation technique can be used to great advantage in the emergency setting. This technique requires access to 100% oxygen at 50 psi and a Luer-Lok connector. The airway is controlled by puncturing the trachea or cricothyroid membrane with a 16-gauge plastic-sheathed needle. The needle is withdrawn, leaving the sheath in the trachea. The sheath is then attached to the high-pressure line through a pressure regulator control, and ventilation

is accomplished using a manual interrupter switch. The patient can be fully ventilated with this technique for at least 30 minutes.

Mini Tracheostomy

Removal of secretions from the tracheobronchial tree is crucial for preventing complications of respiratory therapy in the hospitalized patient. The use of mini tracheostomy, basically an elective cricothyrotomy, for recurrent endotracheal suctioning was first described by Matthews and Hopkinson in 1986.[33] Since then there have been a number of reports which demonstrate the use of mini tracheostomy solely for handling bronchopulmonary secretions. These studies show good clinical results with low morbidity.[2,5,9,24,31,45]

Cricothyrotomy Complications

The reported incidence of complications of cricothyrotomy varies from 6% to 39%, depending on whether the procedure was performed electively or as an emergency.[34] Complications include mediastinal emphysema, misplaced tube into trachea, esophagus or thyrohyoid membrane, hemorrhage, and failure to obtain an airway.

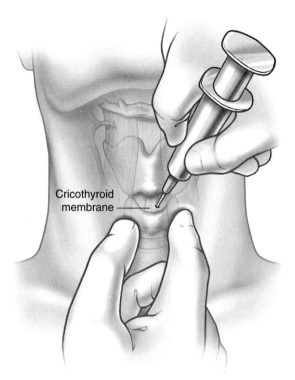

Figure 106-8. Needle cricothyrotomy. A large-gauge needle and cannula with a syringe attached is introduced through the cricothyroid membrane until air can be aspirated.

PERCUTANEOUS DILATIONAL TRACHEOTOMY

Percutaneous dilational tracheotomy (PDT) is the placement of a tracheotomy tube without direct surgical visualization of the trachea. The general consensus is that PDT should be performed only on intubated patients. It is considered to be a minimally invasive, bedside procedure that is easily performed in the intensive care unit or at the patient's bedside, with continuous monitoring of the patient's vital signs. The criteria for PDT are more stringent than those for open surgical tracheotomy.[17] PDT should be performed on patients whose cervical anatomy can be clearly defined by palpation through the skin. The two critically important preoperative criteria are the ability to hyperextend the neck and ensuring that the patient will be able to be reintubated in case of accidental extubation. Obese patients, children, and those with severe coagulopathies should not be considered candidates for this procedure (Table 106-3).[17]

A number of different systems and approaches to performing a percutaneous tracheotomy have been described and marketed since the inception of the idea. Many comprehensive accounts of the evolution of this approach are available in the literature. The controversy surrounding this approach still lingers, but there have been many large series with an acceptable

rate of complications as long as the patient selection and adherence to a procedural protocol is assured.[12]

Ciaglia described a technique in which there is no sharp dissection involved beyond the skin incision.[12] The patient is positioned and prepped in the same way as for the standard operative tracheotomy. The procedure is done under general anesthesia and all steps are done under bronchoscopic vision. A skin incision is made and the pretracheal tissue is cleared with blunt dissection. The endotracheal tube is withdrawn enough to place the cuff at the level of the glottis. The endoscopist places the tip of the bronchoscope such that the light from its tip shines through the surgical wound. The operator then enters the tracheal lumen below the second tracheal ring with an introducer needle. The track between the skin and the tracheal lumen is then serially dilated over a guidewire and stylet. A tracheotomy tube is the placed under direct bronchoscopic vision over a dilator. The placement of the tube is then confirmed again by visualizing the tracheobronchial tree through the tube. The tube is then secured to the skin with sutures and the tracheostomy tape (Figures 106-9 through 106-12).

In the second technique, known as the Shachner (Rapitrac) system, after making a small skin incision, the surgeon passes a dilator tracheotome over the guidewire into the trachea to dilate the tract fully in one step.[41] The tracheotome has a beveled metal core with a hole through its center that accommodates a guidewire. Once inside the trachea, the tracheotome is dilated. A conventional tracheotomy canula, fitted

---

TABLE 106-3

CONTRAINDICATIONS TO PERFORMING A PERCUTANEOUS DILATIONAL TRACHEOTOMY

Relative contraindications
  Children younger than 12 years of age
  Anatomic abnormality of the trachea
  Pulsating palpable blood vessel over the
    tracheotomy site
  Active infection over the tracheotomy site
  Occluding thyroid mass or goiter over the
    tracheotomy site
  Short or obese neck
  Positive end-expiratory pressure greater than
    15 cm H_2O
  Platelet count less than 40,000/mm³
  Bleeding time greater than 10 minutes
  Prothrombin time or partial thromboplastin time
    greater than 1.5 times control
  Limited ability to extend the cervical spine
  History of difficult intubation
Absolute contraindications
  Need for emergency airway access

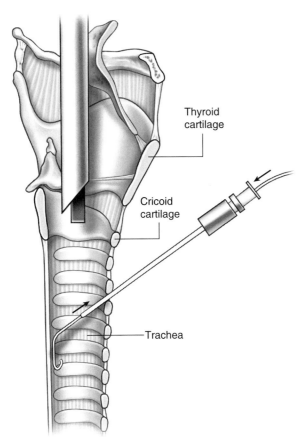

Figure 106-9. Guidewire introduction, with removal of sheath.[17]

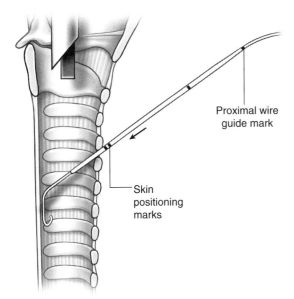

Figure 106-10. Guidewire and catheter are advanced together into the trachea as far as the skin positioning marks on the guide catheter to the skin.[17]

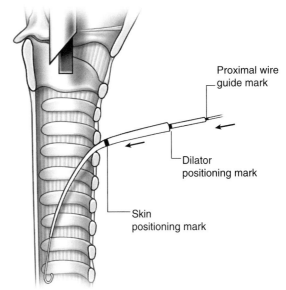

Figure 106-11. Guidewire, guide catheter, and dilator unit are advanced together into the trachea to the skin positioning mark.[17]

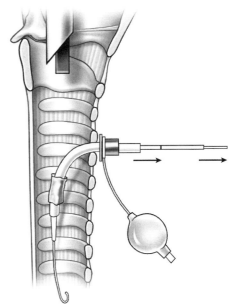

Figure 106-12. The tracheotomy tube is loaded onto a dilator and advanced into the trachea over the guidewire and catheter. The guidewire and catheter are removed, leaving only the tracheostomy tube in the trachea.[17]

with a special obturator, is passed through the tracheal opening. The dilatator and obturator are then removed.

A novel PDT method is called translaryngeal tracheostomy (Fantoni's technique). For Fantoni's tracheostomy, in contrast to the other techniques, the initial puncture of the trachea is carried out with the needle directed cranially and the tracheal cannula inserted with a pull-through technique along the orotracheal route in a retrograde fashion. The cannula is then rotated downward using a plastic obturator. The main advantage of Fantoni's tracheostomy is that there is hardly any skin incision required, and therefore practically no bleeding is observed.[18,38] The procedure can only be carried out under endoscopic guidance, and rotating the tracheal cannula downward may pose a problem, thus demanding that the surgeon have more experience.

The routine use of bronchoscopy during PDT, apart from Fantoni's tracheostomy, is still controversial. There are reports of lower rates of acute complications under endoscopic guidance. Additionally, resultant hypercarbia should be considered when choosing endoscopic-guided PDT for the critically ill or patients with head injuries. However, endoscopic guidance plays a critical role in the training of physicians, during PT on patients with a difficult anatomy, and to remove aspirated blood.

Another consideration that supports the use of bronchoscopy is the ability to better define the exact location of tracheal puncture. A number of cadaver studies on autopsies of patients who had undergone PDT found that the puncture site of the trachea varied greatly. It seems logical that bronchoscopic guidance during PDT can confirm the initial airway puncture site; however, a controlled study is necessary to settle this issue.[44]

PDT's Advantages

The technique of PDT is relatively easy to learn, but it has been repeatedly reported that a learning curve exists, which may be overcome by performing a number of supervised procedures. The time required for performing bedside PDT is considerably shorter than that required for performing an open tracheotomy.[30]

In critical care patients, one of the major advantages of PDT is the elimination of scheduling difficulty associated with the operating room and anesthesiology teams. Bedside PDT also precludes the necessity to schedule the surgery and to transport critically ill patients who require intensive monitoring to and from the operating room. Therefore, PDT actually expedites the performance of the procedure in most cases. Finally, the cost of performing PDT is roughly half that of performing open surgical tracheotomy. The major components of the savings in these series were operating room charges and the anesthesia fees.

REFERENCES

1. Aly A, McIlwain M, Duncavage JA: Electrosurgery-induced endotracheal tube ignition during tracheotomy, *Ann Otol Rhinol Laryngol* 100:31–33, 1991.
2. Au J, Walker WS, Inglis D and others: Percutaneous cricothyroidostomy (minitracheostomy) for bronchial toilet: results of therapeutic and prophylactic use, *Ann Thorac Surg* 48:850–852 1989.
3. Bair AE, Panacek EA, Wisner DH, and others: Cricothyrotomy: a 5-year experience at one institution, *J Emerg Med* 24:151–156, 2003.
4. Behringer EC: Approaches to managing the upper airway, *Anesthesiol Clin North Am* 20:813–832, 2002.
5. Ben-Nun A, Altman E, Best LA: Treatment of sputum retention by minitracheostomy, *Harefuah* 139:195–198, 247, 2000.
6. Benumof JL, Scheller MS: The importance of transtracheal jet ventilation in the management of the difficult airway, *Anesthesiology* 71:769–778, 1989.
7. Bertelsen S, Jensen NM: Innominate artery rupture. A fatal complication of tracheostomy, *Ann Chir Gynaecol* 76:230–233, 1987.
8. Bethea MC, Jackman NT, Carberry DM, and others: Tracheo-innominate fistula: diagnosis and management, *N Y State J Med* 77:1276–1280, 1977.
9. Buckels NJ, Khan ZH, Irwin ST and others: Post-operative sputum retention treated by minitracheostomy—a ward procedure? *Br J Clin Pract* 44:169–671, 1990.
10. Calhoun KH, Weiss RL, Scott B and others: Management of the thyroid isthmus in tracheostomy: a prospective and retrospective study, *Otolaryngol Head Neck Surg* 111:450–452, 1994.
11. Caplan RA, Posner KL, Ward RJ and others: Adverse respiratory events in anesthesia: a closed claims analysis, *Anesthesiology* 72:828–833, 1990.
12. Ciaglia P: Differences in percutaneous dilational tracheostomy kits, *Chest* 117:1823, 2000.
13. Collicott PA, Carrico CJ: *Upper airway management, in advanced trauma life support.* In American College of Surgeons, Chicago, American College of Surgeons, 1984, pp 155–161.
14. Cooper JD: Trachea-innominate artery fistula: successful management of 3 consecutive patients, *Ann Thorac Surg* 24:439–447, 1977.
15. Cormack RS, Lehane J: Difficult tracheal intubation in obstetrics, *Anaesthesia* 39:1105–1111, 1984.
16. Cormack RS, Lehane JR, Adams AP and others: Laryngoscopy grades and percentage glottic opening, *Anaesthesia* 55:184, 2000.
17. Couch ME, Bhatti N: The current status of percutaneous tracheotomy, *Adv Surg* 36:275–296, 2002.
18. Fantoni A, Ripamonti D: A non-derivative, non-surgical tracheostomy: the translaryngeal method, *Intensive Care Med* 23:386–392, 1997.
19. Gillespie MB, Eisele DW: Outcomes of emergency surgical airway procedures in a hospital-wide setting, *Laryngoscope* 109:1766–1769, 1999.
20. Goldenberg D, Ari EG, Golz A and others: Tracheotomy complications: a retrospective study of 1130 cases, *Otolaryngol Head Neck Surg* 123:495–500, 2000.
21. Goldenberg D, Golz A, Netzer A and others: Tracheotomy: changing indications and a review of 1,130 cases, *J Otolaryngol* 31:211–215, 2002.

22. Grillo HC, Moncure AC, McEnany MT: Repair of inflammatory tracheoesophageal fistula, *Ann Thorac Surg* 22:112–119, 1976.

23. Gross ND, Cohen JI, Andersen PE and others: 'Defatting' tracheotomy in morbidly obese patients, *Laryngoscope* 112:1940–1944, 2002.

24. Hart AM, Cashman JN, Baldock GJ and others: Minitracheostomy in the treatment of sputum retention, *Intensive Care Med* 13:81–82, 1987.

25. Heffner JE: The role of tracheotomy in weaning, *Chest* 120:477S–81S, 2001.

26. Jones JW, Reynolds M, Hewitt RL and others: Tracheo-innominate artery erosion: successful surgical management of a devastating complication, *Ann Surg* 184:194–204, 1976.

27. Koh MB, Hunt BJ: The management of perioperative bleeding, *Blood Rev* 17:179–185, 2003.

28. Lai S WG: Tracheostomy: demystifying an ancient technique. *Oper Tech Otolaryngol Head Neck Surg* 14:51–54, 2003.

29. Mallampati SR, Gatt SP, Gugino LD and others: A clinical sign to predict difficult tracheal intubation: a prospective study, *Can Anaesth Soc J* 32:429–434, 1985.

30. Massick DD, Powell DM, Price PD and others: Quantification of the learning curve for percutaneous dilatational tracheotomy, *Laryngoscope* 110:222–228, 2000.

31. Mastboom WJ, Wobbes T, van den Dries A and others: Bronchial suction by minitracheotomy as an effective measure against sputum retention, *Surg Gynecol Obstet* 173:187–192, 1991.

32. Matthews HR, Fischer BJ, Smith BE and others: Minitracheostomy: a new delivery system for jet ventilation, *J Thorac Cardiovasc Surg* 92:673–675, 1986.

33. Matthews HR, Hopkinson RB: Treatment of sputum retention by minitracheotomy, *Br J Surg* 71:147–150, 1984.

34. McGill J, Clinton JE, Ruiz E: Cricothyrotomy in the emergency department, *Ann Emerg Med* 11:361–364, 1982.

35. Milner SM, Bennett JD: Emergency cricothyrotomy, *J Laryngol Otol* 105:883–885, 1991.

36. Myers EN, Carrau RL: Early complications of tracheotomy. Incidence and management, *Clin Chest Med* 12:589–595, 1991.

37. Nelems JM: Tracheo-innominate artery fistula, *Am J Surg* 141:526–527, 1981.

38. Oeken J, Adam H, Bootz F: Fantoni translaryngeal tracheotomy (TLT) with rigid endoscopic control, *Hno* 50:638–643, 2002.

39. Plummer AL, Gracey DR: Consensus conference on artificial airways in patients receiving mechanical ventilation, *Chest* 96:178–180, 1989.

40. Reed MF, Mathisen DJ: Tracheoesophageal fistula, *Chest Surg Clin North Am* 13:271–289, 2003.

41. Samsoon GL, Young JR: Difficult tracheal intubation: a retrospective study, *Anaesthesia* 42:487–490, 1987.

42. Sivarajan M, Stoler E, Kil HK and others: Jet ventilation using fiberoptic bronchoscopes, *Anesth Analg* 80:384–387, 1995.

43. Stock MC, Woodward CG, Shapiro BA and others: Perioperative complications of elective tracheostomy in critically ill patients, *Crit Care Med* 14:861–863, 1986.

44. van Heurn LW, Theunissen PH, Ramsay G and others: Pathologic changes of the trachea after percutaneous dilatational tracheotomy, *Chest* 109:1466–1469. 1996.

45. Wain JC, Wilson DJ, Mathisen DJ: Clinical experience with minitracheostomy, *Ann Thorac Surg* 49:881–886, 1990.

46. Waldron J, Padgham ND, Hurley SE: Complications of emergency and elective tracheostomy: a retrospective study of 150 consecutive cases, *Ann R Coll Surg Engl* 72:218–220, 1990.

47. Walsh ME, Shorten GD: Preparing to perform an awake fiberoptic intubation, *Yale J Biol Med* 71:537–549, 1998.

48. Wang RC, Perlman PW, Parnes SM: Near-fatal complications of tracheotomy infections and their prevention, *Head Neck* 11:528–533, 1989.

49. Wenig BL, Applebaum EL: Indications for and techniques of tracheotomy, *Clin Chest Med* 12:545–553, 1991.

50. Whited RE: A prospective study of laryngotracheal sequelae in long-term intubation, *Laryngoscope* 94:367–377, 1984.

51. Wood DE, Mathisen DJ: Late complications of tracheotomy, *Clin Chest Med* 12:597–609, 1991.

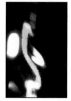

CHAPTER ONE HUNDRED AND SEVEN

ENDOSCOPY OF THE TRACHEOBRONCHIAL TREE

|| Rex C. Yung

INTRODUCTION

Careful consideration of the central and peripheral airways, pulmonary parenchyma, and vasculature is germane to the evaluation of the head and neck. Rapid advances in the realm of imaging are making possible ever more accurate characterization of the anatomic distribution and metabolic properties of normal tissues and pathologic lesions in the head and neck and thoracic structures. Such combined multimodality and multiplanar imaging also makes possible accurate preprocedural planning of diagnostic and therapeutic interventions. However, although there are now many algorithms to deliver such three-dimensional (3D) imaging, including the promise of "virtual endoscopies" through luminal structures such as the tracheobronchial tree, there remains no substitute for tracheobronchial endoscopy in the performance of a detailed examination of the airway surfaces and in directing biopsies and interventional procedures.

Pharyngeal, laryngeal, and thyroid lesions can lead to airway compromise due to direct tracheal and endobronchial extension or extrinsic compression of the central airways. Examples include upper airway malignancies, and also benign but proliferative lesions, such as recurrent respiratory papillomatosis that may extend out to the peripheral lung units.[1] Malignant otolaryngologic lesions have the potential to metastasize to the lungs, and the diagnosis of systemic dissemination will change the overall management. Tobacco-related squamous cell carcinoma of the head and neck region is associated with increased risk for primary bronchogenic carcinoma. Tissue confirmation of synchronous but distinct histologic head and neck and lung primaries that can be independently resected for cure will again confer very different management options and overall prognosis. Compromise of thoracic vascular and neural structures, such as the superior vena cava and the recurrent laryngeal nerves, are additional causes of morbidity.

This chapter reviews the current technology of tracheobronchoscopy with a focus on the advances in flexible bronchoscopy, including incorporation of various ancillary diagnostic technologies such as endobronchial ultrasound (EBUS) and autofluorescence (AF) bronchoscopy. Therapeutic airway interventions for both benign and malignant lesions will also be briefly reviewed.

AIRWAY ANATOMY AND NOMENCLATURE

Although the basic pulmonary function of gas exchange occurs at the level of the alveolus, in the distal acinus beyond respiratory bronchioles, for the purpose of the bronchoscopist, it is more important to recognize the more proximal airway divisions. Distal to the trachea and the mainstem bronchi, the lobar bronchus defines the division of the lobes, and the segmental bronchi the pulmonary lobules. There are thus three lobes in the right lung, with normally ten segmental lobules, although there may be some anatomic variants (Table 107-1). In the left lung, the left upper lobar segments and the lingular subsegments come off the same left upper lobe bronchial division, and this also explains why resection of the left upper lobe often requires inclusion of the lingular and vice versa. Because of the anatomic divisions, the left lung is often divided into nine segmental lobules, although here again anomalies exist and the bronchoscopist should be familiar with the variations. Because of the location of the heart, the right lung usually accounts for 55% to 60% of the total lung parenchyma, and the left lung the smaller remainder. This becomes important when estimating residual pulmonary function after a planned lobar resection or pneumonectomy.

An additional source of frequent confusion in the naming of the segmental and subsegmental bronchi has to do with the frequent but incorrect interchange of the terms *generation* and *order* of the bronchial segments. Standard nomenclature of the human airways

TABLE 107-1	
PULMONARY LOBES AND SEGMENTS	
Right lung	
Right upper lobe (RUL)	RB1 apical segment of RUL
	RB2 posterior segment of RUL
	RB3 anterior segment of RUL
Right middle lobe (RML)	RB4 lateral segment of RML
	RB5 medial segment of RML
Right lower lobe (RLL)	RB6 superior segment of RLL
	RB7 medial basal segment of RLL
	RB8 anterior segment of RLL
	RB9 lateral segment of RLL
	RB10 posterior segment of RLL
Left lung	
Left upper lobe (LUL)	LB1/2 apical posterior segment of LUL
	LB3 anterior segment of LUL
Lingula	LB4 superior segment of lingula
	LB5 inferior segment of lingula
Left lower lobe (LLL)	LB6 superior segment of LLL
	LB7 medial basal segment of LLL
	LB8 anterior segment of LLL
	LB9 lateral segment of LLL
	LB10 posterior segment of LLL

denotes the trachea as the zero-generation airway, with each of the right and left mainstem bronchi being the first generation, lobar bronchi the second generation, lobar segmental bronchi the third generation, and so forth. Conversely, *order* of airway segment refers to the retrograde counting of branching from the "lobular bronchiole," which is the first airway segment with a diameter of less than 0.7 mm. Hence, more central airways of a larger dimension will actually have a higher order.[30,34] However, given the uneven segmentation and subsequent diminution of airways' calibers, there is far less uniformity of which division of airway in the different lobes and lobules will narrow down to 0.7 mm. Finally, without an accurate and consistent way of measuring airway lumen diameters in situ during in vivo bronchoscopy, the respiratory lobule has been defined in vitro in excised tissue with the attendant distortions of fixation and unopposed airway elastic recoil.[30] Hence, the standard textbook description of the 0.7-mm lobular bronchiole located in the 10th- to 14th-generation bronchi does not match the bronchoscopic findings of airways navigable by a bronchoscope significantly wider than 0.7 mm beyond the number of branchings described above.[19,26,34] In summary, it is best to use the term *generation* in the description of sequential airway branchings starting from the central airways. Dr. Shigeto Ikeda, regarded as the founder of modern fiberoptic bronchoscopy, also developed a detailed system of naming segmental and subsegmental airways branchings, but that topic is beyond the scope of this chapter.[15]

INDICATIONS AND PREPARATIONS FOR TRACHEOBRONCHOSCOPY
Indications

Diagnostic and therapeutic indications for tracheobronchoscopy include the evaluation of acute or chronic upper airways and respiratory symptoms including hemoptysis, nonresolving and worsening cough, acute or worsening subacute dyspnea that may be accompanied by wheezing or stridor, pleurisy, chest pain, fever, and other symptoms suggestive of a pulmonary infection. The above symptoms may be accompanied by radiologic abnormalities suggesting an endobronchial lesion or extrinsic compression of the airways by lung masses or focal or diffuse infiltrates. Patients are often also referred for evaluation of asymptomatic lung or mediastinal masses and nonresolving parenchymal lung infiltrates. Pleural effusions usually lead to evaluation of the pleural fluid; however, effusions most often have an underlying parenchymal pulmonary cause, and a nonresolving effusion without an established cause after thoracentesis or thoracoscopy should prompt an examination for endobronchial obstruction and a parenchymal lesion obscured by the atelectatic lung. Bronchoscopy is helpful in assessing the placement of endotracheal tubes, especially in difficult intubation cases or when double-lumen tubes are used. A flexible fiberoptic bronchoscope (FOB) can be used to guide placement of endotracheal (ET) tubes in difficult airways and unstable cervical spine by having the ET tube prepositioned and advanced over the bronchoscope. An FOB can also be used to guide percutaneous tracheostomy. Depending on the findings on radiographs or during a diagnostic bronchoscopy, therapeutic interventions can then be performed to maintain airway patency and improve gas exchange[3,10] (Table 107-2).

After consideration of the appropriateness of the procedure, the next steps of planning should include the multimodality team of radiologists, anesthesiologists, nursing, respiratory therapists, backups in thoracic surgery and interventional radiology if their services may be needed, and not least the patient and family for careful discussion and to obtain informed consent.

Radiology

Given the millimeter-range high resolution and rapid multiplanar reconstruction of the airways achievable with multislice spiral computed tomography (CT) scanners, a preprocedural CT scan can help to pinpoint location and extent of pathology and to reduce

TABLE 107-2

INDICATIONS FOR TRACHEOBRONCHOSCOPY

Diagnostic evaluation
Chronic nonresolving or worsening cough, especially with signs of aspiration
Voice change, hoarseness
Stridor
Wheezing unresponsive to bronchodilator
Hemoptysis
Pulmonary infections: acute processes not responsive to empiric therapy; recurring pneumonias in the same location
Progressive dyspnea
Radiographic abnormalities:
   Volume loss with suggestion of central airways obstruction
   Isolated lung mass(es)
   Infiltrate(s), localized or diffuse
   Mediastinal masses, adenopathy
   Nonresolving atelectasis
   Nondiagnosed pleural effusion with underlying lung consolidation

Interventional
Assist in securing the airway: intubation over the bronchoscope; confirming position of endotracheal tube; assist with double lumen intubation
Removal of foreign body
Therapeutic aspiration of blood clots, inspissated mucus
Relief of central airways obstruction, both benign and malignant causes:
   Thermal ablation and mechanical removal of tumor
   Débridement of benign stenosis
Balloon dilation
Airway stent placement to maintain airway patency
Guide percutaneous tracheostomy

---

the time spent on exploration in patients with respiratory embarrassment and limited cardiopulmonary reserve. A contrast-enhanced CT scan is especially useful to provide the spatial relationship between pathology and vasculature, and hence minimize the risk of accidental and potentially life-threatening vascular injury from interventions such as laser or mechanical débridement. Contrast-enhanced atelectatic lung parenchyma can often also indicate whether there is viable lung tissue beyond central obstruction. 3D measurements of airway stenosis length and diameter facilitate the preselection of balloons for bronchoplasty and airway stents for maintaining patency in an obstructed airway segment. A thoracic surgeon or interventional radiologist should be consulted before the bronchoscopic investigation of massive hemoptysis in case the bleeding source can

only be identified—but not quelled—by bronchoscopic interventions.

Sedation and Airway Management

Maintaining gas exchange is critical during bronchoscopy, together with the desire of minimizing patient discomfort and anxiety. Some degree of sedation, monitoring, and augmentation of oxygenation and ventilation is carried out with the assistance of an anesthesiologist or nursing personnel certified in sedation and airway management. Conscious sedation usually includes intravenous sedation with short-acting benzodiazepines (midazolam is most commonly used) or other anxiolytic agents plus a short-acting narcotic (e.g., fentanyl, meperidine, or morphine sulfate) to help suppress the cough reflex. In the experience of myself and my colleagues, we also find promethazine (Phenergan) useful in patients who are difficult to sedate and those with a strong gag reflex. The medications are given in measured, small boluses and the patient is appropriately monitored with hemodynamics, cardiac rhythm monitors, and pulse oximeters. Not yet routinely used but increasingly available is transcutaneous capnography. Deep sedation with propofol (Diprivan) provides for rapid on-and-off titration of sedation and can be very helpful in some difficult-to-sedate patients. The hemodynamic and respiratory depression can also be much more profound, and hence additional training in deep sedation is recommended. General anesthesia with inhalational anesthetics with or without intravenous sedation provides the greatest control, but this would mandate the use of an ET tube, laryngeal mask airway (LMA) ventilation, rigid endoscopy with side port ventilation, or a previously placed tracheostomy. It is also contingent on the availability of an anesthesiologist or a nurse anesthetist who may not be readily available for bronchoscopies performed in endoscopy units separate from the operating rooms.

For patients undergoing bronchoscopy under conscious sedation, topical anesthetics are commonly used to reduce the amount of systemic sedative-narcotics needed to suppress cough, and also to reduce local discomfort in the nasopharynx during the passage of the bronchoscope. Lidocaine and its derivatives are most commonly used as a solution or gel and applied topically to the nasal passage or the posterior oropharynx as a spray. Solutions with concentrations between 1% and 4% are available, but the operator needs to pay attention to the total dosage applied because systemic lidocaine toxicities, including inadvertent deaths in healthy research subjects, have been reported when more than 500 to 1000 mg is delivered topically in a single session.[25] Therefore, except for spraying to the posterior oropharynx, we limit the use of topical lidocaine injected via the operating channel of the bronchoscope onto the vocal cords and airway mucosa to less than 50 mL of 1% lidocaine (500 mg total dosage). Cocaine is a very effective topical anesthetic and has the advantage of vasoconstricting the nasal mucosa membrane; it is, however, not generally available for use in the average endoscopy suite.

Miscellaneous medications that can be used in bronchoscopy include atropine or glycopyrrolate in patients with excessive secretions. Although it is not always possible to anticipate which patients will benefit from parasympathomimetic agents, chronic bronchitis patients with acute bronchitis and those with preprocedural problems handling bronchial secretions may be good candidates. Caution should be directed toward tachycardia.

Patient Positioning and Route of Bronchoscope Entry

In a consciously sedated patient with or without a previously placed tracheostomy, a flexible bronchoscope can be introduced with the patient supine or in a sitting position. It is generally easier to approach the patient with the bronchoscopist standing at the head of the bed. If choosing a nasal approach, a cotton swab soaked with a lidocaine solution or gel is used to determine which of the nares permit easier passage. Studies have found shorter and smaller patients to experience greater postprocedural nasal discomfort when the same-sized bronchoscope is used; hence, for such patients, an oral approach may be preferable. Conversely, because of the sharper angulation of the bronchoscope at the posterior oropharynx when introduced orally, patients tend to have a greater gag response; therefore, a more thorough application of topical anesthetics to the posterior oropharynx is recommended. Because of the risk of trauma to the teeth and the instrument being used, a properly secured bite block is mandatory in this approach. For rigid bronchoscopy, although the early pioneers performed the procedure on fully conscious patients placed in a sitting position, for all intents and purposes, the procedure should be carried out with the patient supine and the neck extended. The patient is almost always deeply sedated to fully anesthetized with paralysis to facilitate the passage of the rigid bronchoscope. The rigid bronchoscope can most easily be introduced via the oral route. The insertion and maneuvers of the rigid bronchoscope (RB) as well as the proper ventilation and anesthesia for the RB will be covered in a separate section.

Ventilation and oxygenation can be better maintained in a more upright patient under lighter sedation. Using a flexible FOB, the approach is made from the front of the patient. The approach via the nares or an oral passage is similar, although the view on the monitor is inverted because of the position of the bronchoscope tip relative to the approach. Once past the vocal cords, the bronchoscope can easily be turned to regain the familiar view with the ventral or anterior surface of the body facing the top.

In patients under deep sedation or general anesthesia, either flexible FOB or rigid-tube bronchoscopy can be used to examine the airways. For flexible FOB, gas exchange is maintained either with an ET tube or a laryngeal mask; the latter is usually sufficiently large such that bronchoscope size is not a factor in limiting adequate ventilation and oxygenation. For the ET tube, prior discussion with the anesthesiologist will ensure that a sufficiently large ET tube is inserted to permit smooth passage of the bronchoscope. For therapeutic cases using bronchoscopes with a diameter of 6.0 mm or greater, an ET tube of at least 7.5 mm is needed. An additional option is to perform direct suspension laryngoscopy with intermittent ventilation via an ET tube alternating with bronchoscopic examination and intervention.

To facilitate passage of the flexible bronchoscope, water-soluble lubricants are applied to the sheath of the bronchoscope. Lubricant jelly (KY Jelly) has the disadvantage of drying rather quickly, leading to stiffness in maneuvering, especially when the scope is introduced nasally. Lidocaine jelly is a good alternative that also provides some local anesthesia. Newer compounds, such as Endolube, provide excellent lubrication and are ideal when the bronchoscope has a tight fit through devices such as an ET tube. The cost is higher, and caution is necessary to prevent accidental dislodgement from the ventilator because the lubricant also makes slippery the various connections between the ET tube and ventilator tubings. Mineral oil should not be used if at all possible because there is the potential of aspirated oil leading to a lipoid pneumonia, although the quantity of oil is so small as to make this a very unlikely complication.

Patient Discussion and Informed Consent

Well-informed and educated patients and families are more likely to be compliant with therapy. In the case of bronchoscopy, especially in consciously sedated cases, an explanation of the steps will help to alleviate the anxiety over the coughing and gagging that can sometimes lead to premature termination of the procedure. Ancillary diagnostic and therapeutic procedures, especially on hyperemic inflamed or malignant tissue, will often lead to bleeding and postprocedural hemoptysis that should taper off. Similarly, a substantial portion (25%–50%) of patients may experience transient postprocedural fever during the first 24 hours.

The cause need not be infectious and may be more frequent after bronchoalveolar lavage (BAL) that can result in surfactant washout. Informing patients of these two possible minor complications can obviate anxious midnight calls the evening after a procedure. Conversely, they should also be warned about prolonged bleeding and delayed pneumothoraces that may not be detected immediately after the procedure. Therefore, persistent and high spiking fevers, hemoptysis, and worsening dyspnea should prompt a reevaluation with radiograph, physical examination, and other laboratory tests, as indicated.

RIGID BRONCHOSCOPY

RB retains certain important advantages over flexible FOB including the much larger lumen that affords access to larger instruments, which may be necessary to remove foreign bodies, to provide adequate suction in brisk hemoptysis, to place noncompressible Silastic airway stents, and to use the bronchoscope itself to core out tumors and to provide direct tamponade to a bleeding source. However, even though the pioneers of rigid bronchoscopy had performed RB on fully conscious patients placed in various positions including sitting upright, RB today is performed almost exclusively on patients under general anesthesia, and rarely with only topical anesthesia and conscious sedation without paralytics. More commonly intravenous deep sedation, with or without inhalational anesthetics, are used. A variety of ventilatory strategies are used, from intermittent apneic ventilation to spontaneous/assisted ventilation. Oxygenation and ventilation can be provided by tidal volume through a closed system or via an open system of side port Venturi jet ventilation. Before insertion of the RB, either alone or with a telescope lens through the bronchoscope tube to provide a better distal view, the patient must be examined for neck stability and for any loose teeth or dentures. A shoulder roll may give room for added extension of the neck. With or without a teeth guard to protect the upper teeth, the operator's left thumb is placed over the upper teeth and the index finger scissored open to lift up the lower teeth of the relaxed jaw. The bronchoscope with the bevel up is then directed midline and almost perpendicularly toward the hypopharynx until the uvula is passed, and the bronchoscope angle is thereafter slowly leveled towards the horizontal, seeking out the epiglottis while lifting the base of the tongue. When the vocal cords are clearly visualized, the bronchoscope is rotated 90 degrees such that the beveled edge can enter the trachea along the length of the vocal cord, thereby limiting trauma to the cords. Once the tip of the rigid bronchoscope is clearly in the trachea, it is rotated back to its starting position with the bevel up. Left hand and finger positions are maintained to protect the teeth, although it is also necessary to occasionally use the left hand to provide a better seal around the cuffless RB at the level of the cricoid and thyroid cartilages when ventilation is applied. Because larger operative rigid bronchoscopes with diameters of 11 to 12 mm are now available for silicone stent insertion, upper airway and vocal cord edema may be a more severe problem at the end of a prolonged case, hence careful examination of the cords and hypopharynx is important to avoid postprocedural stridor and upper airway obstruction. With the advent of flexible FOB, the number of respiratory disease teaching programs routinely including RB in their training curriculum is also shrinking. Therefore, even though RB should be a skill acquired by all bronchoscopists, generally only those being trained in a thoracic surgical program or a pulmonary program with an active airways interventional program will get adequate exposure and practice.[7]

FLEXIBLE FIBEROPTIC BRONCHOSCOPY

Advances in fiberoptics, illumination, and image capture including the use of true color-chip charged couple device cameras embedded in the distal tip of the FOB have greatly improved the imaging capabilities of the FOB. Most new flexible FOBs are now videoscopes with high-resolution true-color rendition of the image captured by the distal chip. The illumination is still delivered via fiberoptic bundles. The improved imaging quality and the ease of recording areas of interest with digital still images or video segments are offset by the cost of these bronchoscopes, plus the dedicated processor and high-quality video display units. The start-up cost of such a setup with two videobronchoscopes will be in the $60,000 to $80,000 range. Conventional FOBs, in which the image is relayed via fiberoptic bundles and viewed at the proximal end of the FOB by the eyepiece or connected to a video display, continues to have a role. This is especially true for FOBs used at the bedside or during operations to confirm the position of the standard or dual-lumen ET tubes and for the attachment of special illumination and visualization devices such as during autofluorescent bronchoscopy.

Range of Flexible Bronchoscopes and Special Features

Although there remains the tendency to subdivide bronchoscopes into "adult" and "pediatric" categories depending on their outer diameter, this distinction is arbitrary. Because bronchoscopists venture more peripherally with FOB to sample focal lesions, and more interventional procedures via a flexible FOB are performed in the pediatric population, it makes more sense to describe the bronchoscopes and leave their judicious application to the bronchoscopist based on their experience and the situational need.[19,26]

All FOBs have an illumination fiberoptic bundle and imaging fiberoptics or a camera. With the exception of the very few "ultrathin" bronchoscopes, there is also a channel for suction of secretions and blood, for the passage of topical medication and fluid for washing, and for the passage of various instruments for diagnostic retrieval of tissues or for therapeutic procedures (Table 107-3). The "average" diagnostic bronchoscope has an outer diameter of 5.0 to 5.5 mm and an operating channel of 2.0 to 2.2 mm. This caliber channel will admit most cytology brushes, bronchial biopsy forceps, and transbronchial aspiration needles with sheathed outer diameters between 1.8 and 2.0 mm. Smaller bronchoscopes in the range of 3.0 to 4.0 mm at the outer diameter and correspondingly

TABLE 107-3

FLEXIBLE BRONCHOSCOPES, DIMENSIONS, AND FEATURES

Manufacturer/Model Number	Features	Outer/Channel φ	Length
Fujinon			
CHO-SP	Fiber	4.9 / 2.0 mm	40 cm
BRO-YP2	Fiber	4.8 / 2.0 mm	57.5 cm
BRO-Y35	Fiber	5.7 / 2.0 mm	57.5 cm
BRO-YL2	Fiber Therapeutic	6.4 / 2.6 mm	57.5 cm
EB-270S	Video	4.9 / 2.0 mm	60 cm
EB-270T	Video Therapeutic	5.9 / 2.8 mm	60 cm
EB-470S	Video	4.9 / 2.0 mm	60 cm
EB-470T	Video Therapeutic	5.9 / 2.8 mm	60 cm
Karl Storz endoscopy			
11001B11*	Fiber	5.2 / 2.0 mm	55 cm
11004B11*	Fiber Therapeutic	6.4 / 2.8 mm	55 cm
Olympus			
BF-N20	Fiber View only (no operating channel)	2.2 mm	55 cm
BF-XP160F	Video Ultrathin	2.8 / 1.2 mm	60 cm
BF-XP40	Fiber Ultrathin	2.8 / 1.2 mm	60 cm
BF-3C40	Fiber Slim	3.6 / 1.2 mm	55 cm
BF-MP160F	Video Thin	4.0 / 2.0 mm	60 cm
BF-P160	Video	4.9 / 2.0 mm	60 cm
BF-P40	Fiber Slim (older)	5.0 / 2.2 mm	55 cm
BF-160	Video	5.2 / 2.0 mm	60 cm
BF-1T40	Fiber Therapeutic	5.9 / 2.8 mm	55 cm
BF-40	Fiber Standard (old)	6.0 / 2.2 mm	55 cm
BF-1T160	Video Therapeutic	6.0 / 2.8 mm	55 cm
BF-XT160	Video Therapeutic	6.2 / 3.2 mm	60 cm
BF-XT40	Fiber Therapeutic	6.3 / 3.2 mm	55 cm
Pentax			
FB-8V	Fiber Ultrathin	2.7 / 1.2 mm	60 cm
FB-10V	Fiber Thin	3.4 / 1.2 mm	60 cm
FB-15V	Fiber	4.9 / 2.2 mm	60 cm
EB-1530T3	Video 30 series	5.3 / 2.0 mm	60 cm
EB-1570K†	Video K series	5.5 / 2.0 mm	60 cm
FB-18RX	Fiber	5.9 / 2.2 mm	60 cm
FB-18V	Fiber Therapeutic	5.9 / 2.8 mm	60 cm
EB-1830T3	Video Therapeutic	6.0 / 2.6 mm	60 cm
FB-19TV	Fiber Therapeutic	6.2 / 3.2 mm	60 cm
EB-1970K†	Video K Therapeutic	6.3 / 2.8 mm	60 cm

*Built-in filter wheel for tissue autofluorescence and drug-induced autofluorescence examination.
†Pentax's version of advanced color chip camera.

smaller channels are usually given a "P" designation (for pediatrics), but they can of course be used in the adult airways when narrowing is present due to benign strictures or malignant stenosis. Newer generations of "slim" video and FOBs have a 2.0-mm operating channel with a 4.0-mm outer diameter. The one disadvantage of these bronchoscopes is the sacrifice of a smaller image area because of fewer optical bundles. Larger "therapeutic" bronchoscopes (often designated with a "T" in the model number) can of course also be used for diagnostic purposes, but the larger outer diameter can cause greater discomfort and mucosal trauma to a conscious patient and can be harder to pass through an ET or tracheostomy tube, and thus can also impair gas exchange to a greater degree. Such therapeutic bronchoscopes have an outer diameter between 6.0 and 6.3 mm, with operating channel lumen between 2.6 to 3.2 mm. Certain therapeutic instruments, including larger laser fibers, larger electrocautery forceps designed for gastrointestinal endoscopes, cryotherapy probes, and expandable balloons for bronchoplasty will require these larger diameters for their use through FOB. Prototype bronchoscopes with a 9-mm outer diameter and a 5-mm operating channel have been made, the main application of which is to provide access of therapeutic instruments to airway segments that cannot normally be reached by rigid open tube bronchoscopes and telescopes (Figure 107-1). At the other extreme are the ultrathin bronchoscopes, with outer diameters smaller than 3 mm. The production models Olympus BF-XP40 and the video BF-XP160F have outer diameters of 2.8 mm and operating channels of 1.2 mm. Special instruments (e.g., reusable cytology brush and forceps) of the proper caliber are available for tissue sampling (Figure 107-2). Handling of these ultrathin bronchoscopes is often more challenging because the very floppy tips make steering more difficult. Suction via the narrow channels is also much more limited. Nevertheless, with practice and by using small amounts of saline to flush open the distal airways in guiding the bronchoscope forward, the ultrathin bronchoscopes can traverse 12 to 16 generations of airways, and under fluoroscopic or CT guidance, are seen to approach the periphery of the lungs to sample focal lesions.[19,26] The passage of a 2.8-mm instrument beyond the midteens division of the lobular bronchiole measured at 0.7 mm in fixed tissue calls into question some of the accepted measurements of the adult human airways. To permit the greater distance traversed, such ultrathin bronchoscopes usually have an operating length of 60 cm, 5 cm longer than the older bronchoscopes, although the current generation of videobronchoscopes are all built with a 60-cm working length.

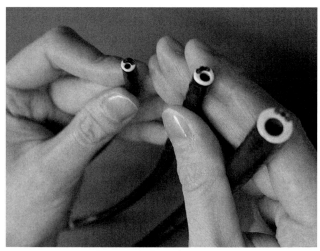

Figure 107-1. Range of FOBs with outer and channel diameters of 4.9/2.0 mm and 6.0/2.8 mm and a prototype therapeutic scope of 9.0/5.0 mm. Note the insulated white ceramic plate, necessary for safe use of electrosurgery.

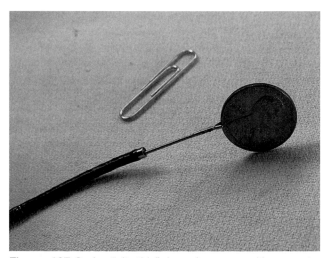

Figure 107-2. An "ultrathin" bronchoscope with an outer diameter of 2.8 mm and working channel of 1.2 mm and a custom forceps holding up a coin for size comparison.

New bronchoscopes manufactured today usually have a white ceramic insulated tip; this is to permit the safe use of electrocautery instruments with reduced risk of retrograde electric shock to the bronchoscopist and damage to the bronchoscope (see Figure 107-1).

Certain bronchoscopes designed for AF imaging have built-in filter wheels that are adjustable to facilitate imaging at specific spectral frequencies. AF bronchoscopy will be briefly mentioned in a latter section of this chapter.

Care of the Flexible Fiberoptic Bronchoscope

Unlike the sturdy open tube RB, the flexible FOB is much more akin to the delicate rigid telescope with glass fiberoptic bundles that can be easily damaged by rough handling or accidental bites by the patient. The narrow operating channel can also be damaged by a number of instruments, especially when these are too large for safe passage. The two especially vulnerable portions of the flexible FOB are the angulated entry port of the working channel and the distal tip of the bronchoscope. Incompletely retracted transbronchial needle aspiration (TBNA) needles are most frequently the culprit, tearing the channel during introduction or retrieval of the instrument by an inexperienced user. Such damages are noted during the "leak test" that should be performed after each use of the bronchoscope and before machine washing. Repair of the bronchoscopes is costly and makes the use of the instrument temporarily unavailable. Therefore, one should always emphasize to the operator and the assistants the need to check the needle before and after each pass, to make sure the tip of the needle is fully retracted into the protective housing. It should also be emphasized that the tip of the bronchoscope should be kept as straight as possible during introduction and retrieval of the instruments. Although the emphasis is on TBNA-associated bronchoscope damage, the same care must be exercised when using the entire range of diagnostic and therapeutic instruments because tears can also occur with biopsy forceps improperly opened within the channel, pushing and pulling of semirigid instruments through the flexed tip of the bronchoscope, burning on the inside of a bronchoscope channel by improper activation of electrocautery instruments, or firing of laser fibers.

There is increasing focus on nosocomial infections resulting from defective endoscopes (loose valves) or from improper cleaning techniques. Thus far, outbreaks of nosocomial bacterial infections (e.g., gram-negative bacilli and mycobacterium) are rare, and there have not been confirmed reports of viral transmission. However, an instrument inadvertently used on a patient subsequently confirmed to have Creutzfeldt-Jakob disease or other prion infections should be considered terminally contaminated and must be discarded. The prevalence of such infections is very low and should not discourage the appropriate performance of bronchoscopy when it can provide important diagnostic information or can aid therapy. There are a number of accepted cleaning techniques ranging from gas sterilization (ethylene oxide) to formaldehyde-based approaches. It is under the purview of the endoscopy unit or operating room director and nursing director to develop quality control measures.

Diagnostic Fiberoptic Bronchoscopy
General Approaches

Although there is usually one primary indication for bronchoscopy, such as obtaining tissue diagnosis of a lung mass, evaluating a focal infiltrate suspected of being infectious, or seeking a source of hemoptysis, an orderly and uniform approach should be taken toward airway examination such that important pathology should not be missed because of impatience to attend to the primary focus. Examination of the nasopharynx, hypopharynx, and vocal cords are covered in much greater detail in other chapters. Starting at the upper trachea, mucosal integrity should be examined. Even when there are no gross endobronchial lesions, the presence of extrinsic tracheal deviation and compression due to paratracheal masses should be noted. TBNA can often successfully provide a tissue diagnosis of extrinsic lesions.[33,35] Still under development is an array of ultrasound devices, balloon probes, and actual dedicated EBUS bronchoscopes that should help in the localization and characterization of such lesions. The posterior membranous portion of the trachea is sometimes the site of airway compromise caused by tracheal malacia or tumor invasion from esophageal cancers and is the site of tracheal-esophageal (TE) fistulas. However, because of inflammation and redundant tissue, the TE fistula may be difficult to locate. Having the patient swallow 15 mL of methylene blue or food coloring immediately preceding bronchoscopy can aid in the localization of the TE tear or fistula. The distal trachea and main carina are important sites for examination because malignant diseases often metastasize to the surrounding mediastinal lymph nodes. The subcarinal (7 and 8 stations), anterior carinal, and low paratracheal lymph nodes bilaterally (4R and 4L stations) are particularly suitable for TBNA.[23,33]

There is no set rule whether the left-sided or right-sided airways should be examined first. In general, unless marginal pulmonary reserve or cardiovascular instability severely limits the time available for bronchoscopic examination, both sides of the lungs should be examined because unexpected radiographically occult airway pathology can occur in up to 10% of primary bronchogenic carcinoma, and a smaller percentage in metastatic diseases. A thorough lobar and segmental review should not take more than 5 to 10 minutes. Countering the instinct to approach the area of suspected pathology, that is, the main region of interest, the bronchoscopic examination should first focus on the contralateral lung. Furthermore, unless the lesion is central and unavoidable, the bronchoscopist should examine apparently uninvolved lobes and segments to look for unexpected pathology. There are several reasons to exhibit this patience. First, once the main pathology is visualized or diagnostic procedures are started, the bronchoscopist is often too distracted to return to a thorough and careful examination of the remainder of the airways. Second, once the site of primary pathology is sampled, bleeding can degrade the quality of the FOB image while coughing and oxygen desaturation will limit the time to complete the procedure. Third, there is a danger that samples retrieved from a secondary site that appear abnormal and are found to contain malignant cells can actually represent contamination from cells dislodged during earlier examination of a primary cancer site. While such false-positive results may have little import in advanced obstructing central airways disease, this confusion could have the devastating effect of overstaging a potentially curable peripheral lesion.

Visual Examination

Less experienced bronchoscopists often regard confirming a positive tissue diagnosis as the main measure of a successful bronchoscopy. One should not, however, discount the value of getting a good "lay of the land" in terms of the dimensions of the airway, any significant anomalies in anatomy, whether these are normal anatomic variants of the number of airway segments and the location of their branchings, or are distortions resulting from prior surgeries or endobronchial or extrinsic pathology. Such a "scouting" bronchoscopy with measurements of the length and the extent of airway compromise is especially important in planning potentially complex interventional procedures.

Bronchial Wash

Most often, some form of specimen is retrieved to diagnose a pathology, or in the case of suspected opportunistic infections, to rule out with a greater certainty pulmonary infection by certain pathogens. Because there are always some airways secretions, and furthermore, aliquots of lidocaine solution and sterile saline are used to numb the airway mucosa and to clear the view of the airway, collecting a bronchial wash entails no more effort than connecting a "trap" in line between the suction port of the bronchoscope and the vacuum source providing suction. Care should be taken to secure the container used as a trap because inadvertent tilting or tipping over of the container with loss of sample easily occurs if it is left dangling loosely. The bronchial wash can be sent for cytology and culture. Concerns that the injected lidocaine may act as a bacteriostatic agent and hence may inhibit bacterial pathogen growth are unwarranted when one considers the overall dilutional effect. A much more valid criticism is that pathology such as

malignancy or infections uncovered from examination of the wash may represent contamination introduced from the oropharynx and upper airways by the passage of the bronchoscope via the nares or oral cavity. For more peripherally located lesions, such as a lung mass or localized infiltrate, the bronchial wash seldom adds to the more specifically targeted sampling techniques listed below.

Bronchoalveolar Lavage

Accounting for the variations in airway compliance and caliber, the standard diagnostic bronchoscope and even the "pediatric" bronchoscopes with an outer diameter of between 3.5 and 5.0 mm can traverse through, at most, 7 to 10 generations of airways. This means that most pulmonary masses and infiltrates will not be directly visualized. With experience, and especially with the aid of radiographic guidance by fluoroscopy or by CT scanning, such lesions can be successfully diagnosed by different transbronchial techniques; however, the yield is always dependent on the skill of the operator and also tends to be lower than that of visible lesions due to sampling errors because of the small size of samples retrieved. BAL is a technique that can provide a larger sample volume and also sampling of a larger lung field.

After identifying the region of the lung of interest, preferably down to the lobar segmental or subsegmental level, the bronchoscope is guided into the segment and "wedged" into place; that is, with gentle forward pressure it is advanced and kept snug against the side walls of a bronchial segment. Maneuvering the bronchoscope tip to obtain the best straightforward view into distal airway segments, aliquots of sterile saline ranging from 20 to 50 mL are gently infused. There should be a slight blanching of the airways. After each aliquot is infused, often with a column of air within the syringe to help propel the lavage fluid distally, suction is applied, either by depressing the suction button that activates the valve or by withdrawing on the syringe recently used to infuse the saline. The initial return will be scant until a certain volume (possibly up to the functional residual capacity) is filled; thereafter, return should be more generous. There is no set "standard" aliquot volume or total volume of normal saline that is used for BAL, and the amount used depends on the amount of return and an estimate of how much sample is required for the desired battery of studies. In general, for the same total volume infused, a larger number of smaller aliquots of 20 to 30 mL (e.g., 4 × 25 mL vs 2 × 50 mL) will yield a higher percentage of total volume recovered. Small-volume lavage return also appears to better reflect the peripheral lung cellular content. This may be the result of a longer dwell time in between aliquots, and a greater number of sequences of infusion and suctioning can cause greater airway turbulence and agitation with better resultant washout of distal conducting airways and alveolar content. In a supine patient, the yield is generally also better with BAL of anterior segments of the lungs, that is, lavage of the lingular and left upper lobe anterior segments and of the right middle lobe and right upper lobe anterior segments. In circumstances in which the infiltrate is in a dependent segment such as the lower lobe superior segments or the posterior segments of the upper lobes, the return can be improved by positioning the patient in an appropriate decubitus position during the BAL. The yield from BAL is higher with infectious causes than for malignancy, although this is contingent on the expertise of the microbiology laboratory or cytology services. For certain infections such as pneumonia caused by *Pneumocystis carinii pneumoniae* (PCP) in the HIV-positive population, cytologic staining of a BAL specimen for PCP has a diagnostic sensitivity of greater than 90%, and therefore transbronchial biopsies are not routinely necessary during the initial study. Conversely, other potential opportunistic organisms such as *Aspergillus* species and cytomegalovirus (CMV) recovered from the BAL may be airway colonizers, and more definitive biopsy proof of tissue invasion may be needed before embarking on toxic therapy. The yield from BAL for malignant invasion of the lung parenchyma by primary bronchogenic or metastatic diseases ranges from 15% to 40% but is generally lower than that of more specifically targeted biopsies.

Complications from BAL are generally self-limited, frequently including increased coughing after the BAL. Whether this is due to induced bronchospasm or to washout of surfactant is unclear, and some practitioners advocate using saline warmed to body temperature to reduce bronchospasm. An excessive amount of lavage volume can potentially aggravate hypoxemia in a diseased lung, although the lung's central and peripheral airspace normally has a great reserve to resorb excess fluid, unless there already exist cardiogenic or noncardiogenic pulmonary edema. As previously mentioned, BAL can also increase the incidence of postbronchoscopy fever that is usually self-limited.

Endobronchial and Transbronchial Biopsies

A number of biopsy forceps are available to biopsy bronchial mucosa, endobronchial lesions, and for transbronchial biopsy of airway and parenchyma beyond direct bronchoscopic vision (Figure 107-3). The catheters are of various diameters and lengths, with larger "therapeutic" forceps fitted with larger forcep cups. The edges of the cups are either smooth-cutting or jagged "alligator" type. A number of the

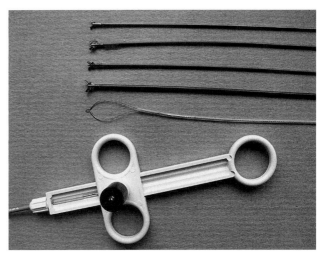

Figure 107-3. Instruments for use with a flexible FOB. From *Top* reusable forceps with steel wire catheter sheath (Olympus USA), disposable forceps with coated catheter (Microvasive, Boston Scientific), disposable needle forceps, large electrocautery forceps, requires a 2.8-mm channel, electrocautery snare, handle with wire attachment for electrosurgical instruments.

larger forceps are designed primarily as forceps for use in upper and lower gastrointestinal endoscopes, and hence they have a cable length that is much longer than the 55 to 60 cm of the bronchoscope working channel. There are additional forceps with a needle or "spike" in the center of the opened jaw near the fulcrum of the opened forceps; this is to aid in the anchoring of the forceps on mucosa, scar tissue, or tumor. These needle forceps are most useful for endobronchial biopsies, especially when the target may be along an airway wall tangential to the bronchoscope and thus cannot be easily grasped by forceps opening at a very shallow angle to the lesion. Some forceps also have an attachment for electrocautery. These may be useful for sampling or removing friable tissue that bleeds because electrocautery can effectively provide thermal hemostasis.

The technique for endobronchial biopsy is fairly straightforward and self-explanatory. After careful positioning of the opened jaws of the forceps, the forceps are advanced toward the target lesion, and closed when the lesion is within grasp. The challenge comes when the target is small, the airways are moving in response to respiration, or the patient is agitated and coughing. The opened jaws of the forceps can further obscure the view from the bronchoscope. Under these circumstances, the resultant tug of a fairly floppy forceps catheter may yield a disappointingly small specimen. One technique to improve the accuracy and yield of the biopsy is to advance with the bronchoscope closer to the target lesion before advancing the biopsy forceps outward. With closure of the forceps cups, one should pull back gently until the forceps are almost but not fully retracted into the bronchoscope channel. The bronchoscope itself should be pulled back slowly but firmly, and the much larger instrument (bronchoscope vs the forceps) will generally help pull out a much larger specimen. Complications from endobronchial biopsies most often involve bleeding due to trauma. Flushing small aliquots (1–2 mL) of a topical vasoconstrictor followed by a saline "chase" of 2 to 3 mL to clear the medication out of the bronchoscope channel will help to stem the bleeding. Tamponade with the tip of the bronchoscope until a clot forms may also help, but this is often less effective and risks further obscuring the view with coagulum. Oxymetazoline (Afrin) 0.05% and lidocaine with epinephrine (1:10,000 dilution) are two vasoconstrictors commonly used for this purpose, although oxymetazoline is preferred because it causes less tachyarrhythmia and hypertension. Airway perforation is a theoretic risk but rarely occurs, except in severely necrotic airways already distorted and destroyed by invasive cancer. Damage to the bronchoscope is a real concern; this can occur if an inexperienced operator attempts to open the forceps while it is still within the channel, or if an incompletely closed forceps or one with a kinked set of cups is forcibly withdrawn back into the channel. When there is any doubt or if there is obvious kinking of the forceps that cannot be corrected within the airways, the entire bronchoscope must be withdrawn and the problem fixed outside the patient's airways.

Transbronchial biopsies (TBBX) use the same instruments, although there is much less reason to use the needle forceps. TBBX is usually directed toward a focal mass lesion most often suspicious for lung carcinoma, or toward focal or diffuse infiltrates suggestive of infection, inflammatory lung processes, fibrotic lung parenchyma, or metastatic carcinoma with lymphangitic or diffuse hematogenous spread. Although it is possible to perform successful TBBX without radiographic guidance, the yield is lowered and the risk of complications increased; therefore, we prefer the availability of fluoroscopy to guide TBBX, especially of smaller, more focal, and more peripheral lesions[9,35] (Figure 107-4).

For more diffuse peripheral disease, whether guided by fluoroscopy or using a "blind" approach, the forceps are advanced slowly in a closed position until gentle resistance is felt or until the tip of the instrument is seen to approach the pleura. Because of the angulation of the segmental airway branchings and the effects of foreshortening, the advancing forceps may not appear to approach the lung periphery on the planar fluoroscope. Once resistance is felt, the forceps

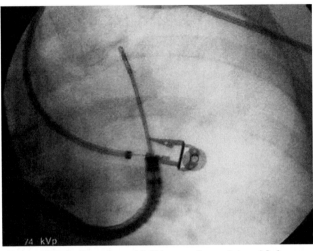

Figure 107-4. Transbronchial biopsy of a peripheral (left upper lobe) lung mass by fluoroscopic guidance.

are retracted about 2 to 3 cm, the cups are opened, and the instrument is gently pushed forward. After firm closure, the position of the forceps is confirmed by fluoroscopy and the instrument withdrawn. In a consciously sedated patient, especially when fluoroscopy is not available, we also ask the patient whether there is chest wall pain, because this would suggest focal pleural irritation caused by the tip of the forceps and would warn us of the increased risk of pneumothorax. The yield from TBBX varies depending on pathology, location and size of lesion, and availability of fluoroscopy. In general, malignant lesions located centrally and larger than 2 cm have a diagnostic yield of about 50% by TBBX, compared with a yield of only 25% for lesions smaller than 2 cm located in the peripheral one third of the lung. Complications of TBBX are bleeding and pneumothorax. As aforementioned, performing fluoroscopy and querying for symptoms of pleurisy will reduce the risk of pneumothorax to less than 10%, with overall rates of 3% to 20% reported in case series.[35] Significant bleeding is not increased in patients taking aspirin and cannot be predicted by routinely ordering platelet counts and coagulation parameters. Nevertheless, in critically ill or pancytopenic patients, an attempt is made to keep the platelet counts above 50,000, to correct coagulopathy if present, and to hold anticoagulation. Bleeding, when brisk, is managed by tamponading the bleeding subsegment with the bronchoscope tip. Depending on operator preference, suction can be applied to collapse the segmental airways to prevent further retrograde bleeding into the central airways, and saline at room temperature or cooled can be lavaged to slow the bleeding. There are no randomized trials to suggest efficacy of one approach over another.

Needless to say, life-threatening hemorrhage from TBBX is rare but reported.

Transbronchial Needle Aspiration

TBNA has traditionally been used to sample mediastinal lymph nodes and cysts. Initial TBNA was performed using needles on a long rigid stem introduced via an RB tube; in fact, the earliest cannulation of the left atrium for measurements of left atrial pressure was performed via this TBNA approach. Diagnosis of benign mediastinal adenopathy (e.g., sarcoidosis) and malignant tissue (e.g., lymphoma, nodal metastases of bronchogenic carcinoma) can be made via rigid TBNA; however, the lymph nodes sampled are often limited to the subcarina and possibly the precarina stations because of the limited angulations achievable with the rigid instruments.

The introduction and refinement of TBNA needles attached to a flexible catheter has permitted sampling of an increased number of lymph node stations, endobronchial lesions in the segmental and subsegmental bronchi, and peripheral endoscopically invisible lesions with a flexible FOB. The majority of the needles are made of stainless steel with calibers ranging from 22 to 19 gauges (Figure 107-5). There remains one plastic needle with a flexible tip (Microvasive Sofcor) that may be bent to facilitate passage into subsegments of the upper lobes (especially RB1 and RB2, LB1/2) and certain lower-lobe subsegments (RB6 and LB6) that are otherwise often not reachable with metal transbronchial needles because the 13- to 15-mm

lengths of these rigid needles reduce the tip angulations of the flexible FOBs.

Although the flexible needles have been divided into smaller gauge (20, 21, and 22 gauge) "cytology" needles and a larger gauge (19-gauge metal and 18-gauge Sofcor) "histology" needles (see Figure 107-5), the choice of the needle depends on operator experience because the larger "histology" needles will still provide tissue for cytologic examination (slide smear or collected for cytospin), and sample aspirated with a smaller "cytology" needles can be spun down into a cell block and cut for histologic examination. The longer needle lengths (15 mm) of the 21-gauge and larger needles offer the advantage of greater depth penetration, but a 19-gauge needle is more unwieldy to maneuver, takes more practice to penetrate the bronchial mucosa, and can potentially cause more trauma. It is often reserved for the sampling of larger lymph nodes suspected of harboring lymphoproliferative tissue (e.g., lymphoma, Castleman's disease) or granulomatous diseases (e.g., sarcoid, mycobacterial, and fungal adenitis) because, with practice, a 21-gauge core sample can be retrieved.

Mediastinoscopy remains the gold standard for examination and sampling of mediastinal lymph nodes; however, access to the subcarina, posterior tracheal, subaortic left-paratracheal/aortopulmonary window and hilar lymph nodes are limited. TBNA via FOB has the advantage of access to a larger number of lymph node stations and of being a less invasive procedure that can be combined with the endoscopic examination of the airways plus as-needed sampling of peripheral lung pathology (see Figure 107-5). Therefore, TBNA may be one of multiple procedures performed in a sequence of "one-stop" diagnosis and staging of thoracic malignancies. There are certain lymph node stations that are also inaccessible to TBNA via FOB; these include the paraesophageal and lateral aortopulmonary-window lymph nodes that can be sampled by endoscopic ultrasound real-time–guided fine-needle aspiration (FNA) via the esophagus and by anterior median-sternotomy (Chamberlain procedure), respectively.

Technical aspects. The "abnormal" lymph node has been classified radiographically as one with a short axis measuring greater than 1 cm. However, thorough lymph node staging of bronchogenic carcinomas has demonstrated a diagnostic sensitivity and specificity of only about 60% to 70% when this rule was applied. 18-Fluorodeoxyglucose positron emission tomography scanning may identify metabolically abnormal lymph nodes and lung nodules even when they do not fulfill this size criterion. After identification of an accessible lymph node suspicious of harboring pathology, a

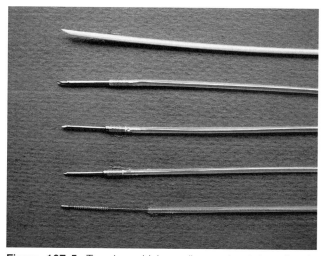

Figure 107-5. Transbronchial needles and cytology brush: from Top 18-gauge Sofcor plastic (Microvasive), 19/21G MW 319 Histology steel; 15-mm length (Bard-Millrose); 21-gauge SW121 cytology steel, 15 mm (Bard-Millrose); 22-gauge MW122/222/522 cytology steel, 13 mm (Bard-Millrose); cytology brush.

TBNA needle with the needle carefully retracted is introduced via the operating channel of the bronchoscope. Regardless of the location of the chosen target, it is best to pass the TBNA through the lumen with the bronchoscope in a fairly central location (i.e., the trachea or mainstem bronchi) with the tip straight or minimally angulated. This is to protect the expensive equipment that can be most easily damaged by instruments at its distal flexible end. With the TBNA needle still in its protective hub, the bronchoscope is then maneuvered into a position proximal to the target lesion. Centering the bronchoscope away from the side-walls, the needle is then deployed and locked in place, and care is taken to avoid mucosal trauma that will cause bleeding and obscuration of the bronchoscopic view. The catheter tips housing the beveled metallic needles usually have a protective metal hub that helps to prevent inadvertent perforation of the bronchoscope channel. During positioning for TBNA, a portion of the needle or the catheter hub should always be visible, otherwise it is possible that the exposed needle was pulled back into the distal bronchoscope tip, again risking damage. If for any reason the needle is not visible, it should be retracted into the catheter and the entire catheter should be removed from the bronchoscope and properly reset for redeployment.

The actual mucosal penetration and spearing of the mediastinal target can be performed by one of two modes, either the "stab" or the "push-jab" technique.[33] The stabbing approach entails holding the bronchoscope in place and stabbing the deployed needle catheter forward, thus traversing the bronchial mucosal into a lymph node or tumor mass. The limitation of this technique is that it is only suited for lesions that are situated directly in the line of sight of the bronchoscope; the needle will more than likely take a somewhat more oblique pathway across the bronchial mucosa, thus leaving less needle length to penetrate the lesion. In a spontaneously breathing patient, subtle airway motion can translate to missing the lesion or having the needle hang up on bronchial cartilage instead of passing through the membranous portion of the mucosa. Finally, if the bronchoscope-needle setup is positioned too far away from the bronchial mucosa point of entry, pushing the flexible TBNA catheter outside the bronchoscope channel will allow the catheter to bend and kink, further limiting its effectiveness. For these reasons, the piggy-back "push-jab" technique is preferred. In this approach, the deployed and locked needle is kept partially withdrawn into the distal bronchoscope and the sharp needle tip is carefully directed toward a selected entry point; the membranous mucosa between cartilage rings is chosen. The bronchoscope tip can be partially flexed such that

the bronchoscope and needle catheter behave as a curved needle set, with the needle anchored at about a 45-degree angle. Control of both the catheter and bronchoscope is obtained, either by the bronchoscopist alone, or with an assistant holding the proximal end of the catheter and readying to advance it on command, and the bronchoscope is pushed forward firmly as the piggy-backed needle-catheter is jabbed forward. With practice, the TBNA needle can be made to traverse the mucosa at a nearly 90-degree angle, thus affording sampling of lesions in the distal left and right paratracheal angles, anterior precarinal space, and right bronchial lymph nodes (Figure 107-6). Once the locked needle catheter set is advanced until the entire length of the needle is buried up to the hub, the clear catheter is pushed from the proximal end until a bit of it is visibly protruding from the distal bronchoscope tip. At this point, inadvertent penetration of one of the major vascular structures, such as the aorta, pulmonary artery branches, superior vena cava, or azygous vein will be obvious by the complete backfill of the distal catheter with blood even without any suction applied. If there is no unexpected return of blood, a cytology or histology sample can be obtained by the forward and backward movement of the needle. Although suction has most often been applied by syringe attached to the proximal end of the TBNA catheters, this is not always necessary because it is really the capillary action plus the regular agitation motion that draws tissue into the lumen of the needle. This is learned from other FNA procedures (e.g., thyroid nodules) where such fine-needle capillary action actually provides a cleaner, less bloody sample than traditional FNA with negative pressure suction applied. This is especially so for looser, less organized malignant tissue, whereas suction may be

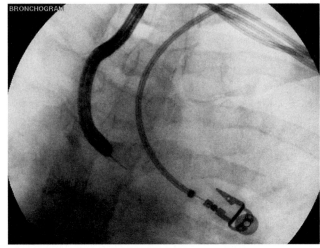

Figure 107-6. Transbronchial needle aspiration of a left paratracheal lymph node. Successful staging of Stage IIIA disease.

required for acquisition of an adequate sample of a denser granulomatous or reactive lymph node.

The same TBNA needles can be used for the transbronchial sampling of peripheral lung masses, although as mentioned earlier, the acute bending of certain lobar segments may preclude successful passage of the TBNA needle into the desired airway segments.[9,35] Contrary to sampling of the central mediastinal lesions or endobronchial pathology, the needle is not deployed until the catheter hub with the protected needle tip is advanced into position as indicated by fluoroscopy or CT scan.

There is some debate as to the ideal method to retrieve the needle-catheter and how to process the sample thereafter. Some experienced practitioners of TBNA will withdraw the still extended and locked needle back into the bronchoscope and out the channel while simultaneously straightening the tip of the bronchoscope. The rationale for not first retracting the needle into the safety of the hubbed tip is to avoid sucking back bronchial epithelial cells that may dilute the presumed pathologic cells of interest within the needle. The obvious risk, however, is the much increased risk of damage wrought on the bronchoscope even if the needle is only pulled back because a rigid needle measuring 13 to 15 mm can scratch and perforate the bronchoscope channel, which can be in a 130- to 180-degree angulation. Current teaching is therefore to always fully retract the needle before pulling the catheter backward, while still straightening the distal tip of the bronchoscope.

The retrieved samples can be prepared and preserved in a number of ways. Generally, more than a single pass is made to ensure adequate sampling, with the maximum yield leveling off after between four and seven passes at a particular site. The samples can be ejected onto a clean labeled slide, and a smear can be made with the edge of a second slide much like the making of a blood smear. If sufficient material is present, a second slide is placed face down on the first, and two slides are made by gently drawing apart them apart. Slides should quickly be placed into alcohol in a jar or air-dried and immediately stained by one of the rapid stains such as Diff-Quik for a bedside review. The presence of rapid on-site evaluation by a pathologist or an experienced cytopathology technician is a helpful adjunct that improves the diagnostic yield of TBNA.[6] The immediate feedback will direct the need for additional TBNA passes. Even when pathology is noted, such as carcinoma or abnormal lymphocytes, extra passes for additional material to be spun down for immunostains or preservation in media for flow analysis may aid in making the identification of a tumor source or cell type with important implications for prognosis and guide for therapy. Additional impor-

tant advantages of bedside cytopathology feedback include improvement of the learning curve of locating bronchoscopically invisible targets and confirmation of which techniques work best for individual operators. In the absence of cytopathology assistance, samples can also be injected into an aliquot of preservative solution such as Saccamanno's preservative and spun down in the laboratory for further analysis. Flushing out the needle with 1 to 2 mL of saline after each pass, as reported earlier, is no longer practiced because this dilutes out small quantities of sample, and the needle loses some of its capillary effect when flushed with liquid. We therefore eject the sample from the needle with an air-filled syringe.

Published series quote a diagnostic yield of 75% to 90% for TBNA sampling of mediastinal lymph nodes, with lower yield for peripheral pulmonary lesions, once again depending on the location and size of the targets.[9,33,35] TBNA, however, remains an underused minimally invasive sampling technique because of uneven teaching of the technique, even at major teaching pulmonary and thoracic programs, and the average low yield of the occasional practitioner of this technique.[7] A number of radiographic techniques have been used or are being developed as adjuncts to help in localization and to guide TBNA sampling of lung pathology. Fluoroscopy can help to image the proper penetration of a lesion in the lung parenchyma, but is generally less useful in accurately localizing mediastinal adenopathy and central masses that may be obscured by the cardiac silhouette and other normal mediastinal structures. Spiral CT scans, either stopped frames or fluoroscopic CT, can be used to help localize and prove TBNA penetration of target lesions, but it is cumbersome to perform these bronchoscopic procedures in the CT scanner, and the patient and staff are exposed to a much higher levels of radiation. The advent of rapid multislice detector CT scanners and the development of software to improve 3D rendering will soon make available a number of high-fidelity "virtual bronchoscopy" programs, including the capability of rendering "transparent" the airway wall and highlighting the adjacent mediastinal structures of interest. The purpose of these programs is not to obviate the need for tissue diagnosis but to guide the approach for procedures such as TBNA and transbronchial biopsies. Another real-time guidance technique is the use of EBUS to localize lymph nodes and other mediastinal structures of interest for tissue sampling.[4,13] Most EBUS uses a radial balloon probe introduced via the working bronchoscope channel. After EBUS imaging is completed, the probe is withdrawn and TBNA is performed. Report of simultaneous imaging and sampling via a double-lumen bronchoscope is not generally applicable due to the rarity of these fiber-bronchoscopes that are largely being phased out and by the imminent introduction of dedicated EBUS bronchoscope with an angled side port for TBNA. EBUS is currently available for clinical use, but is available only at a limited number of centers because of the lack of experienced practitioners and the equipment cost.

Complications from TBNA of mediastinal structures are primarily bleeding into the airways from puncture of vascular structures or vascular tumors. Less commonly, pneumothorax, pneumomediastinum, or hemomediastinum may occur. Bleeding is generally self-limited, and the bronchoscopist should be focused on clearing the airway of blood that would otherwise obscure the bronchoscopist's view and induce coughing and desaturation. Suction should be directed downstream from the TBNA entry site, presenting no interference with the local formation of a small clot. TBNA of peripheral lung lesions entails the same risk as transbronchial biopsies, including bleeding and pneumothoraces.

Bronchoscopic Brush

The use of a cytology brush for the sampling of an endobronchial lesion or under fluoroscopic guidance for the sampling of a peripheral lesion appears obvious and a simple enough procedure. A review of the yield and complications is warranted, however. Because the stiff metallic bristles of the cytology brush can be traumatic over a larger area, bleeding from bronchoscopic brushing can be severe. In spite of a vigorous effort to retrieve sample, the yield can be disappointingly low for carcinoma and generally ranks below directed-forceps biopsies and endobronchial needle aspiration.[9,35] There are multiple explanations for this apparent paradox. Much as with TBNA, in which active negative pressure aspiration can cause more trauma and bleeding than agitation without suction, the nonspecific trauma induced by the bristles leads to a usually bloody sample that can obscure the malignant cells behind a field of red blood cells, fibrin, and other debris. The superficial endobronchial layer of a central tumor can often consist of a biofilm of mucus, necrotic cell debris, and recruited inflammatory cells, thus sampling along the surface with a cytology brush may pick up only these nondiagnostic contaminants and miss the underlying true pathology. The yield of a cytology brush for the sampling of peripheral lesions is equally disappointing, once again because of the sampling issue of picking up mostly normal or inflamed bronchial or bronchiolar epithelial cells. In a number of instances, unless an airway directly leads up into a tumor mass, the catheter of the cytology brush is directed away from the tumor that pushes away adjacent bronchi.[32] In a similar circumstance,

the needle of a TBNA can be extended directly toward a tumor, penetrating the smaller airways as necessary. Therefore, except as a poor substitute for directed-forceps biopsy and TBNA of central endobronchial and peripheral lesions, bronchoscopic brushing for cytology has relatively low merit and rarely adds to the other sampling procedures in cancer diagnosis.

To address the issue of nonspecific bronchial wash or BAL cultures from contamination by upper airways colonizers, a protective microbiologic brush has been developed as an adjunctive method to sample the lower airway. A plastic bristled brush housed within a catheter capped with a plug is introduced into the airway's segment of interest, and the plug is ejected by the deployed brush that will then pick up a "true" lower respiratory tract sample. The brush has furthermore been designed to adsorb a fixed quantity of bronchial secretions (0.1 mL) that can be serially diluted 100-fold in the microbiology laboratory to yield a semiquantitative "protected" microbiologic culture. By this method, growth of 1000 colonies of a particular organism would represent a significant growth. It is advisable to confer with the institution's microbiology staff before embarking on collecting specimens with the protected catheter brush.

With the exception of the protected quantitative culture brush, all of the instruments listed above are available either as single use or reusable forms. The latter are manufactured to withstand chemical cleaning and autoclaving, and cost on average five to 10 times the single-use item. Their longevity depends on many factors, but they seldom last more than 10 uses; this is especially true for instruments used in therapeutic procedures such as electrocautery, as detailed below. Because of the concerns of equipment contamination, breakage and loss of parts in the airways, and general wear and tear that makes the aged instruments function suboptimally (e.g., dulled forceps edges or needle tips), our policy is now to use disposable single-use instruments exclusively.

INTERVENTIONAL BRONCHOSCOPIC PROCEDURES
General Principles

The majority of bronchoscopies performed today are for diagnostic purposes, and most pathologies are managed by systemic therapies such as antimicrobials for infections, chemotherapy, and concurrent radiotherapy for malignancies. Local therapies, when chosen, are most often not directed via the airways but rather involve thoracic surgeries such as resections of localized lesions and drainage of parenchymal-pleural abscesses, or they involve image-guided interventions such as radiofrequency ablation of focal tumor masses or radiology-directed catheter drainage.

The exception is the management of airway narrowing and fistulas, whether acute or subacute in presentation, and whether due to benign or malignant causes. In this section, we shall review the currently practiced bronchoscopic interventional procedures and mention some areas of future development.[2,22,28]

Careful selection of a patient eligible for interventional bronchoscopy is critical to maximize benefit to patients who are in general quite ill. Depending on the particular intervention, the nature of the disease state, and the patient's functional status, the risks associated with interventional procedures can be significant. The majority of our presently performed interventional procedures all strive to maintain airway patency and to reestablish normal gas exchange, or to reestablish as near normal as possible the normal airway structure. These include covering up pathologic openings such as fistulas between the tracheal-bronchial branches and the esophagus or bronchial-mediastinal and bronchial-pleural tears or fistulas.

It is important to recall that for ideal gas exchange to take place, there should be minimal ventilation-perfusion mismatching. Therefore, whereas the removal of a foreign body such as an aspirated object in a toddler or child can lead to immediate and full recovery, in other instances simply reestablishing airway patency may not be sufficient. For thoracic malignancies blocking the airways, whether primary or metastatic, débridement of airway tumor and debris when the accompanying vasculature is also infiltrated and obliterated may simply lead to increased "dead space." Reestablishing ventilation of nonperfused lung segments can in fact worsen hypercapnia and not improve hypoxemia. A good-quality contrast CT scan of the chest is therefore mandatory for review in all cases of airway obstruction, with the exception of those with recent aspiration of a foreign body.

Knowledge of the position of the vasculature is furthermore critical for the interventional bronchologist to avoid potentially life-threatening complications of vascular perforation by laser or mechanical débridement. The intravenous contrast in the CT scan serves another very important purpose. In the cases of known or highly suspected malignancies blocking the central airways, knowledge of whether there is functioning lung distal to the obstruction will help to predict the likelihood of success and whether tenuous patients should be subjected to deep sedation or general anesthesia with mechanical ventilation from which they may not successfully wean. Experienced radiologists will provide a reasonable estimate as to whether viable or necrotic tumorous lungs await the distal aspect of a segment of obstructed central airways—that is, whether an interventional expedition

from within the airway lumen will only reveal disease that is the "tip of the iceberg." They can also comment on the presence of concomitant pleural disease that may portend the very poor prognosis of a "trapped" lung, even when the central airways are reopened and pleural fluid removal attempted.

Preparation of the Patient and Selection of Instruments

Careful history taking should include any use of anticoagulants and antiplatelet agents. Physical examination, review of radiographs (preferably including a recent contrast CT scan), and measurement of platelet counts and other relevant bleeding parameters are routine. Because many of the patients undergoing interventional bronchoscopic procedures often have more advanced pulmonary diseases and possible comorbidities, a baseline electrocardiogram is often requested. Because the purpose of the procedures is often palliative in nature and the procedures are accompanied by higher risk than standard diagnostic bronchoscopies, a detailed discussion of possible complications and the realistic likelihood of achieving subjective relief should be discussed with the patients and their families. In the largest airway interventional series of laser débridement by Cavaliere and others, the overall procedure-related mortality was 0.3% and major complications (including significant hemorrhage, pneumothorax, and pneumomediastinum) was 1.5%.[5]

Most of the interventional procedures discussed below can be performed either via an FOB, an RB, or an FOB introduced via an RB or via direct suspension laryngoscope. There are pros and cons to both approaches, but the operator should be capable of converting a case performed with an FOB into an RB case when the need arises.[2,7] The larger channel of the RB facilitates the use of larger-caliber instruments, and certain rigid silicone stents require rigid instrumentation for their deployment. The bronchoscope itself can be used to core out tumor tissue or to tamponade hemorrhage from the side walls. It is also easier to remove noncancerous foreign bodies and to dilate benign stenotic segments via a larger rigid tube. Conversely, the larger and rigid instruments are more liable to cause trauma to the vocal cords and potentially cause a fistula when used to débride necrotic tissue in distorted airways. The constrained angulation provided by manipulating the patient's head and neck positions can limit the bronchial segments reachable for intervention. The rigid instruments will also mandate the use of general anesthesia. When choosing flexible FOB for interventional procedures, larger-channel "therapeutic" bronchoscopes that can accommodate flexible interventional instruments are selected, but it is often helpful to also have available thinner pediatric bronchoscopes that can be used to bypass critical narrowings.

In the management of airway obstruction, the choice of the specific intervention depends on the location and severity of narrowing. Certain techniques such as cryotherapy, photodynamic therapy, and endoluminal brachytherapy simply do not work on malignant tissue rapidly enough to relieve critical stenosis. The short-term effect is, in fact, tissue edema as tumors undergo cellular death and necrosis. In such instances, mechanical débridement with or without one of the heat thermal therapies will be more appropriate. In significant cases of central airway narrowing, where both mainstem bronchi may be partially compromised, attention should first be directed toward the less affected side, most often also the healthier lung, such that adequate single lung ventilation can be established. Even though the majority of airway interventions will result in improved pulmonary function, the operating team of bronchoscopists, anesthesiologists, and nursing personnel should always be prepared for acute and potentially catastrophic complications. These include turning the patient laterally and keeping the functioning lung upward in case of massive hemorrhage; keeping handy equipment for intubation, including double-lumen ET tubes for split lung ventilation, or at least bronchial blockers to tamponade a bleeding lung; and maintaining the capacity to perform rigid endoscopy if the situation is less dire but larger airway access is needed.

Foreign Body Removal

Although foreign body aspiration (FBA) is classically a pediatric problem, with the highest incidence occurring in children younger than 5 years of age, and a notable cause of accidental deaths in this cohort, this is a problem that can present in adults as well, albeit often with less acute symptoms.[21] The classic signs of witnessed acute choking, wheezing, loss of unilateral breath sounds with corresponding volume loss, or hyperinflation due to air-trapping on the radiographs has a high sensitivity of about 70% but variable specificity for FBA. Other findings of chronic cough, recurrent pneumonias in the same chest region, atelectasis, and even pnemothoraces or pneumomediastinum are more common in adults who may or may not recall an episode of possible aspiration.[2]

The approach in managing suspected FBA differs somewhat between the pediatric and the adult population. RB has been the standard procedure for removal of airway foreign bodies and remains so for pediatric population. Conversely, in adults, a trial of foreign body removal with instruments compatible with a flexible FOB would be reasonable, although

there should always be the backup plan for RB should the aspirated foreign body prove too stubborn for removal by the smaller flexible bronchoscopy instruments. Flexible bronchoscopy is indicated for patients with cervical spine instability and skull and jaw fractures, and such trauma patients may be particularly at risk for the aspiration of broken teeth or dentures, or a preceding aspiration leading to near asphyxiation and loss of consciousness may even be the cause of the subsequent head and neck trauma from a fall or a vehicular accident. Helpful adjuncts in directing the foreign body centrally include repositioning the patient in a Trendelenburg or a decubitus position, movements that would not interfere with flexible FOB but may prove more challenging with an RB. A number of "nonpulmonary" instruments can be adapted to assist in the retrieval of a foreign body; these include a Fogarty catheter pushed distal to the foreign body, then inflated and slowly pulled back, simulating the retrograde clot removal from a vascular lumen. Snares and baskets, such as the Roth basket, developed for gastrointestinal procedures can also be used to retrieve difficult to grasp smooth or rounded items such as peanuts and marbles that are akin in texture and size to biliary stones. Cryotherapy probes used primarily for tumor and granulation tissue ablation can also be used to retrieve a foreign body that has a layer of aqueous condensation or secretions around it by the process of cryoadhesion.[14] Recall the unfortunate child testing this hypothesis on a cold winter's day and getting his tongue stuck to the metal pole.

Hemorrhage can occur as a result of inflammation and granulation formation induced by the foreign body; this is especially true for certain pill fragments and other caustic compounds, oily food such as nuts, and on a more chronic basis, metal pins and other sharp objects. The manipulation of the various instruments can further aggravate this process. Therefore, having the capacity to provide hemostasis with vasoconstrictor compounds and mucosal surface coagulation is desirable. The routine use of corticosteroids to reduce airway edema, either before a scheduled procedure for the removal of a foreign body or subsequent to finding existing edema, has not been rigorously studied but is commonly recommended.

Tissue Débridement
Cold Techniques

The discussion of interventional bronchoscopic approaches in the débridement of malignant or scar tissue causing airway obstruction often become a catalog of technology and devices to deliver these tissue destructive techniques (Table 107-4). However, it is fair to say that the underlying common denominator is mechanical resection assisted by heating, freezing,

TABLE 107-4

FEATURES OF DIFFERENT INTERVENTIONAL BRONCHOSCOPY TECHNIQUES FOR TUMOR ABLATION

Mode of Therapeutic Effects	Mechanical Débridement	Laser	APC	Electrocautery	Cryotherapy	Brachy-therapy	Photo Dynamic Therapy
Immediate	+ + + +	+ + + +	+ + +	+ + +	+	−	−
Prolonged tumor kill	−	−	−	−	−	+ + +	+ + + +
Risk of airway fire	−	+ +	+ +	+ +	−	−	−
Perforation risk	+ +	+ +	+	+	−	−	−
Hemorrhage risk							
Immediate	+ +	+	−	−	−	−	−
Delayed and massive	−	−	−	−	−	+ +	+ +

or biochemical methods of causing cell death. The "cold steel" of an RB with the use of forceps for débridement and the tip of the bronchoscope for coring out tumor therefore remains one of the most effective ways to rapidly reopen the airways. It is less effective for the removal of scarred-in granulation tissue. The length and rigidity of the standard rigid scope limits access to certain lobes and bronchial segments. Cancers and granulation tissues are both hypervascular, and ancillary procedures may be necessary for good hemostasis. Increasingly, powered microdébrider devices designed for use in the sinuses and hypopharynx have been adapted for use below the vocal cords.[8] Unlike laborious tissue removal by conventional forceps biopsy, the rapidly rotating microdébrider blade effectively débrides benign scars and granulation tissues as well as cancers. Longer custom-made blades with a length of 37 cm and curved tips (Xomed Corp) can now gain access to the proximal right and left mainstem bronchi. Directed by rigid telescopes, controlled débridement is rapid and causes surprisingly little bleeding in spite of rapid tissue removal. We have been able to achieve hemostasis in most cases with only the use of topical vasoconstrictors and without the need for additional heat coagulation.[8,36] True cryotherapy involves direct tissue destruction by applying a contact probe onto the surface of or deeper into the tissue to be destroyed. Unlike percutaneous interstitial cryotherapy used in sarcomas or hepatic cancers, a closed system has to be used within the airways so as not to cause asphyxia or unwanted spillage of the cooling agents more distally. Therefore, the current generation of airway cryoprobes uses the Joule-Thomson effect of allowing the sudden expansion of compressed gases (nitrous oxide) or liquid nitrogen to cool the metal cryoprobe tip to −89°C, sufficiently below the −40°C to −50°C needed to cause cell death, cryothrombosis of vessels, and eventual

tissue necrosis. Primarily applied for the destruction of airway cancers, the cyroprobe can also be useful in slowing down the growth of proliferative granulation tissue and is effective in removing hydratable foreign bodies as described above. Cryotherapy units are relatively cheap to purchase and easy to maintain and to use. The safety profile is favorable because there is little risk of airway or vascular wall perforation, and normal nonvascular tissue including bronchial epithelium and the underlying cartilage is cryoresistant and heals almost completely. Conversely, these same effects can be disadvantages because a fairly rapid warming effect of about 10°C for every millimeter from the tip results in limited depth of tissue and tumor kill; slower growing tumors such as carcinoids may be relatively cryoresistant. The delay in clinical response and the need for follow-up débridement of the necrotic debris limits the usefulness of cryotherapy in high-grade central airway obstruction, causing severe symptoms.[2,14]

Thermal Ablation: Hot Techniques

Laser, argon plasma coagulation (APC), and electrocautery are three methods of heat-assisted mechanical resection. There are unique features to each, but there are also common features that will be first discussed. The balance between tissue penetration and cutting vs coagulation can be shifted depending on the power settings, the tools used in electrocautery, and the type of laser chosen. However, all three methods are effective in providing good hemostasis in conjunction with mechanical débridement. There are also common potential complications that warrant caution in their use. Whether the tissue is only charred or actually vaporized, the resulting plume of smoke and particles will reduce vision and contribute to hypoxia, therefore continuous suction via an additional catheter placed within the RB or intermittent suction through the working channel of a therapeutic flexible bronchoscope is necessary. Airway fire, which has been reported, is now less likely because of the phasing out of flammable inhalational anesthetic agents; nevertheless, it is prudent to work closely with anesthesiologists, giving them ample warning to turn down the inspired fraction of oxygen to below 40%, or to perform the heat débridement only during periods of apneic ventilation. There is no consistent need for aluminum wrapping of stiffer red rubber ET tubes, but caution should be exercised when heat is used near potentially flammable material. To avoid costly repairs and even complete destruction of the flexible bronchoscopes, the laser and APC should always be on standby when the catheters are being introduced or withdrawn through the working channel of the bronchoscope. As with all interventional procedures within the airway, but especially for these tissue destructive procedures, it is important to know where the large vessels are located because perforation of the vascular wall can be a fatal complication.

Laser (light amplification of stimulated emission of radiation) light from different elements and compounds has been used in airway débridement of malignant and benign causes of airway obstruction.[2,5] Currently, neodymium:yttrium aluminum-garnet (Nd:YAG) laser is the one most commonly used within the airways. It is a powerful tool, but because of the potential for airway and vascular perforation, the pulses should be delivered in a noncontinuous mode, starting from a lower power setting of 20 to 40 W at the beginning of the case to prevent applying excessive energy density until the tissue response to the laser is established. Laser-safe goggles should be worn by all operating room personnel, and the patient's eyes should also protected. The ready-to-fire laser beam should not be accidentally aimed at personnel or equipment. Nd:YAG laser units are expensive to purchase, but thereafter they are fairly easy to maintain. The same Nd:YAG; KTP; and smaller, less expensive diode lasers capable of delivering focused light in the red 630-nm wavelength can also be used as the light source in the activation of photosensitizing drugs used in photodynamic therapy (PDT) discussed in a later section.

APC is another noncontact method for tissue destruction by heat, achieved by the ignition of a charged argon gas plasma that is generated by a high-voltage, high-frequency electrode. The ionized plasma seeks out conductive tissue and hence can be sprayed onto a surface that may be tangential to the aiming beam. This property allows for its use in cleaning up prostheses, such as airway stents overgrown by granulation tissue or tumor, with much less risk to the nonconductive stent than could be achieved by laser,

which is liable to cut through metal and more likely to ignite a fire. APC has been used on tumors, recurrent respiratory papillomatosis, and granulation scar tissues. One disadvantage is the relatively shallow depth of tissue penetration and a lesser capability to quickly débride bulky tumor. Several specific risks include the danger of air embolism if the jet of ionized argon gas should be blown into an open vascular structure and a potential risk of electrocution if the patient and APC generator are not properly grounded.[2]

Electrocautery, unlike laser and APC, is a direct-contact form of tissue destruction by heat. Monopolar and bipolar instruments are available to affect airway hemostasis and tissue destruction, with the monopolar instruments preferred. There is a wide range of instruments available for use within the flexible bronchoscope, including the blunt-end probe for contact hemostasis, forceps for biopsy and débridement, snare loops of varying diameters for lassoing polypoid lesions, and knife for fine cutting (e.g., radial cuts for an obstructing tracheal web). The patient is always grounded, and because of the risk of retrograde conduction of the high-voltage, high-frequency alternating current, the conducting portions of the electrocautery instruments are kept clear of the insulated surface of the distal end of the bronchoscope (see Figures 107-1 and 107-3).

Photodynamic Therapy and Endobronchial Brachytherapy

PDT is the application of photochemical reactions in generating cytotoxic oxygen radicals that is effective in the destruction of invasive carcinoma and can provide possible cure of preinvasive carcinoma in situ. Three elements are required for PDT: (1) hematoporphyrin-derived photosensitizers (PS) with a selective preference for malignant cells; (2) high-energy photon light source to activate the PS; (3) and molecular oxygen to accept the energy from the excited PS to form singlet oxygen and other oxygen radicals that are highly reactive and that can cause cell death. To minimize cellular damage to normal cells that will also take up PS compounds, a 48-hour interval between drug infusion and light activation is calculated to maximize the tumor–to–normal tissue differential concentration of the drugs. Although the duration of response in maintaining an obstructed airway patent is at least equivalent to laser débridement, the delayed response in PDT (from the time delay between PS injection to light activation and subsequent need for removal of necrotic tissue) means that PDT is not a method for relieving acute and severe airway obstruction. Further disadvantages include systemic photosensitivity for 30 to 60 days and potential allergy to and high unit cost of the PDT compounds. In earlier studies with less tumor-specific PS compounds and with perhaps excessive photon exposure, life-threatening hemoptysis and asphyxiation due to tissue necrosis of the bronchial mucosa and tumor bed led to the suggestion that only small noncircumferential tumors can be safely treated. More recent studies indicate the safe and effective use of PDT in bulky tumors, as long as the patients are closely monitored and emergency airway clearance is possible. Still cautionary is the combination of concurrent treatment of PDT with either radiation or chemotherapy because there may be enhanced toxicities of local edema, bronchitis, and the development of acute or delayed fatal hemoptysis.[2,7,12]

Somewhat similar in response to PDT is endobronchial brachyradiotherapy (EBBT), in that the depth of tumor kill is limited to between 5 and 10 mm from the point source of application. Once again, the response is not immediate, and therefore brachytherapy is not appropriate for very symptomatic central high-grade tumor obstruction. Finally, although brachytherapy may be effective with carcinoma in situ and submucosal spread of invasive cancer, it should not be used in primarily extrinsic tumor narrowing that is not visible by bronchoscopy. *Brachy* is derived from the Greek expression for *short*, hence EBBT is the method of directing over a short distance high-intensity radiation originating from a source placed within the tracheobronchial tree. The temporary bronchoscopic placement of hollow catheters through which a radiation source can be passed later (remote afterloading) has replaced the initial (1922) direct placement of radium implants within the bronchus. This remote-afterloading technique eliminates the risk of radiation exposure to the bronchoscopy room staff. Indications for brachytherapy include treatment of advanced endobronchial cancers in patients who have received the maximal dose of external beam radiation therapy or as a boost to planned external beam radiation therapy in patients with newly diagnosed lung cancers with significant endobronchial compromise.[2,7,24] EBBT has also been applied with curative intent, in small series of patients with carcinoma in situ or a small volume of invasive carcinoma limited to visible portion of the central airways.[29] Although EBBT has been applied almost exclusively to tumor invasion of the airways, there are scattered reports of its application in areas of benign stenosis or where granulation tissue has developed at the site of airway anastomoses or at the ends of airway stents. Lower dosages of EBBT are given after débridement in an attempt to delay the regrowth of granulation tissue. The bronchoscopic procedure of catheter placement is itself simple and entails no greater complexity than directing the passage of the close-ended brachytherapy catheters via the operating channel

into selected airway segments narrowed by endobronchial tumor. Sequential placement of two to four catheters directed into several obstructed airway segments permit more precise treatment of a larger tumor volume of right or left hilar and endobronchial tumors that rarely if ever conform to the cylindrical radiation dosimetry form of a single catheter. High-energy iridium-192 has largely replaced earlier sources of cesium-137, iodine-125, cobalt-60, and radium itself, although the cesium and iodine sources are still occasionally used. The reported dose usually expressed in grays (Gy) is the isodose measured at 1 cm from the radiation source. With current use of iridium-192, a high-intensity high-dose rate (HDR) of more than 2 Gy/min with short treatment times of less than 30 minutes has become the standard, with the low-dose rate (LDR) of less than 2 Gy/h and the intermediate-dose rate (IDR) of 2 to 12 Gy/h applications largely abandoned. Unlike brachytherapy applications in gynecologic, bone, and soft tissue tumors, there has been such a wide variance in the practice of EBBT that there are no consensus guidelines from the American and international endocurietherapy societies as to the ideal dose per fraction, the total number and interval between applications, or the total dose range. The published radiation dose is an applied range from 1 Gy to an upper limit of 15 Gy per treatment, with a single to six fractions separated by 1 week to 1 month, thus reaching a maximal cumulative dose of 50 to 60 Gy.[24] It does not appear that the highest dose per treatment nor the maximal dose range confer survival advantage, therefore the median range adopted by more experienced practitioners is 7 to 10 Gy per application for a total of two to three treatments. Also not yet established are the risks and benefits of concurrent or close sequential combined treatments with external beam radiotherapy, endobronchial PDT, or laser therapies. The most frequent manageable toxicity is radiation bronchitis, but the most severe complication is fatal hemoptysis, which has been reported to occur in between 2% and 25% of case series. Frequently, exsanguination is sudden, occurring some time (weeks to months) after brachytherapy; this may be associated with better symptomatic relief, suggesting that a more vigorous tumor necrosis response may precede the eventual loss of vascular integrity.

Balloon Bronchoplasty and Endobronchial Stent Placement

In addition to reopening an obstructed airway with the various methods described above, there is the additional task of maintaining airway patency. Furthermore, endobronchial débridement will not be useful in instances where the obstruction is extrinsic in nature. Dilation of a narrowed airway segment by mechanical means may be helpful in reestablishing airway patency, albeit temporarily, until more definitive solutions can be instituted. Through a RB or a suspended laryngoscope, metal mechanical dilators can be gently corkscrewed through a length of tracheal stenosis from fibrotic tissue or tumor. However, areas beyond the proximal right or left mainstem bronchi are seldom accessible, and overall, such dilation is no more effective than the use of the RB itself. For more distal portions of the right and left mainstem, and for narrowed lobar and segmental bronchioles, balloon bronchoplasty with fluid-expandable catheter balloons offer another option for mechanical dilation. These balloons were originally designed for endoscopic dilation of the biliary tract and the upper (esophageal and pyloric) or lower (colonic) gastrointestinal tracts. Their diameters at full deployment range from 6 mm (biliary) to 18 mm. The lengths of the balloons are fixed, ranging from 2 cm (biliary) to 8 cm (esophageal and colonic). Because of the balloons' intended original destination within the gastrointestinal tract, the catheters are usually 180 to 240 cm in length, somewhat unwieldy for use via an FOB. More recently, dedicated bronchoscopic balloons with a length of 3 cm mounted on shorter catheters have been introduced. These Controlled Radial Expansion (CRE, Boston Scientific Microvasive) balloons have the additional benefit of being expandable to three sequential diameters (e.g., 8–9–10 mm, 10–11–12 mm, and 12–13.5–15 mm) dependent on the amount of fluid pressure applied, which can be monitored on a manometer supplied with the balloon kit. The fluid can be sterile water or saline, or diluted contrast material that will render the balloon on expansion more visible under fluoroscopy.

In a number of obstructive conditions, such as extrinsic compression or bulky tumor invasion of the airways, débridement with or without dilation will only offer temporary relief. Placement of airway stents may be the definitive treatment or may maintain airway patency long enough for adjunctive treatment to control the underlying disease. A large number of stents have been developed or adapted for airway use over the past 20 years.[2,7,17,28] A detailed discussion of all of the individual types and their variants goes beyond the scope of this chapter. The stents can be grouped into metallic and Silastic-silicone types; most but not all of the metallic stents are self-expanding, whereas most of the latter group are fairly rigid and require RB or direct suspension laryngoscopy for placement.

The earliest airway stent was the Montgomery T-tube, a stiff acrylic polymer tube later replaced by silicone, but its placement required a tracheostomy.

A number of silicone stents, some reinforced with metallic struts embedded circumferentially or three-quarters round to simulate the tracheal cartilage (e.g., Orlowski and Freitag Dynamic Stents, Rusch), are available in various lengths and diameters, plus optional limbs to fit the carina and proximal mainstem. With the exception of a single self-expanding polyester reinforced thinned-walled silicone stent (i.e., Polyflex, Rusch), they require rigid instrumentation for placement. Because of the intrinsic thickness of the stent material and the method of insertion, they are useful primarily for placement within the trachea and first- to second-generation airways only.

The earliest metallic stents used in the airways were Gianturco-Z stents adapted from their intended endovascular application. This type of noncovered stent has to be ballooned open, has no protection against in-growth of tumor, has an unacceptably high rate of inducing severe granulation and airway or vascular perforation. Therefore, it has no role today in endobronchial stenting given the number of dedicated endobronchial stents now available. The current generation of metallic stents is self-expandable, comes packaged in a much slimmer profile, can be delivered over a guidewire into the distal mainstem and lobar segments, and hence can be deployed without the need for rigid instrumentation. These self-expandable metal stents are made from stainless steel (e.g., Wallstent) or the nickel-titanium blend of nitinol (e.g., Ultraflex and Alveolus TB-STS). They are available in a variety of lengths and diameters, with or without an outer polypropylene covering that helps to prevent tumor in-growth. There can still be the problem of tumor or granulation overgrowing the ends of the stents, and proper sizing is important to prevent excessive movement or excessive tension against the airway wall, both of which may promote the proliferation of granulation tissue. Once deployed, the stainless steel Wallstent with the sharp opened prongs is generally fixed in place, whereas the more pliable nitinol stents are maneuverable at least until granulation or tumor overgrows the open ends.

Complications of stent placement include trauma to a compromised airway during the stent insertion, including the inadvertent tears to the tracheal-bronchial mucosa already compromised by tumor invasion. An improperly sized covered stent can occlude functioning airway segments because it is too large or too long, or if it is too small it can subsequently migrate. All stents, covered or otherwise, will interfere with normal mucociliary clearance and, as a foreign body, will promote biofilm formation. Stents can therefore become quickly overgrown with a variety of microorganisms. The problems of granulation and tumor ingrowth have been mentioned. The metallic stents can suffer metal fatigue and undergo fracture and, with the single strand weave of nitinol, can unravel.[27] This problem is especially prominent with tracheal stents in which the constant change in curvature of the posterior tracheal membrane with breathing in and out results in metal fatigue. We have therefore avoided placing self-expandable metal stents in the trachea if we anticipate chronic need of the stent in benign conditions such as tracheobronchomalacia, or if the patient has an anticipated survival beyond several months in malignant conditions.

Esophageal-tracheal and esophageal-bronchial fistulas deserve special mention. The majority of such cases result from malignancies originating from the esophagus and, less commonly, from the bronchus. Fistula formation and poor healing may also be due to radiotherapy. Less commonly, such fistulas are congenital or are caused by acute trauma or chronic erosion from a tracheostomy tube. The most common presenting symptoms are coughing with feeding and other signs of aspiration. Gastrograffin swallow studies and occasionally 3D CT reconstructions may localize the fistula, but failure to demonstrate the defect should be followed by direct visual examination. Having a conscious patient swallow 15 to 30 mL of methylene blue or other dye immediately before the induction of anesthesia may be helpful in pinpointing the site of a small but clinically significant fistula. In the absence of an adequate tracheal replacement and the rarity of being able to resect the length of involved trachea for primary anastomoses, stenting to cover the fistula can provide palliation of symptoms, including aspiration of oral secretions or recurring lower respiratory tract infections, and can allow the patient to swallow for oral gratification in the terminal phase of a malignancy. Either esophageal, tracheal-bronchial, or bilateral stenting with covered self-expanding metallic or silicone stents can be helpful. Close collaboration with an interventional gastroenterologist is necessary.

Nitinol with special properties of elastic memory and maximal tensile strength at body temperature continues to be the favored material in the manufacture of metallic stents. New design techniques allow the formation of a self-expanding stent by lasering a stent from a single tubular piece of nitinol instead of weaving a stent from a long strand of the material. This technique can produce a stent less susceptible to metal fatigue. The focus on endobronchial stent development is on coated stents that can be customized for gene therapy delivery, on coatings with antifibrotic compounds to inhibit granulation tissue, and modifications of the local milieu to reduce formation of biofilms that will promote growth of microorganisms.

INNOVATIONS AND FUTURE DEVELOPMENTS
Autofluorescence Bronchoscopy

Early lung cancer diagnosis is the best hope of improving the current poor overall survival of the 169,000 incidences of lung cancer diagnosed in the United States. Visualization of airway pathology by conventional white-light bronchoscopy has been improved by the introduction of higher-resolution video charged couple device bronchoscopes; however, early preinvasive lung cancer ranging from moderate to severe dysplasia and carcinoma in situ continues to be an elusive finding. It has been recognized that the use of hematoporphyrin-derivative fluorescent compounds can improve the identification of dysplastic airway mucosa, but such diagnostic fluorescent bronchoscopy requires expensive and photosensitizing drugs that come with the attendant adverse effects noted in the section on PDT. Since the early 1990s, trials have been ongoing to test and improve systems to detect tissue AF that is altered in dysplastic and cancerous bronchial tissues. Reduction of tissue AF in precancerous and cancerous tissue result in a change in the green AF of normal bronchial mucosa toward red-brown to blue-black tints. U.S. trials of several systems, including the Xillix LIFE (Laser Imaging Fluorescence Endoscope) and Karl Storz D-Light validate a doubling or higher yield in the detection and localization of severely dysplastic and carcinoma in situ lesions over white-light broncoscopy.[11,18,20]

The examination is carried out with illumination in the violet-blue range of 420 to 450 nm delivered by a cadmium-helium laser or powerful xenon light source, and the AF image is captured by a special filter or camera attachment. A complete AF examination takes an additional 10 minutes, on average. Abnormal AF findings will then direct biopsies. The major cause of false-positive findings is due to mucosal trauma, and blood aspirated from the hypopharynx as blood and mucosal hyperemia will reduce tissue AF, therefore the bronchoscopist has to be cautious in avoiding bronchoscope contact with the mucosa, over-vigorous suctioning, or other maneuvers that will cause coughing. In addition to using AF bronchoscopy to detect early preinvasive lung cancers, AF examination can also help thoracic surgeons planning lung cancer resection by providing an estimate of whether there is submucosal extension of cancer that will mandate more aggressive surgeries such as a sleeve resection or pneumonectomy rather than a simple lobectomy. There are other versions of AF bronchoscopes approved in Europe (e.g., Richard Wolf DAFE) and Japan (e.g., Pentax SAFE), but these have not been validated in U.S. trials and are hence not currently approved for sale in the United States.

Endobronchial Ultrasound

Endoscopic application of ultrasound for characterization and localization of extraluminal structures such as lymph nodes, masses, and blood vessels have been mostly developed in the gastrointestinal field. The adaptation of a balloon-tipped ultrasound probe for use within the airway lumen allows for a more precise localization of regional lymph nodes for tumor staging and for diagnosis of lymphoma and other lymphoproliferative disorders. Ultrasound probes introduced through the working channel of the bronchoscope and directed peripherally have also been used to characterize pulmonary consolidation and may distinguish malignant from nonmalignant causes.[2,4,13] Higher-frequency high-resolution EBUS can also provide additional information about extrabronchial invasion of the serosal surface or submucosal infiltration by cancer, again with prognostic and therapeutic impact. Case reports in abstract form have also described tracheal imaging by EBUS of thyroid malignancies, and these compare EBUS favorably to MRI grading of tumor invasion onto the outer tracheal wall. Currently, sampling by EBUS-directed TBNA requires imaging followed by the removal of the probe and substitution of a sampling needle into the working channel. The next adaptation of ultrasound technology into the airways will be the introduction of a dedicated EBUS bronchoscope with a side-directed radial probe and aspiration port that will allow real-time aspiration. The extra-long needle (4–8-cm working length) can also be used for image-guided interventions, including direct intratumoral injection of antineoplastic agents.

Endoscopic/Bronchoscopic Lung Volume Reduction

There are an estimated 14 million patients with chronic obstructive pulmonary disease (COPD) in the United States today. Advanced emphysema patients may be candidates for lung transplantation, but there is a marked shortage of donor lungs. The National Emphysema Treatment Trial established the benefit of surgical lung volume reduction surgery as an alternative to lung transplantation in select COPD patients. Parallel studies have been undertaken to examine the possibility of affecting lung volume reduction by selective blockage of segmental bronchi leading to regional atelectasis. A number of such endoscopic/bronchoscopic lung volume reduction studies using biologic or synthetic adhesives, such as fibrin glue and removable valves, are currently ongoing. They hold the promise of either being an effective and less invasive method of lung volume reduction surgery or as a less invasive and reversible trial of lung volume reduction before subjecting patients to the rigors of thoracic surgery.[16,31]

Advances in this technology may also find use in the bronchoscopic management of bronchopleural fistulas and in the sealing over of stump dehiscence or tracheobronchial esophageal fistulas.

SUMMARY

Tracheobronchial endoscopy is an integral part of the multimodality examination of aerodigestive tract diseases. The widespread availability of flexible FOBs facilitates an extended examination of the lower respiratory tract with minimal conscious sedation. The introduction of high-resolution and easy to maneuver videobronchoscopes coupled with innovative imaging technologies, such as AF bronchoscopy and endobronchial ultrasound, is advancing the ability of bronchoscopists to identify early airway dysplasia, locate extrabronchial targets such as lymph nodes and mediastinal masses for biopsies, and characterize with greater accuracy the depth and lateral spread of malignancies. Diagnostic bronchoscopy is also aided by the availability of an expanding array of instruments including needles, forceps, brushes, and probes that can be deployed through both the large channel rigid and narrow working channel FOBs to sample visible central endobronchial lesions or, transbronchially, to sample peripheral lesions.

A high yield from diagnostic procedures, especially for tissue sampling and staging of thoracic malignancies, is in part dependent on the fostering of close working relationships with radiologists who can provide sophisticated imaging guidance and with pathologists who can provide bedside confirmation of diagnosis. Therapeutic options to manage both benign fibrotic and malignant distortions of the airways have also grown. Currently, a number of thermal ablative techniques ranging from heat therapies with laser, electrocautery, and argon plasma coagulation to cryotherapy complements mechanical débridement in the reestablishment of airway patency. Some treatments provide immediate relief, whereas others such as cryotherapy, endoluminal brachytherapy, and PDT are less suitable for the urgent relief of critical stenosis, but may provide prolonged action.

The best method of sequencing or combining some of these therapeutic modes remains to be determined. It is often necessary to combine balloon bronchoplasty and airway stenting to maintain the reestablished airway patency. RB and direct-suspension laryngoscopy retains an important role in providing superior access and control for these interventional procedures. We anticipate continual innovations in tracheobronchoscopy, with new imaging modalities, such as optical coherence tomography and spectral analysis, to provide near in vivo airway diagnosis without need for actual biopsies. New stent materials and manufacturing techniques will reduce complications, and coated stents may provide customized therapy. Improved imaging guidance to direct the delivery of high-dose local therapy into central and peripheral airway tumors, as well as the ongoing trials with valves to effect endoscopic lung volume reduction, may introduce a bronchoscopic aspect of minimally invasive thoracic therapy to alleviate illness and palliate symptoms in patients with limited lung reserve and advanced lung diseases.

REFERENCES

1. Bergler W and others: Treatment of recurrent respiratory papillomatosis with argon plasma coagulation, *J Laryngol Otol* 111:381, 1997.
2. Bolliger CT, Mathur PN, editors: *Interventional bronchoscopy.* In *Progress in Respiratory Research,* vol 30, Basel, 2000, S. Karger AG.
3. British Thoracic Society Bronchoscopy Guidelines Committee: British Thoracic Society guidelines on diagnostic flexible bronchoscopy, *Thorax* 56(Suppl 1): i1-21, 2001.
4. Burgers JA and others: Endobronchial ultrasound, *Lung Cancer* 34(Suppl 2):S109, 2001.
5. Cavaliere S and others: Nd:YAG laser therapy in lung cancer:– an 11-year experience with 2,253 applications in 1,585 patients, *J Bronchol* 1:105, 1994.
6. Diette G and others: Utility of on-site cytopathology assessment for bronchoscopic evaluation of lung masses and adenopathy, *Chest* 117:1186, 2000.
7. Ernst A and others: Interventional pulmonary procedures: Guidelines from the American College of Chest Physicians, *Chest* 123:1693, 2003.
8. Flint PW: Powered surgical instruments for laryngeal surgery, *Otolaryngol Head Neck Surg* 122:263, 2000.
9. Gasparini S and others: Integration of transbronchial and percutaneous approach in the diagnosis of peripheral pulmonary nodules or masses: experience with 1,027 consecutive cases, *Chest* 108(1):131, 1995.
10. Guidelines for fiberoptic bronchoscopy in adults. American Thoracic Society. Medical Section of the American Lung Association, *Am Rev Respir Dis* 136:1066, 1987.
11. Haussinger K and others: Autofluorescence detection of bronchial tumors with the D-Light/AF, *Diag Ther Endosc* 5:105, 1999.
12. Hayata Y and others: Photodynamic therapy (PDT) in early stage lung cancer, *Lung Cancer* 9:287, 1993.
13. Herth F and others: Conventional vs endobronchial ultrasound-guided transbronchial needle aspiration: a randomized trial, *Chest* 125:322, 2004.
14. Homasson JP: Bronchoscopic cryotherapy, *J Bronchology* 2:145, 1995.
15. Ikeda S: Flexible bronchofiberscope, *Ann Otol Rhinol Laryngol* 79:916, 1970.
16. Ingenito EP and others: Bronchoscopic lung volume reduction using tissue engineering principles, *Am J Respir Crit Care Med* 167:771, 2003.
17. Jones LM and others: Multidisciplinary airway stent team: a comprehensive approach and protocol for tracheobronchial stent treatment, *Ann Otol Rhinol Laryngol* 109:889, 2000.
18. Kennedy TC and others: Review of recent advances in fluorescence bronchoscopy in early localization of central airway lung cancer, *Oncologist* 6:257, 2001.
19. Kikawada M and others: Peripheral airway findings in chronic obstructive pulmonary disease using an ultrathin bronchoscope, *Eur Respir J* 15:105, 2000.
20. Lam S and others: Localization of bronchial intraepithelial neoplastic lesions by fluorescence bronchoscopy, *Chest* 113:696, 1998.
21. Martinot A and others: Indications for flexible versus rigid bronchoscopy in children with suspected foreign body aspiration, *Am J Respir Crit Care Med* 155:1676, 1997.
22. Mathissen DJ and others: Endoscopic relief malignant airway obstruction, *Ann Thorac Surg* 48:469, 1989.
23. Mountain CF and others: Regional lymph node classification for lung cancer staging, *Chest* 111:1718, 1997.
24. Nag S and others: Survey of brachytherapy practice in the United States: a report of the Clinical Practice Committee of the American Endocurietherapy Society, *Int J Radiat Oncol Biol Phys* 31:103, 1995.
25. Pereira W and others: A prospective cooperative study of complications following flexible fiberoptic bronchoscopy, *Chest* 73(6):813, 1978.
26. Rooney C and others: Ultrathin bronchoscopy as an adjunct to standard bronchoscopy in the diagnosis of peripheral lung lesions, *Respiration* 69:63, 2002.
27. Saad CP and others: Self-expandable metallic airway stents and flexible bronchoscopy: long-term outcomes analysis, *Chest* 124:1993, 2003.
28. Seijo LM and others: Interventional pulmonology, *N Engl J Med* 344:740, 2001.
29. Speiser BL and others: Remote afterloading brachytherapy for the local control of endobronchial carcinoma, *Int J Radiat Oncol Biol Phys* 25:579, 1993.
30. Thurlbeck WM and others: Bronchial dimensions and stature, *Annu Rev Respir Dis* 112:142, 1975.
31. Toma TP and others: Bronchoscopic volume reduction with valve implants in patients with severe emphysema, *Lancet* 361:931, 2003.
32. Tsuboi E and others: Transbronchial biopsy smears for diagnosis of peripheral pulmonary carcinoma, *Cancer* 20:687, 1967.
33. Wang K and others: Flexible transbronchial needle aspiration for staging of bronchogenic carcinoma, *Chest* 84:571, 1983.
34. Weibel ER: *Morphometry of the human lung,* New York, 1963, Academic Press.
35. Yung RC: Tissue diagnosis of suspected lung cancer: selecting between sputum cytology, transthoracic needle aspiration, bronchoscopy, and resectional biopsy, *Respir Care Clin* 9:51, 2003.
36. Yung R and others: Use of a powered instrument for mechanical debridement of bulky endobronchial cancers: oral presentation, *World Congress of Bronchology* June 18, 2002.

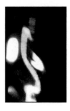

CHAPTER ONE HUNDRED AND EIGHT

DIAGNOSIS AND MANAGEMENT OF TRACHEAL NEOPLASMS

Christine L. Lau
G. Alexander Patterson

OVERVIEW

Tracheal tumors are divided into two types: primary and secondary. Primary tracheal tumors are uncommon. It is estimated that only 2.7 new cases per million per year occur, and therefore only a few centers have acquired expertise with their treatment.[41] Primary tracheal tumors can be either benign or malignant. In adults, few primary tracheal tumors are benign; on the other hand, in children the majority are benign. The preferred treatment for primary tracheal tumors is surgical excision.

Secondary tracheal tumors are, by definition, malignant and involve the trachea either by direct extension or by hematogenous metastases. Direct extension occurs from lung cancer, esophageal cancer, thyroid cancer, mediastinal tumors, and head and neck tumors. Distant metastases from renal cell carcinomas, sarcomas, breast cancer colon cancer, and melanomas are seen.[70] Secondary tracheal tumors are much more common than primary tracheal tumors. Optimal management for this diverse group of tumors depends on their location, natural history of the primary, and comorbidities of the patient.[70] In a subset of lung and thyroid tumors that involve the trachea by direct extension, surgical resection offers a chance for cure. The vast majority of secondary tracheal tumors are treated palliatively.

HISTORICAL REVIEW

Morgagni described the first primary tracheal neoplasm, a fibroma, in 1761.[69] Over 100 years would pass before experimental attempts at tracheal resection with primary end-to-end reconstruction would be described.[14] Kuester performed the first human tracheal resection and primary reconstruction in 1884.[40] Before the 1960s, it was generally believed that tracheal resection was limited to four tracheal rings, about 2 cm, because greater resections would place undue tension on the anastomosis and prevent ade-

quate healing.[3,61] Because of the presumed limits of resection and primary anastomosis, efforts at prosthetic replacement of the trachea were undertaken. In 1950 Belsey[3,4] reported his initial attempt with tracheal reconstruction after resection of an adenoid cystic carcinoma using fascia lata reinforced with stainless wire. Pearson and colleagues[35,55] used heavy Marlex mesh for tracheal replacement in seven patients and reported excellent function of the airway in three patients for several years. Neville and colleagues[50,51] reported extensive experience with the use of a solid silicone tube to replace the trachea; others, however, have reported unacceptable morbidity and mortality with this nonporous material.[66] Over the past several decades, a variety of other foreign materials, nonviable tissue, autogenous tissue, tissue engineering, and transplantation techniques have been attempted, but successful tracheal replacement remains elusive.[21]

Fortunately, the development of techniques for tracheal mobilization[9,22,48] made it possible to perform extensive tracheal resections (>50%) with primary reconstruction. With these techniques the need for tracheal replacement is uncommon. Techniques for tracheal mobilization have allowed significant advances to be made in tracheal surgery, with primary reconstruction after circumferential resection at the subglottal[54] and carinal levels[19] now possible. For the rare occasion when primary anastomosis cannot be performed and replacement is needed, promise lies with tracheal allotransplantation, but long-term immunosuppression requirements will obviously limit its potential uses.[21]

For secondary tumors involving the trachea and carina, surgical techniques have been developed to address those with potential for cure (thyroid and bronchogenic).* Advances in therapeutic bronchoscopy

---

*References 19, 26, 27, 30–32, 40.

offer options for patients who are not candidates for surgical resection. Endoscopic débridement, laser treatment, photodynamic therapy (PDT), cryosurgery, brachytherapy, and stent technology can provide palliation for patients with incurable disease.[70]

PRIMARY TRACHEAL TUMORS

Primary tumors of the trachea are uncommon, but a variety of benign and malignant neoplasms have been described (Table 108-1), often as isolated case reports. Men are slightly more prone to develop tracheal tumors than are women, and the peak age is 50 to 59 years. In adults, approximately 88% of primary tracheal tumors are malignant,[24,55,56,59,60] whereas in children, more than 90% are benign.[17] Primary tumors can originate from any layer in the tracheal wall and morphologically are classified as epithelial or mesenchymal tumors. Although primary tumors can be found anywhere in the trachea, the proximal and distal third of the trachea are most frequently affected, as is the membranous wall. A few large surgical series of primary tracheal tumors have been reported (Table 108-2).[24,55,56,59,60]

TABLE 108-1

CLASSIFICATION OF TRACHEAL TUMORS

Epithelial Neoplasms	Mesenchymal Neoplasms
Benign	**Benign**
Squamous cell papilloma	Fibroma
Papillomatosis	Hemangioma
Pleomorphic adenoma	Granular cell tumor
	Schwannoma
Malignant	Neurofibroma
Squamous cell carcinoma	Fibrous histiocytoma
Adenoid cystic carcinoma	Pseudosarcoma
Carcinoid	Hemangioendothelioma
Mucoepidermoid carcinoma	Leiomyoma
	Chondroma
Adenocarcinoma	Chondroblastoma
Small-cell undifferentiated carcinoma	Lipoma
Secondary malignancies	**Malignant**
Invasion by adjacent malignancy	Leiomyosarcoma
	Chondrosarcoma
Metastases	Paraganglioma
	Spindle-cell sarcoma
Noneoplastic tumors	Lymphoma
Tracheobronchopathia osteochondroplastica	Malignant fibrous histiocytoma
Amyloidosis	Rhabdomyosarcoma
Inflammatory pseudotumor	

(From McCarthy MJ, Rosado-de-Christenson ML: *J Thorac Imag* 10:180, 1995.)

BENIGN PRIMARY TRACHEAL TUMORS

Uncommon in adults, benign primary tracheal tumors are usually well circumscribed, round, soft, and smaller than 2 cm. On chest computed tomography (CT) scanning, these tumors typically do not extend through the tracheal wall. The presence of calcium within the lesion suggests a benign histology.

Squamous Papilloma

Squamous cell papillomas are superficial, sessile, or papillary masses consisting of a connective tissue core covered by squamous epithelium. They may, uncommonly, be seen in adults, developing in association with heavy cigarette smoking. In children, multiple papillomas or juvenile papillomatosis are the most frequent neoplasms seen.[35] These lesions can be found throughout the respiratory tract. Dedo and Yu[10] reported a series of 264 patients with papillomatosis and found the majority of lesions occurred in the larynx (93%). Eleven percent of the patients had papillomatosis in the trachea in addition to the larynx, but only 1.2% had disease isolated to the trachea. Papillomatosis is caused by human papillomavirus (HPV) infection transmitted from mother to fetus during childbirth.[65] Despite being a benign tumor, papillomatosis frequently recurs and is difficult to completely eradicate. Fortunately, it usually regresses spontaneously after puberty.[35] Numerous therapies have been used, including microdébridement, intralesional cidofovir injections, PDT, pulsed dye laser, and indole-3-carbinol.[10] Recently, the carbon dioxide laser has shown promise in the treatment of papillomatosis.[10] Adjuvant treatment with alpha-interferon has been used.[18]

Papillomas rarely undergo malignant transformation to squamous cell carcinoma and verrucous carcinoma, a phenomenon apparently more commonly seen with HPV 11.[58] An incidence of malignant degeneration of 1.6% to 4.0% is reported.[10,38,74]

Granular Cell Tumor

Granular cell tumors were first described by Abrikosoff in 1926.[1] At that time these tumors were thought to be myogenic in origin. Subsequently, granular cell tumors have been found to be neurogenic in origin, probably from the Schwann cell.[5] These tumors develop throughout the body. There appears to be no sex predilection, but the majority of granular cell tumors occur in blacks. They rarely are seen children. Although approximately 50% of granular cell tumors occur in the head and neck region and 10% in the larynx, the trachea is rarely affected.[57] When these tumors do involve the trachea, the cervical portion is the most common location. Multicentric tumors occur in 20% of patients, and these tumors

TABLE 108-2

SUMMARY OF MAJOR RECENT SURGICAL SERIES OF PRIMARY TRACHEAL TUMORS

| | MALIGNANT NEOPLASMS | | | | | BENIGN NEOPLASMS | | | | | ALL | |
	SCC	ACC	Carcin	ME	Misc	Pap	Chon	Leio	GCT	Misc	Total	HM
Pearson and others[55]	9	28	0	0	5	0	1	0	0	1	44	12.8%
Grillo and Mathisen[24]	70	80	11	4	11	5	2	2	2	11	198	5%
Perelman and others[56]	21	66	20	5	13	2	0	1	0	17	144	15%
Regnard and others[60]	94	65	9	5	8	2	5	5	3	12	208	10.5%
Rafaely and Weissberg[59]	5	13	2	0	0	0	0	1	0	1	22	4.5%
Total	199	252	42	14	37	9	8	9	5	42		
% Total	32.3%	40.9%	6.8%	2.3%	6%	1.5%	1.3%	1.5%	0.8%	6.8%		

SCC, squamous cell carcinoma; ACC, adenoid cystic carcinoma; Carcin, carcinoid; ME, mucoepidermoid tumors (low and high grade); Misc, miscellaneous; Pap, papilloma; Chon, chondroma; Leio, leiomyoma; GCT, granular cell tumor; HM, hospital mortality for surgical resection.

tend to be biologically more aggressive.[44] Granular cell tumors are not encapsulated and have a tendency to invade locally. Approximately one-third of these tumors show extraluminal growth, and in a few patients pure extraluminal growth with no endo-bronchial component has been described. Malignant degeneration occurs in 1% to 2% of all granular cell tumors, but it has never been reported for a tracheal granular cell tumor.[5] Daniel and colleagues,[8] after a review of the literature on this tumor, recommend bronchoscopic resection of tumors smaller than or equal to 8 mm in maximal diameter. Granular cell tumors larger than 8 mm have a high likelihood of full-thickness wall involvement and subsequent recurrence after bronchoscopic removal, and these should be managed with segmental tracheal resection.

Chondroma

Chondromas are the most common benign mes-enchymal tracheal tumors.[24,55,56,59,60] These tumors are cartilaginous and they tend to be hard, smooth, broad-based, and covered by intact mucosa. The most common site of origin is the internal aspect of the pos-terior cricoid lamina.[15] Within the trachea, they occur with equal frequency at all levels. Calcification is seen in 75% of patients radiographically, although this will not distinguish a chondroma from its malignant coun-terpart, tracheal chondrosarcoma, into which chon-dromas may degenerate.[62] Incomplete endoscopic resection leads to recurrence, and thus segmental tra-cheal resection is recommended.

Leiomyoma

Tracheal leiomyomas originate from the smooth mus-cle of the tracheal wall, typically from the membra-nous portion of the lower third of the trachea.[12] These tumors grow as a smoothly contoured, polypoid mass and usually have a broad base. Death from bleeding has been reported during bronchoscopic excision, and incomplete resection leads to recurrence.[44] Thus, segmental tracheal resection is recommended.

Hemangioma

Hemangiomas of the airway occur in adults and chil-dren. In adults, cavernous hemangiomas develop in the larynx, whereas capillary hemangiomas originate in the subglottal trachea. Hemangiomas of the trachea occur more often in children, and in children they are the most common subglottal mass causing airway obstruction.[44] These lesions are asymptomatic at birth, but within 6 months most will produce symp-toms of inspiratory stridor. A cutaneous hemangioma is also present in one-half of affected infants.

In the airway, capillary hemangiomas develop within the submucosa and are covered by normal res-piratory epithelium. They are typically located on the posterior or posterolateral aspect of the subglottal tra-chea, are smooth, bluish in color, and project into the airway from a sessile base. Most of these sponta-neously regress by 2 to 3 years of age, and close obser-vation is usually advocated. In highly symptomatic patients, successful shrinkage using radiation, steroids, and laser ablation has been reported.

Miscellaneous Benign Primary Tumors

A variety of other benign tracheal tumors have been reported including adenomas, myoepithelial cell tumors, lipomas, fibromas, schwannomas, neurilemo-mas, hemangiomas, paragangliomas, fibrous histiocy-tomas, neurofibromas, chrondoblastomas, benign mucoepidermoid tumors, angiofibromas, xanthomas, myoblastomas, hamartomas, glomus tumors, intratra-cheal goiters, and chemodectomas.* All combined,

---

*References 7, 24, 34, 55, 56, 59, 60, 63.

these tumors represent fewer than 10% of all primary tracheal tumors. Treatment for these diverse tumors is generally surgical excision, although some may be successfully managed with endoscopic resection.

MALIGNANT PRIMARY TRACHEAL NEOPLASMS

In adults, the majority of primary tracheal tumors are malignant. Typically, malignant lesions have a shorter duration of symptoms than benign lesions, are larger in size, and exhibit an irregular surface. In most large series, more than 80% of primary malignant tracheal neoplasms are histologically either squamous cell carcinoma or adenoid cystic carcinoma.[24,55,56,59,60]

Squamous Cell Carcinoma

In adults, the most common primary tracheal neoplasm is squamous cell carcinoma (Figure 108-1).[16,39,72] However, these lesions are often unresectable at diagnosis, and for this reason in surgical series the majority of malignant tumors are adenoid cystic carcinomas.[24,55,56,59,60] Men are four times more likely to develop this cancer than are women, and the average age of patients is 50 to 60 years. Nearly 100% of those who develop this tumor have a history of cigarette smoking, and synchronous or metachronous respiratory tract malignancies occur in 40% of these patients.[24] Commonly, these tumors demonstrate exophytic growth with ulceration. Sputum cytology results are positive for cancer in nearly one-half of patients. The lateral tracheal wall is often involved by these tumors, although when a squamous cell carcinoma involving the membranous tracheal wall is found, invasion from a primary esophageal tumor should always be considered.

Squamous cell cancers of the trachea are lethal, biologically aggressive tumors that tend to grow rapidly and metastasize early. In the series by Grillo and Mathisen,[24] 45% of patients had tumors that were unresectable, and of those resected, 23% had positive mediastinal lymph nodes. They reported that mediastinal lymph node involvement and the presence of invasive carcinoma at the resection margins were major determinants of poor long-term prognosis. Complete resection with postoperative radiation therapy is the procedure of choice for resectable tumors. Incomplete resection typically leads to recurrence within 2 years and death within 4 years. Overall 5-year survival rate for patients who undergo resection ranges from 13% to 47% in reported series.

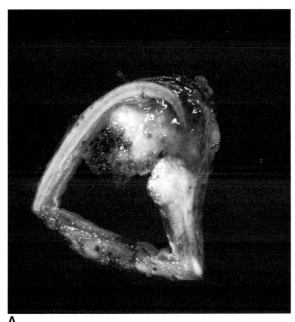
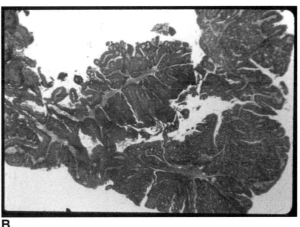

Figure 108-1. A, Cross section of trachea through a tracheal squamous cell carcinoma. The bulk of the mass is intraluminal, with focal growth through the tracheal cartilage and into the adventitial soft tissue. **B,** Histopathologic examination of tracheal squamous cell carcinoma showing a papillary growth pattern, with constituent atypical squamous cells (hematoxylin and eosin, ×40). (Reprinted with permission from *The Journal of Thoracic and Cardiovascular Surgery,* Vol 120 (1), Patterson GA, Campbell DB, Clinical-pathologic conference in thoracic surgery: basaloid squamous carcinoma of the trachea, p. 187–193, 2000.)

Adenoid Cystic Carcinoma

Adenoid cystic carcinomas, previously referred to as *cylindromas,* were first described by Billroth in 1859. These tumors can be seen in all age groups. They usually arise in the trachea or main bronchi and thus frequently are symptomatic, although many patients experience symptoms for more than a year before the diagnosis is secured. There is no association with sex, race, or cigarette smoking. Adenoid cystic carcinomas are nonencapsulated, slow-growing, low-grade malignant tumors that originate from the epithelium of the glands lining the mucosa of the respiratory tract. Adenoid cystic carcinomas are known to push mediastinal structures aside rather than invade them. Despite being slow growing, these tumors unfortunately show a predilection for perineural, submucosal, and distant metastatic spread. Frequently, resection margins are histologically positive well away from grossly apparent tumor. In such circumstances, postoperative radiation therapy has been used and associated with long-term survival.

Treatment consists of surgical resection with preoperative radiation frequently given for large tumors. Complete resection is optimal but can only be performed in approximately 60% of cases. Despite the relentless progression of unresectable residual tumor, prolonged survival with minimal morbidity is often obtainable.[6,29] Although controversial because of the prolonged survival seen even with unresectable disease, pulmonary metastases are not considered a contraindication to tracheal resection in otherwise operable patients.[43,60] Unfortunately, however, even in presumed complete resection, late local recurrence often occurs leading to death. Distant metastases to lung, liver, bone, and brain may be detected. Overall 5-year survival rate is around 70% in the reported series.

Other Malignant Primary Tracheal Tumors

Besides adenoid cystic carcinoma and squamous cell carcinomas, a variety of other malignant trachea tumors have been reported. All combined, these tumors represent approximately 14% of primary tracheal tumors.[24,55,56,59,60] Of this diverse group, carcinoids and mucoepidermoid carcinomas are the most frequent. Less commonly seen malignant primary tracheal tumors are seen in Table 108-1.

Carcinoid Tumors

Carcinoid tumors develop from the argyrophilic Kulchitsky's cells that are present in the airway mucosa. Carcinoids are actually now considered part of a range of neuroendocrine tumors, with small cell lung cancers being the most aggressive. Based on this realization these tumors have been categorized as neuroendocrine grade I (typical carcinoid), grade II (atypical carcinoid), and grade III (small or large cell undifferentiated neuroendocrine carcinoma).[53]

Typical carcinoids are associated with slow growth and infrequent metastases. Atypical carcinoids demonstrate aggressive biologic behavior and characteristic malignant histologic features, including nuclear abnormalities, mitotic activity, and necrosis. The majority of patients with atypical carcinoids will have lymph node or distant metastases at the time of diagnosis. Small cell carcinoma of the trachea is rare and usually unresectable at diagnosis.

The diagnosis of carcinoid tumors depends on histologic confirmation. Bronchoscopy can often be used to obtain tissue; however, these tumors have a tendency to bleed profusely so biopsy in the operating room using a rigid bronchoscope may be preferred. The typical bronchoscopic appearance has been described as "mulberry-like."[29]

The treatment of choice for tracheal carcinoids without mediastinal lymph node involvement is surgical resection. Aggressive atypical carcinoids are often treated as small cell lung cancers, and responses to chemotherapy and radiation therapy have been seen. Small cell carcinoma of the trachea has an extremely poor prognosis despite management with combined chemotherapy and radiation.

Mucoepidermoid Carcinoma

At bronchoscopy, mucoepidermoid carcinomas of the trachea appear as pink, polypoid masses that can be confused with a carcinoid tumor. Mucoepidermoid carcinomas are derived from minor salivary gland tissue of the proximal tracheobronchial tree.[75] Based on mitotic activity, level of necrosis, and nuclear pleomorphism, these tumors are classified as low or high grade. Low-grade tumors behave in a benign fashion, whereas high-grade mucoepidermoid carcinomas progress rapidly. Bronchoscopic biopsy provides the diagnosis, and treatment is surgical resection, when possible. Adenosquamous carcinomas are pathologically similar to mucoepidermoid carcinomas and have an aggressive course.[29]

SECONDARY TRACHEAL TUMORS

Secondary tracheal tumors arise either from direct extension from other primaries or from metastatic spread to the airways. Direct tumor extension from adjacent organs is more frequent than metastatic spread and most commonly occurs from tumors of the lung, esophagus, thyroid, mediastinum, and head and neck. Of the tumors that involve the trachea by direct extension, only lung and thyroid have any chance for cure with surgical resection. Tracheal invasion by thyroid cancer occurs in 1% to 6.5% of patients with thyroid cancer, and airway obstruction represents the most common cause of death in these patients.[49] At the time of thyroidectomy, tumor adherent to the trachea should not be "shaved off" the airway; rather, a complete tracheal resection and reconstruction should be undertaken. Grillo[20] reports effective palliation and occasional cure with aggressive tracheal resection, particularly when the trachea is invaded by well-differentiated thyroid cancer. In a series reported by Ishihara and others,[31] complete resection was associated with an improved 5-year survival rate (78%) compared with those patients who had an incomplete resection (44%), and thus the authors recommended aggressive complete resection whenever possible. This may necessitate cervicomediastinal exenteration, with resection of the involved trachea, larynx, and esophagus, esophageal replacement by colon or stomach, and formation of an end tracheostomy for cure.[49] Anaplastic thyroid cancer and lymphomas with extension to the trachea should not be treated by surgical resection.

Carcinoma of the lung invades the trachea either by proximal extension of a primary tumor within a mainstem bronchus or from involved paratracheal or subcarinal lymph nodes. Aggressive tracheal and carinal resections are warranted in patients without mediastinal lymph node involvement.

Invasion of the trachea by esophageal carcinomas, mediastinal malignant neoplasms, or head and neck cancers are not considered for surgical resection because they have not been shown to benefit from surgical intervention and their outcome is universally poor. Therapy for these tumors is palliative, and management options include radiotherapy, chemotherapy, stents, and other endoscopic techniques.

The most common metastatic tumors to the airway include renal cell carcinoma, sarcomas, breast cancer, and colon cancer.[70] Melanomas can represent a primary tumor of the trachea or more commonly can be metastatic to the trachea. Rarely tumors of the uterus, testes, and adrenal gland have reportedly metastasized to the trachea. Metastatic tumors involving the trachea can cause airway compromise by direct invasion and endoluminal obstruction or by extrinsic compression of the trachea. Determining the cause of the obstruction is crucial in directing treatment. Metastatic lesions to the trachea are incurable and treated palliatively.

DIAGNOSIS
Symptoms, Signs, and Physical Examination

Tracheal masses are often not diagnosed until months or years after the onset of symptoms, and frequently are large when discovered. Tracheal masses grow silently and do not produce symptoms until the lumen

of the airway is narrowed by approximately 75%.[44] Adding to the typical delay in diagnosis is the fact that tracheal tumors are extremely uncommon, and the initial symptoms often mimic those of common disorders such as asthma or chronic bronchitis.

The most common symptom in a patient with a tracheal tumor with significant airway narrowing is exertional dyspnea. Other common symptoms of tracheal lesions include stridor, wheezing, cough, difficulty clearing secretions, recurrent pneumonia, hemoptysis, and hoarseness.[70] Hoarseness is usually the result of reduced air flow across the vocal cords, although it can also indicate recurrent laryngeal nerve involvement. Systemic symptoms including weakness, weight loss, and dysphagia may be seen with metastatic tumors and are a poor prognostic sign.

Physical examination in a patient with a tracheal tumor may be unrevealing, but stridor, wheezing, bronchial breath sounds, increased accessory muscle use, signs of obstructive pneumonia, or subtle alteration in the timber of the voice may be present with significant narrowing of the airway.[70] A clue that the symptoms are not caused by asthma is the primarily inspiratory and often paradoxical nature of the dyspnea, which may occur when the patient lies down, often producing a suffocating sensation. A history of another primary neoplasm in the setting of airway obstructive symptoms suggests direct extension or metastatic spread and should prompt evaluation.

Radiographic Evaluation

In general, the diagnosis of a tracheal tumor requires a high index of suspicion and appropriate confirmatory radiographic studies. A posteroanterior and lateral chest radiograph will identify an obstructing tracheal lesion in one-quarter to one-half of the cases.[44] Findings on a plain chest radiograph suggesting a tracheal tumor include the presence of a mass and narrowing, distortion, or disruption of the tracheal air column (Figure 108-2). Direct extension from an adjacent primary may be detected.

Chest CT scans are an important part of the evaluation of a tracheal tumor. In addition to demonstrating the degree of luminal compromise, CT is excellent for assessing mediastinal tumor extension and nodal or metastatic disease (Figure 108-3). Inspiratory and expiratory CT scans can help clarify dynamic states such as tracheomalacia, and spiral CT with three-dimensional reconstruction is useful in the evaluation and management planning of complex lesions involving the carina.[52]

In many patients, a CT scan can suggest the histologic type of the tumor. The presence of fat and calcification within a tracheal mass is virtually pathognomonic of a hamartoma.[44] Marked enhancement of a tracheal lesion

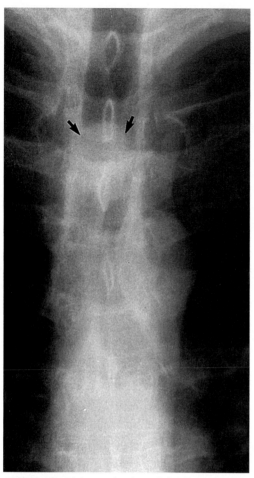

Figure 108-2. Careful examination of the tracheal air column seen in this standard posteroanterior chest radiograph demonstrates an oval mass nearly obstructing the trachea (*arrows*).

after intravenous contrast administration suggests a carcinoid tumor.[37]

In other patients, CT scans may provide clues to the benign or malignant nature of a tracheal tumor. Features suggestive of a benign lesion by CT scan include an intraluminal tumor with limited spread along the tracheal wall, a well-circumscribed lesion with a smooth or lobulated appearance, and a size usually smaller than 2 cm.[68] Calcification suggests a cartilaginous lesion, but it does not rule out malignancy. Features suggestive of a malignant tracheal lesion include an irregular surface with extension over variable lengths of the trachea, extramural extension into the mediastinum, lesions larger than 2 cm, circumferential tracheal involvement, and enlarged mediastinal lymph nodes.[68]

CT scans are unreliable for delineating the submucosal spread of disease, and thus they will underestimate the longitudinal dimensions of a tumor. This is particularly true for adenoid cystic carcinoma, which has a propensity for submucosal spread well beyond the limits of the gross pathologic tumor. Furthermore, since adenoid cystic carcinomas tend to grow slowly and push mediastinal structures away rather than invade them, the CT finding of a loss of fat planes between the tumor and mediastinal structures is a poor predictor of actual invasion with this tumor.[44]

Magnetic resonance imaging (MRI) has been used in the evaluation of tracheal tumors. Coronal, axial, and oblique sagittal planes can demonstrate the superior or inferior extent of a tumor and its relationship to adjacent mediastinal structures. One area in which MRI has shown promise recently has been in the

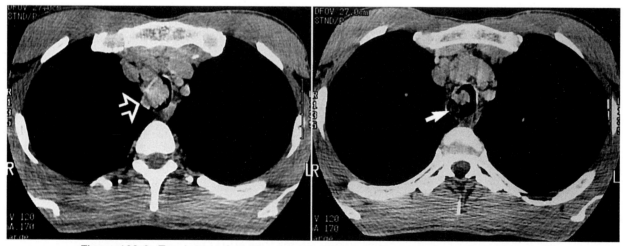

Figure 108-3. Two images from the computed tomography scan of a patient with what proved to be a tracheal hamartoma demonstrate the degree of tracheal luminal obstruction by the tumor and its attachment to the right lateral tracheal wall. Although the right lateral tracheal wall is deformed by the tumor (*open arrow*), there is no invasion beyond the wall. Fat (*closed arrow*) within the tumor suggests the diagnosis of hamartoma.

detection of tracheal invasion by thyroid carcinoma.[67] In general, however, MRI offers little advantage over CT unless vascular or cardiac invasion is suspected.[68]

Pulmonary Function Testing

Pulmonary function tests can suggest an upper airway obstruction and occasionally can lead to the diagnosis of a tracheal lesion. Characteristic findings include a severe reduction in peak expiratory flow rate and maximal breathing capacity, with relative preservation of vital capacity and forced expiratory volume in 1 second.[2] Flow-volume loops may show flattening of the inspiratory or expiratory curve.

Bronchoscopy

Bronchoscopy represents the mainstay of diagnosis for tracheal tumors and is a necessary step in the examination of patients with these neoplasms. Capabilities for rigid bronchoscopy are essential, particularly in those with proximal tracheal tumors. Biopsy and manipulation of a tracheal tumor with flexible bronchoscopy are potentially hazardous because they may precipitate bleeding or total obstruction of an already compromised airway. The combination of flexible and rigid bronchoscopy allows biopsy of the tumor, precise measurement of tracheal length, identification of tumor extension, and determination of the proximity of the tumor to the larynx or carina. Mucosal extension of the tumor may be suggested by evidence of inflammation or erythema above or below the lesion.[70]

Our preference for initial evaluation is transnasal or transoral flexible fiberoptic bronchoscopy using topical anesthesia and intravenous sedation. Patients with nonobstructing distal tracheal tumors can be intubated after the induction of general anesthesia and then can undergo biopsy and evaluation with the flexible bronchoscope. Patients with large proximal tracheal tumors are best treated by the induction of general anesthesia with inhalational agents and intravenous sedatives followed by the evaluation of the airway with a rigid bronchoscope. Rigid bronchoscopy is preferred when tracheal tumors are causing subtotal obstruction because ventilation can be maintained through the bronchoscope. In addition to maintaining ventilation, the rigid bronchoscope can be used to dilate and core-out the malignant lesion, providing stabilization of the airway. Tumor bleeding, although a concern, is rarely a problem with rigid bronchoscopy because the bronchoscope can be used to apply pressure to the site; alternatively, cautery or laser treatment can be used to control bleeding.

TREATMENT

Appropriate treatment of a tracheal tumor begins with a careful assessment of the overall situation. Coexistent medical disorders, especially cardiopulmonary disease, should be evaluated and optimized. Pneumonia should be cleared, and the airway should be stabilized, if necessary, with rigid and flexible bronchoscopic techniques. Importantly, tracheal tumors once symptomatic can rapidly progress to critical airway obstruction. Tracheal luminal diameters larger than 10 mm are typically asymptomatic, even with activities, although exertional dyspnea usually manifests at a tracheal diameter of 8 mm and worsens rapidly with any further decrease in diameter.[2] Stridor is present at rest when the tracheal diameter is narrowed to 5 mm or smaller. Acute decompensation can occur with minimal edema or secretions.

Primary Malignant Tracheal Tumors

The majority of adult tracheal tumors are malignant, and when feasible, surgical excision with circumferential tracheal resection and primary end-to-end reconstruction represents the best therapy. Limitations to resectability include the invasion of critical mediastinal structures and involvement of such an extensive length of trachea that reconstruction would be impossible. Patients with tracheal squamous cell carcinoma who are potential candidates for resection require mediastinoscopy. If metastatic disease is detected in superior mediastinal nodes, the likelihood of complete resection and long-term survival is remote. In these patients, resection should not be undertaken. These patients are treated better with combination chemoradiotherapy. If the results of the mediastinoscopy are negative, resection should proceed immediately. Anterior mobilization of the lower cervical and entire thoracic trachea will already have been accomplished by the mediastinoscopy. In contrast, the presence of metastatic disease in regional mediastinal nodes in patients with adenoid cystic carcinoma does not have a clear impact on survival rate and should not preclude resection. Furthermore, Pearson and colleagues[55] have noted that many patients with adenoid cystic carcinoma remain asymptomatic from pulmonary metastases for years, and thus patients with synchronous pulmonary metastases should not be considered inoperable if their primary tracheal adenoid cystic carcinomas are resectable.

Anesthetic Management

Patients with tracheal tumors present major challenges in airway management. Before surgical resection of tracheal tumors, flexible and rigid bronchoscope techniques are used to stabilize the airway, if necessary. Surgery should then be undertaken in a short time span to prevent the tumor from reobstructing the airway. A mixture of inhalational and intravenous sedation is used, allowing spontaneous ventilation while the airway is secured.[70] Tracheostomy is unwarranted and detrimental in patients with tracheal tumors because stomal placement may interfere subsequently with ideal positioning of the tracheal anastomosis.

After intubation, the next challenge in airway management occurs during tracheal division and reconstruction. After transecting the trachea, ventilation can be maintained by one of three methods: (1) advance the endotracheal tube down into the distal trachea across the transected portion of the airway; (2) pass a small jet ventilation catheter either down the endotracheal tube or across the sterile field and into the distal airway; or (3) directly intubate the distal airway using a sterile, wire-reinforced endotracheal tube connected to sterile, corrugated plastic ventilator tubing brought across the field. For patients with distal tracheal lesions, it may be necessary to intubate the left or right mainstem bronchus individ-

ually, with intermittent inflation of the opposite lung if the oxygen saturation decreases as a result of persistent blood flow through the atelectic lung (shunt). These patients require close monitoring with digital pulse oximetry and frequent arterial blood gases. Cardiopulmonary bypass is hazardous and unnecessary in nearly all patients.[20]

Surgical Management: Tracheal Resection and Primary Reconstruction

A low-collar incision provides access to the cervical and the upper two-thirds of the intrathoracic trachea. If necessary, additional exposure can be obtained by adding a partial or complete sternotomy. Tumors of the distal third of the trachea are approached through a right posterolateral thoracotomy (usually at the fourth interspace) or through a sternotomy. When the carina is involved, a median sternotomy may be preferable for exposure (Figure 108-4).[24,36,55]

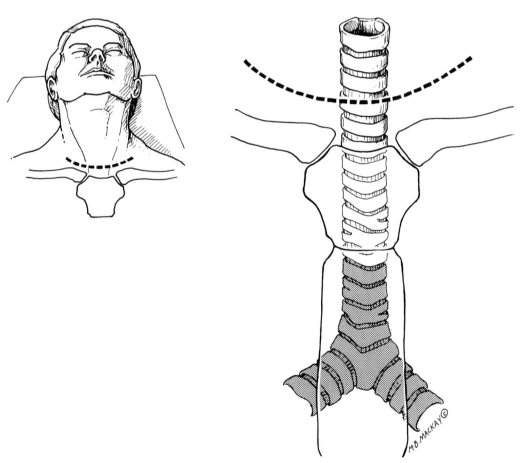

Figure 108-4. Location of cervical incision used for cervical and upper one-half to two-thirds of the mediastinal trachea (unshaded area). The distal trachea and carina (shaded area) requires either a median sternotomy or right posterolateral thoracotomy. (Reprinted with permission from F. Griffith Pearson, Joel D. Cooper, Jean Deslauriers, Robert J. Ginsberg, Clement A. Hiebert, G. Alexander Patterson, & Harold C. Urschel, Jr.: *Thoracic surgery.* Churchill Livingstone , 2002, Figure 19-32; p 407.)

When using a cervical incision, subplatysmal skin flaps are created and the strap muscles are divided in the midline to expose the anterior trachea. The trachea is then mobilized and brought into the incision, and the site of resection is determined. During mobilization of the trachea, care is taken to preserve the blood supply, which enters laterally. In patients with benign tumors, the dissection is kept immediately adjacent to the trachea, and no attempt is made to isolate or identify the recurrent laryngeal nerves. Resections for malignant tumors require identification and preservation of the recurrent laryngeal nerves, if possible. If one recurrent laryngeal nerve is involved with tumor, it should be sacrificed. Sacrifice of both recurrent laryngeal nerves requires concomitant tracheostomy and a subsequent vocal cord-lateralizing procedure. Paratracheal nodes are excised with malignant tumors to the extent possible without compromising the blood supply to the remaining trachea.

Care is taken during resection to prevent anastomotic tension. In optimal circumstances, approximately half the trachea can be resected and a primary anastomosis can still be performed without undue tension,[22] but advanced patient age and prior mediastinal radiation may impose restrictions on tracheal resections because of the loss of tissue resiliency. Before complete division and resection of the involved airway, stay sutures are placed in the remaining proximal and distal ends to facilitate alignment and to gauge tension. The proximal endotracheal tube is pulled back and the distal trachea is intubated for ventilation. Resection margins should be assessed by intraoperative frozen section. Unfortunately, it may not be possible to determine the necessary extent of resection until after the airway is open.

After completion of the tracheal resection, the patient's neck is flexed and a primary anastomosis constructed using interrupted simple sutures (4-0 Vicryl), preferably with the knots on the outside (Figure 108-5). After placement of the posterior membranous sutures, the patient's oral endotracheal tube is readvanced across the anastomosis and the distal endotracheal tube is removed. The anterior tracheal wall sutures are then placed. All intrathoracic anastomoses should be wrapped to interpose tissue between the suture line and adjacent pulmonary or systemic vessels. Frequently, either pedicled pleura or pericardial fat is used, although omentum is recommended when there has been previous mediastinal irradiation.[24] A drain is usually placed alongside the anastomosis and brought out through a separate stab incision in the neck. If there is any doubt about the viability of the anastomosis, a Montgomery T-tube can be placed across it. The incision is then closed by reapproximation of the strap muscles, the platysma, and the skin.

To reduce tension on the anastomosis, cervical flexion is maintained with a heavy (No. 2) monofilament "guardian" stitch between the chin and the anterior chest wall. It is left in place for approximately 7 days and is usually removed after confirmation of anastomotic healing by bronchoscopy (Figure 108-6).

Preferably, and if deemed appropriate, the patient is extubated in the operating room. However, the presence of edema may preclude this, and an uncuffed endotracheal tube should be used in these situations. The patient is taken to the intensive care unit for postoperative management. Yearly follow-up bronchoscopy should be performed for life, particularly in patients with adenoid cystic carcinoma, because recurrences have been identified more than 25 years after tracheal resection.[35]

Release Maneuvers

If it becomes apparent that the necessary amount of tracheal resection will place the anastomosis under tension, various mobilization and release techniques can be performed to provide additional tracheal length. For resections involving the cervical trachea, the easiest maneuver is simple neck flexion and dissection along the anterior trachea in the neck and mediastinum. An additional 2 to 3 cm of tracheal length can be obtained by performing either a suprathyroid[9] or suprahyoid[48] laryngeal release. These procedures allow the larynx to drop down, thus providing additional mobility and tracheal length. Of the two procedures, the suprahyoid is preferred because it involves a lower incidence of swallowing complications postoperatively.[36] For thoracic tracheal and carinal resections, these release maneuvers are generally not very useful. In these cases, dissection of the left main bronchus along its anterior surface (taking care to avoid lateral blood supply) will provide slightly more mobility and is easily performed. Intrapericardial hilar release maneuvers are also used and can be effective in obtaining an additional 2 cm of tracheal length by elevating the carina. The right hilar release is performed by making a U-shaped incision in the pericardium beneath the inferior pulmonary vein and incising the intrapericardial septum, which joins the lateral aspect of the atrium and inferior vena cava to the pericardium (Figure 108-7). Even more mobility can be obtained by incising the pericardium around the hilar vessels. While this release maneuver can be performed on the left, the left mainstem bronchus is relatively fixed by its relationship with the aortic arch. The performance of the maneuver on the left is basically the same, except there is no intrapericardial septum to divide and the ductus arteriosus should be

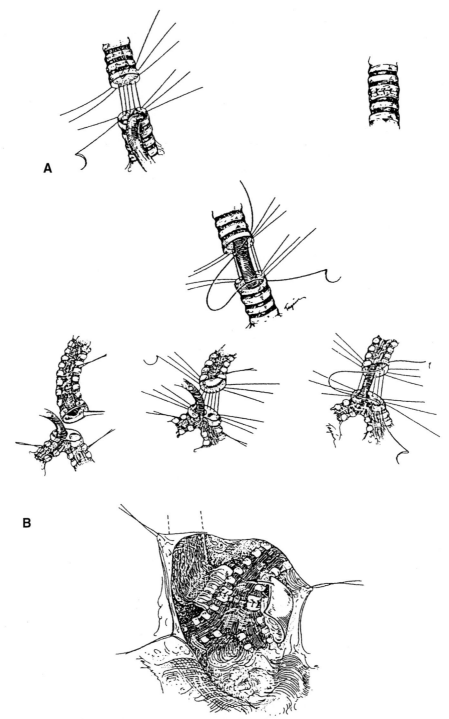

Figure 108-5. A, A tumor of the upper trachea has been excised, and the proximal and distal ends of the trachea are mobilized (although not circumferentially, as suggested in this diagram). Interrupted simple sutures are placed with the knots on the outside. Ventilation is accomplished initially across the field with intubation of the distal airway. Subsequently, as the anastomosis nears completion, the endotracheal tube is advanced across the anastomosis. **B,** A tumor of the distal trachea is excised, and ventilation is maintained by selective intubation of the left mainstem bronchus across the field. After suture placement, the endotracheal tube is advanced across the anastomosis and into the left mainstem bronchus. The completed anastomosis is wrapped with a pleural flap. (From Grillo HC: *Thorax* 28:667, 1973.)

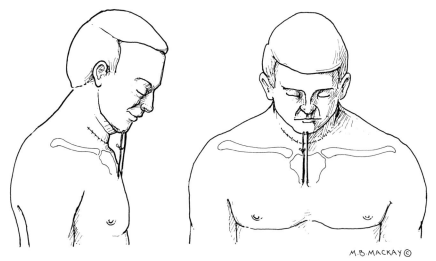

Figure 108-6. Guardian stitch is placed at the end of the operation to maintain neck flexion for the first postoperative week. (Reprinted with permission from F. Griffith Pearson, Joel D. Cooper, Jean Deslauriers, Robert J. Ginsberg, Clement A. Hiebert, G. Alexander Patterson, & Harold C. Urschel, Jr.: *Thoracic surgery,* Churchill Livingstone, 2002, p 411, Figure 19-38.)

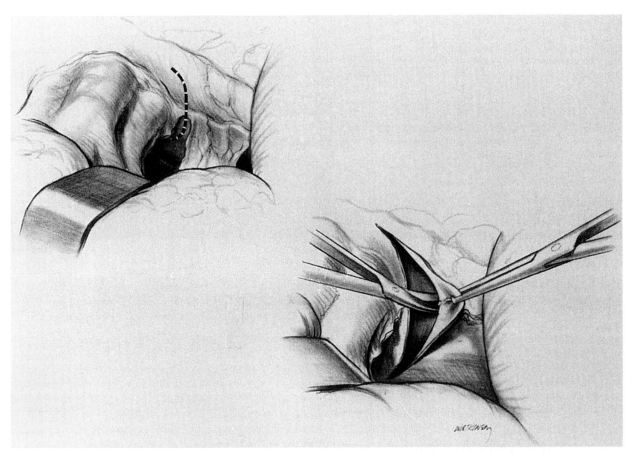

Figure 108-7. Right hilar release is accomplished by creating a U-shaped incision beneath the right inferior pulmonary vein and by then incising the septum joining the lateral aspect of the atrium and inferior vena cava to the pericardium. (Reproduced with permission from Urschel HC Jr., Cooper JD: *Atlas of thoracic surgery*, New York, 1995, Churchill Livingstone.)

transected. Although seldom necessary, an additional 2.7 cm of tracheal length can be obtained through division of the proximal left mainstem bronchus and reimplantation into the bronchus intermedius. Obviously, this increases the complexity and the potential morbidity of the operation.

Subglottal Resections

Tumors that involve the subglottal region require precise surgical intervention to prevent permanent recurrent laryngeal nerve damage and vocal cord injury. In selected patients, tumors of the subglottal airway can be managed by excision of the anterior cricoid arch and the posterior cricoid plate leaving its perichondrium in place. A primary thyrotracheal anastomosis is then performed, usually within 1 cm of the inferior border of the vocal cords with preservation of intact recurrent laryngeal nerves (Figure 108-8).[54] Resectional management of well-differentiated thyroid carcinomas invading the trachea may require complex reconstruction.[26]

Although rarely necessary, techniques for cervical exenteration have been described. Occasionally these techniques may be useful in the palliation of strangulating tumors. Rarely, this drastic technique can be curative.[23]

Carinal Resections

Tumors involving the carinal present major technical challenges. Again, the need for a tension-free anastomosis is critical. In carinal resections, tumors involving more than 4 cm of tracheal length usually preclude resection.[70] The complexities of carinal

resection and the options for reconstruction were well reviewed by Grillo in 1982[19] (Figure 108-9). After carinal resection, the simplest technique for reconstruction involves approximating the medial walls of the right and left mainstem bronchi to fashion a new carina and then anastomosing this to the distal trachea (Figure 108-10). This technique is applicable only with small tumors, which require limited tracheal resection. The fixation of the left mainstem bronchus by the aorta limits the ability to approximate the ends of the airway in most patients. More commonly, the trachea is anastomosed end-to-end to one of the mainstem bronchi, and the other mainstem bronchus is sutured into the lateral wall of the trachea above the first anastomosis (Figure 108-11).

Adjuvant Radiotherapy

Adjuvant radiotherapy is recommended for both squamous cell carcinomas and adenoid cystic carcinomas.[41] Grillo and Mathisen[24] reported that resection combined with irradiation tripled survival time for patients with squamous cell carcinoma and at least tripled survival for adenoid cystic carcinoma. Adenoid cystic carcinomas are especially sensitive to radiation therapy.[24,41] Radiation therapy is usually commenced approximately 4 weeks after surgical resection. Before initiating, radiation bronchoscopy is performed to assess adequacy of healing.[41] Regnard and colleagues[60] reported adjuvant radiotherapy significantly improved survival in patients with an incomplete resection (positive margins). For this reason, they concluded that, given the narrow margins often obtainable with tracheal resection, adjuvant radiation

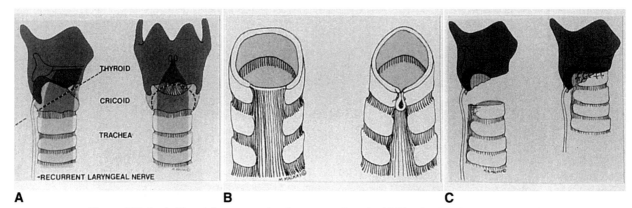

A   **B**   **C**

Figure 108-8. A, The oblique resection line across the cricoid. The line begins anteriorly at the inferior border of the thyroid cartilage and extends posteriorly through the lower border of the cricoid plate below the entry of the recurrent laryngeal nerve. **B,** Diagrammatic appearance of the distal tracheal resection line. The membranous trachea is plicated to approximate the ends of the uppermost tracheal ring and to produce a complete circle of cartilage to replace the resected cricoid ring. **C,** Completed thyrotracheal anastomosis with the distal trachea "telescoped" in front of the shell of residual cricoid cartilage. (From Pearson FG and others: *J Thorac Cardiovasc Surg* 70:806, 1975.)

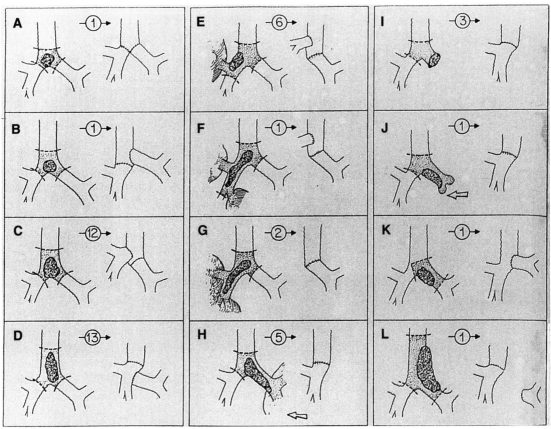

Figure 108-9. Alternatives for carinal resection and reconstruction. Circled number is number of patients. Open arrows indicate side of approach when not conventionally right-sided. **A,** Limited resection permits carinal restitution. **B,** Technique used in initial carinal resection; technique in **A** would now be used. **C,** More extensive resection. **D,** Greater length of trachea. Technique of Barclay and others. **E,** Involvement of right mainstem bronchus and right upper lobe bronchus requires right upper lobectomy. **F,** Middle lobe also removed. Right lower lobe bronchus may be anastomosed to left mainstem bronchus. **G,** Right carinal pneumonectomy. **H,** Left carinal pneumonectomy. **I,** Resection of carina after previous left pneumonectomy. **J,** Resection of carina with extra-long stump. **K,** Wedge removal of left mainstem bronchus from the right. **L,** Tracheocarinal resection with long segment of left mainstem bronchus. Exclusion of remaining left lung from the right. Left pneumonectomy also through bilateral thoracotomy. (From the Society of Thoracic Surgeons: *Ann Thorac Surg* 49:69, 1990.)

should be given to all patients with squamous or adenoid cystic carcinoma. In adenoid cystic carcinomas, Maziak and colleagues[43] reported no significant difference in survival among patients undergoing presumably curative resection with or without radiotherapy. Unfortunately, varying dosages of radiation were used, and even though no difference between the groups was detected, they still concluded it was logical to assume radiotherapy was beneficial.

BENIGN TRACHEAL TUMORS

Most benign tracheal tumors are readily managed with segmental tracheal resection and primary anastomosis. Patients with pedunculated or exophytic tumors or those with benign tumors in anatomic locations that might make resection difficult are potential candidates for endoscopic resection. Current methods of endoscopic resection include coring out and biting off the tumor with a rigid bronchoscope and biopsy forceps, cautery excision, cryoablation, and laser photocoagulation. Benign tumors most amenable to these techniques include lipomas, hamartomas, papillomas, fibromas, and small (≤8.0 mm) granular cell tumors. The base of the tumor should be ablated to reduce the incidence of recurrence, and patients with recurrence detected on a follow-up bronchoscopy should be considered for resection.

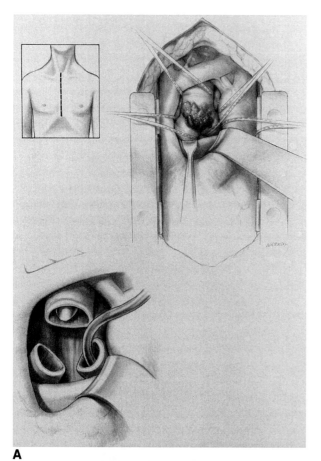

A

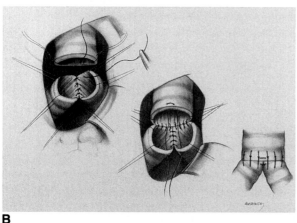

B

Figure 108-10. A, A tumor at the carina is excised. Ventilation is accomplished with a small jet ventilation catheter brought across the field and directed down the left mainstem bronchus. **B,** The medial walls of the right and left mainstem bronchi are anastomosed to form a new carina, which then is sutured to the distal trachea. (From Urschel HC Jr., Cooper JD: *Atlas of thoracic surgery*, New York, Churchill Livingstone, 1995.)

UNRESECTABLE MALIGNANT TRACHEAL TUMORS
Therapeutic Bronchoscopy

Endoscopic procedures including dilatation, mechanical débridement, laser vaporization, PDT, cryotherapy, brachytherapy, or stenting can provide palliation of unresectable obstructing tracheal tumors and metastatic lesions.[70] Of these, only stenting can provide palliation of extrinsic compression of the trachea by a malignant neoplasm; mechanical débridement, laser vaporization, PDT, cryotherapy, and brachytherapy are contraindicated for extrinsic compression. For endotracheal lesions, the optimal choice of endoscopy technique depends on the individual tumor's characteristics, and often a combination offers the best approach.[64,70] Dilation of the narrowed segment, if caused by an endobronchial component, can be dilated by passage of rigid bronchoscopes of increasing size, use of bougies, or, alternatively, balloon dilation. Gentle passage of the rigid bronchoscope past the lesion should be performed to prevent creation of false passage. Dilation, although effective, is temporizing and rarely used as the sole treatment of unresectable endobronchial tumors. One can use the rigid bronchoscope to remove large pieces of an obstructing neoplasm by running the scope against the wall of the trachea and slicing off the tumor. This is referred to commonly as *coring-out* of the tumor or *mechanical débridement.* Bleeding is controlled with compression by the rigid bronchoscope and rarely is a significant problem. If necessary, epinephrine-soaked sponges can be used topically for hemostasis.[42] For lesions that are quite vascular such as metastatic renal cell carcinoma, this technique can be combined with laser vaporization techniques, which aid in hemostasis. Laser vaporization can be used alone as a treatment of unresectable tracheal neoplasms, but this is more time consuming. Besides being hemostatic, an additional advantage of laser vaporization is that it can be performed through a flexible bronchoscope and thus with the patient under topical anesthesia. The most frequently used laser is the neodymium:yttrium-aluminum-garnet (Nd:YAG).[13] Complications with laser vaporization include airway perforation, bronchopulmonary artery fistulas, airway fires, and skin burns.

PDT is an option for endotracheal tumors, but because the edema and exudate initially worsen after a treatment, caution must be used when dealing with highly obstructing lesions. For PDT the patient is given a photosensitizer, dihematoporphyrin ether (DHE), intravenously, which is retained longer in tumor cells but is also taken up by normal cells. After 2 days the patient is then treated with an argon dye laser system (630 nm). The DHE absorbs the light

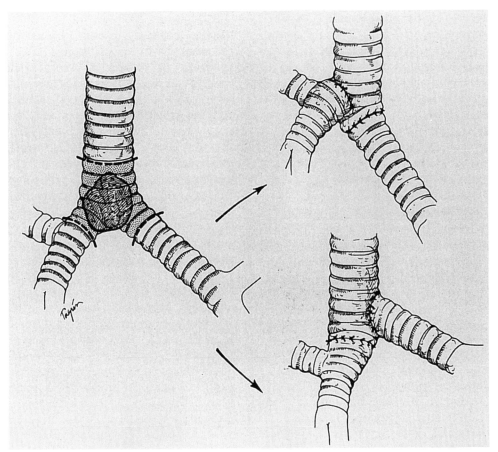

Figure 108-11. Carinal reconstruction after resection. The trachea is anastomosed end to end to either the left (most commonly) or the right mainstem bronchus, and the other bronchus is placed into the lateral wall of the trachea above the first anastomosis. (From Grillo HC: *Ann Thorac Surg* 26:112, 1978.)

energy, radical oxygen species are produced, and the destruction of tumor cells occurs through cell necrosis. PDT results in a wider radial extent of necrosis compared with mechanical débridement and laser vaporization and therefore may result in longer palliation.[11,45,46] Bronchoscopies to remove necrotic débride are usually performed on days 1 and 3 after the treatment. Retreatments can be performed at this time if residual tumor is present; this is often identified when bleeding is seen at the treated tumor sites because the necrotic sites do not bleed. PDT-like laser vaporization is a hemostatic technique causing thrombosis of small vessels and therefore can be used for highly vascular tumors. The disadvantages of PDT are photosensitivity of the patient for up to 8 weeks after DHE injection, scar and stricture formation with multiple treatments, and possibly fistula formation.[46]

Cryotherapy involves a probes placed with either rigid or flexible bronchoscopes to freeze tumor cells, resulting in necrosis. Thus, cryotherapy is similar to PDT in that it does not provide immediate relief and

can initially worsen the obstruction. Repeat bronchoscopy is necessary over the course of the next few days to débride the necrotic exudate. Also similar to PDT, cryotherapy provides extensive radial necrosis, and thus the number of repeat treatments may be lessened. Its major disadvantage lies in its complexity, time requirement, and a lack of familiarity with the procedure among most surgeons.[70]

Brachytherapy delivers high amounts of localized radiation therapy to the tumor with endotracheal catheters that are placed with flexible bronchoscopy. Large, bulky lesions do not respond well to this treatment, but it has been used on unresectable tumors with a curative intent (unlike the other bronchoscopic therapies). It is frequently used in combination with mechanical core-out or laser therapy and provides better palliation than either used alone. Usually iridium-192 is used to deliver 2 Gy/min over several minutes to provide 7 to 15 Gy at a setting. A total of two to four fractions at 1-week intervals are delivered.[73] Brachytherapy has a few significant complications, including radiation bronchitis (10%), stenosis (1%–3%), and massive hemoptysis (5%–20%).[70,73] One study found local failure, persistent malignancy, delivery of laser photocoagulation, and direct contact of the endobronchial brachytherapy applicator and the tracheobronchial walls at the vicinity of the great vessels were the most indicative indicators of a massive hemoptysis.[28]

The extension of unresectable primary malignancies that cause high-grade obstruction by external compression of the trachea are best treated with stenting. After stent placement, palliation of the neoplasm can be undertaken with chemotherapy and radiation therapy. Stenting can also be used to increase the length of palliation for endoluminal lesions treated with one of the above techniques. Different types of stents (silicone and expandable metal) are used after the advantages and disadvantages of each are weighed.[70] Solid silicone stents are more difficult to place than expandable metal stents because they require rigid bronchoscopy. However, these stents are easy to remove and, if necessary, to reposition because they do not incorporate into the surrounding tissues. In comparison, expandable metal stents can be placed with a flexible bronchoscope and they incorporate firmly into tissues and thus are difficult to remove or reposition. Carinal Y stents can provide palliation for lesions involving the distal trachea, carina, and mainstem bronchi. Complications from stent use include stent migration, erosion, ingrowth of granulation tumor, and an inability to effectively clear secretions.[70]

Radiotherapy

Radiation therapy has been used to treat patients with unresectable squamous cell carcinomas and adenoid cystic carcinomas. In a series by Grillo and Mathisen,[24] median survival time with radiation alone was 10 months and 28 months for those with squamous cell and adenoid cystic carcinoma, respectively. Jeremic and colleagues[33] reported a series of tracheal squamous cell carcinomas treated with radiation therapy alone. They use at least 60 Gy of radiation; the reported median survival was 24 months, and 5-year survival was 27%. The presence of metastasis in the mediastinal lymph nodes portended a poor survival.[33] Maziak and colleagues[43] reported six patients with unresectable adenoid cystic carcinomas who underwent primary radiotherapy with mean survivals of 74 ± 64 months. However, in this series, five of the six patients (83%) had local recurrences. Currently, radiotherapy should be considered for primary therapy only in patients with unresectable tumors or in those medically unfit to undergo surgery.

Results

Hospital mortality rates for primary tracheal tumor resection have ranged from 5% to 15%.[24,55,56,59,60] Perelman and colleagues[56] reported anastomotic failure (47%), pneumonia (33%), innominate artery erosion (10%), and pulmonary artery thromboembolism (10%) as causes for postoperative mortality. In their large series, the highest postoperative mortalities occurred in patients undergoing carinal resection and tracheal reconstruction attempts. Regnard and colleagues[60] reported 5- and 10-year survivals of 47% and 36%, respectively, for resected squamous cell carcinomas and 73% and 57% for resected adenoid cystic carcinoma, respectively.

Hospital mortality for patients who underwent tracheal resection for the invasion of a well-differentiated thyroid carcinoma in one series was 9%.[49] Of the 34 patients in this series treated with surgical resection, only two patients had airway recurrence, and 50% of patients remained alive for between 1 month and 14.5 years postoperatively (average, 5.3 years). In a series of 60 tracheal resections for thyroid cancer reported by Ishihara and colleagues,[31] complete resection was possible in 56.7% of patients. Complete resection was associated with improved long-term survival rate (78.1% at 5 years) compared with those who had an incomplete resection (40% at 5 years). Yang and colleagues[71] resected the tumors in eight patients with well-differentiated thyroid carcinoma invading the trachea, and at follow-up ranging from 14 to 183 months, five remained free of disease (three of these were followed up for more than 10 years).

Results for patients with primary lung cancer undergoing carinal resection reveal a 10% operative mortality and 5-year survival of 42%. Patients with no lymph nodes involved have a 51% 5-year survival, whereas those with positive results for mediastinal lymph node disease have only a 12% 5-year survival rate.[47]

Complications

Regnard and colleagues[60] identified four factors that were significantly associated with the development of postoperative complications: an increasing length of resection, the need for laryngeal release, laryngotracheal or carinal resection as opposed to standard tracheal resection, and squamous cell histology.

Common problems after tracheal surgery include atelectasis, retained secretions, pneumonia, and swallowing dysfunction with aspiration. Aspiration is most likely to be a problem in patients with recurrent laryngeal nerve dysfunction and in those who underwent a release procedure of the upper airway (superior laryngeal or suprahyoid technique). In many patients, the problem resolves within a few weeks, either spontaneously or with swallowing modification techniques. Vocal cord dysfunction may be transient or permanent, depending on the nature of the injury to the recurrent laryngeal nerve. Dysfunction of one vocal cord usually produces hoarseness and an impaired cough. Bilateral cord dysfunction can cause airway obstruction requiring tracheostomy.

Wound infections, particularly in the cervical area, are rare. Prompt opening and complete drainage of the wound is essential. Intrathoracic infections are potentially much more serious, particularly when an anastomotic dehiscence produces an air leak or a space within the mediastinum. Urgent and wide drainage is critical to prevent the development of mediastinitis.

Anastomotic dehiscence usually occurs as a result of excessive tension or compromised tracheal blood supply. Excessive tension occurs with overzealous tracheal resection or inadequate mobilization. Ischemia is more likely to occur in patients with previous irradiation to the area and in those who undergo extensive nodal dissection or circumferential mobilization of the airway. Acute separation can be resutured if it occurs early and if there is no necrosis or ischemia.[25] Otherwise, a tracheostomy or T-tube can be inserted across the defect.

An uncommon but lethal complication of airway surgery is tracheal-innominate or tracheal-pulmonary artery fistula formation. Fistulas can result from pressure against the innominate artery by a postoperative tracheostomy tube or by direct abrasion of the anastomosis against the innominate or pulmonary artery. To protect against fistula formation at the airway anastomosis, dissection near the brachiocephalic artery should be performed on the trachea, leaving adjacent soft tissue undisturbed on the artery itself. This will prevent most fistulas. If the artery is bared, vascularized soft tissue such as a pedicled strap muscle should be interposed between the artery and the anastomosis. Within the thorax, soft tissue, like the thymus or pericardium, should be placed between the pulmonary artery and an airway suture line. Some patients will have a "herald" bleed, and prompt exploration with bronchoscopy and opening of the wound may save these patients. Unfortunately, most patients who develop this complication suffer a sudden, fatal hemorrhage into the airway.

Late complications include the development of granulation tissue or stenosis at the anastomosis. Exuberant granulation tissue can often be extracted endoscopically with a biopsy forceps. Occasionally, granulation is a result of infection or necrosis of underlying cartilage and can be a particular problem if it involves the cricoid. When the cricoid is involved, the infection can slowly progress over many months,

and definitive management often requires operative débridement. Anastomotic stenosis developed in 5% of patients survived tracheal or carinal resection and reconstruction in the series by Grillo and Mathisen.[24] Symptomatic stenoses occurred in 14% of patients in the series reported by Regnard and colleagues,[60] and it occurred significantly more frequently among patients who had postoperative locoregional complications such as tracheal dehiscence or mediastinitis. Anastomotic stenoses can often be managed with endoscopic techniques including dilation and T-tube placement. Attempts at resection should be delayed for 4 to 6 months after the initial surgery to allow the acute inflammation to subside.[25] As noted by Grillo and colleagues,[25] the difficulties of tracheal reconstruction increase markedly with each attempt at repair, and thus conditions should be optimal. Every effort should be made at the time of the initial resection and reconstruction to avoid complications that could lead to an anastomotic stenosis.

SUMMARY

Primary tracheal tumors are rare, and in adults, most tumors are malignant. More than 80% of malignant tracheal tumors are either squamous cell carcinoma or adenoid cystic carcinoma. Tracheal tumors are best managed by resection with end-to-end anastomosis. Great care should be taken to avoid excessive tension on the anastomosis by limiting the extent of the resection and, in addition to cervical flexion, performing appropriate release procedures as necessary. Anastomotic ischemia is avoided by limiting the area of circumferential dissection, carefully preserving the lateral blood supply, and being judicious in the extent of the paratracheal lymph node excision.

Adjuvant radiotherapy is probably of benefit after resection of squamous cell and adenoid cystic carcinoma, particularly in those with positive resection margins. Radiotherapy as primary management for malignant tracheal tumors is reserved for patients medically unfit for an operation, those with unresectable airway tumors, and those with metastatic disease. Overall, the 5-year survival rate for patient with adenoid cystic carcinoma (73%) is much greater than for those with squamous cell carcinoma (47%). Management for tumors involving the trachea secondarily is in general palliative, although aggressive tracheal resection for invasive thyroid carcinoma and bronchogenic carcinoma offers a chance for cure.

REFERENCES

1. Abrikosoff AI: Myomas originating from transversely striated voluntary musculature, *Virchows Arch A* 260:215, 1926.
2. Al-Bazzaz F, Grillo HC, Kazemi H: Response to exercise in upper airway obstruction, *Am Rev Resp Dis* 111:631, 1975.

3. Belsey R: Resection and reconstruction of the intrathoraic trachea, *Br J Surg* 38:200, 1950.

4. Belsey R: Stainless steel wire suture technique in thoracic surgery, *Thorax* 1:39, 1946.

5. Burton DM, Heffner DK, Patow MC: Granular cell tumors of the trachea, *Laryngoscope* 102:807, 1992.

6. Conlan A and others: Adenoid cystic carcinoma (cylindroma) and mucoepidermoid carcinoma of the bronchus, *J Thorac Cardiovasc Surg* 76:369, 1978.

7. Cranshaw JH and others: Intramural neurofibroma of the trachea treated by multiple stents, *Thorax* 56:583, 2001.

8. Daniel TM and others: Transbronchoscopic versus surgical resection of tracheobronchial granular cell myoblastomas, *J Thorac Cardiovasc Surg* 80:898, 1980.

9. Dedo H, Fishman N: Laryngeal release and sleeve resection for tracheal stenosis, *Ann Otol Rhinol Laryngol* 78:285, 1969.

10. Dedo HH, Yu KC: CO(2) laser treatment in 244 patients with respiratory papillomas, *Laryngoscope* 111:1639, 2001.

11. Diaz-Jiminez JP and others: Efficacy and safety of photodynamic therapy versus Nd:YAG laser resection in NSCLC with airway obstruction, *Eur Resp J* 14:800, 1999.

12. Douzinas M, Sheppard MN, Lennox SC: Leiomyoma of the trachea: an unusual tumors, *J Thorac Cardiovasc Surg* 37:285, 1989.

13. Duhamel DR, Harrell II JH: Laser bronchoscopy, *Chest Surg Clin North Am* 11:769, 2001.

14. Ferguson DJ, Wild JJ, Wangensteen OH: Experimental resection of the trachea, *Surgery* 28:597, 1950.

15. Frank JL and others: Benign cartilaginous tumors of the upper airway, *J Surg Oncol* 48:69, 1991.

16. Gelder CM, Hetzel MR: Primary tracheal tumours: a national survey [comment], *Thorax* 48:688, 1993.

17. Gilbert J, Mazzarella L, Feit L: Primary tracheal tumors in the infant and adult, *Arch Otolaryngol* 58:1, 1953.

18. Goepfert H and others: Leukocyte interferon in patients with juvenile laryngeal papillomatosis, *Ann Otol Rhinol Laryngol* 91:431, 1982.

19. Grillo HC: Carinal reconstruction, *Ann Thorac Surg* 34:356, 1982.

20. Grillo HC: Notes on the windpipe, *Ann Thorac Surg* 47:9, 1989.

21. Grillo HC: Tracheal replacement: a critical review, *Ann Thorac Surg* 73:1995, 2002.

22. Grillo HC, Dignan EF, Miura T: Extensive resection and reconstruction of mediastinal trachea without prosthesis or graft: an anatomical study in man, *J Thorac Cardiovasc Surg* 48:741, 1964.

23. Grillo HC, Mathisen DJ: Cervical exenteration, *Ann Thorac Surg* 49:401, 1990.

24. Grillo HC, Mathisen DJ: Primary tracheal tumors: treatment and results, *Ann Thorac Surg* 49:69, 1990.

25. Grillo HC and others: Complications of tracheal reconstruction, *J Thorac Cardiovasc Surg* 91:322, 1986.

26. Grillo HC and others: Resectional management of thyroid carcinoma invading the airway, *Ann Thorac Surg* 54:3, 1992.

27. Grillo HC, Zannini P: Resectional management of airway invasion by thyroid carcinoma, *Ann Thorac Surg* 42:287, 1986.

28. Hara R and others: Risk factors for massive hemoptysis after endobronchial brachytherapy in patients with tracheobronchial malignancies, *Cancer* 92:2623, 2001.

29. Harpole DH: *Bronchial adenomas,* ed. 15, vol 1. Philadelphia, Saunders, 1997.

30. Ishihara T and others: Resection of thyroid carcinoma infiltrating the trachea, *Thorax* 33:378, 1978.

31. Ishihara T and others: Surgical treatment of advanced thyroid carcinoma invading the trachea, *J Thorac Cardiovasc Surg* 102:717, 1991.

32. Jensik RJ and others: Tracheal sleeve pneumonectomy for advanced carcinoma of the lung, *Surg Gynecol Obstet* 134:231, 1972.

33. Jeremic B and others: Radiotherapy for primary squamous cell carcinoma of the trachea, *Radiother Oncol* 41:135, 1996.

34. Jones TM and others: Tracheal paraganglioma: a diagnostic dilemma culminating in a complex airway management problem, *J Laryngol Otol* 115:747, 2001.

35. Keshavjee S and others: *Upper airway tumors: primary tumors.* In Pearson FG and others, editors: *Thoracic surgery,* ed. 2, vol 1. New York, 2002, Churchill Livingstone, p 347.

36. Keshavjee S, Pearson FG: *Tracheal resection.* In Pearson FG and others, editors: *Thoracic surgery,* ed. 2, vol 1. New York, 2002, Churchill Livingstone, p 405.

37. Kwong JS, Muller NL, Miller RR: Diseases of the trachea and mainstem bronchi: correlation of CT with pathologic findings, *Radiographics* 12:645, 1992.

38. Lindeberg H, Elbrond O: Malignant tumors in patients with a history of multiple laryngeal papillomas: the significance of irradiation, *Clin Otolaryngol* 16:149, 1991.

39. Manninen MP and others: Treatment of primary tracheal carcinoma in Finland in 1967-1985, *Acta Oncologica* 32:277, 1993.

40. Mathey J and others: Tracheal and tracheobronchial resections; technique and results in 20 cases, *J Thorac Cardiovasc Surg* 51:1, 1966.

41. Mathisen DJ: Tracheal tumors, *Chest Surg Clin North Am* 6:875, 1996.

42. Mathisen DJ, Grillo HC: Endoscopic relief of malignant airway obstruction, *Ann Thorac Surg* 48:469, 1989.

43. Maziak DE and others: Adenoid cystic carcinoma of the airway: thirty-two-year experience, *J Thorac Cardiovasc Surg* 112:1522, 1996.

44. McCarthy MJ, Rosado-de-Christenson ML: Tumors of the trachea, *J Thorac Imag* 10:180, 1995.

45. McCaughan JS Jr.: *Photodynamic therapy versus Nd:YAG laser treatment of endobronchial or esophageal malignancies.* In Spinelli P, Dal-Fante M, Marchesini R, editors: *Photodynamic therapy and biomedical lasers.* New York, 1992, Elsevier, p 23.

46. McCaughan JS Jr., Williams TE: Photodynamic therapy for endobronchial malignant disease: a prospective fourteen-year study, *J Thorac Cardiovas Surg* 114:940, 1997.

47. Mitchell JD and others: Resection for bronchogenic carcinoma involving the carina: long-term results and effect of nodal status on outcome, *J Thorac Cardiovasc Surg* 121:465, 2001.

48. Montgomery W: Suprahyoid release for tracheal stenosis, *Arch Otolaryngol* 99:255, 1974.

49. Muehrcke DD and others: Surgical treatment of thyroid cancer invading the airway, *Surg Rounds* December:669, 1994.

50. Neville WE, Bolanowski JP, Kotia GG: Clinical experience with the silicone tracheal prosthesis, *J Thorac Cardiovasc Surg* 99:604, 1990.

51. Neville WE and others: Replacement of the intrathoracic trachea and both stem bronchi with a molded Silastic prosthesis, *J Thorac Cardiovasc Surg* 63:569, 1972.

52. Newmark GM, Conces DJ, Kopecky KK: Spiral CT evaluation of the trachea and bronchi, *J Comp Assist Tomogr* 18:552, 1994.

53. Paladugu RR and others: Bronchopulmonary Kulchitzky cell carcinoma: a new classification scheme for typical and atypical carcinoids, *Cancer* 55:1303, 1985.

54. Pearson FG and others: Primary tracheal anastomosis after resection of the cricoid cartilage with preservation of recurrent laryngeal nerves, *J Thorac Cardiovasc Surg* 70:806, 1975.

55. Pearson FG, Todd TR, Cooper JD: Experience with primary neoplasms of the trachea and carina, *J Thorac Cardiovasc Surg* 88:511, 1984.
56. Perelman MI and others: Primary tracheal tumors, *Semin Thorac Cardiovasc Surg* 8:400, 1996.
57. Prasad M, Keller JL: Clinical problem solving: pathology. Pathology quiz case 2: granular cell tumor of the trachea, *Arch Otolaryngol Head Neck Surg* 128:593, 2002.
58. Rabah R and others: Human papillomavirus-11-associated recurrent respiratory papillomatosis is more aggressive than human papillomavirus-6-associated disease, *Pediatr Dev Pathol* 4:68, 2001.
59. Refaely Y, Weissberg D: Surgical management of tracheal tumors [comment], *Ann Thorac Surg* 64:1429, 1997.
60. Regnard JF, Fourquier P, Levasseur P: Results and prognostic factors in resections of primary tracheal tumors: a multicenter retrospective study. The French Society of Cardiovascular Surgery, *J Thorac Cardiovasc Surg* 111:808, 1996.
61. Rob CG: Reconstruction of the trachea and cervical oesophagus, *Br J Surg* 37:202, 1949.
62. Salminen US and others: Recurrence and malignant transformation of endotracheal chondroma, *Ann Thorac Surg* 49:830, 1990.
63. Sing TM and others: Chemodectoma of the trachea, *Thorax* 51:341, 1996.
64. Stephens KE Jr., Wood DE: Bronchoscopic management of central airway obstruction, *J Thorac Cardiovasc Surg* 119:289, 2000.
65. Sun JD and others: Mucosal swabs detect HPV in laryngeal papillomatosis patients but not family members, *Int J Pediatr Otorhinolaryngol* 53:95, 2000.
66. Toomes H, Mickisch G, Vogt-Moykopf I: Experiences with prosthetic reconstruction of the trachea and bifurcation, *Thorax* 40:32, 1985.
67. Wang JC and others: Tracheal invasion by thyroid carcinoma: prediction using MR imaging, *AJR Am J Roentgenol* 177:929, 2001.
68. Weber AL, Grillo HC: Tracheal lesions: assessment by conventional films, computed tomography, and magnetic resonance imaging, *Isr J Med Sci* 28:233, 1992.
69. Weber AL, Grillo HC: Tracheal tumors, *Radiol Clin North Am* 16:227, 1978.
70. Wood DE: Management of malignant tracheobronchial obstruction, *Surg Clin North Am* 82:621, 2002.
71. Yang CC and others: Resectional treatment for thyroid cancer with tracheal invasion: a long-term follow-up study, *Arch Surg* 135:704, 2000.
72. Yang KY and others: Revisit of primary malignant neoplasms of the trachea: clinical characteristics and survival analysis, *Jpn J Clin Oncol* 27:305, 1997.
73. Yao MS, Koh WJ: Endobronchial brachytherapy, *Chest Surg Clin North Am* 11:813, 2001.
74. Yoder MG, Batsakis JG: Squamous cell carcinoma in solitary laryngeal papilloma, *Otolaryngol Head Neck Surg* 88:745, 1980.
75. Yousem S, Hochholzer L: Mucoepidermoid tumors of the lung, *Cancer* 60:1346, 1987.

UPPER AIRWAY MANIFESTATIONS OF GASTROESOPHAGEAL REFLUX DISEASE

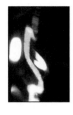

|| Savita Collins

INTRODUCTION

Gastroesophageal reflux (GER) is defined as the movement of gastric material into the esophagus in the absence of belching or vomiting.[26,27,28] *Gastroesophageal reflux disease (GERD)* occurs when GER is associated with symptoms or complications. The American Bronchoesophagological Association (ABEA) promotes the use of the term *extraesophageal reflux (EER)* when discussing nonesophageal manifestations of the regurgitation of gastric contents.[53,95]

It has been estimated that 30% of Americans suffer from GERD, with 7% to 10% of adults experiencing daily heartburn and 29% to 33% having symptoms weekly.[26,41,81,87] Twenty-five to 75 million people in the United States are affected by GERD, with 13% of Americans using indigestion aids at least twice weekly.[87] The incidence of GERD in patients presenting to an otolaryngology practice has been estimated to be 4% to 10%.[93] GERD is not rare in children; it has been described in 18% of children, with a higher incidence in children with esophageal atresia, tracheoesophageal fistula, or neurologic impairment.[104] Unfortunately, accurate estimates of the incidence of EER are not available. Koufman and colleagues[50] showed that 50% of all patients presenting to their center with laryngeal and voice disorders had EER as documented by dual pH probe studies. A retrospective review of patients presenting with common cervical symptoms revealed that GERD was detected in 73% of patients, and symptomatic relief after antireflux medical treatment resulted in symptomatic improvement in 84%.[77] The role and incidence of EER in the development of otolaryngologic disorders is controversial among otolaryngologists. A survey of ABEA members showed that 75% of respondents estimated that less than 50% of their patients had disorders related to EER, and there was a lack of consensus regarding evaluation and treatment modalities.[13] EER has been implicated in several clinical disorders, including chronic laryngitis,[30,49,50] chronic dysphonia,[30,49,50] laryngotracheal stenosis,[97,103] head and neck carcinoma,[17,24,57,88,98] cough,[40,44,45,78,99] asthma,[18,40,78,99] otitis media,[89] dental cares and erosion,[79] laryngeal papilloma,[42] vocal fold granulomas and ulcers,[32,36,39,40] laryngospasm,[5,6,60,65] recurrent croup,[104] and laryngomalacia.[64]

The goals of this chapter are to review the pathophysiology, clinical manifestations, and diagnosis and treatment of EER.

PATHOPHYSIOLOGY

The esophagus is the conduit for the transfer of material from the pharynx to the stomach. The esophagus acts as a vent for the stomach, allowing some normal retrograde flow of gasses and gastric contents.[72] The gatekeepers for the ingress and egress of material are the upper (UES) and lower esophageal sphincters (LES). The four main constituents of the barrier to reflux are the UES, the LES, esophageal acid clearance, and epithelial resistance.[49,95] Head and neck disorders associated with EER are postulated to occur via several mechanisms: direct mucosal damage and direct effect on mucociliary clearance from exposure to gastric contents; GER-related distal esophageal damage that results in vagally mediated referred symptomatology; and laryngeal reflexes mediated by the stimulation of distal esophageal afferents.[5,25,77]

Upper Esophageal Sphincter

The UES is functionally defined as the area of the distal pharynx and proximal esophagus that maintains a closed pharyngoesophageal segment and opens during specific physiologic demands (e.g., swallowing, belching). Anatomically, the UES is made up of the cricopharyngeus, the thyropharyngeus, and the proximal cervical esophagus.[56,72,95] Unlike other muscular sphincters, the UES is not a complete muscular circle but rather a C-shaped sling that attaches to the cricoid cartilage. The pharyngeal plexus innervates the UES and receives contributions from the vagus nerve (superior and recurrent laryngeal nerves), the glossopharyngeal nerve, and the sympathetic nerves from the superior cervical ganglion.[56] The motor neurons that control the cricopharyngeus are found in the brainstem in the nucleus ambiguus, and stimulation of the nucleus tractus solitarius (the afferent nucleus of the vagus) results in contraction of the cricopharyngeus.[56] In canine studies, vagal nerve stimulation produced UES relaxation, and sectioning of both vagus nerves produced severe dysphagia.[49] Sensory information from the UES is transmitted via the glossopharyngeal nerve and the sympathetic nerves.[56]

The UES maintains a closed pharyngoesophageal segment via tonic contraction of the cricopharyngeus.[56,72] During swallowing, UES relaxation occurs, and the cricoid cartilage is pulled upward and anteriorly by the laryngeal musculature, thereby resulting in a stretching of the cricopharyngeus, thus allowing for bolus passage.[72] The UES tonic pressure is increased in response to laryngeal stimulation (laryngo-UES contractile reflex).[81,95] UES pressure is increased with acidification of the distal esophagus.[49,56,95] UES pressure increases with slow balloon distension of the distal esophagus.[56] General anesthetics, sleep state, cigarette smoking, and peppermint consumption are associated with decreased UES pressure.[49,56,95] Koufman[49] and Burke report that smoking and peppermint consumption produced a 50% reduction in UES resting pressure in healthy volunteers within minutes.

The UES is the final gatekeeper in the antireflux barrier, and UES dysfunction may be associated with head and neck manifestations of EER. Deveney, Brenner, and Cohen[22] showed an increased incidence of UES hypotonia in patients with pulmonary problems associated with GERD. In patients with inflammatory lesions of the larynx, they found UES pressures that were somewhat lower than normal.[22] Ulualp and Toohill[95] did not see significant differences in resting UES pressures in patients with posterior laryngitis as compared with normal controls.

Lower Esophageal Sphincter

The LES is the most critical antireflux defense mechanism.[21,26] It is located at the gastroesophageal junction, and it is not as anatomically distinct as the UES. Contraction of the LES results in circular closure that prevents the egress of gastric contents. Relaxation of the LES occurs during swallowing, belching, and vomiting. The LES is anatomically surrounded by the diaphragmatic crura, which mechanically augment the sphincter mechanism and are felt to contribute to 25% of LES competence.[49] Manometric measurements at the LES reflect the combined contributions of the

esophageal LES and the diaphragmatic crura. The intrinsic resting pressure of the LES varies with the phase of the respiratory cycle as a result of differential diaphragmatic contraction.[21] During episodes of straining, there is an increased LES pressure as a result of increased diaphragmatic activity, yielding an increased diaphragmatic squeeze of the LES.[21,72] Hormonal control of LES activity is complex. Gastrin, pitressin, angiotensin II, and motilin increase contractile tone, whereas secretin, cholecystokinin, glucagon, and vasoactive intestinal peptide decrease LES pressure.[21,49]

To prevent GER, the LES must maintain a resting pressure that is higher than the gastric pressure. GER occurs when there is a reversal of this gastric-to-LES pressure gradient.[21,72] Retrograde flow will occur with relaxation of the LES, with chronic hypotonia of the LES, or with increases in gastric pressure that overcome the LES resting pressure. Transient relaxation of the LES occurs in normal healthy adults and children.[21] Recent research has shown that transient relaxation of the LES is the most critical mechanism in the production of GER.[21,94] Dent and colleagues[21] showed that 63% to 74% of GER episodes were associated with transient LES relaxation. Chronic hypotonia of the LES is thought to be associated with GER episodes in a smaller percentage of patients, but it may be associated with more severe esophagitis.[21] Lower LES resting pressures are seen in patients with CREST syndrome, scleroderma, and isolated Raynaud's phenomenon. Although chronic hypotonia of the LES results in more severe reflux, it is an uncommon mechanism for GERD.[21,48] Large hiatal hernias may result in disruption of the relationship of the LES to the diaphragmatic crura; this may impair the ability of the LES to act as an antireflux barrier by removing the additional pressure generated by the squeeze of the diaphragm.[21,49] Although hiatal hernias may play a role in GERD in some patients, not all patients with hiatal hernias have GERD.[26] Table 109-1 lists agents that affect the LES pressure.[26,49]

When gastric pressure exceeds LES pressure, reflux can occur. "Stress reflux" is seen with increased intraabdominal pressure during bending over, heavy lifting, straining, and coughing.[49] Excessive gastric distension resulting in increased gastric pressure can occur postprandially after a large meal and with severe gastroparesis. Impaired gastric emptying is more common in patients with GERD.[48] Pregnancy is a risk factor for GERD as a result of increased abdominal pressure.

Esophageal Acid Clearance

Because some GER is normal, mechanisms exist to clear and neutralize gastric contents when they pass

TABLE 109-1

Increase Lower Esophageal Sphincter Pressure	Decrease Lower Esophageal Sphincter Pressure
Protein	Fat
Bethanecol	Carbohydrates
Metoclopramide	Alcohol
Antacids	Cigarettes
α-adrenergic drugs	Carminatives (peppermint, spearmint)
	Theophylline
	Calcium-channel blockers
	Nitrate drugs
	Atropine
	β-adrenergic drugs
	Dopamine
	Sedatives

into the esophagus. Esophageal peristaltic waves—along with the effect of gravity—act to mechanically clear the esophagus. Weakened or ineffective peristalsis allows for refluxed materials to have increased contact time with esophageal tissues. Knight and colleagues[48] studied 100 subjects with EER and noted that 52% had ineffective esophageal motility. Primary esophageal peristalsis has been shown to be similar to normal controls in patients with GERD and posterior laryngitis.[95] In patients with GERD, secondary esophageal peristalsis was noted to be decreased as compared with normal controls.[95] Increased episodes of GER seen in patients with GERD, when supine, can be partially explained by the loss of gravitational effects. Acidic refluxate left in the esophagus can be neutralized by gastric glandular secretions and buffering agents in saliva.[49] Xerostomia that can be caused by Sjögren's disease, certain medications, and previous radiotherapy may abolish this important antireflux barrier.[49] Although the low pH of gastric material is damaging to epithelium, alkaline pH pancreatic and bile juices, when present, can also result in tissue injury.[26,49]

Epithelial Resistance Factors

When the antireflux barriers fail, the severity of tissue damage will be determined by epithelial resistance factors. There are pre-epithelial, epithelial, and intracellular protective mechanisms. The epithelium is preceded by a mucus layer and an aqueous layer with high bicarbonate content.[49,95] Mucus resists penetration by large molecules such as pepsin, but it does not prevent the ingress of acid. The aqueous layer is alkaline, and it buffers acid material. At the cellular level, the cell membrane and the intracellular junctions resist acid and pepsin.[49] Different tissues have vari-

able epithelial resistance, with esophageal epithelium being more resistant than respiratory epithelium.[22,25,49,77,95] GER to a small degree in the hypopharynx or larynx may cause significant injury, whereas reflux to the same degree in the distal esophagus would be easily resisted.[22,25,49,77,95] Hanson and Jiang[32] postulate that the posterior glottis is especially susceptible to the effect of EER. They theorize that the cilia beat material to the posterior glottis, thereby resulting in increased contact with refluxate and, therefore, more injury to this epithelium.

Mechanisms That Cause Symptomatology as a Result of EER

Head and neck disorders associated with EER are postulated to occur via several mechanisms: direct mucosal damage and direct effect on mucociliary clearance from exposure to gastric contents; GER-related distal esophageal damage that results in vagally mediated referred symptomatology; and laryngeal reflexes mediated by the stimulation of distal esophageal afferents.[5,25,77]

Gaynor[25] studied the effects of direct exposure of gastric contents on rabbit and canine larynges. In the rabbit, direct exposure at a pH of 4.0 resulted in an inflammatory response that involved the submucosa and muscle, and the degree of damage increased with longer durations of exposure. When a pH of 1.4 was used, "severe mucosal ulceration, submucosal and deeper hemorrhage with marked inflammatory response as well as necrosis were noted."[25] In canines, an effect on mucociliary flow (MCF) starting at a pH of 5.0 with no MCF observed at pH of 2.0 was noted. Ciliary activity will persist after the cessation of MCF. Alteration of pH has a direct effect on mucociliary transport and may lead to increased viscosity of the mucus blanket.[25] A reduction in mucociliary transport may result in decreased resistance to infection and has been theorized to contribute to the pathogenesis of subglottic stenosis.[25]

Pepsin, which is found in gastric contents, is maximally active at pH 4.5, and its enzymatic activity produces tissue damage.[49] Koufman[49] demonstrated the importance of pepsin in the production of epithelial damage in canine larynges. He created subglottic mucosal injuries in canines and then compared healing and injury in control, acid-only, and acid- and pepsin-exposed conditions. The acid-only group revealed inflammatory lesions that healed in twice the time it took for the control group. None of the acid- and pepsin-treated animals showed healing, and they were noted to develop ulceration and granulation.[49]

Gaynor[25] monitored ICU patients who were intubated for prolonged periods of time and found that lower pH readings were found and ranged from 2.4 to

7.0. Forty percent of these patients were noted to have reflux episodes of pH less than 4.0. Patients that were treated with antacids or H_2-blockers had pH readings that ranged from 4.7 to 8.9. The work of Koufman[49] and Gaynor[25] supports the use of anti-acid therapy in cases of potential subglottic trauma (e.g., intubation), because it may help prevent irreversible mucosal damage.

Direct stimulation of sensory receptors in the larynx by aspirated or refluxed material can result in reflexive vocal fold adduction or laryngospasm.[5,60,61] This *laryngeal chemoreflex* is associated with bradycardia, central apnea, and hypotension.[104] Partial or complete laryngospasm and cough can also be triggered by GER to the distal esophagus via a vagally mediated reflex.[5,18,26,81] Laryngospasm associated with distal esophageal GER can be associated with bronchospasm, increased secretions, tachycardia, and hypertension.[104] These reflexes have implications for respiratory manifestations of EER and in the mechanisms involved with sudden infant death syndrome and recurrent laryngospasm.[5,25,60,61]

DIAGNOSTIC EVALUATION
Subjective

A good case history is very critical to both the diagnosis and treatment of patients with EER. The clinician must not only identify symptoms but also behavioral and medical risk factors. It is also critical to patient compliance with treatment to actively involve the patient in the identification of the risk factors that he or she can modify. Common symptoms described in association with EER are listed in Table 109-2.*

In a retrospective review of 216 patients with cervical symptoms that were believed to be associated with EER, Rival and colleagues found that the most frequent complaint was cervical dysphagia (33%), followed by globus (19%), sore throat (17%), and chronic throat clearing (14%). The researchers found that 66% of these patients complained of classic symptoms of GERD such as acid regurgitation and heartburn.[77] Fraser, Morton, and Gillibrand[23] prospectively reviewed patients with symptoms believed to be associated with EER who had positive pH probe studies and found cough and hoarseness as the most common symptoms. Seventy-seven percent of their patients also complained of classic symptoms of GERD.[23] Other authors report lower rates of symptomatic GERD in patients with EER, with estimates of 20%,[93] 43%,[49] and 55%.[66] A survey of ABEA members showed that respondents felt that the most common symptoms related to EER were throat clearing, persistent

---

*References 8, 10, 13, 15, 23, 26, 32, 34, 40, 44, 45, 66, 77, 93, 96, 100.

TABLE 109-2
COMMON SYMPTOMS OF EXTRAESOPHAGEAL REFLUX
• Hoarseness/dysphonia (episodic or chronic)
• Globus sensation
• Chronic throat clearing
• Vocal fatigue
• Voice breaks
• Sore throat
• Neck pain
• Excessive throat mucus
• Chronic or nighttime cough
• Dysphagia
• Odynophagia
• Postnasal drip
• Halitosis
• Ear pain
• Laryngospasm
• Asthma exacerbation
• Loss of upper singing range
• Prolonged warmup time in singers
• Heartburn/regurgitation

cough, heartburn/dyspepsia, globus sensation, and voice-quality change findings.[13]

Belafsky, Postma, and Koufman[8,9,10] developed the Reflux Symptom Index (RSI), a self-administered survey of nine questions used to assess patients with EER. They demonstrated that the instrument is reliable and that it provides reproducible and valid findings. Normative data gathered by these authors support that an RSI of more than 10 is associated with a high likelihood of positive dual-channel pH probe study.[11] They prospectively evaluated 40 patients with EER documented by dual pH probe studies and two months of medical management. The RSI was noted to show improvement before changes were seen in the physical examination. The mean RSI at initiation of the study was 19.3, which improved to a mean of 13.9 after 2 months of findings.[8] The RSI is shown in Table 109-3.

Physical Examination/Laryngeal Endoscopy

The physical examination can yield several clues to EER. Observations of the quality of voice, frequent throat clearing, cough or stridor, muscle tension in extralaryngeal musculature, and general body habitus are important to the evaluation. The larynx can be evaluated with indirect laryngoscopy along with rigid and/or flexible laryngoscopy. Videoendoscopy and stroboscopy are very useful, especially for documenting treatment effects and for visualizing subtle signs associated with reflux.

TABLE 109-3

THE REFLUX SYMPTOM INDEX[10]

Within the past month, how did the following problems affect you? Rank them from 0 (no problem) to 5 (severe problem).

1. Hoarseness or a problem with your voice
2. Clearing your throat
3. Excess throat mucus or postnasal drip
4. Difficulty swallowing food, liquids, or pills
5. Coughing after you have eaten or after lying down
6. Breathing difficulties or choking episodes
7. Troublesome or annoying cough
8. Sensations of something sticking in your throat or a lump in your throat
9. Heartburn, chest pain, indigestion, or stomach acid coming up

The majority of laryngeal findings seen in patients with *chronic* laryngitis associated with EER are seen in the posterior larynx. Posterior laryngitis is manifested by edema, increased vascularity and erythema of the posterior commissure, and arytenoids.[29,30,93] Chronic irritation can result in a thickening of the posterior laryngeal mucosa with hyperkeratosis, which is also called *pachydermia laryngeus*.[30,93] Hanson, Kamel, and Kahrilas[30] describe this posterior mucosal thickening with increased granularity and rough cobblestone appearance as "granular mucositis." Increased mucus formation and thickness, along with mucus stranding and pooling, may result from chronic irritation and alterations of mucociliary flow.[25,93] Laryngeal ulceration, granuloma formation, scarring, and stenosis may indicate more severe EER.[30,32,36,42] Cherry and Margulies (1968) first identified extraesophageal reflux of gastric acid as being associated with contact ulcers.[25]

Hanson, Kamel, and Kahrilas[30] examined 233 patients with chronic laryngitis. Videoendoscopic examination revealed that erythema of the posterior larynx was the most prevalent sign and that it was the most reversible with treatment of EER. The authors noted that more severe inflammation or longer duration of symptoms was associated with increasing vascularity and erythema extending into the remainder of the larynx and supraglottis. In their patient population, posterior glottic mucosal thickening was the second most common finding. In some patients with severe EER and cough, the authors noted eschar formation over the posterior glottis that they likened to a "mucosal burn injury." Seven percent of patients were noted to have ulceration of the vocal processes or ulcer formation between the arytenoids, and 3% had granulomas. Patients with prominent throat clearing behavior and chronic cough were more likely

to demonstrate pachydermia laryngeus. The authors used the following grading scale: *mild*—mild posterior glottic erythema; *moderate*—marked erythema, stasis of secretions, and mucosal granularity; and *severe*—ulceration, granulation tissue, or hyperkeratosis of the larynx. Hanson and Jiang[32] digitized endoscopic examinations of a large group of patients with chronic laryngitis and performed digital color analysis. This demonstrated a significant difference between patients and normal controls in the red index, with a significant decrease in the red index after treatment for EER in patients with chronic laryngitis findings.[32]

Habermann and colleagues[29] reviewed the endoscopic findings of 29 patients with chronic dysphonia and chronic laryngitis and showed that abnormalities of the posterior glottic mucosa and reddening of the posterior larynx were the most common findings. The authors noted significant improvement in these changes with therapy. Alteration and reddening of the true vocal fold mucosa and false vocal folds were also noted to improve with treatment. Shaw and Searl[82] assessed 96 patients who had symptoms that were suggestive of EER and noted that posterior glottic edema, nodularity, and erythema were the most "severe and frequent" findings. Only 47% of patients were noted to have ulceration, and three patients were noted to have granulomas. Branski, Bhattacharyya, and Shapiro[14] performed a prospective, randomized, blinded study to assess the reliability of the laryngoscopic evaluation of EER patients. They found that both intra- and interrater reliability were poor; raters demonstrated a poor agreement on the severity of endoscopic findings for laryngopharyngeal reflux (LPR). The authors concluded that using laryngoscopic findings alone for the diagnosis of EER was highly subjective.

Pseudosulcus has been described as a common endoscopic finding of EER.[10,11,37] The term *pseudosulcus* refers to the appearance of edema along the undersurface of the vocal fold from the anterior to the posterior commissure.[10,11,37] By contrast, true sulcus vocalis involves the free edge of the fold and terminates at the vocal process. Belafsky and colleagues evaluated pseudosulcus in 30 patients with EER (i.e., with positive pH probes) and 30 control patients and found pseudosulcus in 70% of patients with EER and in 30% of controls. Patients with pseudosulcus were 2.3 times more likely to have pH-probe documented EER. The sensitivity and specificity of pseudosulcus were estimated to be 70% and 77%, respectively.[11] Hickson, Simpson, and Falcon[37] prospectively studied 20 patients who underwent endoscopic evaluation and were found to have pseudosulcus with dual-channel pH probe studies, and they found positive studies in 18 out of 20 patients. They estimated that the positive predictive value of pseudosulcus for EER was 90%.[37] This study may have overestimated the incidence, because participants were selected from patients who presented to the authors' clinic and required endoscopy as part of their evaluation.

Belafsky and colleagues have developed an endoscopic grading scale for EER. The Reflux Finding Score (RFS) is made up of eight findings that are graded on severity and that yield a score from 0 to 26 (Table 109-4). The authors report that an RFS of more than seven is associated with a high likelihood of dual pH probe positivity.[11] The RFS was tested in 40 controls and 40 patients with positive clinical histories and pH probe studies. This review showed excellent inter- and intraobserver reliability for the RFS. The mean RFS for control subjects was 5.2, whereas the mean RFS at entry for the EER group was 11.5, and an individual with an RFS of more than 7 was noted to have EER, with 95% certainty.[9]

Beaver and colleagues[7] conducted a prospective study of the videostroboscopic images of 49 patients diagnosed with laryngopharyngeal reflux disease on the basis of two or more symptoms (i.e., throat clearing, hoarseness, cough, globus, or excessive mucus) along with physical examination findings of chronic laryngitis. Subjects were evaluated pretreatment and again after 6 weeks of high-dose proton pump inhibitor (PPI) therapy. Ten control patients without any symptoms of EER were included. Three otolaryngologists evaluated the photographs in a blinded manner and in random order and gave each a score using the Laryngopharyngeal Reflux Disease Index (Table 109-5). The mean index value for patients was signif-

icantly higher than that of controls (9.50 vs 2.92), and posttreatment mean scores were significantly lower than pretreatment scores (7.35 vs 9.50). The most useful items on the scoring system were as follows: supraglottic edema and erythema, glottic edema and erythema, and subglottic edema and erythema. Items 7 through 12 were not felt to be as useful, and very few patients had positive scores on these items.

Voice Analysis

Hanson and colleagues[31] reviewed voice quality and measures of jitter, shimmer, and signal-to-noise ratios in 16 patients undergoing treatment for chronic posterior laryngitis. Perceptual analysis did not show correlation with acoustic measures, and it did not show significant change with treatment. The authors did demonstrate that measures of jitter, shimmer, and signal-to-noise ratio improve significantly with antisecretory and antireflux treatment of chronic posterior laryngitis. Shaw and Searl[82] noted significant improvement in measurements of jitter, shimmer, habitual frequency, and frequency range with antireflux treatment in their series of patients with a pretreatment complaint of hoarseness. Hamden and colleagues[34] did not show any change in acoustic parameters in patients with the medical treatment of EER.

Esophagram

Barium esophagram is a convenient, inexpensive, and noninvasive diagnostic test. It is a useful method to diagnose structural and functional abnormalities of the esophagus, including hiatal hernia, erosive esophagitis, strictures, Barrett's esophagus, esophageal rings, extrinsic compression, motility disorders, diverticula,

---

TABLE 109-5

THE LARYNGOPHARYNGEAL REFLUX DISEASE INDEX[7]

Grade each using a scale of 0 to 3 (0, absent; 3, most severe):

1. Edema of posterior supraglottis
2. Edema of vocal folds
3. Edema of subglottis
4. Erythema of posterior supraglottis
5. Erythema of vocal folds
6. Erythema of subglottis

Grade as 1 if present and 0 if absent:

7. Leukoplakia
8. Nodules or prenodules
9. Polyp(s)
10. Posterior pachydermia
11. Web (may be anterior microweb)
12. Contact granuloma

TABLE 109-4

THE REFLUX FINDING SCORE[10]

Pseudosulcus	0, absent; 2, present
Ventricular obliteration	0, none; 2, partial; 4, complete
Erythema/hyperemia	0, none; 2, arytenoids only; 4, diffuse
Vocal fold edema	0, none; 1, mild; 2, moderate; 3, severe; 4, polypoid
Diffuse laryngeal edema	0, none; 1, mild; 2, moderate; 3, severe; 4, obstructing
Posterior commissure hypertrophy	0, none; 1, mild; 2, moderate; 3, severe; 4, obstructing
Granuloma/granulation	0, absent; 2, present
Thick endolaryngeal mucus	0, absent; 2, present

possible malignancy, cricopharyngeal spasm, aspiration, and esophageal shortening.[38,49,91,93,104] Barium studies have significant use for surgical planning for antireflux surgery. Fluoroscopic evaluation is often used to look for the presence of reflux, and it is often combined with provocative maneuvers, such as Valsalva's maneuver, cough, rolling from the supine to the right lateral position, and the water siphon test (the patient drinks 60 mL of water through a straw while supine). The sensitivity of barium esophagram to detect GER is between 20% and 60%, with a specificity of 64% to 90% and accuracy of 69%.[104] Thompson, Koehler, and Richter[91] assessed 117 patients with clinical GERD and compared the results of esophageal pH probe with those of barium esophagram. They demonstrated that barium studies showed unprovoked reflux in 26% of subjects with positive pH probe studies. The addition of the water siphon test increased the sensitivity of barium esophagram in the evaluation of reflux to 70%, with a specificity of 74% and a positive predictive value of 80%.[91]

The relevance of barium esophagography to patients with EER is less clear. In Toohill and Kuhn's[93] series of 286 patients with dysphonia and various laryngeal disorders, 79.9% had abnormal esophagrams. Rival and colleagues[77] showed that 22 out of 73 patients with EER symptoms had normal barium swallow evaluations, with 50% of these patients demonstrating EER on subsequent diagnostic testing. Giacchi, Sullivan, and Rothstein[27] reviewed 28 patients with otolaryngologic manifestations of EER and noted that barium esophagram revealed reflux in 45% of patients and that 50% had normal examinations.

Flexible Endoscopic Evaluation of Swallowing and Sensory Testing

Aviv and colleagues[4] have noted that LPR can be observed during flexible endoscopic evaluation of swallowing and sensory testing (FEEST) examinations. In a prospective pilot study, the authors evaluated 20 dysphagic patients (without neurologic etiology) and 20 controls with FEEST. Eighteen out of 20 of the dysphagic patients were noted to have reflux, whereas no reflux was noted in any of the control subjects. In another prospective study, 54 dysphagic (without neurologic etiology) and 25 healthy controls were evaluated with FEEST.[3] In the dysphagic group, 89% were noted to have posterior glottic edema, 78% had sensory deficits, and 70% were noted to have LPR. Only one out of the 25 control patients had posterior glottic edema, sensory deficits, and LPR. Twenty-three of the patients who were diagnosed by FEEST to have LPR were treated with PPI therapy and were reevaluated by FEEST. Sixty-seven percent were noted to have improved

posterior glottic edema, and 79% had resolution of sensory deficits.[3] The evaluators in this study were not blinded to subject identity or history at the time of evaluation.

Esophageal Endoscopy

Esophagogastroduodenoscopy (EGD) is useful for the direct visualization of the esophagus, along with biopsies and cultures in patients with esophagitis and gastritis. In patients with GERD, it may be valuable in the search for esophageal mucosal irritation and to rule out Barrett's esophagitis. Deveney, Brenner, and Cohen[22] evaluated a small series of patients with laryngeal inflammatory lesions and found that three out of seven (43%) had esophagitis, although none had Barrett's esophagus. Smit and colleagues[84] found pH-probe proved GER in 72% of patients with globus and hoarseness, 35% in patients with hoarseness alone, and 30% in patients with globus alone. Abnormal EGD findings were noted in 65% of the patients in this group who had concurrent GER. On the basis of their findings of a high prevalence of pathologic GER in subjects with globus and hoarseness, the authors recommend that patients with symptomatic EER and concurrent GERD be evaluated with EGD.[84] In a small prospective study in patients with chronic laryngeal symptoms associated with EER and concomitant GER as documented by pH probe study, EGD showed grade II or higher esophagitis in all of the subjects and Barrett's esophagitis or peptic esophageal stricture in 50% of these individuals.[66,67]

Tauber, Gross, and Issing[90] prospectively evaluated the incidence of gastroenterologic diseases in patients presenting with nonspecific laryngopharyngeal symptoms that were felt to be associated with EER. Thirty such patients refused pH probe studies and were evaluated with EGD. GERD was seen in 43%, gastric cultures that were positive for *Helicobacter pylori* were found in 23%, and 73% had some form of gastrointestinal disease diagnosed by EGD and/or biopsy. Medical therapy for reflux and *Helicobacter pylori* (in positive patients) resulted in a 90% therapeutic success rate for symptom resolution.[90]

McMurray and colleagues[65] studied pediatric patients who were undergoing evaluation for airway reconstruction and found that significant reflux as demonstrated in the lower esophageal pH probe did not correlate with positive esophageal endoscopic findings or biopsy-proved inflammation of the upper or lower esophagus. A weak correlation was seen between laryngoscopic findings of EER and postcricoid biopsy findings.[65] The necessity of esophageal endoscopy in patients with EER without GERD is unclear, and the procedure may be unnecessary.[49]

Manometry

The use of manometric evaluation for patients with GERD is well documented. Knight, Wells, and Parrish[48] documented the significance of esophageal dysmotility in patients with EER. They used manometric studies of 100 patients with EER to show that 29% had normal motility, 48% had ineffective motility, 10% had a hypertensive lower esophageal sphincter, 9% had a nutcracker esophagus, and 4% had esophageal achalasia. Rival and others[77] noted low LES pressure in 60% of the patients that they studied who had cervical symptoms of EER. Esophageal manometric evaluation is critical to surgical planning for antireflux surgery.[38] Although manometry is valuable in a certain subset of patients with EER, it may not be useful as a diagnostic test for EER. Because it is only one measurement in time and transient relaxations of the LES are important in the pathogenesis of EER, manometry may not accurately assess patients for the absence of relaxations of the LES and, therefore, EER.[104]

pH Probe

Continuous pH monitoring studies are felt to be the gold standard study for GERD and EER.[49,73,104] Probes that sense pH changes can be placed in different locations in the esophagus, pharynx, or hypopharynx. Probe placement can be verified using manometry, endoscopy, or fluoroscopy. Manometric localization of pH probe location is the most commonly used technique. Single pH probe techniques that involve the use of a probe placed 5 cm above the manometrically determined site of the LES are commonly employed for the evaluation of patients with GERD. With the recognition of extraesophageal symptoms of EER, the importance of adding a second probe above the UES has been elucidated. Postma[73] describes a review of patients with otolaryngologic complaints associated with EER who underwent dual pH probe testing at Wake Forest University in Winston-Salem, NC, where 59% would have been inappropriately assumed to have a negative pH probe when their diagnosis was based solely on the esophageal probe. In these patients, the pharyngeal sensor was needed to document EER.[75] In a similar study, Koufman and colleagues[54] showed that 11% of patients had a positive upper probe with normal esophageal pH probe acid exposure time. Little and others[59] showed the importance of the proximal probe in children and noted that 46% (78 of 168) of subjects demonstrated positive EER by proximal probe in the face of negative lower esophageal probe studies.

Although the advent of dual pH probe studies has added significantly to our diagnostic armamentarium, it is not without its limitations. It is an invasive test,

and its sensitivity is no more than 75% to 80%.[95] Hanson and colleagues[33] state that the false-negative rate may be up to 50%. Noordzij and others[69] compared dual pH probe findings with symptom severity in patients with EER and revealed that dual pH probe positivity had poor predictive value of symptoms or signs of EER. Small variations in technique for probe placement or calibration can significantly affect accuracy.[73] Careful documentation of patient position (supine or upright), diet, and symptoms are equally important during the study. The patient should maintain his or her usual dietary and smoking habits and activity level during the period of the study.[73,83,85]

Although there is a consensus about norms for the distal esophageal pH probe, considerable controversy exists with regard to findings in the proximal pharyngeal probe. Some authors report that a single pharyngeal reflux event as determined by a drop in pH to 4 or below is diagnostic of EER.[73,83] Unfortunately, several studies have documented that a small percentage of normal subjects have proximal probe pH drops below 4.[80,94,96] Vincent and colleagues[96] showed that normal subjects were positive for reflux to the proximal probe (median of one event), with 80.4% of these occurring while the subject was upright. In addition, these authors examined the Reflux Area Index, which incorporates the number and duration of events of pH less than 4. They state that "the reflux area index appears to be the most useful parameter to measure laryngopharyngeal reflux severity."[96] Normative data for pediatric patients is also lacking, and there appears to be considerable age-related variation.[64,104] Bauman and colleagues[6] performed a retrospective review in pediatric patients undergoing pH probe testing at their institution. Sixty-eight patients were noted to have EER symptoms, underwent empiric medical treatment, and were reviewed. Chronic cough, apnea, and recurrent pneumonia were the most commonly documented extraesophageal symptoms. Eight-five percent of subjects were noted by their caretakers to have symptomatic benefit from antireflux therapy. The positive predictive value of the distal esophageal probe was more than 90%, but the negative predictive value was less than 50%. The authors noted that the reproducibility of results on different days was poor; only a small number of subjects had a dual pH probe study, and the mean percentage of time that the pH was less than 4 in the upper probe was 2.6%.[6]

Contencin and Narcy,[16] Hanson and colleagues,[33] and Koufman[49] argue that the criteria of the pH being below 4 may be too stringent. Contencin and Narcy[16] showed that pH drops to 6 or below at the proximal probe in children with laryngotracheitis may be significant. Pepsin, which has been shown to be critical in the pathogenesis of tissue damage, is active at pH levels of up to 5.[49] Hanson and Jiang[32] caution against stringent use of the pH equalling 4 criteria in patients who have had prior radiotherapy, because irradiated tissue may be less resistant to reflux trauma.

Although several authors have shown the importance of a positive proximal pH probe, one must be careful when interpreting a negative study in patients with EER. Many patients with respiratory tract manifestations of EER may not have reflux into the proximal esophagus, but they may have symptoms as a result of a vagally mediated reflex, as discussed previously in this chapter.[83] In addition, there is a potential for sampling error, because EER may potentially cause pathology, but it may be infrequent and therefore not documented in a 24-hour study period.

Many authors support the empiric treatment of EER before obtaining a pH probe study.* Treatment efficacy is well-documented.† These authors state that routine pH probe studies in patients with only laryngitis may be unnecessary, and may instead be reserved for the following indications: patients with symptoms of GERD; patients with partial responses to therapy to assess for the adequacy of acid suppression; continued moderate to severe laryngitis, despite an adequate trial of therapy; when considering antireflux surgery; to evaluate patients after fundoplication who have recurrent or persistent symptoms; and in intubated patients who are in an altered state of consciousness.[22,25,32,33] Although a positive study may be clinically helpful, a negative study does not rule out EER. The American Gastroenterological Association has taken the following position with regard to EER: "There are presently no prospective data showing that ambulatory esophageal pH monitoring can identify either patients with laryngitis or asthmatics that are likely to respond to anti-reflux therapy."[32] There were no significant differences noted on pH probe monitoring that differentiated partial responders from complete responders in patients treated medically for EER.[99] Fraser, Morton, and Gillibrand[23] are proponents of routine pH probe testing before initiating empiric antireflux therapy. In their study, the presence of posterior laryngitis did not predict treatment response. The authors argue that a positive pH probe study may better select patients who will respond to therapy and help to avoid unnecessary treatment in some patients.[23] Further evaluation of pH probe testing in patients with chronic laryngitis is needed to elucidate norms and to demonstrate its utility for identifying patients who will benefit from therapy before this controversy can be resolved.

---

*References 12, 19, 20, 29, 32, 101.
†References 19, 20, 29, 30, 46, 47, 51, 63, 77, 101.

Reflux Scan

Radionuclide scanning involves the oral administration of saline with technetium followed by a gamma scan that looks for reflux. The reflux scan can also be used to quantify delayed gastric emptying.[104] The sensitivity of this test has been found to be between 14% and 90%, and it is considered to have low sensitivity in patients with EER.[49]

Acidification Tests

Acidification tests, such as the Tuttle Test and the Bernstein Test, are rarely used today in clinical practice. The Bernstein Test is used with adult patients and involves delivering saline and variable concentrations of hydrochloric acid to the distal esophagus via a nasogastric tube until symptoms are reproduced or 45 minutes have passed.[49] The Bernstein Acidification Test is a qualitative test that can be used to establish a causal relationship between GER and specific symptoms. The sensitivity of this test for the detection of GERD has been reported to be 32% to 95%.[26,77,104] It is not as useful for the diagnosis of EER, because only a fraction of these patients have concurrent symptoms of GERD.[77] Rival and colleauges[77] studied 146 patients with acid stimulation testing and found that 16% had positive results. However, when they analyzed patients with only cervical symptoms, none had a positive result. The Tuttle Test is performed in children and involves the instillation of an age-dependent concentration of hydrochloric acid into the stomach and measurements of pH in the distal esophagus, with two episodes of the pH level being below 3 considered to be diagnostic of reflux.[104]

Bronchoalveolar Lavage

Bronchoalveolar lavage sampled tracheal aspirates are used to look for lipid-laden macrophages, and is a test for aspiration into the lower respiratory tract. It has been shown to be 85% sensitive, and it becomes positive within 6 hours of the reflux event and stays positive for up to 3 days.[104] Lipid-laden macrophages have been shown to be increased in children with pulmonary complications of EER.[49] The advantage of this test is that it provides the ability to track EER days after the event; the disadvantage is that it requires bronchoscopy to acquire the sample.

TREATMENT
Behavioral Modification

Behavioral changes that are aimed at reducing episodes of reflux may be critical to the successful management of EER. Hanson, Kamel, and Kahrilas[30] have shown that nocturnal reflux precautions alone will result in symptomatic improvement in approximately 50% of patients with posterior laryngitis and chronic dysphonia. Common modifications recommended include the following: avoidance of eating or drinking 3 hours before lying down; avoidance of tobacco products, alcohol, fried foods, fatty foods, chocolate, caffeine, spicy foods and peppermints; avoidance of tight-fitting clothing; and elevation of the head of the bed by 6 to 8 inches.[30,82,95] No controlled studies have evaluated behavioral modifications.[95] Giacchi, Sullivan, and Rothstein[27] evaluated patient compliance with treatment for EER and found that compliance with behavior modification varied widely. The degree of symptomatic improvement positively correlated with both medical therapy and behavior modification. The changes that most significantly correlated with symptom reduction were avoidance of food and liquid before bedtime and elevation of the head of the bed.[27] Multiple authors have shown that there is decreased acid exposure to the lower esophagus with decreased fat intake, decreased smoking, elevation of the head of the bed, and allowing at least 3 hours between eating and lying down.[95] Chewing gum for 1 hour after food intake resulted in reduced acid contact time in both controls and patients with reflux,[2] and it increased esophageal and pharyngeal pH.[86] The benefit was more pronounced in patients with reflux and lasted for up to 3 hours.[2] Avidan and colleagues[2] noted that walking for one hour postprandially had a mild beneficial reduction of acid reflux, but only for a short duration.

Antacids

Multiple antacids are commonly available, they are inexpensive, and they are employed by many Americans before they seek medical attention. Antacids are effective as a result of their acid-neutralizing properties. They neutralize the pH of the refluxate, and they can thereby prevent the tissue damage caused by bile salts and deactivate pepsin at a higher pH.[87] Antacids have been shown to increase LES resting pressure.[26] Gaviscon contains alginic acid and is effective for reducing GER, but it does not appear to change LES pressure. Gaviscon's mechanism of action is not fully understood.[25] Antacids may be used as first-line therapy in patients with minor EER or as an adjunct to other treatment modalities.[76]

H$_2$-Blockers

Several H$_2$-blockers are currently available by prescription and over the counter. These drugs act at the histamine type 2 receptor by competitive binding, and they reduce gastric acid secretion along with pepsin production.[25,87] Some of the H$_2$-blocker effect is on the hepatic metabolism of other drugs, so patients should consult with their physicians and pharmacists to avoid drug-drug interactions. H$_2$-blockers may be used

as first-line therapy in patients with minor EER, as adjunct therapy, or as step-down therapy when weaning patients from PPIs.[76] Of patients with chronic laryngitis who were treated with H$_2$-blockers and behavioral modifications, 54% noted symptomatic relief after six weeks of therapy, with 92% noting some recurrence of symptoms after cessation of H$_2$-blocker therapy.[30] Long-term high-dose H$_2$-blocker therapy was not noted to be as effective or as cost effective as compared with PPI therapy for the treatment of significant esophagitis.[35]

Proton Pump Inhibitors

PPIs act against the enzyme hydrogen-potassium adenosine triphosphatase in the parietal cell, thus blocking the final step of gastric acid production.[25] These drugs are more effective than H$_2$-antagonists for the long-term reduction of basal and stimulated levels of gastric acid production. Postma, Johnson, and Koufman[76] recommend initiating patients with significant EER on twice-daily dosing of PPI therapy, along with behavioral modifications (especially if the patients are positive for GERD or have lower esophageal pH probe positivity); they should then be reevaluated at two-month intervals. H$_2$-blockers may be added to limit nighttime acid breakthrough, but the decision to do this is based on the pattern of reflux seen on dual-channel pH probe study. Patients are assessed with the RFS and RSI, and, when patients have had two consecutive examinations with RFS scores of less than 5 and RSI score of less than 10, the authors recommend tapering PPI therapy. The protocol for tapering medications that the authors recommend involves initially stopping the nighttime do of PPI and substituting an H$_2$-blocker. Two weeks later, the morning medication also becomes an H$_2$-blocker. If the patient experiences breakthrough symptoms, PPI therapy is resumed. For patients who do not show symptomatic improvement at the 4-month mark—despite high-dose PPI therapy—the pH probe study is repeated with the patient taking medication.[76] A significant number of patients with chronic laryngitis on PPI therapy may show relative PPI resistance.[1] Other reasons for treatment failure include poor compliance and breakthrough on acid suppression therapy.[1]

A small, prospective, double-blind, placebo-controlled study of the efficacy of twice-daily dosing of omeprazole for patients with chronic laryngitis and at least four episodes of LPR on pH probe study revealed a placebo effect.[68] Most symptom scores improved over time for both the omeprazole and the placebo groups. The researchers did not see significant changes in endoscopic laryngeal findings in either group. Hoarseness (when scored low) and chronic throat clearing were noted to improve in the omeprazole group. The duration of this study was short; patients were evaluated at one and two months. A long-term, placebo-controlled study of the efficacy of PPI therapy for EER has not as of yet been performed.

Promotility Agents

Metoclopramide is a dopamine antagonist, and it is effective against GER. It increases LES pressure, improves gastric emptying, and may increase esophageal clearance.[25,71] Metoclopramide is the only prokinetic agent that is currently available on the market, although new serotonin agonists are being evaluated by the U.S. Food and Drug Administration. Unfortunately, up to a third of patients may experience side effects from metoclopramide.[25] Patients with diabetes mellitus, dystrophia myotonica, and anorexia nervosa may have significantly delayed gastric emptying and thus may benefit from prokinetic agents.[71] Erythromycin may be used as a prokinetic agent, and it acts as a motilin agonist.[43]

Other Medical Therapy

Sucralfate has been shown to enhance mucosal resistance to trauma, is effective for promoting the healing of duodenal ulcers, and has been shown in animal studies to protect esophageal mucosa against injury from acid.[25] Sucralfate is a salt of sucrose, and it is well tolerated by patients. Its value as a treatment for patients with EER is not well elucidated. Bethanechol is an anticholinergic agent that has been shown to increase LES pressure, decrease GER, and improve salivary flow.[25]

Surgical Treatment

Antireflux surgery involves replacing the LES into the abdomen and then augmenting the LES as an antireflux barrier. The Nissen fundoplication involves the use of a 360-degree wrap of the gastric fundus around the intraabdominal esophagus.[38] Ten-year success rates for the treatment of GERD are quoted to be around 90%, with a mortality rate of 1%.[38] Fundoplication can be performed with an open or a laparoscopic approach. Complications of fundoplication are rare and include bleeding, the need for splenectomy, dysphagia, slippage of the fundoplication into the chest, early satiety, bloating, diarrhea, pneumothorax, and gastric ulceration. Deveney, Brenner, and Cohen[22] assessed 13 patients with persistent laryngeal inflammatory lesions and voice disorders who underwent Nissen fundoplication, and they found that 73% (11 patients) showed a resolution of symptoms and endoscopic changes. Lindstrom and others[58] performed a retrospective review of patients with EER who underwent Nissen fundoplication and found that 25 out of 29 patients had near total symptomatic relief and were

not taking any antireflux medications. Wright and Rhodes[102] reviewed 145 patients with EER symptoms that underwent the laparoscopic Hill repair and saw statistically significant improvement in EER symptoms postoperatively.

OTOLARYNGOLOGIC DISORDERS ASSOCIATED WITH EER
Chronic Laryngitis

Hanson and colleagues[30,31,32] define chronic laryngitis as a three months' or longer history of one or more of the following: hoarseness that worsens with voice use; persistent or recurrent sore throat without throat infection; sensation of postnasal drip; and throat clearing or cough in the absence of lower respiratory tract or pulmonary disease. The authors report that the sensation of chronic postnasal drip is the most common and earliest manifestation of chronic irritative laryngitis, with throat discomfort and dysphonia as the second and third most common symptoms, respectively. The sensation of constant secretions in the back of the throat is thought to be a result of ciliary dysfunction in the posterior larynx and pharynx.[32] Hanson and Jiang[32] studied 182 patients with chronic laryngitis that was felt to be associated with EER. Ninety-six percent of patients experienced relief with antireflux treatment within 12 weeks. Fifty-one percent (93 patients) responded to nocturnal antireflux management alone; 48 patients required the addition of an H_2-blocker nightly, and 34 required the addition of 20 mg of nightly omeprazole. Seven patients in the study required higher dosages of omeprazole, and all of these patients were noted to have severe laryngeal changes at their pretreatment examinations. Symptomatic relapse was common with the discontinuation of therapy. Habermann and colleagues[29] showed that hoarseness, globus pharyngeus, sore throat, heartburn, and coughing were symptoms in patients with chronic laryngitis that showed significant improvement with an empiric 6-week course of a PPI.

Rival and others[77] demonstrated that 84% of patients with cervical symptoms associated with EER had a symptomatic improvement with antireflux therapy. Koufman and colleagues,[52,53] Fraser, Morton, and Gillibrand,[23] and Postma, Johnson, and Koufman[76] point to the need for longer duration of treatment, stating that up to 6 months may be necessary. Koufman and colleagues[53] showed that, with six months of antireflux treatment, 85% of patients with chronic laryngitis showed treatment efficacy. He noted that half of these responders demonstrated an effect in 3 weeks to 3 months, with the remaining patients responding by 6 months.[8,53,76] In a prospective study of patients with chronic laryngitis who were treated with a combination therapy of behavioral modifications, PPI therapy, and cisapride, significant therapeutic benefit was noted in patients with chronic hoarseness, but not in those with intermittent dysphonia.[34]

Contact Ulcer and Laryngeal Granuloma

Proposed etiologies for vocal process granulomas include EER, vocal misuse, intubation trauma, smoking, chronic cough, chronic throat clearing, infection, and allergies.[36] In a retrospective review of 55 patients with vocal fold granulomas, there was a 76% incidence of associated EER or GERD.[36] A 50% recurrence rate was seen with surgical excision alone. Patients that were treated with antireflux measures, medications, and voice therapy showed resolution of granulomas in all but four patients. In the recalcitrant four patients, antireflux surgery resulted in resolution of the granulomas.[36] In a retrospective study of 58 male patients with vocal contact ulcers and granulomas, esophageal dysfunction was found in 74%.[70] Hoffman and colleagues[39] recommend a treatment algorithm for laryngeal granulomas and ulcers that uses surgical intervention as a last step, with the medical management of reflux and voice therapy as the mainstay of treatment; intralaryngeal botulinum toxin is recommended for recalcitrant cases. Surgical management is reserved for cases in which conservative management has failed, in which airway obstructive symptoms are present, or if the diagnosis is in doubt.[39] Figures 109-1 through 109-4 show some clinical examples.

EER and Head and Neck Cancer

Extraesophageal reflux may play a role in the development of head and neck squamous cell carcinoma,

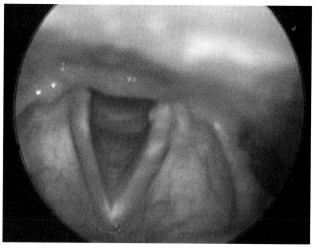

Figure 109-2. The same patient as was seen in Figure 109-1 after 4 months of twice-daily proton pump inhibitor therapy and behavioral modifications.

although it has not been established as a cocarcinogen.[57,88,98] EER may contribute to complications of both surgical management and radiation treatment of head and neck carcinoma.[17] Copper and colleagues[17] prospectively evaluated 24 patients with laryngeal and pharyngeal squamous cell carcinoma and 10 patients who had previously received radiotherapy, with 24-hour dual pH probe studies performed before treatment. Eleven out of 24 patients had pathologic reflux in both probes, and only four patients (17%) were negative according to both probes.[17] Sixty percent of the irradiated patients had pathologic reflux documented by the upper probe, 70% had it according to the lower probe, and 40% positive by both probes.[17] A high incidence of LPR was seen in patients with premalignant and early glottic carcinomas, with 85% having positive

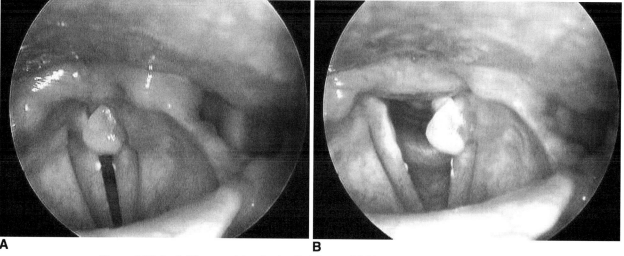

A   B

Figure 109-1. A 60-year-old patient with left vocal fold granuloma before treatment.

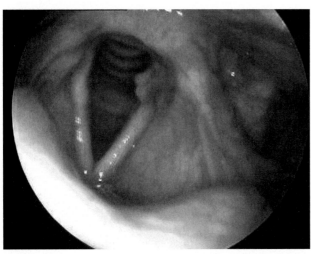

Figure 109-3. A 45-year-old male patient with recalcitrant left vocal fold granuloma. Prior treatment included removal, voice therapy, and high-dose proton pump inhibitor therapy with botulinum toxin injection. Dual pH probe study revealed moderate reflux in both probes.

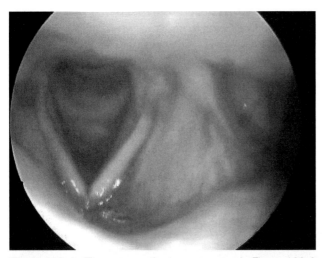

Figure 109-4. The same patient as was seen in Figure 109-3 two months after undergoing an endoscopic antireflux procedure.

pH probe studies.[57] No significant correlations with degree of reflux severity or histologic stage was seen.[57] Sung and colleagues[88] studied the effect of bile acid on cultured human pharyngeal cells. Bile acid is known to be associated with tumor formation in the esophagus through the overexpression of cyclooxygenase-2. Bile salts or acidic conditions were noted to induce cyclooxygenase-2 expression in normal pharyngeal mucosa, which may imply a role in tumorigenesis in the pharynx.[88]

CONCLUSION

There is substantial evidence that many otolaryngologic and respiratory symptoms and disorders can be associated with EER. EER should be considered in patients presenting with laryngeal, pharyngeal, and airway complaints. The evaluation and management of these patients must be individualized. No single diagnostic test available offers us a definitive gold standard; medical management offers these patients substantial symptomatic relief and may require a multidisciplinary approach.

REFERENCES

1. Amin MR and others: Proton pump inhibitor resistance in the treatment of laryngopharyngeal reflux, *Otolaryngol Head Neck Surg* 125:374, 2001.
2. Avidan B and others: Walking and chewing reduce postprandial acid reflux, *Aliment Pharmacol Ther* 15:151, 2001.
3. Aviv JE and others: Laryngopharyngeal sensory deficits in patients with laryngopharyngeal reflux and dysphagia, *Ann Otol Rhinol Laryngol* 109:1000, 2000.
4. Aviv JE and others: Endoscopic evaluation of swallowing as an alternative to 24-hour pH monitoring for diagnosis of extraesophageal reflux, *Ann Otol Rhinol Laryngol* 109:S25, 2000.
5. Bauman NM and others: Reflex laryngospasm induced by stimulation of distal esophageal afferents, *Laryngoscope* 104:209, 1994.
6. Bauman NM and others: Value of pH probe testing in pediatric patients with extraesophageal manifestations of gastroesophageal reflux disease: a retrospective review, *Ann Otol Rhinol Laryngol* 109:S18, 2000.
7. Beaver ME and others: Diagnosis of laryngopharyngeal reflux disease with digital imaging, *Otolaryngol Head Neck Surg* 128:103, 2003.
8. Belafsky PC, Postma GN, Koufman JA: Laryngopharyngeal reflux symptoms improve before changes in physical findings, *Laryngoscope* 111:979, 2001.
9. Belafsky PC, Postma GN, Koufman JA: The validity and reliability of the reflux finding score (RFS), *Laryngoscope* 111:1313, 2001.
10. Belafsky PC and others: Symptoms and findings of laryngopharyngeal reflux, *Ear Nose Throat J* 81(suppl 2):10, 2002.
11. Belafsky PC, Postma GN, Koufman JA: The association between laryngeal pseudosulcus and laryngopharyngeal reflux, *Otolaryngol Head Neck Surg* 126:649, 2002.
12. Bilgin C and others: The comparison of an empiric proton pump inhibitor trial vs 24 hour double-probe pH monitoring in laryngopharyngeal reflux, *J Laryngol Otol* 117:386, 2003.
13. Book DT and others: Perspectives in laryngopharyngeal reflux: an international survey, *Laryngoscope* 112:1399, 2002.
14. Branski RC, Bhattacharyya N, Shapiro J: The reliability of the assessment of endoscopic laryngeal findings associated with laryngopharyngeal reflux disease, *Laryngoscope* 112:1019, 2002.
15. Cohen JT and others: Clinical manifestations of laryngopharyngeal reflux, *Ear Nose Throat J* 81(suppl 2):19, 2002.
16. Contencin P, Narcy P: Gastropharyngeal reflux in infants and children: a pharyngeal pH monitoring study, *Arch Otolaryngol Head Neck Surg*, 118:1028, 1992.

17. Copper MP and others: High incidence if laryngopharyngeal reflux in patients with head and neck cancer, *Laryngoscope* 110:1007, 2000.
18. Cucchiara S and others: Simultaneous prolonged recordings of proximal and distal intraesophageal pH in children with gastroesophageal reflux disease and respiratory symptoms, *Am J Gastroenterol* 90:1791, 1995.
19. de Caestecker J: Medical therapy for supraesophageal complications of gastroesophageal reflux, *Am J Med* 103:138S, 1997.
20. DelGaudio JM, Waring P: Empiric esomeprazole in the treatment of laryngopharyngeal reflux, *Laryngoscope* 113:598, 2003.
21. Dent J: Patterns of lower esophageal sphincter function associated with gastroesophageal reflux, *Am J Med* 103:30S, 1997.
22. Deveney CW, Brenner K, Cohen J: Gastroesophageal reflux and laryngeal disease, *Arch Surg* 128:1021, 1993.
23. Fraser AG, Morton RP, Gillibrand J: Presumed laryngo-pharyngeal reflux: investigate or treat? *J Laryngol Otol* 114:441, 2000.
24. Galli J and others: The role of acid and alkaline reflux in laryngeal squamous cell carcinoma, *Laryngoscope* 112:1861, 2002.
25. Gaynor EB: Gastroesophageal reflux as an etiologic factor in laryngeal complications of intubation, *Laryngoscope* 98:972, 1988.
26. Gaynor EB: Otolaryngologic manifestations of gastroesophageal reflux, *Am J Gastroenterol* 86:801, 1991.
27. Giacchi RJ, Sullivan D, Rothstein SG: Compliance with anti-reflux therapy in patients with otolaryngologic manifestations of gastroesophageal reflux disease, *Laryngoscope* 110:19, 2000.
28. Gumpert L and others: Hoarseness and gastroesophageal reflux in children, *J Laryngol Otol* 112:49, 1998.
29. Habermann W and others: Ex juvantibus approach for chronic posterior laryngitis: results of short-term pantoprazole therapy, *J Laryngol Otol* 113: 734, 1999.
30. Hanson DG, Kamel PL, Kahrilas PJ: Outcomes of antireflux therapy for the treatment of chronic laryngitis, *Ann Otol Rhinol Laryngol* 104:550, 1995.
31. Hanson DG and others: Acoustic measurements of change in voice quality with treatment for chronic posterior laryngitis, *Ann Otol Rhinol Laryngol* 106:279, 1997.
32. Hanson DG, Jiang JJ: Diagnosis and management of chronic laryngitis associated with reflux, *Am J Med* 108:112S, 2000.
33. Hanson DG and others: Role of esophageal pH recording in management of chronic laryngitis, *Ann Otol Rhinol Laryngol* 109:S4, 2000.
34. Hamden AL and others: Effect of aggressive therapy on laryngeal symptoms and voice characteristics in patients with gastroesophageal reflux, *Acta Otolaryngol* 121:868, 2001.
35. Harris RA, Kuppermann M, Richter JE: Proton pump inhibitors or histimine-2 receptor antagonists for the prevention of recurrences of erosive reflux esophagitis: a cost-effective analysis, *Am J Gastroenterol* 92:2179, 1997.
36. Havas TE, Priestley J, Lowinger DS: A management strategy for vocal process granulomas, *Laryngoscope* 109:301, 1999.
37. Hickson C, Simpson CB, Falcon R: Laryngeal pseudosulcus as a predictor of laryngopharyngeal reflux, *Laryngoscope* 111:1742, 2001.
38. Hinder RA and others: The surgical option for gastroesophageal reflux disease, *Am J Med* 103:144S, 1997.
39. Hoffman HT and others: Vocal process granuloma, *Head Neck* 23:1061, 2001.
40. Hogan WJ: Spectrum of supraesophageal complications of gastroesophageal reflux disease, *Am J Med* 103:77S, 1997.
41. Hogan WJ and others: Management issues in supraesophageal complication of GERD. First Multi-Disciplinary International Symposium on Supraesophageal Complications of Gastroesophageal Reflux Disease. Workshop Consensus Reports, *Am J Med* 103:149S, 1997.
42. Holland BW and others: Laryngopharyngeal reflux and laryngeal web formation in patients with pediatric recurrent respiratory papillomas, *Laryngoscope* 112:1926, 2002.
43. Horn JR: Use of prokinetic agents in special populations, *Am J Health Syst Pharm* 53:S27, 1996.
44. Ing AJ: Cough and gastroesophageal reflux, *Am J Med* 103:91S, 1997.
45. Irwin RS and others: Chronic cough due to gastroesophageal reflux, *Chest* 104:1511, 1993.
46. Kamel PL, Hanson DG, Kahrilas PJ: Outcomes of antireflux therapy for the treatment of chronic laryngitis, *Ann Otol Rhinol Laryngol* 104:550, 1996.
47. Kibblewhite DJ, Morrison MD: A double-blind controlled study of the efficacy of cimetidine in the treatment of cervical symptoms of gastroesophageal reflux, *J Otolaryngol* 19:103, 1990.
48. Knight RE, Wells JR, Parrish RS: Esophageal dysmotility as an important co-factor in extraesophageal manifestations of gastroesophageal reflux, *Laryngoscope* 110:1462, 2000.
49. Koufman JA: The otolaryngologic manifestations of gastroesophageal reflux disease (GERD): a clinical investigation of 225 patients using ambulatory 24-pH monitoring and an experimental investigation of the role of acid and pepsin in the development of laryngeal injury, *Laryngoscope* 101:S1, 1991.
50. Koufman JA, Amin MR, Panetti M.: Prevalence of reflux in 113 consecutive patients with laryngeal and voice disorders, *Otolaryngol Head Neck Surg* 123:385, 2000.
51. Koufman JA: Laryngopharyngeal reflux 2002: a new paradigm of airway disease, *Ear Nose Throat J* 81:2, 2002.
52. Koufman JA: Laryngopharyngeal reflux is different from classic gastroesophageal reflux disease, *Ear Nose Throat J* 81:7, 2002.
53. Koufman JA and others: Laryngopharyngeal reflux: position statement of the committee on speech, voice, and swallowing disorders of the American Academy of Otolaryngology–Head and Neck Surgery, *Otolaryngol Head Neck Surg* 127:32, 2002.
54. Koufman JA and others: Prevalence of esophagitis in patients with pH-documented laryngopharyngeal reflux, *Laryngoscope* 112:1606, 2002.
55. Kozarek RA: Complications of reflux esophagitis and their medical management, *Gastroenterol Clin North Am* 19:713, 1990.
56. Lang IM, Shaker R.: Anatomy and physiology of the upper esophageal sphincter, *Am J Med* 103:50S, 1997.
57. Lewin JS and others: Characterization of laryngopharyngeal reflux inpatients with premalignant or early carcinomas of the larynx, *Cancer* 97:1010, 2003.
58. Lindstrom DR and others: Nissen fundoplication surgery for extraesophageal manifestations of gastroesophageal reflux (EER), *Laryngoscope* 112:1762, 2002.
59. Little JP and others: Extraesophageal reflux: 24-hour double probe pH monitoring of 222 children, *Ann Otol Rhinol Laryngol* 169:S1, 1997.
60. Loughlin CJ, Koufman JA: Paroxysmal laryngospasm secondary to gastroesophageal reflux, *Laryngoscope* 106:1502, 1996.
61. Loughlin CJ and others: Acid-induced laryngospasm in canine model, *Laryngoscope* 106:1506, 1996.

62. Maronian NC and others: Association of laryngopharyngeal reflux disease and subglottic stenosis, *Ann Otol Rhinol Laryngol* 110:606, 2001.

63. Mathias S and others: The health related quality of life benefits of treatment with lansoprazole versus omeprazole or erosive reflux esophagitis, *Gastroenterology* 108:A160, 1995.

64. Matthews BL and others: Reflux in infants with laryngomalacia: results of 24-hour double-probe pH monitoring, *Otolaryngol Head Neck Surg* 120:860, 1999.

65. McMurray JS and others: Role of laryngoscopy, dual pH probe monitoring and laryngeal mucosal biopsy in the diagnosis of pharyngoesophageal reflux, *Ann Otol Rhinol Laryngol* 110:299, 2001.

66. McNally PR and others: Evaluation of gastroesophageal reflux as a cause of idiopathic hoarseness, *Dig Dis Sci* 34:1900, 1989.

67. McNally PR and others: Hoarseness and gastroesophageal reflux: what is the relationship? *Gastroenterology* 96:1717, 1990.

68. Noordzij JP and others: Evaluation of omeprazole in the treatment of reflux laryngitis: a prospective, placebo controlled, randomized, double-blind study, *Laryngoscope* 111:2147, 2001.

69. Noordzij JP and others: Correlation of pH probe-measured laryngopharyngeal reflux with symptoms and signs of reflux laryngitis, *Laryngoscope* 112:2192, 2002.

70. Ohman L and others: Esophageal dysfunction in patients with contact ulcer of the larynx, *Ann Otol Rhinol Laryngol* 92:228, 1983.

71. Orihata M, Sarna SK: Contractile mechanism of action of gastroprokinetic agents: cisapride, metoclopramide, and domperidone, *Am J Physiol* 266:G665, 1994.

72. Pope CE: The esophagus for the nonesophagologist, *Am J Med* 103:19S, 1997.

73. Postma GN: Ambulatory pH monitoring methodology, *Ann Otol Rhinol Laryngol* 109:S10, 2000.

74. Postma GN and others: Esophageal motor function in laryngopharyngeal reflux is superior to that in classic gastroesophageal reflux disease, *Ann Otol Rhinol Laryngol* 110:1114, 2001.

75. Postma GN and others: Laryngopharyngeal reflux testing, *Ear Nose Throat J* 81(suppl 2):14, 2002.

76. Postma, G.N., Johnson, L.F., Koufman, J. A.: Treatment of laryngopharyngeal reflux, *ENT* 81(S2):24, 2002.

77. Rival R and others: Role of gastroesophageal reflux disease in patients with cervical symptoms, *Otolaryngol Head Neck Surg* 113:364, 1995.

78. Schiller LR: Upper gastrointestinal motility disorders and respiratory symptoms, *Am J Health Syst Pharm* 53:S13, 1996.

79. Schroeder PL and others: Dental erosion and acid reflux disease, *Ann Intern Med* 122:809, 1995.

80. Shaker R and others: Esophagopharyngeal distribution of refluxed gastric acid in patients with reflux laryngitis, *Gastroenterology* 109:1575, 1995.

81. Shaker R, Lang IM: Reflux mediated airway protective mechanisms against retrograde aspiration, *Am J Med* 103:64S, 1997.

82. Shaw GY, Searl JP: Laryngeal manifestations of gastroesophageal reflux before and after treatment with omeprazole, *South Med J* 90:1115, 1997.

83. Shaw GY: Application of ambulatory 24-hour multiprobe pH monitoring in the presence of extraesophageal manifestations of gastroesophageal reflux, *Ann Otol Rhinol Laryngol* 109:S15, 2000.

84. Smit CF: Gastropharyngeal and gastroesophageal reflux in globus and hoarseness, *Arch Otolaryngol Head Neck Surg* 126:827, 2000.

85. Smit DF and others: Monitoring of laryngopharyngeal reflux: influence of meals and beverages, *Ann Otol Rhinol Laryngol* 112:109, 2003.

86. Smoak BR, Koufman JA: Effects of gum chewing on pharyngeal and esophageal pH, *Ann Otol Rhinol Laryngol* 110:1117, 2001.

87. Sontag SJ: The medical management of reflux esophagitis: role of antacids and acid inhibition, *Gastroenterol Clin North Am,* 19:683,1990.

88. Sung MW and others: Bile acid induces cyclo-oxygenase-2 expression in cultured human pharyngeal cells: a possible mechanism of carcinogenesis in the upper aerodigestive tract by laryngopharyngeal reflux, *Laryngoscope* 113:1059, 2003.

89. Tasker A and others: Is gastric reflux a cause of otitis media with effusion in children? *Laryngoscope* 112:1930, 2002.

90. Tauber S, Gross M, Issing WJ: Association of laryngopharyngeal symptoms with gastroesophageal reflux disease, *Laryngoscope* 112:879, 2002.

91. Thompson JK, Koehler RE, Richter JE: Detection of gastroesophageal reflux: value of barium studies compared with 24-hr pH monitoring, *Am J Radiol* 162:621, 1994.

92. Thurnheer R, Henz S, Knoblauch A: Sleep-related laryngospasm, *Eur Resp J* 10:2084, 1997.

93. Toohill RJ, Kuhn JC: Role of refluxed acid in pathogenesis of laryngeal disorders, *Am J Med* 103:100S, 1997.

94. Ulualp SO and others: Pharyngeal pH monitoring in patients with posterior laryngitis, *Otolaryngol Head Neck Surg* 120:673, 1999.

95. Ulualp SO, Toohill RJ: Laryngopharyngeal reflux: state of the art diagnosis and treatment, *Otolaryngol Clin North Am* 4:785, 2000.

96. Vincent DA and others: The proximal probe in esophageal pH monitoring: development of a normative database, *J Voice* 14:247, 2000.

97. Walner DL and others: Gastroesophageal reflux in patients with subglottic stenosis, *Arch Otolaryngol Head Neck Surg* 124:551, 1998.

98. Ward PH, Hanson DG: Reflux as an etiological factor of carcinoma of the laryngopharynx, *Laryngoscope* 98:1195, 1988.

99. Waring JP and others: Chronic cough and hoarseness in patients with severe gastroesophageal reflux disease, *Dig Dis Sci* 40:1093, 1995.

100. Weiner GM, Batch JG, Radford K: Dysphonia as an atypical presentation of gastro-oesophageal reflux, *J Laryngol Otol* 109:1195, 1995.

101. Wo JM and others: Empiric trial of high-dose omeprazole in patients with posterior laryngitis: a prospective study, *Am J Gastroenterol* 92:2160, 1997.

102. Wright RC, Rhodes KP: Improvement of laryngopharyngeal reflux symptoms after laparoscopic Hill repair, *Am J Surg* 185:455, 2003.

103. Zalzal GH, Choi SS, Patel KM: The effects of gastroesophageal reflux on laryngotracheal reconstruction, *Arch Otolaryngol Head Neck Surg* 122:297, 1996.

104. Zalzal GH, Tran LP: Pediatric gastroesophageal reflux and laryngopharyngeal reflux, *Otolaryngol Clin North Am* 33:151, 2000.

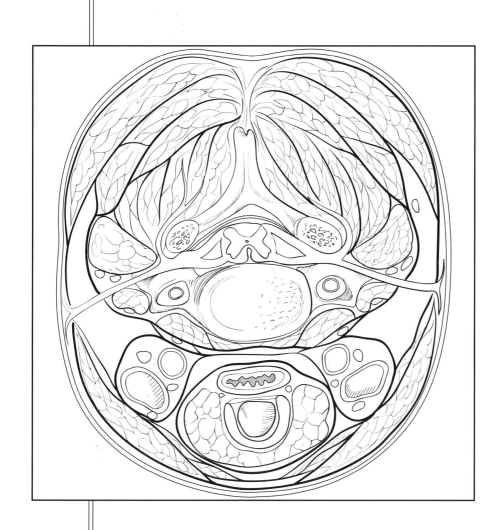

DEEP NECK INFECTION

Harrison G. Weed
L. Arick Forest

INTRODUCTION

Antibiotics have reduced the prevalence and improved the outcomes of deep neck infections; however, deep neck infections continue to be associated with severe illness and death.[3,56] Before the antibiotic era, 70% of deep neck infections evolved from tonsillitis or pharyngitis. Although tonsillitis remains the most common cause of deep neck infections in children,[66] poor dental hygiene and injection drug abuse are now the most common causes of deep neck infections in adults.[43,64] Other causes include trauma, surgical trauma, esophageal perforation, laryngopyocele, infected branchial cleft, and thyroglossal duct cysts,[46] thyroiditis, and mastoiditis with Bezold's (mastoid tip) abscess. Even with such a broad differential diagnosis, there was no apparent cause for 22% of the deep neck infections in one study.[64] Although antibiotic therapy has improved the outcome of deep neck infections, surgery is often necessary for diagnosis and for drainage, especially as infections caused by bacteria that are resistant to many antibiotics become increasingly common.[6,8,14]

MICROBIOLOGY

Deep neck infections are frequently polymicrobial and often caused by oral bacteria. However, although more than 50 species of bacteria can be isolated from a person's mouth, a typical deep neck infection involves only about five different species.[5,13] Anaerobic bacteria, such as Fusobacteria species, pigmented bacteroides species, and anaerobic streptococci (Peptostreptococci species), comprise 90% of the bacteria by weight in the gingival crevice. These anaerobic bacteria are often involved in deep neck infections. Facultatively anaerobic streptococci colonize the tooth and tongue surfaces, and Streptococcus pyogenes (group A streptococcus, the cause of strep throat and erysipelas) adheres well to oral epithelial cells. Streptococci are the organisms most commonly cultured from deep neck abscesses.[17,63,64,66]

Aerobic gram-negative bacilli and staphylococci are not commonly found in the mouth or in deep neck infections, except in injection drug abusers and seriously ill hospitalized patients.[3]

ANATOMY
Lymphatic Vessels

The 10 groups of lymph nodes and their interconnecting vessels constitute routes for physiologic drainage and for potential spread of infection in the neck. The occipital, mastoid, parotid, facial, submandibular, and submental lymph nodes circle the base of the head. They are joined by the sublingual and retropharyngeal lymph nodes to drain into the anterior and, predominantly, the lateral, cervical chains. All lymph nodes in the head and neck ultimately drain into the deep cervical chains along the carotid arteries, providing a potential route for the spread of infection to the deep spaces of the neck and the bloodstream.

Cervical Fascia

An understanding of the layers of the cervical fascia can help in determining the anatomic location of a deep neck infection, in predicting the extent of the infection, and in choosing an approach for surgical drainage. Please see the Radiology chapter for illustrations. The cervical fascia is fibrous connective tissue that envelops muscles and neurovascular bundles, dividing the neck and creating potential spaces. The two major divisions of the cervical fascia are the superficial and the deep. The deep cervical fascia is further divided into the superficial, middle, and deep layers. Where they meet, these layers coalesce and cannot be separated. All three layers of the deep cervical fascia contribute to the carotid sheath, enabling some deep neck infections to track to the great vessels of the neck and, from there, into the skull or the chest.

Superficial Cervical Fascia

The superficial or cervicocephalic fascia is located immediately deep to the dermis. It ensheathes the platysma and the muscles of facial expression. The superficial fascia extends from the epicranium down to the thorax and axilla. The superficial musculoaponeurotic system (SMAS) is part of the superficial cervical fascia. The space between the superficial cervical fascia and the superficial layer of the deep cervical fascia contains adipose tissue, sensory nerves, vessels such as the external and anterior jugular veins, and the superficial lymphatics. Infections limited to this region are not considered deep neck infections and can usually be managed successfully with antibiotics alone or with superficial incision and drainage along Langer's lines.

Superficial Layer of the Deep Cervical Fascia

The superficial layer of the deep cervical fascia also called the anterior layer, the enveloping layer, the external layer, and the investing layer surrounds the neck. It can be described by the "rule of twos." It envelops two muscles and two glands and it forms two spaces. Posteriorly it inserts into the nuchal ridge formed by the spinous processes. The superficial layer of the deep cervical fascia spreads laterally and anteriorly, splitting to envelop both the trapezius and the sternocleidomastoid muscles. It attaches anteriorly to the hyoid bone. The superficial layer of the deep cervical fascia contributes to the lateral aspect of the carotid sheath. Superiorly it envelops both the submandibular and the parotid glands. It fuses with the fascia covering the anterior bellies of the diagastric and mylohyoid muscles, forming the floor of the submandibular space or triangle. At the mandible the superficial layer of the deep cervical fascia splits, and the internal layer covers the medial surface of the pterygoid muscle up to the skull base. The external layer covers the masseter muscle and inserts into the zygomatic arch. Inferiorly, it inserts into the clavicles, sternum, and acromion of the scapula. The two spaces formed by the superficial layer of the deep cervical fascia are the space of the posterior triangle and the suprasternal space of Burns in the anterior midline.

Middle Layer of the Deep Cervical Fascia

The middle layer of the deep cervical fascia is also called the prethyroid fascia and the pretracheal fascia. It is separated into the muscular and the visceral divisions. The muscular division surrounds the sternothyroid, sternohyoid, and thyrohyoid "strap" muscles. Inferiorly this division also inserts into the clavicle and the sternum. Superiorly the middle layer of the deep cervical fascia inserts into the hyoid and thyroid cartilages. Posteriorly it fuses with the alar division of the deep layer of the deep cervical fascia at about the level of the second thoracic vertebra and forms the anterior wall of the retropharyngeal space. The visceral or submucosal division of the middle layer of the deep cervical fascia envelops the thyroid gland, trachea, and esophagus. It extends inferiorly into the upper mediastinum, covering the trachea and the esophagus and joining the fibrous pericardium. The middle layer of the deep cervical fascia also envelops the pharyngeal constrictor and buccinator muscles forming the buccopharyngeal fascia. Superiorly it inserts into the hyoid and thyroid cartilages along with the muscular division. Laterally both divisions of the middle layer contribute to the carotid sheath.

Deep Layer of the Deep Cervical Fascia

At the transverse processes of the cervical spine, the deep layer of the deep cervical fascia separates into a posterior prevertebral division and an anterior alar division. The prevertebral division adheres to the anterior aspect of the vertebral bodies and extends from the skull base down the length of the spine. It extends posteriorly around the spine and the muscles of the deep neck, enveloping the vertebral muscles, deep muscles of the posterior triangle, and scalene muscles. The deep layer of the deep cervical fascia also envelops the vertebral arteries and veins and phrenic nerve. It envelops the brachial plexus and the subclavian vessels, extending laterally as the axillary sheath. The alar division of the deep layer is located between the visceral division of the middle layer and the prevertebral division of the deep layer. The deep layer of the deep cervical fascia delineates the posterior boundary of the retropharyngeal space, extending down to about the level of the second thoracic vertebra, where it fuses with the visceral fascia. Both divisions contribute to the carotid sheath.

Deep Spaces—Clinical Correlation

The layers of the cervical fascia create potential spaces that can be occupied by infection. These spaces can be categorized by location as being: (1) in the face: the buccal, canine, masticator, and parotid spaces; (2) in the suprahyoid neck: the peritonsillar, submandibular, sublingual, and lateral pharyngargeal spaces; (3) in the infrahyoid neck: the anterior visceral space and; (4) extending the length of the neck: the retropharyngeal, "danger," prevertebral, and carotid sheath spaces.[13]

Face

Buccal space infections are usually odontogenic and usually arise from the mandibular or maxillary bicuspid and molar teeth. They usually present with marked cheek swelling, but no trismus, and minimal systemic symptoms. They often can be successfully treated with antibiotics alone. If drainage is required, then it is usually more effective if done extraorally. Canine space infections arise from the canine teeth or the maxillary incisors and present with dramatic swelling of the upper lip, often extending to periorbital edema. Intraoral drainage is usually indicated. The three masticator spaces (masseteric, temporal, and pterygoid) intercommunicate with each other and with the buccal, submandibular, and lateral pharyngeal spaces. Masticator space infections usually arise from molar teeth. They usually present with trismus and with mandibular or preauricular swelling and tenderness. Infection in the space deep to the temporalis muscle may initially present with mild preauricular swelling and tenderness, but can also extend to involve the entire side of the face and the orbit, causing proptosis, optic neuritis, and sixth cranial nerve palsy. Pterygoid space infections abut the lateral pharyngeal wall and therefore can present with mild dysphagia. However, if the lateral wall of the pharynx is displaced medially, then the infection is not limited to the pterygoid space, but has extended into the lateral pharyngeal space. Odontogenic parotid space infections have usually originated in mandibular molars and spread from the masseteric space. Such infections present with marked swelling and pain at the angle of the mandible, but no trismus. Systemic symptoms and signs are often prominent. Because the parotid space abuts the lateral pharyngeal space, parotid space infections can spread into the lateral pharyngeal space and from there into the carotid sheath or the retropharyngeal space.

Suprahyoid Neck

Peritonsillar space infections usually arise from tonsillitis. They are manifested by fever, odynophagia, "hot potato" voice, mild trismus, and bulging of the superior pole of the tonsillar pillar and the adjacent soft palate with deviation of the uvula away from the infection. Antibiotics and aspiration for drainage are usually curative, but peritonsillar infections can spread to deeper neck spaces. Submandibular space infections usually arise from the second and third mandibular molars, but can also be due to trauma, resulting in mandibular fracture or laceration of the floor of the mouth. They should not be confused with infections limited to the submandibular salivary glands or lymph nodes that have different causes and treatments. In submandibular space infections, the mandible is swollen and tender, but trismus is absent or minimal, because the muscles of mastication are not involved. Treatment is extraoral drainage, antibiotics, and dental extraction if the infection is odonto-

genic. The sublingual space is medial to the submandibular space and separated from it by the mylohyoid muscle. Sublingual space infections usually arise from the mandibular incisors and present with erythema and swelling and tenderness of the floor of the mouth that begins near the mandible and spreads medially, sometimes elevating the tongue. Surgical drainage should be intraoral from an incision parallel to Wharton's duct.

Ludwig's Angina

Infections of the submandibular and sublingual spaces are sometimes nonspecifically referred to as Ludwig's angina. It is probably best to limit the diagnosis of Ludwig's angina to infections that fit the classic description of a rapidly spreading, firmly indurated cellulitis that originates intraorally and involves submandibular and sublingual spaces bilaterally, but without abscess or lymphadenopathy. In Ludwig's angina, signs of sepsis are usually present. There is erythema and tender, firm edema of the anterior neck without fluctuance. Tissue fluid is not frankly purulent, but serosanguineous and malodorous. There is non-pitting, firm induration of the entire floor of the mouth, elevating the tongue, impairing chewing and swallowing, and producing the classic "hot potato" voice. If edema extends to the tongue base, it can obstruct the airway. Treatment is intravenous antibiotics, close airway monitoring, often including intubation or tracheotomy. Surgery is an option if needed for debridement of necrotic tissue or for decompression of a compartment. In a series described by Parhiscar and Har-El, 75% of patients with Ludwig's angina required intubation or tracheotomy. In 11 of 20 patients with Ludwig's angina, intubation was unsuccessful, resulting in emergent tracheotomy.[48]

Suprahyoid Neck: The Lateral Pharyngeal Space

The lateral pharyngeal (parapharyngeal or pharyngomaxillary) space lies between the superficial and middle layers of the deep cervical fascia. It extends from the skull to the hyoid bone. The suprahyoid neck is the nexus for the spread of deep neck infections, because it abuts the other spaces, both superficial and deep, and it abuts the carotid sheath. Pharyngitis, tonsillitis, parotiditis, mastoiditis, and otitis can spread to the lateral pharyngeal space. Furthermore, infections in the masticator, the submandibular, and the sublingual spaces can spread to the lateral pharyngeal space. From the lateral pharyngeal space, infections can spread into the spaces that extend the length of the neck or directly into the carotid sheath. The lateral pharyngeal space is divided into anterior and posterior (retrostyloid) compartments. Infections in the anterior compartment of the lateral pharyngeal space are manifest by chills, fever, neck pain, odynophagia, trismus, swelling below the jaw angle, and medial displacement of the lateral pharyngeal wall. Rotating the chin opposite to the infection causes pain from compression of the space by the adjacent sternocleidomastoid muscle. In contrast, infections in the posterior compartment can present with sepsis syndrome and little pain or trismus. Because the posterior compartment is deeper and posterior, pharyngeal swelling is often less evident, but there can be ipsilateral Horner's syndrome and paresis of cranial nerves IX to XII. Sequelae of lateral pharyngeal space infection include airway obstruction from laryngeal edema, internal jugular vein thrombosis (Lemierre's syndrome), and carotid rupture. Lateral pharyngeal space infections should be treated with intravenous antibiotics Abscesses should be drained, and prophylactic tracheotomy should be considered.

Infrahyoid Neck

Anterior visceral space infections are caused by extension of thyroid infections or by penetrating trauma, including surgery. Symptoms of infection are hoarseness, dyspnea, and odynophagia. Physical findings include erythema, edema, tenderness, and crepitation of the anterior neck, and erythema and edema of the hypopharynx that can extend to the glottis.

Length of the Neck

The retropharyngeal space lies between the visceral division of the middle layer of the deep cervical fascia and the deep layer of the cervical fascia. It is posterior to the hypopharynx and the esophagus, is medial to the carotid sheath, and extends inferiorly into the mediastinum as far as the third thoracic vertebral body. Retropharyngeal abscess is predominantly an infection of childhood. It is estimated that half of all retropharyngeal abscesses occur in patients 6 to 12 months old and that more than 90% of these abscesses occur in patients younger than 6 years old. The predominant cause of retropharyngeal abscess in children is bacterial infection of the nasal sinuses or nasopharynx. In children, retropharyngeal abscess presents as irritability, excessive drooling, poor oral intake, and sore throat, accompanied by fever, torticollis, and cervical adenopathy on examination. The predominant causes of retropharyngeal abscess in adults are trauma from instrumentation and extension from an adjacent deep neck infection. In adults, symptoms often include anorexia, nasal obstruction, snoring, neck pain, odynophagia, nasal regurgitation and dyspnea, accompanied by fever, tachypnea, and bulging of the lateral wall of the posterior oropharynx on examination.

Posterior to the retropharyngeal space, in between the alar and the prevertebral divisions of the deep layer of the deep cervical fascia is the danger space, so called because infections in this space extend inferiorly into the mediastinum to the level of the diaphragm. Danger space infections are usually spread from the lateral pharyngeal or the retropharyngeal spaces and they present similarly to retropharyngeal space infections. Computed tomography (CT) or Magnetic resonance imaging (MRI) may be required to differentiate retropharyngeal from danger space infections.

Behind the prevertebral layer of the deep cervical fascia is the prevertebral space. It extends inferiorly along the spine to the coccyx. Infections in this space can be caused by trauma to the pharynx or to the spine. The infection may have spread to the prevertebral space posteriorly from the retropharyngeal or the danger spaces. The infection could also have spread anteriorly from the spine, for example, from a paraspinous or a Pott's abscess.

Infections into the carotid sheath can arise from direct inoculation, such as from injection drug abuse or spread from adjacent neck spaces. Such infections can present with chills, fever, sepsis syndrome, erythema, induration and tenderness of the sternocleidomastoid muscle, nuchal rigidity, contralateral torticollis, ipsilateral Horner's syndrome, and vocal cord paralysis. The complications of carotid sheath infection include internal jugular vein thrombosis (Lemierre's syndrome), which is more common in injection drug abusers. Internal jugular vein thrombosis presents with pulmonary septic emboli and, in patients with a patent foramen ovale, with systemic emboli as well. The dural sinus is often also thrombosed. In addition to intravenous antibiotics, the thrombosed jugular vein must be excised. Whether systemic anticoagulation is beneficial is unknown.

Another complication of carotid sheath infection is carotid artery rupture, which is associated with death in about one-third of patients. The internal carotid artery is most commonly involved. Rupture is often preceded by sentinel bleeding from the ear, nose, or mouth.

EVALUATION OF THE PATIENT
History and Physical Examination

Evaluation of a patient with suspected deep neck infection usually starts with history and physical examination. An appropriate history should include inquiry into the duration and rate of progression of symptoms, with explicit inquiry about any tooth pain. It should also include specific questioning about any oral lesions, upper respiratory infections, blunt or penetrating trauma to the head or neck, including dental procedures and injection drug use. In addition, the physician should inquire about any possible immunosuppression including human immunodeficiency virus (HIV) infection and medications including steroids and chemotherapy. Even mild dyspnea must be thoroughly investigated because, in a patient with deep neck infection, dyspnea may be a manifestation of impending airway obstruction and may be a result of airway compression, laryngeal edema, mediastinitis, or pneumonia. Physical examination should include special attention to the teeth, tonsils, and airway. Fever with focal pain and edema are the hallmark findings of acute deep neck infection. The location and extent of induration and the presence of fluctuance should be explicitly documented and marked on the patient's neck skin for future reference. Transnasal fiberoptic laryngoscopy is often indicated to determine the degree of upper airway obstruction and to look for distortions that might lead to difficulties with intubation.

Radiography
Plain Films

Radiography can be essential for adequately evaluating patients with deep neck infections. Dental radiographs, such as a Panorex oral view, are indicated when a dental infection is suspected. Note that the apices of the mandibular second and third molars extend below the mylohyoid line, providing a direct connection between a root tip abscess and infection in the submandibular space. Lateral cervical plain films can image retropharyngeal soft tissues in the posterior wall of the hypopharynx to assess the retropharyngeal and pretracheal spaces.

Compared with CT, lateral cervical neck films are about 83% sensitive in children.[44] Extremes of neck extension or flexion can produce misleading findings, as can films taken during forced inhalation. Normal prevertebral soft tissue thickness at C2 is 7 mm. At C6 the thickness is 14 mm for children and 22 mm for adults.

A chest radiograph is indicated for all patients with deep neck infection to assess the mediastinal silhouette for evidence of widening. Plain films do not otherwise contribute to patient evaluation because they cannot show the extent or depth of the infection.

Ultrasonography

High-resolution ultrasound has the advantages of being portable and not being ionizing radiation. It is therefore available in many emergency departments and physician's offices. Conversely, the reliability of the findings is operator-dependent, and few studies support its use in diagnosis. Therefore, ultrasound is more commonly used to guide needle aspiration and to follow response to therapy than for diagnosis.[69]

Computed Tomography and Magnetic Resonance Imaging

Either CT or MRI is usually indicated when deep neck abscess is suspected. Findings that indicate a deep neck infection include a mass with an air-fluid interface or a cystic or multiloculated appearance, and edema, or contrast ("ring") enhancement of tissue surrounding the mass.[25] CT or MRI can be invaluable in appropriate surgical management by defining the boundaries of the infection, including involvement of the great vessels. Both methods can also identify specific problems such as tracheal compression, mediastinal spread, and internal jugular vein thrombosis. CT is more widely available and takes less time for imaging than does MRI. With contrast enhancement, CT has been shown to be 91% sensitive and 60% specific in distinguishing superficial cellulitis from abscess.[66] MRI offers better resolution of soft tissues, superior imaging of blood vessels, and no interference by dental fillings. In addition, MRI contrast is less allergenic than CT contrast; however, MRI is more expensive than CT and it requires good patient cooperation, because of longer acquisition times.

TREATMENT
Surgical Management

Ensuring a secure airway is the first priority in the management of a deep neck infection. Therefore, intubation with direct laryngoscopy or tracheotomy should always be considered. Superficial infections, such as cellulitis and, sometimes, even abscesses, can be managed with antibiotic therapy alone.[9,40,45] Furthermore, ultrasound and CT-guided aspiration can be effective.[49,69] However, surgical intervention is indicated for most deep abscesses, especially when there is airway compromise, sepsis syndrome, or no response to antibiotic treatment within 48 hours.[21] Fluid resuscitation should precede surgery if possible, because patients will usually be dehydrated from not eating and from fever-related water loss.

An important principle of surgical drainage of a deep neck abscess is wide exposure. The normal anatomy is often distorted and use of readily identifiable landmarks (such as the medial border of the sternocleidomastoid muscle, greater horn of the thyroid cartilage, hyoid bone, digastric muscle, and cricoid) is often necessary to maintain orientation. Blunt dissection should be used whenever possible. Identifying the carotid sheath early is crucial for avoiding inadvertent damage to it and to the major neurovascular structures it contains. Once the abscess cavity is opened, material should be obtained for Gram stain and for culture of aerobic bacteria, anaerobic bacteria, acid-fast bacteria, and fungi. It is best to avoid the use of swabs. Send pus or tissue to the microbiology laboratory, because fastidious organisms are more likely to be isolated from pus or a tissue specimen than from a swab. If culture swabs must be used, then be sure to submit at least three swabs: one for Gram stain, one for general culture, and one specially designed and handled for anaerobic culture. Remaining tissue specimens should be submitted for pathologic evaluation. The abscess should be completely drained, including blunt avulsion of any loculations. All devitalized tissue must be débrided. If there is extensive tissue necrosis, the débrided wound should not be closed. Instead it should be packed with antimicrobial-soaked dressings and allowed to close by secondary or tertiary intention. Frequent inspection of the wound to assess the need for additional débridement is appropriate. Wounds with less necrosis can be closed with active suction drainage. Large-bore drains (19 French) may be required for irrigation. Complications such as septic emboli, septic shock, and pulmonary aspiration should be anticipated during the recuperative period. More aggressive surgery may be required for complicated deep neck infections. For example, a thrombosed internal jugular vein should be ligated and resected. Infection extending into the mediastinum may require thoracic surgery. Although cervical drainage alone is usually sufficient for infections above the carina and the fourth thoracic vertebral body, an abscess below the level of the carina should be drained transthoracically.[19,67] In mediastinal infections not requiring thoracic drainage, blunt dissection along the carotid sheath and the paratracheal space facilitates evacuation of the abscess, and a drain should be placed in the anterior mediastinum.

Antibiotic Treatment

Consider usual oral flora, local antibiotic susceptibility patterns, and culture results from the patient when selecting an antibiotic for a deep neck infection. Many organisms involved in deep neck infection are fastidious and difficult to culture and not all cultured organisms are equally pathogenic. Therefore, it may be unnecessary to administer antibiotics directed against all of the cultured organisms for effective treatment. Use antibiotic(s) generally effective against streptococci, anaerobes, and beta-lactamase-producing bacteria. Either ampicillin-sulbactam or cefoxitin is appropriate for most patients with deep neck infections (Box 110-1). Clindamycin is an important alternative for penicillin-allergic patients. However, the possibility of *Eikenella corrodens*, a gram-negative facultative anaerobe found in the oral cavity, makes it reasonable to add ciprofloxacin or an aminoglycoside,

---

BOX 110-1

EMPIRIC ANTIBIOTIC MANAGEMENT FOR DEEP NECK INFECTION

Otherwise Healthy Patient

Ampicillin-sulbactam 1.5 to 3 g IV every 6 hours or clindamycin 600 to 900 mg IV every 8 hours or cefoxitin 1 to 2 g IV every 6 hours or ceftriaxone 1 to 2 g IV every 12 hours

Compromised Patient or Pseudomonas Aeruginosa Suspected

Ticarcillin-clavulanate 3 to 0.1 g IV every 4 to 6 hours, or piperacillin-tazobactam 3 to 0.375 g IV every 4 to 6 hours, or imipenem-cilastatin 250–250 to 500–500 mg IV every 6 hours (each + / - an aminoglycoside), or clindamycin 600 to 900 mg IV every 8 hours plus ciprofloxacin 400 mg IV every 12 hours, or plus ceftazidime 1 to 2 g IV every 8 hours

Staphylococcus Aureus Suspected

Add vancomycin 1 g IV every 12 hours (dose adjusted for serum levels)

Necrotizing Cervical Fasciitis

Ceftriaxone 2 g IV every 8 hours plus clindamycin 900 mg IV every 8 hours, or plus metronidazole 500 mg IV every 6 hours

---

such as gentamicin, in penicillin-allergic patients responding poorly to clindamycin alone. The combination of metronidazole plus trimethoprim-sulfamethoxazole is also reasonable antibiotic treatment for deep neck infection.

In compromised or hospitalized patients who are likely to be colonized with facultative gram-negative organisms including *Pseudomonas aeruginosa*, appropriate treatment includes ticarcillin-clavulanate, piperacillin-tazobactam, or imipenem-cilastatin. In compromised, penicillin-allergic patients, the combination of clindamycin plus ciprofloxacin or an aminoglycoside is appropriate. Avoid aminoglycosides in elderly patients and in those at risk for hearing or renal impairment to avoid aminoglycoside ototoxicity and nephrotoxicity. If resistant *Staphylococcus* is suspected (e.g., in a postoperative patient or an injection drug user), then adding vancomycin is appropriate until Gram stain and culture results enable more focused therapy. Traditionally, intravenous antibiotics are continued until the patient remains afebrile for 48 hours. However, in patients with normal gastrointestinal function, the excellent oral bioavailability of amoxicillin-clavulanate, clindamycin, ciprofloxacin, metronidazole, and trimethoprimsulfamethoxazole may enable a more rapid progression to oral antibiotics.

SELECTED SYNDROMES
Immunosuppression

Immunosuppressed patients are increasingly encountered because of the worldwide pandemic of HIV and because of advancements in medical therapy including synthetic insulins for diabetes, chemotherapy for cancer, transplantation for organ failure, and immunosuppression for autoimmune disease. Immunosuppressed patients suffer from the same infections that afflict other patients, but with greater frequency. In addition, immunosuppressed patients are more likely to present with minimal symptoms and signs of infection and to suffer serious complications. Such patients can also be infected with usually nonpathogenic organisms. For example, HIV-infected patients can present with neck infection from *Pneumocystis carinii*.[7,15] Therefore, all physicians should routinely inquire about patients' risk factors for immunosuppression. When caring for immunosuppressed patients, physicians should be vigilant about identifying infection. Closer than usual follow-up and more frequent testing, including invasive tissue sampling, are often appropriate in immunosuppressed patients.[57]

Injection Drug Abuse

Injections into the neck for reasons other than medical care can be a common cause of deep neck infection in some populations. In one inner-city practice, 32% of all neck abscesses had this cause.[64] The most frequent location of infection is the anterior cervical triangle, 43 but a search for additional sites of involvement is recommended. A CT scan of the neck and upper chest may be appropriate. A chest radiograph in full exhalation may also be indicated to rule out pneumothorax caused by perforation of the apical pleura. Although complex syndromes such as mycotic aneurysm of the carotid artery[30] have been described, most infections associated with injection drug abuse are bacterial abscesses. Frequently the abscess surrounds a foreign body, such as a broken needle. The organisms most often cultured from neck abscesses in patients who abuse drugs by injection are gram-positive cocci such as staphylococci and streptococci.[18,31,43,64] The staphylococci are frequently methicillin resistant.[31] Oral anaerobes, Enterobacteriaceae, *Haemophilus* species, and *E. corrodens* are also frequently isolated.[31] Therefore, empiric antibiotic treatment for deep neck infection in patients abusing drugs by injection should cover anaerobes, including *E. corrodens*, Enterobacteriaceae, and gram-positive organisms, including methicillin-resistant staphylococci. Appropriate regimens are the same as for other compromised patients with deep neck infection except that vancomycin should be added (see Box 110-1). In addition, if clindamycin is used to cover anaerobes, then an agent effective against *E. corrodens*, such as ciprofloxacin or an aminoglycoside, should also be used. Antibiotic therapy can often be simplified to focus on specific susceptibilities when Gram stain and culture results become available.

Necrotizing Cervical Fasciitis

Necrotizing cervical fasciitis is a fulminant infection with necrosis of connective tissue spread along fascial planes and high mortality.[4,39,42,59] It is usually polymicrobial and odontogenic and occurs more frequently in immunocompromised and postoperative patients.[22,24,51] Ludwig's angina is the most common type of necrotizing cervical fasciitis. The principles described earlier in this chapter for the evaluation and management of deep neck infections apply to necrotizing cervical fasciitis.

The patient is usually acutely and severely ill with a high fever. The overlying skin may be exquisitely tender, edematous, and erythematous. The erythema associated with necrotizing fasciitis is flat and the transition to adjacent normal skin is indistinct. These findings combined with soft-tissue crepitation from gas are diagnostic. As necrosis progresses, the skin becomes pale and anesthetic, and then dusky. Blisters or bullae form, and sloughing can occur within 48 hours of initial symptoms.

Early surgery is mandated for necrotizing fasciitis. Empiric broad-spectrum intravenous antibiotic therapy, such as a combination of a third-generation cephalosporin (ceftriaxone) plus either clindamycin or metronidazole, should be initiated as soon as possible (see Box 110-1). Relatively benign superficial findings often belie the extensive underlying soft tissue necrosis. Subcutaneous tissues are pale and edematous, with fat liquefaction and "dishwater" drainage. All soft tissue and skin that are no longer viable must be excised. The surgical wound should be left open for continued wound care and packed with antimicrobial-soaked gauze. Daily débridement is indicated until the wound stabilizes. Airway control with tracheotomy is almost always indicated at the time of initial débridement.

Necrotizing cervical fasciitis is life threatening, and all patients with this infection should be monitored in an intensive care setting. Respiratory failure, delirium, mediastinitis, pericardial tamponade, disseminated intravascular coagulopathy, and neuropathy are potential complications. Patients with mediastinitis have a fourfold greater mortality rate than those with only cervical involvement (64% vs 15%).[58] Death often results from sepsis with multiorgan failure and hemodynamic collapse.

Hyperbaric oxygen (HBO) has been proposed as adjunctive treatment for necrotizing fasciitis because high tissue oxygen tension inhibits growth of anaerobic bacteria, improves leukocyte killing of ingested bacteria, and induces neovascularization.[27,34] Some authors report higher survival rates for patients with necrotizing fasciitis who are treated with HBO;[29,35,53] whereas others have not found an improvement in survival.[10] No adverse effects have been described in the management of necrotizing cervical fasciitis with HBO, and the apparent clinical benefit is sometimes impressive. Therefore, the use of HBO should be considered in hemodynamically-stable patients with necrotizing cervical fasciitis.

Actinomycosis

Oral-cervicofacial actinomycosis is an uncommon infection characterized by formation of a soft-tissue mass or a multiloculated abscess, destruction of normal tissue planes, and the presence of macroscopic or microscopic sulfur granules. Actinomycosis classically presents as a slowly growing, painless, firm, possibly suppurating, submandibular mass, but it can also present as a rapidly progressive, painful, fluctuant infection anywhere in the neck or face associated with fever and leukocytosis. The infection is caused by a mixture of oral microbes with a predominance of an actinomycete, such as *Actinomyces israelii*, a large gram-positive, anaerobic bacillus. Actinomycosis is seen more frequently in people with poor oral hygiene and oral mucosal trauma and its incidence has decreased in the antibiotic era.

Management does not always require drainage of the abscess. Prolonged, high-dose, antibiotic therapy with penicillin, tetracycline, erythromycin, or clindamycin is necessary to prevent recurrence. A typical regimen might include penicillin G, 3 million units intravenously every 4 hours for 2 to 6 weeks followed by oral amoxicillin, 1 g orally every 12 hours for 2 to 12 months.[38] Cephalosporins and semi-synthetic penicillins such as nafcillin and dicloxacillin are less active against actinomycetes in vitro and should not be used in treatment.

Cervical Lymphadenopathy

Cervical lymphadenopathy can have many and diverse causes. Local infection with pyogenic organisms and oral microbes is the most common cause, but infection with mycobacteria, or viruses, and even sarcoidosis should be considered in the differential diagnosis (Box 110-2). When there is doubt about the cause, fine-needle aspiration (FNA) can be diagnostic, but excisional biopsy is sometimes necessary.

Pyogenic

Acute, unilateral, pyogenic, cervical lymphadenitis is predominantly an infection of young children (ages 1–5 years) and is usually caused by *S. pyogenes*

BOX 110-2

SOME CAUSES OF CERVICAL LYMPHADENOPATHY

Viruses
Epstein-Barr (infectious mononucleosis)
Human immunodeficiency

Bacteria
Streptococcus pyogenes (group A *Streptococcus*)
Staphylococcus aureus
Mixed oral bacteria, including anaerobes
Mycobacterium tuberculosis
Bartonella henselae (cat–scratch disease)

Protozoans
Toxoplasma gondii

(group A *Streptococcus*) or *Staphylococcus aureus*. The child is usually febrile (37.8–39.6°C) with an elevated leukocyte count (12–25 k/ml). Antibiotic treatment is usually curative.[54]

Mycobacterial

Tuberculous cervical lymphadenitis (scrofula) is the most frequent manifestation of extrapulmonary tuberculosis.[2,12,16] The classic presentation is unilateral, painless, firm, erythematous swelling in the posterior triangle.[32,36] The patient is usually asymptomatic and without other evidence of active tuberculosis; however, children and immunosuppressed adults will often have concurrent pulmonary disease.[1,36] Evaluation of the suspect patient should include a tuberculin skin test and a chest radiograph. The skin test is almost always positive (>10 mm induration).[23] FNA usually shows granulomata, but rarely reveals acid-fast bacilli except in immunosuppressed patients. Culture of the specimen is often crucial for differentiating tuberculous lymphadenitis from that caused by other mycobacteria or fungi. Appropriate management includes antituberculous chemotherapy and complete surgical excision without drains to avoid fistulization. Although the specific chemotherapeutic regimen should be based on local susceptibilities and culture results, a 9-month course of isoniazid and rifampin or a 6-month course of isoniazid, rifampin, and pyrazinamide is sufficient for susceptible organisms.

Cervical lymphadenitis caused by nontuberculous Mycobacteria does not respond to antituberculous chemotherapy. In the United States, the most common nontuberculous mycobacteria isolates from the neck are *Mycobacterium avium* complex (*M. avium* and *Mycobacterium intracellulare*), *Mycobacterium fortuitum*, *Mycobacterium kansasii*, and *Mycobacterium scrofulaceum*.[50,61,65] Cervical lymphadenitis caused by nontuberculous mycobacteria occurs most frequently in the submandibular triangle, upper jugular nodes, or the preauricular nodes of children under the age of 6 years.[61] A tuberculin skin test is frequently positive (10–15 mm induration), but a strongly positive test (> 20 mm) is more consistent with tuberculosis.[23,65] Complete surgical excision can be curative. Recurrence is likely after simple incision and drainage or after incomplete excision.[2,37,55,60,62] However, when complete excision threatens vital structures, such as the marginal mandibular branch of the facial nerve, then curettage can yield acceptable results.[23,26,47,65] Antimicrobial chemotherapy directed against nontuberculous mycobacteria has been used, but is not clearly beneficial. Antituberculous chemotherapy is appropriate while culture results are pending, or when a definitive diagnosis cannot be made.

Cat-Scratch Disease

Bartonella henselae, the agent of cat-scratch disease, is an organism that can cause granulomatous cervical lymphadenitis. This infection may have been originally described as conjunctivitis with preauricular lymphadenopathy (Parinaud's oculoglandular syndrome). Cat-scratch disease is a relatively common infection in young children with a history of exposure to cats, especially to kittens.[11] The diagnosis is established by biopsy, demonstrating small pleomorphic gram-negative rods that can be cultured with enough time and under special conditions. The infection and the adenopathy usually resolve spontaneously over several weeks to months in immunocompetent patients, and antibiotic therapy is not indicated.[69] Patients with acquired immunodeficiency syndrome (AIDS) may require lifelong suppressive therapy with a macrolide (e.g. clarithromycin) or a tetracycline.[28]

Toxoplasmosis

Toxoplasmosis is a cause of cervical lymphadenopathy that can be transmitted to humans by cats. *Toxoplasma gondii* is a protozoan parasite with worldwide distribution in all orders of mammals. Serologic surveys indicate that 3% to 70% of healthy adults in the United States have been infected and 80% to 90% of infections are asymptomatic.[52] The most frequent presentation of infection with *Toxoplasma* organisms in immunocompetent patients is discrete, firm, nontender, not suppurating, less than 3 cm, cervical lymph node enlargement.[41] Enlargement of other lymph nodes, fever, malaise, myalgia, sore throat, rash, hepatosplenomegaly, and circulating atypical lymphocytes may occur. The diagnosis should be considered in all cases of acute cervical lymphadenopathy and is supported by characteristic lymph node morphology on biopsy. The diagnosis can be confirmed by serologic testing and there is an increasing role for polymerase chain reaction isolation of *Toxoplasma species* deoxyribonucleic acid from biopsy material. Treatment is unnecessary in immunocompetent patients. Symptoms and lymphadenopathy resolve spontaneously over weeks to several months. Immunocompromised patients, such as those with AIDS, Can develop fatal encephalitis and require lifelong suppressive therapy.[33]

REFERENCES

1. Alleva M and others: Mycobacterial cervical lymphadenitis: a persistent diagnostic problem, *Laryngoscope* 98:855, 1988.
2. Appling D, Miller RH: Mycobacterial cervical lymphadenopathy: 1981 update, *Laryngoscope* 91:1259, 1981.
3. Baker AS, Montgomery WW: Oropharyngeal space infections, *Curr Clin Top Infect Dis* 8:227, 1987.
4. Balcerak RJ, Sisto JM, Bosak RC: Cervicofacial necrotizing fasciitis, *J Oral Maxillofac Surg* 46:450, 1988.
5. Bartlett JG, O'Keefe P: The bacteriology of perimandibular space infections, *J Oral Surg* 37:407, 1979.
6. Bartlett JG, Froggatt JW III: Antibiotic resistance, *Arch Otolaryngol Head Neck Surg* 121:392, 1995.
7. Biavati MD, Khan A, Kessler C: Disseminated Pneumocystis carinii infection involving the neck and nasopharynx, *Otolaryngol Head Neck Surg* 109:773, 1993.
8. Breiman RF and others: Emergence of drug-resistant pneumococcal infections in the United States, *JAMA* 271:1831, 1994.
9. Broughton RA: Nonsurgical management of deep neck infections in children, *Pediatr Infect Dis J* 11:14, 1992.
10. Brown DR and others: A multicenter review of the treatment of major truncal necrotizing infections with and without hyperbaric oxygen therapy, *Am J Surg* 167:485, 1994.
11. Carithers HA: Cat-scratch disease: an overview based on a study of 1,200 patients, *Am J Dis Child* 139:1124, 1985.
12. Castro DJ and others: Cervical mycobacterial lymphadenitis: medical vs surgical management, *Arch Otolaryngol* 111:816, 1985.
13. Chow AW: Life-threatening infections of the head and neck, *Clin Infect Dis* 14:991, 1992.
14. Coonan KM, Kaplan EL: In vitro susceptibility of recent North American group A streptococcal isolates to eleven oral antibiotics, *Pediatr Infect Dis J* 13:630, 1994.
15. Danahey DG, Kelly DR, Forrest LA: HIV-related Pneumocystis carinii thyroiditis: a unique case and literature review, *Otolaryngol Head Neck Surg* 114:158, 1996.
16. Dietel M and others: Treatment of tuberculous masses in the neck, *Can J Surg* 27:90, 1984.
17. Dodds B, Maniglia AJ: Peritonsillar and neck abscesses in the pediatric age group, *Laryngoscope* 98:956, 1988.
18. Espiritu MB, Medina JE: Complications of heroin injections of the neck, *Laryngoscope* 90:1111, 1980.
19. Estrera AS and others: Descending necrotizing mediastinitis, *Surg Gynecol Obstet* 157:545, 1983.
20. Finch RD, Snider GE, Sprinkle PM: Ludwig's angina, *JAMA* 243:1171, 1980.
21. Gidley PW, Ghorayed BY, Stiernberg CW: Contemporary management of deep neck space infections, *Otolaryngol Head Neck Surg* 116:16, 1997.

22. Greinwald JH Jr, Wilson JF, Haggerty PG: Peritonsillar abscess: an unlikely cause of necrotizing fasciitis, *Ann Otol Rhinol Laryngol* 104:133, 1995.

23. Hawkins DB and others: Mycobacterial cervical adenitis in children: medical and surgical management, *Ear Nose Throat J* 72:733, 1993.

24. Henrich DE, Smith TL, Shockley WW: Fatal craniocervical necrotizing fasciitis in an immunocompetent patient: a case report and literature review, *Head Neck* 17:351, 1995.

25. Holt GR and others: Computed tomography in the diagnosis of deep-neck infections, *Arch Otolaryngol* 108:693, 1982.

26. Kennedy TL: Curettage of nontuberculous mycobacterial cervical lymphadenitis, *Arch Otolaryngol Head Neck Surg* 118:759, 1992.

27. Kindwell EP, Gottlieb LJ, Larson DL: Hyperbaric oxygen therapy in plastic surgery, *Plast Reconstr Surg* 88:898, 1991.

28. Koehler JE and others: Cutaneous vascular lesions and disseminated cat-scratch disease in patients with the acquired immunodeficiency syndrome (AIDS) and AIDS-related complex, *Ann Intern Med* 109:449, 1988.

29. Langford FP and others: Treatment of cervical necrotizing fasciitis with hyperbaric oxygen therapy, *Otolaryngol Head Neck Surg* 112:274, 1995.

30. Ledgerwood AM, Lucas CE: Mycotic aneurysm of the carotid artery, Arch Surg 109:496, 1974.

31. Lee KC and others: Deep neck infections in patients at risk for acquired immunodeficiency syndrome, *Laryngoscope* 100:915, 1990.

32. Lee KC, Schecter G: Tuberculous infections of the head and neck, *Ear Nose Throat J* 74:395, 1995.

33. Luft BJ, Remington JS: Toxoplasmic encephalitis in AIDS, *Clin Infect Dis* 15:211, 1992.

34. Mader JT, Adams KR, Sutton TE: Infectious diseases: pathophysiology and mechanisms of hyperbaric oxygen, *J Hyperbaric Med* 2:133, 1987.

35. Maisel RH, Karlen R: Cervical necrotizing fasciitis, *Laryngoscope* 104:795, 1994.

36. Manolidis S and others: Mycobacterial infections of the head and neck, *Otolaryngol Head Neck Surg* 109:427, 1993.

37. Margileth AM: Management of nontuberculous (atypical) mycobacterial infections in children and adolescents, *Pediatr Infect Dis* 4:119, 1985.

38. Martin MV: The use of oral amoxicillin for the treatment of actinomycosis: a clinical and in-vitro study, *Br Dent J* 156:252, 1984.

39. Mathieu D and others: Cervical necrotizing fasciitis: clinical manifestations and management, *Clin Infect Dis* 21:51, 1995.

40. Mayor GP, Martinez-San Millan J, Martinez-Vidal A: Is conservative treatment of deep neck space infections appropriate? *Head Neck* 23:126, 2001.

41. McCabe RE and others: Clinical spectrum in 107 cases of toxoplasmic lymphadenopathy, *Rev Infect Dis* 9:754, 1987.

42. Meshel RH, Karlen R: Cervical necrotizing fasciitis, *Laryngoscope* 104:795, 1994.

43. Myers EM, Kirkland LS Jr., Mickey R: The head and neck sequelae of cervical intravenous drug abuse, *Laryngoscope* 98:213, 1988.

44. Nagy M, Backstrom J: Comparison of the sensitivity of lateral neck radiographs and computed tomography scanning in pediatric deep-neck infections, *Laryngoscope* 109:775, 1999.

45. Nagy M and others: Deep neck infections in children: a new approach to diagnosis and treatment, *Laryngoscope* 107:1627, 1997

46. Nusbaum AO and others: Recurrence of a deep neck infection: a clinical indication of an underlying congenital lesion, *Arch Otolaryngol Head Neck Surg* 125:1379, 1999.

47. Olson NR: Nontuberculous mycobacterial infections of the face and neck—practical considerations, *Laryngoscope* 91:1714, 1981.

48. Parhiscar A, Har-El G: Deep neck abscess: a retrospective review of 210 cases, *Ann Otol Rhinol Laryngol* 110:1051, 2001.

49. Poe LB, Petro GR, Matta I: Percutaneous CT-guided aspiration of deep neck abscesses, *Am J Neuroradiol* 17:1359, 1996.

50. Pransky SM and others: Cervicofacial mycobacterial adenitis in children: endemic to San Diego? *Laryngoscope* 100:920, 1990.

51. Rapoport Y and others: Cervical necrotizing fasciitis of odontogenic origin, *Oral Surg Oral Med Oral Pathol* 72:15, 1991.

52. Remington JS: Toxoplasmosis in the adult, *Bull NY Acad Med* 50:211, 1974.

53. Riseman JA and others: Hyperbaric oxygen therapy for necrotizing fasciitis reduces mortality and the need for débridements, *Surgery* 108:847, 1990.

54. Saitz EW: Cervical lymphadenitis caused by atypical mycobacteria, *Pediatr Clin North Am* 28:823, 1981.

55. Schaad UB and others: Management of atypical mycobacterial lymphadenitis in childhood: a review based on 380 cases, *J Pediatr* 95:356, 1979.

56. Sethi DS, Stanley RE: Deep neck abscesses—changing trends, *J Laryngol Otol* 108:138, 1994.

57. Shapiro AL, Pincus RL: Fine-needle aspiration of diffuse cervical lymphadenopathy in patients with acquired immunodeficiency syndrome, *Otolaryngol Head Neck Surg* 105:419, 1991.

58. Skorina J, Kaufman D: Necrotizing fasciitis originating from pinna perichondritis, *Otolaryngol Head Neck Surg* 113:467, 1995.

59. Spankus EM and others: Craniocervical necrotizing fasciitis, *Otolaryngol Head Neck Surg* 92:261, 1984.

60. Starke JR: Nontuberculous mycobacterial infections in children, *Adv Pediatr Infect Dis* 7:123, 1992.

61. Stewart MG, Starke JR, Coker NJ: Nontuberculous mycobacterial infections of the head and neck, Arch *Otolaryngol Head Neck Surg* 120:873, 1994.

62. Taha AM, Davidson PT, Bailey WC: Surgical treatment of atypical mycobacterial lymphadenitis in children, *Pediatr Infect Dis J* 4:664, 1985.

63. Thompson JW, Cohen SR, Reddix P: Retropharyngeal abscess in children: a retrospective and historical analysis, *Laryngoscope* 98:589, 1988.

64. Tom MB, Rice DH: Presentation and management of neck abscess: a retrospective analysis, *Laryngoscope* 98:877, 1988.

65. Tunkel DE, Romaneschi KB: Surgical treatment of cervicofacial nontuberculous mycobacterial adenitis in children, *Laryngoscope* 105:1024, 1995.

66. Ungkanont K and others: Head and neck space infections in infants and children, *Otolaryngol Head Neck Surg* 112:375, 1995.

67. Wheatley MJ and others: Descending necrotizing mediastinitis: transcervical drainage is not enough, *Ann Thorac Surg* 49:780, 1990.

68. Yeow KM, Liao CT, Hao SP: US-guided needle aspiration and catheter drainage as an alternative to open surgical drainage for uniloculated neck abscesses, *J Vasc Interv Radiol* 12:589, 2001.

69. Zangwill KM and others: Cat scratch disease in Connecticut: epidemiology, risk factors and evaluation of a new diagnostic test, *N Engl J Med* 329:8, 1993.

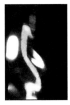

CHAPTER ONE HUNDRED AND ELEVEN

BLUNT AND PENETRATING TRAUMA TO THE NECK

Robert H. Maisel
David B. Hom

INTRODUCTION

As the incidence of violent trauma rises in our society, the rate of penetrating trauma to the head and neck also grows. At present, penetrating neck injury comprises 5% to 10% of all trauma cases. All penetrating neck wounds are potentially dangerous and require emergency treatment.[7]

In the neck, multiple vital structures are vulnerable to injury in a small anatomic area and are not protected by bone. Such vital structures of the neck can be divided into four groups: the air passages (trachea, larynx, pharynx, lung); vascular (carotid, jugular, subclavian, innominate, aortic arch vessels); gastrointestinal (pharynx, esophagus); and neurologic (spinal cord, brachial plexus, peripheral nerves, cranial nerves [CNs]). Signs or symptoms listed in Box 111-1 should alert the otolaryngologist that injury to any of these structures has occurred.

PHYSICAL PROPERTIES OF PENETRATING OBJECTS

Knowledge of the physical properties and ballistics of the penetrating object can help determine a management plan and predict the risk of injury.[36] The location of penetration also predicts risk and helps in planning for management.[17,45] The magnitude of injury is determined by the kinetic energy that is transferred from the projectile to the target tissue: $KE = 1/2M(V_1-V_2)^2$.[45] KE is the kinetic energy of the projectile, M is the mass of the projectile, V_1 is the initial velocity on contact, and V_2 is the exit velocity.[5]

Handgun

Civilian handgun injuries traditionally are from projectiles with low-muzzle velocity (90 m/sec). An impact velocity of 50 m/sec penetrates skin, and an impact velocity of 65 m/sec will fracture bone. These slow-velocity projectiles have been known to push aside vital structures such as arteries. Penetrating wounds caused by small-caliber handguns have a less damaging effect than other projectiles of higher velocity.

Guns are classified by projectile type, speed, and caliber (diameter of muzzle bore). Bullets that travel greater than 610 m/sec are considered high-velocity projectiles. Handguns or pistols (.22 caliber to .45 caliber) have muzzle velocities from 210 to 600 m/sec. Caliber is a term interchangeable with the designation of the cartridge (e.g., 22-caliber pistol). Handguns can develop up to 1000 foot-pounds of energy. A .44-caliber magnum, which has a large powder charge, can create even more hypervelocity. Thus, injury from this gun can cause tissue destruction comparable with that caused by a rifle bullet, a larger projectile.

The yaw of the bullet describes the deflection of the projectile around the axis of travel. If the yaw is minimal (not tumbling), with the bullet entering perpendicular to the body surface, the bullet will pass through the tissues with little energy transmitted. A tumbling bullet causes injury in a wider path. The projectile can follow tissue planes and may not injure vital structures. A bullet also can deflect from bones of the mandible or cervical spine. Unfortunately, civilian gunshot wounds increasingly involve heavier projectiles with higher-velocity handguns. In all cases, a full inspection of the entire naked body and palpation of the head is necessary to reveal all entrance and exit wounds. This information may be useful in predicting damage. Low-velocity bullets are usually lead shielded and often leave a radiographic track. A diagnosis based on physical signs of injury, after full and careful organ system evaluation, is often sufficient for these injuries if all presentations are normal. Radiographic confirmation or surgical exploration should follow any uncertainty or deterioration of physical signs.

Rifle

Most military rifles have a jacket of strong metal, usually copper, that surrounds a lead projectile. This

BOX 111-1

SIGNS AND SYMPTOMS OF PENETRATING NECK TRAUMA

Airway
Reparatory distress
Stridor
Hemoptysis
Hoarseness
Tracheal deviation
Subcutaneous emphysema
Sucking wound

Vascular System
Hematoma
Persistent bleeding
Neurologic deficit
Absent pulse
Hypovolemic shock
Bruit
Thrill
Change of sensorium

Nervous System
Hemiplegia
Quadriplegia
Coma
Cranial nerve deficit
Change of sensorium
Hoarseness

Esophagus/Hypopharynx
Subcutaneous emphysema
Dysphagia
Odynophagia
Hematemesis
Hemoptysis
Tachycardia
Fever

From Stiernberg C and others: Gunshot wounds to the head and neck, *Arch Otolaryngol Head Neck Surg* 118:592, 1992.

permits smoother and longer flight because of less drag and less aerodynamic compression. Similarly, because of the lack of deformation, these military bullets create a clean hole with a through-and-through wound without a lead track to follow. The M16 military rifle has a bullet that is designed to tumble and therefore causes more tissue injury. It is against the terms of the Hague Convention of 1908 for military projectiles to include expanding bullets such as hollow point, softnose, or dumdum bullets. These soft-tip bullets expand on contact and cause greater soft-tissue injury. They create a large wound cavity, may not cause an exit wound, and may fragment, with partial projectiles causing injury far from the primary direct path. Hunting rifles use these expanding bullets, and therefore the civilian wounds caused by these projec-

tiles can be more devastating than a comparable wound inflicted by a military weapon.

Most military rifles have a muzzle velocity of 760 m/sec. High-velocity missiles (>610 m/sec) not only tear tissue but also transmit energy to surrounding tissue. A cavity of up to 30 times the size of the missile may be created and pulsate over 5 to 10 cm, with several waves of contraction and expansion of the tissue[13] (Figure 111-1). This may explain the finding of a punctured viscus without direct penetration and should alert the surgeon to examine the trachea and esophagus, even when a bullet wound is 2 inches away (Figure 111-2).

High-energy missiles are not easily deflected and cause significant destruction along their path as the energy is absorbed by the surrounding tissue. Deer rifles fire a projectile designed to mushroom on impact, causing a large amount of tissue destruction within a small area.

The mortality from all high-velocity rifle injuries inflicted directly on the neck is significant. These patients usually do not survive and are not available for study. In view of the expected severity of injury, all known victims of high-velocity rifle injuries who survive on reaching the hospital merit strong consideration for surgical exploration. For stable patients, angiograms should be considered before surgery. In helping to determine whether mandatory surgical exploration or further preoperative diagnostic tests are needed, knowledge of the size and velocity of the intruding missile is helpful.

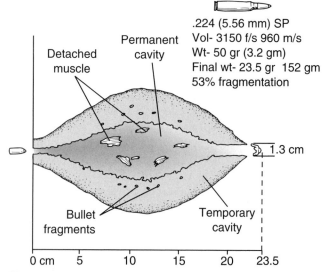

Figure 111-1. Characteristic wound profile of a high-velocity, soft-point rifle bullet. Note characteristic large temporary and permanent cavities with massive tissue disruption. The wound profile of a conventional copper-jacketed, high-velocity bullet would reveal a similar temporary cavity. (From Fackler MA and others: *J Trauma* 28(Suppl):21, 1988.)

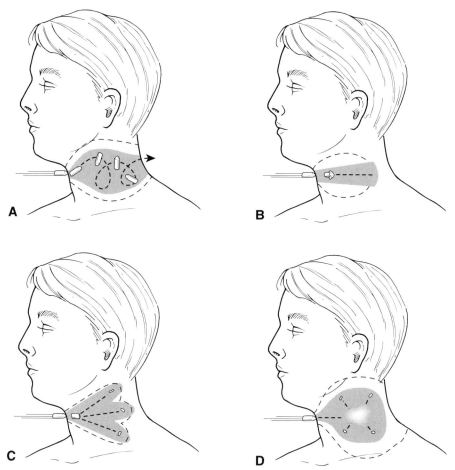

Figure 111-2. Types of injuries caused by different missiles. Both temporary cavity *(dotted line)* and permanent cavity *(stipple area)* are large. **A,** Tumbling missile. **B,** Expanding bullet. **C,** Fragmenting bullet. **D,** Self-exploding bullet. (From Holt GR, Kostohryz G: *Arch Otolaryngol* 109:313, 1983. Copyright 1983, American Medical Association.)

Shotguns

The severity of shotgun wounds largely depends on the distance between the weapon and the victim, the type of weapon used, and the size of the projectile (shot). Pellets have a tendency to scatter as they travel, on the basis of the distance to impact and the interior muzzle diameter (choke) of the shotgun. At close range, the entire charge can act like a single missile with a KE similar to a high-velocity bullet.[10] At further distances, birdshot pellets scatter and act as multiple individual missiles. With larger pellets such as buckshot, significant injuries can occur from individual pellets up to 150 yards away with a standard length barrel. A sawed-off shotgun leads to early spraying of the shot. Shotguns are low-velocity weapons (muzzle velocity of 300 m/sec).

Birdshots are pellets with a diameter ≤3.5 mm (0.13 inch) and are categorized as No. 4 shot or smaller. Buckshots have a diameter >3.5 mm and have a greater range, causing significant injury up to 150 m. This is in contrast to birdshots, which have a 12-m maximum range of serious injury (Tables 111-1 and 111-2). Each pellet injury from a buckshot blast is similar to a bullet injury from a handgun. Buckshot wounds are usually more serious than handgun bullet wounds because of the number of missiles involved.

The gauge of the gun determines how much shot can be included in a single shell. The actual shot varies from 00 buckshot (for deer hunting, which has eight and one-half pellets per ounce with a larger tissue impact) up to 12 buckshot (which has 2400 pellets per ounce, little destructive ability, and is used for target shooting). An 8 buckshot with 400 pellets per ounce is used for shooting small game, such as rabbits and birds.

At close range, shotgun injuries cause as much damage as rifle injuries because of the massive blast effect to the tissues. When the distance between the shooter and the recipient is >6 m, the details of gauge, shot, powder load, and the choke of the gun become more important.[20] Wadding from the shotgun blast also should be searched for and removed from the wound to

TABLE 111-1

SHOTGUN SHELLS

Shot Size	Diameter, *in*	Maximum Range, *yd*	Pellets per Ounce, *n*
12-Gauge round ball	.645	1420	.75
16-Gauge round ball	.610	1340	1.0
10-Gauge round ball	.545	1200	1.25
410-Gauge round ball	.38	850	—
000 Buckshot	.36	—	6
00 Buckshot	.34	748	8
0 Buckshot	.32	704	9
1 Buckshot	.30	660	11
2 Buckshot	.27	—	15
3 Buckshot	.25	—	19
4 Buckshot	.24	—	21
#1 Shot	.16	352	73
#2 Shot	.15	330	90
#3 Shot	.14	308	109
#4 Shot	.13	286	135
#5 Shot	.12	264	170
#6 Shot	.11	242	225
#7 1/2 Shot	.095	209	350
#8 Shot	.09	198	410
#9 Shot	.08	176	585
#12 Shot	.05	110	2385

From Ordog GJ: *Missile wound of the neck.* In Ordog GJ, editor: *Management of gunshot wounds,* New York, 1988, Elsevier.

TABLE 111-2

CLASSIFICATION OF BIRDSHOT SHOTGUN WOUNDS

Type	RANGE* Standard Barrel	Sawed-off Shotgun	Injury	Mortality, %
0	Long >12 m	>4 m	Superficial—pellets in skin only	0
I	Long >12 m	>4 m	Penetrates only subcutaneous tissue	0–5
II	Close 5–12 m	2–4 m	Penetrates beyond deep fascia	15–20
III	Point blank <5 m	0–2 m	Extensive tissue damage	85–90

From Ordog GJ: *Missile wounds of the neck.* In Ordog GJ, editor: *Management of gunshot wounds,* New York, 1988, Elsevier.
*The distance will vary with each type of shotgun and is significantly reduced for sawed-off shotguns.

prevent infection. Radiography is useful for revealing pellets in unexpected locations, such as the intracranial, intrathoracic, or intraorbital cavities. Magnetic resonance imaging (MRI) may be even more valuable than computed tomography (CT) for the stable patient, because metal scatter artifact does not occur.

Miscellaneous Injuries

Knife, icepick, cut-glass, or razor-blade injuries usually proceed along more predictable pathways. However, what seems to be a single-entry wound may be from multiple stab wounds. The history of the attack may be of some help to the physician in determining whether the blow was overhand or underhand, whether both the attacker and the recipient were standing, and other similar details. Compared with gunshot wounds to the neck, cervical stab wounds have a higher incidence of subclavian vessel laceration.[31,38] This is because stabbings to the neck often occur in a downward direction, with the knife slipping over the clavicle and into the subclavian vessels.[32] In gunshot wounds, the direction of the projectile is more perpendicular to the neck; thus, the clavicle can protect the subclavian vessels. In regard to spinal injuries, neck stab wounds have a lower incidence than cervical bullet wounds.[32]

MANDATORY VS ELECTIVE EXPLORATION

Penetrating neck injuries should be differentiated into two basic presentations, depending on whether they are immediately life-threatening or not. The signs of immediate life-threatening injuries include massive bleeding, expanding hematoma, nonexpanding hematoma in the presence of hemodynamic instability, hemomediastinum, hemothorax, and hypovolemic shock. In all of these instances, immediate surgical exploration is mandatory. On the other hand, hemodynamically stable patients who are seen with non–life-threatening features can undergo thorough imaging investigations to determine the extent of injury.

For the stable patient, the choice of management remains controversial: either mandatory exploration for all penetrating neck wounds or selective exploration with observation.[48] A number of retrospective studies have supported both mandatory surgical exploration and selective surgical exploration.[4,16,25] For the selective surgical approach, it is emphasized that the clinical status of the patient should be monitored closely by frequent observation and medical examination with diagnostic radiology and surgical endoscopy. In civilian injury, this is often possible, but in times of war or civilian catastrophe, resources such as radiography and observation beds may not be available for large numbers of casualties.

Until World War II, the mortality of penetrating neck wounds ranged from 7% to 15%. By the end of the Vietnam War, it was reduced to 3% to 6%[25] (Table 111-3). However, mortality remains high if major vascular structures (carotid or subclavian arteries) or the cervical spinal cord is injured. During the Vietnam War, it was customary to explore all patients with penetrating neck wounds below the platysma layer under general anesthesia, regardless of preoperative findings. The idea of mandatory exploration also was advocated by Fogelman and Steward in 1956 for civilian injuries. This philosophy was followed to the mid-1980s by most general trauma centers in large cities in the United States. However, it was realized that in many instances significant injuries to major structures did not occur. This reasoning led some surgeons to follow a more selective approach for these injuries. However, advocates for mandatory exploration believe that exploration has time-proven success. Each of the proponents give arguments that support their views, both medically and economically (Table 111-4).

Classification

Anatomically, the neck can be divided into three major zones to aid in the decision making for diagnostic tests and timing of surgery[45] (Figure 111-3). Zone I is below the cricoid and represents a dangerous area, because the vascular structures in this zone are in close proximity to the thorax. The bony thorax and clavicle act to protect zone I from injury as do other bony structures at the base of the neck. This osseous shield also makes surgical exploration of the root of the neck difficult. In zone I, injuries to the right side are often approached through a median sternotomy, whereas injuries to the left side are often managed by a left anterior thoracotomy to control the hemorrhage. Zone I has a fairly high mortality rate of 12%.[35]

Mandatory exploration is not usually recommended for zone I injuries; angiography is usually suggested to ensure that the great vessels are not injured.

Zone III is located above the angle of the mandible. This area also is protected by skeletal structures and is difficult to explore because of the skull base and the need to divide or displace the mandible. The necessity for craniotomy in exploration and control of high carotid injury in this location makes zone III treacherous. Recognizing injuries to many of the cranial nerves exiting the skull base in zone III is important, because these injuries may be indicative of injuries to the great vessels because of their close proximity. An abnormal neurologic examination would suggest the need for angiography in the stable patient.

In view of the difficult surgical approaches to zone I and zone III, most authors agree that all patients with such injuries who are stable and without evidence of acute airway obstruction, significant bleeding, or expanding hematoma should be evaluated with angiography, with consideration of barium swallow. For zone III injuries, frequent intraoral examination should be performed to observe for edema or expanding hematoma within the parapharyngeal or retropharyngeal spaces.

TABLE 111-3

MORTALITY OF PENETRATING NECK TRAUMA IN WARTIME AND CURRENT CIVILIAN PRACTICE

Incident	Injuries, *n*	Mortality, %
Civil War	4114	15
Spanish-American War	188	18
World War I	594	11
World War II	851	7
Current civilian practice		3–6

From McConnell D, Trunkey D: *Adv Surg* 27:97, 1994.

TABLE 111-4

MANDATORY VS SELECTIVE MANAGEMENT OF NECK WOUNDS

Consideration	Mandatory	Selective
Diagnosis	Potential life-threatening injuries can be missed by the preoperative workup	Most major injuries can be diagnosed preoperatively; routine exploration can miss some injuries
Skill and resources	Selective management requires more skill, manpower, experience, and judgment; additional special diagnostic procedures are also required	Selective care will reduce unnecessary explorations by a surgeon inexperienced with trauma
Hospital stay	Length of stay is similar for observation and negative exploration	No advantage of negative exploration
Delay	If occult injuries are delayed, morbidity and mortality will increase	Delay has not been shown to significantly increase morbidity and mortality of occult injuries
Patient care	Active observation requires continuous availability of experienced trauma medical staff for monitoring the patient	Selective management emphasizes the concept of collaboration among trauma team members and reduces unnecessary surgical exploration

Adapted from Obeid F and others: *Surg Gynecol Obstet* 160:517, 1985.

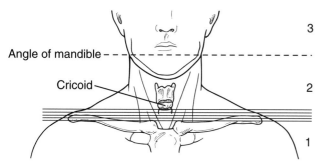

Figure 111-3. The three zones of the neck are seen on this frontal view. The *shaded area* represents the portion that some authors consider zone I but that others label zone II. (From Carducci B and others: *Ann Emerg Med* 15:208, 1986.)

Zone II penetration is the most frequently involved region (60%–75%), and injury in this zone has created a great deal of controversy in the American literature over the past 15 years.[30] There is an ongoing debate about the use of mandatory exploration vs selective exploration with serial examination, endoscopic tests, and angiography. In zone II, isolated venous injuries and isolated pharyngoesophageal injuries are the most common structures missed clinically in the preoperative evaluation.[6] A substantial number of patients can be selectively managed, depending on signs, symptoms, and direction of the trajectory. When patients are stable and lack physical signs of obvious major neck injury, they are evaluated by diagnostic radiologic and endoscopic techniques. All patients are admitted for observation. A hospital with a compre-

hensive trauma service with experienced personnel doing careful and repeated physical examinations and with 24-hour availability of radiologic and endoscopic capability is needed.[32] The leading cause of death from penetrating neck injuries is hemorrhage from vascular structures. In a study by Stone and Callahan,[46] vascular injuries in the neck accounted for 50% of deaths.

One article emphasizes the increased lethal potential of transcervical penetrating neck wounds when the projectile crosses the midline. In this study, all 11 patients with transcervical gunshot and shotgun wounds sustained vascular or aerodigestive injuries and longer hospital stays (14 days) than patients with other gunshot wounds (6.6 days). These authors believe that transcervical injuries should be reported separately from zones I, II, and III injuries, because they tend to be more severe.[3]

Initial Management

The initial care of patients with penetrating neck injuries should follow the basic tenets of trauma care. The emergent management of all penetrating neck trauma requires (1) airway establishment; (2) blood perfusion maintenance; and (3) clarification and classification of the severity of the wound. In the emergency department, satisfactory control of the airway is established by intubation, cricothyroidotomy, or tracheostomy. Direct transcervical tracheal intubation is safer than oral or nasal intubation when the oral cavity, pharynx, or larynx are traumatized and filled with blood. In the setting of a gunshot wound, it may be difficult to fully evaluate the cervical spine until the airway is controlled. Multiple blind intubation attempts will risk enlarging a lacerated piriform sinus wound and extending it iatrogenically into the mediastinum. Similarly, a tracheal tear may be exacerbated by extending the neck, which distracts the proximal and distal segments. The airway must be established, and the hemodynamic status must be stabilized before transporting the patient to the angiography suite. Large-bore intravenous lines are placed, even when the patient is not hypotensive, so that fluids can be rapidly introduced if needed. Particularly in zone II, hemorrhage or an expanding hematoma will respond to direct pressure and should not be managed by indiscriminate clamping through the wound. Under no circumstances should a penetrating neck wound be probed, because clot dislodgement and uncontrollable bleeding can occur.

Every patient with significant neck trauma should have routine anterior and lateral neck and chest radiographs. When a pneumothorax is identified by a radiograph or physical examination, a chest tube should be inserted emergently. In the rare circumstance of an exsanguinating oral hemorrhage, a tracheostomy must be performed immediately, and the pharynx must be packed. In high-volume trauma hospitals, the emergency department usually has an operating theater intended for emergent patients on whom control of a major vessel hemorrhage must be performed immediately. Physical findings of vascular injury are pulse deficit, active bleeding, expanding hematoma, bruit, murmur, neurologic deficit, or hypotension.[14] Patients with acute injury to the spinal cord may have hypotension without tachycardia (spinal shock). Cranial nerve injury is not common; however, when it is evident, documentation of the deficit is helpful in evaluating the direction of the projectile and possible injury to adjacent structures. For instance, if a hypoglossal nerve injury is present, one should be suspicious for a possible carotid artery injury. Horner's syndrome (pupil constriction, upper eyelid ptosis, skin flushing, absence of sweating on the affected side) also may indicate injury to the carotid artery or to structures along the sympathetic chain. Under controlled circumstances, the patient is taken to the operating room, where a wide-apron incision is made from the mastoid tip to the midline of the neck at the cricoid level for definitive exploration.

DIAGNOSTIC EVALUATION

When the patient's stability allows, an orderly history and physical examination are performed, which should include a full examination of the unclothed body to look for entrance or exit wounds. In the conscious patient, a full neurologic examination should be done and a chest radiograph taken. The radiograph should be examined to rule out hemothorax, pneumothorax, or pneumomediastinum. The latter would suggest a punctured viscus and demand further evaluation. Subclavian vessel injury may be first recognized by an abnormal chest radiograph. All patients should be managed assuming potential cervical spine fractures until they undergo radiographic evaluation. On radiographs, all cutaneous wounds can be marked with radiopaque objects to aid in evaluating the site of the injury.

Most trauma centers suggest that personnel and equipment be available 24 hours a day for flexible endoscopy or arteriography, with accessibility for immediate neuroradiologic interpretation.

A hospital trauma team should include an otolaryngologist as part of the surgical team to help evaluate and repair the aerodigestive tract and explore the nerves and branches of the carotid artery in the neck. Patients with significant bleeding or an expanding hematoma need immediate attention with probable emergent exploration in the operating room.

Several series of cases have shown examples of injuries being misdiagnosed, both by angiography and during direct exploration.[29] False aneurysms, external carotid branch lacerations, arteriovenous fistulas, and viscus-vessel fistulas have all been described despite the presence of sophisticated personnel and experienced examiners. Approximately 30% of patients with carotid artery injury have a neurologic deficit.[22,33,50] Arterial injury or propagation of a thrombus into the skull can lead to cerebral ischemia. One-third of the population cannot tolerate complete unilateral carotid occlusion.

The debate over the merits of mandatory vs selective exploration continues. Meyer and others[26] have reviewed their data and suggest that mandatory exploration is appropriate. Others[28,30,37] have used similar data to suggest the advantages of selective exploration.[4,28,30,37] Among patients explored routinely, 50% to 70% have negative explorations with some morbidity and some cosmetic deformity.[5,19]

Several surgeons claim that mandatory exploratory operations are the "gold standard" against which all other procedures should be measured. The rare case of a patient under observation with an underdiagnosed hemorrhage with complications is cited to encourage exploration. However, prospective studies have failed to prove that either choice is clearly better. Many surgical trauma teams, including that of Hennepin Country Medical Center (an American College of Surgeons level I trauma center), are becoming more encouraged by selective management. The preferred management at Hennepin County Medical Center is selective exploration (Figures 111-4 and 111-5). Table 111-5 shows the accuracy of selective evaluation

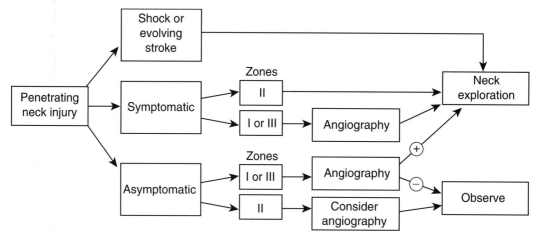

Figure 111-4. Selective management of penetrating neck injury. (Adapted from McConnell D, Trunkey D: *Adv Surg* 27:97, 1994.)

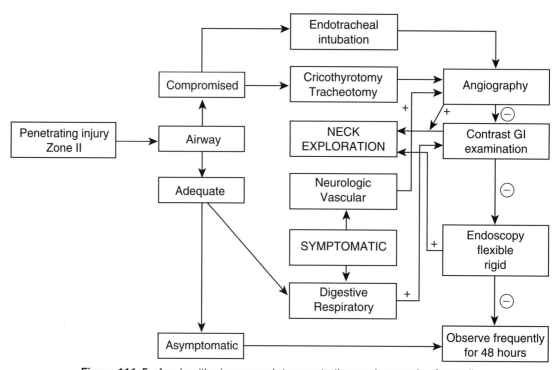

Figure 111-5. An algorithmic approach to penetrating neck wounds of zone II.

techniques with the caveat that using rigid and flexible esophagoscopy together can be more accurate than the use of either one alone.[27] In cases in which the cervical spine has not been cleared, flexible endoscopy is helpful for evaluating injuries of the pharynx and esophagus. Contrast infusion CT scanning can aid in the surgical decision making for zone II penetrating neck injuries.[24]

ANGIOGRAPHY

Angiography is the most urgently performed diagnostic technique, because once the airway has been secured

by intubation or tracheostomy, hemorrhage can be life threatening. A positive angiogram may mandate an immediate trip to the operating room, but evaluation of the upper digestive tract in the radiology suite may be useful if time and the patient's condition permit. Zone I and zone III injuries usually require routine preoperative arteriography on stable patients, because their surgical approach is more difficult than zone II injuries. In addition, when wounds involve both sides of the neck with zone I and zone III injuries, four-vessel angiography (bilateral carotid and vertebral arteries) should be considered in stable but sympto-

TABLE 111-5

ACCURACY OF SELECTIVE EVALUATION TECHNIQUES

Procedure	Indications	Contraindications	Accuracy, %
Angiography	Wounds near vessel in zone I or zone III	Expanding hematoma Profound shock Uncontrolled bleeding	98.5
Barium swallow	Hematemesis Drooling Dysphagia Vocal cord paralysis	Intubated Saliva in wound Unstable patient	90.0
Esophagoscopy	Suspected but unconfirmed injury by barium swallow Intubated Laryngeal or tracheal injury Vascular injury in zone II or zone III	None	86
Direct laryngoscopy and bronchoscopy	Vocal cord paralysis Hoarseness Tenderness or crepitance over larynx Subcutaneous emphysema Hemoptysis	None	100

From Miller RH, Duplechain JK: *Otolaryngol Clin North Am* 24:15, 1991. Used with permission.

matic patients. Zone II wounds are usually easily accessible and a low risk for exploration. Zone II injuries may be evaluated by selective angiography or exploration. Certain indications for an angiogram in zone II injuries include a stable patient who has persistent hemorrhage or neurologic deficits compatible with adjacent vascular structure damage[15] (Figure 111-6). An example of this is Horner's syndrome indicative of sympathetic nerve plexus injury or hoarseness indicating a recurrent laryngeal nerve injury. This neurologic picture suggests that the carotid sheath has been violated, and vascular integrity needs confirmation by angiography, as well as frequent close observation to detect for a lacerated carotid artery, intimal tear, or pseudoaneurysm[42] (Figure 111-7). Arteriography can be accurate diagnostically with good technique and with an experienced radiologist. Patients with negative arteriography and positive physical signs still need exploration. If there is radiographic evidence that a bullet has changed location because of gravitational or positional change of the patient, removal of the bullet should be considered. This is because a migratory bullet can increase the risk of embolic phenomenon.[23]

For asymptomatic zone II penetrating neck injuries, the usefulness of angiography remains controversial. One study showed no statistically significant difference in sensitivities between a clinical examination and angiography for the detection of vascular injury. This study concluded that the clinical examination for zone II injuries may be sufficient to detect significant

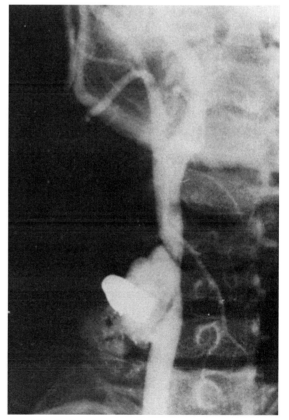

Figure 111-6. Arteriogram demonstrating common carotid artery injury in a 26-year-old man with small hematoma and normal neurologic examination. (From Hiatt JR and others: *J Vasc Surg* 1:860, 1984.)

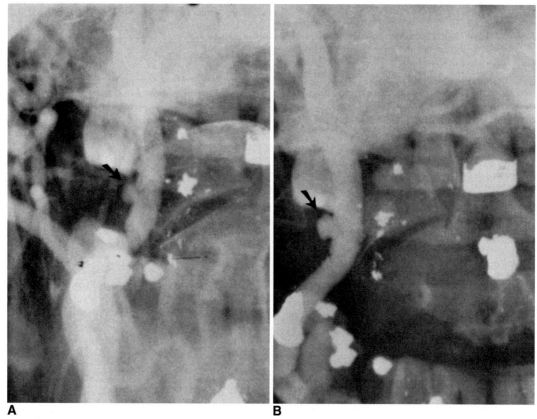

Figure 111-7. A, Anteroposterior view arteriogram of the right common carotid artery reveals a contained extravasation of the internal carotid artery near the base of the skull *(arrow).* Cranial nerve deficits at the jugular foramen (X–XII) accompany this injury. **B,** A follow-up arteriogram of the internal carotid artery 1 week later shows enlargement of the pseudoaneurysm. (From Scalfani SJA and others: *J Trauma* 25:871, 1985.)

vascular lesions unless the trauma is in close proximity to the major vessels.[18] Other studies have supported the use of angiography for stable asymptomatic patients[41] (Figure 111-8). One article has supported the use of color flow Doppler imaging as a promising future alternative to angiography if the radiology department is familiar with the technique.[11]

MANAGEMENT OF VASCULAR PENETRATION

Zone I vascular perforation requires thoracic surgery. Although a low cervical incision may result in sufficient exposure, a mediastinotomy extension or a formal lateral thoracotomy may be needed.

Zone III injuries at the skull base can be temporized by pressure, but once delineated, access to the injury may require mandibulotomy in the midline similar to exposure for a parapharyngeal space tumor. A temporary arterial bypass of the carotid artery may be placed until the lacerated or aneurysmatic vessel can be approached safely.

For controlling distal bleeding from the internal carotid in zone III, Perry[34] has described passing a No. 4 Fogarty catheter through a Pruitt-Inahara shunt.

By passing the Fogarty catheter beyond the injury and inflating the balloon to occlude the lumen, the shunt can then be advanced beyond the injury (Figure 111-9). After removing the Fogarty catheter, proximal shunt placement is performed. To evaluate patency and vascular flow of the artery repair, Doppler probe measurements are conducted with consideration for angiography.

All veins in the neck can be safely ligated to control hemorrhage; if both internal jugular veins are interrupted by the injury, an attempt to repair one is appropriate. All external carotid artery injuries are easily managed by suture ligation, because collateral circulation is good. Common carotid or internal carotid injury in zone II is explored once the diagnosis is made by an approach along the anterior border of the sternocleidomastoid muscle. To find the carotid artery in cases in which the vessel is no longer pulsating (i.e., hematoma injury or proximal interruption), the external carotid branches may be followed retrograde from the facial artery at the submandibular gland or from the superior thyroid artery at the superior cornu of the thyroid cartilage.

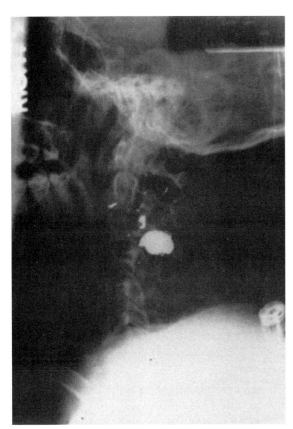

Figure 111-8. This patient had a high cervical cord resection with quadriplegia. No vascular injury was recognized. (From Ordog GJ and others: *J Trauma* 25:238, 1985.)

Techniques of lateral arteriorrhaphy for vascular repair (Fig. 111-10) have been suggested by Dichtel and others and by Calcaterra and Holt.[8,12] End-to-end anastomosis or autogenous grafting is recommended when stenosis is evident by arteriography. Ligation of

the common or internal carotid injuries is generally reserved for irreparable injuries and in patients who are in a profound coma state with bilateral fixed and dilated pupils. Delayed complications from unrepaired vascular injuries include aneurysm formation, dissecting aneurysm, and arteriovenous fistulas.

More recently, interventional radiologists have used angiographic techniques to treat vascular injury. In some instances, embolization procedures can help control arterial disruption. For arterial injuries in zone III, transcatheter arterial embolization can be an effective modality to obtain hemostasis. Penetrating injuries in zone III have a higher incidence of multiple vascular injuries involving the internal carotid artery, internal maxillary artery, and extrarenal carotid artery.[40] In areas of difficult vascular access at the skull base, detachable balloons or steel coils can be placed for carotid occlusion.[43] Embolized bullets

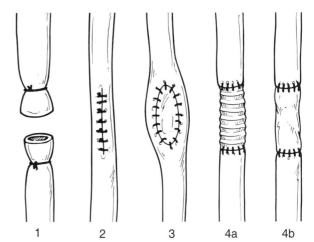

1	2	3	4a	4b

Figure 111-10. Types of vascular repairs. (From Dichtel WJ and others: *Laryngoscope* 94:1142, 1984.)

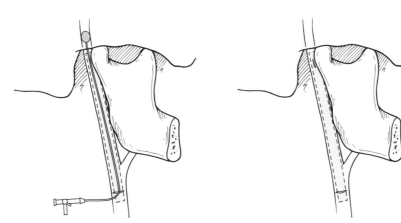

Figure 111-9. No. 4 Fogarty catheter method with shunt placement in an attempt to control bleeding of internal carotid artery near skull base. (Modified from Perry M: *Injuries of the carotid and vertebral arteries.* In Bongard FS, Wilson SE, Perry MO, editors: *Vascular injuries in surgical practice,* Norwalk, Conn, 1991, Appleton & Lange.)

also can be retrieved by angiographic techniques. The possible complications of interventional angiography include blood vessel injury, inadvertent balloon detachment, ischemic events, pseudoaneurysm formation, and treatment failure.

Achieving hemorrhage control of penetrating vertebral artery injuries can be very challenging given their anatomic relationship with the bony structure of the cervical spine and mandible. Because these vertebral artery injuries often result in both neurologic and hemodynamic sequelae, they are frequently associated with higher morbidity and mortality rates. Because their surgical management can be complex, endovascular treatment approaches have been promising.[1]

DIGESTIVE TRACT EVALUATION

In the patient with a possible esophageal perforation, most radiologists recommend Gastrografin swallow as a first-order contrast study, because barium extravasation radiographically distorts soft-tissue planes for other studies and is more toxic. There are mixed reports in the literature[9,29] about which of these methods is more reliable in demonstrating a perforated esophagus or pharynx. A negative Gastrografin study should be followed by a barium swallow if suspicion remains high.[9,29]

Many studies report the use of flexible esophagoscopy to circumvent the need for general anesthesia during rigid endoscopy. Several authors have reported a missed perforation near the cricopharyngeus, as well as the hypopharynx, where flexible endoscopy is least satisfactory because of mucosa redundancy. Missed esophageal tears (Figure 111-11) represent most of the delayed injuries, and, when they progress to mediastinitis, morbidity and mortality are considerable.[44] Meyer and others[26] found a significant incidence of missed esophageal injury in their prospective endoscopic, contrast radiographs, and subsequent mandatory exploration studies. Noyes, McSwain, and Markowitz[29] believe that flexible esophagoscopy is only 86% accurate, and contrast swallow is 90% accurate.

Some surgery services mandate neck exploration for patients who have air in the soft tissues of the neck despite yielding normal endoscopy results. At the time of exploration to rule out pharyngeal and esophageal injuries, a nasogastric tube can be gently pulled up to the level of the neck and methylene blue infused through the nasogastric tube to help localize the injury site. The combination of flexible endoscopy and rigid esophagoscopy to examine the entire cervical and upper thoracic esophagus also has been reported. No perforations were missed in those series that used both techniques on all patients. If suspicion of a pharyngeal perforation remains unconfirmed by examination or even by exploration, the patient is given no food and is observed for several days. Fever, tachycardia, or widening of the mediastinum on serial

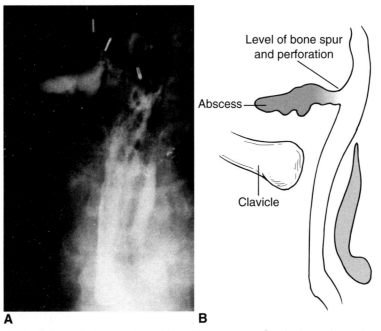

A   **B**

Figure 111-11. This perforation occurred from blunt trauma. Cervical esophageal perforation from flexion-hyperextension injury. **A,** Esophagogram showing perforation at the level of the C5-6 vertebrae. **B,** Level of bone spur and perforation. (From Spenler CW, Benfield JR: *Arch Surg* 111:663, 1986. Copyright 1986, American Medical Association.)

chest radiographs requires that repeat endoscopy or neck exploration be considered. When an esophageal injury is found early, management involves a two-layer closure with wound irrigation, debridement, and adequate drainage. After repair of the mucosa perforation, a muscle flap may be interposed over the esophageal suture line for further protection.[2,47] Miller and Duplechain have shown the value of a muscle flap placed in the bed of a traumatic esophageal and tracheal wound to minimize the risk of a tracheoesophageal fistula[27] (Figure 111-12). If an extensive esophageal injury is present, it may necessitate a lateral cervical esophagostomy and later definitive repair.

The practice at Hennepin County Medical Center has been to perform direct laryngoscopy, bronchoscopy, and rigid esophagoscopy with the patient under anesthesia for penetrating injuries of the neck with air in the soft tissues, hemoptysis, hematemesis, or other suspicious clinical findings. Direct laryngoscopy and rigid bronchoscopy can be combined with flexible airway examination to recognize and stent a lacerated trachea temporarily. In the setting of a cervical spine fracture, rigid esophagoscopy may have to be omitted. Definitive management for any airway compromise is always essential.

If the clinical examination is benign, follow-up examination is done frequently (at least three times

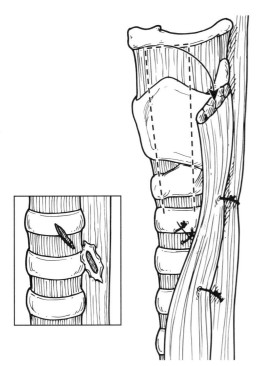

Figure 111-12. Interposition of strap muscle between esophageal and tracheal repair. (From Miller RH: *The surgical atlas of airway and facial trauma*, Philadelphia, 1983, WB Saunders.)

every 24-hour shift) by a physician recording his or her observations. Frequent monitoring of vital signs, as well as examination of the neck and the entry wounds by the nursing staff, is also crucial. A 48- to 72-hour observation period should be used to monitor for changes in physical findings or vital signs that mandate urgent attention. Most vascular injuries that need attention are seen within 48 hours. Careful appraisals show that the patient with a negative physical examination and normal radiograph and endoscopy will most likely have a negative neck exploration, and no significant injury will be discovered. Direct observation can thus be recommended[30] (Figure 111-13).

MANAGEMENT OF LARYNGOTRACHEAL INJURY

Laryngeal mucosal lacerations from penetrating injury should be repaired early (within 24 hours).[39,49] According to Leopold, the time elapsed before repair has an effect on both airway stenosis and on voice.[21]

Significant glottic and supraglottic lacerations and displaced cartilage fractures need surgical approximation. Endoscopy and CT will differentiate between the patients that need only observation (small laceration, shallow laceration, nondisplaced fracture) and those that require a thyrotomy or open fracture reduction and mucosal approximation. A soft laryngeal stent may be needed for badly macerated mucosa. Simple tracheal lacerations that do not detach a tracheal ring or encroach on the airway can be repaired without a tracheostomy. More severe disruptions (gunshot wound directly to the trachea) imply more soft-tissue injury, and a 6-week tracheostomy either below or through the tracheal injury is the safest procedure. Later the stenosis may require sleeve resection, but if the stenosis is soft, it can often be managed by a T-tube tracheostomy tube.

SUMMARY

Emergent surgical exploration is indicated for any immediate life-threatening signs or symptoms from penetrating neck trauma (i.e., massive bleeding, expanding hematoma, nonexpanding hematoma in the presence of hemodynamic instability, hemomediastinum, hemothorax, hypovolemic shock).

For the stable patient, the choice of treatment remains controversial. Knowledge of the neck zone involvement (I, II, or III), mechanism of injury, and velocity of the projectile are helpful in determining the likelihood of vital structure injury. At present, many trauma centers manage stable patients with non–life-threatening penetrating neck trauma with selective exploration; however, this must be supported by on-site angiography, flexible and rigid endoscopy, and closely monitored physical examinations. High-velocity missiles

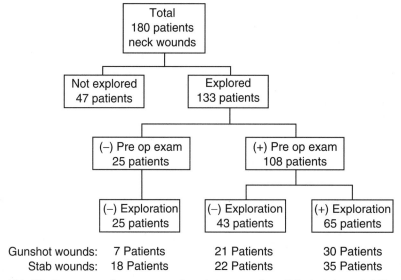

Figure 111-13. Summary of management and preoperative clinical status of 180 patients with penetrating wounds of the neck. (From Obeid FN and others: *Surg Gynecol Obstet* 160:517, 1985.)

inflict a significantly greater amount of damage than low-velocity projectiles. Zone I and zone III injuries usually require arteriography on all stable patents. Stable patients with zone II injuries often require angiography. Because hemorrhage is the leading cause of death for penetrating neck injuries, hemodynamic and neurologic status should always be monitored closely for at least 48 to 72 hours.

REFERENCES

1. Albuquerque FC, Javedan SP, McDougall CG: Endovascular management of penetrating ventral artery injuries, *J Trauma* 53:574, 2002.
2. Armstrong W, Detar T, Stanley R: Diagnosis and management of external penetrating cervical esophageal injuries, *Ann Otol Rhinol Laryngol* 103:863, 1994.
3. Atta HM, Walker ML: Penetrating neck trauma: lack of universal reporting guidelines, Am Surg 64:222, 1998.
4. Beitsch P and others: Physical examination and arteriography in patients with penetrating zone II neck wounds, *Arch Surg* 129:577, 1994.
5. Bishara R and others: The necessity of mandatory exploration of penetrating zone II neck injuries, *Surgery* 100:655, 1986.
6. Reference deleted in pages.
7. Brennan J, Meyers A, Jafek B: Penetrating neck trauma: a 5-year review of the literature, 1983-1988, *Am J Otolaryngol* 11:191, 1990.
8. Calcaterra T, Holt G: Carotid artery injuries, *Laryngoscope* 82:321, 1972.
9. Carducci B, Lowe RA, Dalsey W: Penetrating neck trauma: consensus and controversies, *Ann Emerg Med* 15:208, 1986.
10. Deitch E, Grimes W: Experience with 112 shotgun wounds of the extremities, *J Trauma* 24:600, 1984.
11. Demetriades D and others: Evaluation of penetrating injuries of the neck: prospective study of 233 patients, *World J Surg* 21:41, 1997.
12. Dichtel W and others: Lateral mandibulotomy: a technique of exposure for penetrating injuries of the internal carotid artery at the base of the skull, *Laryngoscope* 94:1140, 1984.
13. Fackler M, Bellamy R, Malinowski J: The wound profile: illustration of the middle-tissue interaction, *J Trauma* 28(Suppl):21, 1988.
14. Hartling R and others: Stab wounds to the neck: role of angiography, *Radiology* 172:79, 1989.
15. Hiatt J, Busuttil R, Wilson S: Impact of routine arteriography on management of penetrating neck injuries, *J Vasc Surg* 1:860, 1984.
16. Hirshberg A and others: Transcervical gunshot injuries, *Am J Surg* 167:309, 1994.
17. Holt R, Kostohryz G: Wound ballistics of gunshot injuries to the head and neck, *Arch Otolaryngol* 109:313, 1983.
18. Jarvik J and others: Penetrating neck trauma: sensitivity of clinical examination and cost-effectiveness of angiography, *Am J Neuroradiol* 16:647, 1995.
19. Jurkovich G and others: Penetrating neck trauma: diagnostic studies in the asymptomatic patient, *J Trauma* 25:819, 1985.
20. Knightly JJ, Swaninathan AP, Rush BF: Management of penetrating wounds to the neck, *Am J Surg* 126:575, 1973.
21. Leopold DA: Laryngeal trauma, *Arch Otolaryngol* 109:106, 1983.
22. Liekweg W, Greenfield L: Management of penetrating carotid arterial injury, *Ann Surg* 188:587, 1978.
23. Mattox K and others: Intravascular migratory bullets, *Am J Surg* 137:192, 1979.
24. Mazolewski PJ an others: Computed tomographic scan can be used for surgical decision making in zone II penetrating neck injuries, *J Trauma* 51:315, 2001.
25. McConnell D, Trunkey D: Management of penetrating trauma to the neck, *Adv Surg* 27:97, 1994.
26. Meyer J and others: Mandatory vs selective exploration for penetrating neck trauma, *Arch Surg* 122:592, 1987.
27. Miller R, Duplechain J: Penetrating wounds of the neck, *Otolaryngol Clin North Am* 24:15, 1991.
28. Narrod J, Moore E: Initial management of penetrating neck wounds: a selective approach, *J Emerg Med* 2:17, 1984.

29. Noyes L, McSwain N, Markowitz I: Panendoscopy with arteriography versus mandatory exploration of penetrating wounds of the neck, *Ann Surg* 204:21, 1986.

30. Obeid F and others: A critical reappraisal of a mandatory exploration policy for penetrating wounds of the neck, *Surg Gynecol Obstet* 160:517, 1985.

31. Ordog G and others: Shotgun "birdshot" wounds to the neck, *J Trauma* 4:491–497, 1988.

32. Ordog G and others: 110 Bullet wounds to the neck, *J Trauma* 25:238, 1985.

33. Pearce W, Whitehill T: Carotid and vertebral arterial injuries, *Surg Clin North Am* 68:705, 1988.

34. Perry M: *Injuries of the carotid and vertebral arteries*. In Bongard FS, Wilson SE, Perry MO, editors: *Vascular injuries in surgical practice*, Norwalk, Conn, Appleton & Lange. 1991.

35. Rao P and others: Penetrating injuries of the neck: criteria for exploration, *J Trauma* 23:47, 1983.

36. Roon A, Christensen N: Evaluation and treatment of penetrating cervical injuries, *J Trauma* 19:391, 1979.

37. Ratlev NK: Penetrating neck trauma: mandatory versus selective exploration, *J Emerg Med* 8:75, 1990.

38. Saletta J, Folk F, Freeark R: Trauma to the neck region, *Surg Clin North Am* 53:73, 1973.

39. Schaefer SD: The treatment of acute external laryngeal injuries, *Arch Otolaryngol* 117:35, 1991.

40. Scalfani AP, Scalafani SJ: Angiography and transcatheter arterial embolization of vascular injuries of the face and neck, *Laryngoscope* 106(2 Pt 1):168, 1996.

41. Sclafani S and others: The role of angiography in penetrating neck trauma, *J Trauma* 31:557, 1991.

42. Sclafani S and others: The management of arterial injuries caused by penetrating of zone III of the neck, *J Trauma* 25:871, 1985.

43. Schwartz T: *Therapeutic angiography in the management of vascular trauma*. In Flanigan DP, Schuler JJ, editors: *Civilian vascular trauma*, Philadelphia, 1992, Lea & Febiger.

44. Spenler C, Benfield JR: Esophageal disruption from blunt and penetrating trauma, *Arch Surg* 111:663, 1976.

45. Stiernberg C and others: Gunshot wounds to the head and neck, *Arch Otolaryngol* 118:592, 1992.

46. Stone H, Callahan G: Soft tissue injuries of the neck, *Surg Gynecol Obstet* 117:745, 1963.

47. Symbas P, Hatcher C, Viasis S: Esophageal gunshot injuries, *Ann Surg* 191:703, 1980.

48. Thal E, Meyer D: Penetrating neck trauma, *Curr Prob Surg* 29(1):1, 1992.

49. Trone T, Schaeffer S, Carder H: Blunt and penetrating laryngeal trauma: a 13-year review, *Otolaryngol Head Neck Surg* 88:257, 1980.

50. Unger S Jr, Mideza M: Carotid arterial trauma, *Surgery* 87:477, 1980.

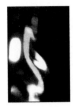

CHAPTER ONE HUNDRED AND TWELVE

DIFFERENTIAL DIAGNOSIS OF NECK MASSES

|| W. Frederick McGuirt, Sr.

INTRODUCTION

The differential diagnosis of a neck mass covers a broad spectrum of diseases and carries implications for management as varied as any area of medicine. All possible diagnoses and means of differentiating them are too numerous for a chapter of this length. Thus, a flowchart is used to help the otolaryngologist make the most logical diagnosis and consider viable options in the management of each problem (Figure 112-1).

GENERAL CONSIDERATIONS

When examining a patient with a neck mass, the physician's first consideration should be the patient's age group: pediatric (15 years of age and younger), young adult (16 to 40 years of age), or older adult (older than 40 years of age). Within each group, the incidence of congenital, inflammatory, and neoplastic disease must be considered because most neck masses fit into one of these three categories (Table 112-1). Pediatric patients generally exhibit inflammatory neck masses more frequently than congenital ones and developmental more than neoplastic masses; this incidence is similar to that found in younger adults. In contrast, the first consideration in older adults should always be neoplasia, with a smaller emphasis on inflammatory masses and even less emphasis on congenital masses.

The next consideration should be the location of the neck mass (Figure 112-2). This is particularly important in the differentiation of congenital and developmental masses because they usually occur in consistent locations. The location of a mass is both diagnostically and prognostically significant. The spread of head and neck carcinoma is similar to inflammatory disease, generally following an orderly lymphatic spread. The appearance and location of a metastatic neck mass may be the key to identifying the primary tumor or source of infection (Figure 112-3).

In addition to recognizing these general background considerations, the physician should evaluate each patient. Specific historic aspects and physical findings that could reduce the possible causes should be sought so that only a limited number of diagnostic tests are needed for differential diagnosis.

DIAGNOSIS
Physical Examination

The most important diagnostic step is the physical examination of the head and neck. Visualization and palpation are the most important components of the physical examination. These help determine the location of the mass according to anatomic lymphatic drainage areas or developmental areas, the size of the lesion and its relationship (fixation or displacement) to surrounding structures, the consistency of the mass, and the presence of any pulsations or thrills. Listening for bruits and detecting the distinct odor of wet keratin and necrotic tumor on the breath are also important.

The physician must not be distracted by the mass and neglect to perform a thorough head and neck evaluation. With the aid of a bright light source, the otolaryngologist should perform an indirect mirror or flexible endoscopic examination of all mucosal surfaces of the upper aerodigestive tract. These areas should also be palpated, even when no lesion can be seen—specifically the primary sites for lymphatic drainage to the location area of the mass in question (see Figure 112-3). A systematic investigation of all mucosal and submucosal areas is central to diagnosing the cause of neck masses. The capability of performing this examination distinguishes the otolaryngologist as the specialist for head and neck disease.

Tests

Often, even the most thorough physical examination only gives the physician a general impression of the derivation of the mass—vascular, salivary, or nodal; inflammatory, congenital, or neoplastic—and not a firm diagnosis. At this point, various tests may be helpful (Box 112-1).

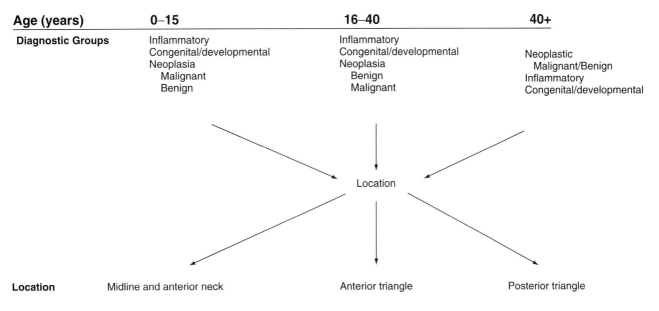

Age (years)	0–15	16–40	40+

Diagnostic Groups	Inflammatory
	Congenital/developmental
	Neoplasia
	  Malignant
	  Benign
		Inflammatory
		Congenital/developmental
		Neoplasia
		  Benign
		  Malignant
			Neoplastic
			  Malignant/Benign
			Inflammatory
			Congenital/developmental

Location

| **Location** | Midline and anterior neck | Anterior triangle | Posterior triangle |

Individual Diagnoses within Groups by Age and Location

Congenital/developmental

Thyroglossal duct cyst
Dermoid
Laryngocele

Congenital/developmental

Branchial cyst
Thymic cyst
Sialadenopathy
  Parotid
  Submaxillary

Congenital/developmental

Lymphangioma

Inflammatory

Adenitis
  Bacterial
  Viral
  Granulomatous

Inflammatory

Adenitis
  Bacterial
  Viral
  Granulomatous
Sialadenitis
  Parotid
  Submaxillary
Thorotrast granuloma

Inflammatory

Adenitis
  Bacterial
  Viral
  Granulomatous

Neoplastic

Thyroid
Lymphoma

Neoplastic

Thyroid
Lymphoma
Metastatic
  Upper jugular
    Oropharynx
    Oral cavity
    Larynx
  Lower jugular
    Hypopharynx
    Thyroid
  Submaxillary
    Oral cavity
    Nasal-sinus
    Face

Primary vascular
  Carotid body
  Glomus
  Hemangioma
Neurogenic
  Neurilemoma
Salivary
  Parotid
  Submaxillary

Neoplastic

Thyroid
Lymphoma
Metastatic
  Jugular
  Posterior
    Nasopharynx
    Scalp
  Supraclavicular
    Infraclavicular
    Primary

Figure 112-1. Neck mass considerations for diagnosis and neck mass occurrence by location.

TABLE 112-1

COMMON NECK MASSES

	Neoplastic	Congenital/Development	Inflammatory
Metastatic	Unknown primary	Sebaceous cysts	Lymphadenopathy
	Epidermoid carcinoma	Branchial cleft cysts	Bacterial
		Thyroglossal duct cysts	Viral
	Primary head and neck	Lymphangioma/hemangioma	Granulomatous
	Epidermoid carcinoma	Dermoid cysts	Tuberculous
	Melanoma	Ectopic thyroid tissue	Cat-scratch
		Laryngocele	Fungal
Primary	Adenocarcinoma	Thymic cysts	Sarcoidosis
	Thyroid		Sialadenitis
	Lymphoma		Parotid
	Salivary		Submaxillary
	Lipoma		
	Glomus vagale		
	Carotid body tumor		
	Rhabdomyosarcoma		

For a patient whose mass is pulsatile or compressible or who has a bruit or thrill, angiographic or ultrasonographic tests can be ordered to differentiate degenerative vascular problems (e.g., aneurysms) from neoplastic conditions (e.g., glomus and carotid body tumors). Ultrasonography can also help to differentiate a solid mass from a cystic mass, or congenital branchial cysts and thyroglossal cysts from solid lymph nodes, neurogenic tumors, and ectopic

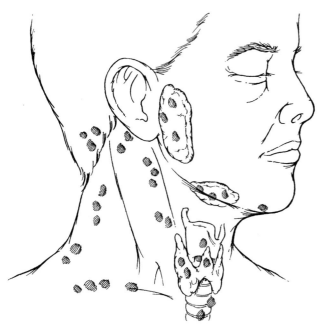

Figure 112-2. Location of common lymphatic and glandular masses of head and neck. *Stippled* areas represent congenital masses.

thyroid tissue.[3] The accuracy of differentiating solid, complex, and cystic lesions with ultrasound ranges is from 90% to 95% when both A-mode and B-mode scans are used.[24,59]

For lesions in the areas of the salivary glands, radionuclide scanning, sialography, and ultrasonography are all valuable.[51] The radionuclide scan or the sialogram usually localizes the mass inside or outside the salivary gland and thus determines whether it has a glandular origin. Similarly, the radionuclide scan shows whether the mass has functioning or nonfunctioning tissue. Positron emission tomography (PET) is a new radionuclide scan that indicates the functional activity of a mass. This has therapeutic implications, especially for a nodal structure identified on computed tomography (CT) or magnetic resonance imaging (MRI) scans, which are equivocal for metastasis. It can also be helpful in differentiating recurrent cancer from postirradiation changes.

PET scanning used as a tool to help determine the primary site for metastatic neck carcinoma of unknown origin can be especially beneficial to the non–head and neck specialist. It is also helpful in locating a primary site beyond the head and neck region or in the identification of concomitant distant metastasis. Because of the results of clinical and endoscopic evaluation by experienced head and neck surgeons, PET scanning is not routinely advocated; its high expense, high false-positive rate due to background salivary activity, and resolution limitations warrant this, unless endoscopy and guided biopsy provides no evidence of a primary lesion.[4,5,19] A more radio-intense mass has greater metabolic activity and is usually neoplastic. False-positive results occur

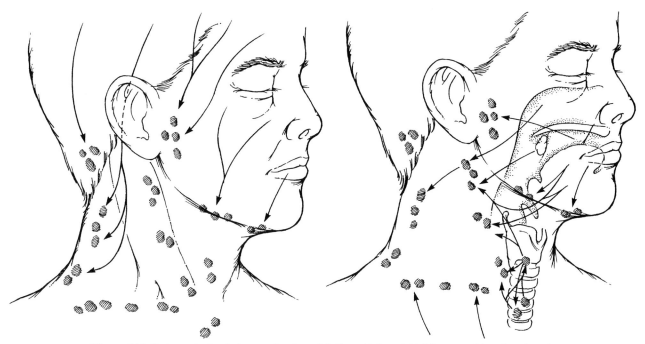

Figure 112-3. Lymphatic drainage of external *(left)* and internal *(right)* areas of head and neck. Arrows indicate lymphatic drainage pathways.

with opposite-side vocal cord paralysis granulomatous adenopathy and with certain salivary tumors such as Warthin's tumors.[22,45,46]

In general, plain radiographs aid little in differentiating masses in the neck. CT and MRI of the neck are currently the most helpful tests, replacing most of the other diagnostic tests. These tests differentiate solid from cystic masses, locate a mass within a glandular structure or within a lymph nodal chain, and differentiate vascular masses. However, CT and MRI remain expensive, and clinical judgment combined with the use of needle biopsy should make their use as purely diagnostic tools for most neck masses infrequent. Magnetic resonance T2-weighted images are often

---

BOX 112-1

DIAGNOSTIC EXAMINATION AND TESTS FOR HEAD AND NECK MASSES

1) Physical examination: Repeated; most important
2) Radionucleotide scanning: Obtain in lesions of anterior neck compartment; helpful in thyroid lesions and in localizing a lesion to be within a salivary gland. PET scan may be helpful in differentiating tumor from postirradiation changes, equivocal adenopathy by CT or MRI exam, and identifying distant metastasis.
3) Ultrasonography: To differentiate solid from cystic masses; especially useful in congenital and developmental cysts; also useful noninvasive technique for vascular lesions
4) Arteriography: For vascular lesions and tumors fixed to the carotid artery
5) Sialography: To diagnose diffuse sialadenopathies or to locate mass within or outside a salivary gland
6) CT and MRI imaging: Single most informative test; differentiates cysts from solid lesions; locates mass within or outside a gland or within a nodal chain; mucosal disease enhancement; provides anatomic relationships
7) X-ray, plain: Rarely of help in differentiating neck masses
8) Antibiotic course: Clinical test for suspected inflammatory bacterial lymphadenopathy; must pursue workup if unresolved after course of antibiotics.
9) Culture with sensitivities: Inflammatory tissue at open biopsy
10) Skin tests: Used when chronic or granulomatous inflammatory lesion is suspected
11) Needle biopsy: Gold standard in diagnosis of a neck mass; use small-gauge needle; obtain flow cytometry of lymphoid population
12) Endoscopy and biopsy: To identify primary tumor as source of metastatic node; use in all patients suspected of having neoplasia
13) Open biopsy: Use only after workup is complete and if diagnosis is not evident; specimen for histologic frozen section; be prepared to do simultaneous neck dissection

helpful in identifying submucosal neoplastic disease as the source of nodal enlargement, especially in the nasopharynx and tongue base. These should be performed before any guided biopsies so there is no confusion in interpreting the scan. Treatment decisions for masses based on findings from imaging studies alone are fraught with danger. These studies should only be viewed as supportive and correlated with the clinical impression and results of biopsy. Imaging by CT or MRI is more helpful in determining the extent of disease and planning surgery than in than in making a correct diagnosis.[58]

For a patient whose diagnosis after examination remains uncertain but who is suspected of having inflammatory adenopathy, a trial of antibiotic therapy and observation, not to exceed 2 weeks, is acceptable as a clinical test.

If the mass in question persists or increases in size after a trial course of antibiotics, additional investigational testing is necessary. Biopsy with pathologic examination is the definitive diagnostic test of preference. Open biopsy should be performed, however, only after the physician has performed a complete head and neck examination using direct and indirect methods and has performed an initial fine-needle aspiration (FNA) biopsy, which is the standard of care for initial biopsy. This is especially necessary for adults. The biopsy should generally include the following: (1) progressively enlarging nodes; (2) a single asymmetric nodal mass; (3) a persistent nodal mass without antecedent active signs of infection; and (4) actively infectious conditions that do not respond to conventional antibiotics and in which routine bacteriologic determinations are unsuccessful, so that a tissue sample is needed for further bacteriologic studies.

UNKNOWN NECK MASS WORKUP PROTOCOL

If the history, physical examination, and routine diagnostic tests do not lead to a definitive diagnosis, any unknown neck mass, particularly a unilateral, asymptomatic mass corresponding to the location of known lymph node groups, must be considered a metastatic neoplastic lesion until proven otherwise.

Fine-Needle Aspiration and Open Biopsy

An FNA biopsy is performed before endoscopy but after a thorough head and neck examination. The technique of obtaining multiple aspirations with a 25-gauge needle is recommended. Experience in collection and slide preparation is needed to guarantee maximal information. The onsite presence of a cytopathologist ensures the acquisition of adequate and representative tissue and enhances the yield and accuracy of FNA biopsies.[13] FNA biopsy has become standard in making both diagnostic and management

decisions on neck masses. Microamounts of tissue obtained by FNA have been studied by flow cytometry for lymphoma diagnosis and polymerase chain reaction (PCR) to identify the Epstein-Barr virus (EBV) for diagnosis of primary nasopharyngeal carcinoma.[14,60]

FNA biopsy is also used in a patient with a known distant malignancy in whom confirmation of metastases is needed for staging and planning therapy, in a patient with a head and neck primary tumor who is not a candidate for surgery but for whom the physician needs to make a tissue diagnosis to initiate nonsurgical therapy, and in a patient with an unknown neck mass.

FNA biopsy can usually readily differentiate a cystic lesion from inflammatory tissue. It is quite helpful in an overly anxious patient for whom the clinical index of suspicion for a neoplasm is low and the head and neck examination workup results are negative, and whose physician wishes to prevent an open biopsy or more extensive workup. Negative needle biopsy results may allay the patient's fear of cancer and allow the physician time to follow the mass more confidently.

FNA can be cost effective and helpful in differentiating lymphoma from carcinoma in adult patients. This distinction avoids an endoscopic examination, guided biopsy and general anesthesia for a diagnosis of lymphoma.

Occasionally, in high-risk patients who are chronic users of tobacco or alcohol and who have a solid neck mass but no obvious primary head and neck mucosal tumor, the FNA biopsy may have inconclusive or negative results. In this group, endoscopy and open biopsy for confirmation are still required because the index of suspicion is high.

Endoscopy and Guided Biopsy

The search for the primary lesion must include a second, thorough—direct and indirect—examination of the oral cavity, nasopharynx, hypopharynx, larynx, thyroid, salivary glands, and skin of the scalp and face (see Box 112-1). Chest and abdominal images are frequently ordered but are usually of minimal help in differentiating neck masses found in locations other than the supraclavicular region. FNA biopsy is the standard of evaluation after a complete office physical examination. If the nature of the mass or the source of a metastasis identified by FNA remains elusive, the aerodigestive tract should be examined endoscopically, especially in the area from which primary lymphatic drainage to the mass occurs (see Figure 112-3). An obvious lesion should be biopsied; when no lesion is seen or palpated, guided (not "blind") biopsies should be performed of the most logical areas for the silent primary tumor based on known lymphatic drainage.[18] These areas are usually the nasopharynx around Rosenmüller's fossa, the tonsil (in which case a tonsillectomy replaces an incisional biopsy),[52] the base of the tongue, and the pyriform sinus. The rationale for the guided biopsy when an obvious lesion is not present is that the primary tumor is often submucosal or arises deep in the crypts of the palatine tonsil or the folds of the lingual lymphoid tissue.

Open Excisional Biopsy

Similarly, when the FNA biopsy specimen tests positive for carcinoma and the clinical examination and endoscopy do not reveal a primary tumor site, open excisional biopsy is the next step in confirming or diagnosing the mass. When open excisional biopsy is performed, immediate examination by frozen section should be obtained and further therapeutic decisions made on the basis of that report (see Box 112-1). Specifically, if the diagnosis is squamous cell carcinoma, melanoma, or adenocarcinoma (unless the mass is supraclavicular), a radical neck dissection should be performed, which requires appropriate preoperative counseling and the patient's permission.

Biopsy in Younger Age Groups

In children and young adults in whom inflammatory and nonspecific reactive adenopathy is common, frequent, repeated examinations and nonsurgical management are the norm. Nodal masses that are solitary and asymmetric, located in the supraclavicular area, progressively increasing in size, or associated with other worrisome historical or physical findings should stimulate a consideration of surgical interventional therapy. Most nodal masses do not have these characteristics and can be followed clinically in patients in the younger age groups.[25] This more conservative approach to the neck mass in children is supported by the findings of Knight, Malne, and Vassy,[30] who found that diagnostic lymph node biopsy evaluation with culture showed a specific cause in only 41% of 234 children under the age of 16 years, but 16% were found to have malignant adenopathy. Supraclavicular adenopathy tested positive for malignancy in 60% (14 of 23) of the children. Because a significant number of children with a neck mass will have a malignancy, they must not all be diagnosed as having inflammatory or reactive adenopathy when they present with a neck mass.

Among those in the younger age groups, which carry a lower incidence of malignancy, needle biopsies are still often useful for sampling the mass, thereby allaying the physicians', patients', and families' fears of malignancy, temporizing any premature open biopsy, and allowing time for appropriate clinical follow-up examinations. Even patients with negative needle biopsy results must be followed up for other signs of neoplasia because of the difficulty in correctly interpreting lymphomas (the largest group of tumors in these age groups) by needle biopsy. Small quantities of nodal tissue obtained by FNA showing lymphocyte predominance should be studied by flow cytometry to aid in a diagnosis of lymphoma.[6] In a child, if an adequate FNA biopsy cannot be obtained in the office and anesthesia is needed for biopsy, an excisional biopsy is preferable to needle biopsy because of the larger amount of tissue and information obtained. Again, the main indications for biopsy should be: (1) progressively enlarging nodes; (2) a single asymmetric nodal mass; (3) a persistent nodal mass without antecedent active signs of infection; and (4) actively infectious conditions that do not respond to conventional antibiotics.

MANAGEMENT
Unknown Primary Lesions

Any neck mass in an adult patient must be approached as being neoplastic and possibly malignant.[7,37,41] In fact, it is the fear of cancer that usually brings the patient to the physician.[27,49]

In 1952, Martin and Romieu[36] reviewed 1300 primary tumors of the head and neck manifested by a cervical lump in 12.4% of cases. They stated, "Asymmetric enlargement of one or more cervical lymph nodes in an adult is almost always cancerous and usually is due to metastasis from a primary lesion in the mouth or pharynx." This principle remains sound today. The key to its validity lies in the words *enlarged lymph node, asymmetric,* and *adults.* If the physician remembers that primary cervical malignancy is rare and that almost all malignant cervical tumors except for lymphomas are metastatic, and if the history and physical examination are thorough, the physician should not confuse metastatic malignant cervical tumors with inflammatory lymphadenopathy, cysts, or benign neck tumors.

A study by Lee and Helmus[33] supports the theory that an asymmetric neck mass in the adult should be considered malignant until proven otherwise. They reviewed biopsy specimens of neck masses in 163 patients seen consecutively in a community hospital; of patients older than 40 years, 29.4% had carcinoma and 21.4% had lymphoma. Those figures agree closely with the 50% incidence of neoplasia reported by Slaughter, Majarakis, and Southwick[55] and Mayo and Lee.[37] The incidence of malignant disease in a neck mass rose to 80% in the Slaughter series when benign thyroid nodules were excluded.

A second principle regarding unknown primary lesions is that the immediate removal of an enlarged lymph node for diagnostic purposes is a disservice to

TABLE 112-2

CORRELATION OF WOUND NECROSIS, LOCAL AND DISTAL RECURRENCE, TIME OF BIOPSY

Variable Examined	Biopsy Before Definitive Treatment No. of Patients (Incidence)	Biopsy at Time of Definitive Treatment No. of Patients (Incidence)	No Biopsy No. of Patients (Incidence)
Wound necrosis	13/64 (20.3%)	5/46 (10.9%)	98/605 (12.9%)
Regional neck recurrence	21/64 (32.8%)	11/46 (23.9%)	116/600 (19.5%)
Distant metastasis	25/63 (39.7%)	11/46 (23.9%)	131/598 (21.9%)

the patient with metastatic cervical carcinoma.[2,44] Distant metastases and late regional recurrences are more frequent in patients who have had pretreatment biopsies than in those with the same stage of disease who have not (Table 112-2).[29] The pretreatment biopsy group also has a higher incidence of local wound complications. These findings suggest that disruption of lymphatic drainage and manipulation of a metastasis decrease the chances for clean surgical excision and cure. Lymphangiographic studies of the neck clearly document this disruption of the normal lymphatic drainage pattern by incisional therapy.[15]

Gooder and Palmer[20] have similarly confirmed this increased incidence of neck recurrence and wound complications in patients having previously received biopsies. Robbins and others[53] have disputed this incidence of increased metastasis, complications, and recurrence. However, the series on which they base their statement is weighted toward unknown primary tumors and nasopharyngeal and tonsillar tumors of Waldeyer's ring, as well as tumors that may well have natural histories and responses to management different from those of other mucosal squamous cell carcinomas. Indeed, their figures for distant metastasis were notably higher for tongue and hypopharyngeal primary tumors, which had neck node violation. Similarly, their incidence of local neck recurrence was nearly double that of matched controls in patients having incisional biopsies.

Probably no surgical condition is detected more easily in early physical examination, yet is most often inappropriately diagnosed and initially managed, than a malignant tumor of unknown primary origin located in the neck. The attempt to diagnose and cure this problem should begin with a careful examination of the oral cavity, nasopharynx, hypopharynx, larynx, thyroid, salivary glands, and skin of the head and neck. Historically, 50% to 67% of patients diagnosed by nodal examination have had their primary tumor site identified by the initial head and neck examination.[28,29,35]

In a patient who presents with a neck mass and in whom prior routine physical examination of the head and neck is negative, an independent second survey of the less visible areas of the upper digestive and respiratory tracts is the most cost-effective diagnostic tool (Table 112-3). If the results of the second examination are negative, an FNA biopsy should be performed. FNA biopsy results that are positive or equivocal for cancer, or even negative in a high-risk patient (e.g., tobacco or alcohol user) should stimulate further diagnostic evaluation. Direct endoscopic examination should be performed after appropriate scans are obtained.[12] The T2-weighted MRI is preferred because of its better delineation of submucosal disease.[58] If endoscopy provides no evidence of a primary lesion, the sites most likely to contain an occult tumor should be biopsied. A 16% incidence of identification of the primary site with endoscopy has been reported.[29]

The location of the lymph nodes involved should guide the surgeon to the appropriate sites for biopsy (Figure 112-3). Enlarged nodes high in the neck or in the posterior triangle suggest a nasopharyngeal lesion, whereas enlarged jugulodigastric nodes point to the tonsils, the base of the tongue, and the supraglottic larynx. The ipsilateral tonsil should be removed and examined for upper jugular adenopathy.[52] When the enlarged nodes are in the supraclavicular area or the lower third of the neck, the surgeon must consider the whole length of the digestive tract, the tracheobronchial tree, the breast, the genitourinary tract, and the thyroid gland as potential sites of the lesion. When the mass is located in the supraclavicular triangle, only a thorough physical examination and radiographic imaging are recommended to screen those areas before proceeding to biopsy if the workup findings are negative.

If the workup for an enlarged neck node is thorough and the site of the primary lesion is still not apparent, an open excisional biopsy of the cervical node should be performed. The patient should know that a complete neck dissection may be necessary. The biopsy should

TABLE 112-3

Workup of Head and Neck Asymmetric, Unilateral "Nodal" Mass

1. Complete repeated physical examination of:	Oral cavity Nasopharynx Hypopharynx Larynx Thyroid Salivary glands Skin of head and neck
2. Needle biopsy	
3. Imaging	Chest Upper aerodigestive tract/neck after FNA, if positive
4. Panendoscopy with guided biopsy based on location of nodal mass	Nasopharynx Base of tongue Tonsillectomy
5. Open biopsy of cervical mass with:	Frozen section diagnosis if no primary found Epidermoid carcinomas, melanoma, upper neck adenocarcinoma: simultaneous neck dissection Lymphoma: close and stage before radiation therapy, chemotherapy, or both Adenocarcinoma: close; pursue primary lesion if supraclavicular Granuloma or inflammation: culture and close

be done through an incision along a line acceptable for a radical neck dissection and only if the surgeon is prepared and capable of doing this dissection when the frozen section indicates this course. Other findings dictate the course outlined previously (Table 112-3). When adenocarcinoma is found, most patients (86%) have other distal metastases as well, and the cure rate is not affected by treatment of the neck. The exception may be an adenocarcinomatous node found above the level of the cricoid.[32] Approximately 5% of all cancer patients whose diagnoses start out as an unknown lesion and who undergo this diagnostic workup require an open biopsy.

For a patient with an unknown primary metastatic squamous cell carcinoma, postoperative irradiation of the nasopharynx, ipsilateral tonsil, base of the tongue, and contralateral side of the neck is frequently advocated after radical neck dissection.

This practice of prophylactic irradiation is still controversial.* Arguments against prophylactic irradiation include:

1. A percentage of unknown primary lesions are from infraclavicular sites or are metastases of a previously excised skin lesion that cannot be proved or assumed to be the source of malignancy. These lesions would not benefit from such irradiation.

2. Prophylactic irradiation therapy can compromise management of mucosal carcinoma appearing later.
3. Prophylactic irradiation can induce later mucosal carcinoma.
4. Such therapy can also cause major prolonged morbidity in the form of xerostomia, dysphagia, and dental caries.
5. Cure rates have been reported to be higher with surgery to the neck alone than with wide-field irradiation therapy alone. These factors should be weighed against the increase in cure rates reported from postoperative irradiation, and the reports and results are varied.[34,61,62]

If the head and neck area, including Waldeyer's ring, is managed with radiotherapy, the incidence of late-appearing primary disease is reported to be as high as 30%, but the consensus is that the incidence decreases to roughly one-half that (12%) without radiotherapy.[23,26] Jesse, Perez, and Fletcher[28] reported this figure with adjuvant radiotherapy to be as low as 5.7%. Nordstrom, Tewfik, and Latourette[50] and Weir and others[62] reported it to be only 2%.

The best candidates for postoperative irradiation to control recurrence in the neck are patients whose nodal mass is staged N_1 with nodal capsular penetration, N_2, or N_3. Controversy exists over how to manage patients with N_1 disease not extending through the nodal capsule. There are advocates for surgery to the

*References 18, 22, 36, 44, 52, 54, 58.

neck only, for local nodal excision plus irradiation, and for complete neck dissection plus radiotherapy.

Clinicians not supporting postoperative irradiation rely on careful follow-up examination and management of the primary lesion when it is found. This approach requires a compliant and easily examined patient.

Regardless of whether postoperative irradiation therapy is used, patients with malignant metastatic cervical nodes and unknown primary lesions must be reexamined frequently. Only careful, periodic follow-up examinations can ensure early detection and management of the primary malignancy.

In the past, the most common site of a silent primary lesion was the nasopharynx because it was the most difficult area to examine. PCR used to detect EBV in metastatic nodal carcinoma is now being used to help identify primary nasopharyngeal carcinoma.[14,60] Today, with flexible endoscopic instruments in the office, MRI, and PET scans, the most common locations of these small, silent tumors are in the tonsils and the base of the tongue.[11]

The use of PET scanning to detect unknown primary tumors remains unsettled. For head and neck tumor teams of experienced surgeons and radiologists, these have not proven significantly additive to clinical examination, CT/MRI imaging, and endoscopic biopsy.[22]

Known Primary Lesions

The neck mass in a patient with a known primary neoplasm of the head and neck should be managed according to the principles described for each primary site. In general, when clinically positive cervical lymph node metastases are present, a complete cervical lymphadenectomy should be done along with removal of the primary tumor. When the primary lesion is not in the head or neck, excisional biopsy of the metastatic cervical mass for confirmation and staging is indicated, with further management dictated by the primary lesion. However, care must be taken to follow the suggestions for an unknown primary lesion to be certain that the mass in question is not a manifestation of a second, independent primary lesion of the head or neck. This is also true for a patient with a known primary head and neck tumor and neck mass. The rate of occurrence for a second, synchronous primary lesion is significant in patients who have a head or neck neoplasm. A 6% incidence of silent synchronous tumors is found only by prospective panendoscopic examinations.[40]

Knowledge of a second lesion might affect management decisions and allow better prognostic counseling to the patient. Correlations of concomitant tumor sites include larynx-lung, tonsil-esophagus, and oral cavity–oral cavity.

Primary Tumors

Thyroid neoplasms, both benign and malignant, are a leading cause of anterior-compartment neck masses in all age groups and, along with lymph node malignancies, are the most common neoplastic lesions in the pediatric and young adult age groups. In the pediatric group, thyroid neoplasms frequently show a male predominance as well as an increased incidence of malignant disease. In contrast, the young adult and older groups show a greater incidence of benign conditions and a female predominance.

Lymph node metastasis is the initial symptom in about 15% of cases of papillary carcinoma; up to 40% of patients with malignant thyroid nodules have neck nodes that test clinically positive, and up to 90% have neck nodes that prove to be histologically positive when they are operated on.[39] Ultrasound, thyroid scans, and thyroid function tests can be considered for patients having an anterior compartment neck mass. Thyroid mass lesions found to be cystic by ultrasound should be aspirated. Solid lesions should be managed according to their activity on nuclear scan. Functioning nodules should be managed by suppression, and all nonfunctioning cold nodules should be explored with appropriate concomitant therapeutic measures being taken on the basis of histology and extent of disease. When scans are obtained, 20% to 25% of solitary cold nodules will prove to be cystic, and 20% to 25% will prove to be cancerous.[20] Initial FNA of all thyroid mass lesions, skipping both the nuclear scan and the sonogram, has become the standard of care because it yields a more rapid, economical, and definitive answer as to the nature of the mass. This approach requires the services of an expert cytopathologist.

Lymphomas, Hodgkin's disease, and lymphosarcomas occur in persons in all age groups but are more likely to occur and form a greater percentage of all neoplasms among those in the pediatric and young adult age groups.[17] These lesions alone account for up to 55% of all pediatric cancers. Among children with lymphosarcoma or Hodgkin's disease, as many as 40% and 80%, respectively, have at least one neck mass.

Except for progressive enlargement of lymph node tissue, local head and neck symptoms are usually absent, but systemic and other organ system findings should be sought. Lymphomas are usually discrete, rubbery, and nontender.

Specimens from a suspicious-appearing mass (single, dominant, supraclavicular, asymmetric) can initially be biopsied by FNA and studied by flow cytometry if the child is cooperative. When the child will not allow an FNA biopsy in the office or the FNA and flow cytometry results are equivocal or negative but suspicion for large cell lymphoma (which may often be negative on FNA) exists, the next diagnostic step should be open biopsy for complete histocytopathologic examination, followed by appropriate staging procedures.[6] The immediate biopsy in these younger patients following complete physical examination is permissible because of the rarity of mucosal primary carcinoma in these age groups. If routine physical examination or laryngopharyngoscopy yields an abnormality of Waldeyer's ring, biopsy of that abnormality is necessary for staging at the time of the neck node biopsy.[10,56] Extranodal lymphomas can be associated with gastrointestinal or central nervous system involvement and require appropriate evaluation.

Salivary neoplasms must be considered whenever an enlarging solid mass lies in front of and below the ear, at the angle of the mandible, or in the submandibular triangle. Benign salivary lesions are usually asymptomatic. Pain, rapid growth, cranial nerve (CN) VII symptoms, or skin fixation suggest malignancy. Diagnostic radiographic studies (e.g., sialography, nuclear scans, CT scans) indicate whether the mass is salivary in origin, but they are no better than physical examinations in differentiating benign from malignant lesions.[45] The diagnostic test of preference is open biopsy in the form of complete submandibular gland removal or superficial parotidectomy.

In the case of the unknown primary tumor, for which the principle is: "The surgeon planning to do a node biopsy must be prepared to perform an immediate neck dissection," the surgeon approaching masses in and around the ear should be prepared to perform a total parotidectomy and facial nerve dissection. Any approach less complete will lower the patient's chance for a complete cure because there is a high risk of implantation and seeding of benign mixed tumors, which make up two-thirds of all salivary tumors.

Carotid body tumors and *glomus tumors* classically occur in the upper anterior triangle around the carotid bifurcation and are pulsatile, compressible masses that rapidly refill on the release of pressure. Carotid body tissue can be moved from side to side but not up or down. Both a bruit and a thrill are present, and with glomus vagale tumors, the ipsilateral tonsil may pulsate and be deviated toward the midline. The diagnosis is made angiographically. Small tumors in young patients should be resected.[42] In elderly patients or for extensive tumors in patients who are at high risk for functional disability from cranial nerve damage by resection, management by irradiation to arrest the growth with a good long-term outcome is permissible.[4,31] The use of arterial embolization for larger lesions aids in tumor clearance in a more expedited fashion with less blood loss.[48]

Schwannomas or *neurilemomas* are solid, neurogenic tumors that occur most commonly in the parapharyngeal space and will usually cause medial tonsillar displacement. They have no diagnostic characteristics, although their origin from the vagus nerve can cause hoarseness, and their origin from the sympathetic chain may be associated with Horner's syndrome. Routine evaluation for an unknown primary tumor is indicated before surgical exploration and excision are done.

Lipomas are ill-defined soft masses that occur in various neck locations most commonly in patients older than 35 years. These tumors are asymptomatic and have no specific diagnostic characteristics. On a CT scan, a lipoma appears as a fat-air density.

Congenital and Developmental Disorders

Branchial cleft cysts most commonly occur in late childhood or early adulthood.[38] They frequently follow an upper respiratory tract infection, and often appear initially as an inflammatory mass with pain, swelling, tenderness, and fever. After management with appropriate antibiotics these cysts may resolve, but more frequently they persist as soft, doughy, variably sized masses occurring in characteristic locations in the anterior triangle of the neck. The second branchial cleft cyst occurs deep to and along the anterior edge of the sternocleidomastoid muscle, sometimes having a remnant tract that courses between the carotid branches anterior to CN IX and CN XII to enter the oropharynx. The less common first branchial cleft cyst occurs along the inferior mandible, at the angle of the mandible, or just below the ear lobule. A remnant tract can be found going to the external auditory canal. Ultrasonic scans can be helpful in identifying the lesions as cystic rather than solid. Aspiration of the contents yields a milky, mucoid, or brownish fluid, which often contains cholesterol crystals.

Management involves initial control of local infection followed by surgical excision of the cyst and its entire tract. For first branchial cleft cysts, this means having the skill to perform a total parotidectomy with facial nerve dissection and preservation. Due to its proximity to CN XI, resection of a second branchial cleft cyst also should be done without administering muscle relaxants to the patient. Proper identification of the nerve during the surgical resection is important.

Thyroglossal duct cysts are anterior neck, midline structures that, like branchial cleft cysts, often appear after an upper respiratory tract infection. Once the acute infection has been controlled through the use of antibiotics, ultrasonography can be used to differentiate the persistent mass from a lymph node, a dermoid cyst, or thyroid tissue. A pathognomonic sign is vertical motion of the mass with swallowing and tongue protrusion. In the past, radionuclide scanning was advocated in the workup of thyroglossal duct cysts. Due to its low yield, however, it is no longer performed routinely, being reserved for cysts in the tongue base, which must be differentiated from undescended lingual thyroid tissue. The cyst tract should be completely removed, along with the midportion of the hyoid bone, as described by Sistrunk.[54] All thyroglossal cysts and tracts should be examined histologically for the rare instance of concomitant neoplastic disease, especially when the patient has received prior neck irradiation.[43]

Lymphangiomas usually occur in the pediatric population; most are present at birth, and over 90% are evident within the first year of life. Lymphangiomas in the neck most commonly appear in the posterior triangle. The cervical lymphangioma is a fluctuant, diffuse, soft, spongy mass, often having indiscrete margins. It is believed to arise from incomplete development and obstruction of the normal lymphatic system. Its extent is often much greater than is apparent. Transillumination is diagnostic, along with the physical appearance and the characteristics on palpation.

The lesion should be excised if it is easily accessible or is affecting vital functions. It should not be removed if its removal would require a mutilating procedure for limited benefits. Sclerotherapy represents an option in extensive lesions with a high risk of recurrence or complications especially for large cavity lesions.[21]

Hemangiomas, like lymphangiomas, are usually considered congenital because they are either present at birth or they appear within the first year of life. Their bluish-purple coloration, increased warmth, compressibility followed by refilling, bruit, and thrill help distinguish them from other head and neck masses. Traditional management of lymphangiomas has consisted of observation only unless rapid growth, thrombocytopenia, or involvement of vital structures occurs. Most of these congenital lesions, however, resolve spontaneously. Increasingly, interventional management with lasers is being advocated. Newer pulse-dye lasers are superior and are being accepted as appropriate management in speeding resolution and improving the curative outcome over that with argon and neodymium:yttrium-aluminum-garnet (Nd:YAG) lasers.[47] Local resection of some lesions is also advocated for better end-result cosmesis.

Dermoid cysts occur most commonly in pediatric patients and young adults in the same cervical areas as branchial and thyroglossal duct cysts. Dermoid cysts slowly enlarge because of accumulation of their sebaceous content, but unlike epidermal or sebaceous cysts they lie deep to the cervical fascia and the skin moves freely over them. No specific diagnostic tests

exist. These cysts are cured by simple complete excision.

Inflammation

Lymphadenitis occurs in nearly every person at some point in life, especially during the first decade of life.[25] Lymphadenopathy, caused by bacterial or viral infections of the upper respiratory tract, is so common that it is an expected sign. The source of the reactive lymphadenopathy is usually identified easily by reviewing the source of drainage to the nodal area in question (Figure 112-3) and by using specific culture and sensitivity tests to determine the preferred antibiotic treatment. A physician waiting for test results should administer an antibiotic that covers a broad spectrum of head and neck pathogenic organisms.

Granulomatous inflammatory disease affects specific age groups and locations; the physician should remember this when evaluating a patient with a neck mass (Table 112-4). Excisional biopsy in these lesions is usually diagnostic and curative. Incisional biopsy should be avoided due to the sequelae of a chronic draining fistula from the residual neck infection.[1]

Acquired Immunodeficiency Syndrome

Cervical lymph node hyperplasia is ubiquitous in human immunodeficiency virus (HIV)–positive patients, and nodal masses in these patients infrequently need to be considered for biopsy. The physician should perform a biopsy only if there is a single rapidly enlarging node, a newly tender node, a node that has enlarged concomitant with a change in systemic systems, or a single enlarged (>3 cm) node in a chain of nodes.[5] When node biopsy is indicated in an HIV-positive patient, it is preferably done by FNA. Tender enlarging nodes should make one suspicious of tuberculous or *Nocardia* species infections, whereas nontender enlarging head and neck nodes often indicate Kaposi's sarcoma or Burkitt's lymphoma.

TABLE 112-4

GRANULOMATOUS ADENOPATHY

Disease	Age Group	Location
Cat-scratch disease	Pediatric	Preauricular and submandibular
Actinomycosis	Adult	Submandibular and upper jugular
Tuberculosis	Adult	Posterior triangle
Atypical tuberculosis	Pediatric	Anterior triangle

Trauma

Sequelae of trauma occasionally present as a neck mass. In pediatric patients, neck trauma, especially when related to forceps delivery, can result in a mass in the anterior neck within the sternocleidomastoid muscle. This hematoma, with organization, can easily be confused with a desmoid or sarcoma and should not be overtreated. Heat, massage, and observation are often associated with resolution. Continued growth or increasing torticollis indicate surgical exploration.[57]

Pseudoaneurysms of major vessels are occasionally associated with blunt neck trauma. These are pulsatile masses that may have systemic emboli or neurologic sequelae. Ultrasound or infused MRI or magnetic resonance angiography can be diagnostic, obviating the need for an angiogram.

Neuromas are small neck masses that are found after surgery, especially radical neck dissections. They occur from sensory nerve endings that are found most commonly in the posterior triangle. The great auricular nerve (C2-3) is the most common nerve of origin. Neuromas are tender, associated with sharp shooting pains on palpation, and are quite slow in growth. Systomatology or consideration of recurrent cancer dictates their excision.

SUMMARY

Many head and neck disease processes manifest themselves as neck masses. These conditions are managed by surgical excision except for some inflammatory masses, and these often must be excised for diagnostic reasons.

The real question is when to excise the lesion to expedite management in a cost-effective manner. In general, when signs of inflammation are associated with the mass, antibiotic management with observation for up to 2 weeks is acceptable. Persistence of the mass beyond that time or an increase in mass size during that time suggests that surgical intervention should be considered. The timing of intervention may be tempered by the age group. A more prolonged period of observation (monitoring for growth or the development of other associated symptoms of malignancy) is appropriate in children because of their low incidence of malignant tumors.

In children, if a biopsy of the mass is deemed appropriate because of progressive growth, the isolated nature or asymmetry of the mass, the location (supraclavicular), the development of symptoms associated with lymphoma (fever and hypertrophy of the spleen, liver, or Waldeyer's ring), or the static size (if >3 cm), excisional biopsy alone (without further workup) is performed. This excisional biopsy in younger patients can be carried out once a complete examination of the head and neck and special tests yield no further information. This procedure is acceptable because of the rarity of mucosal carcinoma (and its lymphatic spread with worsening of prognosis by biopsy) in children. Other mass lesions in this age group do not appear to have their prognoses adversely affected by biopsy, but thyroid neoplasia, regardless of the patient's age, should be managed definitively (based on the frozen section diagnosis) at the time of biopsy.

In adult patients beyond the fourth decade of life, complete, repeated head and neck physical examination is mandatory. After examination, needle biopsy of the mass is the current standard of care if no cause has been found for the mass. Benign cystic lesions or lymphomas indicate the need for excision, either as definitive management or for diagnostic purposes. If the needle biopsy results are positive for carcinoma, equivocal, or even negative in the presence of a high index of suspicion for metastatic squamous cell carcinoma, an endoscopic examination is mandatory before open excision biopsy of the mass and excisional removal of the mass with frozen section examination are performed. If no discrete lesion is seen, guided biopsy of the upper aerodigestive tract is performed before open excisional biopsy. If, on excision, the mass proves to be metastatic carcinoma, a concomitant neck dissection should be performed.

REFERENCES

1. Altman RP, Margileth AM: Cervical lymphadenopathy from atypical mycobacteria: diagnosis and surgical treatment, *J Pediatr Surg* 10:419, 1975.
2. Birchall MA, Stafford ND, Walsh-Waring GP: Malignant neck lumps: a measured approach, *Ann R Coll Surg Eng* 73:91, 1991.
3. Blei CI, Gooding GAW, Rector W: Ultrasonic and fluorescent scanning: a combined noninvasive diagnostic approach to extrathyroidal neck lesions, *Am J Surg* 134:369, 1977.
4. Bungaard T and others: Treatment of glomus tumours: a retrospective survey, *Clin Otolaryngol* 14:155, 1989.
5. Burton F, Patete ML, Goodwin WJ: Indications for open cervical node biopsy in HIV-positive patients, *Otolaryngol Head Neck Surg* 107:367, 1992.
6. Cannon CR, Richardson LD: Value of flow cytometry in the evaluation of head and neck fine needle lymphoid aspirations, *Otolaryngol Head and Neck Surg,* 124:544-548, 2001.
7. Coker DD and others: Metastases to lymph nodes of the head and neck from an unknown primary site, *Am J Surg* 134:517, 1977.
8. Coster JR and others: Cervical nodal metastasis of squamous cell carcinoma of unknown origin; indications for withholding radiation therapy, *Int J Radiat Oncol Biol Phys* 23:743, 1992.
9. Davidson BJ and others: Cervical metastases of occult origin: the impact of combined modality therapy, *Am J Surg* 168:395, 1994.
10. DeVita VT Jr, Jaffe ES, Hellman S: *Hodgkin's disease and the non-Hodgkin's lymphomas.* In DeVita VT Jr, Hellman S, Rosenberg SA, editors: *Cancer: principles and practice of oncology,* Philadelphia, 1985, JB Lippincott.

11. Dictor M and others: Determination of nonendemic nasopharyngeal carcinoma by in situ hybridization for Epstein-Barr virus EBER1 RNA: sensitivity and specificity in cervical node metastases, *Laryngoscope* 105:407, 1995.

12. Dillon WP, Harnsberger HR: The impact of radiologic imaging on staging of cancer of the head and neck, *Semin Oncol* 18:64, 1991.

13. Eisele DW and others: Utility of immediate on-site cytopathological procurement and evaluation in fine needle aspiration biopsy of head and neck masses, *Laryngoscope* 102:1328, 1992.

14. Feinmesser R and others: Diagnosis of nasopharyngeal carcinoma by DNA amplification of tissue obtained by fine-needle aspiration, *N Engl J Med* 326:17, 1992.

15. Fisch U: *Cervical lymph flow following surgery in the neck.* In *Lymphography of the cervical lymphatic systems,* Philadelphia, 1968, WB Saunders.

16. Freeman D and others: Unknown primary squamous cell carcinoma of the head and neck: is mucosal irradiation necessary? *Int J Radiat Oncol Biol Phys* 23:889, 1992.

17. Giles FJ, Timmis HH Jr: *Hodgkin's disease and the non-Hodgkin's lymphomas: diagnosis, staging, and therapy.* In Shockley WW, Pillsbury HC III, editors: *The neck: diagnosis and surgery,* St Louis, 1994, Mosby.

18. Gluckman JL, Robbins KT, Fried MP: Cervical metastatic squamous carcinoma of unknown or occult primary source, *Head Neck* 12:440, 1990.

19. Gobien RP: Aspiration biopsy of the solitary thyroid nodule, *Radiol Clin North Am* 17:543, 1979.

20. Gooder P, Palmer M: Cervical lymph node biopsy: a study of its morbidity, *J Laryngol Otol* 98:1031, 1984.

21. Greinwald JH Jr and others: Treatment of lymphangioma in children: an update of picibanil (OK 432) sclerotherapy, *International Journal of Pediatric Otolaryngol* 65:1-6, 2002.

22. Greven K, McGuirt WF: The emerging role of positron emission tomography in the management of head and neck cancer, *Curr Opin Otol-HNS* 7(2):48-51, 1999.

23. Harper CS and others: Cancer in neck nodes with unknown primate site: role of mucosal radiotherapy, *Head Neck* 12:463, 1990.

24. Hassani S, Bard R: Proceedings of the 23rd Annual Meeting of the American Institute for Ultrasound in Medicine and 7th Annual Meeting American Society of Ultrasound Technology Specialists, San Diego, Calif, 1978, Mercury Press.

25. Herzog LW: Prevalence of lymphadenopathy of the head and neck in infants and children, *Clin Pediatr* 22:485, 1983.

26. Jacques DA: *Metastases to lymph nodes of the head and neck from an unknown primary site,* American College of Surgeons Postgraduate Course No. 10, 1979.

27. Jakobsen J and others: Lymph node metastases in the neck from unknown primary tumor, *Acta Oncol* 31:653, 1992.

28. Jesse RH, Perez CA, Fletcher GH: Cervical lymph node metastasis: unknown primary cause, *Cancer* 31:854, 1973.

29. Jones AS and others: Squamous carcinoma presenting as an enlarged cervical lymph node, *Cancer* 71:1756, 1993.

30. Knight PJ, Malne AF, Vassy LE: When is lymph node biopsy indicated in children with enlarged peripheral nodes? *Pediatrics* 69:391, 1982.

31. Konefal JB and others: Radiation therapy in the treatment of chemodectomas, *Laryngoscope* 97:1331, 1987.

32. Lee NK and others: Metastatic adenocarcinoma to the neck from an unknown primary source, *Am J Surg* 162:306, 1991.

33. Lee SG, Helmus C: Cervical lymph node biopsy, *Mich Med* 69:581, 1970.

34. Marcial-Vega VA and others: Cervical metastases from unknown primaries: radiotherapeutic management and appearance of subsequent primaries, *Int J Radiat Oncol Biol Phys* 19:919, 1990.

35. Martin H, Morfit M: Cervical lymph node metastasis as the first symptom of cancer, *Surg Gynecol Obstet* 78:133, 1994.

36. Martin H, Romieu C: The diagnostic significance of a lump in the neck, *Postgrad Med* 11:491, 1952.

37. Mayo CW, Lee MJ Sr: Significance of tumor of the neck, *Lancet* 70:420, 1950.

38. McGuirt WF: *Asymptomatic mass in anterior triangle of neck in a 13-year-old boy.* In McGuirt WF, editor: *Pediatric otolaryngology: case studies,* ed. 2. New Hyde Park, New York, 1984, Excerpta Medica.

39. McGuirt WF: Management of occult metastatic cervical disease from well-differentiated thyroid carcinoma, *Ear Nose Throat J* 68:170, 1989.

40. McGuirt WF: Panendoscopy as a screening examination for simultaneous primary tumors in head and neck cancer: a prospective sequential study and review, *Laryngoscope* 92:569, 1982.

41. McGuirt WF: The unknown primary in metastatic head and neck cancer: a clinical approach, *NC Med J* 39:299, 1978.

42. McGuirt WF, Harker LA: Carotid body tumors, *Arch Otolaryngol* 101:58, 1975.

43. McGuirt WF, Marshall RB: Postirradiation carcinoma in a thyroglossal duct remnant: follicular variant of papillary thyroid carcinoma, *Head Neck Surg* 2:420, 1980.

44. McGuirt WF, McCabe BF: Significance of node biopsy before definitive treatment of cervical metastatic carcinoma, *Laryngoscope* 88:594, 1978.

45. McGuirt WF and others: A comparative diagnostic study of head and neck nodal metastases using positron emission tomography, *Laryngoscope* 105:373, 1995.

46. McGuirt WF and others: Preoperative identification of benign versus malignant parotid masses: a comparative study including positron emission tomography, *Laryngoscope* 105:579, 1995.

47. Morelli JG and others: Tunable dye laser (577 nm) treatment of port wine stains, *Lasers Surg Med* 6:94, 1986.

48. Murphy TP, Brackmann DE: Effects of preoperative embolization on glomus jugulare tumors, *Laryngoscope* 66:1244, 1989.

49. Nguyen C and others: Metastatic squamous cell carcinoma to cervical lymph nodes from unknown primary mucosal sites, *Head Neck* 16:58, 1994.

50. Nordstrom DG, Tewfik HH, Latourette HB: Cervical lymph node metastases from an unknown primary, *Int J Radiat Oncol Biol Phys* 5:73, 1979.

51. Odette J, Szymanowski RT, Nichols RD: Multiple head and neck malignancies, *Trans Am Acad Ophthalmol Otolaryngol* 84:805, 1977.

52. Righi PD, Sofferman RA: Screening unilateral tonsillectomy in the unknown primary, *Laryngoscope* 105:548, 1995.

53. Robbins KT and others: The violated neck: cervical node biopsy prior to definitive treatment, *Otolaryngol Head Neck Surg* 94:605, 1986.

54. Sistrunk WE: Technique of removal of cysts and sinuses of the thyroglossal duct, *Surg Gynecol Obstet* 46:109, 1928.

55. Slaughter DP, Majarakis JD, Southwick HW: Clinical evaluation of swellings in the neck, *Surg Clin North Am* 36:3-9, 1956.

56. Snow JB Jr: Neoplasms of the head and neck in children, *Ad Otolaryngol* 23:115, 1978.

57. Tom LWC and others: Torticollis in children, *Otolaryngol Head Neck Surg* 105:1, 1991.

58. Underhill T, McGuirt WF, Williams DW: Advances in imaging in head and neck tumors, *Current Opinions in Otol-HNS,* 8:91-97, 2000.
59. Walfish PG and others: Application of special diagnostic techniques in the management of nodular goitre, *Can Med Assoc J* 115:35, 1976.
60. Walter MA, Menarguez-Palanca J, Peiper SC: Epstein-Barr virus detection in neck metastases by polymerase chain reaction, *Laryngoscope* 102:481, 1992.
61. Wang RC and others: Unknown primary squamous cell carcinoma metastatic to the neck, *Arch Otolaryngol Head Neck Surg* 116:1388, 1990.
62. Weir L and others: Radiation treatment of cervical lymph node metastases from an unknown primary: an analysis of outcome by treatment volume and other prognostic factors, *Radiother Oncol* 35:206, 1995.

SUGGESTED READING

Martin H, Morfit HM, Ehrlich H: The case for branchiogenic cancer (malignant branchioma), *Ann Surg* 132:867, 1950.

PRIMARY NEOPLASMS OF THE NECK

Terry A. Day
John K. Joe

INTRODUCTION

Primary neoplasms of the neck include those tumors that arise from, rather than metastasize to, lymphovascular structures of the neck, as well as those tumors originating from the soft tissues of the neck. These neoplasms may be either benign or malignant and, although they are less commonly the cause for a lump of the neck, one should always consider these tumors in the differential diagnosis of a neck mass. The following chapter will be divided into benign and malignant sections and provide the reader with a comprehensive review of neoplasms that may originate in the neck.

DIAGNOSTIC EVALUATION

The diagnosis of neoplasms of the neck involves the standard practice of the complete history and physical examination. Importantly, the patient should be questioned regarding prior neoplasms, family history, systemic signs, and symptoms in addition to the risk factor of prior radiation therapy to the head and neck region. The comprehensive head and neck examination should include the ear and temporal bone, sinonasal cavity, nasopharynx, oropharynx, hypopharynx, and larynx in addition to the full cranial nerve examination. If the neck mass in not pulsatile or vascular in nature, a fine-needle aspiration should be performed. Only when the fine-needle aspiration is nondiagnostic or inadequate should excisional biopsy be performed, and at that time, the surgeon should be prepare to proceed with appropriate neck dissection with margin analysis if necessary.

Radiologic Studies

Both computed tomography (CT) scan and magnetic resonance imaging (MRI) may be useful in the evaluation of soft tissue tumors of the head and neck region with particular advantages of each technique varying by type of tumor, location, regional disease, and proximity to vital structures. Although radiographic findings may provide clues to the diagnosis within the broad differential, accurate diagnosis cannot be confirmed without histologic evaluation. CT scanning is particularly useful in evaluating bone detail in addition to calcification within tumor. In addition, CT-directed biopsy of tumors that are difficult to access, such as the parapharyngeal space, may provide diagnostic tissue. MRI has surpassed CT in evaluating soft tissue extent and relationships in the head and neck region. It is generally recommended in the majority of soft tissue tumors or tumors adjacent to vital structures of this region. Positron emission tomograph (PET) scanning to evaluate primary tumors and metastatic disease has been described, but further studies will be necessary to determine the overall indications for its use in head and neck malignancies.[45,57,94,170]

BENIGN NEOPLASMS OF THE NECK

Benign neoplasms of the neck are often misdiagnosed as infectious in etiology (e.g., lymphadenitis) or congenital (e.g., branchial cleft cyst) on initial examination. Thus, the diagnosis of all neck masses requires a vigilant approach using the history, physical examination, radiologic studies, and fine-needle aspiration biopsy. Because these tumors are uncommon, a review of the diagnostic approach is vital to the clinician's evaluation and management of each case. Benign primary neoplasms of the neck include vascular tumors, such as paragangliomas; peripheral nerve neoplasms, such as schwannomas or neurofibromas; and lipomas. The following discussion of these benign neoplasms will be categorized by tissue of origin.

Vascular Neoplasms

Paragangliomas compose the most common class of benign vascular neoplasm of the neck. Paragangliomas arise from extraadrenal paraganglionic cells derived from the neural crest.

Pathology

The paraganglionic system denotes a collection of neuroectoderm-derived chromaffin cells in extraadrenal sites. The system is vital as a source of catecholamines in fetal development, until the formation of the adrenal medulla.

Normal paraganglia contain two types of cells: type I, chief cells or granular cells; and type II, the supporting or sustentacular cells. Type I cells contain dense-core granules filled with catecholamines, a property that places them in the amine precursor and uptake decarboxylase (APUD) system. Type II, or sustenacular cells, are elongated cells that closely resemble Schwann cells. Their function is not entirely clear.

Tumors of paraganglia, such as carotid body tumors, contain both type I and II cells. Type I cells predominate and are arranged in an organized-nested pattern, known as *Zellballen*, surrounded by sustentacular cells in a fibrous stoma. These nests of Zellballen are illustrated in Figure 113-1. Type I chief cells tend to be polygonal shaped with abundant granular eosinophilic cytoplasm. They are peripherally surrounded by type II sustentacular cells, which are difficult to identify by light microscopy and appear as spindle-shaped basophilic cells. Nuclear pleomorphism and cellular hyperchromatism are common in paragangliomas and should not be considered evidence of malignancy.

Immunohistochemistry aids the diagnosis and differential diagnosis of this neoplasm. Type I cells stain positively with neuron-specific enolase, chromogranin

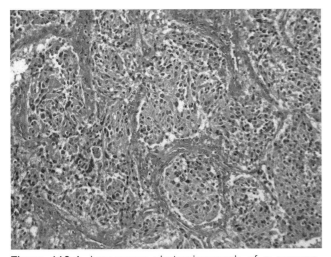

Figure 113-1. Low-power photomicrograph of a paraganglioma demonstrating nests of Zellballen within a fibrous stroma (hematoxylin and eosin stain). To view this image in color, please go to *www.ototext.com* or the Electronic Image Collection CD, bound into your copy of Cummings Otolaryngology—Head and Neck Surgery, 4th edition.

A, and synaptophysin. Type II cells stain with S-100 and focally with glial fibrillary acidic protein.

Nomenclature

The controversy over the proper nomenclature of paragangliomas has been confusing. Historically they have been referred to as *glomus tumors, chemodectomas,* and *non-chromaffin tumors.*

The correct terminology of paragangliomas is based on location, that is, there are "carotid paragangliomas," "jugulotympanic paragangliomas," and "vagal paragangliomas," although the terms *carotid body tumor, glomus tympanicum,* and *glomus jugulare* still persist.

Other terms such as *chemodectoma, glomus tumor,* and *non-chromaffin tumor* are less accurate terms and should be avoided. *Chemodectoma* is an inaccurate term to describe all paragangliomas of the head and neck because carotid and aortic bodies are the only known paraganglia of the head and neck that behave as chemoreceptors. The term *glomus tumor* more accurately describes benign cutaneous tumors arising from neuromyoarterial cells surrounding arteriovenous anastomoses. Designation as a non-chromaffin tumor relates to histologic staining characteristics. An early histologic staining technique using the chromaffic reaction failed to show the presence of catecholamines; paragangliomas were therefore described as non-chromaffin tumors. Newer techniques, however, have detected catecholamines in small quantities.[91] The chromaffin reaction is a highly insensitive method on which to classify these tumors.[61]

Epidemiology

Approximately 90% of tumors arising from the paraganglion system are in the adrenal gland, and these tumors are termed *pheochromocytoma*. The remaining 10% arise from extraadrenal sites with 85% arising in the abdomen, 12% in the thorax, and the remaining 3% in the head and neck area.

The most common paraganglioma of the head and neck is the carotid body, followed by jugulotympanic paragangliomas and vagal paragangliomas. Other sites include the larynx, nasal cavity, orbit, trachea, aortic body, lung, and mediastinum. It has been estimated that paragangliomas constitute 1 in 30,000 head and neck tumors.[109] However, the true incidence of paragangliomas may be unknown, since previous reports have confused paragangliomas with neuroendocrine tumors.[7] Further complicating an accurate estimate is the multicentricity of these tumors, particularly in familial paragangliomas.

Types of Paragangliomas

Carotid paragangliomas. Carotid paragangliomas are the most common type of paragangliomas and will serve as the template of discussion of the history, physiology, and etiologic factors relevant to paragangliomas.

History. The anatomist von Haller first described the carotid body in 1743; its function, however, was unknown at the time. Histologic studies of the carotid body revealed glandular acini, and so the carotid body was renamed the *carotid gland*. Von Luschka[176] first described a tumor of the carotid body in 1862. In 1880, Reigner performed the first resection of a carotid body tumor, but the patient did not survive. Six years later, Maydl resected a carotid body tumor; the patient survived but had postoperative hemiplegia and aphasia.

In 1889, Albert was the first surgeon to successfully resect a carotid body without ligating the carotid vessels. The first successful removal of a carotid body tumor in the United States was reported by Scudder in 1903.[157] The term *paraganglion* was first used by histologist Kohn in 1903[93] to describe the carotid body. This term was most appropriate because cells of the carotid body originate from the neural crest and migrate in close association with autonomic ganglion cells, hence the name *paraganglionic*. In 1950, Mulligan described, in the dog, neoplastic degeneration of the carotid body as chemodectoma, due to the chemoreceptor function of the carotid body.[123]

Anatomy and physiology. The carotid body is located in the adventitia of the posteromedial aspect of the bifurcation of the common carotid artery.

The normal carotid body measures 3 to 5 mm in diameter but is often larger in persons living at higher altitudes. The average weight of the normal adult gland is 12 mg, with a wide range previously reported as 1 to 47 mg.[71] On inspection, the carotid body is a small, reddish-brown to tan, ovoid structure attached to the carotid vessels at the bifurcation by Mayer's ligament through which the feeding vessels run, primarily from the external carotid artery. Blood flow and oxygen consumption of the carotid body, gram for gram, exceed those of the brain or thyroid gland.[59] Sensory innervation is from Hering's nerve, a branch of the glossopharyngeal nerve that originates approximately 1.5 cm distal to the jugular foramen.

The carotid body has a chemoreceptor role by modulating respiratory and cardiovascular function in response to fluctuations in arterial pH, oxygen, and carbon dioxide tension. Acidemia, hypoxia, or hypercapnia stimulates the carotid body to initiate an autonomic reflex that leads to increased respiratory rate and depth as well as increased heart rate, blood pressure, and cerebral cortical activity. It is this close association with respiratory drive and the sympathetic nervous system response that have prompted investigation of the carotid body's role in disease processes such as obstructive sleep apnea and sudden infant death syndrome. Although no clear conclusions can be drawn at this time, the carotid body and its response to intermittent hypoxia appear to be related to the systemic hypertension seen in obstructive sleep apnea. It has also been shown that some children with sudden infant death syndrome had either small carotid bodies or a decreased ratio of mature type I to type II cells. It is hypothesized that this may attenuate the child's response to a hypoxic crisis.

Etiology. The etiology of paragangliomas appears to be multifactorial. Most paragangliomas are solitary. Multiple pheochromocytomas and paragangliomas are seen in familial syndromes, mainly multiple endocrine neoplasia types IIA and IIB. Other syndromes associated with paragangliomas are neurofibromatosis type 1 and von Hippel-Lindau disease, which is characterized by retinal angiomas, and cerebellar hemoangioblastomas. Carney's triad demonstrates the association of paraganglioma, pulmonary chondroma, and gastric leiomyosarcoma.[24]

In addition to these associations, a syndrome of familial paragangliomas characterized by multiple paragangliomas, especially in the head and neck region, has been described and occurs in approximately 10% of cases, most commonly as bilateral carotid body tumors. The familial nature of carotid body tumors was first suggested by Chase in 1933 in his description of two sisters with carotid body tumors.[27] Genetic mapping reveals this syndrome to be linked to the long arm of chromosome 11. The inheritance pattern for familial paragangliomas is autosomal dominant modified by genomic imprinting. Genomic imprinting in paragangliomas was described by van der Mey and colleagues[174] after reviewing data from 15 large Dutch pedigrees. The imprintable gene is transmitted in a mendelian manner, but the expression of the gene is determined by the sex of the transmitting parent. With paragangliomas, the gene results in the development of a tumor when it is paternally inherited. The offspring of male carriers were observed to demonstrate a 50% incidence of tumors, whereas children of female carriers never developed tumors. Huntington's disease and myotonic dystrophy represent other genetic diseases associated with genomic imprinting.

An increased incidence of carotid body tumors has been suggested in individuals living at altitudes greater than 2000 meters,[149] having atmospheric hypoxia, or with conditions causing chronic arterial hypoxemia such as cyanotic heart conditions and chronic lung disorders.[97,98] In fact, animals such as cattle, dogs, rabbits, and guinea pigs living in higher altitudes have been demonstrated to have heavier and larger carotid bodies, with an increased incidence of carotid body tumors, than those living at sea level.[3,46] Stimulation of the carotid body by chronic hypobaric hypoxia was thought to be the inciting mechanism.

Clinical presentation and diagnosis. The characteristic feature of carotid body tumors is slow growth rate, which is reflected clinically by the delay between the first symptoms and the diagnosis, averaging between 4 and 7 years.

A carotid body tumor usually presents as a lateral cervical mass, which is mobile laterally but less mobile in the craniocaudal direction because of its adherence to the carotid arteries. This physical finding has been called a positive Fontaine sign.[181] Alternatively, a carotid body tumor may present as a parapharyngeal mass. Many carotid body tumors are pulsatile by transmission from the carotid vessels or, less commonly, they expand themselves, reflecting their extreme intrinsic vascularity. Sometimes, a bruit can be heard by auscultation but can disappear with carotid compression. The consistency varies from soft and elastic to firm, and they are generally nontender. As these tumors enlarge, progressive symptoms of dysphagia, odynophagia, hoarseness, and other cranial nerve (IX–XII) deficits appear. Carotid sinus syndrome syncope has been described in association with carotid body tumors.[151] The syndrome refers to a loss of consciousness accompanied with a reflex bradycardia and hypertension. Inciting stimuli include spontaneous movement of the head or following pressure applied to the tumor. Rarely, paraganglioma of the head and neck may present as a functional neuropeptide-secreting tumor.

Paragangliomas have the capacity to produce neuropeptides. This production pathway begins with tyrosine, which is obtained from the diet or synthesized from phenylalanine in the liver. Tyrosine is converted to L-dopa by tyrosine hydroxylase. The next step in the pathway converts L-dopa to dopamine. Dopamine is then converted to norepinephrine. The final conversion of norepinephrine to epinephrine is catalyzed by the enzyme phenylethanolamine-N-methyltransferase. This enzyme exists only in the adrenal medulla and in small numbers of neurons in the central nervous system (CNS). Because this enzyme does not occur in paragangliomas of the head and neck, these tumors do not accumulate or secrete epinephrine. Instead, paragangliomas tend to accumulate norepinephrine. Other neurotransmitters may also be produced, including serotonin, vasoactive intestinal peptide, and neuron-specific enolase.

The capacity for catecholamine synthesis in head and neck paragangliomas, however, does not translate immediately to clinical findings. Although all paragangliomas have neurosecretory granules, only 1% to 3% are considered functional.[108] Glenner and Roberts[61]

first described a functional carotid body tumor-secreting norepinephrine in 1962. Patients should be asked about signs and symptoms indicating elevated catecholamine levels. Complaints of headaches, palpitations, flushing, and perspiration should be evaluated. In these patients, a 24-hour urine collection is examined for norepinephrine and its metabolites, including vanillylmandelic acid and normetanephrine. Excess epinephrine or metanephrine should prompt suspicion of an adrenal pheochromocytoma because head and neck paragangliomas lack the enzyme to convert norepinephrine to epinephrine (phenylethanolamine-N-methyltransferase). An abdominal CT scan should be performed to rule out a concomitant adrenal pheochromocytoma. α and β-adrenergic blocking is undertaken if a tumor is found to be functional preoperatively. This decreases the risk from sudden catecholamine release that can occur with tumor manipulation in surgery. Routine screening for urinary metanephrines, vanillylmandelic acid, and serum catacholamines is probably only indicated for multiple or familial paragangliomas or in the presence of catecholamine-related symptoms.[84] However, considering the hazards associated with operating on a previously unsuspected, metabolically active tumor, an argument can be made for obtaining these studies in all cases.

Multicentricity. The carotid body tumor is the most common paraganglioma in the head and neck, and the most frequent combination of multiple tumors is bilateral carotid body tumors. The overall incidence of multiple tumors is reported in the literature to be approximately 10%; some of these may be unrecognized familial genetic mutations. If a familial pattern is recognized, the incidence of multiple tumors is reported to be between 30% and 50%.

Malignancy. Cellular criteria for malignancy, however, have not been established. Harrington and Dockerty[69] attempted to classify malignant tumors of the carotid body, including as criteria for malignancy mitoses with giant cells, nuclear pleomorphism, and capsular invasion. Using these criteria, 50% of the 20 tumors studied would be considered malignant. Batsakis[13] concurred that increased mitotic rate and capsular invasion should not be considered as determinants of malignancy. Other authors have hypothesized that all carotid body tumors demonstrate some degree of capsular invasion.[16] Malignancy is determined by metastasis, which must be proved with biopsy, because paragangliomas may exhibit multicentricity. There are no histologic criteria for malignancy. In fact, previous reports have described metastatic carotid body tumors without mitoses.[190] The diagnosis of malignancy should be made by evidence of spread to regional lymph nodes or distant sites (most common being lung and bones).[30,168]

Malignant paragangliomas have been reported in 6% of carotid body paragangliomas by Batsakis.[13]

Accurate 5-year survival rates are not available because of the low malignancy rate of an uncommon tumor. Data from the literature (National Cancer Data Base) suggest a 60% 5-year survival rate based on 59 reported cases in which regional metastases were found. Distant metastases had a worse prognosis.

Imaging studies. There are various diagnostic imaging modalities available in the workup of carotid body tumors. Noninvasive duplex ultrasonography demonstrates a hypervascular mass and the tumor's relationship to the carotid artery. Ultrasonography may also delineate any intrinsic carotid artery disease.

CT scanning with intravenous contrast demonstrates a hypervascular mass at the carotid bifurcation, splaying the internal and external carotid arteries. CT angiography may be performed to demonstrate the relationship of the carotid vessels to the enhancing neck mass.

MRI may be the most useful imaging study for evaluating carotid body tumors because it offers triplanar views and superior soft tissue contrast without the need for ionizing radiation, compared with CT scanning. Figure 113-2 demonstrates the superior soft tissue delineation provided by MRI scanning. MRI is sensitive for tumors as small as 0.8 cm.[125] Note the splaying of the carotid arteries. Paragangliomas larger than 2 cm in diameter typically demonstrate on T2-weighted images with a salt-and-pepper appearance, as shown in this Figure 113-2, with areas of hemorrhage accounting for the salt appearance and flow voids contributing to the pepper appearance.[130] As illustrated in Figure 113-3, MRI also provides for MR angiography, a noninvasive study for these vascular tumors, requiring fewer contrast loads than does CT angiography. Carotid body tumors demonstrate a characteristic lyre sign shown in Figure 113-4, a bowing and displacing of the internal and external carotid arteries. Radiographic evaluation should be sufficient to make the diagnosis of carotid body tumor.

Carotid angiography has been replaced by MR angiography, but carotid angiography is useful when preoperative embolization is necessary. The use of preoperative embolization is controversial, but many authors have recommended its use for large tumors to decrease blood loss.[182] Preoperative embolization can also be used in those rare instances where malignant carotid body may be suspected. If preoperative embolization is planned, surgery should be planned 24 to 48 hours subsequently to avoid revascularization, edema, or local inflammation. Additionally, angiography with temporary balloon occlusion using clinical and electroencephalographic monitoring, combined

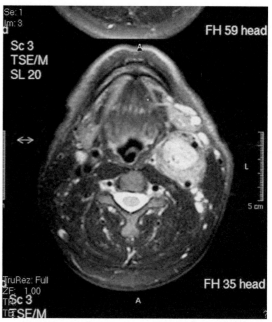

Figure 113-2. Axial MRI (T2-weighted) of left carotid paraganglioma resulting in splaying of the internal and external carotid arteries. Note the characteristic salt-and-pepper appearance, with areas of hemorrhage (salt) and flow voids (pepper).

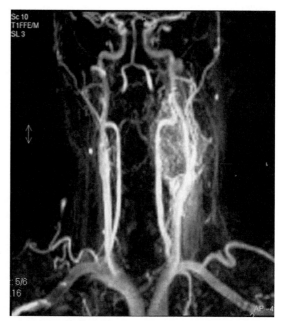

Figure 113-3. Coronal MR angiography of left carotid paraganglioma.

with xenon cerebral blood flow scanning, can provide specificity as to the tolerance of collateral cerebral circulation across in the circle of Willis in select cases.

The high density of somatostatin receptors in paragangliomas provides for newer functional nuclear medicine imaging techniques, including metaiodobenzylguanidine (MIBG) scanning and octreotide scanning.

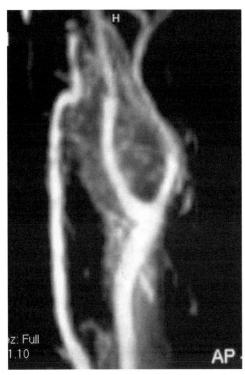

Figure 113-4. Coronal MR angiography (close-up) of carotid paraganglioma demonstrating the characteristic "lyre" sign from splaying of the internal and external carotid arteries.

MIBG scanning uses iodine-131–labeled tracer, which is concentrated in intracellular storage vesicles of paragangliomas.[177] Octreotide scanning uses a labeled somatostatin analog indium-111 octreotide to diagnose primary tumors of the APUD system, as well as their metastases.[89] These functional imaging studies have been recommended as a possible screening test for familial paragangliomas for patients at risk.[124]

Classification. Although not universally adopted in the literature on carotid body tumors, a classification system has been previously proposed for carotid body tumors. In 1971, while he was a surgery resident at the Mayo clinic, Shamblin[160] described a classification system used to grade the difficulty of resection in carotid body tumors. Group I tumors were defined as localized, relatively small, and minimally attached to the carotid vessels. Surgical excision was described as carried out without difficulty in this group. Group II encompassed tumors adherent to or partially surrounding the vessels, with moderate arterial attachment. These tumors were described as amenable to careful surgical removal. Group III carotid body tumors completely encased the carotids. Shamblin and his colleagues recommended approaching these tumors with great care and with consideration for vessel replacement.

Management. Surgery remains the mainstay of treatment for carotid body tumors. However, controversy persists in certain cases, particularly as it relates to multicentric tumors or for patients with advanced disease or significant comorbidities.

Surgery. In a report from Memorial by Lack and others,[99] 39 of 43 patients with carotid body tumors were treated surgically; one patient received definitive radiation therapy, and three others were observed but not treated. In this cohort of patients, 24 of 39 patients were free of disease after surgery, at an average follow-up interval of 12 years (6 months to 38 years). Local recurrence occurred in 4 of 39 patients (10%). Regional or distant metastases occurred in four of 39 patients (10%). All 4 of these patients were dead of disease within 6 years.

The incidence of permanent cranial nerve impairment as a complication of surgery has been reported in the literature to occur in approximately 20% of cases. In this report by Lack and colleagues,[99] cranial nerve sacrifice of the vagus or hypoglossal nerve was necessary in 15% (6 of 39) of patients. An additional patient developed Horner's syndrome postoperatively. Although not quantified, the superior laryngeal nerve, supplying sensory innervation to the larynx and motor innervation to the cricothyroid muscle, may be the nerve most frequently injured during carotid body resection. Paralysis of one superior laryngeal nerve can result in some degree of aspiration, although isolated palsy of one superior laryngeal nerve typically requires no additional rehabilitation. Furthermore, denervation of one cricothyroid muscle can result in pitch changes in singers, but changes in voice may not be perceptible. Injury to the cervical sympathetic chain will result in Horner's syndrome, with ipsilateral ptosis, miosis, and anhydrosis. Netterville and others[125] have described first bite syndrome resulting from injury to the cervical sympathetic chain, causing loss of sympathetic input to the parotid gland. Patients with first bite syndrome complain of severe cramping in the parotid area when they take the first bite of food, particularly with the first meal of the day. The pain generally subsides over the next several bites, but is more intense with strong sialogogues, such as tart or bitter foods. The physiologic mechanism behind first bite syndrome is likely due to denervation supersensitivity of the sympathetic receptors that control the myoepithelial cells in the parotid gland. With oral intake, parasympathetic neurotransmitters are released and cross-stimulation of the sympathetic receptors causes a supramaximal response of the myoepithelial cells. Treatment includes restriction to bland foods and oral carbamazepine (100–200 mg bid) with severe pain.

Anand and colleagues[1] reviewed 1181 published cases of carotid body tumors treated with surgical resection. Internal carotid artery injury was identified in 275 cases (23%), with an overall occurrence of CNS complications of 26%. This subcategory of internal carotid artery injury was further examined. In 62 cases (23%), internal carotid artery repair was accomplished simply with suture or patch repair, with a CNS complication rate of 3%. The internal carotid artery was reconstructed in 125 cases (45%), with a CNS complication rate of 10% and a mortality rate of 2%. It was necessary to ligate the internal carotid artery in 89 cases (32%), resulting in a CNS complication rate of 66% and a mortality rate of 46%.

Minimizing surgical complications requires a multidisciplinary approach using head and neck surgeons familiar with cervical neurovascular anatomy for approaching the tumor and the vascular surgeon for assistance in resection and vascular repair, if necessary. The keys to successful surgery are careful preoperative planning, proximal and distal control of the vasculature with vessel loops, careful identification and preservation of neural structures, such as the vagus nerve and hypoglossal nerve, and dissection in the periadventitial plane with meticulous attention to hemostasis. Occasionally, ligation of the external carotid artery is necessary to resect the carotid body tumor; however, typically, it can be preserved. Larger tumors may require bisection of the tumor to separate it from the internal and external carotid artery branches. The surgeon should be prepared for vascular reconstruction of the internal carotid artery, if necessary, with suture repair, patch grafting, or interposition saphenous vein graft. Routine intraoperative shunting is not recommended and should be used only as necessary in those rare instances where internal carotid artery resection and reconstruction is required in patients who do not tolerate preoperative balloon occlusion testing. Shunts cause vascular complications, including hemorrhage and thrombosis, and are associated with a 6% incidence of CNS complications and a 2% mortality rate.

Few reports address the issue of coexistent paragangliomas in the face of significant carotid artery stenosis. Although a paucity of data exist to suggest the best management, previous reports have recommended carotid endarterectomy at the time of carotid body tumor resection.[5,43,79] The same indications for performing a carotid endarterectomy without a tumor should also apply for those instances where tumor resection is planned. In these cases, carotid artery occlusion is necessary and shunting with EEG monitoring should be considered.

Controversy of surgery for multicentric tumors.
In the patient with bilateral paraganglioma, every effort must be made to save at least one vagus nerve and its laryngeal branches. Should a patient present with bilateral carotid body tumors, the case may be made to resect the smaller carotid body tumor first, with the intent of preserving the vagus and hypoglossal nerves on the less challenging side, before embarking on resecting the larger tumor of the other side. At a planned second stage, resection of the larger carotid body tumor can be undertaken. In the case of bilateral carotid body tumors with unilateral preexisting cranial nerve palsy, such as that affecting the vagus nerve (whether caused by surgery or the natural course of the tumor), the functional side should undergo tumor resection only if growth has been observed clinically or radiologically. In these cases, further bilateral cranial nerve damage must be prevented. In the case of enlarging tumor, radiation therapy may be an option and some authors are advocating this therapy.

Another recently described and rarely recognized problem after bilateral carotid body excision is baroreflex failure syndrome.[125] The clinical manifestations are caused by bilateral denervation of the carotid sinus. The carotid sinus is situated in the adventitia of the carotid bulb, and serves as a baroreceptor to decrease systemic blood pressure. Bilateral baroreceptor dysfunction causes unopposed sympathetic outflow, resulting in marked fluctuations in blood pressure and a sustained tachycardia postoperatively. Over time, compensation occurs, but it is variable and unpredictable. Compensation may occur by baroreceptor fibers in the aorta or through neural regrowth at the carotid sinus. Therapy consists of sodium nitroprusside in the early recovery phase to prevent excessive hypertension. Long-term control can be accomplished using oral antihypertensives, such as clonidine or phenoxybenzamine. Clonidine is an α_2-agonist, and it results in decreased release of norepinephrine into synaptic clefts and stimulation of parasympathetic outflow, slowing the heart rate. Phenoxybenzamine is an α_1- and α_2-antagonist that decreases peripheral resistance and increases cardiac output.

Radiation therapy. Carotid body tumors were originally thought not to be radiosensitive because the effects of radiation therapy were cytostatic but not cytotoxic. Radiation therapy for paragangliomas will arrest growth but not shrink tumor size. Furthermore, potential tumor regrowth after radiation therapy remains a possibility. Risks associated with radiation therapy for paragangliomas include carotid atherosclerosis, radiation-induced malignancy, and associated morbidity, including mucositis.

Radiation oncologists at the University of Florida have described effective local control of 23 carotid and vagal paragangliomas using definitive radiotherapy.[50] In their study, 15 patients with 23 carotid or vagal paragangliomas were treated with radiotherapy between 1981 and 1995. Nineteen tumors were treated with radiation therapy alone, and four were treated with surgery and postoperative radiation therapy. For benign tumors, total doses ranged from 35 to 48.5 Gy. The two malignant tumors received 64.8 and 70 Gy. Follow-up ranged from 1.5 to 10 years. Local control was achieved in 96% of tumors at 5 years. Five-year disease-specific survival was 89%, with one patient dead of locally recurrent disease 5 years after radiation therapy. This patient had been previously treated with surgery and radiation therapy before treatment by the authors. Another patient died of atherosclerotic disease 13.5 years after radiation therapy. There were no patients with regional or distant failure after treatment. Complications reported by these authors included one patient experiencing a delayed transient CNS syndrome. No other complications were reported.

Valdagni and Amichetti[173] reported seven patients with 13 carotid body tumors treated with radiation therapy between 1968 and 1987. Treatment consisted of radiotherapy alone for 10 tumors, and surgery plus radiation therapy for three tumors. Total doses ranged from 46 to 60 Gy at 1.8 to 2.5 Gy per fraction. Follow-up ranged from 1 to 19 years. Local control was achieved in all patients. Acute adverse effects were minimal. No short- or long-term toxicities were reported.

Even proponents of radiation therapy for carotid body tumors concur with surgical resection as the preferred modality of treatment for most lesions.[115] Definitive radiation therapy may be reserved for patients who are poor surgical candidates due to debilitated medical condition and for locally advanced tumors where anticipated postoperative morbidity may preclude consideration for surgical resection. Adjuvant radiation therapy may be considered after surgery for malignant carotid body tumors for locoregional control.

Observation. Using sequential radiologic imaging, Jansen and colleagues[83] have estimated the median tumor doubling time for 20 carotid body tumors as 7.1 years, including 12 cases without detectable growth. Farr[53] has estimated a growth rate for carotid body tumors, plotting tumor size against years of symptom duration, calculating a growth rate of 2 cm in 5 years.

Serial scanning at selected intervals may be considered for those patients who are not suitable candidates for surgery or radiation therapy. This highly select group of patients includes those individuals whose medical condition is so poor that both

surgery and radiation therapy are contraindicated, or those patients of such advanced age that the carotid body tumor may have minimal impact on their life expectancy or quality of life. This group may also include those patients with malignant carotid body tumors with distant metastases where locoregional treatment would be only palliative in intent.

Vagal paragangliomas. Vagal paragangliomas are tumors derived from paraganglionic tissue associated with one of the ganglia of the vagus nerve.[179] Vagal paragangliomas most commonly arise from the inferior vagal ganglion, also referred to as the *nodose ganglion*. Tumors arising from the superior vagal ganglion, or jugular ganglion, may be dumbbell-shaped and may extend from the neck intracranially through the jugular foramen.

Clinical presentation and diagnosis. Vagal paragangliomas, like carotid body tumors, may present as a palpable neck mass that is more mobile in a lateral direction than a craniocaudal orientation. Paralysis of the ipsilateral true vocal cord or Horner's syndrome, from involvement of the ipsilateral sympathetic chain, may be present as the tumor grows in size. True vocal cord paralysis can result in hoarseness with or without aspiration of liquids from glottic incompetence. Large tumors arising from the jugular ganglion may be associated with cranial neuropathies of cranial nerves IX, XI, and XII. Diagnostic imaging studies previously described in this chapter may demonstrate anterior displacement of the carotid artery from the tumor present in the posterior carotid sheath. Unlike carotid body tumors, the internal and external carotid arteries do not manifest a splayed configuration.

Management. The treatment strategies used for carotid paragangliomas described in the previous section apply to the management of vagal paragangliomas as well. Most are treated by surgical resection, and the discussion pertinent to preoperative embolization described above is germane to vagal paragangliomas, as well. Patients should be counseled preoperatively as to the fact that complete resection of the vagal paraganglioma typically necessitates sacrifice of the vagus nerve. The resultant ipsilateral true vocal cord paralysis can be addressed in the postoperative period as needed, based on the patient's deficits. Vagal paragangliomas arising from the nodose ganglion are usually approached by a transcervical approach, whereas more superiorly located tumors of the jugular ganglion may require a combined transmastoid-transcervical approach, with possible craniotomy should there be intracranial extension. Indications for definitive radiation therapy or observation alone, which have been previously described for carotid paragangliomas, are applicable to vagal paragangliomas as well.

Jugular paragangliomas. Jugular paragangliomas may present as one of two types, traditionally referred to as *glomus tympanicum* and *glomus jugulare*. Glomus tympanicum typically arises from a branch of either the glossopharyngeal nerve (tympanic branch of Jacobson) or the vagus nerve (posterior auricular branch of Arnold). Glomus jugulare originates from the jugular bulb.

Clinical presentation and diagnosis. Patients with jugular paragangliomas may present with pulsatile tinnitus, hearing loss, or with cranial neuropathies of cranial nerves IX, X, XI, or XII. Otoscopic examination may demonstrate a vascular mass in the middle ear.

CT scans with thin sections of the temporal bone should be obtained in axial and coronal orientations to delineate the extent of tumor. Evaluation of intracranial extension is best obtained by MRI, which provides information relevant to the neurovascular anatomy. The indications for preoperative embolization described above for carotid paragangliomas apply to jugular paragangliomas as well.

Staging. Staging systems for jugular paragangliomas developed by Oldring and Fisch[128] and by Glasscock and Jackson[128] are listed in Tables 113-1 and 113-2, respectively. The staging system advocated by Glasscock and Jackson divides into groups glomus tympanicum and glomus jugulare.

Management. A comprehensive review of the surgical tenets applicable to resection of jugular paragangliomas is beyond the scope of this text, but tantamount to the approach to these tumors is a multidisciplinary team effort among the head and neck surgeon, neurotologist, and neurosurgeon. The approach is tailored to the location and extent of the tumor, with preoperative discussion addressing potential temporary and permanent cranial neuropathies.

As described above in the section for carotid paragangliomas, radiation therapy has been advocated to arrest tumor growth in those patients who are not deemed appropriate surgical candidates either because of antecedent comorbidities or due to expected complications from postoperative cranial neuropathies. It should be reiterated, however, that although tumor growth arrest is the intended goal of radiation therapy as single modality treatment, the paraganglioma does not shrink in size, and the potential exists for tumor regrowth after radiation treatment.

Paragangliomas of other sites in the head and neck. Other sites of the head and neck where paragangliomas may arise include the orbital, sinonasal, laryngeal, and aroticopulmonary regions.[99] Paragangliomas of these sites are rare.

Peripheral Nerve Neoplasms

In addition to tumors of vascular origin, other primary tumors of the neck include those derived from peripheral nerves. Benign tumors of the head and neck arising from peripheral nerves include schwannomas and neurofibromas.

TABLE 113-1

FISCH CLASSIFICATION OF GLOMUS TUMORS OF THE TEMPORAL REGION

Type A - Tumors limited to the middle ear cleft
Type B - Tumors limited to the tympanomastoid area with no infralabyrinthine compartment involvement
Type C - Tumors involving the infralablyrinthine compartment of the temporal bone and extending to the petrous apex
Type D1 - Tumors with an intracranial extension less than 2 cm in diameter
Type D2 - Tumors with an intracranial extension larger than 2 cm in diameter

---

TABLE 113-2

GLASSCOCK-JACKSON CLASSIFICATION OF GLOMUS TUMORS

Glomus Tympanicum	Glomus Jugulare
Type I - Small mass limited to the promontory	Type I - Small tumor involving the jugular bulb, middle ear, and mastoid
Type II - Tumor completely filling the middle ear	Type II - Tumor extending under the internal auditory canal; may have intracranial extension
Type III - Tumor filling the middle ear and extending into the mastoid	Type III - Tumor extending into the petrous apex; may have intracranial extension
Type IV - Tumor filling the middle ear, extending into the mastoid or through the tympanic membrane to fill the external auditory canal; may extend anterior to the internal carotid artery	Type IV - Tumor extending beyond the petrous apex into the clivus or infratemporal fossa; may have intracranial extension

Schwannomas

Schwannomas, also called *neurilemmomas*, are typically well-encapsulated, slowly growing tumors that arise from Schwann cells of peripheral nerves. These tumors are typically solitary, but may be multiple, and as many as one half occur in the head and neck region.[35] Schwannomas may arise from cranial nerves, such as VIII (i.e., acoustic neuromas) or X; the sympathetic chain; cervical nerve roots; or the brachial plexus.

Clinically, schwannomas of the lateral neck may present as a painless neck mass. The clinical presentation of acoustic neuromas is covered elsewhere in this text. Radiologically, schwannomas typically present as well-circumscribed masses that enhance on contrast. Histologically, schwannomas demonstrate a characteristic cellular pattern of alternating regions containing compact spindle cells called *Antoni type A areas,* and more loosely arranged, hypocellular zones called *Antoni type B areas.* Rows of nuclear palisading may be observed, and such arrangements are referred to as *Verocay bodies.* The treatment of choice of schwannomas of the neck typically involves surgical resection. Malignant transformation of schwannomas is rare.

Neurofibromas

Neuofibromas are benign nerve sheath tumors that may present either as a solitary neck mass or as multiple tumor nodules in association with the autosomal dominant disorder von Recklinghausen's disease. In contrast to schwannomas, neurofibromas are unencapsulated and histologically demonstrate an interlacing bundle of spindle cells. Like schwannomas, solitary neurofibromas undergo malignant transformation uncommonly and are best treated by complete surgical resection. Neurofibromatosis associated with von Recklinghausen's disease is more difficult to treat, in light of the multiple number of infiltrative tumors that are not well defined. Surgery for neurofibromatosis is typically reserved for those lesions that are painful, those that may cause compressive symptoms from their large size, or lesions that are malignant. Malignant transformation of neurofibromatosis occurs more commonly than solitary neurofibromas.

Lipomas

Lipomas are benign tumors derived from adipose tissue. They are the most common soft tissue tumor of the neck and typically present as a soft, painless neck mass. Their histologic appearance is consistent with a lobular pattern of mature adipocytes. Lipomas are best treated by complete surgical resection for compressive or aesthetic reasons. The case can be made for observation of asymptomatic, small lipomas.

MALIGNANT PRIMARY NEOPLASMS OF THE NECK

Primary neoplasms of the neck are rare entities. Few studies have elucidated the true incidence of primary neoplasms of the neck because they are often described in case reports or small series or not reported at all. Thus, our knowledge and data are based on these limited publications and reports on non–head-and-neck–related soft tissue tumors. In the larger series of reports of these tumors of the entire head and neck region, only approximately four to 20 cases are listed per year.[54,82] The following discussion will provide the reader with an overview of the differential diagnosis, evaluation, and management of malignant tumors of the neck.

As malignant primary neoplasms of the neck are rare, it is imperative that consideration be given to the most common neoplasms that are often misdiagnosed before definite biopsy and treatment. Thus, before addressing the "primary" tumors in this region, a brief discussion will include the unknown primary, metastatic lesions from the region and distant sites to provide the physician with the necessary foundation from which he or she can then address primary malignancies of this complicated area.

Metastatic Lesions to the Neck
Unknown Primary

The unknown primary metastatic lesion is considered a squamous cell carcinoma identified in the lymphatic structures of the neck that has not originated from a known primary site. This tumor is usually identified by a mass in the neck and is expected to be diagnosed by a fine-needle aspiration biopsy. Typically, this diagnosis reminds the physician to repeat a more thorough head and neck examination to include the entire upper aerodigestive tract, the most common site of these primary lesions.[145] When a patient undergoes excisional biopsy of a cervical lymph node, frozen-section analysis revealing squamous cell carcinoma should lead the surgeon to consider simultaneous neck dissection. There is evidence that survival is lower in patients that have radiation after an excisional biopsy than in those radiated after neck dissection.[144]

The location of the neck mass signals a clue regarding the primary site due to the well-known lymphatic drainage routes in the head and neck region and the updated classification system of neck lymph node levels (see Figure 113-4). When the mass presents in the supraclavicular region, esophageal and pulmonary primary sites should be considered in addition to abdominal and pelvic locations.[40]

Usually, the primary site is identified during this examination or during operative endoscopy, at which time biopsies confirm the location and histology of the primary site. When the primary site cannot be identified, imaging techniques including CT, MRI, PET scanning, or a combination of these have been used with varying degrees of success.[36,66,86]

The treatment of unknown primary cancers of the neck remains controversial but consideration should be given to neck dissection and radiation therapy to bilateral necks and the mucosa of the aerodigestive tract. This is discussed in more detail in other chapters and sections of this text.

Regional

Aside from the unknown primary metastatic lesion and the far more common squamous cell carcinomas of the aerodigestive tract, it is important to not overlook the possibility of metastatic disease from other sites in the head and neck region. Common primary sites of metastatic disease include the skin of the ear, face, scalp, and neck that often can present with an enlarged lymph node in the parotid, cheek, submandibular, or cervical region. The major and minor salivary glands may present with a primary neoplasm that initially appears to be a metastatic lesion to the neck manifesting as a level 1 or 2 neck mass. The surprising diagnosis of adenocarcinoma can lead one to an exhausting search for a primary site in the lower digestive tract only to surmise eventually that this is a primary salivary gland tumor. Another common primary site that may be diagnosed first as a primary neck neoplasm is the thyroid gland, which not uncommonly initially presents as a neck mass.[29]

Distant

Any neck mass determined to be malignant should also be considered as originating at a distant site. Although hundreds of neoplasms have been described to metastasize to the neck, the more common distant sites include pulmonary, esophageal, renal, ovarian, cervical, and prostatic regions.[14]

Primary Malignant Tumors of the Neck

The following discussion will include those rare malignancies that arise in the neck region without known primary sites and are considered to be isolated primary malignancies. The following neoplasms are not all inclusive but include those that most practitioners should consider in the differential diagnosis of a malignant mass in this region.

Malignant Paragangliomas

Obviously, any neck mass should be palpated and auscultated if necessary to ensure that it is not attached to or arising from a vascular structure. Most paragangliomas do not require tissue for accurate diagnosis, as described in the earlier section. The potential for

malignancy of paraganglioma correlates with the site of origin, 2% to 19% of these neoplasms have been reported to be malignant, with glomus jugulare tumors at the low end and vagal tumors at the high end of these percentages. Approximately 6% of carotid body tumors are malignant, although histologic analysis is considered insufficient to determine malignancy.[102] Rather, this is a diagnosis that is predicated on tumor behavior such as lymph node or distant metastases.[118,129,137]

Parapharyngeal Space Neoplasms

Numerous histologic types of primary malignancies of the parapharyngeal space have been reported, including malignant salivary gland tumors (adenoid cystic carcinoma, carcinoma ex-pleomorphic adenoma, acinic cell carcinoma), malignant neurogenic tumors, lymphoma, liposarcoma, fibrosarcoma, malignant meningioma, and others.[25,76,129,133,137]

Sarcomas. The neck and parotid have been described as the most common head and neck site involved by sarcomas, although they represent fewer than 1% of all head and neck malignancies.[180] In the United States, fewer than 5000 cases are reported annually, with approximately 80% diagnosed in adults. Of these, only 15% to 20% are identified in the head and neck region, with soft tissues of the neck and paranasal sinus region the most common sites identified. Although the etiology has not been determined, these neoplasms arise from mesenchymal cells, which may include endothelial cells, muscle, cartilage, and supporting connective tissue. More than 80% of sarcomas are derived from soft tissue, whereas approximately 20% arise within bone.

When all anatomic sites are considered, the most common histologic type is malignant fibrous histiocytoma (MFH). In the head and neck, the most common sarcoma in children is rhabdomyosarcoma (RMS); in adults, osteosarcoma, angiosarcoma, MFH, and fibrosarcoma are most common.

RMS is the most common sarcoma in children and is also the most common sarcoma of the head and neck region. Overall, however, MFH is considered the most common type of sarcoma.

Classification and staging. Sarcomas have generally been classified and named according to the tissue of origin rather than "site" of origin. Many "soft tissue" sarcomas such as MFH can be diagnosed within bone, but the diagnosis depends on the histologic material for confirmation. The staging system is now separated by bone and soft tissue sites for origin of the sarcoma. The listing of types of soft tissue sarcomas is provided in Table 113-3A, and the AJCC staging is shown in Table 113–3B for the soft tissue histologies.

The listing of bone histologies and AJCC staging can be found in Tables 113-4A and 113-4B.

The American Joint Commission for Cancer (AJCC) staging system for soft tissue sarcoma is shown in Table 113-3, although other staging systems have been described particularly for some of the various types of tumors. In addition, fibrosarcoma grade I (fibromatosis or desmoid tumor) and dermatofibrosarcoma are not listed under sarcoma staging. Other changes effective in 2003 included the addition of subdivisions of tumor (T) category into superficial (T_a) and deep (T_b) lesions. In general, the tumor should be described pathologically by grade as G_1-G_4 with tumor size as smaller than 5 cm (T_1) or larger than 5 cm (T_2). The types of soft tissue sarcomas included in the AJCC staging system include those listed in Table 113-4.

The AJCC staging system for bone sarcoma is shown in Table 113-5, although other staging systems

---

TABLE 113-4

ALVEOLAR SOFT PART SARCOMA

Angiosarcoma
Epithelioid sarcoma
Extraskeletal chondrosarcoma
Extraskeletal osteosarcoma
Fibrosarcoma
Leiomyosarcoma
Liposarcoma
Malignant fibrous histiocytoma
Malignant hemangiopericytoma
Malignant mesenchymoma
Malignant schwannoma
Rhabdomyosarcoma
Synovial sarcoma

TABLE 113-3

AMERICAN JOINT COMMITTEE ON CANCER (AJCC) STAGING SYSTEM FOR SOFT TISSUE SARCOMAS (2003)

Stage	Definition
Primary tumor	
T_x	Primary tumor cannot be assessed
T_0	No evidence of primary tumor
T_1	Tumor <5 cm in greatest dimension (T_{1a}, superficial; T_{1b}, deep)
T_2	Tumor >5 cm in greatest dimension (T_{2a}, superficial; T_{2b}, deep)
Regional lymph nodes	
N_x	Lymph nodes cannot be assessed
N_0	No regional lymph nodes metastasis
N_1*	Regional lymph nodes metastasis
Distant metastases	
M_x	Distant metastasis cannot be assessed
M_0	No distant metastasis
M_1	Distant metastasis present
Histopathologic grade	
G_x	Grade cannot be assessed
G_1	Well differentiated
G_2	Moderately differentiated
G_3	Poorly differentiated
G_4	Poorly differentiated or undifferentiated
Combined	
IA - G_{1-2}, T_{1a-b}, N_0, M_0	Low-grade, small, and superficial or deep tumor
IB - G_{1-2}, T_{2a}, N_0, M_0	Low-grade, large, and superficial tumor
IIA - G_{1-2}, T_{2b}, N_0, M_0	Low-grade, large, and deep tumor
IIB - G_{3-4}, T_{1a-b}, N_0, M_0	High-grade, small, and superficial or deep tumor
IIC - G_{3-4}, T_{2a}, N_0, M_0	High-grade, large, and superficial tumor
III - G_{3-4}, T_{2b}, N_0, M_0	High-grade, large, and deep tumor
IV - any G, any T, N_1, M_0	Any metastasis

TABLE 113-5

AMERICAN JOINT COMMITTEE ON CANCER (AJCC) STAGING SYSTEM FOR BONE SARCOMAS (2003)

Stage	Definition
Primary tumor	
T_x	Primary tumor cannot be assessed
T_0	No evidence of primary tumor
T_1	Tumor confined within the cortex
T_2	Tumor invades beyond the cortex
Regional lymph nodes	
N_x	Lymph nodes cannot be assessed
N_0	No regional lymph nodes metastasis
N_1	Regional lymph nodes metastasis
Distant metastases	
M_x	Distant metastasis cannot be assessed
M_0	No distant metastasis
M_1	Distant metastasis present
Histopathologic grade	
G_x	Grade cannot be assessed
G_1	Well differentiated (low grade)
G_2	Moderately differentiated (low grade)
G_3	Poorly differentiated (high grade)
G_4*	Poorly differentiated or undifferentiated (high grade)

*Ewing's sarcoma, considered G_4.

have been described particularly for some of the various types of tumors. In addition, malignant lymphoma, leukemia, and multiple myeloma are not listed in the bone sarcoma staging system. Unlike the soft tissue sarcomas, the bone sites do not include subdivisions by depth of tumor as superficial or deep. Instead, T_1 tumors are confined to within the cortex, and T_2 tumors invade beyond the cortex. The tumors that can be classified and staged within this category are listed in Table 113-6.

Treatment. The treatment of sarcomas involving the head and neck region involves a multidisciplinary approach, evaluation, and planning in order to provide the optimal chance of cure and rehabilitation. The treatment should always include consultation with a head and neck surgeon, medical oncologist,

TABLE 113-6

BONE SARCOMAS

Osteosarcoma
Chondrosarcoma
Mesenchymal chondrosarcoma
Malignant giant cell tumor
Ewing's sarcoma

and radiation oncologist in close cooperation with a head and neck pathologist and neuroradiologist familiar with these neoplasms. Other specialists often involved in the care of these patients include dental oncologists, maxillofacial prosthodontist, and speech and swallowing therapist in addition to rehabilitation specialists. The histology, evaluation, and treatment of each histologic type of sarcoma and site of origin will vary, and thus, will be discussed according to the cell of origin.

Types of sarcomas

Alveolar soft part sarcoma. Alveolar soft part sarcoma is a rare tumor that is stated to involve the head and neck region in approximately 25% of cases, although it represents fewer than 1% of all sarcomas. The cell of origin has not been elucidated, although muscular and neural differentiation have been identified. The common sites affected in the head and neck include the tongue and the orbit, with the orbit having the best prognosis. Alveolar soft part sarcoma rarely involves the neck and is reported to metastasize to the neck from head and neck primary sites in fewer than 10% of cases, making elective neck dissection unwarranted. Distant metastatic disease does occur and may not present for years or decades after the primary site was treated. Surgery remains the mainstay of treatment, although local recurrence is common. More recent reports have shown success with multimodality treatment including chemotherapy. Overall survival is approximately 65% at 5 years but drops to 50% at 10 years.*

Angiosarcoma. Angiosarcoma is another rare sarcoma representing fewer than 1% of all sarcomas, although up to half involve the head and neck. There remains consideration that this disease involves both vascular and lymphatic vessels, hence the differentiation from lymphangiosarcoma. The etiology remains unclear although trauma, radiation, and lymphedema have been associated with some cases.

Treatment is primarily surgical, although wide margins are necessary due to the multicentric nature of these tumors and local recurrence rate nearing 50%. Postoperative radiation therapy is also generally recommended, although there is limited experience using chemotherapy in these neoplasms. Metastatic disease commonly occurs in the lung and liver, whereas regional metastatic disease is common in lesions of the scalp. Elective neck dissection is recommended for clinically and radiographically evident disease or primary lesion involving the scalp. The 5-year survival rate remains low, with most reporting less than 25%.†

---

*References 12, 15, 77, 131, 140, 163, 167.
†References 22, 28, 42, 48, 51, 55, 64, 73, 106, 110, 122, 134.

Epithelioid hemangioendothelioma. This tumor is extremely rare and is described to involve the head and neck region in only approximately 10% to 15% of the cases. These lesions are found to be derived from a epitheliod or histiocytoid type of endothelial cell.[185] It does manifest in a wide spectrum of biologic behavior ranging from a benign form to an extremely aggressive form of the disease, although all are vascular in nature. There has recently been described a more "benign" variant without distant metastases.[19] Another form has been described as spindle cell hemangioendothelioma but is now thought to be a benign process; it was suggested that this variant be referred to as *spindle cell hemangioma for solitary lesions.*[138] Those variants that are more aggressive and similar to angiosarcoma most often arise in the thyroid, submandibular, and neck soft tissues, although mucosal and skin sites have been described including the paranasal sinuses, larynx, and temporal bone.* Treatment typically has included surgical excision with possible radiation therapy. Recurrence and metastatic potential correlates with biologic aggressiveness with the more epithelioid lesions having a better prognosis, whereas the sarcomatous lesions have a higher metastatic potential and a poorer prognosis.[116,183]

Chondrosarcoma. Although chondrosarcoma is typically found in the maxillary and mandibular region of the head and neck, presentation in the neck or origin in soft tissues can occur.[60,92] Histologically, evidence of cartilage formation exists with varying degrees of differentiation and grade. These tumors are typically classified as osseous or extraosseous and may be subtyped into conventional, myxoid, and mesenchymal with mesenchymal being much more common in children and young adults. Prognosis does seem to be related to the subtype, with myxoid having the worst prognosis followed by mesenchymal and conventional. There has been some controversy surrounding the histologic separation of osteoblastic chondrosarcoma from osteosarcoma. According to the National Cancer Database (NCDB) report, the average age of patients with chondrosarcoma of the head and neck is 51 years, although over 32% were younger than age 40. There is a slight male predominance, and ethnicity reveals that non-Hispanic white persons constitute over 86% of cases. There appears to be only a small percentage with regional or distant metastases at diagnosis with 5.6% and 6.7%, respectively, in the NCDB report.[92] Treatment includes wide surgical resection, although consideration of postoperative radiation may be entertained, particularly in high-grade tumors. Survival rates in the NCDB report

reveal a surprisingly high survival of patients with head and neck chondrosarcomas at 87.2% 5-year and 70.6% 10-year survival with 59.5% undergoing surgery alone, while 21.0% had adjuvant radiation therapy.

Osteosarcoma. Osteosarcoma of the head and neck primarily involves the mandible and maxilla, with the mandible having a slightly higher incidence. The tumor rarely involves the soft tissues of the neck, although isolated regional metastases have been reported in addition to several reports involving the hyoid and larynx.[2,34,139] The treatment of these lesions has primarily included surgical resection with or without radiation therapy and chemotherapy. The incidence of cervical metastases is reported to be less than 10%, making routine neck dissection unwarranted.[11] The poor prognosis of soft tissue osteosarcomas of the larynx may encourage multimodality treatment for these sites in the future.

Fibrosarcoma. The neck is the second most common site of presentation of head and neck fibrosarcoma, after the paranasal sinus region. Although it can occur at any age, it is more common in adults between 40 and 70 years of age, although there exists a subset of children diagnosed before the age of 2 years. This neoplasm originates from the fibroblast and usually arises spontaneously but is known to arise in areas of prior burn scars and radiation therapy.[65,107] Histologically, they are identified by a malignant fibroblastic proliferation with variable amounts of collagen and reticulin forming a "herringbone" pattern. These lesions have a broad differential diagnosis, and the well-differentiated types are commonly confused with fibromatosis and other benign processes. They typically present in the neck as a painless enlarging firm mass and have a low rate of lymphatic metastasis, thus making routine neck dissection unwarranted. There tends to be a high local recurrence rate up to 50% despite radical surgical excision with a survival rate of 50% to 75% and possibly higher in young children.[32,58,65,111,158] Adjuvant treatment should be based on the size of the tumor, tumor grade, and status of surgical margins.[111] A review of the literature on these tumors should be undertaken with caution due to changes in histochemical diagnosis that may alter the inclusion of certain tumors previously classified as fibrosarcoma in earlier series.

Leiomyosarcoma. Leiomyosarcoma is a neoplasm that generally affects older adults, although it can occur at any age. It represents 6% of all sarcomas, and 3% involve the head and neck region where the oral cavity followed by the sinonasal region and then subcutaneous areas are the most common sites.[9] Although the scalp and face are the most common site of occurrence of the subcutaneous lesions, there are

---

*References 62, 75, 155, 171, 186, 189.

reports involving the superficial and deep tissues of the cervical region.[39,159,165] The neoplasm develops from smooth muscle origin and histologically has a typical appearance of fascicles arranged in a perpendicular fashion with the cigar-shaped nuclei, eosinophilic cytoplasm, and paranuclear vacuoles. Most also expressed muscle-specific actin, smooth muscle actin, and desmin.[121] These can be differentiated from fibrosarcomas by their "cigar-shaped" nuclei rather than the "pointy" nuclei of fibrosarcomas. The most common presentation is a nodular dark blue or black lesion involving the dermis and epidermis that may be tender to palpation. Those that arise in the subcutaneous tissues have a higher local recurrence, metastatic rate, and worse prognosis.[154] Of those originating in the oral cavity, there was a high rate of local recurrence in addition to metastatic disease to the cervical nodes, lungs, and subcutaneous tissues.[9] Deep neck masses should also be considered in the differential, even without skin involvement. The treatment includes wide resection with negative margins. Neck dissection may be indicated due to the potential for regional and distant metastases.[80,119] The prognosis varies greatly with site of origin and histologic variations, thus making the accurate estimation of survival of each site difficult.

Liposarcoma. Although considered the most common soft tissue sarcoma of adults, constituting 12% to 18% of cases, involvement in the head and neck region is rare, occurring in an estimated 3% to 6%.[114] Although a relationship to previous lipoma and traumatic events has been considered, there is not yet enough evidence to confirm the relationship to the development of liposarcoma. In a review of head and neck liposarcomas, Barnes[9] identified the larynx and hypopharynx to be the most common site followed closely by the neck, although others report the neck to be more commonly involved.[63] The prognosis appears to be dependent on site and classification with the well-differentiated and myxoid having a better prognosis (75%–100%) than the round cell and pleomorphic varieties (12%–30%).[9,63,114,132] The liposarcoma is considered to occur more often in deeper soft tissue locations than the lipoma or atypical lipoma; cervical metastases are rare, and distant metastases have been reported primarily to the lung and liver.

Atypical lipoma. Although histologically and behaviorly benign, the atypical lipoma or pleomorphic lipoma may be misdiagnosed as liposarcoma because of the histologic similarity. These are typically more superficial, and radical treatment is not necessary if wide surgical margins are obtained. Similarly, the spindle cell lipoma has also been described and behaves in a similar fashion to the atypical lipoma.

Both of these processes are more common in men during adulthood.[49]

Malignant fibrous histiocytoma. Most consider MFH the most common soft tissue sarcoma in adults. It rarely involves the head and neck region, although the sites described include the soft tissues of the paranasal sinuses, neck, skull base, and parotid gland. Of 88 fibrous histiocytomas (benign and malignant) of the head and neck analyzed, the neck was the second most common site after the sinonasal region.[52] Etiologic factors include prior radiation therapy and historical use of silica as injection material. The cell of origin has received much discussion, although consideration of fibroblastic or primitive mesenchymal cell has emerged as the leading theories.[52,187] Microscopically, these tumors tend to reveal histiocytes, fibroblasts, giant cells, spindle cells, and collagen with the storiform-pleomorphic form the most common. MFH is considered a high grade sarcoma and is classified into numerous subtypes providing for a separation from the standard staging for sarcomas. There is evidence that the survival and course of the disease is related to the size and depth of these tumors.[184] The treatment is surgical with wide margins, and elective treatment of the neck is not indicated due to the low incidence of cervical metastases, although there is some evidence to suggest that oral cavity MFH has a higher metastatic potential for regional lymph nodes.[10,21] Local recurrence rates approach 30% with overall lymph node metastases near 10% and distant metastases approximately 35% with most metastases occurring within the first 2 years.[10,184] Recurrence seems to result in a lower surgical salvage rate for head and neck MFH than in extremities, and overall survival also is poorer for head and neck sites.[188] Survival approaches 75% for patients without local recurrence after surgery and drops to 38% with local recurrence for an overall 5-year survival of approximately 51%.[188]

Malignant hemangiopericytoma. Hemangiopericytoma arises from the cells of Zimmerman, which occur around capillaries and postcapillary venules. The majority of hemangiopericytomas of the head and neck are found in the paranasal sinuses, although due to the cell of origin, nearly any tissue could be involved, including the neck.[38,156,178] The tumor primarily affects adults, although there is a subset of children (usually younger than 5 years) that can be affected. The treatment is surgical because hemangiopericytomas have been shown to be relatively radioresistant, and the highly vascular nature of these tumors may require preoperative embolization. Adjuvant radiation therapy has been recommended for those with high-grade features or positive margins. Neck dissection is not necessary because lymphatic spread is rare, although there are varying reports of distant metastases that seem to correlate with histologic pattern, mitotic figures, and proliferation indices.[18,23,95] The 5-year survival rate is near 70%, and distant metastases usually portend recurrence at the primary site.

Malignant peripheral nerve sheath tumor. The term *malignant peripheral nerve sheath tumor* (MPNST) refers to a type of neurosarcoma that represents nearly 10% of all sarcomas, behaves in an aggressive fashion, and carries a poor prognosis. The tumor appears to have varying distribution by gender and is typically a disease of adults.[44,175] The tumor typically arises in the neck in up to half of the head and neck cases, although the sinonasal region, parapharyngeal space, parotid, and thyroid have been involved. These tumors are generally considered to occur in two settings: de novo, and within the setting of a neurofibroma, particularly neurofibromatosis 1 (NF-1). Those arising in the latter typically occur at a younger age (fourth decade of life) and have a worse prognosis.[26,88,105] It is stated that for patients diagnosed with NF-1, the risk of developing a MPNST is 2%.[88]

The typical presentation is of a progressive swelling, and many present with pain in the region. Those with a history of NF-1 may describe a long history of a mass with a recent rapid enlargement. Associated neurogenic symptoms of weakness or paresthesias may be associated. Microscopically, they typically reveal atypical spindle cells similar to Schwann cells that are closely associated with a peripheral nerve. There remains significant controversy and variability in the histopathologic diagnostic criteria. The treatment includes wide resection with clear margins and postoperative radiation with margin status and tumor size correlating with survival.[4,74,105] The prognosis is poor despite aggressive treatment, with over 40% developing local recurrence, although the presence of lymphatic metastases is rare.[4,67,166,175]

Malignant mesenchymoma. Malignant mesenchymoma is an extremely rare tumor with only a handful of cases reported involving the head and neck with sites ranging from the skin of the face to the orbit, mandible, maxilla, and larynx.* These tumors are considered high-grade sarcomas that have a variable histologic pattern, and Barnes suggests that they be diagnosed with the additional comment to include, "rhabdomyosarcoma with chondrosarcoma."[9,126]

Rhabdomyosarcoma. RMS is a malignancy that is derived from mesenchymal cells associated with skeletal muscle differentiation. It represents the most

common soft tissue sarcoma in children and also accounts for 20% of all sarcomas. Over 45% of rhabdomyosarcomas arise in the head and neck region, with the highest incidence in the first decade and another peak occurring in the second and third decade. The most common sites in the head and neck from a recent series of 50 cases include the face, orbit, nasal cavity, neck, paranasal sinuses, and parameningeal sites.[72] Metastatic disease was present in 33% of cases, with the most common sites being bone marrow, cerebrospinal fluid, peritoneal fluid, and lung.[72] Other reports reveal the neck soft tissue to be involved in almost 14% of adult head and neck RMS.[9]

These tumors are categorized by the Intergroup Rhabdomyosarcoma Study (IRS) into the following subtypes, embryonal, embryonal-botryoid variant, embryonal-spindle cell variant, alveolar-classic, and solid variants, undifferentiated and anaplastic. These are also commonly classified as embryonal, alveolar, pleomorphic, and mixed types. The embryonal represents the most common RMS in both children and adults and microscopically reveals small spindle cells with a central nucleus, although round cells often resembling lymphocytes may be seen. The botryoid variant grows in a polypoid, grape-like fashion and differs microscopically from the classic embryonal by a subepithelial condensation of tumor cells. The alveolar type occurs primarily in the teenage and young adult population and is identified histologically by an alveolar pattern of loosely arranged cells with hyperchromatic nuclei. The pleomorphic type represents approximately 17% of the adult RMS and fewer than 5% of pediatric cases. These lesions are found to have large, pleomorphic cells with eosinophilic cytoplasm. Immunohistochemistry has provided valuable diagnostic techniques to the histologic diagnosis of these lesions with antidesmin staining in 94%, 77% positive for desmin, 78% positive for muscle specific actin, and 30% for myoglobin.[136]

The treatment of RMS has continued to improve since the development of the IRS and now often involves combined modality treatment to include surgery, chemotherapy, and radiation therapy. Therapy has been based on the site categories that the IRS delineated as: (1) orbit; (2) parameningeal; and (3) other head and neck. Primary treatment often includes induction chemotherapy followed by radiation therapy, although concomitant therapy can be used. Surgery is typically reserved for debulking or for tumors that can be resected entirely without functional or cosmetic deformity. Neck dissection is warranted in cases of obvious neck involvement or in clinically enlarged adenopathy. The survival rates for each of these sites were 92%, 69%, and 81%, respectively.[33,112,113,148] IRS III and IV analysis does

---

*References 17, 20, 90, 103, 153, 169.

show an overall 83% 5-year survival and a better prognosis in N_0 patients than those with N_1 disease.[135] Prognosis correlates with patient age, site of disease, histological type, size of tumor, and metastases with botryoid and spindle associated with a better prognosis than embryonal, which is better than alveolar and pleomorphic.[127] Long-term follow-up has identified significant morbidity related to these treatments and long-term functional outcomes should be considered in addition to locoregional control and survival.[142] Lymphatic metastases are found to occur in 3% to 20% of RMS, although hematogenous spread may also occur.[100,161] Staging of RMS is commonly based on the IRS, which incorporates the extent of disease with metastases and surgical results. It was also recommended by the IRS that staging systems for this disease require continuous evaluation due to the loss of the prognostic correlation in early-stage tumors[101,136] (Table 113-7).

TABLE 113-7

RMS INTERGROUP STAGING SYSTEM

TNM PRETREATMENT STAGING SYSTEM (IRSG)

Stage	Sites	T	Tumor Alae	N	M
I	Orbit Head and neck (excluding parameningeal) GU-Nonbladder/Nonprostate	T_1 or T_2	a or b	N_0 or N_1 or N_2	M_0
II	Bladder/Prostate Extremly Head and neck parameningeal Other (including trunk, retroperitoneum, etc.)	T_1 or T_2	a	N_0 or N_X	M_0
III	Bladder/Prostate Extremly Head and neck parameningeal Other (including trunk, retroperitoneum, etc.)	T_1 or T_2	a b	N_1 N_0 or N_1 or N_X	M_0
IV	All	T_1 or T_2	a or b	N_0 or N_1	M_1

DEFINITIONS OF T, N, AND M CLASSIFICATIONS IN PRETREATMENT STAGING

Classification	Description
Tumor	
T_1	Confined to anatomic size of origin
a	<5 cm in diameter
b	≥5 cm in diameter
T_2	Extension and/or fixation to surrounding tissue
a	<5 cm in diameter
b	≥5 cm in diameter
Regional lymph nodes	
N_0	Regional lymph nodes not clinically involved
N_1	Regional lymph nodes clinically involved by neoplasm
N_1	Clinical status of regional lymph nodes unknown (especially with sites that preclude lymph node evaluation)
Metastasis	
M_0	No distant metastasis
M_1	Metastasis present

IBSG, Intergroup Rhabdomyosarcoma Study Group; GU, genitourinary.

TABLE 113-7		

RMS Intergroup Staging System—cont'd

Survival of IRS-II and IRS-III Patients by IRSG Pretreatment Stage

| | Estimated 5-year survival | |
Pretreatment Stage	IRS-II	IRS-III
I	91%	09%
II	73%	06%
III	52%	69%
IV	23%	30%

IRS, Intergroup Rhabdomyosarcoma Study.

Synovial sarcoma. Synovial sarcoma composes 6% to 10% of all soft tissue sarcomas and 3% to 10% of all head and neck sarcomas. This neoplasm has been described to arise in the periarticular regions of the body, although the sites of the head and neck are not usually in these areas. This tumor typically arises in people aged 20 to 40 years, with the hypopharyngeal and retropharyngeal regions the most likely site of the head and neck. It is thought to be derived from a pluripotential mesenchymal cell with both epithelioid and spindle differentiation. Microscopically, the tumor is found to have a predominant spindle cell component with cuboidal and columnar cells surrounding glandular areas and may have calcifications in up to 30% of cases.[70,152] Prognosis appears related to tumor size, mitotic indices, high grade, local recurrence, and tumor necrosis, although the absence of calcifications and ploidy may also be related.[47,70]

The symptoms on presentation are usually related to mass effect, although a painful mass may be identified. The treatment requires wide surgical resection; however, chemotherapy may also be potentially beneficial when used preoperatively according to recent reports.[47,87] Neck dissection is not necessary due to the absence of cervical metastases. The 5-year survival is 47% to 58% with up to 40% incidence of local recurrence.[9,152,162]

Malignant giant cell tumor. The malignant giant cell tumor (MGCT) of the head and neck region is extremely rare and may be considered to be radiation induced after patients are treated for a benign GCT. MGCTs account for fewer than 10% of all GCTs. The sinonasal region and the mandible are the most common sites where these occur in the head and neck.[120,141] The secondary MGCT appears to be more common than primary MGCT, which arises de novo without prior evidence of a benign GCT. The overall 5-year survival rate of secondary MGCT was reported as 32%.[147] Metastatic lesions of GCT are usually identified in the lungs.[146]

Ewing's sarcoma. Ewing's sarcoma represents a malignancy derived from primitive neuroectoderm and is the second most common bone tumor in children. Of 70 cases described at a single institution, only five (7.1%) occurred in the head and neck region.[172] They are separated into osseous and extraosseous types with approximately 75% occurring in the first two decades of life. Primitive neuroectodermal tumor is a diagnosis that has many overlapping features with extraosseous Ewing's sarcoma and may be related.[9] Primitive neuroectodermal tumor occurs in the paraspinous regions in approximately 50% of cases. The most common head and neck sites for these tumors includes the mandible, maxilla, skull, and sinonasal region, although soft tissue sites have been described.[85] The incidence of lymphatic spread to the cervical nodes is uncommon. Treatment involves multimodality therapy, including chemotherapy, while surgery may be necessary for complete control of the primary site and for reconstructive considerations. Radiation may be beneficial in combination with these other modalities.

Desmoplastic small round cell neoplasm. The desmoplastic round cell tumor is an extremely rare tumor that typically presents in the abdomen, although reports in the head and neck exist.[117] The tumor appears to be highly aggressive and may be chemosensitive, although overall survival has been poor. Recent reports suggest that combined modality including surgery, radiation, and chemotherapy may be necessary to improve prognosis.[104]

Other solitary fibrous tumor. There exists a wide range of benign and malignant fibrous tumors with varying degrees of local, regional, and metastatic growth potential. The one that deserves mention due to the frequency in the head and neck, particularly in children, is desmoid fibromatosis. These tumors have a wide range of behavior and a very low mortality rate.

Treatment includes wide resection due to the high local recurrence rate of 21% to 47%.[8,31,37]

Lymphoma. Lymphoma deserves mention due to the common presentation in enlarged cervical lymph nodes but will be presented in detail in Chapter 114.

Melanoma. Although melanoma has been identified to arise or metastasize to the neck without a known primary site, a thorough evaluation should be undertaken to identify the primary site. A review of 300 cases of melanoma by Balm and others[6] revealed 17 (5.7%) presented with a cervical lymph node without a known primary site. The treatment included surgery and the 5-year disease-specific survival was 48%, with a median of 36 months (which correlated with other patients with a stage II cutaneous melanoma).[6]

In a large series of head and neck melanoma, elective neck dissection and therapeutic neck dissection did not appear to improve survival over patients undergoing delayed neck dissection for regional metastases developing more than 3 months after primary treatment. There was, however, a high incidence of distant metastatic disease in patients that did develop regional metastatic disease.[56]

Squamous cell carcinoma arising in a branchial cleft cyst. Although rare, squamous cell carcinomas have been documented to arise within branchial cleft cysts of the neck. Cytopathologic diagnosis is difficult, but it should be considered in the differential diagnosis of a cystic neck mass. Final confirmation of the diagnosis should follow the criteria proposed in differentiating these tumors from cystic squamous cell carcinoma of cervical lymph nodes.[164]

Carcinoma arising within a thyroglossal duct cyst. This extremely rare occurrence has been described, providing evidence for cytologic examination of thyroglossal duct cysts in suspicious cases.[41,68,96,143]

Although it is understood that many soft tissue tumors can metastasize or originate in the neck region, the most common remains squamous cell carcinoma of the head and neck aerodigestive tract. A broad differential is required when evaluating the neck mass, particularly in children, making a systematic approach essential to the diagnosis. Due to the limited number of prospective and retrospective studies of nonsquamous malignancies involving the neck, it is essential that the clinician remain updated on the optimal treatment and incorporate a multidisciplinary approach to these tumors.

SUMMARY

Primary neoplasms of the neck are rare but must be considered in the differential diagnosis of any neck mass to allow for optimal evaluation and management. The well-known diagnostic algorithm should be followed for any neck mass, and when suspicious cells are identified on fine-needle aspiration biopsy or unusual findings are found on radiologic studies, a primary tumor of the neck region should be considered. The ultimate diagnosis often requires surgical resection, which may entail simultaneous wide resection with confirmed clear margins and neck dissection to afford the patient the best chance for cure. A review of the existing literature for rare tumors including sarcomas and consideration of clinical trials will allow for long-term improvement in locoregional response and survival.

The authors wish to extend their appreciation to Mrs. Ann Durgun and Dr. Jennifer Schnellman for their expertise and assistance in the preparation of this manuscript.

REFERENCES

1. Anand VK, Alemar GO, Sanders TS: Management of the internal carotid artery during carotid body tumor surgery, *Laryngoscope* 105(3 Pt 1):231–235, 1995.
2. Anderson TD, Kearney JJ: Osteosarcoma of the hyoid bone, *Otolaryngol Head Neck Surg* 126:81–82, 2002.
3. Arias-Stella J, Bustos F: Chronic hypoxia and chemodectomas in bovines at high altitudes, *Arch Pathol Lab Med* 100:636–639, 1976.
4. Bailet JW and others: Malignant nerve sheath tumors of the head and neck: a combined experience from two university hospitals, *Laryngoscope* 101:1044–1049, 1991.
5. Ballard J, Smith L: *Carotid body paragangliomas: diagnosis, prognosis, and surgical management.* In Moore WS, editor: *Surgery for cerebrovascular disease.* Philadelphia, 1996, WB Saunders, pp 432–439.
6. Balm AJ and others: Lymph node metastases in the neck and parotid gland from an unknown primary melanoma, *Clin Otolaryngol* 19:161–165, 1994.
7. Barnes L: Paraganglioma of the larynx: a critical review of the literature, *ORL J Otorhinolaryngol Relat Spec* 53:220–234, 1991.
8. Barnes L: *Tumors and tumorlike lesions of the soft tissues.* In Barnes L, editor: *Surgical pathology of the head and neck.* New York, 1985, Marcel Dekker.
9. Barnes L: *Tumors and tumor-like lesions of the soft tissues.* In Barnes L, editor: *Surgical pathology of the head and neck.* New York, 2001, Marcel Dekker, pp 889–1048.
10. Barnes L, Kanbour A: Malignant fibrous histiocytoma of the head and neck: a report of 12 cases, *Arch Otolaryngol Head Neck Surg* 114:1149–1156, 1988.
11. Barnes L and others: *Diseases of the bones and joints.* In Barnes L, editor: *Surgical pathology of the head and neck.* New York, 2001, Marcel Dekker, pp 1049–1232.
12. Batsakis JG: Alveolar soft-part sarcoma, *Ann Otol Rhinol Laryngol* 97(3 Pt 1):328–329, 1988.
13. Batsakis JG: *Paragangliomas of the head and neck.* Baltimore, Williams and Wilkins, 1979, pp 369–380.

14. Batsakis JG, McBurney TA: Metastatic neoplasms to the head and neck, *Surg Gynecol Obstet* 133:673–677, 1971.

15. Batsakis JG, Regezi JA, Rice DH: The pathology of head and neck tumors: fibroadipose tissue and skeletal muscle, Part 8, *Head Neck Surg* 3:145–168, 1980.

16. Bestler JM, Toomey JM: Malignant carotid body tumor: report of a case, *Arch Otolaryngol* 89:752–755, 1969.

17. Beuerlein ME, Schuller DE, DeYoung BR: Maxillary malignant mesenchymoma and massive fibrous dysplasia, *Arch Otolaryngol Head Neck Surg* 123:106–109, 1997.

18. Billings KR and others: Hemangiopericytoma of the head and neck, *Am J Otolaryngol*, 21:238–243, 2000.

19. Billings SD, Folpe AL, Weiss SW: Epithelioid sarcoma-like hemangioendothelioma, *Am J Surg Pathol* 27:48–57, 2003.

20. Brannan PA and others: Malignant mesenchymoma of the orbit: case report and review of the literature, *Ophthalmology* 110:314–317, 2003.

21. Bras J, Batsakis JG, Luna MA: Malignant fibrous histiocytoma of the oral soft tissues, *Oral Surg Oral Med Oral Pathol* 64:57–67, 1987.

22. Bullen R and others: Angiosarcoma of the head and neck managed by a combination of multiple biopsies to determine tumor margin and radiation therapy: report of three cases and review of the literature, *Dermatol Surg* 24:1105–1110, 1998.

23. Carew JF, Singh B, Kraus DH: Hemangiopericytoma of the head and neck, *Laryngoscope* 109:1409–1411, 1999.

24. Carney JA and others: The triad of gastric leiomyosarcoma, functioning extra-adrenal paraganglioma and pulmonary chondroma, *N Engl J Med* 296:1517–1518, 1977.

25. Carrau RL, Johnson JT, Myers EN: Management of tumors of the parapharyngeal space, *Oncology (Huntingt)* 11:633–640, 642, 1997.

26. Chang SM, Ho WL: Malignant peripheral nerve sheath tumor: a study of 21 cases, *Zhonghua Yi Xue Za Zhi (Taipei)* 54:122–130, 1994.

27. Chase W: Familial and bilateral tumors of the carotid body, *J Pathol Bacteriol* 36:1–12, 1933.

28. Cochran JH Jr, Fee WE Jr: Angiosarcoma of the head and neck, *Otolaryngol Head Neck Surg* 87:409–416, 1979.

29. Coleman SC and others: Long-standing lateral neck mass as the initial manifestation of well-differentiated thyroid carcinoma, *Laryngoscope* 110(2 Pt 1):204–209, 2000.

30. Conley J: The management of carotid body tumors, *Surg Gynecol Obstet* 117:722, 1963.

31. Conley J, Healey WV, Stout AP: Fibromatosis of the head and neck, *Am J Surg* 112:609–614, 1966.

32. Conley J, Stout AP, Healey WV: Clinicopathologic analysis of eighty-four patients with an original diagnosis of fibrosarcoma of the head and neck, *Am J Surg* 114:564–569, 1967.

33. Crist W and others: The Third Intergroup Rhabdomyosarcoma Study, *J Clin Oncol* 13:610–630, 1995.

34. Dahm LJ and others: Osteosarcoma of the soft tissue of the larynx: report of a case with light and electron microscopic studies, *Cancer* 42:2343–2351, 1978.

35. Das Gupta TK and others: Benign solitary Schwannomas (neurilemomas), *Cancer* 24:355–366, 1969.

36. de Braud F, al-Sarraf M: Diagnosis and management of squamous cell carcinoma of unknown primary tumor site of the neck, *Semin Oncol* 20:273–278, 1993.

37. Dehner LP, Askin FB: Tumors of fibrous tissue origin in childhood. A clinicopathologic study of cutaneous and soft tissue neoplasms in 66 children, *Cancer* 38:888–900, 1976.

38. DelGaudio JM and others: Hemangiopericytoma of the oral cavity, *Otolaryngol Head Neck Surg* 114:339–340, 1996.

39. de Saint Aubain Somerhausen N, Fletcher CD: Leiomyosarcoma of soft tissue in children: clinicopathologic analysis of 20 cases, *Am J Surg Pathol* 23:755–763, 1999.

40. DeSanto LW, Neel HB 3rd: Squamous cell carcinoma: metastasis to the neck from an unknown or undiscovered primary, *Otolaryngol Clin North Am* 18:505–513, 1985.

41. Deshpande A, Bobhate SK: Squamous cell carcinoma in thyroglossal duct cyst, *J Laryngol Otol* 109:1001–1004, 1995.

42. De Silva BD, Nawroz I, Doherty VR: Angiosarcoma of the head and neck associated with xeroderma pigmentosum variant, *Br J Dermatol* 141:166–167, 1999.

43. Dickinson PH and others: Carotid body tumour: 30 years experience, *Br J Surg* 73:14–16, 1986.

44. Ducatman BS, and others: Malignant peripheral nerve sheath tumors. A clinicopathologic study of 120 cases, *Cancer* 1986. 57:2006–2021, 1986.

45. Eary JF and others: Quantitative [F-18]fluorodeoxyglucose positron emission tomography in pretreatment and grading of sarcoma, *Clin Cancer Res* 4:1215–1220, 1998.

46. Edwards C and others: The carotid body in animals at high altitude, *J Pathol* 104: 231–238, 1971.

47. el-Naggar AK and others: Synovial sarcoma: a DNA flow cytometric study, *Cancer* 65:2295–2300, 1990.

48. el-Sharkawi S: Angiosarcoma of the head and neck, *J Laryngol Otol* 111:175–176, 1997.

49. Enzinger FM, Harvey DA: Spindle cell lipoma, *Cancer* 36:1852–1859, 1975.

50. Evenson LJ and others: Radiotherapy in the management of chemodectomas of the carotid body and glomus vagale, *Head Neck* 20:609–613, 1998.

51. Fakih MG and others: Unusual tumors involving the head and neck region: case 1. Angiosarcoma of the scalp, *J Clin Oncol* 19:4173–4174, 2001.

52. Fang CY and others: Malignant fibrous histiocytoma of the left ventricle: a case report, *Changgeng Yi Xue Za Zhi* 19:187–190, 1996.

53. Farr HW: Carotid body tumors: a 40-year study, *CA Cancer J Clin* 30:260–265, 1980.

54. Farr HW: Soft part sarcomas of the head and neck, *Semin Oncol* 8:185–189, 1981.

55. Favia G and others: Angiosarcoma of the head and neck with intra-oral presentation: a clinico-pathological study of four cases, *Oral Oncol* 38:757–762, 2002.

56. Fisher SR: Elective, therapeutic, and delayed lymph node dissection for malignant melanoma of the head and neck: analysis of 1444 patients from 1970 to 1998, *Laryngoscope* 112:99–110, 2002.

57. Folpe AL and others: (F-18) fluorodeoxyglucose positron emission tomography as a predictor of pathologic grade and other prognostic variables in bone and soft tissue sarcoma, *Clin Cancer Res* 6: 1279–1287, 2000.

58. Frankenthaler R and others: Fibrosarcoma of the head and neck, *Laryngoscope* 100:799–802, 1990.

59. Frey CF, Karoll RP: Management of chemodectomas, *Am J Surg* 111:536–542, 1966.

60. Gadwal SR and others: Primary chondrosarcoma of the head and neck in pediatric patients: a clinicopathologic study of 14 cases with a review of the literature, *Cancer* 88:2181–2188, 2000.

61. Glenner GG, Crout JR, Roberts WC: A functional carotid body-like tumor secreting levarterenol, *Arch Pathol Lab Med* 73:230–240, 1962.

62. Goldstein WS, Bowen BC, Balkany T. Malignant hemangioendothelioma of the temporal bone masquerading as glomus tympanicum, *Ann Otol Rhinol Laryngol* 103:156–159, 1994.

63. Golledge J, Fisher C, Rhys-Evans PH: Head and neck liposarcoma, *Cancer* 76:1051–1058, 1995.

64. Grady AM, Krishnan V, Cohen L: Postirradiation angiosarcoma of the head and neck: report of a case, *J Oral Maxillofac Surg* 60:828–831, 2002.

65. Greager JA and others: Fibrosarcoma of the head and neck, *Am J Surg* 167:437–439, 1994.

66. Greven KM and others: Occult primary tumors of the head and neck: lack of benefit from positron emission tomography imaging with 2-[F-18]fluoro-2-deoxy-D-glucose, *Cancer* 86:114–118, 1999.

67. Guccion JG, Enzinger FM: Malignant Schwannoma associated with von Recklinghausen's neurofibromatosis, *Virchows Arch A Pathol Anat Histol* 383:43–57, 1979.

68. Hanna E: Squamous cell carcinoma in a thyroglossal duct cyst (TGDC): clinical presentation, diagnosis, and management, *Am J Otolaryngol* 17:353–357, 1996.

69. Harrington SW, Dockerty MB: Tumors of the carotid body: clinical and pathological considerations of 20 tumors affecting 19 patients, *Ann Surg* 114:820–833, 1941.

70. Hasegawa T and others: Prognostic significance of histologic grade and nuclear expression of beta-catenin in synovial sarcoma, *Hum Pathol* 32:257–263, 2001.

71. Heath D, Edwards C, Harris P: Post-mortem size and structure of the human carotid body, *Thorax* 25:129–140, 1970.

72. Hicks J, Flaitz C: Rhabdomyosarcoma of the head and neck in children, *Oral Oncol* 38:450–459, 2002.

73. Hodgkinson DJ, Soule EH, Woods JE: Cutaneous angiosarcoma of the head and neck, *Cancer* 44:1106–1113, 1979.

74. Hoffmann DF and others: Malignant nerve sheath tumors of the head and neck, *Otolaryngol Head Neck Surg* 99:309–314, 1988.

75. Hori Y: Malignant hemangioendothelioma of the skin, *J Dermatol Surg Oncol* 7:130–136, 1981.

76. Hughes KV 3rd, Olsen KD, McCaffrey TV: Parapharyngeal space neoplasms, *Head Neck* 17:124–130, 1995.

77. Hunter BC and others: Alveolar soft part sarcoma of the head and neck region, *Ann Otol Rhinol Laryngol* 107(9 Pt 1):810–814, 1998.

78. Hyams VJ: Differential diagnosis of neoplasia of the palatine tonsil, *Clin Otolaryngol* 3:117–126, 1978.

79. Iafrati MD, O'Donnell TF Jr: Adjuvant techniques for the management of large carotid body tumors: a case report and review, *Cardiovasc Surg* 7:139–145, 1999.

80. Izumi K and others: Primary leiomyosarcoma of the maxilla with regional lymph node metastasis: report of a case and review of the literature, *Oral Surg Oral Med Oral Pathol Oral Radiol Endod*, 80:310–319, 1995.

81. Jackson CG, Glasscock ME 3rd, Harris PF: Glomus tumors: diagnosis, classification, and management of large lesions, *Arch Otolaryngol* 108:401–410, 1982.

82. Jaffe BF: Pediatric head and neck tumors: a study of 178 cases, *Laryngoscope* 83:1644–1651, 1973.

83. Jansen JC and others: Estimation of growth rate in patients with head and neck paragangliomas influences the treatment proposal, *Cancer* 88:2811–2816, 2000.

84. Johnson JT: *Parapharyngeal space masses: diagnosis and management.* In Paparella M and others, editors: *Otolaryngology.* Philadelphia, 1991, W.B. Saunders, p 2584.

85. Jones JE, McGill T: Peripheral primitive neuroectodermal tumors of the head and neck, *Arch Otolaryngol Head Neck Surg* 121:1392–1395, 1995.

86. Jungehulsing M and others: 2[F]-fluoro-2-deoxy-D-glucose positron emission tomography is a sensitive tool for the detection of occult primary cancer (carcinoma of unknown primary syndrome) with head and neck lymph node manifestation, *Otolaryngol Head Neck Surg* 123:294–301, 2000.

87. Kampe CE and others: Synovial sarcoma: a study of intensive chemotherapy in 14 patients with localized disease, *Cancer* 72:2161–2169, 1993.

88. Kapadia SB: *Tumors of the nervous system.* In Barnes L, editor: *Surgical pathology of the head and neck.* New York, 2001, Marcel Dekker, pp 787–888.

89. Kau R, Arnold W: Somatostatin receptor scintigraphy and therapy of neuroendocrine (APUD) tumors of the head and neck, *Acta Otolaryngol* 116:345–349, 1996.

90. Kawashima O and others: Malignant mesenchymoma of the larynx, *J Laryngol Otol* 104:440–444, 1990.

91. Kersing W: Demonstration of hormonal activity of a glomus jugulare tumour by catecholamine determination; *Arch Otolaryngol* 217: 463–473, 1977.

92. Koch BB and others: National cancer database report on chondrosarcoma of the head and neck, *Head Neck* 22:408–425, 2000.

93. Kohn A: *Die paraganglien. Arch Mikr Anat* 62, 1903.

94. Kole AC and others: Detection of local recurrence of soft-tissue sarcoma with positron emission tomography using [18F]fluorodeoxyglucose, *Ann Surg Oncol* 4: 57–63, 1997.

95. Kowalski PJ, Paulino AF: Proliferation index as a prognostic marker in hemangiopericytoma of the head and neck, *Head Neck* 23:492–496, 2001.

96. Kwan and others: Concurrent papillary and squamous carcinoma in a thyroglossal duct cyst: a case report, *Can J Surg* 39:328–332, 1996.

97. Lack EE: Carotid body hypertrophy in patients with cystic fibrosis and cyanotic congenital heart disease, *Hum Pathol* 8: 39–51, 1977.

98. Lack EE: Hyperplasia of vagal and carotid body paraganglia in patients with chronic hypoxemia, *Am J Pathol* 91:497–516, 1978.

99. Lack EE and others: Paragangliomas of the head and neck region: a clinical study of 69 patients, *Cancer* 39:397–409, 1977.

100. Lawrence W Jr, Hays DM, Moon TE: Lymphatic metastasis with childhood rhabdomyosarcoma, *Cancer* 39:556–559, 1977.

101. Lawrence W Jr and others: Pretreatment TNM staging of childhood rhabdomyosarcoma: a report of the Intergroup Rhabdomyosarcoma Study Group. Children's Cancer Study Group. Pediatric Oncology Group, *Cancer* 80:1165–1170, 1997.

102. Lee JH and others: National Cancer Data Base report on malignant paragangliomas of the head and neck, *Cancer* 94:730–737, 2002.

103. Leong HK and others: Malignant mesenchymoma of the retropharyngeal space, *J Laryngol Otol* 107:1165–1168, 1993.

104. Lippe P and others: Desmoplastic small round cell tumour: a description of two cases and review of the literature, *Oncology* 64:14–17, 2003.

105. Loree TR and others: Malignant peripheral nerve sheath tumors of the head and neck: analysis of prognostic factors, *Otolaryngol Head Neck Surg* 122:667–672, 2000.

106. Lydiatt WM, Shaha AR, Shah JP: Angiosarcoma of the head and neck, *Am J Surg* 168:451–454, 1994.

107. Mahmoud NA: Radiation-induced fibrosarcoma of the head and neck, *J Laryngol Otol* 94:231–242, 1980.

108. Manolidis S and others: Malignant glomus tumors, *Laryngoscope* 109:30–34, 1999.

109. Mariman EC and others: Fine mapping of a putatively imprinted gene for familial non-chromaffin paragangliomas

to chromosome 11q13.1: evidence for genetic heterogeneity, *Hum Genet* 95:56–62, 1995.

110. Mark RJ and others: Angiosarcoma of the head and neck: the UCLA experience 1955 through 1990, *Arch Otolaryngol Head Neck Surg* 119:973–978, 1993.

111. Mark RJ and others: Fibrosarcoma of the head and neck: the UCLA experience, *Arch Otolaryngol Head Neck Surg* 117:396–401, 1991.

112. Maurer HM and others: The Intergroup Rhabdomyosarcoma Study: I. a final report, *Cancer* 61:209–220, 1988.

113. Maurer HM and others: The Intergroup Rhabdomyosarcoma Study: II, *Cancer* 71:1904–1922, 1993.

114. McCulloch TM, Makielski KH, McNutt MA: Head and neck liposarcoma. A histopathologic reevaluation of reported cases, *Arch Otolaryngol Head Neck Surg* 118:1045–1049, 1992.

115. Mendenhall WM and others: Treatment of paragangliomas with radiation therapy, *Otolaryngol Clin North Am* 34: 1007–1020, 2001.

116. Mentzel T and others: Epithelioid hemangioendothelioma of skin and soft tissues: clinicopathologic and immunohisto-chemical study of 30 cases, *Am J Surg Pathol* 21:363–374, 1997.

117. Mihok NA, Cha I: Desmoplastic small round cell tumor presenting as a neck mass: a case report, *Diagn Cytopathol* 25:68–72, 2001.

118. Miller FR and others: Magnetic resonance imaging and the management of parapharyngeal space tumors, *Head Neck* 18:67–77, 1996.

119. Mindell RS, Calcaterra TC, Ward PH: Leiomyosarcoma of the head and neck: a review of the literature and report of two cases, *Laryngoscope* 85:904–910, 1975.

120. Mintz GA and others: Primary malignant giant cell tumor of the mandible. Report of a case and review of the literature, *Oral Surg Oral Med Oral Pathol* 51:164–171, 1981.

121. Montgomery E, Goldblum JR, Fisher C: Leiomyosarcoma of the head and neck: a clinicopathological study, *Histopathology* 40:518–525, 2002.

122. Morrison WH and others: Cutaneous angiosarcoma of the head and neck. A therapeutic dilemma, *Cancer* 76:319–327, 1995.

123. Mulligan R: Chemodectoma in the dog, *Am J Pathol* 26: 680, 1950.

124. Myssiorek D, Palestro CJ: 111Indium pentetreotide scan detection of familial paragangliomas, *Laryngoscope* 108: 228–231, 1998.

125. Netterville JL and others: Carotid body tumors: a review of 30 patients with 46 tumors, *Laryngoscope* 105:115–126, 1995.

126. Newman PL, Fletcher CD: Malignant mesenchymoma. Clinicopathologic analysis of a series with evidence of low-grade behaviour, *Am J Surg Pathol* 15:607–614, 1991.

127. Newton WA Jr and others: Classification of rhabdomyosar-comas and related sarcomas: pathologic aspects and proposal for a new classification—an Intergroup Rhabdomyosarcoma Study, *Cancer* 76:1073–1085, 1995.

128. Oldring D, Fisch U: Glomus tumors of the temporal region: surgical therapy, *Am J Otol* 1:7–18, 1979.

129. Olsen KD: Tumors and surgery of the parapharyngeal space, *Laryngoscope* 104(5 Pt 2 Suppl 63):1–28, 1994.

130. Olsen WL and others: MR imaging of paragangliomas, *AJR Am J Roentgenol* 148:201–204, 1987.

131. Ordonez NG: Alveolar soft part sarcoma: a review and update, *Adv Anat Pathol* 6:125–139, 1999.

132. Otte T, Kleinsasser O: Liposarcoma of the head and neck, *Arch Otorhinolaryngol* 232:285–291, 1981.

133. Pang KP, Goh CH, Tan HM: Parapharyngeal space tumours: an 18 year review, *J Laryngol Otol* 116:170–175, 2002.

134. Panje WR and others: Angiosarcoma of the head and neck: review of 11 cases, *Laryngoscope* 96:1381–1384, 1986.

135. Pappo AS and others: Treatment of localized nonorbital, nonparameningeal head and neck rhabdomyosarcoma: lessons learned from intergroup rhabdomyosarcoma studies III and IV, *J Clin Oncol* 21:638–645, 2003.

136. Parham DM and others: Immunohistochemical study of childhood rhabdomyosarcomas and related neoplasms: results of an Intergroup Rhabdomyosarcoma study project, *Cancer* 67:3072–3080, 1991.

137. Pensak ML, Gluckman JL, Shumrick KA: Parapharyngeal space tumors: an algorithm for evaluation and management, *Laryngoscope* 104:1170–1173, 1994.

138. Perkins P, Weiss SW: Spindle cell hemangioendothelioma: an analysis of 78 cases with reassessment of its pathogenesis and biologic behavior, *Am J Surg Pathol* 20:1196–1204, 1996.

139. Pinsolle J and others: Osteosarcoma of the soft tissue of the larynx: report of a case with electron microscopic studies, *Otolaryngol Head Neck Surg* 102:276–280, 1990.

140. Portera CA Jr and others: Alveolar soft part sarcoma: clinical course and patterns of metastasis in 70 patients treated at a single institution, *Cancer* 91:585–591, 2001.

141. Potter GD, McClennan BL: Malignant giant cell tumor of the sphenoid bone and its differential diagnosis, *Cancer* 25:167–170, 1970.

142. Raney RB and others: Late complications of therapy in 213 children with localized, nonorbital soft-tissue sarcoma of the head and neck: A descriptive report from the Intergroup Rhabdomyosarcoma Studies (IRS)-II and - III. IRS Group of the Children's Cancer Group and the Pediatric Oncology Group, *Med Pediatr Oncol* 33:362–371, 1999.

143. Ranieri E, D'Andrea MR, Vecchione A: Fine needle aspiration cytology of squamous cell carcinoma arising in a thyroglossal duct cyst: a case report, *Acta Cytol* 40:747–750, 1996.

144. Reddy SP, Marks JE: Metastatic carcinoma in the cervical lymph nodes from an unknown primary site: results of bilateral neck plus mucosal irradiation vs. ipsilateral neck irradiation, *Int J Radiat Oncol Biol Phys* 37:797–802, 1997.

145. Rice DH, Hybels RL: The mass in the neck, *Am Fam Physician* 17:187–189, 1978.

146. Rock MG, Pritchard DJ, Unni KK: Metastases from histologically benign giant-cell tumor of bone, *J Bone Joint Surg Am* 66:269–274, 1984.

147. Rock MG and others: Secondary malignant giant-cell tumor of bone. Clinicopathological assessment of nineteen patients, *J Bone Joint Surg Am* 68:1073–1079, 1986.

148. Rodary C and others: Prognostic factors in 951 nonmetastatic rhabdomyosarcoma in children: a report from the International Rhabdomyosarcoma Workshop, *Med Pediatr Oncol* 19:89–95, 1991.

149. Rodriguez-Cuevas H, Lau I, Rodriguez HP: High-altitude paragangliomas diagnostic and therapeutic considerations, *Cancer* 57: 672–676, 1986.

150. Rosen G and others: Synovial sarcoma: uniform response of metastases to high dose ifosfamide, *Cancer* 73:2506–2511, 1994.

151. Rosenkranz L, Schell AR: Carotid body tumor as reversible cause of recurrent syncope, *NY State J Med* 1984. 84:38–39, 1984.

152. Roth JA, Enzinger FM, Tannenbaum M: Synovial sarcoma of the neck: a followup study of 24 cases, *Cancer* 35:1243–1253, 1975.

153. Samandari F, Mersol VF: Malignant mesenchymoma of the soft palate, *Ear Nose Throat J* 55:250–251, 1976.

154. Samlali R and others [Leiomyosarcoma of the larynx. Review of the literature apropos of a case], *Bull Cancer* 83:882–885, 1996.

155. Schmid U, Eckert F: Malignant thyroid hemangioendothelioma, *Am J Surg Pathol* 14:1170–1171, 1990.

156. Schwartz MR, Donovan DT: Hemangiopericytoma of the larynx: a case report and review of the literature, *Otolaryngol Head Neck Surg* 96:369–372, 1987.

157. Scudder C: Tumor of the intercarotid body: A report of one case, together with all cases in literature, *Am J Med Sci* 126:384–389, 1903.

158. Swain RE, Sessions DG, Ogura JH: Fibrosarcoma of the head and neck in children, *Laryngoscope*, 86:113–116, 1976.

159. SenGupta SK, Nag S: Cervical paravertebral leiomyosarcoma mimicking a nerve sheath tumor, *Hum Pathol* 23:708–710, 1992.

160. Shamblin WR and others: Carotid body tumor (chemodectoma): clinicopathologic analysis of ninety cases, *Am J Surg* 122:732–739, 1971.

161. Shimada H and others: Pathology of fatal rhabdomyosarcoma: report from Intergroup Rhabdomyosarcoma Study (IRS-I and IRS-II), *Cancer* 59:459–465, 1987.

162. Shmookler BM, Enzinger FM, Brannon RB: Orofacial synovial sarcoma: a clinicopathologic study of 11 new cases and review of the literature, *Cancer* 50:269–276, 1982.

163. Simmons WB and others: Alveolar soft part sarcoma of the head and neck. A disease of children and young adults, *Int J Pediatr Otorhinolaryngol* 17:139–153, 1989.

164. Singh B and others: Branchial cleft cyst carcinoma: myth or reality? *Ann Otol Rhinol Laryngol* 107:519–524, 1998.

165. Snowden RT and others: Superficial leiomyosarcoma of the head and neck: case report and review of the literature, *Ear Nose Throat J* 80:449–453, 2001.

166. Sordillo PP and others: Malignant schwannoma: clinical characteristics, survival, and response to therapy, *Cancer* 47:2503–2509, 1981.

167. Spector RA, Travis LW, Smith J: Alveolar soft part sarcoma of the head and neck, *Laryngoscope* 89:1301–1306, 1979.

168. Staats EF, Brown RL, Smith RR: Carotid body tumors, benign and malignant, *Laryngoscope* 76:907–916, 1966.

169. Sterns EE, Haust MD, Wollin DG: Malignant mesenchymoma of the mandible, *Can J Surg* 12:444–449, 1969.

170. Stokkel MP, Draisma A, Pauwels EK: Positron emission tomography with 2-[18F]-fluoro-2-deoxy-D-glucose in oncology. Part IIIb: Therapy response monitoring in colorectal and lung tumours, head and neck cancer, hepatocellular carcinoma and sarcoma, *J Cancer Res Clin Oncol* 127:278–285, 2001.

171. Triplet I, Vankemmel B, Madelain M: [Malignant hemangioendothelioma of the larynx with subcutaneous metastases], *Lille Med* 19:743–745, 1974.

172. Vaccani JP and others: Ewing's sarcoma of the head and neck in children, *Int J Pediatr Otorhinolaryngol* 48:209–216, 1999.

173. Valdagni R, Amichetti M: Radiation therapy of carotid body tumors, *Am J Clin Oncol* 13:45–48, 1990.

174. van der Mey AG and others: Genomic imprinting in hereditary glomus tumours: evidence for new genetic theory, *Lancet* 2:1291–1294, 1989.

175. Vege DS and others: Malignant peripheral nerve sheath tumors of the head and neck: a clinicopathological study, *J Surg Oncol*, 1994. 55:100–103, 1994.

176. Von Luschka H: Uber de drusenartige natur des sogennten ganglion intercaroticum, *Archive fuer Anatomie, Physiologie und Wissenschaftliche* 405–414, 1862.

177. Von Moll L and others: Iodine-131 MIBG scintigraphy of neuroendocrine tumors other than pheochromocytoma and neuroblastoma, *J Nucl Med* 28:979–988, 1987.

178. Walike JW, Bailey BJ: Head and neck hemangiopericytoma, *Arch Otolaryngol* 93:345–353, 1971.

179. Walsh RM and others: Malignant vagal paraganglioma, *J Laryngol Otol* 111:83–88, 1997.

180. Wanebo HJ and others: Head and neck sarcoma: report of the Head and Neck Sarcoma Registry. Society of Head and Neck Surgeons Committee on Research, *Head Neck* 14:1–7, 1992.

181. Wang SJ and others: Surgical management of carotid body tumors, *Otolaryngol Head Neck Surg* 123:202–206, 2000.

182. Ward PH and others: Embolization: an adjunctive measure for removal of carotid body tumors, *Laryngoscope* 98:1287–1291, 1988.

183. Weiss SW, Enzinger FM: Epithelioid hemangioendothelioma: a vascular tumor often mistaken for a carcinoma, *Cancer* 50:970–981, 1982.

184. Weiss SW, Enzinger FM: Malignant fibrous histiocytoma: an analysis of 200 cases, *Cancer* 41:2250–2266, 1978.

185. Weiss SW and others: Epithelioid hemangioendothelioma and related lesions, *Semin Diagn Pathol* 3:259–287, 1986.

186. Wesley RK, Mintz SM, Wertheimer FW: Primary malignant hemangioendothelioma of the gingiva: report of a case and review of the literature, *Oral Surg Oral Med Oral Pathol* 39:103–112, 1975.

187. Wood GS and others: Malignant fibrous histiocytoma tumor cells resemble fibroblasts, *Am J Surg Pathol* 10:323–335, 1986.

188. Wu X, Qi Y, Tang P: [A comparison of malignant fibrous histiocytoma of head, neck and extremities], *Chin Med J (Engl)* 113:532–535, 2000.

189. Yasuoka T and others: Hemangioma and malignant hemangioendothelioma of the maxillary sinus: case reports and clinical consideration, *J Oral Maxillofac Surg* 48:877–881, 1990.

190. Zbaren P, Lehmann W: Carotid body paraganglioma with metastases, *Laryngoscope* 95:450–454, 1985.

LYMPHOMAS PRESENTING IN THE HEAD AND NECK

Nancy Price Mendenhall
Ilona M. Schmalfuss
Matthew C. Hull

INTRODUCTION

Lymphomas in the head and neck fall into the basic categories of Hodgkin's lymphoma (HL) and non-Hodgkin's lymphoma (NHL). NHL occurs more than five times as frequently as HL and is the second most common type of cancer occurring in the head and neck.

NON-HODGKIN'S LYMPHOMAS

NHLs are a heterogeneous group of diseases arising in nodal or extranodal lymphoid tissue. A favored presentation site is the head and neck, where between one-third and two-thirds of all extranodal NHLs arise. The full spectrum of heterogeneity in the morphology, phenotype, genotype, presentation, natural history, response to treatment, and prognosis of NHLs is represented in the various clinicopathologic entities occurring in the head and neck. The spectrum of biologic behavior in head and neck lymphomas ranges from indolent tumors, present for years before diagnosis, to rapidly growing tumors that double in size over days. The difficulty in classification of NHLs is reflected in the many classification systems devised over the past 30 to 40 years. Even with the use of modern molecular genetic tools for pathologic classification, the natural history and response to treatment in a given lymphoma cannot always be predicted reliably based on tissue examination, so it is incumbent on the clinician to recognize the repertoire of natural histories associated with different patterns of presentation in the NHLs and to be familiar with the relevant therapeutic tools available.

Epidemiology

In the United States, NHL accounts for approximately 4.5% of all cancer diagnoses. The incidence of NHL in the United States has been increasing over the past decade, and the American Cancer Society estimates that in 2003 there will be approximately 53,400 new cases and 23,400 deaths due to this disease.[1] There is a slight male predominance and the median age of patients is 65 years,[20] with certain types of lymphomas represented throughout the age groups and others correlated with a specific age group, sex, site, or predisposing factor.

A viral association has been clearly documented in two types of NHL. Epstein-Barr virus has been detected in the lymphoma cells of 90% of children with African Burkitt's lymphoma,[43,57,61] and HTLV-1 has been identified in tumor cells of an aggressive form of peripheral T-cell lymphoma.[60] There is an increased incidence of the more aggressive subtypes of NHL in immunocompromised patients,[54] including iatrogenic immunocompromise associated with organ transplantation,[10] the viral-induced immunocompromise of acquired immuno deficiency syndrome,[49] and congenital disorders associated with immunocompromise such as ataxia telangiectasia[69] and Wiskott-Aldrich syndrome.[41] There is also an association between lymphoma and prior autoimmune and inflammatory disorders such as Sjögren's[2,39,76,80,85] and Hashimoto's thyroiditis.[31,33] Occasionally, the diagnosis of a lymphoma is preceded by a sentinel infectious or inflammatory event or preceding waxing and waning lymphadenopathy, suggesting the possibility that proliferative immune or reparative responses may trigger an underlying genetic capacity for lymphoma development.

Pathology

The Rappaport, Lukes-Collins, and Kiel (Lennert) classification systems used before 1982 were based primarily on tumor morphology. The Working Formulation system,[56,73] which was proposed in 1982, was based on both morphology and natural history and included 10 separate entities that were grouped as low-grade (small lymphocytic, follicular predominantly small cleaved cell, and follicular mixed small cleaved and large cell lymphomas), intermediate-grade (follicular predominantly large cell, diffuse small cleaved cell, diffuse mixed small and large cell, and diffuse large cell), and high-grade lymphomas (small non-cleaved or Burkitt's, lymphoblastic, and immunoblastic). Over the next decade, chromosomal analysis, immunohistochemical staining, and molecular genetic techniques revealed specific phenotypic and genotypic patterns among the lymphomas, which were correlated with natural history. The Revised European and American Lymphoma (REAL)[27] classification, and later the World Health Organization (WHO) classification,[35] are attempts to move beyond the limits of morphologic classification in lymphomas by incorporating immunohistochemical, kinetic, and molecular genetic information. In the new systems, a number of new entities were described that have predictable natural histories and treatment responses, such as large cell anaplastic lymphoma, NK/T-cell lymphomas of the sinonasal tract, mantle cell lymphomas, and marginal zone lymphomas including the mucosa-associated lymphoid tissues (MALT). Table 114-1 shows a summary of diagnostic criteria for the most common clinicopathologic NHL entities occurring in the head and neck area, along with typical sites of presentation, and expected clinical behavior.[78]

Evaluation, Staging, and Prognostic Factors

Fine-needle aspiration can be sufficient to confirm recurrence in an already well-characterized lymphoma and will occasionally be sufficient to secure initial diagnosis, but excisional biopsy is generally preferred to afford assessment of nodal or extranodal tissue architecture. Morphologic assessment is no longer sufficient for definitive diagnosis in many lymphomas, if supporting documentation of the patterns of surface antigens is not available (see Table 114-1). Flow cytometry is useful in correlating cell size not only with cell surface phenotype but also with the proportion of cells in S phase, which is indicative of biologic behavior.

Once a diagnosis is made, extent of disease must be assessed for staging. Because radiation therapy is generally used as part of the management of most lymphomas, knowledge of the anatomic extent of disease is required for treatment planning. Computed tomography (CT) of the head and neck, chest, abdomen, and pelvis is indicated in essentially all low-, intermediate-, and high-grade lymphomas to evaluate all nodal and extranodal lymphoid structures. Lymphomas differ from the more common carcinomas occurring in the head and neck area in that they tend to push, compress, or surround rather than invade anatomic structures such as arteries, bone, muscle, and mucosa.

Central necrosis in a node or mass usually occurs only with high-grade lymphomas or in immunocompromised patients. Neurotropic spread is rare but has been reported in marginal zone lymphomas occurring in the head and neck.[19] Most lymphomas are homogeneous, are slightly hyperintense on CT, show a slightly increased signal on magnetic resonance imaging (MRI), and enhance with CT and MRI contrast agents. Certain clinicopathologic entities may require additional studies to assess particular potential patterns of involvement: upper gastrointestinal series, barium enema, endoscopy, or colonoscopy may be indicated in patients with Waldeyer's ring, thyroid, and salivary gland MALToma. MRI of the brain may be helpful in patients with vitreous, paranasal sinus, parapharyngeal space, pterygopalatine fossa, and orbit involvement. MRI may also be useful in identifying areas of perineural and bone marrow involvement. Bone marrow biopsy is indicated in most lymphomas other than localized asymptomatic MALTomas and other marginal zone lymphomas. Both follicular and more aggressive lymphoma subtypes show a 2-deoxy-2-[F-18]-fluoro-D-glucose (FDG) uptake, making positron emission tomography (PET) potentially useful in staging and response assessment. Studies have documented excellent 2-deoxy-2-[F-18]-fluoro-D-glucose-PET sensitivity and specificity for nodal staging.[65,82] FDG is not reliably taken up by some lymphoma subtypes, such as MALT, but other agents such as ^{111}In-DTPA-D-Phe(1)-octreotide, which is taken up by somatostatin receptors, may be of use in dealing with MALT tumors.[64]

The Ann Arbor staging system is used for NHLs (Table 114-2).[1] Many other factors besides stage have been shown to have potential prognostic significance in NHL, including histologic type, immunophenotype, tumor bulk, site of extranodal presentation, age and sex of the patient, performance status, hemoglobin, number of involved nodal and extranodal sites, proliferation indices, interleukin 6 level, lactate dehydrogenase (LDH), β_2-microglobulin, and phenotypic variants indicated by expression of human leukocyte antigen-DR (HLA-DR), CD44 antigen, B-cell CLL/lymphoma 2 (BCL-2), and B-cell CLL/lymphoma 6 (BCL-6). An international group of NHL investigators proposed a tool called the International Prognostic Index (IPI), which was based on a multivariate analysis of factors associated with prognosis in patients with aggressive NHL treated with doxorubicin-based combination chemotherapy on phases II and III trials.[58] The IPI includes five unfavorable prognostic factors: stage (III–IV), age (>60 years), performance status (ECOG 2–4), number of extranodal sites (>1), and LDH (>1 × normal). The IPI categorizes patients into four risk categories based on the number of risk

TABLE 114-1

DIAGNOSTIC CRITERIA FOR COMMON LYMPHOMAS OF THE HEAD AND NECK

Histologic Subtype	Cell Type	Additional CD Markers	Associated Oncogene	Translocation (Incidence in Subtype)	Cellular Activity	Typical Head and Neck Site	Typical Behavior
Small lymphocytic lymphoma	B*	CD5+, CD10-, CD23+	ND	ND	ND	Anterior orbit, nodes	Indolent
Follicular	B*	CD5-, CD43-, CD10+, CD23±	BCL-2	t(14;18)(q32;q11) (90%)	Suppression of apoptosis	Nodes, Waldeyer's ring, salivary glands	Indolent
Diffuse large cell	B*	CD5-, CD10+, CD23±, CD43-, CD30-	BCL-2	t(14;18)(q32;q11) (20%)	Suppression of apoptosis	Waldeyer's ring, nodes, salivary glands, thyroid, orbit, sinonasal tract	Aggressive
			BCL-6	3q27 (40%)	Zinc finger transcription factor		
			BCL-8	t(14;15)(q32;q11-13) (3%-4%)	Transcription factor		
MALT	B*	CD5-, CD10-, CD23	ND	t(11;18)(q21;q21) (35%)	ND	Salivary glands, orbit, thyroid, Waldeyer's ring	Indolent
Marginal zone (monocytoid)	B*		ND	ND	ND	Nodes, neurotropic presentation	Indolent
Mantle	B*	CD5+, CD10±, CD23-, CD43+	BCL-1 (cyclin-D)	t(11;14)(q13;q32) (70%)	G1/S progression	Waldeyer's ring, nodes	Aggressive
Burkitt's	B*		C-MYC	8q24 (100%)	Transcription activation; cell cycle control	Waldeyer's ring, parapharyngeal site	Aggressive
Primary system C or primary cutaneous anaplastic large cell	T*	CD30+	ALK/NPM	t(2;5) (p23;q35) (ND)	Tyrosine kinase	Skin	Variable
Angiocentric lymphoma (AKA) lethal midline granuloma, nasal T-cell lymphoma, nasal (T-NK cell) lymphoma	T*	CD56+, CD4+	ND	ND	ND	Sinonasal tract	Aggressive

*Pan B-cell markers are CD19+, CD20+, and CD22; Pan T-cell markers are CD2+, CD3+, CD4+, CD7+, and CD8+.
ND, no data.
(Modified from Tsang RW, Gospodarowicz MK: *Non-Hodgkin's lymphoma.* In Gunderson LL, Tepper JE, editors: *Clinical radiation oncology,* Philadelphia, 2000, Churchill Livingstone, pp 1158–1188.)

TABLE 114-2

AMERICAN JOINT COMMITTEE ON CANCER/ANN ARBOR STAGING SYSTEM FOR NON-HODGKIN'S LYMPHOMA

Hodgkin and Non-Hodgkin Lymphoma

Staging	
Stage I	Involvement of a single lymph node region (I); or, localized involvement of a single extralymphatic organ or site in the absence of any lymph node involvement (IE) (rare in Hodgkin lymphoma)
Stage II	Involvement of two or more lymph node regions on the same side of the diaphragm (II); or, localized involvement of a single extralymphatic organ or site in association with regional lymph node involvement with or without involvement of other lymph node regions on the same side of the diaphragm (IIE); the number of regions involved may be indicated by a subscript, as in, for example, II_3
Stage III	Involvement of lymph node regions on both sides of the diaphragm (III), which also may be accompanied by extralymphatic extension in association with adjacent lymph node involvement (IIIE), by involvement of the spleen (IIIS), or both (IIIE,S)
Stage IV	Diffuse or disseminated involvement of one or more extralymphatic organs, with or without associated lymph node involvement; or, isolated extralymphatic organ involvement in the absence of adjacent regional lymph node involvement, but in conjunction with disease in distant site(s); any involvement of the liver or bone marrow, or nodular involvement of the lung(s)
A and B Classification (Symptoms). Each stage should be classified as either A or B according to the absence or presence of defined constitutional symptoms.	1. *Fevers:* unexplained fever with temperature above 38°C 2. *Night sweats:* drenching sweats that require change of bedclothes 3. *Weight loss:* unexplained weight loss of more than 10% of the usual body weight in the 6 months before diagnosis

(Data from the 2002 American Joint Committee on Cancer: *AJCC cancer staging handbook*, ed 6, New York, 2002, Springer.)

factors present. In this group of patients, 5-year survival rates for patients with low risk (0 or 1 factor) were 73%; low-intermediate risk (2 factors), 51%; high-intermediate risk (3 factors), 43%; and high risk (4 or 5 factors), 26%. Because of the prognostic significance of the IPI score, it is a useful tool for guiding the intensity of therapy and important in providing a standard for comparison of therapeutic outcomes.

Therapy

The generally indolent natural history of low-grade lymphomas (which may include transient spontaneous remissions, transformation to rapidly lethal high-grade lymphomas, or both) make evaluation of various treatment approaches difficult. There is no convincing evidence of cure in low-grade lymphoma with systemic therapy, although there may be excellent responses with a variety of agents including monoclonal antibodies, radioimmunolabeled antibodies,

biologic agents such as interferon, single-agent purine analogs and alkylating agents, combination chemotherapy, and high-dose ablative chemotherapy with stem cell rescue. The low-grade lymphomas are almost always responsive to radiation therapy, and they are potentially curable in a high proportion of cases, depending on stage, histology, site, and disease extent. In contrast to squamous cell carcinoma, for which radiation doses of 60 to 76 Gy are necessary, low-grade NHLs require only 20 to 30 Gy.[38] Typical outcomes with radiation therapy include freedom-from-disease-progression rates at 10 years of approximately 80%, 60%, and 40% for stages I, II, and III, respectively.[51] Because of the indolent natural history, management options also include delay of treatment until the disease becomes symptomatic. At symptomatic progression, many options for palliation exist, including the systematic approach listed above. Radiation therapy should provide long-term disease control in the sites applied, as well as a potential for cure if the disease is still limited.

Intermediate-grade NHLs, most commonly diffuse large B-cell lymphomas, are usually treated with three to six cycles of CHOP-R-based chemotherapy regimens (cyclophosphamide, doxorubicin, vincristine, prednisone, rituxan) followed by involved field radiation therapy with expected freedom-from-disease-progression or relapse rates of approximately 80%, 60%, and 40% for stages I, II, and III, respectively.[17] Radiation doses in intermediate-grade NHL range from 30 to 50 Gy, depending on response to chemotherapy and size of tumor.[21,38,52] Because of the indolent natural history, management options also include delay of treatment until the disease becomes symptomatic.

High-grade lymphomas typically have such a high growth fraction that localized therapy may be of little benefit; consequently most patients with Burkitt's lymphoma and lymphoblastic lymphoma are treated primarily with chemotherapy. Radiation therapy can be used in patients with incomplete responses to chemotherapy and for treatment of sanctuary sites at high risk for recurrence after chemotherapy such as the central nervous system and, occasionally, the testicles. Most lymphomas in children are high grade and are treated with chemotherapy alone.[44]

Some clinicopathologic entities may require more specific treatment approaches, as detailed below.

Most Common Clinicopathologic Entities in NHL

Although both aggressive and indolent NHLs may occur in any tissue, the following patterns represent the most common presentation of NHL occurring in the head and neck.

Waldeyer's Ring

Waldeyer's ring is a band of lymphoid tissue encircling the entryway from the oral and nasal cavities to the aerodigestive track and includes lymphoid tissue in the tonsils, adenoids, base of the tongue, and nasopharynx. Whether the lymphoid tissue in Waldeyer's ring should be considered nodal or extranodal is debatable. The presence of primarily IgG-secreting resident plasma cells and the absence of a prominent marginal zone in the tissue support the argument for a nodal origin. However, the location along the aerodigestive tract and the lack of afferent lymphatics are evidence for an extranodal origin. Fifty percent to 60% of stages I and II extranodal NHLs of the head and neck occur in Waldeyer's ring, with nearly half arising in the tonsil.[14,23,71] Patients with primary tonsil lymphomas have a significant incidence (20%–30%) of synchronous or metachronous gastrointestinal involvement.[8,26] The most common histology is diffuse large B-cell lymphoma, followed by follicular lymphoma,

extranodal marginal zone B-cell lymphoma (MALT type), and Burkitt's lymphoma.[14] Waldeyer's ring is considered a single site because of the frequent involvement of more than one part of it. Common symptoms include persistent sore throat, otalgia, dysphagia, and airway obstruction. Common appearance on physical examination is tonsil enlargement, bulging of the mucosa in the nasopharynx or base of the tongue, and displacement or bulging of the soft palate; mucosal ulceration is not common. Rubbery, matted lymphadenopathy is common, frequently involving not just internal jugular chain nodes, but also the spinal accessory chain. Occasionally submental, submandibular, parotid, preauricular, and occipital nodes may be involved. Treatment for stages I and II is radiation therapy alone for low-grade lymphomas and radiation therapy preceded by three to six cycles of CHOP-R-based chemotherapy in intermediate-grade lymphomas. Five-year survival rates range from 60% to 90%.[5,17,21,53] Figures 114-1 through 114-4 demonstrate the common radiographic appearance of tonsil, base of tongue, and nasopharyngeal NHL.

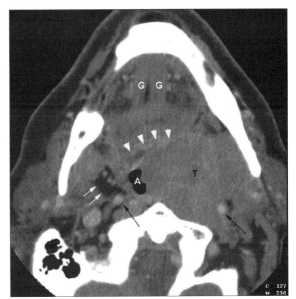

Figure 114-1. Diffuse large B-cell lymphoma in an HIV-positive 68-year-old man. Contrast-enhanced axial CT image of an HIV-positive patient show a large tumor *(T)* in the oropharynx, probably originating in the tonsil, involving the lateral pharyngeal wall and parapharyngeal space on the left. The mass significantly compromises the upper airway *(A)*. Notice the complete obliteration of the parapharyngeal fat planes on the left when compared with the right *(white arrows)*. The internal carotid artery *(black arrow on each side)* is partially surrounded along its medial aspect by tumor without evidence of luminal narrowing. Notice also the marked anterior displacement of the soft palate on the left as nicely seen as oblique position of the fat plane within the soft palate *(arrowheads)*. G, genioglossus muscle; A, airway.

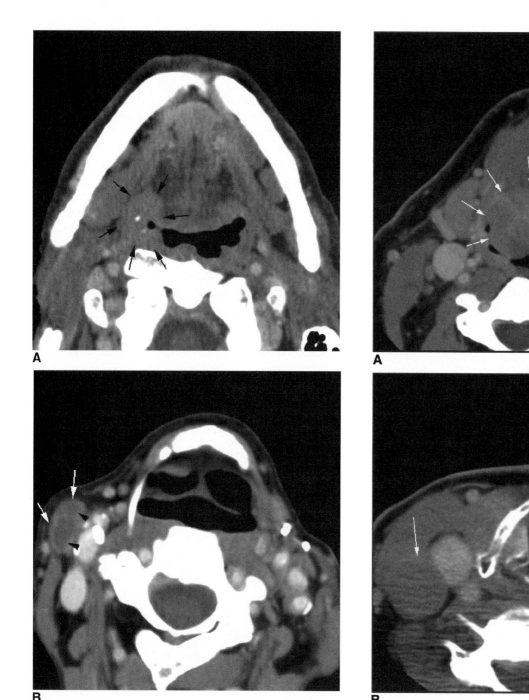

A

B

A

B

Figure 114-2. A small lymphocytic lymphoma of the tonsil in an 83-year-old man. **A,** Axial contrasted CT image in a patient with small lymphocytic lymphoma shows a mass *(black arrows)* in the tonsillar fossa on the right with deep infiltration. The focal calcifications are often seen in normal tonsillar tissues, particularly if the patient has history of chronic tonsillitis. **B,** The contrasted axial CT image performed at the level of the hyoid bone shows a slightly enlarged lymph node at the junction of groups 2 and 3 on the right *(white arrows)* with focal areas of decreased density *(arrowheads)* suggestive of necrosis. Such an appearance is atypical for lymphoma but can be seen in very aggressive types of lymphoma, lymphomas in significantly immunocompromised patients, and after treatment.

Figure 114-3. Low-grade T-cell lymphoma of the base of the tongue in a 65-year-old man. **A,** Contrast-enhanced axial CT image through the level of the tongue base shows significant hypertrophy of the lymphoid tissue *(arrows)*, worse on the right, with signs of deep infiltration. **B,** In addition, there is an enlarged group 3 lymph node on the right *(arrow on right)* showing homogenous attenuation as typically seen in lymphoma. Notice the normal-sized group 3 lymph node on the left *(arrow)*. Low-grade T-cell lymphoma in Waldeyer's ring is unusual. A, airway.

Salivary Glands

Salivary gland lymphoma is uncommon, accounting for 2% to 5% of all salivary gland neoplasms and between 5% to 10% of all NHLs of the head and neck region.[34] Patients with lymphoepithelial sialoadenitis

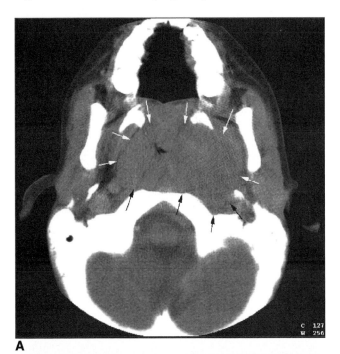

A

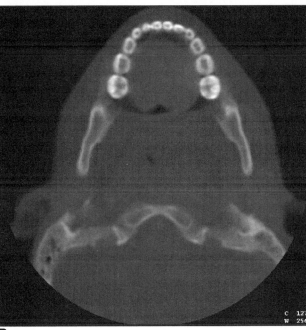

B

Figure 114-4. Diffuse large B-cell lymphoma in an 8-year-old boy with AIDS. **A,** Axial contrasted CT image of a patient with AIDS reveals a huge mass *(arrows)* in the nasopharynx bilaterally, worse on the left. **B,** The bone window image at the similar level shows no signs of bone invasion despite the large tumor size. This is typical for lymphoma in contrast to squamous cell carcinomas of the nasopharynx.

of Sjögren's syndrome (LESA) have a 44-fold increased risk of developing salivary gland or extrasalivary lymphoma.[2,39,76,85] Lymphoma may arise either in the extranodal parenchyma of the parotid or submandibular glands or within the intraparotid or periparotid nodes. The most common salivary gland nodal histology is follicular, whereas the most common extranodal salivary gland histology is marginal zone lymphoma of the MALT type. Other B-cell lymphomas of the salivary glands include diffuse large B-cell, mantle cell, lymphoplasmocytic, and small lymphocytic lymphomas. Primary salivary T-cell lymphoma is very rare in the Western population, with only a few cases reported.[30] The most common presenting symptom is painless swelling of the involved salivary gland. Radiographic evaluation may reveal either an intraparenchymal mass (Figure 114-5) or intraglandular nodal enlargement which is often multifocal, bilateral, or both. Most salivary gland NHLs are low grade and present with an indolent course. Rapid progression may represent de novo intermediate- or high-grade NHL or, alternatively, transformation from a preceding low-grade NHL to a high-grade NHL. Localized low-grade

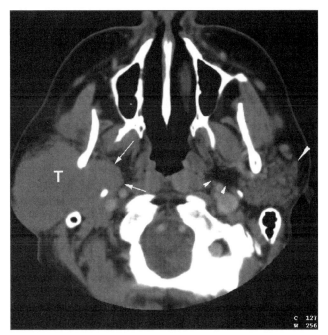

Figure 114-5. Diffuse large B-cell lymphoma in a 30-year-old woman with Sjögren's syndrome. Contrast-enhanced axial CT image through the parotid glands in a patient with Sjögren's disease demonstrates a large mass *(T)* in the right parotid gland. Almost the entire parotid gland is infiltrated. The deep extension of the mass displaces and partially obliterates the fat pad within the parapharyngeal space on the right *(arrows on right)* when compared to the left *(small arrowheads on left)*. Notice the multinodular appearance of the parotid gland on the left *(large white arrowhead)* reflecting the typical appearance of the parotid gland in Sjögren's disease.

NHL is treated with radiation therapy alone and intermediate-grade with chemotherapy followed by radiation therapy.

Orbit

Lymphomas account for up to half of all orbital tumors, and the incidence appears to be increasing. Lymphoma in the orbit may occur in the posterior orbit, vitreous, conjunctiva, eyelid, or lacrimal glands* as either primary localized disease or as a manifestation of systemic disease.[12,19,47,75,84] The vast majority of orbital lymphomas are B-cell NHL, with primary T-cell NHL representing only 1% to 3% of all ocular adnexal NHL.[4,11,29,36] The most common histology in both anterior structures as well as the posterior orbit is MALT, followed by diffuse large B-cell, follicular lymphomas. Diffuse large B-cell lymphomas are more likely to occur in the posterior orbit than in anterior tissues. Other histologies in orbital lymphoma include marginal zone, mantle zone, and diffuse small-cleaved cell lymphoma. In the past, some MALT lymphomas were classified as small lymphocytic lymphomas or pseudolymphomas.

Orbital MALT lymphoma usually presents with painless unilateral orbital swelling, occasionally proptosis, ptosis, blurred vision, and diplopia; 10% to 20% of cases may be bilateral.[11,40,50,70,81] Conjunctival involvement is bilateral in approximately 45% of cases.[72] The presenting symptoms and signs of conjunctival lymphoma include a scratchy, sandpaper sensation in the eye and a fleshy, salmon-pink proliferation in the conjunctiva, often projecting over sclerae from the medial or lateral conjunctival recesses. Rarely, the optic nerve may be encased and compressed by low-grade NHL, particularly low-grade marginal zone lymphomas,[19] resulting in visual field deficit or blurred vision. High-grade NHL of the orbit can destroy bone and invade the central nervous system and the sinonasal tract. Isolated vitreous involvement is a rare presentation of intermediate- to high-grade NHL, which is frequently associated with concurrent or subsequent central nervous system NHL.[22,51,79] Figure 114-6 shows an example of orbital lymphoma. Low-grade orbital lesions are treated with radiation therapy alone with excellent disease control; localized intermediate- and high-grade NHL require chemotherapy and radiation therapy.[6]

Thyroid

Only 5% of thyroid malignancies are primary lymphomas,[46,68] but many tumors classified in the past as "anaplastic carcinoma" have in fact been reclassified

---

*References 4, 6, 11–13, 29, 36, 40, 46, 47, 50, 55, 70, 72, 75, 81, 84.

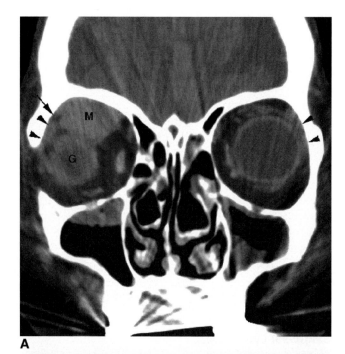

A

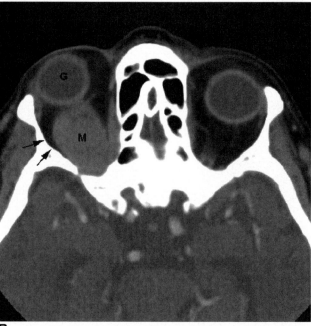

B

Figure 114-6. Low-grade B-cell lymphoma of the orbit in a 74-year-old woman. Coronal **(A)** and axial **(B)** CT images performed after IV contrast administration illustrate a mass (*M*) in the upper midorbit in extraconal location. This mass is separate from the lacrimal gland (*arrowheads* in **A**) as seen by a thin preserved fat plane (*arrow* in **A**) between the mass (*M*) and the lacrimal gland (*arrowheads* in **A**). Notice also the preserved fat plane (*arrows* in **B**) between the lateral wall of the orbit and the mass itself. G, globe.

as lymphoma due to more sophisticated immunochemical and molecular genetic diagnostic tools.[32,83] There is a striking 8:1 female to male predominance in thyroid lymphoma* and a strong association with prior Hashimoto's thyroiditis.[31,33,59] The median patient age at presentation is between 65 and 75 years. The most common histologic subtypes occurring in the thyroid are diffuse large cell and MALT.[23] T-cell lymphoma of the thyroid occurs primarily in Asia and appears to carry a worse prognosis. Most patients visit health care facilities exhibiting a painless mass in the thyroid region that grows rapidly, resulting in dysphagia, hoarseness, and dyspnea. Regional lymph node involvement is common, and about half of patients have abnormal thyroid function studies (Figure 114-7 shows thyroid NHL). Early-stage MALT is treated with radiation therapy with expected freedom from relapse rates of more than 90%.[3,42,77] Localized diffuse large cell lymphomas are treated with chemotherapy and radiation therapy and have an expected freedom from relapse of 50% to 70%, depending on prognostic factors.[25]

Sinonasal Lymphoma

Lymphoma accounts for approximately 10% of all sinonasal cancers[24] and, sinonasal lymphomas account for about 2% of all NHLs in the western world.[15,16,24,67] In Asia, sinonasal lymphoma is more common, accounting for 7% of all NHLs, and it is more likely to

be of the NK/T-cell variety rather than B-cell.[8,25] The distinction in cell type is important because of significant differences in natural history and response to treatment. Both B-cell and NK/T-cell lymphomas in this location are aggressive, but NK/T-cell tumors are more likely to arise in the nasal cavity, affect younger patients, and have an aggressive local course with an extremely poor prognosis.[28,63] Presenting symptoms depend on the site of origin within the sinonasal tract and include nasal passage obstruction, epistaxis, ulceration, cranial nerve deficits, facial swelling, proptosis, and pain. Figure 114-8 shows an example of a sinonasal lymphoma. Sinonasal lymphomas are

---

*References 7, 9, 37, 45, 59, 62, 74, 83.

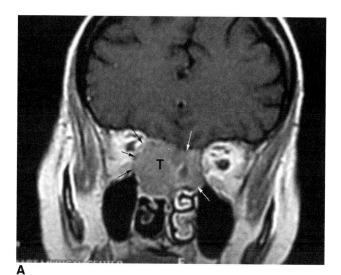

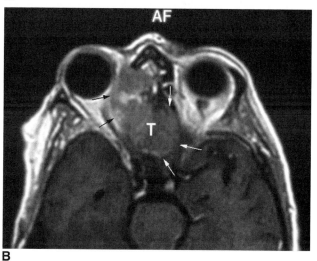

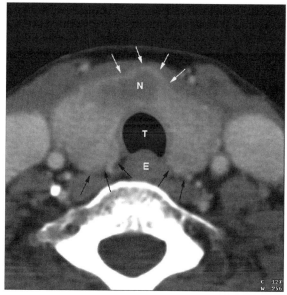

Figure 114-7. Diffuse large B-cell lymphoma of the thyroid in a 62-year-old woman. The thyroid gland including the isthmus *(arrowheads)* is enlarged, inhomogeneous, and extending posteriorly into the tracheoesophageal grooves bilaterally *(arrows)*. Focal areas of decreased enhancement are seen *(N)*, possibly representing focal necrosis. T, trachea; E, esophagus.

Figure 114-8. Diffuse large B-cell lymphoma of the ethmoid sinus in a 70-year-old woman. Coronal **(A)** and axial **(B)** T1-weighted images following gadolinium administration demonstrate a tumor *(T)* centered in the ethmoid air cells on the right extending the midline to the left *(white arrows)*. Laterally, the tumor involved the medial aspect of the orbit *(black arrows)*.

treated with chemotherapy and radiation therapy. Because of the particularly aggressive local course, radiation can be given concurrently or before chemotherapy in NK/T-cell lymphoma.[66]

Nodes

Lymphoma can arise at any nodal site in the head and neck, including jugular, spinal accessory, submental and submandibular, facial, buccal, canine fossa, parotid, preauricular, postauricular, and occipital nodes. The most common histologies are follicular, diffuse large cell, and mantle cell. Tissue evaluation and staging are essentially the same for nodal presentations as for extranodal presentations. Treatment is determined by histologic subtype, stage, and IPI.

Other Sites

NHL may occur in any tissue containing lymphoid cells. Rare cases have been reported in the larynx (Figure 114-9), buccal mucosa, and soft tissues of the face. In addition, some lesions may be neurotropic, infiltrating and thickening the nerve or depositing tumor nodules along the track of a nerve (Figure 114-10).[19] The skin may be the primary site for several broad categories of lymphoma, including indolent systemic cutaneous T-cell lymphomas (e.g., mycosis

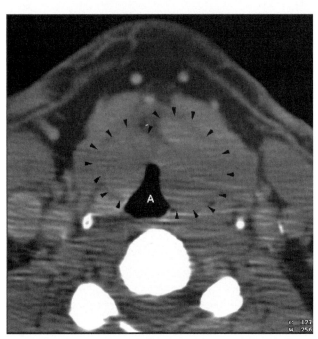

Figure 114-9. MALT lymphoma of the larynx in a 58-year-old man. Contrasted axial CT images through the larynx in a patient with low-grade B-cell NHL demonstrate diffuse infiltration of the aryepiglottic folds *(arrowheads)*. Other primary tumors, typically squamous cell carcinomas, are usually more focal. Endoscopic evaluation revealed that the tumor was submucosal in location. A, airway.

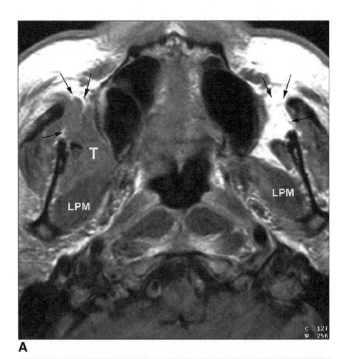

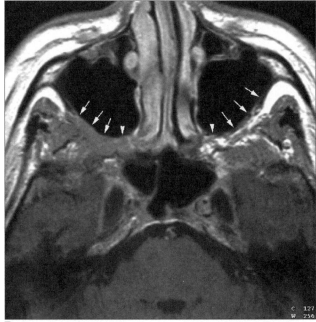

Figure 114-10. MALT lymphoma of the masticator space in a 65-year-old man. Axial gadolinium-enhanced **(A** and **B)** and coronal fat-suppressed T2-weighted **(C)** images through the mid-face demonstrate a mass *(T)* centered in the masticator space on the right. Inferiorly, the mass also involves the buccal space seen as obliteration of the buccal fat pad *(arrows* in **A)** on the right when compared to the left. The tumor *(T)* partially infiltrates the lateral pterygoid muscle and shows no significant involvement of the medial pterygoid muscle; see the normal lateral *(LPM)* and medial *(MPM)* pterygoid muscles on the left side for comparison **(A** and **C).**

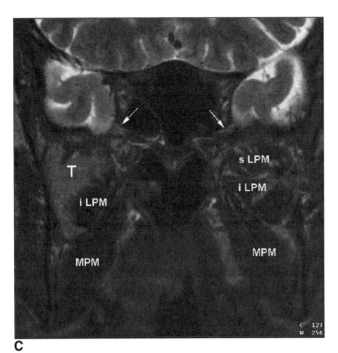

C

Figure 114-10, cont'd The mass also extends along the posterior wall of the maxillary sinus—reflected as obscuration of the fat plane (*arrows* in **B**) on the right when compared with the left—into the pterygopalatine fossa (*arrowhead* in **B**). The involvement of the latter is clearly identified as obliteration of the fat plane within the pterygopalatine fossa by a soft tissue mass on the right when compared with the left (*arrowheads* in **B**). The tumor continues superiorly via the pterygopalatine fossa and inferior orbital fissure into the foramen rotundum to involve the second division of the trigeminal nerve on the right (*white arrow* in **C**).

fungoids), large cell T-cell lymphomas (e.g., anaplastic large cell), and cutaneous B-cell lymphoma (e.g., follicular, marginal-zone, and diffuse large cell). Occasionally, chronic lymphocytic leukemia will present with chloromas (lymphoid deposits in the skin). These lesions all tend to be sensitive to radiation therapy and, in the early stages, can be curable.

HODGKIN'S LYMPHOMA

HL arises almost exclusively in nodal tissue. In the head and neck region, two scenarios are likely: (1) enlarged rubbery painless nodes in the low neck and/or supraclavicular fossa, or (2) above the hyoid in the submental, submandibular, periauricular, or periparotid nodes. Patients, particularly those with bulky disease, may have constitutional "B" symptoms including fevers higher than 101°F (38°C), unexplained weight loss of more than 10% of body weight in the preceding 6 months, and drenching night sweats. The disease spreads in an orderly fashion to contiguous nodal regions. The median patient age is in the low to mid-20s, with half of the patients between 15 and 30 years

of age; HL is rare in patients younger than age 10 and after age 60. The age distribution is bimodal with a peak in the low 20s and a second peak in the low 40s. Evaluation is similar to that in NHL, with morphologic and immunohistochemical examination of diagnostic tissue and CT imaging of the head and neck, chest, abdomen, and pelvis, which are all areas at risk for involvement. Patients with clinical stage III or IV disease, B symptoms, or abnormal blood indices also require a bone marrow biopsy. The Ann Arbor staging system is used (see Table 114-2). The presence of B symptoms is an independent negative prognostic factor indicated in the Ann Arbor staging system by a postscript. The presence of extranodal disease is indicated by a postscript of E and splenic disease by a postscript of S. Prognostic factors other than stage include tumor bulk, presence of large mediastinal adenopathy, extranodal disease, number of sites involved, sedimentation rate, complete blood count, and patient age. Both chemotherapy and radiation therapy are effective treatments for HL, and most patients receive both. The overall survival rate in HL approaches 90% with standard therapy.

REFERENCES

1. American Joint Committee on Cancer: *AJCC cancer staging manual*, ed 6. New York, Springer, 2002.
2. Anderson LG, Talal N: The spectrum of benign to malignant lymphoproliferation in Sjögren's syndrome, *Clin Exp Immunol* 10:199–221, 1972.
3. Aozasa K and others: Malignant lymphomas of the thyroid gland: analysis of 79 patients with emphasis on histologic prognostic factors, *Cancer* 58:100–104, 1986.
4. Auw-Haedrich C and others: Long term outcome of ocular adnexal lymphoma subtyped according to the REAL classification. Revised European and American Lymphoma, *Br J Ophthalmol* 85:63–69, 2001.
5. Aviles A and others: Treatment of non-Hodgkin's lymphoma of Waldeyer's ring: radiotherapy versus chemotherapy versus combined therapy, *Eur J Cancer B Oral Oncol* 32B:19–23, 1996.
6. Bolek TW and others: Radiotherapy in the management of orbital lymphoma, *Int J Radiat Oncol Biol Phys* 44:31–36, 1999.
7. Butler JS, Jr., Brady LW, Amendola BE: Lymphoma of the thyroid: report of five cases and review, *Am J Clin Oncol* 13:64–69, 1990.
8. Chan JK and others: Most nasal/nasopharyngeal lymphomas are peripheral T-cell neoplasms, *Am J Surg Pathol* 11:418–429, 1987.
9. Compagno J, Oertel JE: Malignant lymphoma and other lymphoproliferative disorders of the thyroid gland: a clinico-pathologic study of 245 cases, *Am J Clin Pathol* 74:1–11, 1980.
10. Costes-Martineau V and others: Anaplastic lymphoma kinase (ALK) protein expressing lymphoma after liver transplantation: case report and literature review, *J Clin Pathol* 55:868–871, 2002.
11. Coupland SE and others: Lymphoproliferative lesions of the ocular adnexa: analysis of 112 cases, *Ophthalmology* 105:1430–1441, 1998.

12. Dunbar SF and others: Conjunctival lymphoma: results and treatment with a single anterior electron field; a lens sparing approach, *Int J Radiat Oncol Biol Phys* 19:249–257, 1990.

13. Esmaeli B and others: Clinical presentation and treatment of secondary orbital lymphoma, *Opthal Plast Reconstr Surg* 18:247–253, 2002.

14. Ezzat AA and others: Localized non-Hodgkin's lymphoma of Waldeyer's ring: clinical features, management and prognosis of 130 adult patients, *Head Neck* 23:547–558, 2001.

15. Freeman C, Berg JW, Cutler SJ: Occurrence and prognosis of extranodal lymphomas, *Cancer* 29:252–260, 1972.

16. Frierson HF, Jr, Mills SE, Innes DJ, Jr.: Non-Hodgkin's lymphomas of the sinonasal region: histologic subtypes and their clinicopathologic features, *Am J Clin Pathol* 81:721–727, 1984.

17. Fuller LM and others: Significance of tumor size and radiation dose to local control in stage I-III diffuse large cell lymphoma treated with CHOP-Bleo and radiation, *Int J Radiat Oncol Biol Phys* 31:3–11, 1995.

18. Garcia-Serra A and others: Carcinoma of the skin with perinerual invasion, *Head Neck* 25:1027–1033, 2003.

19. Garcia-Serra A and others: Management of neurotropic low-grade B-cell lymphoma: report of two cases, *Head Neck* 25:972–976, 2003.

20. Glass AG, Karnell LH, Menck HR: The National Cancer Data Base report on non-Hodgkin's lymphoma, *Cancer* 80: 2311–2320, 1997.

21. Glick JH and others: An ECOG randomized phase III trial of CHOP vs. CHOP + radiotherapy (XRT) for intermediate grade early stage non-Hodgkin's lymphoma (NHL) [abstract], *Proc Annu Meet Am Soc Clin Oncol* 14:391, 1995.

22. Goldey SH and others: Immunophenotypic characterization of an unusual T-cell lymphoma presenting as anterior uveitis: a clinicopathologic case report, *Arch Ophthalmol* 107: 1349–1353, 1989.

23. Gospodarowicz MK, Sutcliffe SB: The extranodal lymphomas, *Semin Radiat Oncol* 5:281–300, 1995.

24. Grau C and others: Sino-nasal cancer in Denmark 1982-1991: a nationwide survey, *Acta Oncol* 40:19–23, 2001.

25. Ha CS, Shadle KM, Medeiros LJ: Localized non-Hodgkin lymphoma involving the thyroid gland, *Cancer* 91:629–635, 2001.

26. Hanna E and others: Extranodal lymphomas of the head and neck: a 20-year experience, *Arch Otolaryngol Head Neck Surg* 123:1318–1323, 1997.

27. Harris NL and others: A revised European-American classification of lymphoid neoplasms: a proposal from the International Lymphoma Study Group, *Blood* 84:1361–1392, 1994.

28. Hatta C and others: Non-Hodgkin's malignant lymphoma of the sinonasal tract: treatment outcome for 53 patients according to REAL classification, *Auris Nasus Larynx* 28: 55–60, 2001.

29. Henderson JW, Banks PM, Yeatts RP: T-cell lymphoma of the orbit, *Mayo Clin Proc* 64:940–944, 1989.

30. Hew WS and others: Primary T cell lymphoma of salivary gland: a report of a case and review of the literature, *J Clin Pathol* 55:61–63, 2002.

31. Holm LE, Blomgren H, Lowhagen T: Cancer risks in patients with chronic lymphocytic thyroiditis, *N Engl J Med* 312: 601–604, 1985.

32. Holting C and others: Immunohistochemical reclassification of anaplastic carcinoma reveals small and giant cell lymphoma, *World J Surg* 14:291–294, 1990.

33. Hyjek E, Isaacson PG: Primary B cell lymphoma of the thyroid and its relationship to Hashimoto's thyroiditis, *Hum Pathol* 19:1315–1326, 1988.

34. Jaehne M and others: The clinical presentation of non-Hodgkin lymphomas of the major salivary glands, *Acta Otolaryngol* 121:647–651, 2001.

35. Jaffe ES and others: World Health Organization classification of neoplastic diseases of the hematopoietic and lymphoid tissues: a progress report, *Am J Clin Pathol* 111:S8–S12, 1999.

36. Jenkins C and others: Histological features of ocular adnexal lymphoma (REAL classification) and their association with patient morbidity and survival, *Br J Ophthalmol* 84:907–913, 2000.

37. Junor EJ, Paul J, Reed NS: Primary non-Hodgkin's lymphoma of the thyroid, *Eur J Surg Oncol* 18:313–321, 1992.

38. Kamath SS and others: The impact of radiotherapy dose and other treatment-related and clinical factors on in-field control in stage I and II non-Hodgkin's lymphoma, *Int J Radiat Oncol Biol Phys* 44:563–568, 1999.

39. Kassan SS, Thomas TL: Increased risk of lymphoma in sicca syndrome, *Ann Intern Med* 89:888–892, 1978.

40. Knowles DM and others: Lymphoid hyperplasia and malignant lymphoma occurring in the ocular adnexa (orbit, conjunctiva, and eyelids): a prospective multiparametric analysis of 108 cases during 1977 to 1987, *Hum Pathol* 22:959–973, 1990.

41. Kumar S, Pruthi RK, Nichols WL: Acquired von Willebrand's syndrome: a single institution experience, *Am J Hematol* 72:243–247, 2003.

42. Laing RW, Hoskin P, Hudson BV: The significance of MALT histology in thyroid lymphoma: a review of patients from the BNLI and Royal Marsden Hospital, *Clin Oncol* 6:300–304, 1994.

43. Lindahl T and others: Relationship between Epstein-Barr virus (EBV) DNA and the EBV-determined nuclear antigen (EBNA) in Burkitt lymphoma biopsies and other lymphoproliferative malignancies, *Int J Cancer* 13:764–772, 1974.

44. Link MP and others: Results of treatment of childhood localized non-Hodgkin's lymphoma with combination chemotherapy with or without radiotherapy, *N Engl J Med* 322:1169–1174, 1990.

45. Logue JP and others: Primary malignant lymphoma of the thyroid: a clinicopathological analysis, *Int J Radiat Oncol Biol Phys* 22:929–933, 1992.

46. Mannami T and others: Clinical, histopathological, and immunogenetic analysis of ocular adnexal lymphoproliferative disorders: characterization of malt lymphoma and reactive lymphoid hyperplasia, *Mod Pathol* 14:641–649, 2001.

47. Margo CE, Mulla ZD: Malignant tumors of the orbit. Analysis of the Florida Cancer Registry, *Ophthalmology* 105:185–190, 1998.

48. Matsuzuka F and others: Clinical aspects of primary thyroid lymphoma: diagnosis and treatment based on our experience of 119 cases, *Thyroid* 3:93–99, 1993.

49. Mbulaiteye SM and others: Immune deficiency and risk for malignancy among persons with AIDS. *J Acquir Imm Defic Synd* 32:527–533, 2003.

50. McNally L, Jakobeic FA, Knowles DM II: Clinical, morphologic, immunophenotypic, and molecular genetic analysis of bilateral ocular adnexal lymphoid neoplasms in 17 patients, *Am J Ophthalmol* 103:555–568, 1987.

51. Mendenhall NP, Lynch JW, Jr.: The low-grade lymphomas, *Semin Radiat Oncol* 5:254–266, 1995.

52. Miller TP and others: Chemotherapy alone compared with chemotherapy plus radiotherapy for localized intermediate- and high-grade non-Hodgkin's lymphoma, *N Engl J Med* 339:21–26, 1998.

53. Miller TP and others: Three cycles of CHOP (3) plus radiotherapy (RT) is superior to eight cycles of CHOP (8) alone for localized intermediate and high grade non-Hodgkin's

lymphoma (NHL): a Southwest Oncology Group study [abstract], *Proc Annu Meet Am Soc Clin Oncol* 15:411, 1996.

54. Moshous D and others: Partial T and B lymphocyte immunodeficiency and predisposition to lymphoma in patients with hypomorphic mutations in Artemis, *J Clin Invest* 111:381–387, 2003.

55. Nakata M and others: Histology according to the Revised European-American Lymphoma Classification significantly predicts the prognosis of ocular adnexal lymphoma, *Leuk Lymphoma* 32:533–543, 1999.

56. National Cancer Institute sponsored study of classification of non-Hodgkin's lymphomas: summary and description of a working formulation for clinical usage. The Non-Hodgkin's Lymphoma Pathologic Classification Project, *Cancer* 49: 2112–2135, 1982.

57. Niller HH and others: The in vivo binding site for oncoprotein c-Myc in the promoter for Epstein-Barr virus (EBV) encoding RNA (EBER) 1 suggests a specific role for EBV in lymphomagenesis, *Med Sci Monit* 9:HYI-9, 2003.

58. A predictive model for aggressive non-Hodgkin's lymphoma: the International Non-Hodgkin's Lymphoma Prognostic Factors Project, *N Engl J Med* 329:987–994, 1993.

59. Pederson RK, Pederson NT: Primary non-Hodgkin's lymphoma of the thyroid gland: a population based study, *Histopathology* 28:25–32, 1996.

60. Poiesz BJ and others: Detection and isolation of type C retrovirus particles from fresh and cultured lymphocytes of a patient with cutaneous T-cell lymphoma, *Proc Natl Acad Sci USA* 77:7415–7419, 1980.

61. Preciado MV and others: Epstein Barr virus-associated lymphoma in HIV-infected children, *Pathol Res Pract* 198:327–332, 2002.

62. Pyke CM and others: Non-Hodgkin's lymphoma of the thyroid: is more than biopsy necessary? *World J Surg* 16:604–609, 1992.

63. Quraishi MS and others: Non-Hodgkin's lymphoma of the sinonasal tract, *Laryngoscope* 110:1489–1492, 2000.

64. Raderer M and others: Somatostatin-receptor scintigraphy for staging and follow-up of patients with extraintestinal marginal zone B-cell lymphoma of the mucosa associated lymphoid tissue (MALT)-type, *Br J Cancer* 85:1462–1466, 2001.

65. Reske SN, Kotzerke J: FDG-PET for clinical use. Results of the 3rd German Interdisciplinary Consensus Conference, "Onko-PET III," 21 July and 19 September 2000, *Eur J Nucl Med* 28:1707–1723, 2001.

66. Ribrag V and others: Early locoregional high-dose radiotherapy is associated with long-term disease control in localized primary angiocentric lymphoma of the nose and nasopharynx, *Leukemia* 15:1123–1126, 2001.

67. Robbins KT and others: Primary lymphomas of the nasal cavity and paranasal sinuses, *Cancer* 56:814–819, 1985.

68. Rosai J: *Malignant lymphoma*. In Rosai J, editor: *Atlas of tumor pathology, tumors of the thyroid gland*. Washington, DC, 2003, AFIP.

69. Sandoval C, Swift M: Hodgkin disease in ataxia-telegiectasia patients with poor outcomes, *Med Pediatr Oncol* 40:162–166, 2003.

70. Sasai K and others: Non-Hodgkin's lymphoma of the ocular adnexa, *Acta Oncol* 40:485–490, 2001.

71. Saul SH, Kapadia SB: Primary lymphoma of Waldeyer's ring: clinicopathologic study of 68 cases, *Cancer* 56:157–166, 1985.

72. Shields CL and others: Conjunctival lymphoid tumors: clinical analysis of 117 cases and relationship to systemic lymphoma, *Ophthalmology* 108:979–984, 2001.

73. Simon R and others: The Non-Hodgkin Lymphoma Pathologic Classification Project: long-term follow-up of 1153 patients with non-Hodgkin lymphomas, *Ann Intern Med* 109:939–945, 1988.

74. Skarsgard ED, Connors JM, Robins RE: A current analysis of primary lymphoma of the thyroid, *Arch Surg* 126:1199–1203, 1991.

75. Takamura H and others: A case of orbital solitary fibrous tumor, *Jpn J Opthalmology* 45:412–419, 2001.

76. Talal N, Sokoloff L, Barth WF: Extrasalivary lymphoid abnormalities in Sjogren's syndrome (reticulum cell sarcoma, "pseudolymphoma," macroglobulinemia), *Am J Med* 43:50–65, 1967.

77. Thieblemont C and others: Primary thyroid lymphoma is a heterogeneous disease, *J Clin Endocrinol Metab* 87:105–111, 2002.

78. Tsang RW, Gospodarowicz MK: *Non-Hodgkin's lymphoma*. In: Gunderson LL, Tepper JE, editors: *Clinical radiation oncology*. Philadelphia, 2000, Churchill Livingstone, pp 1158–1188.

79. Tuaillon N, Chan CC: Molecular analysis of primary central nervous system and primary intraocular lymphomas, *Curr Mol Med* 1:259–272, 2001.

80. Varoczy L and others: Malignant lymphoma-associated autoimmune diseases: a descriptive epidemiological study, *Rhuematol Int* 22:233–237, 2002.

81. White WL and others: Ocular adnexal lymphoma: a clinicopathologic study with identification of lymphomas of mucosa-associated lymphoid tissue type, *Ophthalmology* 102:1994–2006, 1995.

82. Wirth A and others: Fluorine-18 fluorodeoxyglucose positron emission tomography, gallium-67 scintigraphy, and conventional staging for Hodgkin's disease and non-Hodgkin's lymphoma, *Am J Med* 112:262–268, 2002.

83. Wolf BC and others: Immunohistochemical analysis of small cell tumors of the thyroid gland: an Eastern Cooperative Oncology Group study, *Hum Pathol* 23:1252–1261, 1992.

84. Wotherspoon AC and others: Primary low-grade B-cell lymphoma of the conjunctiva: a mucosa-associated lymphoid tissue type lymphoma, *Histopathology* 23:417–424, 1993.

85. Zulman J, Jaffe R, Talal N: Evidence that the malignant lymphoma of Sjogren's syndrome is a monoclonal B-cell neoplasm, *N Engl J Med* 299:1215–1220, 2003.

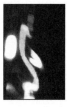

RADIATION THERAPY AND MANAGEMENT OF THE CERVICAL LYMPH NODES

Bernard Cummings
John Kim
Brian O'Sullivan

INTRODUCTION

Management of the regional lymph nodes is integral to the overall treatment of malignant tumors of the head and neck. This chapter considers several aspects of radiation therapy specific to management of the lymph nodes. Many of the concepts described were established several decades ago on the basis of the findings of clinical examination and standard histopathologic sectioning of nodes removed surgically. The rapid evolution over the past decade of anatomic and functional imaging, and histopathology and molecular pathology, has provided new insights into many aspects of neck node management, although there has not yet been time to assess fully the impact of these new techniques. There has also been major progress in the technical aspects of radiation treatment, allowing revision of long-established concepts of the tolerance of normal tissues to radiation and permitting consideration of the delivery of higher and more effective radiation doses.

ANATOMY AND PATHOLOGY

When considering management of the cervical lymph nodes, it is essential to understand the normal anatomic distribution of nodes, the pattern of metastases associated with different malignancies, and the difficulties in determining whether nodes are involved by metastatic cancer. Also, certain features peculiar to lymph node metastases may affect prognosis and influence the choice of management.

Normal Anatomic Patterns

Approximately one-third of the more than 500 lymph nodes in the body lay above the clavicles. The lymphatics and nodes are found within the cellular and fatty connective tissue around the muscles, neurovascular structures, and organs. The pathways of lymph flow have been studied directly by techniques such as lymphography[61,102] and indirectly by review of the patterns of lymph node metastases observed in cancers arising in different sites.[31,109,125,165] In general, malignant tumors that arise laterally, away from the midline, spread to ipsilateral lymph node groups. However, tumors that arise at or close to the midline and those originating anywhere in the nasopharynx or posterior third of the tongue may spread contralaterally as a result of the patterns of development and lymphatic flow determined in the embryo.[61] If normal pathways are interrupted, abnormal patterns of node metastases may occur. Some structures, such as the vocal cords and the mucosal lining of the paranasal sinuses, have few lymphatics.

In the lymphographic studies, deep lymphatic vessels underneath the superficial cutaneous fascia in the retroauricular region[61] or lymphatics in the tongue or floor of the mouth[102] were cannulated and injected. The investigative procedure of sentinel node biopsy uses injection of tracer substances closely adjacent to the tumor.[168] Lymphography shows that the normal pattern of lymph flow in the neck is downward and medial[61] (Figure 115-1). Lymphography and neck dissection specimens identify a group of 20 or more lymph nodes in the upper neck near the angle of the jaw. This group constitutes a junctional area from which lymph flows downward in the neck to nodes along the jugular vein and spinal accessory nerve. This junctional node group receives the regional drainage from much of the nasopharynx, oropharynx, and upper part of the larynx and hypopharynx. These nodes receive the efferent lymphatic vessels from the circle of lymph nodes that lie where the head and neck merge (this circle includes the submental, submandibular, retropharyngeal, parotid, retroauricular,

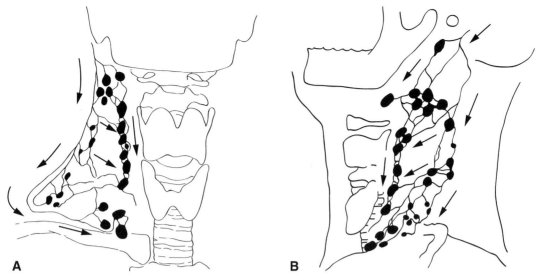

Figure 115-1. Cervical lymph flow as visualized by lymphography. **A,** Anteroposterior projection. **B,** Lateral projection. (From Fisch U: *Lymphographische untersuchungen uber das zervikale Lymphsystem*, Basel, 1968, S. Karger.)

and occipital groups). These junctional nodes are often termed the jugulodigastric lymph nodes. The lymph nodes in the retropharyngeal, paralaryngeal, and paratracheal regions are not visualized by subcutaneous lymphography, suggesting that lymph from these regions normally flows laterally into the jugular system or downward into the mediastinum. Inferiorly, the lymph from the jugular and spinal accessory systems drains to the confluence of the jugular and subclavian veins or into the thoracic duct on the left and lymphatic duct on the right.

Although groups of lymph nodes are generally named according to the structures to which they lie adjacent, for example, jugular nodes, these groupings seem to have anatomic rather than functional significance. A variety of nomenclature has been used to describe the distribution of nodes. The International Union Against Cancer (UICC) grouped the principal lymph nodes of the neck into 12 groups to assist with staging.[173] An important and widely used standardized classification for neck dissection introduced in 1991, and updated in 2002, divided the nodes of the neck into six basic levels, some of which are subdivided.[157] In this classification, the lymph nodes are related to landmarks identifiable at neck dissection and do not include node groups not routinely removed by radical neck dissection (for example, the retropharyngeal nodes). A comparison of the UICC grouping and Robbins' revised classification is shown in Table 115-1. There have also been efforts to harmonize the anatomic landmarks and boundaries used in radiology and surgery of the neck.[172] Radiation oncologists are also adopting this standardized termi-

nology and incorporating it into their planning protocols.[82,134,192]

Patterns of Cervical Node Metastases from Squamous Cell Cancers

Several authors have cataloged the locations of lymph node metastases identified by physical and radiologic examination, although the full impact of modern imaging techniques has not yet been integrated into these patterns. A summary of some of those studies is shown in Table 115-2. Most abnormal nodes are found in level II, the upper jugular level. The highest proportion of contralateral nodes is also found in level II. The authors whose reports form the basis of Table 115-2 did not identify the number of patients with midline cancers, so that the potential for contralateral spread from a well-lateralized primary cancer cannot be deduced from the table. It is generally considered that the pattern of nodal metastases from any cancer is similar in both the ipsilateral and contralateral neck.

The data in Table 115-2 are organized according to the levels used to categorize nodes removed at neck dissection.[157] Hence, metastases to nodes such as the preauricular or retropharyngeal groups are not included. Imaging with modern computed tomography (CT) or magnetic resonance imaging (MRI) techniques has shown good correlation with the occasional studies that have included pathologic examination of the retropharyngeal nodes. The retropharyngeal nodes lay between the skull base and cervical C3 to C4 level. Metastases to these nodes are associated particularly with nasopharyngeal cancer (approximately 30% of

TABLE 115-1

COMPARISON BETWEEN THE TNM ATLAS TERMINOLOGY AND THE REVISED ROBBINS' CLASSIFICATION OF THE LYMPH NODES OF THE NECK

TNM Atlas (1992)		Robbins' Classification (2002)	
Group number	Descriptor	Level	Descriptor
1	Submental	IA	Submental
2	Submandibular	IB	Submandibular
3	Cranial jugular	IIA (anterior)	Upper jugular
		IIB (posterior)	Upper jugular
4	Medial jugular	III	Middle jugular
5	Caudal jugular	IV	Lower jugular
6	Dorsal cervical along the spinal accessory nerve	VA (superior)	Spinal accessory
7	Supraclavicular	VB	Transverse cervical and supraclavicular
8	Prelaryngeal and paratracheal	VI	Anterior compartment
9	Retropharyngeal		
10	Parotid		
11	Buccal		
12	Retroauricular and occipital		

Modified from Gregoire V and others: *Radiother Oncol* 56:135, 2000.

TABLE 115-2

DISTRIBUTION OF CLINICAL METASTATIC NECK NODES FROM HEAD AND NECK SQUAMOUS CELL CARCINOMA

Tumor Site	Patients with N+ (%)	Distribution of Metastatic Lymph Nodes per Level (percentage of the node-positive patients)				
		I	II	III	IV	V
Oral cavity (n = 787)	36	42/3.5*	79/8	18/3	5/1	1/0
Oropharynx (n = 1479)	64	13/2	81/24	23/5	9/2.5	13/3
Hypopharynx (n = 847)	70	2/0	80/13	51/4	20/3	24/2
Supraglottic larynx (n = 428)	55	2/0	71/21	48/10	18/7	15/4
Nasopharynx (n = 440)	80	9/5	71/56	36/32	22/15	32/26

*Ipsilateral/contralateral nodes.
Adapted from Gregoire V and others: *Radiother Oncol* 56:135, 2000.

cases) and posterior wall oropharyngeal or hypopharyngeal cancers (approximately 25%), predominantly in patients with more advanced primary cancers and node metastases elsewhere in the neck.[43,136]

Although clinical observation suggests that metastatic involvement of the various lymph node regions usually progresses from superior to inferior in the neck, lymph node groups may be bypassed even on normal lymphography.[61,102] Discontinuous, or "skip," patterns of metastases were described in from 3% (2 of 64)[175] to 10% (9 of 90)[30] of patients below dissected areas that were pathologically node negative.

The risk of lymph node involvement by metastatic squamous cell carcinoma varies according to the site of origin, size, and histologic grade of the primary tumor. For most sites in the oral cavity, soft palate, glottic larynx, nasal cavity, and paranasal sinuses, the risk increases as the size of the primary tumor increases.[32,109] The association between the size of the primary tumor and nodal status is not so pronounced for other sites. For primary carcinomas of the oropharynx, the risk of lymph node involvement is 50% or more, and the likelihood of nodal disease increases only moderately as the primary cancer enlarges.[15,109] Carcinomas of the supraglottic larynx, hypopharynx, and nasopharynx are associated with a progressively greater risk of lymph node metastases (approximately 50%, 75%, and 85%, respectively), and even small primary carcinomas arising in these sites are frequently accompanied by lymph node metastases.[109]

Review of both therapeutic and elective radical neck dissection specimens shows that the patterns of nodal metastases generally mirror those found by clinical examination. Gregoire and others[82] analyzed several publications from the Memorial Sloan-Kettering Cancer Center.[37,38,164,165] In patients who underwent therapeutic neck dissection, there was typically pathologic infiltration of one nodal level beyond that apparent clinically. This subclinical infiltration was found most frequently in distal node groups, but up to 15% of clinical N_0 patients with oropharyngeal cancers had involvement of submandibular (level I) nodes, suggesting retrograde spread, and similar patterns of limited retrograde spread were observed for other primary tumor sites.

Assessment of the Neck Nodes

Errors in assessing the status of the cervical nodes may arise from several causes. Normal lymph nodes vary in size from 0.1 to 3 cm.[56,57] Sako[160] suggested that the lower limit of palpability for a lymph node is approximately 0.5 cm in diameter in superficial areas of the neck and 1 cm in deeper areas. The limits of resolution of currently available techniques of CT scanning, MRI, and ultrasonography are in the range of 0.5 to 1 cm.[40] Although improvements in imaging have increased the detection of node metastases, the criteria of abnormality, typically size, the appearance of necrosis, abnormalities of contrast enhancement, and evidence of extracapsular spread still lack the precision of histopathologic examination.[179] However, even histologic examination of the nodes is not free from potential error. Sampling errors, insensitive histopathologic techniques, and skip metastases are possible explanations why 4% to 8% of patients have tumor recurrence in the neck after nodal dissection, although no carcinoma was identified on histologic examination of radical neck dissection specimens.[51,52]

By use of traditional histopathologic techniques, histologically positive nodes have been found in from 4%[22] to 60%[111] (usual range, 20%–40%) when the neck was considered negative on palpation. In one series,[52] a clinically negative neck was equally likely to contain multiple histologically positive nodes (13%) and a single positive node (16%). Not all enlarged nodes harbor metastatic cancer, although fewer false-positive results occur (8%–35%) than false-negative results.[22,160] The rate of false-positive results decreases when lymph node masses are larger than approximately 3 cm.[69] DeSanto and others[52] found that 14% (49 of 359) of patients with a single enlarged node and 4% (8 of 188) of those with multiple clinically abnormal nodes had negative histologic findings. In the series reviewed by Gregoire and others,[82] the overall sensitivity and specificity of the clinical examination of the neck (not augmented by modern imaging

techniques) was 85% and 62%, respectively. Serial sections,[193] immunohistochemical, and molecular pathology techniques[168,179] may disclose small deposits of cancer in nodes that would otherwise be overlooked. In one typical study, micrometastases (defined as <3 mm) were found in 21 of 96 (22%) elective neck dissection specimens.[179] In 9 of the 36 (25%) tumor-positive specimens, and 9 of the 96 (9%) specimens overall, only micrometastases were found. The clinical significance of micrometastases in lymph nodes discovered during neck dissection, or by sentinel node biopsy techniques, remains uncertain, and many studies are in progress. When micrometastases are included in the statistics for sentinel node biopsy in head and neck cancer, the overall sensitivity of this technique is said to be approximately 90%, similar to that of staging neck dissection.[159,168]

The staging of neck node metastases at this time is divided broadly into clinical and pathologic classifications.[79,171] There are, as yet, insufficient data from newer imaging and pathologic techniques to allow development of a "minimum" set of required evaluations. Accordingly, there is considerable variation in the information used to stage patients, both within and between treatment centers. It must be assumed that substantial "stage shifting" is occurring. Any comparisons between the series discussed in this chapter, particularly between current and older series, should be made with more than the usual circumspection attached to such comparisons.

Prognostic Factors

Prognosis correlates with the presence or absence of lymph node metastases and is invariably worse for all primary tumor sites when lymph nodes are involved. As noted earlier, the significance of micrometastases is not established. Clinical staging systems most commonly subdivide lymph node metastases according to size (currently at 3 cm and at 6 cm) and whether the metastatic nodes are unilateral or bilateral, single or multiple, and by location in the neck. For head and neck squamous cell cancers and adenocarcinomas, the definition of the nodal (N) staging categories is the same for all head and neck sites except nasopharynx and thyroid.[79,171] This likely reflects a lack of relevant data rather than true uniformity of biologic behavior of metastases arising from different primary cancer sites.

Histopathologic features with prognostic discriminative value have also been described, including in particular extranodal extension of cancer, the presence of which significantly worsens the prognosis, particularly for recurrence in the neck and for survival (Table 115-3). Cachin[32,33] found capsular rupture

TABLE 115-3

CORRELATION BETWEEN LYMPH NODE INVOLVEMENT AND CLINICAL COURSE OF CARCINOMA OF THE UPPER RESPIRATORY AND DIGESTIVE TRACTS

	N–	N+	N+R–	N+R+
3-Year survival*	65%	25%	33%	16%
Primary tumor recurrence[†]	20%	19%	19%	19%
Neck recurrence[†]	14%	22%	14%	27%
Distal metastases[†]	4%	10%	8%	11%
Total recurrence[†]	38%	51%	41%	57%

Adapted from Cachin Y and others: *Otolaryngol Clin North Am* 12:145, 1979.
N, Lymph node; R, capsular rupture; –, absent; +, present.
*Based on 601 cases.
[†]Based on 944 cases.

with carcinomas of all sites and with all grades of squamous cell carcinomas. Rupture in even a single node was as significant as rupture in multiple nodes. Extension of cancer outside the lymph node was found in 40% of histologically involved nodes <2 cm in size and in 80% of those 4 cm or more. Capsular rupture has also been found in up to 16% (18 of 109) of patients with clinically negative necks who had elective node dissection.[3] Carter and others[39] found that the risk of recurrence in the neck was nearly 10 times greater in patients with macroscopic transcapsular tumor spread than in those with microscopic or no extracapsular extension. Some have measured the extent of extracapsular spread in millimeters and have reported worse prognosis with extension >2 mm.[60,80]

In a multifactorial study of 1330 patients, it was found that, irrespective of T classification, the presence of extracapsular tumor extension, of three or more positive lymph nodes, or of lymph node involvement in level IV had a similar impact on prognosis, with a risk of nodal recurrence two times higher and a risk of distant metastases three times higher compared with patients without one of these three features of nodal involvement.[106]

Reviewers of large databases suggest that the probability of control of the primary tumor decreases as the extent of cervical node metastases increases. However, in general, more extensive nodal metastases are associated with larger primary tumors.[17,114,119,187] Other prognostic factors associated with lymph node metastases include the observation that necrotic nodes are less chemoresponsive and radioresponsive,[126] presumably because of poor blood supply and hypoxia. Direct measurement of oxygen levels has

shown that nodes that were poorly oxygenated before irradiation were more likely to contain apparently viable residual tumor cells at later neck dissection.[27] Also, there was a significant correlation between the median measured Po_2 of primary tumors and their neck metastases.[21] Locoregional failure was more common in patients in whom the median of the measured Po_2 values was <2.5 mm Hg.[131]

Several molecular markers of potential prognostic value have been identified, although the relative importance of assay of these markers in the primary tumor and in metastatic nodes is not yet known.[151,156,180]

ADVANCES IN TECHNICAL RADIATION THERAPY AND RADIATION RESPONSE MODIFYING DRUGS

There have been substantial advances in engineering and computing over the past two decades that have led to improvements in radiation dose distribution within the body. As a result, many of the limitations of the techniques with which the clinical results described in this chapter were achieved have now been overcome. It is anticipated that the morbidity of treatment of the cervical nodes will decrease, and the effectiveness of radiation treatment will improve. The introduction of three-dimensional (3D) conformal techniques, intensity-modulated radiation therapy (IMRT), and other techniques still in development has allowed relative sparing of the parotid salivary glands, such that permanent xerostomia need no longer be an inevitable accompaniment of the treatment of many head and neck cancers.[54] An example of the radiation dose distributions achievable is shown in Figure 115-2. Because critical structures can now be excluded with confidence from the high-dose radiation volume, studies to confirm the anticipated effectiveness of higher tumor doses can be undertaken.[108]

In parallel to these technical advances is the development of drugs that act as radiation protectors of normal tissue, thereby reducing morbidity and possibly allowing the delivery of higher radiation doses. Although none of these drugs is yet in general clinical use, the prototype, amifostine, has shown the potential for pharmacologic manipulation of radiation response.[5,149] There have also been extensive studies of concurrent radiation and cytotoxic chemotherapy protocols, and although it remains unclear whether most drugs simply provide additional cytotoxicity or act also as radiosensitizers, this is a major field of current research.[149]

SQUAMOUS CELL CARCINOMAS
Elective Irradiation of Clinically Normal Lymph Nodes

Elective regional lymph node irradiation (ENI) is used frequently because of the relatively high incidence of

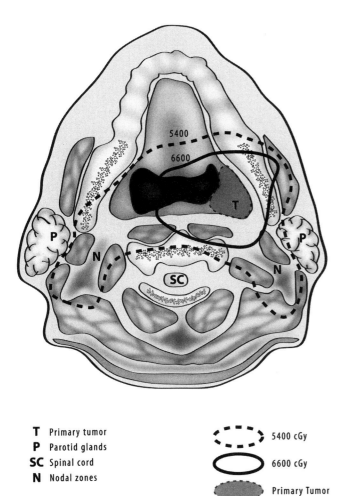

T   Primary tumor
P   Parotid glands
SC Spinal cord
N   Nodal zones

- - - - 5400 cGy

⬭ 6600 cGy

▬ Primary Tumor

Figure 115-2. Line drawing of axial-computed tomography plan for intensity-modulated radiation treatment of a stage T_2N_0 cancer of the tonsil. The dose to the primary tumor is 6600 cGy; the dose to the lymph node regions is 5400 cGy; the dose to the parotid glands is <2600 cGy; the dose to the spinal cord is <4500 cGy.

histologically positive nodes present in patients with clinically normal nodes and because during follow-up of patients in whom only the primary tumor was treated, an appreciable proportion eventually show neck node metastases. The risk of node involvement at some time is at least 15% to 20% for most primary cancer sites in the head and neck, although wide variation exists among different series (Table 115-4). Prophylactic management of clinically normal lymph nodes depends on the premise that elective treatment is more effective than the management necessary for patients in whom neck node metastases become apparent after control of the primary cancer is achieved.

In three randomized trials, elective treatment of the neck was compared with observation and therapeutic management of patients in whom node metastases later became apparent. Mature results are available for only two of those trials. Neither had the

TABLE 115-4

THE RISK OF LYMPH NODE METASTASES IN PATIENTS WITH SQUAMOUS CELL CARCINOMA

Site	Node Positive at Presentation (%)	Node Negative Followed by Node Positive (%) if Not Treated*
Nasopharynx	77–90	50
Oropharynx		
Soft palate	37–56	16–25
Tonsillar fossa	58–76	13–40
Base of tongue	50–83	
Pharyngeal walls	50–71	
Hypopharynx	52–72	33
Oral cavity		
Lip	1–2	5–7
Buccal mucosa	9–42	16–30
Floor of mouth	30–59	20–35
Oral tongue	13–65	38–52
Gingiva	18–52	17
Hard palate	13–36	
Retromolar trigone (faucial pillar)	39–56	
Larynx		
Supraglottic	31–54	33
Glottic	7–12	
Subglottic	10	
Paranasal sinuses	10–17	9–17
Nose		
Nasal cavity	10–13	5
Nasal vestibule	6	5

*Includes patients with uncontrolled primary carcinoma in some series.
Adapted from Mendenhall WM and others: *Int J Radiat Oncol Biol Phys* 14:249, 1988; additional data from Chung CK and others: *Int J Radiat Oncol Biol Phys* 5:191, 1979; Fitzpatrick PJ: *J Otolaryngol* 13:32, 1984; Fletcher GH: *Textbook of radiotherapy*, ed 3, Philadelphia, Lea & Febiger, 1980; Harwood AR and others: *Int J Radiat Oncol Biol Phys* 5:899, 1979; Jorgensen K and others: *Acta Radiol; Ther Phys Biol* 12:177, 1973; Payne DG: *J Otolaryngol* 12:197, 1983; Pietrantoni L and others: *Laryngoscope* 52:151, 1962; Ratzer ER and others: *Am J Surg* 119:294, 1970; Robin PE, Powell DJ: *J Laryngol Otol* 94:301, 1980; Strong EW: *Cancer Treat Symp* 2:5, 1983; Vegers JWM and others: *Arch Otolaryngol Head Neck Surg* 105:192, 1979; Wong CS, Cummings BJ: *Acta Oncol* 27: 203, 1988.

power to evaluate all relevant end points adequately. Pointon and Gleave[150] compared ENI with observation and therapeutic neck dissection. The management of the neck was randomly determined in patients with oral cavity carcinomas after radiotherapy for the primary cancer. In those who received ENI, the ipsilateral neck nodes received 5000 cGy in 15 fractions in 3 weeks. At 2 years, the failure rate in the neck was 20% in the 100 patients in the ENI group compared with 35% in the 105 patients managed by observation and therapeutic neck dissection. This difference was not statistically significant. The 2-year survival rate in each group was approximately 75%. Vandenbrouck and others[181] treated primary carcinomas of the oral tongue in 75 patients with radiation. Six weeks later, the patients were randomly assigned to elective or therapeutic radical neck dissection. When nodes were positive on histologic examination, postoperative radiotherapy was given to the neck. In the group managed by elective dissection, 19 of 39 (49%) had histologically positive nodes. In those treated by therapeutic dissection, nodes became enlarged in 19 of 36 patients and were histologically abnormal in 17 (47%). The rate of lymph node capsular rupture increased from 13% in those who underwent elective surgery to 25% in the therapeutic dissection group, but this normally poor prognostic feature was not reflected in the survival rates, which were almost identical in the two groups. These two trials suggest that if patients remain under regular observation so that therapeutic dissection can be carried out without delay, there may be no survival advantage to elective treatment of the neck nodes. The early results of a third randomized trial in India, in which prophylactic and therapeutic neck dissection were compared in 98 patients with early stage carcinoma of the oral tongue, favored prophylactic dissection,[58] but a final report on this trial has not been published. Despite the two negative trials described, opinion in many centers favors elective treatment of negative neck nodes for a variety of reasons, including possible difficulty in achieving control of enlarged nodes and an association of distant metastases and clinical node metastases.

When an expectant policy is followed, from 25% to 35% of patients will have clinical metastases in neck nodes. It has been estimated that two-thirds of these patients will achieve control in the neck by treatment at that time. This suggests that even in patients who attend for regular reviews, the risk of uncontrolled neck disease after a policy of therapeutic rather than elective treatment is approximately 8% to 12%, or about twice that of elective treatment. Many authors also consider that the procedures required to manage clinically detectable nodes are often associated with greater morbidity than those of elective procedures performed in the absence of enlarged nodes. The counter arguments to elective treatment include the morbidity and financial costs of treatment of the two-thirds of patients who do not have subclinical node metastases.

The presence of clinically detectable nodes in the neck is associated with an increase in the incidence of distant metastases,[107] and it has been suggested, although not proven, that eradication of neck node metastases at the earliest possible time may reduce the risk of distant failure. Jesse and others[95] found distant metastases in 11% of patients who had late node metastases develop after being seen with a clinically negative neck compared with only 3% in patients who were seen with a single enlarged neck node at the time of initial treatment of the primary tumor and neck and did not experience later recurrence in the neck.

In a review of the surgical literature, Nahum and others[128] concluded that the possible benefits of elective neck dissection had not been clearly defined and that, in most cases, no more that 5% of patients would benefit from elective neck dissection. The mortality attributed to neck dissection is from 1% to 3%.[103,128,145] In the many reports of nonrandomized series, opinions on the merits of elective dissection vary widely. Farr and Arthur[59] reported a 5-year survival rate of 33% in patients with histologically positive nodes at the time of elective dissection, a rate similar to what they found in patients with ipsilateral clinically positive nodes at presentation and in patients in whom clinical node involvement became evident after initial management. However, Lee and Krause[103] described a 48% 5-year survival rate in patients with positive lymph nodes at elective radical neck dissection compared with 33% after therapeutic dissection of node metastases diagnosed at first presentation and 33% after secondary dissection of late-developing nodes. Piedbois and others[145] reported a series of 233 patients with early stage oral cavity cancer. Ten-year survival was 37% in the 110 patients who underwent elective neck dissection, and 31% of the 123 followed expectantly, of whom 21 (17%) relapsed in the neck and were treated at that point. Multivariate analysis showed that the patients in the elective neck dissection group had a significantly lower probability of death from cancer.

The choice of elective nodal irradiation assumes that ENI is at least as effective as elective lymph node dissection and is not associated with any greater morbidity. In the case of radiotherapy, it is anticipated that early elective treatment should be more effective because there are fewer tumor cells, and conditions associated with reduced effectiveness of radiation, such as extracapsular spread and tissue hypoxia, become more common as nodes grow.

Elective neck irradiation has been found to reduce late relapse in initially clinically negative regions of the neck in two situations. First, when the patient is seen without clinical lymph node metastases and, after ENI, never had node failure develop. Second, in patients who are seen with one or more abnormal nodes, and whose initial management includes ENI to the clinically uninvolved areas of the neck, no further cancer is seen in cervical node groups that were clinically free of disease at first presentation.

The decision to recommend ENI depends in part on how the primary cancer is to be managed and whether the patient is considered to be at significant risk of nodal metastasis. It is often suggested that a single treatment modality be used for both primary tumor and lymph nodes when possible for patient convenience and economic reasons, although this is not essential. What constitutes a "significant risk" remains a matter of physician preference. Weiss and others[190] developed a decision analysis model for planning a management strategy for the stage N_0 neck. They concluded that treatment of the neck was warranted if the probability of node metastasis was >20%. However, Gregoire and others[82] considered that this level was too high and that in most European centers the neck would be treated electively when the probability of occult metastases was >5% to 10%. A guideline grid to the risk of nodal metastases for the more common primary sites is shown in Figure 115-3. Many centers would include at least some category T_1 cancers, shown as "low risk" in the grid, in ENI protocols, and most would include all intermediate[4] and "high-risk" cancers.

Selected results of ENI in patients who had no clinically abnormal nodes at presentation are shown in Table 115-5. None of these studies was randomized, various primary tumor sites and stages were included, and the neck was subjected to differing doses of radiation. However, ENI seems to be equally effective for all primary sites. The reasons why only some patients received ENI were usually not stated, and policies differed over the extent of the neck irradiated. Despite those caveats, few patients had late lymph node metastases develop after ENI. On the basis of the series surveyed in Table 115-5, late neck node metastases were found in only 5% who received ENI to the entire neck and in only 10% in whom part of the neck was treated compared with a failure rate of approximately 35% when the neck nodes were not irradiated. This continues to be the general experience today. However, not all investigators have reported similar levels of success in reducing the risk of late nodal relapse by ENI. Node failure has been reported in as many as 40% of cases (23 of 57).[64] The most likely reason for the failure of ENI to eradicate all subclinical nodal metastases is inadequate coverage of the nodes at risk and use of a radiation dose that is not adequate to sterilize a relatively bulky, but undetected, node metastasis. Reseeding from an uncontrolled primary tumor may also lead to neck failure.

The lymph node groups irradiated are determined by the need to encompass adequately in the volume irradiated either the untreated primary carcinoma or the site of that cancer after surgery, by the patterns of lymph node metastases usually associated with different primary cancers, and by the philosophy adopted with regard to entire or partial neck irradiation.

Risk Groups for Subclinical Node Metastases

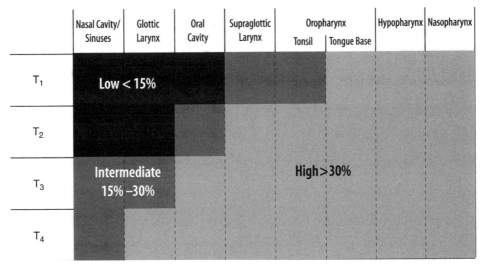

Figure 115-3. Grid showing risk of subclinical lymph node metastases for various primary sites by T category.

2598 Part Eight NECK

TABLE 115-5

EFFECT OF ELECTIVE IRRADIATION ON INCIDENCE OF LATE NECK NODE METASTASES IN PATIENTS WITH INITIALLY CLINICALLY NEGATIVE NODES

Study	Sites	Radiation Dose (cGy)	Entire Ipsilateral or Bilateral Neck Irradiation (n)	Partial Neck Irradiation (n)	No Neck Irradiation (n)
Horiuchi and Adachi[91]*	Oral tongue	4000/3–4 weeks	–	1/21	6/16
Barkley and others[12]†	Supraglottic larynx, hypopharynx tonsillar fossa, base of tongue	>5000–6000/5–6 weeks >6000/6 weeks plus 5000/5 weeks in lower neck	1/24 0/26	3/54 10/31	16/29 –
Bataini and others[20]†	Supraglottic larynx	5000–5500/5 weeks	1/66	–	–
Million[124]	Oral tongue, floor of mouth	4500–5000/5 weeks 2000–3000/2–3 weeks	–	0/9 6/16	2/8
Goffinet and others[76]‡	Oral cavity, tonsil, posterior tongue, supraglottic region	5500/5 weeks	13/87	7/53	7/18
Rabuzzi and others[152]†	Oral cavity, oropharynx hypopharynx, larynx, nasopharynx	5000/5 weeks	5/126	–	–
Decroix and Ghossein[51]†	Oral tongue >4.5 cm	5000/5 weeks	7/50	–	–
Mantravadi and others[113]†	Oral cavity, oropharynx, hypopharynx, larynx, nasopharynx	55 patients <5000/5 weeks 132 patients >5000/5 weeks	– –	2/154	–
Meoz and others[121]†	Oral tongue	2000/1 week 5000/5 weeks	– 2/13	9/27 10/30	–
Mendenhall and others[118]†	Oral cavity, oropharynx, hypopharynx, larynx, nasopharynx	>4500–7000/5–8 weeks	2/74 18/379 5%	6/88 46/409 11%	6/28 24/65 37%

*Primary tumor status not given.
†Primary tumor controlled.
‡Primary tumor not controlled in 18 of 20 irradiated patients.

Contralateral lymph node metastases developed in only 3% (8 of 237) of patients who received bilateral neck irradiation compared with 25% (53 of 215) of patients who had unilateral nodes from primary carcinomas in similar sites but were not managed with ENI.[12,65] Berger and others[22] described node metastases in new areas of the neck in 13% (22 of 163) of patients who underwent ENI to part of neck but in only 3% (7 of 227) in whom the entire neck was irradiated. These results are not an indication that bilateral irradiation to the entire neck is always necessary. O'Sullivan and others[137] found that treatment of selected well-lateralized cancers of the tonsil with homolateral radiation techniques did not increase significantly the risk of failure in the contralateral neck (contralateral node relapse in 0 of 133 N_0 and 5 of 56 N_1 cases). Analysis of tumor failure patterns suggests that extending radiation volumes to include the mediastinal lymph nodes is not advantageous.[123] The results of the few randomized trials that have attempted to study the relative merits of ENI to different volumes of the neck are not widely accepted. In a small randomized trial in Hong Kong of patients with stage I (T_1N_0) nasopharyngeal cancers, no patient relapsed in the neck when the upper neck had not been irradiated, and only 1 of 34 relapsed after ENI.[90] However, most North American and European centers recommend ENI to the entire neck in all patients with nasopharyngeal cancer, including those with stage I disease.

The most effective radiation dosage for ENI has not been studied systematically. However, analysis of results such as those in Table 115-5 has led to the recommendation of doses in the range of 4500 to 5000 cGy in 4.5 to 5.5 weeks.[194] There is some uncertainty about the minimum effective dose, but doses <3000 cGy in 3 weeks to 4000 cGy in 4 weeks seem to be relatively ineffective.[91,124]

Elective irradiation of the neck nodes is accompanied by little morbidity apart from damage to the salivary glands. Significant xerostomia is usually seen only after bilateral irradiation of primary nasopharyngeal or oropharyngeal cancers. Recently developed techniques such as 3D conformal treatment and IMRT[54] have shown that the incidence of xerostomia can be greatly reduced without compromise in tumor control rates.

Few data exist on the possible influence of ENI on survival. Most publications do not allow analysis of this important end point. Although multivariate analysis of some retrospective series indicates a survival advantage after elective management of the neck,[49] the suggestion that ENI changes only the pattern of disease and not survival has not been refuted.

Management of a patient treated with ENI who subsequently has recurrence of the primary cancer is not compromised. It is presumed that the cervical nodes are at risk of reseeding by cancer, and the possibility of late regrowth in the neck of cancer cells not sterilized by the initial course of ENI cannot be excluded. There is some evidence that the risk of cervical node metastases from a recurrent primary cancer is decreased in patients who have previously had ENI.[120] It is usually advisable to perform neck dissection together with resection of the recurrent primary cancer, even in patients who remain clinically free of node metastases.

Therapeutic Irradiation of Cancerous Lymph Nodes

For most primary tumors in the head and neck, the relative 5-year survival rate in the United States when clinically detectable cervical nodes were present at diagnosis was for many years only approximately 20% to 35%.[169] Advances in modern diagnosis and treatment have improved relative overall survival to approximately 40%, but most patients still die of their disease.[81] The recognition that no inherent major differences exist in radioresponsiveness and radiocurability between the primary carcinoma and its lymph node metastases led to the use of megavoltage radiotherapy as the sole method of management of cervical node metastases in some patients, although, more commonly, it was combined with neck dissection. Recent advances in multimodality treatment, incorporating varied combinations of altered radiation fractionation, cytotoxic chemotherapy, and surgery will potentially lead to further improvements in survival and locoregional control rates.

Radiation Alone

Wizenberg and others[196] reported the successful use of radiation in 113 patients, all of whom had histologic proof of lymph node involvement on needle biopsy. The overall control rate for the primary tumor and nodes was 52%; failure occurred in the lymph nodes alone in 8%. Similarly, Hanks and others[83] failed to control large, multiple, or fixed lymph nodes in only 1 of 69 patients when the primary tumor was controlled. These and other early studies showed that radiation could successfully sterilize some lymph node metastases.

Radiation doses similar to those used for the primary carcinoma are required to treat grossly involved lymph nodes. Fewer than 10% of enlarged nodes were controlled by 4000 cGy in 3 to 4 weeks.[91] Fewer than 50% of single nodes of 3 cm or less in diameter were controlled with 5000 cGy in 5 weeks.[133] Ninety percent were controlled by a dose equivalent to 6500 cGy in 6 weeks, with no apparent increase in control above that level.[18,163] Bernier and Bataini[23] examined dose/response relationships in cervical node metastases from oropharyngeal, hypopharyngeal, and lateral epilaryngeal cancers. There was no clear-cut dose-control relationship for nodes <3 cm with doses from 5500 to 8000 cGy in 6 weeks. The overall control rate was 90% (498 of 551). For nodes 3 to 6 cm in diameter, control was achieved in 86% (77 of 90) with doses of 7000 to 8500 cGy in 6 weeks, and 65% (9 of 14) with <7000 cGy. For nodes >6 cm, the control rate was about 75% (32 of 43) for doses more than 7500 cGy, and 50% (10 of 20) for doses from 5500 to 7500 cGy in 6 weeks. However, although Bataini and others[16,17] successfully used high-dose radiation to eradicate neck metastases and reported neck surgery could be performed after such doses without undue morbidity, the risks of surgical complications after very high radiation doses prompted most centers to manage patients with large nodes with from 5000 cGy in 5 weeks to 7000 cGy in 8 weeks (a less intense schedule than the same dose in 6 weeks) followed by neck dissection. This policy of planned surgery after radiation for patients who have clinical node metastases is being reevaluated in light of the demonstrated effectiveness and tolerability of high doses delivered by modern techniques.[112,144] The role of planned surgery with altered fractionation radiotherapy schedules or chemoradiation requires further evaluation.

Central to any reliance on radiation alone to eradicate metastatic nodes is confidence in the accuracy of techniques used to assess the neck after irradiation. Several groups have studied the rate of regression of cervical nodes after radiation. Bataini and others[16] found that the clearance rate of the primary tumor was significantly higher than that for the nodal metastases at the completion of radiotherapy, but that the percentage of cases with residual disease at the primary or nodal sites was almost the same 2 months after treatment. The larger the node, the slower the observed clearance rate. At 2 months after radiation, 83% of nodes (422 of 507) <3 cm had regressed completely compared with 63% of nodes (94 of 148) 3 to 6 cm in size, and 45% of nodes (30 of 67) >6 cm. Postradiation fibrosis may make clinical evaluation difficult. Fibrosis is usually greater in patients who have had bulky node metastases. This is not solely caused by higher radiation doses but may be related to cancer extension beyond the capsule of the lymph nodes and infiltration and adhesion to other structures in the neck.

Because some large nodes regress relatively slowly after irradiation, Bataini[16] suggested that salvage surgery be considered no earlier than approximately 2 months after conventional radiation when the initial size of the node was <6 cm and at 4 to 5 months when the nodes were >6 cm. When nodes regress completely, the risk of later nodal failure in some series is low (5%–17%).[14,16,144] However, others found that up to 50% of patients with no residual palpable tumor after the irradiation of large node masses still had apparently intact cancer cells if dissection was performed.[77,133] This may be due to differences in radiation doses given, different intervals between completion of radiation and surgery, and the phenomenon by which radiation damage to chromosomes is manifest only when a cell progresses to mitosis, so that cells that have not yet reached mitosis may appear intact when examined microscopically after

exposure to radiation. Many authors recommend at least limited dissection of the node masses and preferably radical or modified radical dissection of the entire ipsilateral neck after irradiation of large or multiple lymph nodes, without consideration of the degree of regression clinically. This approach is not indicated in patients with nasopharyngeal carcinomas for whom such surgery does not seem to be necessary if the nodes regress completely,[93] and node metastases from tonsillar fossa cancers are also relatively readily controlled by radiation alone.[14,42,66]

Although progress in imaging has been considerable, the resolution of CT scanning, MRI, and ultrasonography does not allow identification of residual tumor masses smaller than approximately 0.5 cm.[40] The potential of functional imaging such as positron emission tomography (PET) scanning to identify residual cancer after irradiation of neck node metastases has not yet been determined. At this time, consideration of planned node resection is still advisable after irradiation of nodal metastases categorized as N_2 or greater.

For some patients, even limited surgical resection of the residual node is not possible. If further management is considered appropriate, palliative radiation by implantation of radioactive isotopes is sometimes an option.[89,188]

The alternative to radiotherapy is neck dissection. After radical neck dissection alone for metastatic squamous cell carcinomas, tumor recurrence in the neck is reported in approximately 20% to 30% of patients in whom the primary tumor remains controlled.[52,176] This recurrence rate is related to the number of lymph nodes involved and the presence of capsular rupture.[33,176] Recurrences in the neck after previous dissection are rarely cured.[68,141] The appearance of contralateral nodal metastases after unilateral dissection may also be a problem from primary carcinomas in sites such as hypopharynx and supraglottic larynx.[115]

Planned Combined Radiation and Surgery

Because neck dissection and radiation each are of limited effectiveness, many centers prefer planned combinations of radiotherapy and resection of the neck nodes. Radiotherapy may be given before or after neck surgery, but the timing is to some extent influenced by the choice of management of the primary cancer. Preoperative radiotherapy reduces the size of the carcinomatous deposits and decreases the likelihood of regrowth locally and beyond the neck by any irradiated tumor cells not removed at surgery. Preoperative radiotherapy may be given to a restricted volume that encompasses only the lymph node groups at risk and adjacent tissues, depending on the center's philosophy with respect to management of clinically negative neck nodes. High-dose preoperative radiotherapy may increase the morbidity of surgical resection. Increased complication rates for pharyngeal anastomoses were reported after doses greater than approximately 5000 cGy in 5 weeks[115] and for soft-tissue healing after subcutaneous doses greater than approximately 6000 cGy in 6 to 7 weeks.[118] When the primary cancer is managed by radiotherapy, there is no evidence that preoperative radiotherapy of clinically positive nodes followed by neck dissection adversely affects the likelihood of successful resection should cancer recur later at the primary site.[120] Postoperative radiotherapy is intended to control any carcinoma that remains after surgery and lies within the volume irradiated. Postoperative radiotherapy should encompass all tissues disturbed at surgery, because carcinoma cells may have implanted anywhere within that volume. The volume irradiated after surgery is usually larger than that for preoperative management, and sensitive structures such as the larynx and spinal cord may be more difficult to shield. Also, some neck tissues may have diminished blood supply after resection, and, as a result, residual tumor cells in those areas may be relatively hypoxic and less radiosensitive than well-oxygenated cells. The relative merits of preoperative and postoperative radiotherapy have not been resolved, and there is no agreement that combined modality management is better than single-modality management.

It has been suggested that combined therapy may be particularly beneficial when carcinoma has extended through the lymph node capsule[14,32] and that failure to stratify patients by this parameter may confound the interpretation of studies of combined therapy.[39,96] Many authors regard nodal extracapsular tumor extension as an indication for radiotherapy after neck dissection,[32] although others regard any positive findings in a neck dissection as significant and recommend postoperative irradiation to the entire neck with an additional boost to areas where the capsular rupture was found.[93,143,181] The delivery of radiation after a neck dissection in which histologically involved lymph nodes are found seems to reduce the risk of neck recurrences in most series. Lundahl and others[110] retrospectively compared the results from 95 irradiated patients to a cohort of unirradiated patients matched according to age, gender, pN stage, number of nodes, and presence of a desmoplastic lymph node pattern. These authors reported reduced cancer-related death and improved overall survival rates with postoperative neck irradiation. The apparent ability of bilateral elective neck irradiation to prevent the appearance of new nodal metastases in the contralateral neck has been discussed earlier; elective neck irradiation provides a useful alternative to synchronous or staged bilateral neck dissections.

The recommended preoperative radiation dose is 5000 cGy in 5 weeks, although higher doses may be needed for large or fixed nodes. The recommended postoperative dose has frequently been approximately 6000 cGy in 6 weeks to the upper neck and not <5000 cGy in 5 weeks to the lower neck; the higher dose is intended to counter any relative hypoxia in the tissues disturbed by surgery and is possible because problems with postoperative healing are not a consideration. The dose for postoperative management was studied systematically by Peters and others.[143] In a report of a randomized trial involving 302 patients, the authors concluded that, at radiation doses of 180 cGy/day, a minimum dose of 5760 cGy to the entire operative bed should be delivered, with a boost to 6300 cGy for sites of increased risk, especially regions of extracapsular nodal disease. A dose of 5400 cGy was recommended for undissected areas potentially harboring subclinical disease. The authors concluded that at a dose of 180 cGy/day, escalation above 6300 cGy would not improve the therapeutic ratio because of toxicity.

The optimum interval between surgery and radiotherapy is not known, although intuition suggests this interval should not be excessive. Vikram and others[184] reported that when radiotherapy was started within 6 weeks after surgery, only 2% of patients (1 of 53) who had pathologically proven node metastases subsequently had neck recurrence develop. When radiotherapy did not begin until >6 weeks after surgery, 22% (9 of 41) had a recurrence develop. Peters and others[143] reported 2-year locoregional control rates of 64% and 77% in patients beginning radiotherapy more than or less than 6 weeks after surgery. Although this difference was not statistically significant, the authors advised that radiotherapy be started as soon as possible after surgery to minimize the proliferation of residual tumor. The most effective interval between preoperative radiotherapy and surgery has not been studied systematically. After a short 1-week course of radiation, the interval is usually a few days.[176] After higher doses, such as 5000 cGy in 5 weeks, it is more usual to allow 4 to 8 weeks to elapse, so that the nodes and primary may regress and the acute inflammatory reaction induced by radiation settle. With the finding that there may be an increased proliferation rate of surviving tumor clonogens during or after irradiation,[142,195] this strategy should be reassessed. Neck dissection has been performed successfully and without undue morbidity 3 weeks after 6000 cGy in 6 weeks to the neck nodes and primary cancer.

It would be helpful to resolve the various claims for improved control from combined therapy and to establish the optimal radiation doses and timing in controlled clinical trials. In one trial intended to do this, the Radiation Therapy Oncology Group (RTOG) randomly assigned patients to preoperative radiotherapy (5000 cGy in 5 weeks, surgery 4–8 weeks later) or to postoperative radiotherapy (6000 cGy to the primary site, 5000 cGy in 5 weeks to the lower neck, beginning within 4 weeks of surgery).[101] For all tumor sites combined, in 277 evaluable patients, locoregional control was significantly better after a median follow-up of 60 months for patients assigned to receive postoperative radiotherapy (65% vs 48% P = .04), and survival also showed a trend in favor of postoperative radiotherapy (P = .10). Rates of severe surgical and radiotherapy complications were similar overall. This trial lacked the power to resolve several key issues related to the management of different tumor sites and stages.

Some investigators believe that the addition of radiation does not improve the results of neck dissection.[52] High rates of locoregional recurrence have been reported despite postoperative radiotherapy for some patients.[8,45,46] Cooper and others[45] retrospectively analyzed risk factors predictive of locoregional recurrence in patients with locally advanced head and neck cancer treated with postoperative radiotherapy alone. Patients with microscopically positive surgical margins had a 5-year risk of locoregional recurrence of 61%, whereas patients with negative margins but two or more metastatic lymph nodes and extracapsular tumor extension had a risk of 27%. More favorable risk factors of fewer than two lymph nodes, no extracapsular tumor extension, and negative margins were associated with a locoregional recurrence risk of 17% at 5 years. Ang and others[8] reported a prospective evaluation of risk factors for locoregional recurrence in patients with advanced squamous cell carcinoma of the oral cavity, oropharynx, larynx, and hypopharynx. In this study, 151 high-risk patients with extracapsular tumor extension or two or more involved lymph nodes were randomly assigned to receive 6300 cGy in 5 weeks (concomitant boost) vs 6300 cGy in 7 weeks (conventional fractionation). Intermediate-risk patients with one adverse pathologic feature excluding extracapsular tumor extension (oral cavity primary, fewer than two lymph node metastases, microscopically positive margins, or perineural invasion) received 5760 cGy in 6.5 weeks. Patients with no adverse risk factors did not receive postoperative radiotherapy. Low-risk, intermediate-risk, and high-risk patients had a 5-year risk of locoregional recurrence of 10%, 6%, and 32%, respectively. Five-year survival rates were 83%, 66%, and 42% for the low-, intermediate-, and high-risk groups, respectively. The high-risk patient group had a worse outcome than the lower risk groups, despite receiving higher doses of postoperative radiation. Unfortunately, primary site and nodal patterns of failure were not reported separately in either of these studies.[8,45]

The order in which radiotherapy and surgery are undertaken is based on a joint decision of the management group. Sometimes, for example, the policy for tumor sites such as the larynx and hypopharynx has generally been one of delayed combined management,[87] with surgical resection being deferred to permit observation of the primary carcinoma and preservation of organs such as the larynx to the greatest extent possible; radiation is the initial modality. For cancers of the oral cavity, this sequence is reversed, because good function can be obtained by reconstructive surgery, and it has been thought that such surgery may be easier in unirradiated tissues.

Progress in Treatment of Advanced Neck Disease

The effectiveness of fractionated radiation depends on the dose and schedule and the number and size of involved lymph nodes. Recently, unconventional dose-fractionation schedules (*altered fractionation*) and concurrent chemotherapy (*chemoradiation*) have been shown in some instances to improve locoregional control compared with conventional fractionation alone for patients with locally advanced disease.

Altered radiation fractionation. Conventional head and neck radiotherapy delivers daily fraction sizes of 180 to 250 cGy. In the United States, 180 to 200 cGy per fraction is typical. Unconventional dose-fractionation radiotherapy schedules (*altered fractionation*) have been used to improve the biologic effectiveness of radiation to eradicate both primary cancers and metastases in lymph nodes.[130] *Hyperfractionation* is a strategy used to escalate the total radiation dose while limiting normal tissue toxicity by decreasing the dose per fraction below conventional fraction sizes. Hyperfractionation seeks to exploit the differential sensitivity of cancer and normal tissues to lower fractional doses of radiation, particularly for critical organs such as the spinal cord. Doses are generally reduced to the range of 110 to 160 cGy. Two or more doses are given each day, with an interval of at least 6 hours between fractions to permit substantial repair of cellular radiation damage. The overall treatment time is the same as that of conventional fractionation. *Accelerated fractionation* is designed to reduce the overall treatment time to counteract the tumor repopulation that may occur during a standard course of fractionated radiotherapy.[130] In this strategy, the fractional doses are at conventional or near-conventional levels. Many schedules used clinically combine hyperfractionation and accelerated fractionation.

Whether altered fractionated radiation schedules improve nodal control compared with conventional fractionation is often unclear, both because many studies have failed to present detailed failure analyses and because metastatic nodes may be resected. Ang[6] observed that the several trials of hyperfractionated radiation in which the total dose was increased by 10% to 15% over a conventional regimen of 6600 to 7000 cGy in 7 weeks resulted in a 10% to 15% increase in the control rate of the primary cancers without any increase in serious late complications. The benefit was greatest in intermediate-sized rather than very large tumors, and the effect on control of lymph node metastases seemed minor.

When trials of accelerated radiation were considered, a shortening of the overall treatment time by 1 to 1.5 weeks also resulted in an approximately 15% higher control rate, predominantly of the primary cancer. Acceleration of treatment can be achieved in several ways. The most popular are by delivering six fractions a week, either by treating on 6 days rather than the usual 5 or by treating twice on 1 weekday; another approach is the concomitant boost technique, in which two fractions are given twice a day for 1 to 2 weeks of the schedule; the second fraction usually is slightly less than the conventional dose and the volume treated is also reduced. Peters and others[144] described a series of patients with primary oropharyngeal cancer treated with a concomitant boost schedule. Complete regression of metastatic nodes occurred in 62 of 75 patients (83%) assessed clinically and radiologically. Failure in the neck occurred later in three patients. Overgaard and others[139] treated patients with an accelerated schedule that delivered six fractions per week and compared the results with those of the standard five fractions per week. With this accelerated regimen, 6600 to 6800 cGy could be delivered in approximately 9 days less than with conventional fractionation. In a retrospective analysis of pooled patients from three randomized protocols (DAHANCA 2, 5, and 7) that included 333 patients treated with the accelerated protocol, an improvement at 5 years was found with the accelerated regimen in local control but not in nodal control. Waldron and others[186] investigated a treatment approach in which the high-dose radiation volume, delivered with an accelerated and hyperfractionated schedule (160 cGy twice a day, 5 days per week, for 4 weeks, to 6400 cGy), was limited to the primary site only. A lower dose was given to the neck node regions (200 cGy once a day to 4000 cGy). In this phase II study, neck dissection was planned for patients with lymph node metastases >3 cm or for nodes that could not be treated to the same dose as the primary tumor without increasing the volume of normal air and food passages irradiated. Control in the neck was achieved in 95%, and there was no increase in surgical morbidity (Waldron J: Personal communication, June 2003). Kaanders and others[98] concluded that with accelerated radiation, relative to a conventional schedule of 7000 cGy in 7 weeks, the achievable acceleration in treatment time is about 2 weeks, with the mucosa being the limiting tissue. Further acceleration requires a reduction in total dose. A number of strategies are being investigated to overcome this limitation. A randomized trial of continuous hyperfractionated accelerated radiation therapy (CHART) conducted by Dische and others,[53] in which patients received 54 Gy in 36 fractions, three times 150 cGy per day, for 12 consecutive days, failed to identify any improvement in the control of regional node metastases compared with 6600 cGy in 33 daily fractions over 6.5 weeks. A recently reported large randomized study compared conventional fractionation of 7000 cGy in 7 weeks with two accelerated regimens, one a concomitant boost design and the other a split course accelerated fractionation design.[74] Both of the accelerated regimens showed improved locoregional control rates at 2 years relative to conventional radiation. However, the nodal failure rates at 2 years were 32%, 27%, and 33% in the standard fractionation, hyperfractionation, and concomitant boost arms, respectively. Neck dissection was allowed for nodes that were >3 cm before irradiation and likely contributed to this similarity in nodal control rates.

A meta-analysis of 6515 patients treated by hyperfractionated and/or accelerated radiation schedules compared with conventional fractionated radiation found small, but significant, improvements in survival and locoregional control from all altered fractionation regimens.[25] The greatest benefits were found in trials in which the altered fractionation scheme allowed an increase in total radiation dose (hazard ratio [HR] of death, 0.78; HR of locoregional failure, 0.76). The impression gained from the trials of altered fractionation reported to date is that benefit is more likely to be seen in control of the primary cancer than in that of the regional node metastases. The use of postradiation neck dissection on an individual basis makes interpretation of the effect of altered fractionation on node metastases difficult.

Radiation and chemotherapy. Meta-analyses have shown an absolute improvement in overall survival of from 8% to 12% with concurrent chemotherapy and radiation compared with radiation alone in the management of locally advanced head and neck carcinomas.[28,55,127,147] Adjuvant and neoadjuvant regimens have shown insignificant improvements of no more than 1% to 2%.[147] As a result, much of the emphasis in current research is on concurrent radiation and chemotherapy regimens.[9] The optimal concurrent chemotherapy regimen is unknown. Cisplatin seems to be the most active agent in combination with radiation[28] and is frequently given at the dose of 100 mg/m[2] each 21 days. Overall survival at 5 years is approximately 40% with concurrent chemotherapy protocols.[147] A number of trials have reported an improvement in locoregional control with concurrent modality protocols.* As with the data relating to altered fractionation, identification of any benefit in eradication of nodal disease is affected by the lack of detailed site of failure analyses and the widespread inclusion of neck dissection in these protocols.

The management of unresectable metastatic nodes remains problematic. Patients with unresectable nodes were eligible for a recent randomized trial in which standard radiation therapy and two schedules of concurrent chemotherapy were compared as treatment for unresectable squamous cell cancer of the head and neck.[1] The chemoradiation schedules included either bolus cisplatin or infusional 5-fluorouracil plus bolus cisplatin. The addition of concurrent high-dose (100 mg/m[2] each 3 weeks) cisplatin to conventional single daily fractionation radiation (7000 cGy in 7 weeks) significantly improved survival (37% vs 23% at 3 years, $P = .014$) but with increased acute toxicity. Approximately equal numbers underwent neck dissection in each arm of the trial, but the number of patients with initially unresectable nodes was not described.

Two collaborative groups have reported the preliminary results of large phase III trials investigating the addition of concurrent cisplatin to postoperative radiotherapy.[24,47] The European Organization for the Research and Treatment of Cancer (EORTC) group randomly assigned head and neck cancer patients at high risk of locoregional recurrence to receive a postoperative radiation dose of 6600 cGy in 6.5 weeks alone or radiation plus three doses of concurrent cisplatin (100 mg/m[2] on days 1, 22, and 43 of radiation). Three-year rates of disease-free survival (41% vs 59%, $P = .0096$) and overall survival (49% vs 65%, $P = .0057$) favored the chemoradiation arm.[24] The RTOG/Intergroup conducted a similar trial in 459 patients with two or more involved lymph nodes, extracapsular tumor extension, and/or microscopically positive margins. Patients received either 6000 to 6600 cGy in 6 to 6.5 weeks postoperatively alone or in combination with three doses of concurrent cisplatin by a dose schedule similar to the EORTC trial. There was no difference in the 2-year locoregional recur-

rence rate (74% vs 79%, $P = .16$) for radiation and chemoradiation, respectively. Detailed site of failure analyses are not yet available for either study.

Nguyen and Ang[130] suggest that concurrent chemotherapy and radiation is to be preferred for the nonsurgical treatment of patients with locally advanced carcinoma and that altered fractionation is best considered for patients with intermediate stage tumors or who are medically unsuitable for chemotherapy. They recommend that combinations of altered fractionation with chemotherapy be used only within formal studies. Institutional policies are usually guided by patient preferences, local experience, local bias, and available multidisciplinary expertise.

Neck Node Metastases from an Unidentified Primary Cancer

Despite detailed clinical and radiologic investigations, the primary site remains unidentified in up to approximately 3% of patients who are seen with metastatic cervical lymphadenopathy.[78] The most common histologic finding is squamous cell carcinoma. There has been considerable progress in imaging and other studies that can assist in identifying the site of the primary cancer.[129] In exploratory studies, the finding of Epstein-Barr virus (EBV) in a metastatic node suggested origin from the nasopharynx,[105] and human papillomavirus (HPV) was found most frequently in oropharyngeal cancers.[148] Molecular techniques may also eventually be helpful in localizing potential primary sites.[36]

A single enlarged node was present in the jugulodigastric region in 60% to 75% of patients in several large series of patients in whom a primary tumor could not be found.[19,94,155,189] The jugulodigastric and midjugular regions account for >50% of metastatic node sites in most series. Bilateral nodes were found in <10% of patients with an occult primary carcinoma.[71,94,189] Molinari and others[125] reviewed the files of >2500 patients with carcinomas of the head and neck and 600 patients with lymphomas or malignant tumors of sites other than the head and neck. From these records, they calculated the statistical probabilities of finding clinically abnormal lymph nodes in each of several zones in the neck. Table 115-6 shows the results of Molinari's analysis for the probabilities of a single enlarged node from a squamous cell carcinoma in each zone. The most commonly affected zone, the jugulodigastric, was involved with almost equal frequency by nasopharyngeal, oral cavity, oropharyngeal, or hypopharyngeal carcinomas. An upper or midposterior triangle node was most likely to be from a nasopharyngeal carcinoma. A single supraclavicular node was more likely to be associated with a primary bronchogenic carcinoma than with a head and neck primary site.

---

*References 2, 26, 35, 92, 122, 192.

TABLE 115-6

PRIMARY TUMOR SITES ASSOCIATED WITH SINGLE CERVICAL NODE METASTASES

Lymph Node Groups	Oral Cavity	PRIMARY TUMOR SITES (%)					
		Tonsil and Oropharynx	Base of Tongue	Nasopharynx	Hypopharynx	Larynx	Lung
Jugular chain							
Submaxillary	71	14	7				
Subdigastric	22	10	18	12	15	9	
Midjugular		10	11	7	21	13	
Low jugular		5	8	12	25	13	
Posterior cervical chain							
Upper posterior cervical		18	8	58	8	5	
Midposterior cervical		17	12	55	12		
Low posterior cervical		15		24	25		
Supraclavicular							90

Adapted from data in Molinari R and others: *Tumori* 63:267, 1977.
Only probabilities of a single lymph node metastasis of 5% or more and primary sites giving rise to squamous cell carcinoma have been included.

Any generalization about the most appropriate choice of management on the basis of published reports is impossible because of the disparities in the clinical material and the selection of subsets for reporting. Nieder and others[129] recently reviewed selected series (Table 115-7). Patients managed by surgery only in the series reviewed in general had a single small node and no indication for postoperative radiation therapy. Prognosis seemed to be related to lymph node factors similar to those considered when the primary cancer site is known. Thus, prognosis was worse for more advanced N categories, when there were multiple nodes, when nodes were larger than approximately 3 cm, or when there was evidence of extracapsular extension. When the node was in the supraclavicular fossa, survival rates ranged from 3% to 20% at 3 years.[63,75,94] The prognosis was poor in patients with metastatic adenocarcinoma, wherever the nodes were located.[13,104] Additional prognostic factors identified in a large national review included performance status, gender (women had better cause-specific survival), and hemoglobin.[78]

Proponents of radiotherapy argue that inclusion in the volume treated of the most likely primary mucosal cancer sites and the remainder of the cervical lymph node fields reduces the risk of later emergence of the primary cancer or of low or contralateral cervical node metastases. Treatment by neck dissection may sometimes avoid the need for radiation and its side effects but may be associated with higher rates of late primary cancer and contralateral nodal disease (Table 115-8). In practice, combined therapy is often recommended, either because nodes fail to regress completely after radiation or because surgery reveals one or more of the adverse nodal features noted earlier. Chemotherapy is sometimes included in the management regimen, especially for patients with bulky node metastases,[50] although any long-term advantage from this has not yet been demonstrated.

TABLE 115-7

REPORTED RESULTS OF TREATMENT OF CERVICAL LYMPH NODE METASTASES FROM OCCULT SQUAMOUS CELL CARCINOMA

End point	Unilateral RT (6 series)	Comprehensive RT (12 series)	Surgery (4 series)
Median mucosal primary emergence rate (range)	8% (5–44)	10% (2–13)	25%
Median neck relapse rate (range)	52% (31–63)	19% (8–49)	34%
Median distant metastases rate (range)	38% (1 series)	19% (11–23)	–
Median 5-year overall survival rate (range)	37% (22–41)	50% (34–63)	–

Adapted from Nieder C and others: *Int J Radiat Oncol Biol Phys* 50:727, 2001.

Opinions differ about whether the later emergence of a primary carcinoma in the head and neck worsens prognosis. Jesse and others[94] found a 3-year survival rate of 31% in patients in whom a primary tumor later appeared compared with 58% in those in whom the primary site was never found. The data collected in Table 115-7 that also suggest this may well reflect patient selection. Pooled data from several series indicate that subsequent primary tumors emerged in all sites, but predominantly in the oral cavity and oropharynx.[72] Possible "second primaries" could not be excluded. In the series surveyed by Fu,[72] the late emerging primary cancer was controlled in only 39 of 92 (42%) patients. Relapse in the neck is more common than later emergence of a mucosal primary cancer.

Two different radiation treatment strategies are followed, each with its proponents. The first is comprehensive irradiation of the abnormal node site together with the clinically uninvolved ipsilateral and contralateral node regions and all compartments of the laryngopharynx. Selective shielding, or tailoring of the radiation volume to avoid low-risk mucosal sites, may be undertaken if there are clinical or histologic features that point to a particular primary tumor site. The radiation dose delivered to the mucosa is generally that appropriate for a category T_1 cancer (typically 6000 to 6500 cGy in 6 weeks, or equivalent). Some authors have suggested a lower dose, analogous to that used to treat clinically uninvolved regions of the neck (5000 cGy in 5 weeks or equivalent).[84] The second approach is to treat only the ipsilateral nodes. There are also variants of this latter philosophy, with some authors favoring concentration of treatment on the lymph node basins only, for example, with electron beam therapy, and others opting to include the ipsilateral mucosal walls of the oropharynx and hypopharynx.

The wide variety of approaches to these patients may be resolved, at least in part, by a current randomized trial being led by the EORTC. In this trial, patients who are seen with unilateral cervical node metastases of squamous cell carcinoma undergo comprehensive neck dissection and are then randomly assigned to irradiation of the ipsilateral neck or to extensive irradiation of the nasopharyngeal, oropharyngeal, hypopharyngeal, and laryngeal mucosa plus the bilateral neck nodes.[129] Improvements in radiation therapy technique that permit substantial sparing of the parotid glands, thereby reducing the severity of postradiation xerostomia, are likely to encourage treatment of all potential primary tumor sites rather than ipsilateral node regions only, although it would clearly be preferable that this decision be buttressed by the result of the randomized trial.

SALIVARY GLAND CARCINOMAS

Postoperative radiotherapy reduces the risk of local recurrence at the site of primary salivary gland cancers in high-risk patients.[11,73,99,116,132] There do not seem to be any major differences in radiation response between the different histologic types of malignant salivary gland tumors.[73,99] These observations form the basis for the use of radiation treatment in the management of the cervical nodes. Lymph node metastases are a poor prognostic factor, although often their influence cannot be separated from factors related to an uncontrolled primary tumor. In one series, the 5-year survival rate was only 9% in patients who had lymph node metastases at admission and 17% in those who later had node metastases develop compared with 74% in patients who never had spread to nodes.[174]

There is considerable variation in the frequency of nodal metastasis from malignant salivary gland tumors, determined by the salivary gland in which the tumor arises and by the histologic type and grade. Most series are small, and management protocols that might identify node metastases have often varied over time. The overall incidence of lymph node metastases at the time of presentation reported by Rafla-Demetrious[153] was 24% (43 of 179); there were cervical node metastases from 24% (16 of 66) of parotid carcinomas, 38% (8 of 21) of submandibular and sublingual gland carcinomas, and 20% (19 of 92) of minor salivary gland carcinomas. There were very few node metastases from salivary gland carcinomas that arose in the palate or paranasal sinuses. Some series have reported a lower rate of node metastases, for example, 16% for parotid cancers and 8% for submandibular and sublingual tumors.[10]

Node metastases from parotid cancers were found predominantly in levels II, III, IV, and from submandibular cancers in levels I, II, and III.[10] The risk of involvement of posterior triangle (level V) nodes was small. Contralateral metastases from lateralized salivary gland cancers, even from sublingual gland tumors, were very uncommon. The risk of both clinically detectable and occult lymph node metastases was related to histologic type (higher risk in adenocarcinomas and in anaplastic, epidermoid, and salivary duct cancers); tumor grade (higher risk in high grade); and primary tumor size (higher risk with larger tumors).[10,70,73,174] Low-grade mucoepidermoid, acinic cell, malignant mixed tumors, and, in many series, adenoid cystic cancers carried a very low risk of nodal metastases, generally 5% or less.[10,70,73] Elective neck dissection has been performed infrequently and is generally believed not to be necessary.[117,182] In one retrospective review of 99 patients with primary parotid malignancies who underwent elective dissection for a clinically disease-free neck, 12 patients

TABLE 115-8

LATE DISEASE AND SURVIVAL AFTER MANAGEMENT OF NECK NODES CONTAINING METASTATIC SQUAMOUS CELL CARCINOMA FROM AN UNIDENTIFIED PRIMARY TUMOR

	NODAL DISEASE (N/N (%))			
Initial Management	Initially Managed Side	Contralateral Side	Head and Neck Primary Tumor Found After Neck Management	Survival 3-yr Disease Free
Surgery	25/104 (24)	16/97 (16)	21/104 (20)	59/104 (57)
Radiotherapy	11/52 (21)	0/39 (0)	3/52 (6)	25/52(48)
Combined	4/28 (14)	0/28 (0)	4/28 (14)	13/28 (47)

*Includes patients salvaged by secondary management.
Modified from Jesse RH: *Cancer* 31:854, 1973.

(12%) had pathologically positive nodes.[70] Multivariate analysis indicated that, of preoperatively assessable factors, tumor type, high tumor grade, and facial nerve paralysis were most predictive of occult nodal disease. Extension of the analysis to include operatively or histopathologically assessable characteristics added perilymphatic invasion and extraparotid tumor extension as significant predictive factors.[70] Factors predictive of occult nodal metastases were reviewed also by Medina[117] and vanderPoorten and others.[182]

Decreased locoregional failure rates, sometimes with improved survival rates, in patients who have cervical node metastases and who, after neck dissection, received postoperative radiation compared with rates in those who were not irradiated were reported in a matched-pair analysis[11] and in comparison with historical controls.[99,132,100] No randomized trials have addressed this issue. Armstrong[11] reported a 5-year locoregional control rate of 69% in 23 patients with node metastases who received radiation to the neck and 40% in 16 patients treated with surgery only. The survival rates for these two patient groups were 49% and 19%. The significance of parameters such as number of abnormal nodes and extracapsular extension are not well defined for salivary gland cancer metastases, and many authors recommended postoperative radiotherapy if any node metastasis is found.

The relatively low risk of subclinical nodal metastases in unselected patients and the varied factors used to select patients for elective treatment do not permit comparison of the relative efficacy of elective neck dissection and elective nodal irradiation. The generally accepted criteria for postoperative radiotherapy to the primary tumor bed are similar to the factors that predict a high risk of occult neck metastases. If it is assumed that a risk of subclinical lymph node metastases of approximately 15% to 20% justifies elective radiation of the regional lymph nodes, a management policy may be formulated as follows.

Systematic irradiation of the neck nodes is not necessary after complete resection of low-grade mucoepidermoid carcinomas or in patients with small malignant mixed carcinomas, acinic cell carcinomas, or adenoid cystic carcinomas who have no evidence of cervical lymph node metastases. Irradiation of the ipsilateral neck nodes is recommended for patients who have:

- Indications for postoperative irradiation to the primary site for any histologic findings (for example, tumor unresectable or grossly or microscopically incompletely resected; ulcerated or fixed; >4 cm; multiple tumor nodules; adherent to cranial nerve VII or nerve dysfunction caused by cancer; extension to extraglandular tissues; perilymphatic or perineural invasion).
- Undifferentiated carcinomas, epidermoid carcinomas, grade II or III mucoepidermoid cancers, adenocarcinomas, or salivary duct cancers.
- After dissection of histologically positive nodes.

The entire ipsilateral neck is usually irradiated. The radiation doses commonly recommended are 6000 cGy in 6 weeks to the primary site and upper neck (levels I, II, and III) and 5000 cGy in 5 weeks to the lower neck (levels IV and VB) or equivalent doses. Additional boost treatment is given to known residual tumor or areas at high risk.

MELANOMAS

Melanomas are not radioresistant, although the role of radiotherapy in the management of primary and metastatic melanomas is debated. Several radiobiologic and clinical studies have suggested that many melanomas respond better to higher-than-standard fractional doses of radiation.[138] However, this observation was not confirmed by a randomized trial in which patients with measurable melanomatous masses received four 800 cGy doses at 7-day intervals (21 days overall, total 3200 cGy) or more conventional 20 fractions of 250 cGy in 26 to 28 days overall (total 5000 cGy) at the rate of five treatments per week.[162] The complete response (CR) and partial response (PR) rates to each regimen were similar (CR 24% vs 23%; PR 36% vs 34%). Nevertheless, most radiation oncologists favor managing melanomas with fractional radiation doses of at least 300 cGy or more.

Melanomas of the skin of the head and neck represent approximately 20% of all cutaneous melanomas. Melanomas also arise, although less commonly, from the mucosa, especially of the oral cavity, nasal cavity, and paranasal sinuses. The likelihood of regional lymph node metastases varies with the type of melanoma: approximately 0% to 1% for lentigo maligna, 10% for lentigo maligna melanoma, 30% to 50% for nodular cutaneous melanoma, and 50% or more for oral cavity and other mucosal primary sites.[41,85] The patterns of lymph node metastases from cutaneous melanomas of the head and neck were studied by Shah and others,[166] who reviewed 111 radical neck dissection specimens and noted that the distribution of metastases was less predictable than for squamous cell carcinoma arising in the mucosa. They concluded that radical neck dissection incorporating parotidectomy would frequently be the most appropriate management, particularly when the primary melanoma arose on the ear, face, or anterior scalp. Their conclusion has considerable implications for the design of adjuvant radiotherapy treatment fields. However, others have not found irregular patterns of metastasis.[185] Evaluation of sentinel lymph node status is of help in deciding the first lymph node groups at risk[178] but has not been used directly to assist the design of radiation fields. There is some evidence that the risk of regional recurrence can be reduced by the type of neck surgery performed, possibly to a greater extent than might be achievable by adjuvant radiation.[161,167]

The risk of recurrence in the lymph node basin after neck dissection for metastatic melanoma is generally reported to be in the range of 15% to 30%,[34,135,167,170] although rates as high as 50% have been described.[29] The factors predictive of recurrence after surgery include extracapsular extension and involvement of multiple nodes. There have been several nonrandomized studies of postoperative adjuvant radiation to all or part of the neck, with subsequent recurrence rates of from approximately 10% to 20%,[7,86,135] about one-half of those of many surgery-only studies. Large fractional dose radiation schedules were used. Ang and others[7] reported neck recurrence in only 3 of 95 patients who were treated by neck dissection coupled with preoperative or, more usually, postoperative radiotherapy. Radiation consisted of

3000 cGy in 2.5 weeks, delivered in fractions of 600 cGy twice a week. The treatment was designed so that the spinal cord dose did not exceed 2400 cGy. Shen and others[167] described 217 patients, only 21 of whom received adjuvant postoperative irradiation. The cervical recurrence rate was 14% in each group. A higher proportion of those irradiated had adverse prognostic factors. Shen and others[167] concluded that postoperative radiation should be considered only for those with extracapsular melanoma extension. Although a randomized trial of adjuvant radiation after regional lymphadenectomy for melanoma of the trunk and extremities showed some delay in the median time to recurrence in patients who received radiation, no other advantages were found.[48] The radiation schedule in that trial of 5040 cGy in 28 fractions of 180 cGy over 10 weeks (split course) has been criticized as suboptimal. In a current randomized trial conducted by the Eastern Cooperative Oncology Group (ECOG), patients receive adjuvant interferon-alpha after metastatic node dissection and are randomly assigned to receive adjuvant radiotherapy or no additional treatment.

Elective neck dissection reveals subclinical node metastases in approximately 20% to 30% of patients, a rate similar to the development of clinical neck node metastases in those who do not undergo elective dissection.[4] Many patients in whom subclinical metastases are found are treated similarly to those with overt nodal metastases and receive postoperative radiation. It is difficult to determine from the literature the outcome in this subset of patients. Similarly, the information on the possible use of elective neck irradiation as an alternative to elective surgery is largely anecdotal, and this approach has not been studied systematically. Ang and others[7] described 79 patients who received elective irradiation of the neck after wide local excision of cutaneous melanomas 1.5 mm or more thick. Regional recurrence was seen in only five patients (6%).

Although most authors agree that the role of radiation treatment of the neck would be best resolved by randomized trials, in melanoma, as in other malignancies, accrual to such studies has often been disappointing.

SUMMARY

The various patterns of lymph node metastases in the neck and the radiation fields necessary to encompass these nodes are well defined. Techniques that allow the delivery of effective radiation doses without undue toxicity are available. There is good evidence that elective irradiation of clinically normal nodes in high-risk patients and therapeutic irradiation of clinically metastatic lymph nodes can influence the patterns of tumor failure in patients with squamous cell carcinomas. Radiation improves the control of regional metastases from salivary gland carcinomas and probably also from melanomas. The influence of cervical node irradiation on survival rates is more difficult to determine, because survival depends also on successful management of the primary tumor (which is often considered in reports together with the cervical nodes), on the risk of more distant metastases, and on deaths from intercurrent disease.

The role of surgery and radiation therapy, as single modalities or in combination, in the management of cervical node metastases has been argued vigorously and inconclusively. However, with advances in technical radiation therapy and in cancer control rates by altered radiation fractionation and by combination of radiation and chemotherapy, the debate has moved to identifying the most effective multimodality schedules. It seems probable that advances in imaging and molecular pathology will assist in selection of the most effective regimens. The number of formal clinical trials conducted has increased greatly over the past two decades, and these studies provide the best evidence of improvements in clinical outcome. Many traditional concepts of the role of radiation in the management of the neck nodes are being reexamined within the context of these trials.

REFERENCES

1. Adelstein DJ and others: An intergroup phase III comparison of standard radiation therapy and two schedules of concurrent chemoradiotherapy in patients with unresectable squamous cell head and neck cancer, *J Clin Oncol* 21:92, 2003.
2. Adelstein DJ and others: A phase III randomized trial comparing concurrent chemotherapy and radiotherapy with radiotherapy alone in resectable stage III and IV squamous cell head and neck cancer: preliminary results, *Head Neck* 19:567, 1997.
3. Alvi A, Johnson JT: Extracapsular spread with clinically negative neck: implications and outcome, *Otolaryngol Head Neck Surg* 114:65, 1996.
4. Ames FC, Sugarbaker EV, Ballantyne AJ: Analysis of survival and disease control in stage I melanoma of the head and neck, *Am J Surg* 132:484, 1976.
5. Andreassen CN, Gran C, Lindegaard JC: Chemical radioprotection: a critical review of amifostine as a cytoprotector in radiotherapy, *Semin Radiat Oncol* 13:62, 2003.
6. Ang KK: Altered fractionation trials in head and neck cancer, *Semin Radiat Oncol* 8:230, 1998.
7. Ang KK and others: Postoperative radiotherapy for cutaneous melanoma of the head and neck region, *Int J Radiat Oncol Biol Phys* 30:795, 1994.
8. Ang KK and others: Randomized trial addressing risk features and time factors of surgery plus radiotherapy in advanced head-and-neck cancer, *Int J Radiat Oncol Biol Phys* 51:571, 2001.
9. Argiris A: Update on chemotherapy for head and neck cancer, *Curr Opin Oncol* 14:323, 2002.
10. Armstrong JG and others: The indications for elective treatment of the neck in cancer of the major salivary glands, *Cancer* 69:615, 1992.
11. Armstrong JG and others: Malignant tumors of major salivary gland origin, *Arch Otolaryngol Head Neck Surg* 116:290, 1990.
12. Barkley HT and others: Management of cervical lymph node metastases in squamous cell carcinomas of the tonsillar fossa, base of tongue, supraglottic larynx, and hypopharynx, *Am J Surg* 124:462, 1972.
13. Barrie JR, Knapper WH, Strong EW: Cervical nodal metastases of unknown origin, *Am J Surg* 120:466, 1970.
14. Bartelink H, Breur K, Hart G: Radiotherapy of lymph node metastases in patients with squamous cell carcinoma of the head and neck region, *Int J Radiat Oncol Biol Phys* 8:983, 1982.
15. Bataini JP and others: Natural history of neck disease in patients with squamous cell carcinoma of the oropharynx and pharyngolarynx, *Radiother Oncol* 3:245, 1985.
16. Bataini JP and others: Impact of neck node radioresponsiveness on the regional control probability in patients with oropharynx and pharyngolarynx cancers managed by definitive radiotherapy, *Int J Radiat Oncol Biol Phys* 13:817, 1987.
17. Bataini JP and others: Impact of cervical disease and its definitive radiotherapeutic management on survival: experience in 2013 patients with squamous cell carcinomas of the oropharynx and pharyngolarynx, *Laryngoscope* 100:716, 1990.
18. Bataini JP and others: *Size/dose relationships and local control of oro- and hypopharyngeal cancer treated by radiotherapy*. In Karcher KH, editor: *Progress in radio-oncology*, ed 2, New York, Raven Press, 1982.
19. Bataini JP and others: Treatment of metastatic neck nodes secondary to an occult epidermoid carcinoma of the head and neck, *Laryngoscope* 97:1080, 1987.
20. Bataini JP and others: Treatment of supraglottic cancer by radical high-dose radiotherapy, *Cancer* 33:1253, 1974.
21. Becker A and others: Oxygenation of squamous cell carcinoma of the head and neck: comparison of primary tumors, neck node metastases, and normal tissue, *Int J Radiat Oncol Biol Phys* 42:35, 1998.
22. Berger DS and others: Elective irradiation of the neck lymphatics for squamous cell carcinomas of the nasopharynx and oropharynx, *Am J Roentgenol* 111:66, 1971.
23. Bernier J, Bataini JP: Regional outcome in oropharyngeal and pharyngolaryngeal cancer treated with high dose per fraction radiotherapy: analysis of neck disease response in 1646 cases, *Radiother Oncol* 6:87, 1986.
24. Bernier J: Chemo-radiotherapy, as compared to radiotherapy alone, significantly increases disease-free and overall survival in head and neck cancer patients after surgery: results of EORTC Phase III trial 22931 [abstract], *Int J Radiat Oncol Bio Phys* 51(Suppl):1, 2001.
25. Bourhis J and others: Conventional vs modified fractionated radiotherapy. Meta-analysis of radiotherapy in head and neck squamous cell carcinoma: a meta-analysis based on individual patient data [abstract], *Int J Radiat Oncol Biol Phys* 54(Suppl):71, 2002.
26. Brizel DM and others: Hyperfractionated irradiation with or without concurrent chemotherapy for locally advanced head and neck cancer, *N Engl J Med* 338:1798, 1998.
27. Brizel DM and others: Oxygenation of head and neck cancer: changes during radiotherapy and impact on treatment outcome, *Radiother Oncol* 53:113, 1999.
28. Browman GP and others: Choosing a concomitant chemotherapy and radiotherapy regimen for squamous cell head and neck cancer: a systematic review of the published literature with subgroup analysis, *Head Neck* 23:579, 2001.

29. Byers RM: The role of modified neck dissection in the treatment of cutaneous melanoma of the head and neck, *Arch Surg* 12:1338, 1986.

30. Byers RM and others: Frequency and therapeutic implications of 'skip metastases' in the neck from squamous carcinoma of the oral tongue, *Head Neck* 19:14, 1997.

31. Byers RM, Wolf PF, Ballantyne AJ: Rationale for elective modified neck dissection, *Head Neck Surg* 10:160, 1988.

32. Cachin Y: *Management of cervical nodes in head and neck cancer*. In Evans PHR, editor: *Head and neck cancer*, New York, Alan R. Liss, 1983.

33. Cachin Y and others: Nodal metastasis from carcinomas of the oropharynx, *Otolaryngol Clin North Am* 12:145, 1979.

34. Calabro A, Singletary SE, Balch CM: Patterns of relapse in 1001 consecutive patients with melanoma nodal metastases, *Arch Surg* 124:1051, 1989.

35. Calais G and others: Randomized trial of radiation therapy versus concomitant chemotherapy and radiation therapy for advanced-stage oropharynx carcinoma, *J Natl Cancer Inst* 91:2081, 1999.

36. Califano J and others: Unknown primary head and neck squamous cell carcinoma: molecular identification of the site of origin, *J Natl Cancer Inst* 91:599, 1999.

37. Candela FC, Kothari K, Shah JP: Patterns of cervical node metastases from squamous carcinoma of the oropharynx and hypopharynx, *Head Neck* 12:197, 1990.

38. Candela FC and others: Patterns of cervical node metastases from squamous carcinoma of the larynx, *Arch Otolaryngol Head Neck Surg* 116:432, 1990.

39. Carter RL and others: Radical neck dissections for squamous carcinomas: pathological findings and their clinical implications with particular reference to transcapsular spread, *Int J Radiat Oncol Biol Phys* 13:825, 1987.

40. Castelijns JA, van den Brekel MW: Imaging of lymphadenopathy in the neck, *Eur Radiol* 12:727, 2002.

41. Chaudry AP, Hampel A, Gorlin RJ: Primary malignant melanoma of the oral cavity: a review of 105 cases, *Cancer* 11:923, 1958.

42. Chow E and others: Enhanced control by radiotherapy of cervical lymph node metastases arising from nasopharyngeal carcinoma compared with nodal metastases from other head and neck squamous cell carcinomas, *Int J Radiat Oncol Biol Phys* 39:149, 1997.

43. Chua DT and others: Retropharyngeal lymphadenopathy in patients with nasopharyngeal carcinoma. A computed tomography–based study, *Cancer* 79:869, 1997.

44. Chung CK and others: Squamous cell carcinoma of the hard palate, *Int J Radiat Oncol Biol Phys* 5:191, 1979.

45. Cooper JS and others: Precisely defining high-risk operable head and neck tumors based on RTOG #85-03 and #88-24: targets for postoperative radiochemotherapy? *Head Neck* 20:588, 1998.

46. Cooper JS and others: Validation of the RTOG recursive partitioning classification for head and neck tumors, *Head Neck* 23:669, 2001.

47. Cooper JS and others: Patterns of failure for resected advanced head and neck cancer treated by concurrent chemotherapy and radiation therapy: analysis of RTOG 9501/Intergroup Phase III trial. [abstract], *Int J Radiat Oncol Biol Phys* 54 (Suppl):2, 2002.

48. Creagan ET and others: Adjuvant radiation therapy for regional nodal metastases from malignant melanoma: a randomized prospective study, *Cancer* 42:2206, 1978.

49. Dearnaley DP and others: Interstitial irradiation for carcinoma of the tongue and floor of mouth: Royal Marsden Hospital experience 1970-1986, *Radiother Oncol* 21:183, 1991.

50. de Braud F and others: Metastatic squamous cell carcinoma of unknown primary localized to the neck: advantage of an aggressive treatment, *Cancer* 54:510, 1989.

51. Decroix Y, Ghossein NA: Experience of the Curie Institute in treatment of cancer of the mobile tongue: II. Management of the neck nodes, *Cancer* 47:503, 1981.

52. DeSanto LW and others: Neck dissection: is it worthwhile? *Laryngoscope* 92:502, 1982.

53. Dische S and others: A randomized multicentre trial of CHART versus conventional radiotherapy in head and neck cancer, *Radiother Oncol* 44:123, 1997.

54. Eisbruch A and others: Salivary gland sparing and improved target irradiation by conformal and intensity modulated irradiation of head and neck cancer, *World J Surg* 27:832, 2003.

55. El-Sayed S, Nelson N: Adjuvant and adjunctive chemotherapy in the management of squamous cell carcinoma of the head and neck region. A meta-analysis of prospective and randomized trials, *J Clin Oncol* 14:838, 1996.

56. Fajardo LF: Lymph nodes and cancer: a review, *Front Radiat Ther Oncol* 28:1, 1994.

57. Fajardo LF: Effects of ionizing radiation on lymph nodes: a review, *Front Radiat Ther Oncol* 28:37, 1994.

58. Fakih AR, Rao RS, Patel AR: Prophylactic neck dissection in squamous cell carcinoma of the oral tongue: a prospective randomized study, *Semin Surg Oncol* 5:327, 1989.

59. Farr HW, Arthur K: Epidermoid carcinoma of the mouth and pharynx, 1960-1964: elective radical neck dissection, *Clin Bull* 1:130, 1971.

60. Ferlito A and others: Prognostic significance of microscopic and macroscopic extracapsular spread from metastatic tumour in lymph nodes, *Oral Oncol* 38:747, 2002.

61. Fisch U: *Lymphography of the cervical lymphatic system*, Basel, S Karger, 1968.

62. Fitzpatrick PJ: Cancer of the lip, *J Otolaryngol* 13:32, 1984.

63. Fitzpatrick PJ, Kotalik JF: Cervical metastases from an unknown primary tumor, *Radiology* 110:659, 1974.

64. Fitzpatrick PJ, Tepperman BS: Carcinoma of the floor of the mouth, *J Can Assoc Radiol* 33:148, 1982.

65. Fletcher GH: Elective irradiation of subclinical disease in cancers of the head and neck, *Cancer* 29:1450, 1972.

66. Fletcher GH: The role of irradiation in the management of squamous-cell carcinomas of the mouth and throat, *Head Neck Surg* 1:441, 1979.

67. Fletcher GH: *Textbook of radiotherapy*, ed 3, Philadelphia, 1980, Lea & Febiger.

68. Fletcher GH, Evers WT: Radiotherapeutic management of surgical recurrences and postoperative residuals in tumors of the head and neck, *Radiology* 95:185, 1970.

69. Fletcher GH, Lindberg RD: *Radiation therapy of tumors of the neck*. In Thawley SE and others, editors: *Comprehensive management of head and neck tumors*, Philadelphia, 1987, WB Saunders.

70. Frankenthaler RA and others: Predicting occult lymph node metastases in parotid cancer, *Arch Otolaryngol Head Neck Surg* 119:517, 1993.

71. Fried MP and others: Cervical metastasis from an unknown primary, *Ann Otol Rhinol Laryngol* 84:152, 1975.

72. Fu KK: Neck node metastases from unknown primary: controversies in management, *Front Radiat Ther Oncol* 28:66, 1994.

73. Fu KK and others: Carcinoma of the major and minor salivary glands: analysis of treatment results and sites and causes of failures, *Cancer* 40:2882, 1977.

74. Fu KK and others: A Radiation Therapy Oncology Group (RTOG) phase III randomized study to compare hyperfractionation and two variants of accelerated fractionation to standard fractionation radiotherapy for head and neck squamous cell carcinomas: first report of RTOG 9003, *Int J Radiat Oncol Biol Phys* 48:7, 2000.

75. Glynne-Jones RGT and others: Metastatic carcinoma in the cervical lymph nodes from an occult primary: a conservative approach to the role of radiotherapy, *Int J Radiat Oncol Biol Phys* 18:289, 1990.

76. Goffinet DR and others: Irradiation of clinically uninvolved cervical lymph nodes, *Can J Otolaryngol* 4:927, 1975.

77. Goodwin WJ Jr., Chandler JR: Indications for radical neck dissection following radiation therapy, *Arch Otolaryngol Head Neck Surg* 104:367, 1978.

78. Grau C and others: Cervical lymph node metastases from unknown primary tumours. Results from a national survey by the Danish Society for Head and Neck Oncology, *Radiother Oncol* 55:121, 2000.

79. Greave FL and others, editors: *AJCC cancer staging manual*, ed 6, New York, 2002, Springer.

80. Greenberg JS and others: Extent of extracapsular spread: a critical prognostic factor of oral tongue cancer, *Cancer* 97:1464, 2003.

81. Greenlee RT and others: Cancer statistics, 2000, *Ca Cancer J Clin* 50:7, 2000.

82. Gregoire V and others: Selection and delineation of lymph node target volumes in head and neck conformal radiotherapy. Proposal for standardizing terminology and procedure based on surgical experience, *Radiother Oncol* 56:135, 2000.

83. Hanks GE, Bagshaw MA, Kaplan HS: The management of cervical lymph node metastasis by megavoltage radiotherapy, *Am J Roentgenol* 105:74, 1969.

84. Harper CS and others: Cancer in neck nodes with unknown primary site: role of mucosal radiotherapy, *Head Neck Surg* 12:463, 1990.

85. Harwood AR: *Melanoma of the head and neck*. In Million RR, editor: *Management of head and neck cancer: a multidisciplinary approach*, Philadelphia, 1984, JB Lippincott.

86. Harwood AR, Cummings BJ: Radiotherapy for malignant melanoma: a reappraisal, *Cancer Treat Rev* 8:271, 1981.

87. Harwood AR, Keane TJ: General principles of irradiation therapy as applied to head and neck cancer, *J Otolaryngol* 11:69, 1982.

88. Harwood AR and others: Management of advanced glottic cancer, *Int J Radiat Oncol Biol Phys* 5:899, 1979.

89. Hilaris BS, Nori D: *New approaches to brachytherapy*. In Devita VT, Hellman S, Rosenberg SA, editors: *Important advances in oncology*, Philadelphia, 1987, JB Lippincott.

90. Ho JHC: An epidemiologic and clinical study of nasopharyngeal carcinoma, *Int J Radiat Oncol Biol Phys* 4:183, 1978.

91. Horiuchi J, Adachi T: Some considerations on radiation therapy of tongue cancer, *Cancer* 28:335, 1971.

92. Jeremic B and others: Radiation therapy alone or with concurrent low-dose daily either cisplatin or carboplatin in locally advanced unresectable squamous cell carcinoma of the head and neck: a prospective randomized trial, *Radiother Oncol* 43:29, 1997.

93. Jesse RH, Fletcher GH: Treatment of the neck in patients with squamous cell carcinoma of the head and neck, *Cancer* 39:868, 1977.

94. Jesse RH, Perez CA, Fletcher GH: Cervical lymph node metastasis: unknown primary cancer, *Cancer* 31:854, 1973.

95. Jesse RH and others: Cancer of the oral cavity: is elective neck dissection beneficial? *Am J Surg* 120:505, 1970.

96. Johnson JT and others: The extracapsular spread of tumors in cervical node metastasis, *Arch Otolaryngol Head Neck Surg* 107:725, 1981.

97. Jorgensen K, Elbrond O, Andersen AP: Carcinoma of the lip: a series of 869 cases, *Acta Radiol Ther Phys Biol* 12:177, 1973.

98. Kaanders JH, van der Kogel AJ, Ang KK: Altered fractionation: limited by mucosal reactions, *Radiother Oncol* 50:247, 1999.

99. King JJ, Fletcher GH: Malignant tumors of the major salivary glands, *Radiology* 100:381, 1971.

100. Kirkbride P, Liu FF, O'Sullivan B and others: Outcome of curative management of malignant tumours of the parotid gland, *J Otolaryngol* 30:271, 2001.

101. Kramer S and others: Combined radiation therapy and surgery in the management of advanced head and neck cancer: final report of study 73-03 of the Radiation Therapy Oncology Group, *Head Neck Surg* 10:19, 1987.

102. Larson DL and others: Lymphatics of the mouth and neck, *Am J Surg* 110:625, 1965.

103. Lee JG, Krause CJ: Radical neck dissection: elective, therapeutic, and secondary, *Arch Otolaryngol Head Neck Surg* 101:656, 1975.

104. Lee NK and others: Metastatic adenocarcinoma to the neck from an unknown primary source, *Am J Surg* 162:306, 1991.

105. Lee WY and others: Epstein-Barr virus detection in neck metastases by in-situ hybridization in fine-needle aspiration cytologic studies: an aid to differentiating the primary site, *Head Neck* 22:336, 2000.

106. Lefebvre JL and others: *Oral cavity, pharynx, and larynx cancer*. In Gospodarowicz MK and others, editors: *Prognostic factors in cancer*, ed 2, New York, 2001, Wiley-Liss.

107. Leibel SA and others: The effect of local-regional control on distant metastatic dissemination in carcinomas of the head and neck: results of an analysis from the RTOG head and neck database, *Int J Radiat Oncol Biol Phys* 21:549, 1991.

108. Levendag PC and others: Local tumor control in radiation therapy of cancers in the head and neck, *Am J Clin Oncol* 19:469, 1996.

109. Lindberg R: Distribution of cervical lymph node metastases from squamous cell carcinoma of the upper respiratory and digestive tracts, *Cancer* 29:1446, 1972.

110. Lundahl RE and others: Combined neck dissection and postoperative radiation therapy in the management of the high-risk neck: a matched-pair analysis, *Int J Radiat Oncol Biol Phys* 40:529, 1998.

111. Lyall D, Schetlin CF: Cancer of the tongue, *Ann Surg* 135:489, 1952.

112. Mak AC and others: Base of tongue carcinoma: treatment results using concomitant boost radiotherapy, *Int J Radiat Oncol Biol Phys* 33:289, 1995.

113. Mantravadi R and others: Radiation therapy for subclinical carcinoma in cervical lymph nodes, *Arch Otolaryngol Head Neck Surg* 108:108, 1982.

114. Marcial V, Marcial-Vega VA: Treatment of neck in head and neck mucosal squamous cell carcinoma: what our experience teaches, *Front Radiat Ther Oncol* 28:51, 1994.

115. Marks JE and others: Carcinoma of the pyriform sinus: an analysis of treatment results and patterns of failure, *Cancer* 41:1008, 1978.

116. McNaney D and others: Postoperative irradiation in malignant epithelial tumors of the parotid, *Int J Radiat Oncol Biol Phys* 9:1289, 1983.

117. Medina JE: Neck dissection in the treatment of cancer of major salivary glands, *Otolaryngol Clin North Am* 31:815, 1998.

118. Mendenhall WM, Million RR, Cassisi NJ: Squamous cell carcinoma of the head and neck treated with radiation therapy: the role of neck dissection for clinically positive neck nodes, *Int J Radiat Oncol Biol Phys* 12:733, 1986.

119. Mendenhall WM and others: Squamous cell carcinoma of the head and neck treated with radiation therapy: the impact of neck stage on local control, *Int J Radiat Oncol Biol Phys* 14:249, 1988.

120. Mendenhall WM and others: Squamous cell carcinoma of the head and neck treated with radiotherapy: does planned neck dissection reduce the chance for successful surgical management of subsequent local recurrence, *Head Neck Surg* 10:302, 1988.

121. Meoz RT, Fletcher GH, Lindberg RD: Anatomical coverage in elective irradiation of the neck for squamous cell carcinoma of the oral tongue, *Int J Radiat Oncol Biol Phys* 8:1881, 1982.

122. Merlano M and others: Five-year update of a randomized trial of alternating radiotherapy and chemotherapy compared with radiotherapy alone in treatment of unresectable squamous cell carcinoma of the head and neck [comment], *J Natl Cancer Inst* 88:583, 1996.

123. Merino OR, Lindberg RD, Fletcher GH: An analysis of distant metastases from squamous cell carcinoma of the upper respiratory and digestive tracts, *Cancer* 40:145, 1977.

124. Million RR: Elective neck irradiation for squamous carcinoma of the oral tongue and floor of mouth, *Cancer* 34:149, 1974.

125. Molinari R and others: A statistical approach to detection of the primary cancer based on the site of neck lymph node metastases, *Tumori* 63:267, 1977.

126. Munck JN and others: Computed tomographic density of metastatic lymph nodes as a treatment-related prognostic factor in advanced head and neck cancer, *J Natl Cancer Inst* 83:569, 1991.

127. Munro AJ: An overview of randomized controlled trials of adjuvant chemotherapy in head and neck cancer, *Br J Cancer* 71:83, 1995.

128. Nahum AM, Bone RC, Davidson TM: The case for elective prophylactic neck dissection, *Laryngoscope* 87:588, 1977.

129. Neider C, Gregoire V, Ang KK: Cervical lymph node metastases from occult squamous cell carcinoma: cut down a tree to get an apple? *Int J Radiat Oncol Biol Phys* 50:727, 2001.

130. Nguyen LN, Ang KK: Radiotherapy for cancer of the head and neck: altered fractionated regimens. *Lancer Oncol* 3:693, 2002.

131. Nordsmark M, Overgaard M, Overgaard J: Pretreatment oxygenation predicts radiation response in advanced squamous cell carcinoma of the head and neck, *Radiother Oncol* 41:31, 1996.

132. North CA and others: Carcinoma of the major salivary glands treated by surgery or surgery plus postoperative radiotherapy, *Int J Radiat Oncol Biol Phys* 18:1319, 1990.

133. Northrop M and others: Evolution of neck disease in patients with primary squamous cell carcinoma of the oral tongue, floor of mouth, and palatine arch, and clinically positive neck nodes neither fixed nor bilateral, *Cancer* 29:23, 1972.

134. Nowak PJ and others: A three-dimensional CT-based target definition for elective irradiation of the neck, *Int J Radiat Oncol Biol Phys* 45:33, 1999.

135. O'Brien CJ and others: Adjuvant radiotherapy following neck dissection and parotidectomy for metastatic malignant melanoma, *Head Neck* 19:589, 1997.

136. Okumura K and others: Retropharyngeal node metastasis in cancer of the oropharynx and lymphopharynx: analysis of retropharyngeal node dissection regarding preoperative radiographic diagnosis [English abstract], *Nippon Jibiinkoka Gakkai Kaiho* 101:573, 1998,

137. O'Sullivan B and others: The benefits and pitfalls of ipsilateral radiotherapy in carcinoma of the tonsillar region, *Int J Radiat Oncol Biol Phys* 51:322, 2001.

138. Overgaard J and others: Some factors of importance in the radiation treatment of malignant melanoma, *Radiother Oncol* 5:183, 1986.

139. Overgaard J and others: Importance of overall treatment time for the response to radiotherapy in patients with squamous cell carcinoma of the head and neck, *Rays* 25:313, 2000.

140. Payne DG: Carcinoma of the nasopharynx, *J Otolaryngol* 12:197, 1983.

141. Pearlman NW: Treatment outcome in recurrent head and neck cancer, *Arch Surg* 114:39, 1979.

142. Peters LJ and others: Accelerated fractionation in the radiation treatment of head and neck cancer: a critical comparison of different strategies, *Acta Oncol* 27:185, 1988.

143. Peters LJ and others: Evaluation of the dose of postoperative radiation therapy of head and neck cancer: first report of a prospective randomized trial, *Int J Radiat Oncol Biol Phys* 26:3, 1993.

144. Peters LJ and others: Neck surgery in patients with primary oropharyngeal cancer treated by radiotherapy, *Head Neck* 18:552, 1996.

145. Piedbois P and others: Stage I-II squamous cell carcinoma of the oral cavity treated by iridium-192: is elective neck dissection indicated? *Radiother Oncol* 21:100, 1991.

146. Pietrantoni L, Agazzi C, Fior R: Indications for surgical treatment of cervical lymph nodes in cancer of the larynx and hypopharynx, *Laryngoscope* 52:1511, 1962.

147. Pignon JP and others: Chemotherapy added to locoregional treatment for head and neck squamous cell carcinoma: three meta-analyses of updated individual data, *Lancet* 355:949, 2000.

148. Pintos J and others. Human papillomavirus and prognosis of patients with cancers of the upper aerodigestive tract, *Cancer* 85:1903, 1999.

149. Poggi MM, Coleman CN, Mitchell JB: Sensitizers and protectors or radiation and chemotherapy, *Curr Probl Cancer* 25:334, 2001.

150. Pointon RC, Gleave EN: *Lymphatic spread.* In Sikora K, Halnan KE, editors: *Treatment of cancer,* ed 2, London, 1990, Chapman and Hall.

151. Quon H, Liu FF, Cummings BJ: Potential molecular prognostic markers in head and neck squamous cell carcinomas, *Head Neck* 23:147, 2001.

152. Rabuzzi DD, Chung CT, Sagerman RH: Prophylactic neck irradiation, *Arch Otolaryngol Head Neck Surg* 106:454, 1980.

153. Rafla-Demetrious S: *Mucous and salivary gland tumors,* Springfield, Ill, Charles C Thomas, 1970.

154. Ratzer ER, Schweitzer RJ, Frazell EL: Epidermoid carcinoma of the palate, *Am J Surg* 119:294, 1970.

155. Richard JM, Micheau C: Malignant cervical adenopathies from carcinomas of unknown origin, *Tumori* 63:249, 1977.

156. Ritter MA: Determination of tumor kinetics: strategies for the delivery of radiotherapy and chemotherapy, *Curr Opin Oncol* 11:177, 1999.

157. Robbins KT and others: Neck dissection classification update: Revisions proposed by the American Head and Neck Society and the American Academy of Otolaryngology-Head and Neck Surgery, *Arch Otolaryngol* 182:751, 2002.

158. Robin PE, Powell DJ: Regional node involvement and distant metastases in carcinoma of the nasal cavity and paranasal sinuses, J *Laryngol Otol* 94:301, 1980.

159. Ross GL and others: The First International Conference on Sentinel Node Biopsy in mucosal head and neck cancer and adoption of a multicentre trial protocol, *Ann Surg Oncol* 9:406, 2002.

160. Sako K and others: Fallibility of palpation in the diagnosis of metastases to cervical nodes, *Surg Gynecol Obstet* 118:989, 1964.

161. Santini H, Byers RM, Wolf PF: Melanoma metastatic to cervical and parotid nodes from an unknown primary site, *Am J Surg* 150:510, 1985.

162. Sause WT and others: Fraction size in external beam radiation therapy in the treatment of melanoma, *Int J Radiat Oncol Biol Phys* 20:429, 1991.

163. Schneider JJ, Fletcher GH, Barkley HT Jr: Control by irradiation alone of nonfixed clinically positive lymph nodes from squamous cell carcinoma of the oral cavity, oropharynx, supraglottic larynx, and hypopharynx, *Am J Roentgenol* 123:42, 1975.

164. Shah JP: Cervical node metastases-diagnostic, therapeutic, and prognostic implications, *Oncology* 4:61, 1990.

165. Shah JP: Patterns of cervical lymph node metastasis from squamous carcinomas of the upper aerodigestive tract, *Am J Surg* 160:405, 1990.

166. Shah JP and others: Patterns of regional lymph nodes metastases from cutaneous melanomas of the head and neck, *Am J Surg* 162:320, 1991.

167. Shen P, Wanek LA, Morton DL: Is adjuvant radiotherapy necessary after positive lymph node dissection in head and neck melanomas? *Am Surg Oncol* 7:554, 2000.

168. Shoaib T, Soutar DS: Sentinel node biopsy in head and neck cancer, *Curr Opin Otolaryngol Head Neck Surg* 9:79, 2001.

169. Silverberg E: Cancer statistics, 1977, *Ca Cancer J Clin* 27:26, 1977.

170. Singletary SE and others: Prognostic factors in patients with regional cervical nodal metastases from cutaneous malignant melanoma, *Am J Surg* 152:371, 1986.

171. Sobin LH, Wittekind C, editors: *TNM classification of malignant tumors*, ed 6, New York, 2002, Wiley-Liss.

172. Som PM, Curtin HD, Mancuso AA: An image-based classification for the cervical nodes designed as an adjunct to resect clinically based nodal classifications, *Arch Otolaryngol* 125:388, 1999.

173. Spiessl B, Beahrs OH, Hermanek P, editors: *TNM atlas, illustrated guide to the TNM/pTNM classification of malignant tumors*, rev 2, Berlin, 1992, Springer.

174. Spiro RH, Huvos AG, Strong EW: Cancer of the parotid gland: a clinicopathologic study of 288 primary cases, *Am J Surg* 130:452, 1975.

175. Spiro JD and others: Critical assessment of supraomohyoid neck dissection, *Am J Surg* 156:286, 1988.

176. Strong EW: Preoperative radiation and radical neck dissection, *Surg Clin North Am* 49:271, 1969.

177. Strong EW: Sites of treatment failure in head and neck cancer, *Cancer Treat Symp* 2:5, 1983.

178. Thompson JF and others: Sentinel lymph node status as an indicator of the presence of metastatic melanoma in regional lymph nodes, *Melanoma Res* 5:255, 1995.

179. Van den Brekel MW and others: The incidence of macrometastases in neck dissection specimens obtained from elective neck dissections, *Laryngoscope* 106:987, 1996.

180. van Houten JM and others: Molecular diagnosis of head and neck cancer, *Recent Results Cancer Res* 157:90, 2000.

181. Vandenbrouck C and others: Elective versus therapeutic radical neck dissection in epidermoid carcinoma of the oral cavity, *Cancer* 46:386, 1980.

182. Vander Poorten VL, Balm AJ, Hilgers FJ: Management of cancer of the parotid gland, *Curr Opin Otolaryngol Head Neck Surg* 10:134, 2002.

183. Vegers JWM, Snow GB, Van der Waal C: Squamous cell carcinoma of the buccal mucosa, *Arch Otolaryngol Head Neck Surg* 105:192, 1979.

184. Vikram B and others: Failure in the neck following multimodality treatment for advanced head and neck cancer, *Head Neck Surg* 6:724, 1984.

185. Vreeburg GC and others: Cutaneous melanoma of the head and neck, *Eur J Surg Oncol* 14:165, 1988.

186. Waldron JN and others: A phase II study of hyperfractionated accelerated radiation delivered with integrated neck surgery (HARDWINS) for advanced squamous cell carcinoma of the head and neck [abstract], *Int J Radiat Oncol Biol Phys* 48(Suppl):320, 2000.

187. Wall TJ and others: Relationship between lymph node status and primary tumor control probability in tumors of the supraglottic larynx, *Int J Radiat Oncol Biol Phys* 11:1895, 1985.

188. Wang CC: *Brachytherapy for selected cancers of the head and neck*. In Chretien PB and others, editors: *Head and neck cancer*, vol 1, Philadelphia, Mosby, 1985.

189. Weir L and others: Radiation treatment of cervical lymph node metastases from an unknown primary: an analysis of outcome by treatment volume and other prognostic factors, *Radiother Oncol* 35:206, 1995.

190. Weiss MH, Harrison LB, Isaacs RB: Use of decision analysis in planning a management strategy for the stage N_0 neck, *Arch Otolaryngol Head Neck Surg* 120:699, 1994.

191. Wendt TG and others: Simultaneous radiochemotherapy versus radiotherapy alone in advanced head and neck cancer: a randomized multicenter study, *J Clin Oncol* 16:1318, 1998.

192. Wijers OB and others: A simplified CT-based definition of the lymph node levels in the node negative neck, *Radiother Oncol* 52:35, 1999.

193. Wilkinson EJ, Hause L: Probability in lymph node sectioning, *Cancer* 33:1269, 1974.

194. Withers HR, Peters LJ, Taylor JM: Dose-response relationship for radiation therapy of subclinical disease, *Int J Radiat Oncol Biol Phys* 31:353, 1995.

195. Withers HR, Taylor JM, Maciejewski B: The hazard of accelerated tumor clonogen repopulation during radiotherapy, *Acta Oncol* 27:131, 1988.

196. Wizenberg MJ and others: Treatment of lymph node metastases in head and neck cancer: a radiotherapeutic approach, *Cancer* 29:1455, 1972.

197. Wong CS, Cummings BJ: The place of radiation therapy in the treatment of squamous cell carcinoma of the nasal vestibule, *Acta Oncol* 27:203, 1988.

CHAPTER ONE HUNDRED AND SIXTEEN

NECK DISSECTION

K. Thomas Robbins
Sandeep Samant

INTRODUCTION

The terms *neck dissection* and *cervical lymphadenectomy* refer to the systematic removal of lymph nodes with their surrounding fibrofatty tissue from the various compartments of the neck. This procedure is used to eradicate cancer metastases to the regional lymph nodes of the neck. In most patients, these metastases originate from primary lesions involving mucosal sites of the upper aerodigestive tract, particularly the oral cavity, the pharynx, and the larynx.

The propensity for spread to the regional lymph nodes by carcinomas of the upper aerodigestive tract is variable and is associated with several factors, such as histology, T classification, and location of the primary tumor. For example, if the histology shows perineural invasion or invasion of the tumor's microcirculation, the risk is higher. In general, the more advanced the T classification, the higher the likelihood of nodal spread. Certain subsites, such as the oral tongue, the floor of the mouth, the piriform sinus, and the supraglottic larynx, are associated with high rates of metastases as compared with such subsites as the buccal mucosa, the lip, the nasal cavity, the paranasal sinuses, and the glottic larynx. Although the anatomic distribution of the surrounding lymphatic channels may explain some of this variation, inherent differences in the biologic behavior among these cancers also are likely. Thus, the indications for cervical lymphadenectomy depend not only on the presence of palpable disease but on factors that increase the risk of occult disease, such as the size and characteristics of the primary tumor. The term *therapeutic neck dissection* applies to the former condition, whereas the term *elective neck dissection* applies to the latter situation. Other factors that are important when deciding whether cervical lymphadenectomy is indicated relate to the overall treatment plan. For example, if the treatment of choice for the primary tumor is radiation rather than surgery, it may also be preferable to radiate the regional nodes when the clinical staging of the nodal disease is N_0 or N_1. If surgical transgression of the regional lymphatics is required to resect the primary tumor, cervical lymphadenectomy should also be included.

HISTORICAL PERSPECTIVE

In publications that came out before the 20th century, little attention was given to the indications or techniques for treating cervical lymph node metastases. The first conceptual approach for removing nodal metastases was made by Kocher in 1880[26]; he described the removal of the lymph node that bore contents of the submandibular triangle to gain access to tongue cancer. Later, Kocher recommended that nodal metastases should be removed more widely through a Y-shaped incision, with the long arm extending from the mastoid to the level of the omohyoid at its junction with the anterior border of the sternocleidomastoid muscle. Around the same time, Parkard supported the concept of removing the surrounding lymph nodes for lingual cancer.[45]

Without decreasing the importance of the contributions by these pioneer surgeons, the major individual to be credited with developing and reporting the fundamentals of cervical lymphadenectomy is George Crile.[16] Crile believed that distant (hematogenous) metastases were uncommon in head and neck cancer and that metastases more commonly occurred in the neck through the permeation of lymphatics. His description of a block resection encompassing all of the cervical nodal groups from the level of the mandible above to the clavicle below became the basis for the radical neck dissection we know today. Relevant to the modifications of radical neck dissection that were subsequently made, Crile recommended preservation of the internal jugular vein and the sternocleidomastoid muscle for patients in whom there were no palpable nodes. In addition, his technique was to remove only the regional lymph nodes that were known to drain the field of the original focus of disease when metastases could not be seen. It also is interesting to note that, in the accompanying illustrations of the more radical en bloc resections, the spinal accessory nerve was preserved.

The philosophy held by head and neck surgeons during the first half of the 20th century regarding the indications and techniques of cervical lymphadenectomy was based on the descriptions of Crile and perpetuated by others. Blair and Brown[6] and Martin[33] were strong proponents of the radical en bloc technique, which was similar to the radical surgery that had evolved for breast cancer. Martin in particular categorically insisted that the spinal accessory nerve, the internal jugular vein, and the sternocleidomastoid muscle should be removed as part of all cervical lymphadenectomies. During this time, one should remember that radiotherapy had not been developed as an effective adjuvant modality, and radical surgery represented the only hope for cure.

Associated with the procedure of the radical neck dissection was the presence of significant postoperative morbidity related to shoulder dysfunction; the operation also had limitations as a bilateral procedure.[40] In the 1950s, Ward and Robben[75] reported that the neck dissection could be modified in some circumstances by sparing the spinal accessory nerve and thereby preventing postoperative shoulder drop. Later, Saunders, Hirata, and Jaques[55] compared the functional results of cases undergoing radical neck dissection with those in whom the spinal accessory nerve was spared; this demonstrated that shoulder symptoms were only mild or moderate in more than 80% of the patients who had the nerve preserved or cable grafted. The concept of conservation neck surgery was further popularized during the 1960s by Suarez[71] in Argentina and promoted by Bocca and Pignataro,[7] who independently described an operation that removed all of the lymph node groups while sparing the spinal accessory nerve, the sternocleidomastoid muscle, and the internal jugular vein. They emphasized that fascial compartments surrounding the lymphatic contents of the neck could be removed without sacrificing the nonlymphatic structures, as mentioned.

Other authors reported the sparsity of nodal disease within the posterior triangle for carcinoma of the oral cavity, the pharynx, and the larynx, thus setting the stage for dissection modifications directed toward preserving lymph node groups.[31,36,64,73] These observations paved the way for another type of neck dissection modification, in which there was selective preservation of one or more lymph node groups.[9,50,61] Some of the initial proponents of this concept were the surgeons at MD Anderson Cancer Center, who called the procedure "modified neck dissection."[3,23] Two of the variations of the modified neck dissection were also called "supraomohyoid" and "anterior" neck dissections.[9] The term *selective neck dissection* (SND) subsequently became associated with the concept of preserving lymph nodes in one or more of the neck levels through the American Academy of Otolaryngology's classification.[50,52] The lymph node groups removed are based on the pattern of metastases, which are predictable relative to the primary site of cancer.

TERMINOLOGY OF NECK DISSECTION

The evolution of cervical lymphadenectomy procedures during the 20th century has provided the modern head and neck surgeon with a repertoire of surgical techniques for removing nodal metastases. Concurrent with this expansion has been the emergence of a multitude of terms used to describe these procedures. Originally proposed by authors without any uniformity of terminology, this lack of standardization unfortunately resulted in redundancy, misinterpretation, and even confusion among clinicians. Realizing the importance for standardizing the diverse nomenclature, the Committee for Head and Neck Surgery and Oncology of the American Academy of Otolaryngology–Head and Neck Surgery convened a special task force in 1988 to address terminology problems related to cervical lymphadenectomy. The specific objectives of the group were as follows: (1) to recommend terminology that adhered to more traditional terms, such as "radical" and "modified radical" neck dissection, and to avoid the use of eponyms and acronyms; (2) to define which lymphatic structures and other nonlymphatic structures should be removed or preserved relative to the radical neck dissection; (3) to provide standard nomenclature for the lymph node groups and the nonlymphatic structures; (4) to define the boundaries of resection for lymph node groups; (5) to use terms for the neck dissection procedures that are basic and easy to understand; and (6) to develop a classification based on the biology of the cervical metastases and the principles of oncologic surgery.[50]

Ten years after the initiation of the neck dissection classification project, the Committee for Neck Dissection Classification of the American Head and Neck Society reviewed and updated the 1991 neck dissection classification system (Table 116-1).[53,55] The new version included modifications of the original classification in an effort to remain contemporary and to keep with the current philosophy of managing lymph node metastases.

TABLE 116-1

CLASSIFICATION OF NECK DISSECTION

1991 Classification	2001 Classification
1. Radical neck dissection	1. Radical neck dissection
2. Modified radical neck dissection	2. Modified radical neck dissection
3. Selective neck dissection a) Supraomohyoid b) Lateral c) Posterolateral d) Anterior	3. Selective neck dissection: each variation is depicted by "SND" and the use of parentheses to denote the levels or sublevels removed
4. Extended neck dissection	4. Extended neck dissection

CERVICAL LYMPH NODE GROUPS

The patterns of spread of cancers from various primary sites in the head and neck to the cervical lymph nodes have been documented by retrospective analyses of large series of patients undergoing neck dissection.[9,31,62] The nodal groups at risk for involvement are widespread throughout the neck, extending from the mandible and skull base superiorly to the clavicle inferiorly and from the posterior triangle of the neck laterally to the midline viscera and to the contralateral side of the neck. It now is recommended that the lymph node groups in the neck be categorized according to the level system originally described by the Sloan-Kettering Memorial Group (Figure 116-1).[61]

Level I: There are two important lymph node groups within level I: the submental group and the submandibular group. The *submental nodes* are defined as those that are contained within the boundaries of the submental triangle (i.e., the anterior belly of the digastric muscles and the hyoid bone). The *submandibular lymph node group* refers to the nodes lying within the boundaries of the submandibular triangle (i.e., the anterior and posterior bellies of the digastric muscle and the body of the mandible). Because many of these lymph node groups lie in close proximity to the submandibular gland, this structure is removed to ensure thorough exenteration of all of the lymph nodes within this triangle. Thus, the boundaries of level I lymph nodes include the body of the mandible, the anterior belly of the contralateral digastric muscle, and the anterior and posterior bellies of the ipsilateral digastric muscle and the stylohyoid muscle. It should be noted that the perifacial lymph nodes, including the buccinator nodes, are located outside of this triangle superior to the mandibular body. These nodes may contain metastatic disease when the primary site involved is the lip, the buccal

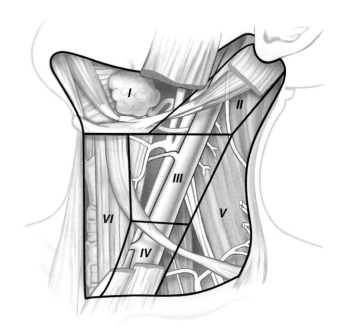

Figure 116-1. The six levels of the neck for describing the location of lymph nodes in the neck. Level I, submental and submandibular group; level II, upper jugular group; level III, middle jugular group; level IV, lower jugular group; level V, posterior triangle group; and level VI, anterior compartment group. (Courtesy of Douglas Denys, M.D.)

mucosa, the anterior nasal cavity, or the soft tissue of the cheek. Thus, the neck dissection performed for nodal disease associated with primary lesions of these sites should be modified to encompass the perifacial nodes.

Level II is defined as the region containing the upper jugular lymph nodes. These are located around the upper third of the internal jugular vein and adjacent to the spinal accessory nerve, extending from the level of the carotid bifurcation (surgical landmark) or hyoid bone (clinical landmark) inferiorly to the skull base superiorly. The lateral boundary is the posterior border of the sternocleidomastoid muscle, and the medial boundary is the lateral border of the sternohyoid muscle and the posterior belly of the digastric muscle and stylohyoid muscle.

Level III contains the middle jugular lymph node group. These nodes are located around the middle third of the internal jugular vein, extending from the carotid bifurcation superiorly (surgical landmark) or the level of the hyoid bone (clinical landmark) to the junction of the omohyoid muscle with the internal jugular vein (surgical landmark) or the lower border of the cricoid arch (clinical landmark) inferiorly. The lateral boundary is the posterior border of the sternocleidomastoid muscle, and the medial boundary is the lateral border of the sternohyoid muscle.

Level IV contains the lower jugular lymph node group. These nodes surround the lower third of the internal jugular vein, extending from the omohyoid muscle (surgical landmark) or cricoid arch (clinical landmark) superiorly to the clavicle inferiorly. The lateral boundary is the posterior border of the sternocleidomastoid muscle, and the medial or anterior boundary is the lateral border of the sternohyoid muscle.

Level V encompasses all lymph nodes contained within the posterior triangle, and these are collectively referred to as the *posterior triangle group*. The boundaries include the anterior border of the trapezius muscle laterally, the posterior border of the sternocleidomastoid muscle medially, and the clavicle inferiorly. The nodes in this triangle comprise three predominant lymphatic pathways: nodes located along the spinal accessory nerve as it traverses the posterior triangle; nodes located along the transverse cervical artery as it courses along the lower third of the triangle; and the supraclavicular nodes located immediately above the clavicle. The supraclavicular nodes also extend under the clavicle to include one particular node of importance: the sentinel—or Virchow's—node.

Level VI encompasses the lymph nodes of the anterior compartment of the neck.[52,61] This group is made up of nodes that surround the midline visceral structures of the neck, extending from the level of the hyoid bone superiorly to the suprasternal notch inferiorly. On each side, the lateral boundary is formed by the medial border of the carotid sheath. Located within this compartment are the perithyroidal lymph nodes, the paratracheal lymph nodes, lymph nodes along the recurrent laryngeal nerves, and the precricoid (Delphian) lymph node. These lymph nodes and their connecting lymphatic channels represent pathways of spread from primary cancers originating in the thyroid gland, the apex of the piriform sinus, the subglottic larynx, the cervical esophagus, and the cervical trachea.

Division of Neck Levels by Sublevels

The 2001 report of the American Head and Neck Society's Neck Dissection Committee recommended the use of sublevels for defining selected lymph node groups within levels I, II, and V on the basis of the biologic significance, independent of the larger zone in which they lay.[52] These are outlined in Figure 116-2 as sublevels IA (submental nodes), IB (submandibular nodes), IIA and IIB (together composing the upper jugular nodes), VA (spinal accessory nodes), and VB (transverse cervical and supraclavicular nodes). The boundaries for each of these sublevels are defined in Table 116-2.

The risk of nodal disease in sublevel IIB is greater for tumors arising in the oropharynx as compared with the oral cavity and larynx. Thus, in the absence

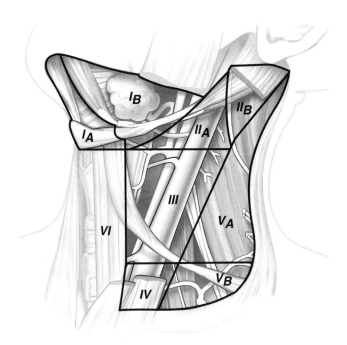

Figure 116-2. The six sublevels of the neck for describing the location of lymph nodes within levels I, II, and V. Level IA, submental group; level IB, submandibular group; level IIA, upper jugular nodes along the carotid sheath, including the subdigastric group; level IIB, upper jugular nodes in the submuscular recess; level VA, spinal accessory nodes; and level VB, the supraclavicular and transverse cervical nodes. (Courtesy of Douglas Denys, M.D.)

of clinical nodal disease in sublevel IIA, it is likely not necessary to include sublevel IIB for tumors arising in these latter sites. The dissection of the node-bearing tissue of sublevel IIB (submuscular recess) creates a risk of morbidity. Adequate exposure necessitates significant manipulation of the spinal accessory nerve and may account for trapezius muscle dysfunction observed in a significant minority of patients after a SND. Sublevel IA is a zone from which many surgeons do not remove lymph nodes unless the primary cancer involves the floor of the mouth, the lip, or structures of the anterior midface or there is obvious lymphadenopathy.

Level V is the third region that has been subdivided, into levels VA and VB. The superior component, level VA, primarily contains the spinal accessory lymph nodes, whereas level VB contains the transverse cervical nodes and the supraclavicular nodes, which carry a more ominous prognosis when positive for aerodigestive tract malignancies.

Correlation of Neck Level Boundaries with Anatomic Markers Depicted Radiologically

Radiologists have now identified landmarks that more accurately identify the location of lymph nodes according to the level system (Table 116-3).[67] Using

TABLE 116-2

LYMPH NODE GROUPS FOUND WITHIN THE SIX NECK LEVELS AND THE SIX SUBLEVELS

Lymph Node Group	Description
Submental (sublevel IA)	Lymph nodes within the triangular boundary of the anterior belly of the digastric muscles and the hyoid bone; these nodes are at the greatest risk of harboring metastases from cancers arising from the floor of the mouth, the anterior oral tongue, the anterior mandibular alveolar ridge, and the lower lip (see Figure 116-2).
Submandibular (sublevel IB)	Lymph nodes within the boundaries of the anterior belly of the digastric muscle, the stylohyoid muscle and the body of the mandible, including the pre- and postglandular nodes and the pre- and postvascular nodes. The submandibular gland is included in the specimen when the lymph nodes within this triangle are removed. These nodes are at greatest risk for harboring metastases from cancers arising from the oral cavity, the anterior nasal cavity, and the soft-tissue structures of the midface and the submandibular gland (see Figure 116-3).
Upper jugular (includes sublevels IIA and IIB)	Lymph nodes located around the upper third of the internal jugular vein and the adjacent spinal accessory nerve, extending from the level of the skull base above to the level of the inferior border of the hyoid bone below. The anterior (medial) boundary is the stylohyoid muscle (the radiologic correlate is the vertical plane defined by the posterior surface of the submandibular gland), and the posterior (lateral) boundary is the posterior border of the sternocleidomastoid muscle. Sublevel IIA nodes are located anterior (medial) to the vertical plane defined by the spinal accessory nerve. Sublevel IIB nodes are located posterior (lateral) to the vertical plane defined by the spinal accessory nerve. The upper jugular nodes are at greatest risk for harboring metastases from cancers arising from the oral cavity, the nasal cavity, the nasopharynx, the oropharynx, the hypopharynx, the larynx, and the parotid gland (see Figure 116-3).
Middle jugular (level III)	Lymph nodes located around the middle third of the internal jugular vein, extending from the inferior border of the hyoid bone above to the inferior border of the cricoid cartilage below. The anterior (medial) boundary is the lateral border of the sternohyoid muscle, and the posterior (lateral) boundary is the posterior border of the sternocleidomastoid muscle. These nodes are at greatest risk for harboring metastases from cancers arising from the oral cavity, the nasopharynx, the oropharynx, the hypopharynx, and the larynx (see Figure 116-3).
Lower jugular (level IV)	Lymph nodes located around the lower third of the internal jugular vein, extending from the inferior border of the cricoid cartilage above to the clavicle below. The anterior (medial) boundary is the lateral border of the sternohyoid muscle, and the posterior (lateral) boundary is the posterior border of the sternocleidomastoid muscle. These nodes are at greatest risk of harboring metastases from cancers arising from the hypopharynx, the thyroid, the cervical esophagus, and the larynx (see Figure 116-3).
Posterior triangle group (includes sublevels VA and VB)	This group is composed predominantly of the lymph nodes located along the lower half of the spinal accessory nerve and the transverse cervical artery. The supraclavicular nodes are also included in the posterior triangle group. The superior boundary is the apex formed by the convergence of the sternocleidomastoid and trapezius muscles; the inferior boundary is the clavicle, the anterior (medial) boundary is the posterior border of the sternocleidomastoid muscle, and the posterior (lateral) boundary is the anterior border of the trapezius muscle. Sublevel VA is separated from sublevel VB by a horizontal plane marking the inferior border of the anterior cricoid arch. Thus, sublevel VA includes the spinal accessory nodes, whereas sublevel VB includes the nodes that follow the transverse cervical vessels and the supraclavicular nodes (with the exception of Virchow's node, which is located in level IV). The posterior triangle nodes are at greatest risk for harboring metastases from cancers arising from the nasopharynx, the oropharynx, and cutaneous structures of the posterior scalp and neck (see Figure 116-3).

TABLE 116-2

LYMPH NODE GROUPS FOUND WITHIN THE SIX NECK LEVELS AND THE SIX SUBLEVELS—cont'd.

Lymph Node Group	Description
Anterior compartment group (level VI)	Lymph nodes in this compartment include the pre- and paratracheal nodes, the precricoid (Delphian) node, and the perithyroidal nodes, including the lymph nodes along the recurrent laryngeal nerves. The superior boundary is the hyoid bone, the inferior boundary is the suprasternal notch, and the lateral boundaries are the common carotid arteries. These nodes are at greatest risk for harboring metastases from cancers arising from the thyroid gland, the glottic and subglottic larynx, the apex of the piriform sinus, and the cervical esophagus (see Figure 116-2).

TABLE 116-3

ANATOMIC STRUCTURES THAT DEFINE THE BOUNDARIES OF THE NECK LEVELS AND SUBLEVELS

Level	Superior	Inferior	Anterior (Medial)	Posterior (Lateral)
IA	Symphysis of the mandible	Body of the hyoid	Anterior belly of the contralateral digastric muscle	Anterior belly of the ipsilateral digastric muscle
IB	Body of the mandible	Posterior belly of the digastric muscle	Anterior belly of the ipsilateral digastric muscle	Stylohyoid muscle
IIA	Skull base	Horizontal plane defined by the inferior body of the hyoid bone	Stylohyoid muscle	Vertical plane defined by the spinal accessory nerve
IIB	Skull base	Horizontal plane defined by the inferior body of the hyoid bone	Vertical plane defined by the spinal accessory nerve	Lateral border of the sternocleidomastoid (SCM) muscle
III	Horizontal plane defined by the inferior body of the hyoid	Horizontal plane defined by the inferior border of the cricoid cartilage	Lateral border of the sternohyoid muscle	Lateral border of the sternocleidomastoid or sensory branches of the cervical plexus
IV	Horizontal plane defined by the inferior border of the cricoid cartilage	Clavicle	Lateral border of the sternohyoid muscle	Lateral border of the sternocleidomastoid or sensory branches of the cervical plexus
VA	Apex of the convergence of the sternocleidomastoid and trapezius muscles	Horizontal plane defined by the lower border of the cricoid cartilage	Posterior border of the sternocleidomastoid muscle or sensory branches of the cervical plexus	Anterior border of the trapezius muscle
VB	Horizontal plane defined by the lower border of the cricoid cartilage	Clavicle	Posterior border of the sternocleidomastoid muscle or sensory branches of the cervical plexus	Anterior border of the trapezius muscle
VI	Hyoid bone	Suprasternal notch	Common carotid artery	Common carotid artery

radiologic landmarks, level I includes all of the nodes above the level of the lower body of the hyoid bone, below the mylohyoid muscles, and anterior to a transverse line drawn on each axial image through the posterior edge of the submandibular gland. Level IA represents those nodes that lie between the medial margins of the anterior bellies of the digastric muscles, above the level of the lower body of the hyoid bone, and below the mylohyoid muscle (these were previously classified as submental nodes). Level IB represents the nodes that lie below the mylohyoid muscle, above the level of the lower body of the hyoid bone, posterior and lateral to the medial edge of the ipsilateral anterior belly of the digastric muscle, and anterior to a transverse line drawn on each axial image tangent to the posterior surface of the submandibular gland on each side of the neck (these are also referred to as submandibular nodes). Level II extends from the skull base at the lower level of the bony margin of the jugular fossa to the level of the lower body of the hyoid bone. Level II nodes lie anterior to a transverse line drawn on each axial image through the posterior edge of the sternocleidomastoid muscle, and they lie posterior to a transverse line drawn on each axial scan through the posterior edge of the submandibular gland. However, any nodes that lie medial to the internal carotid artery (ICA) are retropharyngeal and thus not level II.

Level III nodes lie between the level of the lower body of the hyoid bone and the level of the lower margin of the cricoid cartilage. These nodes lie anterior to a transverse line drawn on each axial image through the posterior edge of the sternocleidomastoid muscle. Level III nodes also lie lateral to the medial margin of either the common carotid artery or the ICA. On each side of the neck, the medial margin of these arteries separates level III nodes, which are lateral, from level VI nodes, which are medial.

Thus, the revised classification uses the horizontal plane defined by the inferior border of the hyoid bone instead of the carotid bifurcation to delineate the boundary between level II and III. Similarly, the revised classification uses the horizontal plane defined by the inferior border of the cricoid cartilage instead of the junction between the superior belly of the omohyoid muscle to delineate the boundary between level III and level IV. However, from a surgical perspective, it is important to note the significance of the anatomic relationship between the omohyoid muscle and the internal jugular vein, because lymph nodes usually are located in this region. These nodes would be included in level III.

NECK DISSECTION CLASSIFICATION

The classification for neck dissection recommended by the American Head and Neck Society's committee

is based on the following rationale: (1) that radical neck dissection is the standard basic procedure for cervical lymphadenectomy, and all other procedures represent one or more modifications of this procedures; (2) when the modification of the radical neck dissection involves the preservation of one or more nonlymphatic structures, the procedure is called *modified radical neck dissection*; (3) when the modification involves the preservation of one or more lymph node groups that are routinely removed in the radical neck dissection, the procedure is called *SND*; and (4) when the modification involves the removal of additional lymph node groups or nonlymphatic structures relative to the radical neck dissection, the procedure is called *extended radical neck dissection* (see Table 116-1).

Radical Neck Dissection

Definition. This procedure includes the removal of all ipsilateral cervical lymph node groups extending from the body of the mandible superiorly to the clavicle inferiorly and from the lateral border of the sternohyoid muscle, the hyoid bone, and the contralateral anterior belly of the digastric muscle anteriorly to the anterior border of the trapezius muscle posteriorly.[53] Included are all lymph node groups from levels I through V, the spinal accessory nerve, the internal jugular vein, and the sternocleidomastoid muscle (Figure 116-3). It does not include the removal of the postauricular and suboccipital nodes, the periparotid nodes (except for a few nodes located in the tail of the

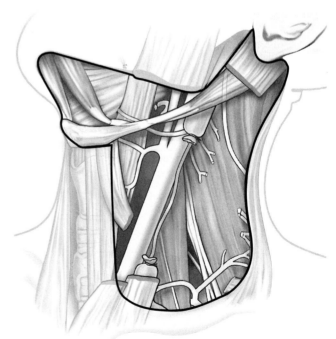

Figure 116-3. Radical neck dissection; the boundaries of dissection are depicted by the heavy line. (Courtesy of Douglas Denys, M.D.)

parotid gland), the perifacial and buccinator nodes, the retropharyngeal nodes, and the paratrachealnodes.

Indications. The radical neck dissection is primarily indicated for patients with extensive lymph node metastases or extension beyond the capsule of the node or nodes to involve the spinal accessory nerve and the internal jugular vein. The procedure has also been traditionally applied to patients with lymph node disease surrounding the spinal accessory nerve without gross evidence of invasion of the spinal accessory or the internal jugular vein. In this latter setting, many surgeons would prefer to do a modified radical neck dissection if there is no gross pathologic evidence of direct invasion of the nonlymphatic structures. However, it is empiric that a surgical violation of tumor-bearing nodes should not be risked for the purpose of preserving any of the aforementioned nonlymphatic structures.

Technique

Positioning. The patient is positioned supine on the table with the shoulder roll placed to optimally extend the neck. The skin is prepped and draped to allow for full exposure of both sides of the neck with clear visualization of surrounding landmarks (e.g., the

lower face including the mentum, both mastoid processes, and earlobes) and the clavicles and suprasternal notch inferiorly. In this way, the incision may be mapped in an accurate fashion, and, throughout the procedure, overall orientation may be maintained.

Incision planning. The incision is planned for optimal exposure of all lymph node levels to be dissected (levels I–V) and to preserve as much blood supply as possible. The neck flaps raised should be broadly based, either superiorly or inferiorly, and preferably to avoid any trifurcations, particularly overlying the carotid sheath. Incisions that best fit these criteria are the hockey stick and boomerang patterns; the McFee incision; and, in patients undergoing bilateral neck dissection, the apron incision, which is a bilateral hockey stick incision (Figure 116-4). Other incisions use trifurcations that overlie the carotid sheath, although modifications of the Schobinger incision include placing the trifurcation more laterally based. Although the boomerang incision may be somewhat less aesthetically pleasing, it is an excellent alternative to use in conjunction with oral cavity and oropharyngeal tumors wherein exposure of the primary site involves extending the incision through the lip for a mandibulotomy approach.

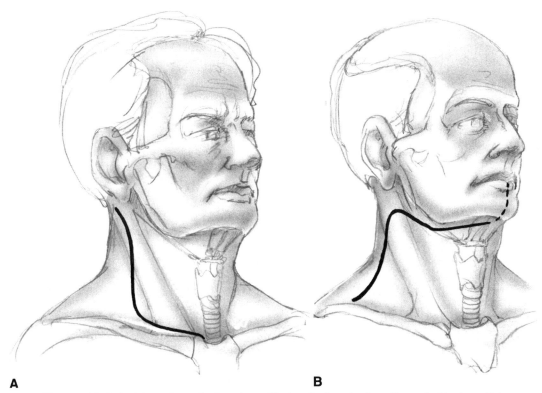

A   **B**

Figure 116-4. Incisions for radical and modified radical neck dissections. **A,** Hockey stick. **B,** Boomerang.

Continued

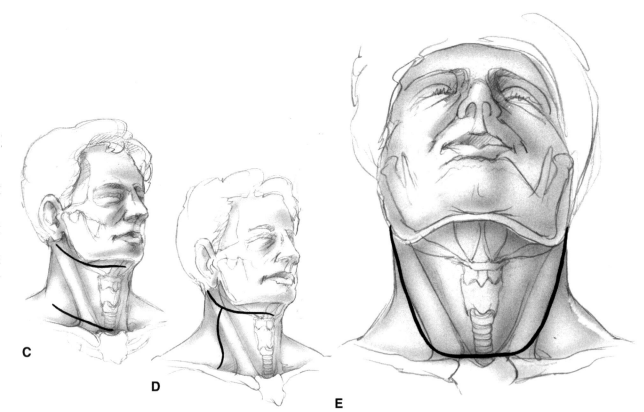

Figure 116-4, cont'd C, McFee. **D,** Modified Schobinger. **E,** Apron or bilateral hockey stick.

Flap elevation. The initial incision is carried through skin and platysma muscle, although the platysma is deficient in the midline and the lateral-most parts of the incision. The flap is raised in the subplatysmal plane so that the external jugular vein and the greater auricular nerves are not included in the flap (Figure 116-5, *A*). Although these structures ultimately will be sacrificed in the radical neck dissection, in SND procedures, these structures are routinely preserved. When there is gross pathologic evidence of tumor extension through the platysmal muscle, with or without skin involvement, the area of disease involvement also should be removed, and modifications of the skin flap may be required. After there has been complete elevation of the skin flap superiorly and inferiorly to expose all of the lymph node levels of the neck, identification of the mandibular branch of the facial nerve is performed next. It is recommended that the anterior facial vein be ligated and retracted superiorly to protect the ramus mandibularis only after the superior skin flap is raised. This allows proper assessment of the prevascular and postvascular lymph nodes in the submandibular triangle, which will need to be removed. Therefore, it is best to incise the submandibular fascia at the lower border of the submandibular gland and to

carefully raise this fascia off of the submandibular gland superiorly to the level of the lower border of the mandible as a separate flap. Usually the mandibular branch of the facial nerve may be seen as this fascia is raised (Figure 116-5, *B*).

Dissection of the posterior triangle. The subsequent order of dissection is a matter of individual preference, although there is some oncologic rationale for dissecting from below upward rather than from above downward. Thus, the next step is to expose the anterior border of the trapezius muscle from its superior aspect, where it converges with the posterior border of the sternocleidomastoid muscle, to its inferior aspect, where it approaches the clavicle (Figure 116-5, *C*). The fibrofatty tissue is then incised along its anterior border beginning superiorly and working inferiorly to expose the muscular floor of the posterior triangle. In so doing, the spinal accessory nerve will be severed at the point at which it enters the trapezius muscle in the lower aspect of the posterior triangle. After this step has been completed, the floor of the posterior triangle at its inferior extent is next exposed by incising through the fibrofatty tissue immediately above the superior border of the clavicle. This requires incising through the inferior belly of the omohyoid muscle and the fibrofatty tissue overlying

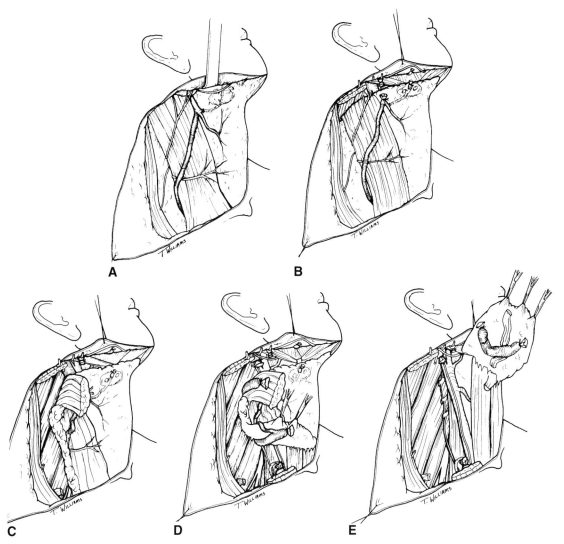

Figure 116-5. Steps of the radical neck dissection.

the brachial plexus. In this region, the transverse facial artery will be encountered immediately overlying the muscular floor of the triangle; this artery should be preserved unless there is gross disease involving the region. The fibrofatty contents of the posterior triangle are then mobilized anteriorly, lifting them away from the floor of the neck, which, in this region, is formed by the splenius capitis, the levator scapulae, and the scalene muscles. It is important to remain superficial to the prevertebral fascia during this step of the operation to prevent injury to the phrenic nerve and the brachial plexus. As the fibrofatty tissue is swept in a lateral-to-medial direction, the sensory branches of the cervical plexus will be encountered and divided.

Anterior triangle dissection. As the fibrofatty tissue is elevated medially toward the carotid sheath, it will be necessary to incise the mastoid attachment of

the sternocleidomastoid muscle and the clavicular attachments (Figure 116-5, *D*). The carotid sheath will be exposed, and identification of the common carotid artery and vagus nerve may be made. Attention should be given to preserving the cervical sympathetic chain, which is closely applied to the prevertebral fascia behind the carotid sheath. The plane of dissection will be carried between the vagus nerve and the carotid artery below and the internal jugular vein above. Thus, the internal jugular vein may be mobilized from the skull base superiorly to its inferior aspect near the clavicle; ties may then be placed around the upper and lower ends of the internal jugular vein, thereby allowing ligation and complete mobilization. When incising the soft-tissue contents of the lower medial aspect of the neck, lymphatic channels will be encountered, particularly on the left side. It is imperative to precisely identify these and ligate them immediately as they are encountered. The thoracic duct is located to the right of and behind the left common carotid artery and the vagus nerve. From here, it arches upward, forward, and laterally, passing behind the internal jugular vein and in front of the anterior scalene muscle and the phrenic nerve; it then opens into the internal jugular vein, the subclavian vein, or the angle formed by the junction of these two vessels. The duct is anterior to the thyrocervical trunk and the transverse cervical artery. To prevent a chyle leak, the surgeon should also remember that the thoracic duct may be multiple in its upper end and that, at the base of the neck, it usually receives the jugular trunk, a subclavian trunk, and maybe other minor lymphatic trunks that should be individually divided and ligated or clipped.

After ligation of the lower part of the internal jugular vein, the contents of the mobilized specimen are retracted superiorly and medially. Dissection is carried along the common carotid artery and medially as far as the sternohyoid muscle. Further elevation of the contents exposes the carotid bifurcation. As this is done, the branches of the internal jugular vein require identification and ligation. Specifically, these are the middle and superior thyroid veins and the retromandibular vein. Further superior elevation of the fibrofatty contents away from the upper part of the carotid sheath exposes the hypoglossal nerve lying lateral to the external carotid artery and the spinal accessory nerve extending from above downward.

At this point, the posterior belly of the digastric muscle is identified, and the soft-tissue attachments of the neck contents lying superior to the muscle are divided, including the sternocleidomastoid muscle as it attaches to the mastoid process, vascular channels extending into the postauricular region and parotid gland, the tail of the parotid gland that extends downward inferior to the level of the digastric muscle, and soft-tissue attachments to the angle of the mandible. After completion of this part of the dissection, all of the lower contents of the neck dissection specimen should be freely mobile, and the only remaining attachments are the upper end of the internal jugular vein and the undissected contents of the submandibular triangle and the submental triangle (Figure 116-5, *E*).

Dissection of the upper neck compartments.
Excision of level I lymph nodes is begun by dividing the soft tissue overlying the body of the mandible, including the facial artery and vein as they emerge above the submandibular gland and extend lateral to the body of the mandible. The anterior bellies of the ipsilateral and contralateral digastric muscles are skeletonized, thereby delineating the boundaries of the submental triangle. After the fibrofatty tissue has been removed from occupying this space, the fibrofatty contents of the anterior portion of the submandibular triangle are removed from the underlying mylohyoid muscle until its lateral border may be identified. The posterior border of the muscle is retracted anteriorly, exposing the deep contents of the submandibular triangle; this allows for visualization of the lingual nerve, the submandibular duct, and the hypoglossal nerve. The submandibular duct is isolated, divided, and ligated. Next, the submandibular ganglion should be clamped and divided, thus allowing the lingual nerve to retract superiorly away from the area of dissection. Care is taken to not injure the hypoglossal nerve and its venae comitantes in the deep portion of the triangle. The last attachment of the contents of the submandibular triangle is the proximal end of the facial artery as it courses deep to the submandibular gland. It is important to remember that complete excision of all contents of the submandibular triangle within its muscular boundaries—and not just the submandibular gland—is required.

Variations in the approach to the radical neck dissection should be made, depending on the location of the disease and its degree of mobility. For example, it is best to mobilize the areas that are least involved with a tumor that is difficult to remove, which will enhance the exposure of the anatomic structures that may be directly invaded by the disease itself.

Neck drains are inserted and brought through separate stab incisions through the most dependent areas of the dead space. Closure of the incisions are usually performed in two layers, including approximation of the platysma anteriorly and the subcutaneous tissue laterally and the second layer approximating the skin.

Modified Radical Neck Dissection

Definition. A *modified radical neck dissection* is defined as the en bloc removal of lymph-node–bearing tissue from one side of the neck (levels I–V). The dissection extends from the inferior border of the mandible above to the clavicle below and from the lateral border of the strap muscles medially to the anterior border of the trapezius muscle laterally. Unlike the radical neck dissection, there is preservation of one or more of the following structures in the modified radical dissection: the spinal accessory nerve, the internal jugular vein, and the sternocleidomastoid muscle (Figure 116-6). The major purpose of these modifications relates to the morbidity encountered when the spinal accessory nerve is removed. Although the degree of morbidity is less for removal of the sternocleidomastoid muscle and the internal jugular vein, this issue becomes far more important if bilateral neck dissections are required. Simultaneous sacrifice of both

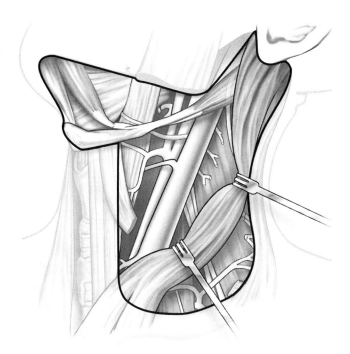

Figure 116-6. Boundaries of the modified radical neck dissection, in which there is preservation of the spinal accessory nerve, the sternocleidomastoid muscle, and the internal jugular vein. (Courtesy of Douglas Denys, M.D.)

internal jugular veins may result in severe swelling of the face with increased intracranial pressure.

Indications. The major indication for a modified radical neck dissection is to remove probable or grossly pathologic visible lymph node disease that is not directly infiltrating or fixed to the nonlymphatic structures. Because the spinal accessory nerve is rarely directly invaded by metastatic disease, it is difficult to justify its sacrifice when the hypoglossal nerve or the vagus nerve, which also lie in the same proximity to the nodal disease, are spared.

Technique. Knowledge of the surgical anatomy of the spinal accessory nerve is essential to preserve this structure. Below the jugular foramen, the spinal accessory nerve is located deep to the digastric and stylohyoid muscles and lateral or immediately posterior to the internal jugular vein; it then runs obliquely downward inferiorly and posteriorly to reach the medial surface of the sternocleidomastoid muscle near the junction of the superior and middle third. It traverses this muscle, giving off a major branch to it. The remaining part of the nerve then exits the posterior border of the sternocleidomastoid muscle near the point wherein the greater auricular nerve turns around it, which is known as Erb's point. From Erb's

point the nerve courses through the posterior triangle of the neck to enter the anterior border of the trapezius muscle approximately 2 cm above the superior border of the clavicle.

The incisions and skin flaps are raised for modified radical neck dissection as similarly described for the radical neck dissection. The same procedure is followed to identify and protect the mandibular branch of the facial nerve in level I.

Unlike what is found in the radical neck dissection procedure, the next step is to identify the spinal accessory nerve. This is initially done in the posterior triangle from which the nerve exits at or around Erb's point (Figure 116-7, *A*). The nerve lies superficially in the fibrofatty contents of the posterior triangle and usually may be identified by careful spreading of the fibrofatty tissue; the use of a nerve stimulator may facilitate this process. Once located, the nerve is isolated and dissected away from the underlying fibrofatty contents from Erb's point medially to the point at which it enters the anterior border of the trapezius muscle laterally (Figure 116-7, *B*). The nerve is next isolated in its superior third, which is done by incising the anterior border of the sternocleidomastoid muscle from its attachment superiorly at the mastoid to its lowermost attachment at the sternal head. The sternocleidomastoid muscle is retracted laterally and mobilized as the fibrofatty soft-tissue contents, with its vessels, are divided. This part of the procedure mobilizes the anterior aspect of the sternocleidomastoid muscle along its full extent. As the muscle is retracted laterally in its upper portion, the spinal accessory nerve is seen entering its anterior border (Figure 116-7, *C*). Thus, the nerve may be isolated from the point of its entry into the sternocleidomastoid muscle superiorly to the skull base. When performing this superior isolation maneuver, the digastric muscle is also identified, and its inferior border may be mobilized to retract it superiorly and to provide optimal exposure of the spinal accessory nerve and the underlying internal jugular vein at the skull base. The only portion of the spinal accessory nerve that has not been mobilized is the portion that branches within the sternocleidomastoid muscle. Thus, the posterior border of the sternocleidomastoid muscle may be incised in a vertical fashion from its mastoid attachment above to its clavicular attachment below. Dissection is carried underneath this muscle so that it may be fully mobilized and elevated as a bipedicle flap. The spinal accessory nerve is now completely mobilized from its lowermost attachment to the anterior border of the trapezius muscle to its superior extent at the skull base.

The fibrofatty tissue in the posterior triangle is separated from the entire anterior border of the trapezius

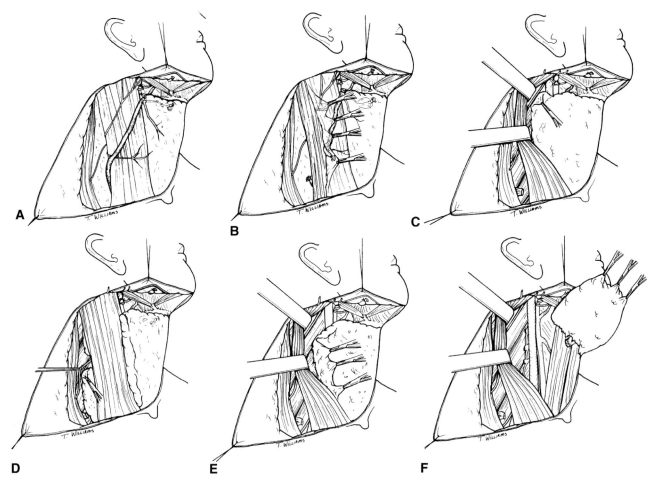

Figure 116-7. Steps of the modified radical neck dissection, in which there is preservation of the spinal accessory nerve, the internal jugular vein, and the sternocleidomastoid muscle.

muscle and is mobilized from a lateral to a medial direction. Tissue lying superficial to the spinal accessory nerve as it courses across the posterior triangle should be divided immediately above the spinal accessory nerve so that it may be passed along with its deep component beneath the nerve and the elevated sternocleidomastoid muscle (Figure 116-7, *D*). After the fibrofatty contents have been dissected and swept over the carotid artery, the vagus nerve, and the internal jugular vein, the sternocleidomastoid muscle may be retracted laterally and the contents passed underneath the muscle for subsequent dissection of the anterior triangle of the neck (Figure 116-7, *E*). Careful sharp dissection will allow for separation of these contents from the carotid artery and the jugular vein. This dissection is continued until the sternohyoid muscle, which is the medial boundary of anterior triangle contents in the lower neck, is reached. The branches of the internal jugular vein usually are ligated to allow a thorough clean out of the anterior triangle contents. Dissection is carried superiorly to remove the fibrofatty tissue attachments overlying the

internal jugular vein at the level of the skull base. The retromandibular vein may be preserved, but the anterior facial vein needs to be ligated (Figure 116-7, *F*). Subsequent dissection is then performed to remove the contents of the submandibular and submental triangles.

Sacrifice of one or two of the nonlymphatic structures of the neck (i.e., the spinal accessory nerve, the sternocleidomastoid muscle, and the internal jugular vein) may become necessary as a result of gross pathologic involvement intraoperatively, although the operation continues to be called a modified radical neck dissection as long as at least one of these structures is preserved (Figure 116-8).

Selective Neck Dissection

Definition. SND is performed for patients who are at risk for early lymph node metastases. The procedure consists of the en bloc removal of one or more lymph node groups that are at risk for harboring metastatic cancer, an assessment that is based on the location of the primary tumor. Thus, the levels removed depend

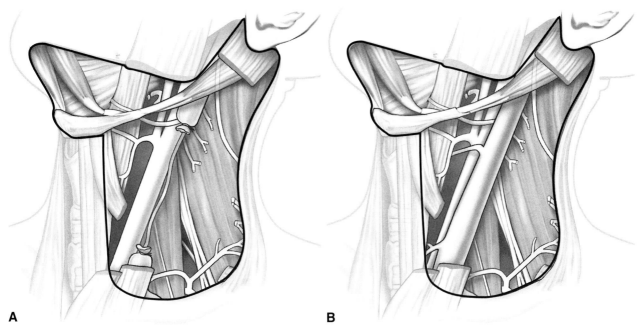

A   **B**

Figure 116-8. Modified radical neck dissection in which there is **A,** preservation of the spinal accessory nerve only, and **B,** preservation of the spinal accessory nerve and internal jugular vein. (Courtesy of Douglas Denys, M.D.)

on the location of the primary lesion and its known pattern of spread.

Rationale. Although the concept of SND dates back to procedures used for treating lip cancer, the further adoption of this concept was through the surgeons at MD Anderson Cancer Center.[23] It was based on removing lymph node groups that were at highest risk for patients with N_0 nodal disease. Studies have shown that this procedure has the same therapeutic value as more extensive procedures[9]; it is also intended to preserve functionally and cosmetically relevant structures as a secondary goal.

The topographic distribution of lymph node metastases appears to be predictable in patients with previously untreated squamous cell carcinoma of the head and neck, particularly in those with early disease. The basic anatomic studies of Rouviere[56] and Fisch and Sigel[19] showed that the lymphatic drainage of the mucosal surfaces of the head and neck follow relatively constant and predictable routes. The clinical study by Lindberg in 1972[31] showed that the lymph node groups most frequently involved in patients with carcinoma of the oral cavity are the jugulodigastric and midjugular nodes. In addition, the nodes in the submandibular triangle frequently are involved in patients with carcinoma of the floor of the mouth, the anterior oral tongue, and the buccal mucosa. Lindberg also noted that tumors frequently metastasize to both

sides of the neck and may skip the submandibular and jugulodigastric nodes, metastasizing first to the midjugular region. The Lindberg study showed that, in the absence of metastases to the first echelon nodes, tumors of the oral cavity and oropharynx rarely involve the lower jugular and posterior triangle nodes. Similar findings were reported by Skolnik in 1976,[64] who, in a study of radical neck dissection specimens, found no metastases in the nodes of the posterior triangle of the neck in radical neck dissections, regardless of the site of the primary tumor or the presence or absence of metastases in the jugular nodes. Further evidence subsequently has been provided by Shah[62] in a retrospective study of radical neck dissection specimens performed for patients with oral cavity and larynx or laryngopharyngeal metastases. Shah demonstrated that tumors of the oral cavity metastasize most frequently to neck nodes in levels I, II, and III, whereas carcinomas of the pharynx, hypopharynx, and larynx involve mainly the nodes in levels II, III, and IV. Whenever nodes were found in other areas, there was also positive disease in the areas of highest risk.

Some authorities believe that SND is, in essence, a procedure for staging the necks of patients whose tumors are amenable to treatment with surgery alone. In patients who have this procedure done in conjunction with the excision of the primary tumor, further information about the status of the nodal disease is provided. If there is evidence of multiple lymph node metastases or extracapsular spread in the neck dissection contents, then postoperative radiotherapy is indicated. Byers[12] also reported a lower rate of regional recurrence among patients with N_1 disease if postoperative radiation therapy was administered. More intensive therapy may be used for patients who have more aggressive tumors.

Selective neck dissection for oral cavity cancer
Definition and rationale. The procedure of choice is SND (levels I–III) and is often called the supraomohyoid neck dissection. The procedure involves the removal of lymph nodes contained in the submental and submandibular triangles (level I), the upper jugular lymph nodes (level II), and the midjugular lymph nodes (level III). The cutaneous branches of the cervical plexus and the posterior border of the sternocleidomastoid muscle mark the posterior limit of the dissection. The inferior limit is the junction between the superior belly of the omohyoid muscle and the internal jugular vein.

SND is recommended for patients with oral cavity cancer who are at risk of harboring occult nodal disease (Figure 116-9). Tumors originating in this region, particularly in the subsites of the oral tongue and the floor of the mouth, have a high propensity to metastasize early, regardless of size and differentiation. Primary echelons for nodal spread include the submental, submandibular, upper jugular, and middle jugular groups. In patients with tongue cancer, the lower jugular lymph node groups are also at risk. Even when there is no clinical evidence of nodal disease, there is at least a 20% risk for occult disease associated with these lesions. Unless the management of choice for the primary lesion is radiotherapy, elective neck dissection with removal of levels I through III (level IV for those with tongue cancer) is the minimal recommended treatment for patients with squamous cell carcinoma of the oral cavity associated with N_0 nodal disease. In the case of oral tongue cancer, there is evidence that indicates that level IV is also at risk.[11] Thus, some authorities recommend the SND procedure for this subsite within the oral cavity to include levels I through IV. If there is palpable nodal disease, it is also usually necessary to remove levels IV and V as well. One exception is in those patients with nodal disease confined to level I and II. In these patients, selective removal of levels I through IV is an appropriate alternative. With the exception of a solitary metastatic node without extracapsular extension, postoperative radiation therapy is usually indicated for all patients undergoing SND who have positive pathologic nodes in the specimen.[12] Elective cervical lymphadenectomy of the

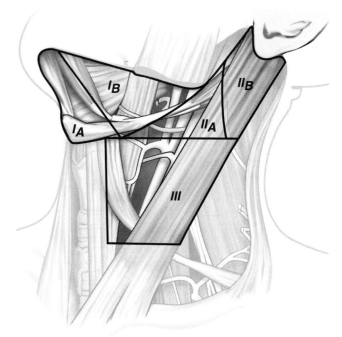

Figure 116-9. Boundaries of the selective neck dissection for oral cavity cancer, SND (I-III) or supraomohyoid type. (Courtesy of Douglas Denys, M.D.)

contralateral neck is indicated for patients with primary lesions involving the floor of the mouth or the ventral surface or with midline involvement of the tongue, in whom ipsilateral neck dissection is planned and in whom there are no definite indications for postoperative radiotherapy. Contralateral therapeutic neck dissection is indicated for patients with clinically N_{2c} disease.

Technique. When an ipsilateral supraomohyoid neck dissection is planned, a modified apron incision is made to provide adequate exposure of levels I through III (Figure 116-10, *A*). If bilateral neck dissection is needed, the horizontal component of the apron incision is carried across the midline to the other side of the neck (bilateral apron incision; Figure 116-10, *B*). The ipsilateral and bilateral apron incisions also are appropriate for exposure of the primary disease when a pull-through exposure is indicated. When it is necessary to split the lip for access to the primary tumor, the medial component of the ipsilateral apron incision may be extended for this purpose. If bilateral neck dissection is planned and a lip-splitting incision is also required, a bilateral boomerang incision is substituted for the bilateral apron incision (Figure 116-10, *C*). This neck incision pattern is also preferred for those with more advanced nodal disease associated with oral cavity primaries in whom it is necessary to dissect all five levels of the ipsilateral neck. The boomerang incision is also preferred

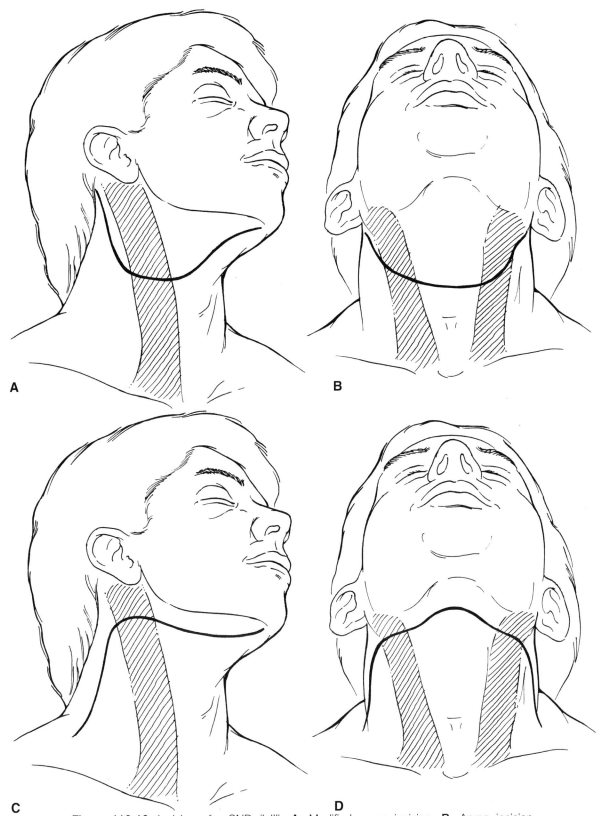

A

B

C

D

Figure 116-10. Incisions for SND (I–III). **A,** Modified apron incision. **B,** Apron incision. **C,** Boomerang incision. **D,** Bilateral boomerang incision.

for patients with stage N_{2c} disease, because it may be extended across the midline for exposure of all levels of the contralateral lymph nodes (Figure 116-10, *D*).

For the removal of levels I through III, the modified apron skin flap is raised in the subplatysmal plane until there is exposure of the upper two-thirds of the anterior border of the sternocleidomastoid muscle, the mastoid process, the body of the mandible, and the mandibular symphysis (Figure 116-11, *A* and *B*). It is preferred not to raise the fascia off of the submandibular gland until the subplatysmal flap is first elevated to the level of the body of the mandible, which permits a more accurate assessment of the submandibular triangle for assessing tumor involvement of the superficial layer of the deep cervical fascia. After this possibility is excluded, the fascia overlying the submandibular gland is carefully raised as a separate flap to avoid injuring the mandibular branch of the facial nerve. This branch is often seen within the superficial layer of the deep cervical fascia, but, with careful dissection of this layer, the nerve may be protected and preserved.

Next an incision is made in the investing layer of the deep fascia at the anterior border of the sternocleidomastoid muscle. Care is taken to not injure the external jugular vein and branches of the greater auricular nerve that lie lateral to the sternocleidomastoid muscle but posterior to the fascial incision being made. Because lymph nodes associated with the external jugular vein are almost never involved with aerodigestive tract carcinomas, these structures are left undisturbed. The fibrofatty contents of the anterior triangle are peeled away first from the anterior border and then from the medial aspect of the sternocleidomastoid muscle all the way from a point close to the mastoid process above down to the level of the omohyoid muscle below, stopping when the posterior border of the muscle is reached. Although the upper third of the sternocleidomastoid muscle is being separated, the spinal accessory nerve comes into view as it enters the muscle (Figure 116-11, *C*). This nerve is dissected free of its surrounding fibrofatty tissue from the level of the skull base adjacent to the internal jugular vein to its point of entry into the sternocleidomastoid muscle. It is necessary to dissect along the inferior border of the posterior belly of the digastric muscle and to retract it supralaterally to provide adequate exposure of the upper carotid sheath near the skull base. Fibrofatty tissue is also dissected away from the inferior border of the posterior belly of the digastric muscle as far posteriorly as the attachment of the mastoid process. This triangle formed by the digastric muscle, the spinal accessory nerve, and the sternocleidomastoid muscle outlines the triangu-

lar packet of tissue-bearing lymph nodes belonging to level II. It is important to separate this triangular packet from the underlying paraspinal muscles and to pass it under the spinal accessory nerve (Figure 116-11, *D*). The dissection is continued inferiorly by incising along the fibrofatty tissue corresponding with the posterior border of the sternocleidomastoid muscle to the level of the omohyoid muscle. Care is taken to not cut across the sensory branches of the cervical plexus as the incision is carried down to the muscular floor. When the sensory branches of the cervical plexus are encountered, the fibrofatty tissue is dissected in a plane that is superficial to these nerves (Figure 116-11, *E*). At this point in the procedure, it is important to carefully inspect and palpate the lower jugular chain and the posterior triangle for evidence of nodal disease. If found, the dissection of the lymph-node–bearing tissue would have to be extended to encompass level IV and the posterior triangle (level V), thus converting the operation to a modified radical neck dissection. For this purpose, a lower cervical flap would then be raised for adequate exposure of the clavicle and the anterior border of the trapezius.

After completion of the lateral boundary of dissection, the lymph-node–bearing tissue is swept medially in a plane immediately above the fascia of the paraspinal muscles. The sensory branches of the cervical plexus may be preserved only when level V dissection is not performed. This maneuver allows the lymph-node–bearing tissue to be swept over the carotid sheath and permits exposure of its structures from the level of the clavicle or omohyoid muscle below to the skull base above. Sharp dissection is used to remove the fascia overlying the sheath, which usually includes preserving the internal jugular vein if a tissue plane can be readily identified. Next, the superior belly of the omohyoid muscle is skeletonized along its superior border to the level of the hyoid bone. The hyoid bone is also skeletonized medially, as is the anterior belly of the contralateral digastric muscle; this completes the medial boundary of dissection. The fibrofatty tissue is dissected from below at the level of the omohyoid muscle in a superior direction toward the submandibular triangle. After the lymph-node–bearing tissue in the submental triangle has been cleared, the contents of the submandibular triangle are removed to complete the neck dissection (see Figure 116-11). To ensure complete removal of all lymph nodes from this region, it is important to dissect along the fascial planes of the muscles within this triangle rather than enucleating the submandibular gland only, which includes dissecting the preglandular nodes underneath the anterior belly of the digastric muscle and the prevascular and postvascular nodes along the

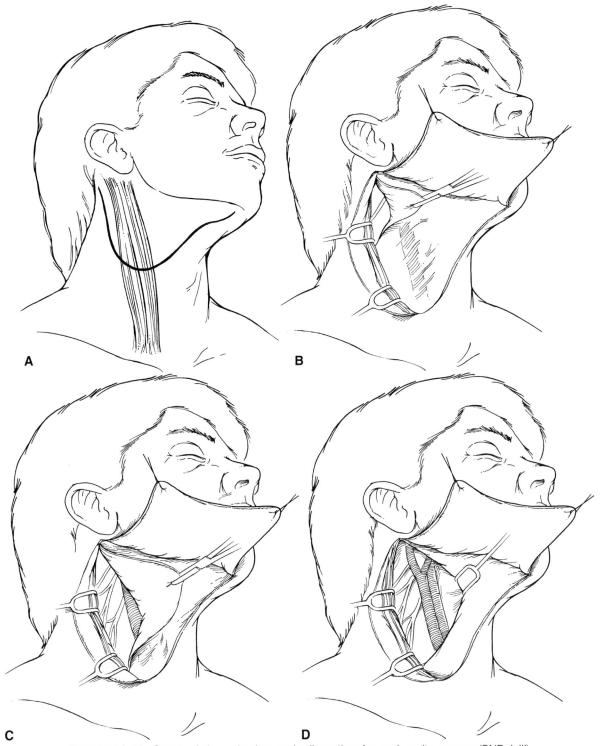

Figure 116-11. Steps of the selective neck dissection for oral cavity cancer (SND I–III). **A,** Modified apron incision. **B,** Flap raised in the subplatysmal plane to expose the upper two-thirds of the carotid sheath and the submandibular and submental triangle; exposure of the upper third of the spinal accessory nerve and dissection of the submuscular recess (level IIB). **C,** Dissection of level III and preservation of the cervical plexus. **D,** Completion of the dissection of levels III and IIA.

Continued

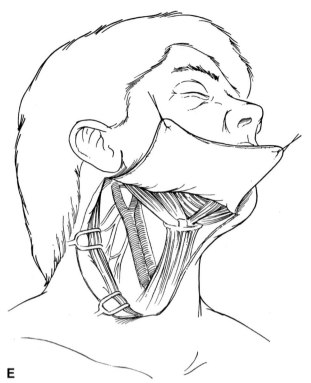

E

Figure 116-11, cont'd E, Dissection of level I.

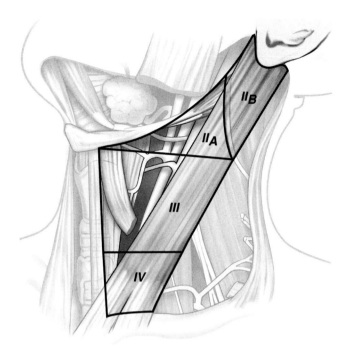

Figure 116-12. Boundaries of the selective neck dissection for oropharyngeal, laryngeal, and hypopharyngeal cancer, SND (II–IV) or lateral type. (Courtesy of Douglas Denys, M.D.)

lower border of the body of the mandible. It is usually not necessary to remove the perifacial nodes lying lateral to the mandibular body, unless the primary cancer involves the buccal mucosa, the upper gum, or the upper lip. Dissection of this latter nodal group increases the risk of injury to the mandibular branch of the facial nerve. After completion of the dissection, the excised tissue is separated according to the level of the lymph node groups, each level being submitted separately for pathologic evaluation. Before closing the incisions, a single drain is placed in the surgical bed extending inferiorly from the digastric muscle above to a separate cutaneous puncture site made at the most dependent region below the skin incision. The drain is placed on continuous suction, and a bulky pressure dressing is applied for 24 hours. A second drain is placed in the contralateral neck for bilateral procedures. The drain is usually removed 3 days after surgery, if the fluid collection is less than 20 mL/24 hours.

Selective neck dissection for oropharyngeal, hypopharyngeal, and laryngeal cancer

Definition and rationale. The procedure of choice for these anatomic sites is SND (levels II–IV), and its boundaries are outlined in Figure 116-12; it is also called *lateral neck dissection*. The procedure refers to the removal of the upper jugular lymph nodes

(level II), the midjugular lymph nodes (level III), and the lower jugular lymph nodes (level IV). The superior limit of dissection is the skull base, and the inferior limit is the clavicle. The anterior (medial) limit is the lateral border of the sternohyoid muscle and the stylohyoid muscle. The posterior (lateral) limit of the dissection is marked by the cutaneous branches of the cervical plexus and the posterior border of the sternocleidomastoid muscle. In the case of cancers involving the oropharynx and the hypopharynx, there is evidence indicating that the lateral retropharyngeal nodes are also at risk. Level IIB is at greater risk for metastases associated with oropharyngeal lesions relative to laryngeal and hypopharyngeal cancers. Thus, if level IIB is excluded (as is sometimes done for laryngeal and hypopharyngeal cancers), the procedure would be designated SND (IIA, III, and IV). When lymphatic metastases occur bilaterally, the procedure of choice is a bilateral SND (II–IV). If the retropharyngeal lymph nodes are included, as in the case of cancers involving the pharyngeal wall, the procedure is designated SND (II–IV, retropharyngeal nodes). If the nodes in level VI are removed, as in the case of laryngeal and hypopharyngeal cancers extending below the level of the glottis, the procedure is designated SND (II–IV and VI).

Technique. The incision should allow for adequate exposure of levels II through IV and, should occult disease be found, exposure of level V as well. The hockey stick incision as described for radical and modified radical neck dissection is useful for this purpose; it also may be extended across the midline and carried along the contralateral neck as a broadly based apron flap or bilateral hockey stick incision (Figure 116-13). After the neck flaps have been raised, the fibrofatty contents of the anterior triangle are removed en bloc, including the lymph nodes lying along the internal jugular vein from the skull base superiorly to the clavicle inferiorly. The dissection proceeds by incising along the anterior border of the sternocleidomastoid muscle and by separating it from its underlying attachments to the fibrofatty tissue. Care is taken to identify the spinal accessory nerve as it enters the anterior aspect of the sternocleidomastoid muscle. It then is skeletonized from its entry point into the muscle inferiorly and into the skull base superiorly, wherein it lies deep to the posterior belly of the digastric muscle and lateral to the internal jugular vein. As described for the supraomohyoid neck dissection, the fibrofatty tissue deep to the sternocleidomastoid muscle is incised and separated from the underlying splenius and levator muscles. The sensory branches of the cervical plexus may also be preserved by limiting the mobilization of fibrofatty tissue to the region superficial to these nerve branches. The contents then are swept medially over the internal jugular vein, thereby exposing the full length of the vein from the skull base above to the clavicle below. At the lower end, care should be taken to meticulously identify and ligate any lymphatic channels encountered. On the left side, the thoracic duct will frequently be encountered; this structure must be carefully separated away from the fibrofatty tissue, avoiding any injury. If injury occurs, a repair must immediately be performed with fine, nonabsorbable suture material (e.g., silk, monofilament synthetic); occasionally this will necessitate ligation of the duct. After the internal jugular vein has been completely skeletonized, the remainder of the fibrofatty contents of the anterior triangle is mobilized by skeletonizing the medial border of the sternohyoid muscle and the stylohyoid muscle. The branches of the internal jugular vein in the neck may be sacrificed to facilitate this process, although the communicating branch to the anterior facial and retromandibular veins may be easily preserved.

Selective neck dissection for cutaneous malignancies

Definition and rationale. The operation of choice depends on the location of the lesion and the adjacent

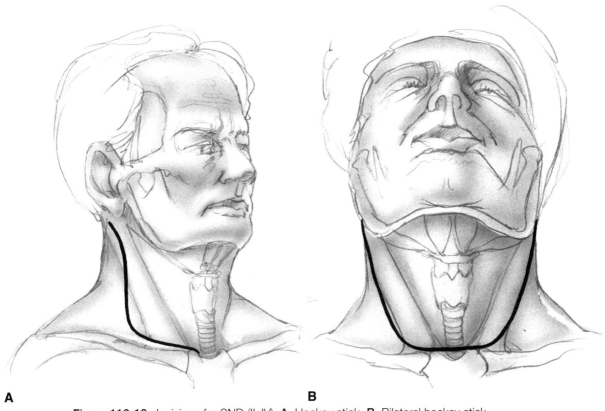

A **B**

Figure 116-13. Incisions for SND (II–IV). **A,** Hockey stick. **B,** Bilateral hockey stick.

lymph node groups, which are most likely to harbor metastatic disease. In the case of cancers involving the posterior scalp and upper neck, the procedure of choice is SND (II–V, postauricular, and suboccipital) (Figure 116-14). This particular version is also called the *posterolateral neck dissection;* it is primarily used to eradicate nodal metastases associated with cutaneous malignancies and soft-tissue sarcomas.[55]

It involves the removal of the suboccipital lymph nodes, the retroauricular lymph nodes, the upper jugular lymph nodes (level II), the middle jugular lymph nodes (level III), the lower jugular lymph nodes (level IV), and the nodes of the posterior triangle of the neck (level V). The superior limit of dissection is the skull base anteriorly and the nuchal ridge posteriorly, and the inferior limit is the clavicle. The medial (anterior) limit is the lateral border of the sternohyoid muscle and the stylohyoid muscle; the lateral (posterior) limit is the anterior border of the trapezius muscle inferiorly and the midline of the neck superiorly. It is common to all sites that the lymphatic pathways for the seeding of tumor to the first and secondary echelon nodes involve the posterior auricular, occipital, posterior triangle, and jugular groups (Figure 116-14). Thus the dissection is designed to encompass the lymph-node–bearing fibrofatty tissue of the posterior and lateral compartments of the neck. In addition, it is important to remove the intervening subdermal fat and underlying fascia between the lymph node groups and the primary dis-

ease, which ensures the removal of smaller nests of metastasizing tumor cells that are characteristic of malignancies originating in cutaneous soft tissue. For cutaneous malignancies arising on the preauricular, anterior scalp, and temporal regions, the elective neck dissection of choice is SND (parotid and facial nodes, levels IIA, IIB, III, and VA, and the external jugular nodes). For cutaneous malignancies arising on the anterior and lateral face, the elective neck dissection of choice is SND (parotid and facial nodes, levels IA, IB, II, and III). The development of techniques of lymphatic mapping may have a future role in specifically defining nonpredictable lymphatic echelons of risk for cutaneous malignancies.

Technique. The optimal incision for posterolateral neck dissection is one that allows exposure along the nuchal ridge to the occiput and the posterior triangle and exposure of the upper, middle, and lower jugular lymph node groups; this may usually be accomplished with a lazy **S** pattern or the combination of the hockey stick pattern with a horizontal extension from its upper aspect along the nuchal ridge. The patient should be placed in the lateral decubitus position to allow for adequate exposure of the posterior scalp and occiput. In patients with midline posterior scalp lesions, the procedure should encompass the nodal groups on both sides of the neck. In this latter situation, the patient should be placed in the prone position to allow access to both sides. The skin flaps are raised in the subplatysmal plane anteriorly and the subdermal plane posteriorly. The posterior auricular

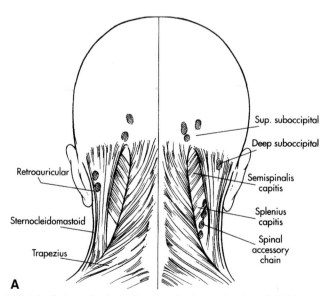

A

Figure 116-14. A, Localization of retroauricular and suboccipital lymph nodes.

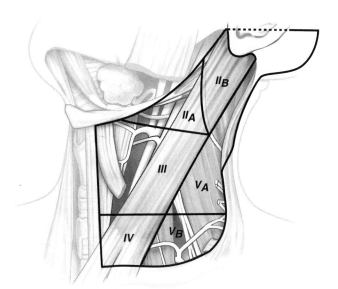

Figure 116-14, cont'd B, Selective neck dissection for posterior scalp and upper posterolateral cutaneous malignancies, SND (II–V, postauricular, suboccipital) or posterolateral neck dissection. (Courtesy of Douglas Denys, M.D.)

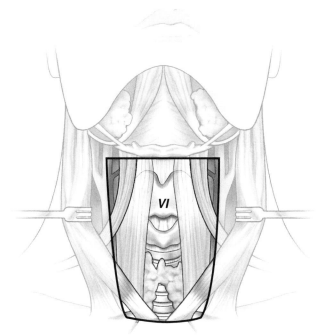

Figure 116-15. Boundaries of the selective neck dissection for thyroid cancer, SND (VI) or anterior neck dissection. (Courtesy of Douglas Denys, M.D.)

and suboccipital nodes are removed by incising the soft tissue overlying the fascia of the upper neck muscles that attach to the nuchal ridge and occiput. In addition, the upper part of the trapezius muscle that attaches to the skull base should be divided to allow for complete exposure of the suboccipital nodes; these nodes lie along the occipital artery as it courses laterally along the skull base. After completing this part of the dissection, the posterior triangle is cleared in the fashion that has already been described for the modified radical neck dissection. The spinal accessory nerve is routinely identified and preserved unless there is direct tumor extension into the soft tissue surrounding it. The technique for locating and preserving the spinal accessory nerve has already been described. The remainder of the procedure involves mobilizing the fibrofatty contents of the anterior triangle, thereby removing the upper, middle, and lower jugular groups of lymph nodes. The technique for this procedure has already been described.

Selective neck dissection for cancer of the midline structures of the anterior lower neck

Definition and rationale. The procedure of choice is SND (level VI) and is often called the *anterior neck dissection* or the *central compartment dissection* (Figure 116-15). The procedure is most often indicated with or without dissection of other neck levels for thyroid cancer, advanced glottic and subglottic larynx cancer, advanced piriform sinus cancer, and cervical esophageal/tracheal cancer. This refers to the

removal of the lymph nodes within the central compartment of the neck, including the paratracheal, precricoid (Delphian), and perithyroidal nodes and the nodes located along the recurrent laryngeal nerves. The superior limit of dissection is the body of the hyoid bone, and the inferior limit is the suprasternal notch; the lateral limits are defined by the medial border of the carotid sheath (the common carotid artery). This neck dissection does not have a contralateral counterpart, and it assumes that the lymph nodes are removed on both sides of the trachea. In the case of metastases extending below the level of the suprasternal notch, dissection of the superior mediastinal nodes may be indicated, in which case the procedure is designated SND (VI, superior mediastinal nodes). Exposure of this latter region requires removing the manubrium and possibly one or both sternal heads.

In the case of thyroid cancer in which there is evidence of nodal metastases into level V, the procedure of choice would include the jugular nodes as well as the posterior triangle nodes and would be designated SND (VI, II–V).

In patients with unilateral laryngeal and hypopharyngeal lesions, the dissection of level VI may be confined to one side of the compartment, provided that there is no evidence of nodal metastases involving the contralateral side. In this way the morbidity of disrupting the blood supply to the parathyroid glands or reimplanting them may be avoided.

Technique. If there is an indication to dissect the lateral and posterior neck compartments, this procedure is done first. Then the strap muscles are either divided near the attachments at the sternum or mobilized and retracted laterally. The carotid artery is skeletonized along its medial border as far superiorly as the superior thyroid artery (Figure 116-16, *A*). The ipsilateral lobe of the thyroid gland is mobilized along its lateral border by dividing the fascia and its arterial and venous supply (Figure 116-16, *B*). The recurrent laryngeal nerve is identified inferiorly as it courses the tracheoesophageal groove. If the larynx is to be removed, protection of the nerve is unnecessary. The fibrofatty contents of each side of the anterior compartment then may be removed by excising all of the loose areolar tissue located between the carotid artery laterally and the trachea medially (Figure 116-16, *C*); the thyroid lobe also is removed as part of this en bloc resection (Figure 116-16, *D*). The parathyroid glands should be identified and reimplanted into the sternocleidomastoid muscle. If it is necessary to completely remove nodal-bearing tissue from the entire anterior compartment, the procedure is completed on the contralateral side of the trachea. Thus, a total thyroidectomy is performed, and all of the parathyroid glands are reimplanted. The dissection is carried superiorly as far as the hyoid bone and inferiorly as far as the suprasternal notch. If there is evidence of nodal disease at the lower end of the trachea, a more thorough clean out of the superior mediastinum may be achieved by splitting the sternum or removing the manubrium and one or more clavicular heads.

Extended Neck Dissection

Any of the neck dissections described previously may be extended to remove either lymph node groups or vascular, neural, or muscular structures that are not routinely removed in a neck dissection. A neck dissection may be extended to remove the retropharyngeal lymph nodes on one or both sides when the primary tumor originates in the pharyngeal walls. Ballantyne[4] found a 44% incidence of retropharyngeal node involvement in a group of patients with carcinomas of the pharyngeal wall who were treated surgically. Tumors of the base of the tongue, the tonsil, the soft palate, and the retromolar trigone may also spread

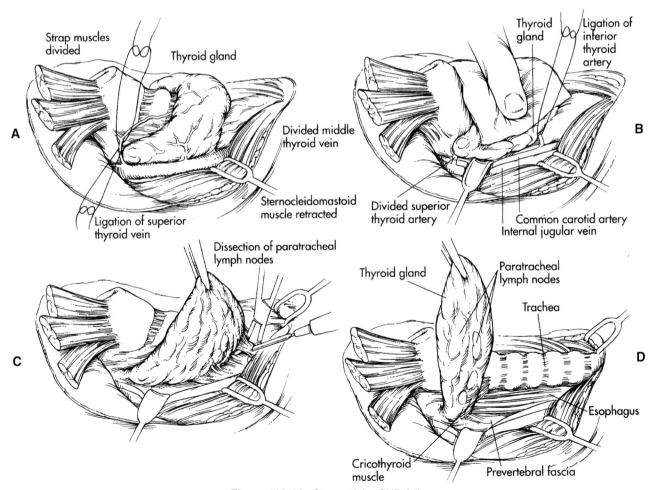

Figure 116-16. Steps of the SND (VI).

to these lymph nodes when they involve the lateral or posterior walls of the oropharynx. Adequate removal of a metastatic tumor in the neck may dictate the need to extend a neck dissection to resect structures such as the hypoglossal nerve, the levator scapulae muscle, or the carotid artery.

Controversy still exists about the advisability of resecting the common or the internal carotoid artery (ICA) (Figure 116-17). Some surgeons believe that it is not justified to resect these arteries in patients with squamous cell carcinoma of the upper aerodigestive tract because of the associated morbidity and because the prognosis of patients with disease in the neck that is extensive enough to warrant such a resection is dismal.[13] For example, Moore and Baker[38] observed a mortality rate of 30% and a cerebral complication rate of 45% among patients who underwent carotid ligation; it should be noted that these figures included elective and emergency ligation. In a study of 28 patients who had tumors grossly excised by "peeling" them off of the carotid artery, Kennedy, Krouse, and Lovey[25] found that only 18% developed a recurrence in the neck without distant metastases; this observation led the authors to state that only this small group of patients may have benefitted from carotid resection. Goffinet, Paryani, and Fee[20] reported encouraging results for patients with large cervical metastases attached to the carotid artery who were treated by the resection of the tumor and intraoperative iodine[125] seed-sutres suture implants over the remaining carotid artery. Tumor control was obtained in the

neck in 77% of the patients, although only 15% of them were alive and free of disease after 1 year. There are surgeons who advocate resecting the common artery or the ICA when the extent of disease dictates it; they believe that current methods of assessing the adequacy of cerebral circulation on the basis of the contralateral carotid system allow for better preoperative patient selection.[5,37,74] These beliefs—coupled with improved techniques for vascular and soft-tissue reconstruction—have made it possible to resect the carotid artery with acceptable morbidity. McCready and others[34] reported their observations in 16 patients who underwent carotid artery resection for the management of advanced carcinomas of the head and neck. Only two patients (12%) developed postoperative cerebrovascular complications, and seven patients (45%) were free of disease at 1 year. Others have reported similar results.[5,74] Patients with frank involvement of the carotid wall whose preoperative examination indicates intolerance of carotid ligation should have carotid resection and reconstruction. Saphenous vein grafts are preferred over prosthetic grafts for reconstruction, and, if the skin has been heavily radiated or a portion of the skin over the carotid is resected, a myocutaneous flap should be used to cover the graft.[43,66]

If carotid artery resection is considered preoperatively, then endovascular balloon occlusion of the ICA with physiologic assessment will strongly predict the potential for stroke and the need for revascularization.[21,59]

An angiogram is performed, and an intravascular balloon placed in the ICA. The patient is heparinized, and the balloon is inflated to occlude the ICA. A second catheter in the contralateral carotid artery is used for an intracranial angiogram to assess the patency of collateral flow through the circle of Willis to the hemisphere in jeopardy. The demonstration of an excellent crossover flow through a patent anterior communicating artery, along with symmetric venous filling bilaterally, is predictive of a very low probability of stroke if the ICA is sacrificed, and there is no indication for revascularization. If the angiogram is questionable, then occlusion may be maintained for 30 minutes, hypotension induced, and the patient observed clinically. Alternatively, a functional cerebral blood flow study can be performed, such as intraarterial xenon, xenon inhalation computed tomography scan, or single photon emission computed tomography scan, to assess functional cerebral blood flow to the hemisphere in jeopardy. If studies suggest that the patient will not tolerate ICA sacrifice, then consideration should be given to surgery designed to salvage the ICA, or a revascularization procedure should be employed.

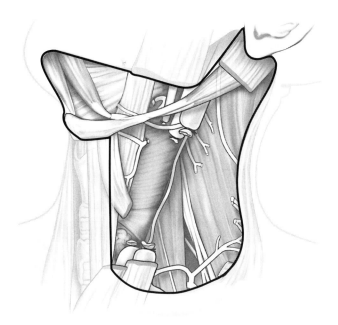

Figure 116-17. Extended radical neck dissection, with resection of the common carotid artery. (Courtesy of Douglas Denys, M.D.)

Revascularization procedures may be within the bed of the tumor resection if proximal and distal ends of the carotid artery and ICA remain. Artificial versus saphenous vein interposition grafts can be used, depending on previous or future radiation therapy and wound infection potential. ICA revascularization procedures continue to be practiced in select neurosurgical cases, particularly in those involving extracranial to intracranial bypass grafting, with good results seen at select centers.[21,59]

Patients with significant atheromatous disease pose an interesting dilemma with regard to planned cervical dissections. A history of any embolic symptoms will increase the risk of stroke with carotid vessel manipulation at surgery. If carotid salvage is planned as a part of the procedure, then preoperative stenting should be considered before cervical dissection, or endarterectomy should be performed at the time of surgery, if anatomy allows. Asymptomatic carotid bifurcation disease should be managed by careful intraoperative manipulation, with vessel preservation dictated by the surgical expectations.

RESULTS OF NECK DISSECTION
Radical Neck Dissection

Obviously the best results reported for patients undergoing radical neck dissection are those in whom the presence of histologically positive metastatic disease is not evident. In this scenario, 3% to 7% of patients will have disease recur in the ipsilateral neck.[29] When radical neck dissection is used as a therapeutic procedure, there is a range of regional control rates. An appropriate analysis of results should, therefore, involve the consideration of several factors related to the degree of nodal involvement and whether the primary tumor remains under control.

The presence of extracapsular spread is an important prognostic factor with regard to recurrence in the neck after neck dissection.[24,65] In addition, the degree of extracapsular involvement is also important. For example, Carter[13] reported a 44% recurrence rate for macroscopic extracapsular spread vs a 25% rate for microscopic extracapsular spread. In addition, the number of lymph nodes involved by tumor has also been found to correlate with the rate of recurrence. Patients with four or more involved nodes had a dramatically worse 4-year survival rate than patients with only one involved node.[42] Strong also reported that the level of nodal involvement had prognostic importance, observing a recurrence rate in the neck of 36.5% in patients with positive nodes in one level vs 71% in patients with positive nodes in multiple levels.[70] Remember that the use of adjuvant radiotherapy is considered by most to improve the rate of control in the neck after neck dissection.[29,68]

Modified Radical Neck Dissection

The rate of recurrence in the neck after modified radical neck dissection depends on the amount of disease to which the procedure was applied. When used as an elective procedure for patients with clinically N_0 disease, the rate of recurrence varies between 4% to 7%. However, when this procedure is used therapeutically for patients with clinically positive disease, the recurrence rate in the dissected neck varies between 0% and 20%. In some of these reports, preoperative or postoperative radiation was also used. These results indicate that, in selected patients, modified radical neck dissection is an attractive alternative to radical neck dissection.[9,29]

Selective Neck Dissection

Data indicating the effectiveness of SND for the control of regional metastases related to upper aerodigestive tract carcinoma are available. For supraomohyoid neck dissection, Byers[9] reported a regional recurrence rate of 5.8% for 154 patients with pathologic N_0 disease, 24 of whom received postoperative radiotherapy. The rate of regional disease control for 80 patients with pathologic positive nodal disease was 15%; 62 of these patients had multiple positive nodes, and 61% had postoperative radiotherapy. In a later review of the MD Anderson experience, Medina and Byers[37] found the recurrence rate to be 5% among patients with pathologic N_0 disease, 10% when a single nodal metastases without extracapsular spread was found, and 24% when multiple positive nodes or extracapsular spread was found. Postoperative radiotherapy decreased the recurrence rate to 15% in the group with multiple nodes or extracapsular spread.

For patients undergoing lateral neck dissection, Byers[9] reported a regional recurrence rate of 3.9% among 256 patients with pathologic N_0 disease, 126 of whom received postoperative radiotherapy. Among the 41 patients with pathologic positive nodal disease, 37 of whom had postoperative radiotherapy, 7.3% had regional recurrences.

The data indicating relatively low regional recurrence rates for patients with clinical N_0 neck disease support the effectiveness of SND procedures for patients with upper aerodigestive tract carcinoma. Of greater controversy is whether the procedures are effective for patients with node-positive disease. Pelliteri, Robbins, and Neuman[46] found the regional recurrence rate for patients with pathologic positive nodal disease to be 11.1% among 27 patients undergoing a supraomohyoid neck dissection and 4.8% among 21 patients who had a lateral neck dissection. These results, along with those reported by Byers[9] and Medina and Byers,[37] indicate that the SND is feasible for a defined subset of patients with positive nodal disease. Postoperative radiotherapy is recommended for patients with multiple nodal disease or extracapsular spread. More recently, the efficacy of SND for clinically positive neck disease has been demonstrated by others.[1,14,27] In 2002, Andersen and colleagues[2] reported about a 10-year, multiinstitutional, retrospective review of pooled data from 106 previously untreated clinically and pathologically node-positive patients undergoing 129 SNDs and followed for a minimum of 2 years or until patient death. Overall, nine patients experienced disease recurrence in the neck, for a regional control rate of 94.3%. Six of these recurrences were in the areas of the neck that had been dissected during the SND. The authors concluded that these results support the use of SND in carefully selected patients with clinically positive nodal metastasis from head and neck squamous cell carcinoma (HNSCC). Regional control rates comparable with those achieved with the radical and modified radical neck dissections could be achieved in appropriately selected patients. The main advantages of the use of SND are that surgical time is shortened and morbidity—especially with regard to shoulder dysfunction—is decreased.

Among patients previously treated with radiotherapy or other types of neck surgery, most surgeons prefer to perform neck dissections that encompass all five neck levels when salvage surgery is feasible. However, there is emerging data to support the use of SND as part of the planned treatment for patients with bulky neck disease whose primary tumor and regional nodes were initially treated with definitive radiation therapy or chemoradiation.[18,22] Nigauri and others[41] failed to find evidence of skip metastases outside of levels II and III among 217 patients with squamous cell carcinoma of the oropharynx who were treated with radiation therapy. These authors recommended SND for patients with N_1 disease, whereas modified radical neck dissection or radical neck dissection was recommended for patients with N_2 or N_3 disease. Boyd and colleagues[8] analyzed 25 patients with squamous cell carcinoma of the oropharynx, the nasopharynx, the hypopharynx, and the supraglottic larynx who had been treated with radiation therapy. Among the 28 necks dissected (all but one patient had N_2 or N_3 disease), only one had tumor outside of levels II through IV. On the basis of this, SND was recommended for patients with disease in all pharyngeal sites who required salvage or planned neck surgery after radiation therapy. Efficacy of targeted chemoradiation and planned SND to control bulk nodal disease in advanced neck cancer has been reported by Robbins and colleagues.[51] In addition, Clayman and colleagues[15] have used SND after chemoradiotherapy for oropharyngeal cancer in patients with advanced nodal

disease. Thus, it may be that, in the future, SND will play a more definitive role in the overall management of patients with initial bulky neck node disease with head and neck cancer that has been treated with nonsurgical modalities; however, further evidence is needed.

Lymphoscintigraphy-Directed Neck Dissection

A potentially powerful adjunct to surgical treatment of the neck is lymphoscintigraphy and sentinel lymph node biopsy. This technique, which was pioneered by Morton and others[39] for use in detecting the lymphatic spread of cutaneous melanoma, capitalizes on the ability of nuclear radiography to identify primary, secondary, and tertiary echelons of lymphatic drainage basins and to identify the index or "sentinel" lymph node associated with primary regions within the head and neck. It is minimally invasive, and it possesses the capacity to accurately stage the clinically occult neck in a number of different neoplasms.[44] Linking this diagnostic and staging modality to lymphadenectomy or other elective treatment of the neck in mucosal carcinomas represents an attractive concept that has recently been explored by Pitman and others[47] at the University of Pittsburgh. These investigators examined the feasibility of identifying the sentinel lymph node in primary echelons of drainage from known primary neoplasms though lymphoscintigraphy and sentinel lymph node biopsy, thus enabling one to stage the N_0 neck in a minimally invasive manner and to direct elective neck therapy accordingly. On the basis of findings with both N_0 and N_+ patients, the investigators thought that lymphoscintigraphy and lymphatic mapping would offer the ability to stage neck disease and provide information about the presence of atypical basins of lymphatic flow from upper aerodigestive tract primary sites that would not typically be addressed by the more classic anatomic regions outlined for SND. Accordingly, patients undergoing this procedure would have lymphatic flow patterns uniquely defined according to neck anatomy and the effects of previous treatment. In addition, findings from the study suggested that lymphoscintigraphy in the N_+ or previously treated neck demonstrated the potential for defining unpredictable cervical nodal levels at risk for metastasis. Studies such as this indicate that the use of lymphatic mapping for the treatment of HNSCC may ultimately provide the surgeon with the ability to adequately stage the N_0 neck and direct elective therapy or assess the neck with recurrence in a minimally invasive manner to determine the extent of salvage required. The place of lymphatic mapping for avoiding a neck dissection remains inadequately defined at this time in terms of therapeutic efficacy, practical application, and health-related quality of life. Lymphatic mapping in HNSCC is probably best considered an investigational technique; as such, it has not yet achieved the status of "standard of care" for the treatment of head and neck carcinoma patients.[48]

SEQUELAE OF NECK DISSECTION

The most notable sequela observed in patients who have undergone a radical neck dissection is related to the removal of the spinal accessory nerve. The resulting denervation of the trapezius muscle, which is one of the most important shoulder abductors, causes destabilization of the scapula, with progressive flaring of this bone at the vertebral border (drooping of the scapula and lateral and anterior rotation of it). The loss of the trapezius function decreases the patient's ability to abduct the shoulder above 30 degrees at the shoulder. These physical changes result in the recognized shoulder syndrome of pain, weakness, and deformity of the shoulder girdle that is commonly associated with radical neck dissection.

For the past few years, it has been debated in the literature whether there is a major difference in postoperative shoulder dysfunction after a radical neck dissection that preserves the spinal accessory nerve. Using patient questionnaires, Schuller and others[60] compared symptomatology and the ability to return to preoperative employment of patients who underwent either a radical neck dissection or a modified radical neck dissection. Although they found no statistically significant difference between the two groups, Sterns and Shaheen[69] and others using similar methods found that the majority of patients who had a nerve-sparing procedure did not have postoperative pain or shoulder dysfunction.[63,76]

Only recently has objective data about shoulder dysfunction after neck dissection been gathered prospectively. Leipzig and others[30] studied 109 patients who had undergone various types of neck dissections using preoperative and postoperative observations of shoulder movement made by the surgeons who rated the degree of shoulder dysfunction. The researchers concluded that any type of neck dissection may result in an impairment of function of the shoulder. They also noted that dysfunction occurred more frequently among those patients in whom the spinal accessory nerve was extensively dissected or resected.

In 1985, Sobol and others[66] performed a prospective study in which preoperative and postoperative measures of shoulder range of motion were compared. In addition, postoperative electromyograms (EMGs) were obtained in some patients. Shoulder range of motion was better in patients who underwent a nerve-sparing procedure than in patients who had a radical

neck dissection. In addition, the type of nerve-sparing procedure was found to have an influence on the degree of shoulder disability. Patients who had undergone a modified radical neck dissection, in which the entire length of the nerve was dissected, had no dramatic difference in shoulder range of motion as compared with those patients who had a radical neck dissection 16 weeks after surgery. Patients who underwent a supraomohyoid neck dissection, in which there was less-extensive dissection of the spinal accessory nerve, performed significantly better ($P > .05$) than either of the other groups in terms of shoulder range of motion and EMG findings for the trapezius muscle. Interestingly, 16 weeks after surgery, moderate to severe EMG abnormalities were noted in as many as 65% of the patients in whom the spinal accessory nerve was dissected along its entire length (i.e., modified radical neck dissection). Although no severe abnormalities were noted in the group undergoing supraomohyoid neck dissection, 22% of these patients showed moderate abnormalities. Several patients from each group had repeat studies at approximately 1 year after surgery. Unlike patients who had a radical neck dissection, patients in whom the nerve was spared showed evidence of improvement in all parameters studied.

A prospective study by Remmler and others[49] revealed that patients who had a nerve-sparing procedure had a serious but temporary spinal accessory nerve dysfunction. In this study, preoperative strength, range-of-motion measures, and EMG of the trapezius muscle were compared with postoperative measures obtained at 1, 3, 6, and 12 months. The groups studied consisted of patients undergoing nerve-sparing procedures and those who had the nerve resected. Most of the patients in the nerve-sparing group had supraomohyoid neck dissections. Patients who underwent radical neck dissections had a major decrease in trapezius muscle strength on EMG at 1 month; these parameters did not improve with time. Interestingly, patients in the nerve-sparing group had a small but significant reduction in trapezius muscle strength and evidence of trapezius muscle denervation at 1 and 3 months, which improved by 12 months. More recently, Weymuller and others reported reduced quality-of-life scores among patients after neck dissection, with the worst scores being associated with radical neck dissection and the best scores with SND.

Hence, the evidence indicates that even procedures involving minimal dissection of the spinal accessory nerve may result in shoulder dysfunction.[28] It is only appropriate, therefore, to make every effort to avoid undue stretch or trauma to the nerve when a nerve-sparing procedure is performed. In addition, it is imperative that every patient who undergoes a neck dissection be questioned about the function of the shoulder and be examined by a physical therapist early during the postoperative period. If any deficit is detected, the patient should be properly counseled and coached to ensure proper rehabilitation of the shoulder.

COMPLICATIONS OF NECK DISSECTION

In addition to the various medical complications that may occur after any surgical procedure in the head and neck region, a number of surgical complications may be related solely or in part to the neck dissection. If the course of a patient who has undergone a neck dissection as part of the surgical treatment of cancer of the head and neck region is followed, several complications may arise.

Air Leaks

Circulation of air through a wound drain is a common complication that is usually encountered 1 day after surgery. The point of entrance of air may be located somewhere along the skin incision, although, if the drains are connected to suction in the operating room near the completion of the wound closure, such an air leak usually becomes apparent then and may be corrected. Other points of entrance may not become apparent until after surgery, when the position of the neck changes or when the patient begins to move. A typical example of this situation is the improperly secured suction drain that gets displaced, thereby exposing one or more of the drain vents. A similar situation occurs frequently when a lateral trapezius flap is used in conjunction with a neck dissection. The slightest movement of the shoulder may produce an air leak into the neck wound through the extensive donor defect, even after meticulous tacking of the skin edges to the underlying tissues and painstaking suturing of a skin graft. This problem may be prevented by using an adhesive vinyl drape applied over the defect and surrounding skin to seal any possible air leak instead of using the bolster of gauze that is traditionally used to immobilize the skin graft.

Air leaks with potentially more serious consequences are those that occur through a communication of the neck wound with the tracheostomy site or through a mucosal suture line. In these patients, it is likely that, in addition to air, contaminated secretions are circulated through the wound. Thus, early identification of the site of leakage is desirable, although it may not be a simple task, and correcting it may require revision of the wound closure in the operating room.

Bleeding

Postoperative hemorrhage usually occurs immediately after surgery. External bleeding through the incision, without distortion of the skin flaps, often originates in a subcutaneous blood vessel. In most patients, this may be readily controlled by ligation or infiltration of the surrounding tissues with an anesthetic solution containing epinephrine. Pronounced swelling or ballooning of the skin flaps immediately after surgery, with or without external bleeding, should be attributed to a hematoma in the wound. If a hematoma is detected early, "milking" the drains occasionally may result in evacuation of the accumulated blood and the problem will resolve. If this is not accomplished immediately or if blood reaccumulates quickly, it is best to return the patient to the operating room, explore the wound under sterile conditions, evacuate the hematoma, and control the bleeding. Attempting to do this in the recovery room or at the bedside is ill advised, because lighting and surgical equipment may be inadequate, and sterile conditions may be precarious. Failure to recognize or manage a postoperative hematoma properly may predispose the patient to the development of a wound infection. Although bulky pressure dressings may be useful for curtailing postoperative edema and they do not prevent hematomas, they may delay their recognition as well.

Chylous Fistula

In a recent review of 823 neck dissections performed by the surgeons at Memorial Hospital in New York City that included the removal of the lymph nodes in level IV, Spiro, Spiro, and Strong[68] found that 14 patients (1.9%) developed a chyle fistula. In this and other studies,[17] a chylous leakage was identified and apparently controlled intraoperatively in the majority of patients who developed the complication. These observations remind the surgeon to not only avoid injury to the thoracic duct proper but also to ligate or clip any visualized or potential lymphatic tributaries in the area of the thoracic duct. This may be accomplished with relative ease if the operative field is kept bloodless when dissecting in this area of the neck. In addition, as soon as the dissection of this area is completed and again before closing the wound, the area should be observed for 20 or 30 seconds while the anesthesiologist increases the intrathoracic pressure; even the smallest leak of chylous material should be pursued until it is arrested. Indiscriminate clamping and ligating may be difficult and sometimes counterproductive because of the fragility of the lymphatic vessels and the surrounding fatty tissue. Hemoclips are ideal to control a source of leakage that is clearly visualized; otherwise it is preferable to use suture ligatures with pliable material, such as No. 5-0 silk, which are tied over a piece of hemostatic sponge to avoid tearing.

Despite the surgeon's best efforts to avoid it, a postoperative chylous fistula occurs after 1% to 2% of neck dissections. Management of this complication depends on the time of onset of the leak and the amount of chyle drainage in a 24-hour period and on the physician's ability to prevent accumulation of chyle under the skin flaps. When the daily output of chyle exceeds 600 mL (especially when the chyle fistula becomes apparent immediately after surgery), conservative closed wound management is not likely to succeed. In such patients, early surgical exploration is preferred, before the tissues exposed to the chyle become markedly inflamed and before the fibrinous material that coats these tissues becomes adherent, thus obscuring and jeopardizing important structures, such as the phrenic and vagus nerves.

Chylous fistulas that become apparent only after enteral feedings are resumed and, particularly those that drain less than 600 mL of chyle per day, are initially managed conservatively with closed wound drainage, pressure dressings, and low-fat nutritional support. Parenteral alimentation through a central line can further reduce chylous output and may be considered for high-output or intractable fistulas.

Facial/Cerebral Edema

Synchronous bilateral radical neck dissections, in which both internal jugular veins are ligated, may result in the development of facial edema, cerebral edema, or both. The facial edema, which sometimes may be dramatically severe, appears to be caused by an inadequacy of venous drainage, which usually resolves to a variable extent with time as collateral circulation is established. Facial edema appears to be more common and more severe in patients who had previous radiation to the head and neck and in those patients in whom the resection includes large segments of the lateral and posterior pharyngeal walls. Massive facial edema may be prevented by preserving at least one external jugular vein whenever a bilateral radical neck dissection is anticipated. The external jugular is usually separated from the tumor in the neck by the sternocleidomastoid muscle and may be dissected free between the tail of the parotid and subclavian veins.

The development of cerebral edema may be at the root of the impaired neurologic function and even coma that may occur after bilateral radical neck dissection. Ligation of the internal jugular veins leads to increased intracranial pressure.[57,72] It has been shown experimentally that the increased cerebral venous pressure that occurs as a result of ligating both internal jugular veins in dogs is associated with inappro-

priate secretion of antidiuretic hormone.[35] It may then be speculated that the resulting expansion of extracellular fluids and dilutional hyponatremia aggravate the cerebral edema and create a vicious cycle. In practice, these observations behoove the surgeon and the anesthesiologist to curtail the administration of fluids during and after bilateral radical neck dissections.[77] In addition, perioperative management of fluid and electrolytes in these patients should not be guided solely by their urine output but rather by the monitoring of central venous pressure, cardiac output, and serum and urine osmolarity.

Blindness

Visual loss after bilateral neck dissection is a rare but catastrophic complication. To date, there have been five cases reported in the literature.[32] In one report, histologic examination revealed intraorbital optic nerve infarction, which suggests intraoperative hypotension and severe venous distension as possible etiologic factors.[42]

Carotid Artery Rupture

The most feared and the most commonly lethal complication after surgery of the neck is the exposure and rupture of the carotid artery; therefore, every effort should be made to prevent it. If the skin incisions have been designed properly, seldom does the carotid artery become exposed in the absence of a salivary fistula. Fistula formation and flap breakdown are more likely to occur in the presence of malnutrition, diabetes, infection, and previous radiotherapy, which impair healing capacity and compromise vascular supply. Faced with any of these risk factors, the surgeon should use flawless surgical techniques in the closure of oral and pharyngeal defects. The use of free and pedicled vascularized flaps (which provide skin for the closure of mucosal defects) has rendered nearly obsolete the use of "protective" measures such as dermal grafts, levator scapulae muscle flaps, and controlled pharyngostomies.

Management of the exposed carotid artery depends on the likelihood of rupture based on the length of the exposed segment, the condition of the surrounding tissues, and the size of the oropharyngocutaneous fistula. Large cutaneous defects or large, high-output fistulas in previously irradiated patients are not likely to heal by secondary intention in a timely manner. The likelihood of rupture of the carotid artery in these patients is extremely high. Therefore, an attempt should be made to repair the defect and to cover the carotid using well-vascularized tissue before the vessel has been irreversibly damaged. Whenever the carotid is exposed, it is advisable to take "carotid precautions," which include warning and instructing

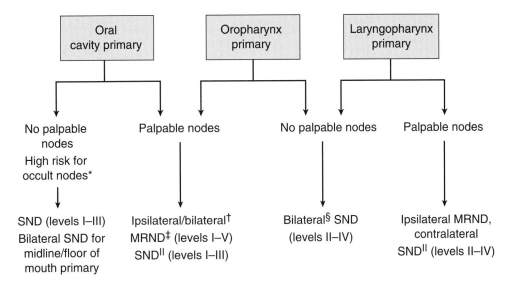

*T_1–T_4 oral tongue; T_{2-4} other sites; perineural/lymphatic invasion
†Bilateral neck dissection for N_{2c} disease
‡RND if gross tumor invasion of nonlymphatic structures
§Ipsilateral neck dissection for oropharyngeal primaries if postoperative radiotherapy is planned
‖ SND for nodes confined to one level

Figure 116-18. Algorithm for cervical lymphadenectomy options in patients with carcinomas of the upper aerodigestive tract, assuming that cervical lymphadenectomy is the treatment of choice for these regional lymph nodes. SND, Selective neck dissection; MRND, modified radical neck dissection.

nursing personnel and house staff about the possibility of a carotid rupture, the site of potential rupture, and the steps to be taken in the event of bleeding; having compatible blood available; and keeping appropriate surgical instruments at the bedside.

When a carotid artery rupture occurs, it is usually possible to stop the bleeding with manual pressure while blood and fluids are administered to restore and maintain the patient's blood pressure; only then is the patient taken to surgery. Attempts to repair the area of rupture are futile. Introduction of Fogarty catheters through the area of rupture is helpful for controlling the bleeding temporarily while the artery is exposed and ligated proximally and distally to the area of rupture.

SUMMARY

Neck dissection is an operative procedure that is designed to remove metastases involving the regional cervical lymph nodes. The gold standard procedure is the radical neck dissection, which, for most patients, is too extensive and results in excessive morbidity. Modifications of the radical neck dissection procedure, which have been designed to reduce morbidity by sparing nonlymphatic structures (modified radical neck dissection) and to treat early nodal disease by removing only the lymph node groups at greatest risk for harboring metastases (SND), have now evolved. To help the reader determine which type of neck dissection is most appropriate for the management of nodal disease associated with the three major sites of the upper aerodigestive tract, an algorithm is provided (Figure 116-18).

REFERENCES

1. Ambrosch P and others: Efficacy of selective neck dissection: a review of 503 cases of elective and therapeutic treatment of the neck in squamous cell carcinoma of the upper aerodigestive tract, *Otolaryngol Head Neck Surg* 124:180, 2001.
2. Andersen PE and others: Results of selective neck dissection in management of the node-positive neck, *Arch Otolaryngol Head Neck Surg* 128:1180, 2002.
3. Ballantyne AJ: *Classical and functional neck dissection.* In Ariyan S, editor: *Cancer of the head and neck.* St Louis, 1987, Mosby.
4. Ballantyne AJ: Significance of retropharyngeal nodes in cancer of the head and neck, *Am J Surg* 108:500, 1964.
5. Biller HF and others: Carotid artery resection and bypass for neck carcinoma, *Laryngoscope* 98:181, 1988.
6. Blair VP, Brown JP: The treatment of cancerous or potentially cancerous cervical lymph nodes, *Ann Surg* 98:650, 1933.
7. Bocca E, Pignataro O: A conservation technique in radical neck dissection, *Ann Otol Rhinol Laryngol* 76:975, 1967.

8. Boyd TS and others: Planned postradiotherapy neck dissection in patients with advanced head and neck cancer, *Head Neck* 20:132, 1998.

9. Byers RM: Modified neck dissection: a study of 967 cases from 1970 to 1980, *Am J Surg* 150:414, 1985.

10. Byers RM, Ballantyne AJ: Selection criteria for modified neck dissection with postoperative irradiation for N3 staged metastases. In Chretien PB and others, editors: *Head and neck cancer*. Philadelphia, 1985, Mosby.

11. Byers RM and others: Frequency and therapeutic implications of "skip metastases" in the neck from squamous carcinoma of the oral tongue, *Head Neck* 19:14, 1997.

12. Byers RM and others: Selective neck dissections for squamous carcinoma of the upper aerodigestive tract: patterns of regional failure, *Head Neck* 21:499, 1999.

13. Carter RL and others: Transcapsular spread of metastatic squamous cell carcinoma from cervical lymph nodes, *Am J Surg* 150:495, 1985.

14. Chepeha DB and others: Selective neck dissection for the treatment of neck metastasis from squamous cell carcinoma of the head and neck, *Laryngoscope* 112:434, 2002.

15. Clayman GL and others: The role of neck dissection after chemoradiotherapy for oropharyngeal cancer with advanced nodal disease, *Arch Otolaryngol Head Neck Surg* 127:135, 2001.

16. Crile G: Excision of cancer of the head and neck, *JAMA* 47:1780, 1906.

17. Crumley RL, Smith JD: Postoperative chylous fistula prevention and management, *Laryngoscope* 86:804, 1976.

18. Doweck I, Robbins KT and others: Neck level-specific nodal metastases in oropharyngeal cancer: is there a role for selective neck dissection following definitive radiation therapy? *Head Neck* 25:960, 2003.

19. Fisch UP, Sigel ME: Cervical lymphatic system as visualized by lymphography, *Ann Otol Rhinol Laryngol* 73:869, 1964.

20. Goffinet DR, Paryani SB, Fee WE: *Management of patients with N3 cervical lymphadenopathy and/or carotid artery involvement.* In Chretien PB and others, editors: *Head and neck cancer,* Philadelphia, 1985, Mosby.

21. Grubb RL and others: Importance of hemodynamic factors in the prognosis of symptomatic carotid occlusion, *JAMA* 280:1055, 1998.

22. Hehr T and others: Selective lymph node dissection following hyperfractionated accelerated radio-(chemo-)therapy for advanced head and neck cancer, *Strahlenther Onkol* 178:363, 2002.

23. Jesse RH, Ballantyne AJ, Larson D: Radical or modified neck dissection: a therapeutic dilemma, *Am J Surg* 136:516, 1978.

24. Johnson JT and others: The extracapsular spread of tumor in cervical-node metastases, *Arch Otolaryngol* 107:725, 1981.

25. Kennedy JT, Krause CJ, Lovey S: The importance of tumor attachment to the carotid artery, *Arch Otolaryngol* 103:70, 1977.

26. Kocher: Ueber radicalheilung des krebses, *Dtsch Z Chir* 13:134, 1880.

27. Konsulov SS and others: Selective neck dissection in treatment of node-positive neck cases, *Folia Med (Plovdiv)* 43:27, 2001.

28. Kuntz AL, Weymuller EA Jr: Impact of neck dissection on quality of life, *Laryngoscope* 109:1334, 1999.

29. Leemans CR and others: The efficacy of comprehensive neck dissection with or without postoperative radiotherapy in nodal metastases of squamous cell carcinoma of the upper respiratory and digestive tracts, *Laryngoscope* 100:1194, 1990.

30. Leipzig B and others: Functional evaluation of the spinal accessory nerve after neck dissection, *Am J Surg* 146:526, 1983.

31. Lindberg R: Distribution of cervical lymph node metastases from squamous cell carcinoma of the upper respiratory and digestive tracts, *Cancer* 29:1446, 1972.

32. Marks SC and others: Blindness following bilateral radical neck dissection, *Head Neck Surg* 12:342, 1990.

33. Martin H: The treatment of cervical metastatic cancer, *Ann Surg* 114:972, 1941.

34. McCready RA and others: What is the role of carotid arterial resection in the management of advanced cervical cancer? *J Vasc Surg* 10:274, 1989.

35. McQuarrie DG and others: A physiologic approach to the problem of simultaneous bilateral neck dissection, *Am J Neurosurg* 134:455, 1977.

36. McGavran MH, Bauer WC, Ogura JH: The incidence of cervical lymph node metastases from epidermoid carcinoma of the larynx and their relationship to certain characteristics of the primary tumor, *Cancer* 14:55, 1961.

37. Medina JE, Byers RM: Supraomohyoid neck dissection: rationale, indications and surgical technique, *Head Neck Surg* 11:111, 1989.

38. Moore O, Baker HW: Carotid artery ligation in surgery of the head and neck, *Cancer* 80:712, 1955.

39. Morton DL and others: Technical details of the intraoperative lymphatic mapping for early stage melanoma, *Arch Surg* 127:392, 1992.

40. Nahum AM, Mullally W, Marmor L. A syndrome resulting from radical neck dissection, *Arch Otolaryngol* 74:82, 1961.

41. Nigauri T and others: [Treatment strategy for cervical node metastasis from squamous cell carcinoma of the oropharynx], *Nippon Jibiinkoka Gakkai Kaiho* 103:803, 2000.

42. O'Brien CJ and others: Neck dissection with and without radiotherapy: prognostic factors, patterns of recurrence, and survival, *Am J Surg* 152:456, 1986.

43. Olcott C and others: Planned approach to the management of malignant invasion of the carotid artery, *Am J Surg* 142:123, 1981.

44. Pan D, Narayan D, Ariyan S: Merkel cell carcinoma: five case reports using sentinel lymph node biopsy and a review of 110 new cases, *Plast Reconstr Surg* 110:1259, 2002.

45. Parkard JH: *A system of surgery, theoretical and practical in treatises by various authors,* ed 1. Philadelphia, Henry C. Lea's Sons & Co, 1881.

46. Pelliteri PK, Robbins KT, Neuman T: The expanded application of selective neck dissection with regard to nodal status, *Head Neck* 19:260, 1997.

47. Pitman KT and others: Sentinel lymph node biopsy in head and neck squamous cell carcinoma, *Laryngoscope* 112:2101, 2002.

48. Pitman KT and others: Sentinel lymph node biopsy in head and neck cancer, *Oral Oncol* 39:343, 2003.

49. Remmler D and others: A prospective study of shoulder disability resulting from radical and modified neck dissections, *Head Neck Surg* 8:280, 1986.

50. Robbins KT and others: Standardizing neck dissection terminology, *Arch Otolaryngol* 117:601, 1991.

51. Robbins KT and others: Efficacy of targeted chemoradiation and planned selective neck dissection to control bulky nodal disease in advanced head and neck cancer. *Arch Otolaryngol Head Neck Surg* 125:670, 1999.

52. Robbins KT and others: *Neck dissection classification and TNM staging of head and neck cancer.* In Robbins KT, editor: *Pocket guide to neck dissection classification and TNM*

staging of head and neck cancer, ed 2. Alexandria, Virginia, 2001, American Academy of Otolaryngology.

53. Robbins KT and others and the Committee for Head and Neck Surgery and Oncology, American Academy of Otolaryngology–Head and Neck Surgery: *Neck dissection classification update.* Revisions proposed by the American Head and Neck Society and the American Academy of Otolaryngology–Head and Neck Surgery, *Arch Otolaryngol Head Neck Surg* 128:751, 2002.

54. Robbins KT: *Classification for neck dissection,* ed 2, monograph, American Academy of Head and Neck Surgery, 2001.

55. Rochlin DB: Posterolateral neck dissection for malignant neoplasms, *Surg Gynecol Obstet* 115:369, 1962.

56. Rouviere H: *Anatomy of the human lymphatic system.* Ann Arbor, Michigan, Edward Brothers, 1938.

57. Royster MP: The relation between internal jugular vein pressure and pressure in the operation of radical neck dissection, *Ann Surg* 13:831, 1953.

58. Saunders JR Jr, Hirata RM, Jaques DA: Considering the spinal accessory nerve in head and neck surgery, *Am J Surg* 150:491, 1985.

59. Schmiedek P and others: Improvement of cerebrovascular reserve capacity by EC-IC arterial bypass in patients with ICA occlusion and hemodynamic cerebral ischemia, *J Neurosurg* 81:236, 1994.

60. Schuller DE and others: Analysis of disability resulting from treatment of radical neck dissection or modified neck dissection, *Head Neck* 6:551, 1983.

61. Shah JP and others: Neck dissection: current status and future possibilities, *Clin Bull* 11:25, 1981.

62. Shah JP: Patterns of lymph node metastases from squamous carcinomas of the upper aerodigestive tract, *Am J Surg* 160:405, 1990.

63. Short SO and others: Shoulder pain and function after neck dissection without preservation of the spinal accessory nerve, *Am J Surg* 14:482, 1984.

64. Skolnik EM and others: The posterolateral triangle in radical neck surgery, *Arch Otolaryngol* 102:1, 1976.

65. Snow GB, Larson DL, Guillamondegui OM and others: *Prognostic factors in neck node metastasis.* In *Cancer of the neck.* New York, 1986, MacMillin Publishing.

66. Sobol S and others: Objective comparison of physical dysfunction after dissection, *Am J Surg* 150:503, 1985.

67. Som PM, Curtin HD, Mancuso AA: The new imaging-based classification for describing the location of lymph nodes in the neck with particular regard to cervical lymph nodes in relation to cancer of the larynx, *ORL J Otorhinolaryngol Relat Spec* 62:186, 2000.

68. Spiro JD, Spiro RH, Strong EW: The management of chyle fistula, *Laryngoscope* 100:771, 1990.

69. Sterns MP, Shaheen OH: Preservation of the accessory nerve in dissections, *J Otol Rhinol Laryngol* 95:1141, 1981.

70. Strong EW: Preoperative radiation and neck dissection, *Surg Clin Am* 49:271, 1969.

71. Suarez O: El problema de las metastasis linfáticas y alejadas del cancer de laringe e hipofaringe, *Rev Otorhinolaringol* 23:83, 1963.

72. Sugarbaker ED, Wiley HM: Intracranial pressure studies incident resection of the internal jugular vein, *Cancer* 4:242, 1951.

73. Toker C: Some observations on the distribution of metastatic squamous cell carcinoma within cervical lymph nodes, *Ann Surg* 157:419, 1963.

74. Urken M and others: Salvage surgery for recurrent neck carcinoma modality therapy, *Head Neck Surg* 8:332, 1986.

75. Ward GE, Robben JO: A composite operation for radical neck dissection and removal of cancer of the mouth, *Cancer* 4:98, 1951.

76. Weitz JW, Weitz SL, McElhinney AJ: A technique for preserving spinal accessory nerve function in radical neck dissection, *Heart Surg* 5:75, 1982.

77. Wenig BL, Heller KS: The syndrome of inappropriate secretion diuretic hormone (SIADH) following neck dissection, *Laryngoscope* 97:467, 1987.

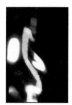

CHAPTER ONE HUNDRED AND SEVENTEEN

SURGICAL COMPLICATIONS OF THE NECK

|| Carol M. Bier-Laning

INTRODUCTION

Complications relating to surgery of the neck depend on factors broadly classified as surgical factors and patient factors. Surgical factors include the type of procedure, choice of incisions, surgeon's experience, length of surgery, and other details that are often difficult to quantify. Patient factors consist of the general health and nutritional status of the patient, body habitus, the extent of the neoplasm, and other conditions that may or may not be possible to modify preoperatively. Although any combination of surgical factors and patient factors may exist in a single case, this chapter focuses primarily on neck dissection for squamous cell carcinoma. The risk factors for these malignancies include use of tobacco products and heavy alcohol consumption. Because of this, when assessing patient factors, it is important to consider other medical ramifications of tobacco and alcohol use, including pulmonary disease, cardiovascular disease, hepatic disease with possible associated coagulation defects, and malnutrition.

Despite these many variables, complications of surgery of the neck are well known. Some complications are specific to structures in the neck, whereas others, such as hematoma and infection, occur in all parts of the body. Some complications are a necessary result of complete tumor extirpation. This chapter outlines and identifies the most common avoidable complications resulting from neck surgery to aid in their prevention.

WOUND COMPLICATIONS
Incisions

Well-planned incisions may not prevent wound complications, but poorly chosen incisions can lead to flap necrosis, wound breakdown, and carotid exposure. Important factors to consider are the location of the tumor, exposure of the primary tumor when a combined procedure is planned, previous incisions, and the need to resect incisions from previous biopsies or other involved skin. A study of 184 neck dissections in 166 patients showed a statistically significant increase in the incidence of wound dehiscence (but not other complications such as seroma, hematoma, wound infection, or fistula formation) when a triradiate incision was used compared with an apron flap incision (11% vs 0%). In addition, these authors noted an increase in wound dehiscence in previously irradiated necks, but the increase was significant only for the triradiate incision.[56] On the basis of these findings, they recommend the use of the apron vs the modified MacFee incision in previously irradiated necks, because they believe the former gives easier access to important neck structures.[56] Because neck dissection is generally indicated only for malignancy, only secondary emphasis may be given to cosmesis as it relates to the incision. Once the issues of appropriate cancer treatment have been addressed, consideration may be given to improving the appearance of the neck dissection defect. The deep plane neck lift has been described to offset the cosmetic defect of a radical neck dissection.[17]

Various neck incisions have been described (Figure 117-1). A general principle for any neck incision is elevation in a subplatysmal plane. This plane is avascular and therefore aids in surgical dissection. Separate limbs of the incision should meet at right angles to decrease the risk of flap tip necrosis. Any limb should avoid running along the carotid artery and, in particular trifurcation points, should avoid the carotid artery in the event of wound breakdown. Lesser procedures than neck dissection should include the same careful planning in the event that a neck dissection is necessary in the future.

Infection

When considering neck dissection, a distinction must be made between a neck dissection performed as a separate procedure and one combined with resection of the primary tumor involving contamination of the

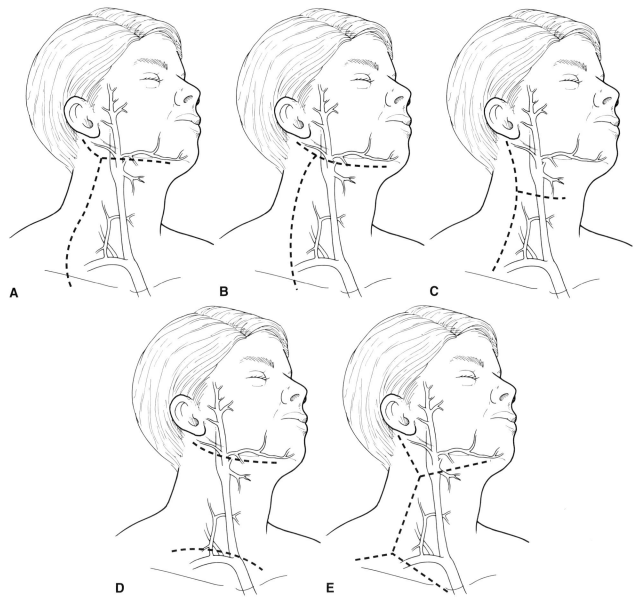

Figure 117-1. Incisions for major head and neck oncologic surgery should provide good exposure and viable coverage for underlying structure: **A,** Conley incision; **B,** Schobinger incision; **C,** modified H incision; **D,** MacFee incision. **E,** T incision.

wound with oral flora. As a separate procedure, a neck dissection is considered a clean procedure, and therefore the risk of wound infection is relatively low. In a review of 438 patients who underwent clean procedures of the neck (thyroidectomy, parotidectomy, or submandibular gland excision), only three had a wound infection; one of these three received prophylactic antibiotics.[23] Although the risk of wound infection in a clean, uncontaminated neck dissection is believed to be low, it may be affected by the use of perioperative antibiotics. In a retrospective study of 192 patients undergoing clean, uncontaminated neck

dissection,[10] 10% of patients who did not receive antibiotics had a subsequent wound infection develop. This represented approximately three times as many wound infections vs the number of wound infections in the group of patients who received prophylactic antibiotics. This finding did not achieve statistical significance because of the sample size. In fact, the type II error ($\beta > 0.2$) indicated that there was a 20% chance that a real difference existed but was not seen because of the sample size. A sample size of more than 700 patients would be needed to show a significant difference between wound infection rates in

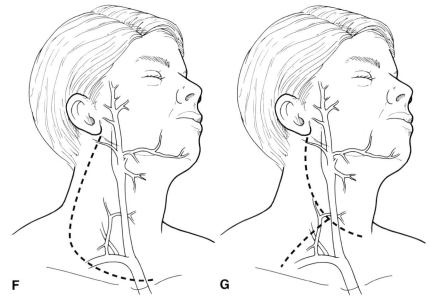

F   **G**

Figure 117-1, cont'd F, Martin incision; **G,** utility incision; and **H,** Frazier incision. (From Everts EC, Cohen JI, McMenomey SO: *Surgical complications.* In Cummings CW and others, editors: *Otolaryngology—Head and Neck Surgery,* ed 2, St Louis, 1992, Mosby.)

those treated with prophylactic antibiotics and those untreated.[6] Because this number of patients cannot be achieved in a single institution, the conclusion can only be made that there is a *trend* favoring antibiotic prophylaxis in patients undergoing neck dissection.

Because there are no prospective data on the efficacy of prophylactic antibiotic use for decreasing wound infection rates in neck dissections, and because a prospective trial would require a prohibitively large population to have the power to show significance, it is useful to examine other data to make a decision regarding the usefulness of prophylactic antibiotics for a neck dissection. In a cost analysis study published in 1995,[6] it was found that the cost in extra hospital days alone for treating three patients with wound infection after neck dissection was more than twice the cost of one preoperative and three postoperative doses of antibiotics (clindamycin or cefoperazone) for 100 patients. Furthermore, in a study that included 201 clean head and neck cases, it was found that the rate of wound infection for radical neck dissection was significantly higher that other clean procedures (13% vs 1%, P = .001).[11] Although the explanation for this difference is not known, but may include such patient related factors as malnutrition and microvascular disease related to tobacco use, it seems prudent to strongly consider the use of 24 hours of antibiotic prophylaxis in patients undergoing neck dissection.

Although any neck procedure may be associated with subsequent wound infection and breakdown, the risk of wound infection rises significantly when the operative bed is contaminated with oral secretions from a concomitant resection of a lesion involving the upper aerodigestive tract. This rate of wound infections, which may be as high as 87%,[5] dramatically decreases with the use of perioperative antibiotic prophylaxis.[5,8,22,32] Current controversies revolve around the types and duration of the antibiotic regimen. In general, the antibiotics should cover the common pathogens that colonize the skin, namely *Staphylococcus* and *Streptococcus* species and oral anaerobes. Consideration may be given to broader coverage of gram-negative bacilli if the patient was hospitalized or in a nursing home before surgery, in which case the oral flora may include these organisms. If a patient is diagnosed with a wound infection, the purulent material should be cultured to identify a predominant organism and identify drug sensitivities so that specific antibiotic coverage can be used.

At present, shorter management courses are favored (e.g., 24–48 hours), because longer courses seem to select resistant organisms. In support of this, a retrospective study of patients undergoing neck dissections,[48] found that 24 hours of perioperative antibiotics was as effective at controlling postoperative wound infection rates as continuing antibiotics until suction drains were discontinued. Similarly, another study that looked at 201 clean head and neck cases, as well as 207 clean-contaminated head and neck cases, found no difference in either group in the incidence of wound infections between patients who received prolonged (5 days in the clean group, 7 days in the clean-contaminated group) antibiotics and those who received 1 day of postoperative antibiotic coverage.[11]

Although there is generalized agreement toward decreasing the length of prophylactic antibiotic regimens, there continues to be controversy as to the optimum antibiotics to be used. In general, for a clean case, normal skin flora should be covered. For cases in which the upper aerodigestive tract is entered, coverage should be broader and include oral flora, specifically anaerobes. There is disagreement as to the need for gram-negative coverage. One group has found that the rate of infection with gram-negative organisms in patients undergoing head and neck cancer surgery was higher in a group who received prophylactic clindamycin than in a group who received prophylactic sulbactam-ampicillin.[9] There are data to support the presence of gram-negative bacteria in the oral flora of head and neck cancer patients in general[4] and specifically in patients with prolonged nasogastric tube feeding.[28] Ideally, antibiotic coverage should be tailored to the organisms most commonly responsible for wound infections at the institution where the surgery is performed, with attention paid to the antibiogram of these organisms (Table 117-1).

Wound Bleeding

Wound bleeding and hematoma formation are uncommon after neck dissection. In a large series,[36] wound bleeding complicated 12 of 885 cases of neck dissection combined with other procedures (1.3%) and 6 of 534 cases of neck dissection alone (1.1%). Wound bleeding is identified by high drain output, bleeding from suture lines, or the formation of a hematoma as evidenced by elevation of the skin flaps. Complications resulting from wound bleeding can include significant blood loss, disruption of suture lines, airway compromise, compromise of the vascular pedicle of a flap used for reconstruction, and wound infection.

Bleeding and hematoma formation can be handled differently. Matory and Spiro[36] recognized that patients who had postoperative wound bleeding had a prolonged hospital stay. The shortest increase was noted in patients who went to the operating room for reexploration compared with those explored at the bedside or observed. In 31 patients returned to the operating room and explored, a bleeding vessel was identified in only 14. In 13 patients explored at the bedside, a bleeding vessel was identified in 5.

Although identifying factors that predispose to wound bleeding can be difficult, several guidelines are useful. It is important to identify patients who are receiving anticoagulant or platelet-inhibiting drugs preoperatively so that these drugs can be discontinued or modified (e.g., warfarin should be converted to heparin, which can be discontinued for the procedure). Good surgical practice involves careful observation and attention to hemostasis at the end of the case, with the patient's blood pressure in the range of normal. Drains should be placed in a dependent position. The drains should be placed to suction immediately and constantly to prevent the formation of a clot around the drain, rendering it useless. Finally, communication with the anesthesiologist aids in the patient emerging from general anesthesia as smoothly as possible to avoid acute hypertension and struggling.

Radiation and Chemotherapy Effects

Both radiation and chemotherapy have effects on tissue that can have an impact on wound healing. Although controversy exists as to whether these effects impact the risk of complications in all cases, these effects may

TABLE 117-1

EXAMPLES OF ANTIBIOTIC REGIMENS BASED ON SURGICAL PROCEDURE AND LIKELY CONTAMINANTS OF SURGERY

Type of Surgery	Organisms to be Covered	Example of Antibiotic Regimen
Neck dissection	Skin flora (gram-positive bacteria)	First-generation cephalosporin[6,11] Clindamycin[6] Penicillins[6]
Clean-contaminated case	Skin flora (gram-positive bacteria), oral flora (anaerobes)	Cefazolin and metronidazole[52] Clindamycin[11]
Clean-contaminated case when gram-negative coverage is deemed important	Skin flora (gram-positive bacteria), oral flora (anaerobes, probability of gram-negative bacteria)	Sulbactam-ampicillin[9] Cefazolin and aminoglycoside[11] Clindamycin and aminoglycoside[44]

sometimes be significant. Knowledge of these effects can be used to modify procedures on patients previously exposed to these forms of management.

Radiation dose is calculated in grays (Gy), which measure the amount of energy deposited in tissue per unit mass. One gray equals 1 J of energy per kilogram of tissue. Thus 1 Gy equals 100 rad, and 1 cGy equals 1 rad.[38]

Dose alone gives incomplete information on the biologic effect of the radiation.[20] Total dose, dose per fraction, and the time over which the total dose is given are the important parameters that describe the effect of radiation. Radiation causes both early and late effects. The early effect is caused by the DNA damage and cell death in rapidly dividing cells. The most important factor affecting the risk of injury to early-responding tissues is the overall treatment time.[20] The late effect is thought to be caused by microvascular damage and the depletion of slowly dividing cells. The important factor affecting the risk of injury to late-responding tissues is the fraction dose.[20] Because of these principles, there are characteristic early and late injury patterns in the head and neck. Acute injury manifests as mucositis, xerostomia, and decreased taste. Chronic injury manifests as dilation and obliteration of capillaries and increased fibrous tissue within the submucosal and subcutaneous tissue planes.[20] This decreased vascularity and increased fibrosis leaves irradiated tissue more susceptible to trauma, including the trauma of surgery, infection, and irritation.

Radiation has been shown to affect wound healing. A single dose of 300 cGy or less anytime does not affect wound healing, but a dose of 1000 cGy or more given within 3 weeks of injury retards wound healing.[16] In a study of 34 patients who underwent planned neck dissection after treatment with chemoradiotherapy or radiotherapy alone, there was a significant difference in the incidence of skin flap necrosis between those patients who had received <70 Gy of preoperative radiotherapy (0% incidence of skin flap necrosis) and those who received >70 Gy of radiation (33% incidence of skin flap necrosis).[14] When salvage or other surgery is performed in previously irradiated tissue, these effects should be considered. The decreased vascularity and increased fibrosis may increase the chances of postoperative infection and wound breakdown with possible salivary contamination and carotid artery exposure. Other complications including the need for tracheotomy, nerve transection and paresis, and permanent hypocalcemia were seen in 16% of 69 patients who underwent neck dissection after chemoradiotherapy.[51] The effects of previous radiation are especially important to consider when concomitant conditions that may affect vascularity (e.g.,

diabetes, hypertension) are present. Closure without tension, well-planned surgical incisions, and the use of nonirradiated distant tissue for closure or vascular coverage, such as pedicled flaps or free-tissue transfer, are important considerations in these patients.

Empiric studies have given some guidance on the timing of radiation relative to surgery. With regards to preoperative radiation, a large study of 69 patients who underwent preoperative chemoradiotherapy before neck dissection found an acceptable incidence of wound healing complications (10%) in patients who underwent neck dissection in the range of 5 to 17 weeks after completion of therapy.[51] The authors suggest that this time frame is a "window" between the acute and chronic phases of chemoradiotherapy injury. Postoperative radiotherapy is generally considered safe to begin 3 to 6 weeks after surgery. Although radiotherapy given 1 week after injury showed no detectable clinical effects on healing or tensile strength,[16] this time course is generally impractical given the overall condition of the patient. With appropriate precautions and good nutritional support, patients with open neck wounds undergoing postoperative radiotherapy did not experience serious complications.[21] In fact, 10 of 13 patients in this study ultimately healed the open wound, with 6 of 10 experiencing spontaneous healing.

Chemotherapy seems to impact wound healing by its effect on white blood cells. Wound healing occurs on a continuum: (1) inflammation involves polymorphonuclear cells and monocytes and the release of various humoral factors; (2) proliferation involves capillary formation and fibroblast proliferation; and (3) maturation involves decreased fibroblasts and macrophages and increased collagen and wound tensile strength.[16] Chemotherapy may cause transient neutropenia, which limits the patient's ability to heal, presumably by interfering with the inflammatory phase of healing. Because the effects of chemotherapy are transient, the timing of injury relative to the administration of chemotherapy seems important. An absolute neutrophil count of <500 cells/mL is thought to be detrimental to wound healing, and the critical period for wound-healing difficulty seems to be within the first 5 to 7 days after injury.[16] The general recommendation is to allow the patient's white count to increase before surgery if possible. Chemotherapy causing a significant decrease in the white count should be avoided within approximately 1 week of a surgical procedure.

Chyle Leak

Chyle leak is an uncommon complication of neck dissection, occurring in approximately 1% to 2% of cases.[13] Most chyle leaks occur in the left side of the neck because of the anatomy of the thoracic duct. This structure ascends through the chest cavity and carries fats in the form of chylomicrons absorbed from the gut. It empties into the left subclavian vein, near the entrance of the left internal jugular vein. Because of this position, it is at risk for injury at the time of neck dissection. The lymphatic duct is a somewhat analogous structure in the right side of the neck. It is a shorter structure, draining lymph fluid from the right side of the head, neck, upper extremity, right side of the chest, and the convex surface of the liver. The lymphatic duct empties into the right subclavian vein, near the junction of the right internal jugular vein. This structure also may be injured during neck dissection and, although its origin is different, can cause a chylous leak. Up to 25% of chyle leaks after neck dissection have occurred in the right side of the neck.[13]

During dissection in the region of the lower jugular vein, the thoracic or lymphatic duct should be carefully ligated if identified. To ensure that no injury has occurred or to verify adequate repair, positive airway pressure should be applied for 30 seconds or more. If milky or oily-appearing fluid emanates from the jugular stump, repair and ligation should be continued until this finding is no longer noted. Nonabsorbable suture, Surgicel, and sclerosing agents (e.g., tetracycline) have been recommended for this use.[47]

Identification of a chylous leak in the postoperative period is usually heralded by high-output milky drainage. Other causes can account for increased drain output, such as bleeding, serous drainage, or salivary fistula. This may make identification of a chylous fistula difficult. Rodgers and others[43] analyzed drain output from uncomplicated neck dissections and found that the normal triglyceride content of neck drainage is <100 mg/dL. In addition, the presence of chylomicrons does not necessarily imply the presence of a chyle fistula, because uncomplicated neck drainage showed up to 4% chylomicrons, even after centrifugation.

Once a chylous fistula is recognized, conservative therapy may be attempted. This consists of head elevation, continued suction drainage, pressure dressings, and replacement of fluid lost through the fistula, which can reach up to 4 L/day.[47] In addition, nutritional modification consisting of a medium chain triglyceride (MCT) enteral diet or total parenteral nutrition (TPN) should be instituted. The rationale for the former is that long-chain triglycerides are broken down into their components, fatty acids and glycerol. The fatty acids are packaged into chylomicrons and absorbed into the lymphatic duct. Medium-chain fatty acids are, however, absorbed directly into the portal system and bypass the lymphatics. The use of MCTs

through an enteral pathway has been shown to be effective in the management of postoperative chylous fistula and has prevented the need for parenteral hyperalimentation, with its associated morbidity.[34]

When conservative measures fail, reoperation is necessary. Patients in whom chylous drainage is >600 mL/24 hours are likely to have conservative therapy fail. Early reoperation in this group is thought to decrease the overall morbidity and hospital stay.[50] In a recent series of 15 patients treated at a single institution, it was noted that conservative medical management ultimately failed in three patients.[41] Review of these patients revealed that each was identified by a peak 24-hour drainage >1000 mL that did not promptly respond to medical management. These three patients each responded to reoperation. More problematic were two patients who had prolonged low-output fistulas that ultimately responded to medical management lasting >10 days but had complications related to their prolonged medical management.[41] A variety of surgical approaches have been suggested, including fibrin glue, use of muscular flaps, and tetracycline or doxycycline as a sclerosing agent; these latter agents are known to be neurotoxic.[41]

Chylothorax is an uncommon complication after a chylous fistula in the neck. The cause of this complication is debatable. Two theories have been proposed: (1) fluid extravasates through the wall of the thoracic duct in the mediastinum because of increased pressure in the system after the duct is ligated in the neck; and (2) fluid continues to leak after unsuccessful ligation in the neck but passes downward into the mediastinum.[27] This complication has been successfully treated by chest drainage and TPN,[24] although a new method of treatment with subcutaneous somatostatin injections for 1 week was successful along with other conservative measures in treating bilateral chylothorax after neck dissection.[2] In fact, this treatment may become a useful adjunct to the conservative management of chylous fistula after neck dissection, because use of a somatostatin analog was successful in the case of a cervical thoracic duct fistula after revision thyroidectomy and neck dissection.[54]

VASCULAR COMPLICATIONS
Internal Jugular Vein

When performed as classically described, modified and functional neck dissections, which have been popularized since the 1960s, include preservation of the internal jugular vein. Although left intact, this vessel is at risk for associated complications, namely thrombosis and rupture. Few studies have examined the integrity of the jugular vein after selective neck dissection, so accurate assessment of their incidence is impossible.

An advantage to performing a neck dissection with preservation of the internal jugular vein is to avoid the complications associated with bilateral jugular vein occlusion if a contralateral radical neck dissection is performed synchronously or in the future. These serious complications include facial and cerebral edema and blindness, which has been reported as a rare complication after bilateral radical neck dissection.[1,3,33] Notably, blindness is a reported complication after head and neck surgery, as well as surgery in distant areas of the body, despite the preservation of one or even both jugular veins.[19,31] The etiology of blindness in these cases may be due to increased cerebrospinal fluid pressure caused by thrombosis of the internal jugular vein or head positioning. The etiology may also be related to ischemia caused by anything that may affect the perfusion pressure of the posterior ciliary arteries, including atherosclerotic disease and intraoperative hypotension.[31] Late jugular vein occlusion after treatment of head and neck cancer is also known to occur. One report describes the use of endovascular stents in the unoperated neck in the case of a patient who had severe facial and cerebral edema develop, leading to loss of consciousness 2 years after unilateral radical neck dissection.[26]

The rationale for jugular preservation is only valid if the retained jugular vein actually remains patent. One series examined 79 preserved jugular veins between 11 days and 113 weeks after neck dissection.[12] Computed tomography (CT) or magnetic resonance imaging (MRI) was used to assess for recurrence or as follow-up. Of the 79 veins, 68 (86%) were found to be patent by CT or MRI criteria. Of the 11 occluded or significantly compressed veins, 7 seemed to be caused by recurrent tumor. Four patients required a pectoralis major musculocutaneous flap for reconstruction, and three of these four had an occluded ipsilateral jugular vein. The final patient with an occluded vein received preoperative radiotherapy. Of 69 patients who received preoperative or postoperative radiation, however, only one experienced occlusion, excluding those patients whose veins were compressed by tumor or a flap.

In another series, 27 internal jugular veins were evaluated by retrograde venography within 90 days of surgery.[29] Nineteen were found to be patent. Of eight thrombosed veins, four occurred in the face of a postoperative salivary fistula, and another occurred after a severe wound infection. Notably, two patients who had a fistula develop were noted to have a patent jugular vein. The remaining three thrombosed veins were not associated with any identifiable risk factor, including the use of a myocutaneous flap. In fact, two patients with flaps maintained patency, and three patients with flaps who had thrombosed veins had other complications.

The question has been raised as to whether radiotherapy after a jugular-preserving neck dissection negatively impacts the patency of the vein. One series used ultrasound to examine jugular veins after neck dissection.[15] Data regarding the jugular vein at rest and its distensibility with Valsalva's maneuver were assessed. Seventeen patients who received both neck dissection and radiotherapy were identified. Of these patients, 13 had a simultaneous free tissue transfer with the venous anastomosis involving the jugular system on the side of the surgery. Three patients had normal jugular veins bilaterally, seven had normal or reduced sized veins with an abnormal Valsalva's response, and seven had decreased or absent flow in the ipsilateral jugular vein. The abnormal Valsalva's response is hypothesized to be a result of increased fibrosis of the tissues around the jugular vein secondary to the radiotherapy effect. Despite these abnormalities, no vascular problems were noted with the free tissue transfers. The ability to perform a successful long-term microvascular venous anastomosis seems to be a clear and attainable benefit of jugular vein preservation.

A rare complication of jugular vein-preserving neck dissection is jugular vein rupture. An 8-year retrospective review at a major institution revealed only four cases of jugular blowout.[53] These cases were complicated by a pharyngocutaneous fistula, and one patient also had a carotid artery rupture. Patients who suffer jugular vein rupture present with multiple, generally small bleeding episodes that may be aggravated by coughing. Life-threatening hemorrhage can occur, however. Management of this complication is surgical exploration and ligation of the jugular vein, distant from the site of the fistula. The carotid artery should also be carefully inspected, because the risk factors for jugular vein rupture are the same as those for carotid artery blowout. Preservation of the sternocleidomastoid muscle would be expected to provide some protection; however, two of four patients in this study had jugular rupture despite the preservation of this muscle.

In some cases, preservation of a single internal jugular vein (IJV) is impossible because of the extent of the cancer. Reconstruction of the IJV can be accomplished by an external jugular vein (EJV) to IJV anastomosis or by use of a saphenous vein interposition graft of the IJV itself or as an interposition graft between the IJV and the EJV.[25] When considering cases in which the disease demands bilateral sacrifice of the IJV, the gravity of the presence of significant bilateral neck disease must be considered. A review of 193 bilateral neck dissections[30] revealed that in the six patients in this series who required bilateral radical neck dissections, none survived for 5 years.

Carotid Artery

Stimulation of the carotid sinus can occur during surgery or manipulation in the area of the carotid bulb. The carotid sinus, a blood pressure–regulating area, is found as a dilation of the proximal internal carotid and may involve the common carotid.[39] Stimulation of this area results in a compensatory drop in blood pressure, heart rate, or both. It is important for the surgeon to communicate with the anesthesiologist so that manipulation can stop immediately if this reflex is triggered. It has been suggested that this reflex can be blocked by the injection of 1% lidocaine without epinephrine in a subadventitial plane in the area of the carotid bulb.[47]

Repair vs ligation of the carotid system secondary to trauma is controversial. Injury to the internal or common carotid system during neck dissection, however, should be repaired at the time of damage. Primary closure is generally sufficient, but the surgeon may wish to consult a vascular surgical colleague if in doubt.

One of the most feared complications of neck surgery is postoperative carotid rupture. The incidence of this complication is 3% to 7%, but the mortality rate from spontaneous rupture can be as high as 50%.[47] Wound breakdown, wound infection, and salivary fistula formation with carotid exposure and contamination are associated with this problem. Previous radiation is considered a risk factor for these problems, which are often, but not inevitably, associated with surgery in a previously radiated bed. Surgical technique also is important in preventing this complication. Careful handling of the carotid artery and preservation of the adventitia, which contains the vasa vasorum (the blood supply to the vessel wall), are important. If the sternocleidomastoid muscle will not be preserved, consideration may be given to protection of the carotid artery with another muscle flap or coverage with a dermal graft if the neck dissection is performed with a concomitant procedure that enters the pharynx and places the patient at risk for a fistula.

If wound breakdown causing a fistula has occurred, it is important to attempt to divert the salivary flow away from the carotid artery. This may require wide opening of other areas of the incision, because saliva takes the path of least resistance in the most dependent area of the neck. It is also important to keep the vessel moist to prevent desiccation. Some dressing materials absorb and retain moisture. These dressings, or a wet-to-wet dressing, are preferable to a wet-to-dry dressing. As important as prevention is the recognition of an impending carotid artery rupture. This complication should be considered whenever the carotid artery is exposed to saliva, infection, or air.

In the presence of a significant wound breakdown, the carotid often may be visualized. Desiccation of the vessel should alert the surgeon to possible rupture in the near future. Sentinel bleeding is a classic warning sign of impending blowout. Although much less dramatic than an actual carotid rupture, it should be given appropriate attention, and elective ligation should be considered.

Once the carotid has ruptured, it should be considered as any other site of hemorrhage. Direct pressure should be applied, and the operating room should be readied. Blood should be immediately cross-matched, and the patient's intravascular volume should be supported. Generally, the blowout is at or near the carotid bulb and is pinpoint in size. Finger pressure and gauze are usually sufficient to maintain pressure, although in this urgent situation, much more material may be placed in the neck and may interfere with appropriate control. If control is not adequate, excess dressing material and the blood clot should be cleared to allow for directed pressure and to prevent excessive pressure on the entire carotid, which may further decrease cerebral blood flow.

Although repair of the rupture is usually futile, because the vessel has obviously been damaged by the surrounding hostile conditions, endovascular stents have been described to repair carotid rupture or impending carotid rupture.[55] Ligation away from the contaminated area is a more traditional approach to treating carotid rupture. The vessel ends can be buried in local tissue for further protection. Significant differences have been noted in the risk of neurologic sequelae after elective vs emergency ligation. Moore, Karlan, and Sigler[40] reported a 23% risk of neurologic complications after elective ligation vs 50% after emergency ligation. The risk of death was 17% vs 38%, respectively. Martinez[35] also found a large difference in mortality. Of 11 patients with emergency ligation, 64% died compared with 14% of 7 patients with elective ligation. This difference is thought to be secondary to the hemodynamic compromise frequently associated with a sudden carotid rupture. This evidence should be considered when counseling a patient who is at risk for carotid blowout about possible carotid ligation.

NEURAL COMPLICATIONS

In general, nerve damage is caused by surgical inexperience with incomplete knowledge of the surgical anatomy or by the need to sacrifice structures in proximity to or involved by the malignancy. The best way to avoid injury is to be familiar with the anatomy. If a nerve is divided, inadvertently or intentionally, repair may be attempted primarily. If tension exists, a cable graft also may be considered, depending on the importance of the nerve, time constraints, and other factors.

Trigeminal Nerve

Branches of the mandibular division of the trigeminal nerve are at risk during a neck dissection. The inferior alveolar nerve and its terminal extension, the mental nerve, are at risk when standard neck dissection is combined with a procedure on the mandible. If the mandible must be sacrificed, the inferior alveolar nerve also will be lost. If, however, the mandible is only to be split, elevating the soft tissues medial to the mental foramen preserves the mental nerve and sensory innervation to the mental area.

The lingual nerve, another branch of the mandibular division of the trigeminal nerve, supplies sensation to the floor of mouth and the anterior two-thirds of the ipsilateral tongue. It also carries parasympathetic fibers, which convey taste sensation from the anterior two-thirds of the tongue, and fibers that innervate the submandibular gland. This nerve is at risk during dissection of the submandibular triangle. When the gland is dissected free from its surrounding attachments and retracted inferiorly, the nerve can be identified. The submandibular ganglion can be clamped and ligated near the gland to prevent injury to the lingual nerve. This maneuver further frees the gland and allows the lingual nerve to return to its position medial to the mandible.

Facial Nerve

In standard neck dissection, the only branches of the facial nerve at risk are the marginal mandibular and cervical branches. Only if the neck dissection is extended in a more superior aspect than normal would the main trunk of the nerve, as it exits the stylomastoid foramen lateral to the styloid process, be at risk. If this extension is necessary, the nerve should be identified as for a parotidectomy.

The cervical branch of the facial nerve innervates the platysma. Because this muscle is divided during elevation of the flaps, and therefore has questionable function after neck dissection, and because it is thought to be a vestigial muscle, sacrifice of this branch is not considered significant. The marginal mandibular branch of the facial nerve innervates the depressor muscles of the mouth. Because of this, sacrifice of this branch is noticeable during movement of the mouth and sometimes at rest. Patients also may complain of a lack of oral competence when this nerve is nonfunctional. This nerve follows a course along the inferior mandible and down into the neck before turning superiorly back toward the facial musculature. It is particularly susceptible to injury in the region of the angle of the mandible and the area of

the submandibular triangle. This branch is deep to the platysma but superficial to the fascia over the submandibular gland. It may be protected, therefore, by elevating the fascia of the submandibular gland along with the neck flaps. The nerve also runs superficial to the facial vein. Therefore, ligation of this vein and superior retraction should aid in protecting this branch.

Vagus Nerve

The vagus nerve exits the base of the skull through the jugular foramen and descends in the neck within the carotid sheath. The first branch is the superior laryngeal nerve, which travels in close association with the superior thyroid artery. This nerve innervates the cricothyroid muscle through its external branch and supplies sensation to the supraglottic larynx through its internal branch. Damage to this branch may increase the risk of aspiration and can affect the singing voice but has little effect on the speaking voice.[47]

The recurrent laryngeal nerve arises from the vagus nerve and has a different course in the right and left neck. In the right neck, the nerve loops around the subclavian artery and ascends in the tracheoesophageal groove. In the left neck, the recurrent laryngeal nerve branches from the vagus, loops around the arch of the aorta, and ascends in the neck in the tracheoesophageal groove. The recurrent laryngeal nerve innervates the intrinsic muscles of the larynx (except for the cricothyroid). Damage to this nerve results in unilateral vocal cord paralysis, which leads to varying degrees of breathy voice, ineffective cough, and risk of aspiration. This nerve is most at risk during thyroidectomy. The main trunk of the vagus may incur injury during neck dissection if the contents of the carotid sheath are not clearly identified or during ligation of the internal jugular vein at the skull base.

Spinal Accessory Nerve

The spinal accessory nerve exits the skull through the jugular foramen. It innervates the trapezius muscle. It can be located at the base of the skull adjacent to the jugular vein. It also can be located in the posterior triangle of the neck based on three landmarks: (1) the distance between the clavicle and the point at which the nerve passes under or pierces the trapezius is 2 to 4 cm; (2) the accessory nerve may be found within 2 cm above the point at which the greater auricular nerve curves forward from the posterior border of the sternocleidomastoid muscle across the muscle; and (3) the accessory nerve can usually be found along the top half of the posterior border of the sternocleidomastoid muscle.[49]

Much controversy exists in the literature regarding sacrifice vs preservation of this nerve during neck dissection. The constellation of symptoms associated with sacrifice of this nerve is known as the eleventh nerve syndrome and was first described by Ewing and Martin.[18] This syndrome includes a dull ache, stiffness or soreness, drooping of the shoulder, aberrant scapular rotation, limited forward shoulder flexion, and limited active shoulder abduction. Radical neck dissection in which the accessory nerve is sacrificed does not uniformly result in shoulder complaints,[46] and conversely modified neck dissections that preserve this nerve can still result in disability.[7] Some of this discrepancy may be explained by the theory that adhesive capsulitis of the shoulder may be the cause of persistent shoulder problems in patients, even after recovery of a preserved spinal accessory nerve.[42]

Preservation of the spinal accessory nerve generally relies on many factors, including location and extent of tumor, patient factors, and preference of the surgeon. Inadvertent damage to this nerve should be avoided in situations in which exposure is limited and the goal may not be tumor extirpation (e.g., biopsy of a neck mass in the posterior triangle). The spinal accessory nerve may be monitored to assist with its preservation,[34] but it is not clear whether monitoring this nerve is superior to knowledge of surgical anatomy and good surgical technique.

Hypoglossal Nerve

The hypoglossal nerve, which exits the skull base through the foramen of the same name, provides motor innervation to the tongue. It runs in close proximity to the carotid artery at its bifurcation and to the greater cornu of the hyoid. It thus is at risk during procedures involving these areas, such as carotid endarterectomy or laryngectomy.

Sympathetic Trunk

The sympathetic trunk runs deep to the carotid sheath along the prevertebral fascia (Figure 117-2). Injury to this nerve causes an ipsilateral Horner's syndrome.

Phrenic Nerve

The phrenic nerve receives contributions from cervical roots C3, C4, and C5. The nerve runs deep to the fascia overlying the scalene muscles and innervates the ipsilateral diaphragm. Injury to this nerve can be prevented by preserving this fascial layer. In addition, the sensory branches from C3 to C5 should be sacrificed well away from the phrenic nerve to avoid traction or other injury.

Sensory Nerves

As in any surgery, neck dissection results in some loss of sensation in the operative area. Attempts can be made to preserve certain sensory nerves such as the great auricular nerve. A study that looked at the sensory deficit after selective neck dissection[45] found that the defect after selective neck dissection in which the cervical rootlets were preserved resulted in a sensory

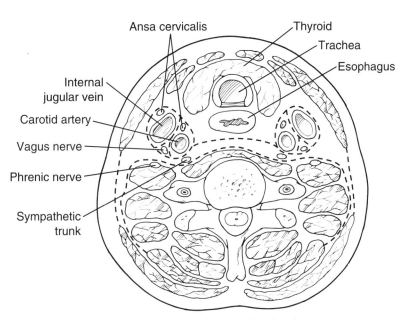

Figure 117-2. Anatomy of the cervical sympathetic trunk: phrenic nerve; vagus nerve; cervical sympathetic trunk; anterior scalene muscle; internal jugular vein; carotid sheath; common carotid artery; thyroid gland; and prevertebral fascia. (From Shockley WW, McQueen CT, Postma GN: *Complications of neck surgery.* In Weissler MC, Pillsbury HC III, editors: *Complications of Head and Neck Surgery*, New York, 1995, Thieme.)

defect of the upper anterior neck more than in any other region. In selective neck dissections in which the cervical rootlets were not spared, patients complained of numbness throughout the ipsilateral neck that was more likely to remain numb in all regions except the upper anterior neck compared with patients who underwent nerve-sparing neck dissection.

REFERENCES

1. Ahn C, Sindelar WF: Bilateral radical neck dissection: report of results in 55 patients, *J Surg Oncol* 40:252, 1989.
2. Al-Sebeih K, Sadeghi N, Al-Dhahri S: Bilateral chylothorax following neck dissection: a new method of treatment, *Ann Oto Rhino Laryngol* 110:381, 2001.
3. Ballantyne AJ, Jackson GL: Synchronous bilateral neck dissection, *Am J Surg* 144:452, 1982.
4. Barry B: Pharyngeal flora in patients undergoing head and neck oncologic surgery, *Acta Otorhinolaryngol Belg* 53:237, 1999.
5. Becker GD, Parell GJ: Cefazolin prophylaxis in head and neck cancer surgery, *Ann Otol Rhinol Laryngol* 88:183, 1979.
6. Blair EA, Johnson JT, Wagner RL and others: Cost analysis of antibiotic prophylaxis in clean head and neck surgery, *Arch Otolaryngol Head Neck Surg* 121:269, 1995.
7. Blessing R, Mann W, Beck C: How important is preservation of the accessory nerve in neck dissection, *Laryngol Rhinolotologie* 65:403, 1986.
8. Brand B and others: Prophylactic perioperative antibiotics in contaminated head and neck surgery, *Otolaryngol Head Neck Surg* 90:315, 1982.
9. Callender DL: Antibiotic prophylaxis in head and neck oncologic surgery: the role of gram-negative coverage, *Int J Antimicrob Agents* 1(12 Suppl):S21, 1999.
10. Carrau RL and others: Role of prophylactic antibiotics in uncontaminated neck dissections, *Arch Otolaryngol Head Neck Surg* 117:194, 1991.
11. Coskun H, Erisen L, Basut O: Factors affecting wound infection rates in head and neck surgery, *Otolaryngol Head Neck Surg* 123:328, 2000.
12. Cotter CS and others: Patency of the internal jugular vein following modified radical neck dissection, *Laryngoscope* 104:841, 1994.
13. Crumley RL, Smith JD: Postoperative chylous fistula prevention and management, *Laryngoscope* 86:804, 1976.
14. Davidson BJ, Newkirk KA, Harter KW and others: Complications from planned, posttreatment neck dissections, *Arch Otolaryngol Head Neck Surg* 125:401, 1999.
15. Docherty JG, Carter R, Sheldon CD and others: Relative effect of surgery and radiotherapy on the internal jugular vein following functional neck dissection, *Head Neck* 15:553, 1993.
16. Drake DB, Oishi SN: Wound healing considerations in chemotherapy and radiation therapy: postoncologic reconstruction, *Clin Plast Surg* 22:31, 1995.
17. Ducic Y, Hilger PA: The use of unilateral deep plane neck lifting to improve the aesthetic appearance of the neck dissection deformity, *Am J Otolaryngol* 21:202, 2000.
18. Ewing MR, Martin H: Disability following "radical neck dissection," *Cancer* 5:873, 1952.
19. Fenton S, Fenton JE, Browne M and others: Ischaemic optic neuropathy following bilateral neck dissection, *J Laryngol Otol* 115:158, 2001.
20. Hom DB, Adams GL, Monyak D: Irradiated soft tissue and its management: wound healing for the otolaryngologist head and neck surgeon, *Otolaryngol Clin North Am* 28:1003, 1995.
21. Isaacs JH Jr., Thompson WB, Cassisi NJ and others: Postoperative radiation of open head and neck wounds, *Laryngoscope* 97:267, 1987.
22. Johnson JT, Myers EN, and others: Antimicrobial prophylaxis for contaminated head and neck surgery, *Laryngoscope* 94:46, 1984.
23. Johnson JT, Wagner RL: Infection following uncontaminated head and neck surgery, *Arch Otolaryngol Head Neck Surg* 113:368, 1987.
24. Jortay A, Bisschop P: Bilateral chylothorax after left radical neck dissection, *Acta Otorhinolaryngol Belg* 55:285, 2001.
25. Katsuno S, Ishiyama T, Nezu K and others: Three types of internal jugular vein reconstruction in bilateral radical neck dissection, *Laryngoscope* 110:1578, 2000.
26. Kwei S, Ohki T, Beitler J and others: Complicated emergent endovascular repair of a life-threatening bilateral internal jugular vein occlusion, *J Vasc Surg* 32:397, 2000.
27. LaHei ER, Menzie SJ, Thompson JF: Right chylothorax following left radical neck dissection, *Aust N Z J Surg* 63:77, 1993.
28. Leibovitz A, Plotnikov G, Habot B and others: Saliva secretion and oral flora in prolonged nasogastric tube-fed elderly patients, *Isr Med Assoc J* 5:329, 2003.
29. Leontsinis TG, Currie AR, Mannell A: Internal jugular vein thrombosis following functional neck dissection, *Laryngoscope* 105:169, 1995.
30. Magrin J, Kowalski L: Bilateral radical neck dissection: results in 193 cases, *J Surg Oncol* 75:232, 2000.
31. Mamede RCM, Figueiredo DLA, Mamede FV: Blindness after laryngectomy and bilateral neck dissection in a diabetic patient: case report, *Sao Paulo Med J* 119:181, 2001.
32. Mandell-Brown M, Johnson JT, Wagner RL: Cost-effectiveness of prophylactic antibiotics in head and neck surgery, *Otolaryngol Head Neck Surg* 92:520, 1984.
33. Marks SC, Jaques DA, Hirata RM and others: Blindness following bilateral radical neck dissection, *Head Neck* 12:342, 1990.
34. Martin IC, Marinho LH, Brown AE and others: Medium chain triglycerides in the management of chylous fistulae following neck dissection, *Br J Oral Maxillofac Surg* 31:236, 1993.
35. Martinez SA, Oller DW, Gee W and others: Elective carotid artery resection, *Arch Otolaryngol Head Neck Surg* 101:744, 1975.
36. Matory YL, Spiro RH: Wound bleeding after head and neck surgery, *J Surg Oncol* 53:17, 1993.
37. Midwinter K, Willatt D: Accessory nerve monitoring and stimulation during neck surgery, *J Laryngol Oto* 116:272, 2002.
38. Monyak D, Levitt S: *Radiation therapy of head and neck cancer.* In Paparella MM, Shumrick DA, Gluckman JL and others, editors: *Otolaryngology, vol III, Head and Neck,* Philadelphia, WB Saunders, 1991.
39. Moore KL: *Clinically oriented anatomy,* ed 2, Baltimore, Williams & Wilkins, 1985.
40. Moore OS, Karlan M, Sigler L: Factors influencing the safety of carotid ligation, *Am J Surg* 118:666, 1969.
41. Nussenbaum B, Liu JH, Sinard RJ: Systematic management of chyle fistula: the Southwestern experience and review of the literature, *Otolaryngol Head Neck Surg* 122:31, 2000.
42. Patten C, Hillel AD: The 11th nerve syndrome: accessory nerve palsy or adhesive capsulitis, *Arch Otolaryngol Head Neck Surg* 119:215, 1993.
43. Rodgers GK, Johnson JT, Petruzzelli GJ and others: Lipid and volume analysis of neck drainage in patients undergoing neck dissection, *Am J Otolaryngol* 13:306, 1992.

44. Rodrigo JP, Alvarez JC, Gomez JR and others: Comparison of three prophylactic antibiotic regimens in clean-contaminated head and neck surgery, *Head Neck* 19:188, 1997.

45. Saffold SH, Wax MK, Nguyen A and others: Sensory changes associated with selective neck dissection, *Arch Otolaryngol Head Neck Surg* 126:425, 2000.

46. Saunders JR, Hirata RM, Jaques DA: Considering the spinal accessory nerve in head and neck surgery, *Am J Surg* 150:491, 1985.

47. Shockley WW, McQueen CT, Postma GN: *Complications of neck surgery*. In Weissler MC, Pillsbury HC III, editors: *Complications of Head and Neck Surgery*, New York, Thieme, 1995.

48. Slattery WH, Stringer SP, Cassisi NJ: Prophylactic antibiotic use in clean, uncontaminated neck dissection, *Laryngoscope* 105:244, 1995.

49. Soo KC, Hamlyn PJ, Pegington J and others: Anatomy of the accessory nerve and its cervical contributions in the neck, *Head Neck Surg* 9:111, 1986.

50. Spiro JD, Spiro RH, Strong EW: The management of chyle fistula, *Laryngoscope* 100:771, 1990.

51. Stenson KM, Haraf DJ, Pelzer H and others: The role of cervical lymphadenectomy after aggressive concomitant chemoradiotherapy: the feasibility of selective neck dissection, *Arch Otolaryngol Head Neck Surg* 126:950, 2000.

52. Strauss M, Saccogna PW, Allphin AL: Cephazolin and metronidazole prophylaxis in head and neck surgery, *J Laryngol Otol* 111:631, 1997.

53. Timon CVI, Brown D, Gullane P: Internal jugular vein blowout complicating head and neck surgery, *J Laryngol Otol* 108:423, 1994.

54. Valentine CN, Barresi R, Prinz RA: Somatostatin analog treatment of a cervical thoracic duct fistula, *Head Neck* 24:810, 2002.

55. Warren FM, Cohen JI, Nesbit GM and others: Management of carotid 'blowout' with endovascular stent grafts, *Laryngoscope* 112:428, 2002.

56. Yii NW, Patel SG, Williamson P and others: Use of apron flap incision for neck dissection, *Plast Reconstr Surg* 103:1655, 1999.

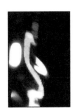

PART NINE

THYROID/PARATHYROID

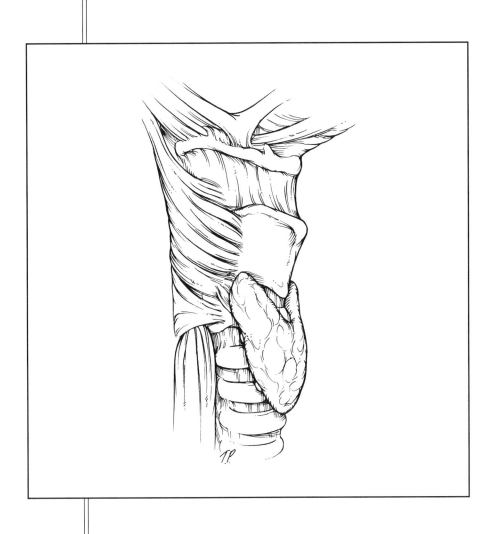

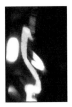

CHAPTER ONE HUNDRED AND EIGHTEEN

DISORDERS OF THE THYROID GLAND

Phillip K. Pellitteri
Steven Ing

INTRODUCTION

Thyroid diseases are relatively common. They occur in the form of abnormalities in the size and shape of the thyroid gland (goiter) and of abnormalities of thyroid secretion. Nonthyroidal illness is accompanied by any alteration in thyroid physiology that can complicate the evaluation of thyroid status.

The scope of problems relating to thyroid disease can be so complex and encompassing as to create a major challenge to the diagnostic capabilities of the clinician. The patient may have such a variety of seemingly unrelated signs and symptoms as to lull the practitioner into a suspicion of hypochondriasis. This is especially true in our current "cost-effective" frame of mind in which screening batteries of diagnostic tests are no longer in vogue, and time is of the essence. The patient's symptoms can be confusing and bizarre, leading the physician at times to nonspecific diagnoses, such as psychological problems with depression or anxiety, chronic fatigue syndrome, cardiac failure, fibromyalgia, and a host of other nonspecific entities. The dilemma is more than simply one of hyperfunction vs hypofunction or nodular vs diffuse or benign vs malignant. Nor should the examination be merely one of placing the thumb on the lower neck while the patient swallows a few sips of water and answers a couple of quick questions about heat intolerance, weight changes, and gastrointestinal function.

In reality, the thyroid gland controls body metabolism and has a profound effect on all bodily functions. In addition, the peculiarities of development and the strategic location of the thyroid gland may produce symptom complexes that divert the physician's attention away from the thyroid gland and toward the symptoms itself. To be proficient in the management of thyroid disease, the physician must be knowledgeable about all phases of the embryology, anatomy, endocrine function, genetic implications, and environmental issues that may affect the thyroid, and he or she must be keenly suspicious of all the patient's signs and symptoms.

The patient's history and review of symptoms should be comprehensive. Generalized symptoms relating to hypothyroidism include weakness and fatigue with cold intolerance; weight gain; hair loss; edema of the hands and face; thick, dry skin and hair; and a decreased tendency to sweating. Otolaryngologic symptoms may include hearing loss, dizziness, tinnitus, voice aberrations, middle ear effusion, and slurred speech with an enlarged tongue. The gastrointestinal symptoms include constipation, anorexia, intermittent nausea and vomiting, and dysphagia and bloating. Dysphagia is especially common if there is external compression on the esophagus by a circumferential or enlarged thyroid gland. Genitourinary symptoms include menstrual disorders and a tendency toward polyuria. Cardiovascular symptoms include bradycardia, some elevation of the blood pressure, intermittent angina, at times pericardial effusion, and peripheral edema. Central nervous system symptoms may include daytime somnolence but insomnia at night, headaches and dizziness, mental and physical slowness, delayed reflexes, and psychological symptoms suggestive of depression or anxiety. Pulmonary symptoms may include shortness of breath if there is tracheal compression or pleural effusion. Finally, musculoskeletal symptoms include arthritis and stiffness of the joints with muscle cramps and weakness.

The general symptoms of hyperthyroidism commonly include a rapid heartbeat or perceptible palpitations, irritability, anxiety, easy fatigue, increased number of bowel movements with weight loss, and heat intolerance. Physical findings may include tachycardia with or without arrhythmia, moist warm skin, a fine tremor of the fingers, and the thyroid on many occasions is enlarged. Eye signs may be present including lid lag, eyelid retraction, and exophthalmos.

The thyroid gland is strategically located in the lower anterior neck in close relationship to the larynx, the trachea, the esophagus, the carotid sheath structures, the sympathetic chain, the recurrent laryngeal nerve, and the mediastinal structures. Diffuse or nodular enlargement, whether benign or malignant, may cause compression or invasion of these adjacent structures. Resulting symptoms may include dysphagia, dyspnea, voice aberration, vocal cord paralysis, Horner syndrome, superior vena cava syndrome, and at times pericardial or pleural effusions.

The medical history may disclose a history of thyroid agenesis, prior thyroidectomy surgery, therapeutic irradiation with iodine-131 (^{131}I), external radiation therapy, Hashimoto's thyroiditis, history of laryngeal cancer or laryngectomy surgery, a history of cancer elsewhere with possible metastasis to the thyroid, and a history of other recent head and neck infections, which may have resulted in an inflammatory process within the thyroid gland.

PHYSICAL EXAMINATION

Facility with the examination of the thyroid and surrounding structures is essential for accurate diagnosis and appropriate management of malignant and benign thyroid disease. The patient is initially observed anteriorly. Some findings may be obvious, whereas others may be subtle. The clinical patient with hypothyroidism will usually seem more lethargic, perhaps somewhat overweight, and slower in response. Skin and hair may appear dry and coarse.

Conversely, the hyperthyroid patient may seem more anxious, thinner, somewhat more apprehensive with moist, warm skin and perhaps a visible tremor noted in his or her fingers. Eye signs may or may not be present. These may include exophthalmos, lid lag, or lid retraction.

In either the hypothyroid or the hyperthyroid patient, a diffuse or nodular goiter may not uncommonly be visible in the neck on simple inspection. The patient may have some aberration of the voice. The patient with hypothyroidism with myxedematous infiltration of the vocal cords will have a husky, raspy type voice. On the other hand, the patient whose recurrent laryngeal nerve is compromised by pressure or tumor infiltration will elicit the voice of a paralyzed vocal cord, which will be breathy, barely audible, and inefficient as far as air use is concerned. In other circumstances, the voice may have a guttural quality signifying obstruction of the aerodigestive passageway, usually at the level of the tongue base. This, of course, would suggest a lingual thyroid that has failed to descend along normal developmental pathways. Horner syndrome may be present with either benign or malignant thyroid disease. The patient may seem

to have a hearing deficit in normal conversational situations. This may be the result of middle ear effusions that can be drained and reversed. On the other hand, inner ear myxedematous changes involving the cochlear or vestibular structures may contribute to a sensorineural type of hearing loss accompanied by tinnitus and vertigo. Facial swelling or plethora and the distention of the jugular veins may signify obstruction of the superior vena cava from benign or malignant substernal thyroid disease. Pemberton's sign should be elicited in patients with large goiters. Pemberton's sign is elicited by having the patient extend both arms above the head observing for facial erythema, swelling, and/or distention of the jugular veins indicating cervicothoracic inlet obstruction.

After careful observation of the patient's general appearance, the neck is examined. The thyroid should be examined from behind the patient. The thyroid is palpated initially for gross pathology. The patient is then asked to swallow several sips of water. This will move the thyroid cephalad and make the lower portion of the thyroid more easily approached. If the patient extends the neck less fully, the more inferior aspects of the thyroid (especially in patients with substernal goiter or kyphosis) may be easily and accurately examined. Moderate pressure in the tracheal groove on one side will facilitate more accurate palpation of the contralateral lobe. The examiner will note the size relative to a normal thyroid gland. Similarly, the size and locations of its nodules should be accurately recorded. A pyramidal lobe of the thyroid can sometimes be palpated in patients, especially those with Graves' or Hashimoto's disease. A thyroid nodule with recent hemorrhage may be moderately tender, whereas an acute, suppurative, or subacute viral thyroiditis is usually exquisitely tender to palpation. Not uncommonly, the pain from the thyroid will radiate to the ipsilateral ear.

The texture of the thyroid may suggest the etiology of the disease. Autoimmune thyroid disease often is seen as a firm, bosselated (cobblestone-like) gland. This, in conjunction with a low or elevated serum thyroid-stimulating hormone (TSH) level, should strongly suggest Graves' disease or Hashimoto's thyroiditis, respectively. Smooth nodularity of the thyroid usually represents colloid goiter. Although firm nodules may represent thyroid cancer, this clinical characteristic is not diagnostic.

Attention is next turned to the areas of lymphatic drainage of the thyroid. The superior pole and the lateral lobes drain superiorly and laterally toward the jugular lymph nodes, whereas the isthmus and lower poles of the thyroid drain inferiorly along the tracheoesophageal groove and into the mediastinum. Each side of the neck should be examined methodically from the mandible to the supraclavicular notch.

Once the observation of the external surfaces, as well as examination of the external neck, is accomplished, attention is turned to the internal examination of the aerodigestive system. Intraorally, the tongue in the myxedematous patient may be enlarged and thickened. Careful examination of the base of the tongue should be done to rule out a lingual thyroid gland. If present, this would indicate a developmental anomaly. The lingual thyroid can enlarge during periods of increased hormonal demand such as puberty and pregnancy. When this occurs, the guttural qualities of the voice may be even more profound. In addition, bleeding may occur from the lingual thyroid, and finally enlargement of the lingual thyroid may continue to the point of dysphagia and airway obstruction that may precipitate a semi-emergent condition. Most commonly, hormonal treatment will reduce the size of the mass on the back of the tongue. Occasionally, surgical intervention is required to ensure a safe airway. This area of the oropharynx and tongue base is usually readily examined with the aid of a tongue blade and a laryngeal mirror. However, in patients with an extremely active gag reflex, a better examination is usually obtained with the fiberoptic nasopharyngolaryngoscope.

Assessment of the etiology of the patient's hoarseness is determined with the fiberoptic nasopharyngolaryngoscope to obtain a dynamic examination of the hypopharynx and larynx. In the hypothyroid patient, the vocal cords are mobile. However, they may exhibit myxedematous changes, causing them to be thickened and at times even polypoid along the edges of the vocal folds. The voice in these instances is quite harsh and raspy. The airway may become partially compromised by the thickened myxedematous polypoid tissue, and at times it is necessary to surgically trim this back to ensure an adequate airway.

When one vocal cord is paralyzed, the airway initially becomes incompetent. The patient may cough or choke on liquids or secretions unless careful swallowing is followed. The larynx is inefficient and will produce only two or three words per each breath of air. The voice is of an exaggerated, forced, whispered quality. As time passes, the larynx will compensate somewhat by having the mobile vocal cord cross the midline to partially close the deficit in the airway. This will improve speech and swallowing almost to normal levels. It is important that preoperative laryngeal examination be done before thyroid surgery to establish the mobility of the vocal cords. Because it is possible to have a nearly normal sounding voice with one cord paralyzed, it is important for the operating surgeon to know that there is a paralyzed cord, because injury to the opposite cord would then precipitate the more emergent situation of bilateral vocal cord paralysis and the probable need for subsequent tracheostomy and/or thyroplasty. Paralysis of the vocal cords usually implies compromise of the recurrent laryngeal nerve on the ipsilateral side. This may be secondary to pressure on the nerve but more likely is caused by infiltration of the nerve by malignancy.

External compression on the trachea and/or esophagus by thyroid masses can lead to severe dyspnea and/or dysphagia. It is important to know whether the airway and esophageal involvement are secondary to external compression alone or whether there is an element of tumor infiltration within these organs. Therefore, internal examination with a bronchoscope and an esophagoscope is necessary to determine the status of these organs. At times, radiographic studies are necessary to complement the examinations and to aid in planning of surgery. Under such circumstances, barium swallow of the esophagus may outline the areas of obstruction.

In summary, elucidating the various etiologies of thyroid disease is often accomplished by considering the aggregate data available on the patient's history, clinical examination, by chemical and imaging studies, and by specific diagnostic examinations.

PHYSIOLOGY OF THE THYROID GLAND

The thyroid gland produces two hormones, 3,5,3′-tri-iodothyronine (T_3) and 3,5,3′,5′-tetraiodothyronine or thyroxine (T_4). Both are iodinated derivatives of tyrosine. Hormone production is dependent on an external iodine supply and on intrathyroidal mechanisms for concentrating ingested iodide and then incorporating it into the tissue specific protein, thyroglobulin (Tg). The thyroid gland is unique within the endocrine system in having a large extracellular space, the follicular lumen, which is used for storage of the hormones and their precursors. As hormone is needed by the organism, Tg is retrieved by the cell, where the biologically active hormones are released from Tg before being passed into circulation (Figure 118-1).

Iodide Transport

A daily dietary intake of at least 100 µg of iodine per day is required in man to ensure adequate production of thyroid hormone. In North America, the average daily intake is somewhat higher than this, largely because of the use of iodine as a food additive.[55] In many parts of the world, however, consumption is significantly below the minimum level, and iodine deficiency is the leading cause of thyroid-related disorders.

The thyroid normally concentrates iodide some 20-fold to 40-fold over the extracellular space and

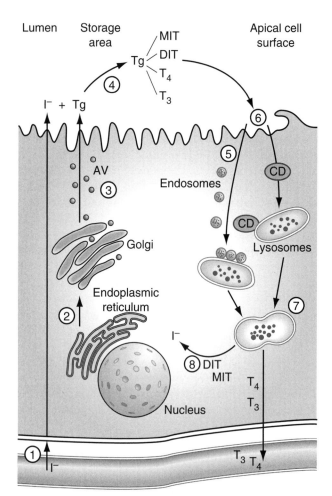

Figure 118-1. Synthesis and release of thyroid hormone. (1) Iodide transported into the thyrocyte at the basal cell membrane by the symporter (NIS) travels down its electrochemical gradient to the apical surface. (2) Tg's polypeptide chain is synthesized on the surface of the endoplasmic reticulum (ER) then translocated into its lumen. Here synthesis of carbohydrate units begins, and conformational changes transform the polypeptide chains into stable dimmers. Tg enters the Golgi where carbohydrate units are completed. (3) Uniodinated Tg travels to the apical surface in small vesicles (AV). (4) Here, Tg is iodinated and iodotyrosyls coupled to form T_4 and T_3 by thyroperoxidase in the presence of H_2O_2. (5) Tg, retrieved by micropinocytosis enters the endosome-lysosomal pathway, where proteolysis and hormone release occurs. (6) Alternatively, Tg, retrieved by macropinocytosis travels to lysosomes in colloid droplets (CD). (7) Thyroid hormones and precursors leave the lysosomes, and T_4 and T_3 enter the bloodstream. (8) MIT and DIT are deiodinated, and released iodide is recirculated. (From Dunn AD: In Pellitteri PK, editor: *Endocrine surgery of the head and neck*, New York, 2003, Delmar Publishing, p 50.)

against an electrical gradient of approximately 40 mV. Key to this trapping action is a protein located in the basal membrane of the thyroid cell known as the sodium/iodide symporter (NIS).[102] NIS couples with the influx of Na^+ down its electrochemical gradient with the simultaneous influx of I^- up its electrochemical gradient. An Na^+/K^+-ATPase acts to maintain the Na^+ gradient. Iodide then travels down its electrochemical gradient to the apical surface of the thyrocyte, where it is incorporated into Tg. Recent evidence suggests an apical membrane protein, pendrin, aids in releasing iodide into the follicular lumen.[143] Mutations in the gene and coding for this protein are responsible for the common hereditary disorder known as Pendred's syndrome, which is associated with mild hypothyroidism, goiter, and hearing loss.[143] Mutations in the gene coding for NIS have been identified in patients with iodide trapping defects, a relatively rare cause of congenital hypothyroidism.[102]

Thyroglobulin

Thyroglobulin is essential to thyroid physiology. It is a tissue-specific protein that serves both as matrix for the synthesis of hormone and as a vehicle for its storage.[56] The human Tg gene has been cloned and is located on the long arm of chromosome 8Q24. Tg is a large dimeric glycoprotein of approximately 660 kDa consisting in man of two identical polypeptide chains each of 2750 amino acids. About 10% of its weight is carbohydrate, and about 0.1% to 1% is iodine. Synthesis and maturation of Tg follow a pathway typical of proteins destined for secretion. The polypeptide chain is synthesized on the surface of the rough endoplasmic reticulum. As that passes through a series of intracellular compartments, it undergoes important posttranslational modifications before reaching the follicular lumen.[90] Carbohydrate units are added to the polypeptide chain as it is translocated into the lumen of the rough endoplasmic reticulum. Folding and dimerization of the polypeptide chain occurs within this compartment, aided by folding enzymes and a group of proteins known as molecular chaperones. Any perturbations of this process result in block of protein transport beyond this point and cause congenital hypothyroidism.[90] Under normal circumstances, the properly folded Tg dimers migrate to the Golgi complex, where processing of the carbohydrate units are completed. Mature but as of yet uniodinated Tg is transferred from the Golgi complex to the apical cell surface in small vesicles.

Iodination and Thyroperoxidase

Newly formed Tg and iodide meet at the apical cell surface, where hormone synthesis occurs. This process includes (1) the oxidation of iodide; (2) its subsequent transfer to thyrosyl residues on Tg, producing monoiodotyrosine (MIT) and di-iodotyrosine (DIT); and (3) coupling of two iodotyrosine molecules, either one each of MIT and DIT to form T_3 or two of DIT to form T_4. Thyroperoxidase (TPO), an enzyme present in the apical cell membrane, is responsible for each of these steps.[124] Hydrogen peroxide, required in the iodinating and coupling reactions, is generated at the apical membrane by an reduced nicotinamide adenine dinucleotide phosphate (NADPH) oxidase.[118] Mutations in the TPO gene have been found in patients with congenital hypothyroidism caused by defective organification. Abnormalities in hydrogen peroxide (H_2O_2) generation seem to be more rare.

Under normal circumstances, iodide, once trapped, is rapidly incorporated into Tg so that little free iodide exists within the thyroid gland at any given time. The extent to which Tg is iodinated depends on the thyroid's iodide supply. At a level of 0.5% iodine, the Tg dimer in man contains on average 5 residues of MIT, 5 of DIT, 2.5 of T_4, and 0.7 of T_3 of a total of 132 residues of tyrosine.[56]

Hormone formation involves the coupling of two residues of iodotyrosine within the Tg polypeptide chain. At the hormonogenic site, the "acceptor" diiodotyrosyl receives the iodinated phenol ring of the "donor" iodothyrosyl (either MIT or DIT) located at some distal site on the polypeptide chain. In the process, the alanine side chain of the donor remains behind, now presumably in the form of hydroalanine. Iodination in vitro of low iodine human Tg indicates that certain thyrocele sites are favored for early iodination and that three or four major sites exist for hormone formation. The most important hormonogenic site is located five residues from the amino terminal Tg, whereas a second major site is located three residues from the carboxy terminal. The locations of donor thyrosyls are incomplete. To date, only one has been identified in human Tg, and this resides in the amino terminal region of the molecule.[56]

Storage and Release of Hormone

Most mature iodinated Tg is stored in the colloid as soluble dimers, although some (approximately 10%) highly iodinated molecules associate as tetramers. The colloidal nature of the follicular lumen is caused by its high concentration of protein. This intracellular space thus contains a large supply of both iodine and hormone available to the organism, which protects it against times of iodine deprivation.

Hormone release is initiated by the retrieval of Tg from the follicular lumen. Under stimulatory conditions in some species, this process may occur by macropinocytosis. Pseudopods form at the thyrocytes' apical surface and engulf Tg as large colloid droplets. However, under physiologic conditions in most species, including man, Tg is retrieved by micropinocytosis into

small vesicles. It is then passed through the endosome-lysosomal system, where the combined action of several acid proteases including cathepsins B, D, and L, and lysosomal dipeptidase 1, release the hormones and their iodotyrosine precursors from the polypeptide backbone.[56] Evidence suggests the iodo amino acids may be preferentially cleaved first, but ultimately Tg is broken down into amino acids or small peptides within the lysosomes.

Once released from Tg, the thyroid hormones and their precursors enter the cytosol; there MIT and DIT are deiodinated by an iodotyrosine specific deiodinase, and the released iodide reenters the iodine pool. Some T_4 is deiodinated to T_3 before it is released into the circulation by 5'-iodothyronine deiodinase similar to that found in peripheral tissue.[93] The mechanism by which T_4 and T_3 are released from the thyrocyte is not known, but recent evidence suggests a carrier protein may be involved.[38]

Circulating Thyroid Hormones

Less than 1% of circulating thyroid hormones exist as free iodo amino acids. The remainder are bound in reversible, noncovalent linkage to one of several plasma proteins.[152] In man, the most important of these is thyroxine binding protein (TBG), accounting for approximately 70% of circulating hormone. The TBG molecule has one hormone-binding site with a very high infinity for T_4 and somewhat lower infinity for T_3. A second plasma protein transthyretin accounts for approximately 10% of circulating T_4 and T_3. Each transthyretin molecule has two hormone binding sites, but the infinity of the first is somewhat lower than that of TBG, and that of the second site is very low for both hormones. Albumin also serves as a thyroid hormone transport protein. Although it has low infinity, its abundance allows it to account for 10% to 20% of bound circulating hormone.

The bound hormones are in equilibrium with the minute fraction of free circulating hormone that is available for use in peripheral tissue. Under euthyroid conditions, approximately 0.2% of T_4 and about 0.3% of T_3 in circulation is unbound. The larger free/bound ratio of T_3 relative to T_4 is caused by the lower infinity of TBG for T_3.[154] To date, no change in thyroid state has been attributed to abnormalities in these hormone-binding proteins, despite their apparent role in thyroid function homeostasis.

Metabolism of Thyroid Hormones

Thyroxine must first be deiodinated to T_3 to exert most of its biologic actions. Because relatively little T_3 is directly synthesized on thyroglobulin, this transformation becomes an important step in hormonogenesis. Three iodothyronine deiodinases are present in mammals.[93] These are membrane-bound enzymes that are closely related structurally and are distinguished by the presence of selenocysteine at their active sites. Each has distinctive substrate preferences, activity characteristics, inhibitor sensitivities, and relative tissue specificity. Types I and II deiodinases, through their combined action, are responsible for generating approximately 80% of the total T_3 production. Type I deiodinase is the primary source of circulating T_3 and is found in liver, kidney, and thyroid (where it is activated by TSH) tissues, and to a lesser extent in other tissues. Type I deiodinase is positively regulated by thyroid hormones and is greatly reduced under pathophysiologic states such as starvation and nonthyroidal illnesses. It is inhibited by the antithyroid drug propylthiouracil. Type II deiodinase is present primarily in the central nervous system, the pituitary, the placenta, the skin, and has recently been found also in the thyroid.[146] Its major role is thought to be in the local production of T_3, but it may also contribute to circulating T_3. In contrast to type I deiodinase, the type II enzyme is negatively regulated by thyroid hormone and is unaffected by propylthiouracil. Type III deiodinase inactivates T_4 and T_3 by inner ring deiodination in the five position, forming, respectively, reversed T_3. The enzyme is present in the adult brain, skin, and placenta and is also present in high levels in fetal tissues, where it is thought to be important in protecting developing tissue from excess levels of thyroid hormone.[11]

Control of Thyroid Function

The anterior pituitary is the primary internal regulator of thyroid function, influencing virtually all phases of thyroid metabolism.[178] It secretes TSH, also known as thyrotropin, which is a 28- to 30-kDa lipoprotein consisting of two subunits, alpha and LH. The alpha subunit is common to the pituitary hormones follicle-stimulating hormone (FSH) and LH and to chorionic gonadotropin. The β-subunit, however, is unique to TSH and is responsible for the binding of the hormone to its receptor in the basal membrane of the thyroid cell. On interaction with TSH, the receptor, a member of a family of G protein coupled receptors, undergoes conformational changes that activate one or two regulatory pathways. Most TSH effects are mediated by the activation of the cyclic adenosine monophosphate (cAMP) pathway; others involve the Ca^{2+}/phosphatidylinositol cascade. The pathway used to elicit a given effect may vary among species. TSH stimulates both the efflux of iodide into the follicle and the resorption of colloid into the cell within minutes. Later effects include increased expression of the NIS, Tg, and TPO genes; stimula-

tion of hydrogen peroxide production; promotion of glycosylation; and increased production of T_3 relative to T_4.

Circulating levels of TSH are controlled by the opposing influences of thyroid hormone and of thyrotropin-releasing hormone (TRH) from the hypothalamus.[151] The latter is a modified tripeptide secreted to the anterior pituitary by way of the hypothalamo-hypophyseal portal system. TRH binds to the plasma membrane of the thyrotrope and stimulates both the release of TSH and the expression of its gene. Levels of circulating TSH are under strict control by the thyroid in a classic negative feedback system. As levels of thyroid hormone rise in response to TSH stimulation, T_4 and T_3 block the TRH stimulated release of TSH in the thyrotrope. The thyroid hormones also act indirectly by inhibiting TRH gene expression in the hypothalamus.

Iodine supply is the major external factor influencing the thyroid state. Autoregulatory mechanisms present in the thyroid help to compensate for variations in iodide intake. In response to increasing doses of iodine, the thyroid initially increases hormone synthesis but then reverses this process as intrathyroidal levels of iodide reach a critical level and further organification is inhibited.

Withdrawal of iodide from the diet leads to a rapid decrease in serum T_4 and an increase in serum TSH. Serum T_3 levels initially are unaffected but eventually fall with prolonged withdrawal. In response to TSH stimulation, the thyroid increases iodide uptake and organification, alters the distribution of iodo amino acids within Tg by increasing the ratios of MIT/DIT and T_3/T_4, and increases the intrathyroidal conversion of T_4 to T_3 by types 1 and 2 deiodinases.[93] With prolonged iodine deficiency, TSH-stimulated cell proliferation eventually leads to goiter.

Antithyroid Agents

Antithyroid drugs can inhibit thyroid hormone synthesis secretion or metabolism.[44] Some of the more common agents and their major actions are summarized in Table 118-1. A number of agents used in the treatment of nonthyroidal illnesses may have profound effects on thyroid hormone production. Notable among these are the iodinated radiocontrast agents that are potent inhibitors of thyroid hormone deiodination and can also interfere with hepatic uptake of T_4 and binding of T_3 to nuclear receptors.[50] The antiarrhythmic agent amiodarone, which is also heavily iodinated, elicits similar alterations in thyroid hormone metabolism and action. Lithium, used in the treatment of bipolar illness, is a potent inhibitor of thyroid hormone release and acts by blocking thyroglobulin endocytosis.[100]

TABLE 118-1

Drugs Used in Hyperthyroidism

Drug	Usual Starting Dose
Propylthiouracil (PTU)	200 mg PO tid
Methimazole (MMI)	20 mg PO bid
Propranolol	10–40 mg PO qid
Saturated solution of potassium iodide (SSKI)	1–2 ggts PO qd-tid
Compound solution of iodine (Lugol's solution)	2–5 ggts PO qd-tid
Dexamethasone	2 mg PO qid
Prednisone	40–60 mg po qd
Ipodate	1 g PO qd
Lithium	300–450 mg PO tid
Perchlorate	1 g PO qd
Cholestyramine	2–4 g PO bid-qid
Colestipol	5 g PO 1–5 times a day
Octreotide	50–100 μg sq bid-tid
Diltiazem	120 mg PO tid

PO, by mouth; sq, subcutaneously; ggts, drops; bid, twice a day; tid, three times a day; qid, four times a day; qd, every day.

Thyroid Hormone Mechanism of Action

The thyroid has multiple effects on development, growth, and metabolism. The first named are widespread phylogenetically and can be dramatically observed during the course of amphibian metamorphosis. The appropriate levels of thyroid hormone during fetal and neonatal stages in man are critical for the normal maturation of the central nervous system, as well as for muscle, bone, and lung. In severe cases of thyroid hormone deficiency during this period, the syndrome of cretinism results with its associated mental retardation, deafness, mutism, and stunted growth.[22] Similarly, an excess of thyroid hormone during these critical developmental periods can also result in neurologic abnormalities. The metabolic effects of thyroid hormone seem to be confined to birds and mammals, presumably evolving in response to the increased metabolic pressures of thermogenesis. Oxygen consumption and the metabolism of proteins, carbohydrates, and fats are all under thyroid hormone control.

Most effects of thyroid hormone are now believed to be exerted by interactions with specific nuclear thyroid hormone receptors, resulting in the altered expression of specific genes.[23] Thyroxine has little infinity for the nuclear receptors and must be first converted to T_3 to be effective. The receptors themselves belong to a large superfamily of nuclear receptors, which includes the steroid hormones, retinoic acid, and vitamin D. The thyroid hormone receptors are closely related isoforms, despite being encoded by two different genes (alpha and beta).

The thyroid hormones may have some nongenomic actions, including plasma and mitochondrial membrane transport, familiarization of actin in astrocytes, and modulation of the activities of several enzymes including type II deiodinase. Such nongenomic effects tend to occur rapidly and, unlike nuclear events, T_4 may be as effective or more so than T_3.

THYROID FUNCTION STUDIES

Thyroid function may be assessed by measuring circulating thyroid hormone levels, serum TSH concentrations, and thyroidal ^{123}I uptake.

Circulating Thyroid Hormone Measurement

Radioimmunoassay remains the standard method for measuring serum total T_4, although isotopic methods may also be used. Previous methods, none of which are used today, include the protein-bound iodine test, the butanol extraction iodine test, and T_4 measurement by column or by competitive protein binding. Although the serum total T_4 measurement generally reflects the functional status of the thyroid gland, a number of factors may alter total T_4 levels without changing the individual's thyrometabolic status. The most common of these, in the ambulatory individual, is a change in concentration of TBG. High or low TBG states, with their respective increases and decreases in total T_4 concentrations, do not affect metabolic status.

Elevated total T_4 levels may also occur when there is production of endogenous antibodies to T_4, especially in patients with Hashimoto's thyroiditis or other autoimmune disorders and also occasionally in patients with Waldenstrom macroglobulinemia associated with a benign monoclonal gammopathy.[145]

Another condition of elevated total T_4 level is peripheral resistance to thyroid hormone. Individuals with this condition may have goiter, and they may also be hyperactive.[137] Patients with this disorder are euthyroid, and although rarely found, it has led to inappropriate treatment for hyperthyroidism.

The most widely used measurement of thyrometabolic status is measurement of serum free T_4 by equilibrium dialysis.[121] When measured by the dialysis method, the free T_4 is not affected by changes in binding protein concentrations or by nonthyroidal illness. This method is cumbersome and expensive, and it is therefore not routinely performed. Commercial free T_4 levels are most commonly measured by immunoassay techniques, but their reliability is less than optimal, because they may be affected by illness or significant changes in binding proteins.[158] Thus, the clinical usefulness of free T_4 measurements by any method may be limited.[87]

Although the thyrometabolic status is best reflected by the free T_4 level, from a clinical standpoint, an index or estimate of free T_4 is generally adequate. The free T_4 index is obtained by multiplying the serum total T_4 and an indirect assessment of thyroglobulin. Serum thyroglobulin is generally estimated by one of two methods, one termed the thyroid uptake test (TU) and the other the T_3 uptake test (T_3U).[87] The TU is directly proportional to thyroglobulin levels in serum, whereas the T_3U is inversely proportional to thyroglobulin levels.[99] The result, by use of either method, is that variances in serum thyroglobulin levels are largely eliminated, and the calculated free T_4 index accurately reflects actual free T_4 status.

It should be noted that extreme changes in thyroglobulin levels, or the presence of the severe nonthyroidal illness, may result in poor correlation between calculated and measured free T_4 levels.

T_3 is measured in serum by radioimmunoassay. Like T_4, T_3 is bound to thyroglobulin, although less avidly. Alterations in thyroglobulin levels result in changes in total T_3 (but not free T_3) concentrations. Therefore, as with serum T_4, an estimate or index of free T_3 may be obtained by use of the same formula used in calculating the free T_4 index.

Because most T_3 is derived from peripheral metabolism of T_4, clinical states or pharmacologic agents that impair normal T_4 metabolism result in lower T_3 levels.

The principles used for obtaining the serum T_3 are to determine the severity of hyperthyroidism and to confirm the diagnosis of suspected thyrotoxicosis in which serum T_4 levels are normal or equivocal. In addition, the serum T_3 may be indicated in evaluating patients with autonomously functioning thyroid adenomas, in whom so-called T_3 toxicosis may be present. Such patients may have normal or borderline elevated serum T_4 levels along with suppressed serum TSH levels.[20]

Serum Thyrotropin Measurement

Until approximately 10 years ago, virtually all clinical TSH assays were performed by radioimmunoassay. By the mid 1980s, many commercial laboratories began using more sensitive immunometric TSH methods with either monoclonal or polyclonal antibodies. Functional sensitivity of these assays represented a 10-fold improvement in sensitivity over radioimmunoassay methods. Recently, nonisotopic immunometric TSH assays have been developed with a chemiluminescent label. These newer assays have a 10-fold greater sensitivity than the early immunometric TSH assays and are 100 times more sensitive than radioimmunoassay methods. These latest TSH assays, with a sensitivity of 0.01 mU/L, are currently termed *third-generation TSH assays* and represent the most sensitive method for detecting thyrotropin level.[159]

The clinical application of thyrotropin detection may be summarized as follows:

1. *The diagnosis of primary hypothyroidism.* The presence of an elevated TSH is confirmation of primary hypothyroidism. The degree of hypothyroidism may be determined by obtaining a serum T_4 level. TSH levels are also elevated in patients with subclinical hypothyroidism, in which total serum T_4 is normal or borderline low.

2. *Guidance of thyroid hormone replacement therapy.* The goal of treatment of primary hypothyroidism with levothyroxine is normalization of both serum T_4 and TSH levels. Current TSH assays may detect over-replacement with levothyroxine, because TSH concentrations will be low. Chronic over-replacement with levothyroxine may be associated with cardiac abnormalities, including ventricular arrhythmias and ventricular septal hypertrophy, as well as bone demineralization, especially in postmenopausal women.[91,141,150]

3. *Determination of TSH suppression in treating thyroid cancer.* Thyroid suppressive therapy is part of the routine management of certain patients with well-differentiated thyroid carcinoma, because growth of these tumors may be TSH responsive. Treatment with levothyroxine is titrated to suppress TSH while attempting to avoid clinical hyperthyroidism. With few exceptions, suppressed TSH levels, when measured in third-generation assays, correlate with absent TSH response.[163]

4. *Determination of suppressive therapy for nodular goiter.* TSH measurements are useful for following patients with either solitary or multinodular goiter, in whom suppressive thyroid hormone therapy may be used. Although the efficacy of levothyroxine suppression for benign goiter is not uniformly agreed on, it is still frequently used.

5. *Diagnosis of subclinical hyperthyroidism.* Patients with few or equivocal symptoms and signs of hyperthyroidism, with normal or borderline elevated total T_4 and total T_3 levels, and with suppressed serum TSH levels have subclinical hyperthyroidism.[140] Before the development of more sensitive TSH assays, these individuals usually went undiagnosed.

The fact that serum TSH is abnormal in both hypothyroidism and hyperthyroidism would seem to make it ideally suited as a screen of thyroid status, because, with rare exceptions, a normal TSH level would suggest normal thyroid hormone homeostasis. Experience in ambulatory individuals suggests that a normal TSH virtually excludes the possibility of thyroid dysfunction.[41] In addition, the serum TSH level is more sensitive than the serum T_4 level as a test for thyroid dysfunction, because TSH can detect subclinical thyroid disorders in which serum total T_4 (and T_3) is usually normal. Thus, as a result of advances in TSH methodology, measurement of circulating thyroid hormones may become assigned to a second line of assessment of suspected thyroid dysfunction. A number of investigators believe that the serum TSH is preferable as a screening method for thyrometabolic status.[91,154] Figure 118-2 illustrates a suggested algorithm for the use of TSH level in the evaluation of thyroid function.

Serum Thyroglobulin Measurement

Thyroglobulin is elevated in the serum of patients with nearly all types of thyroid disorders, thus limiting its usefulness as a diagnostic test. Its greatest clinical value is in the management of patients with well-differentiated thyroid carcinoma. An elevated or rising thyroglobulin level (after initial surgical and ablation therapy) suggests persistence or recurrence of tumor.[160] Thyroglobulin is measured by either radioimmunoassay or immunometric technique. Although antithyroid antibodies may cause interference with accurate thyroglobulin measurement in up to 10% of individuals, in these patients measurements of both thyroglobulin and antithyroglobulin antibodies may be used concurrently to provide information regarding the tumor status.[160]

Thyroid Antibody Status

Circulating antithyroid antibodies, specifically antimicrosomal (AMA) and antithyroglobulin (ATA) antibodies, are usually present in patients with autoimmune thyroid disease.[26] Since the introduction of immunoassay techniques, the term antithyroperoxidase (anti-TPO) has become interchangeable with AMA. Antimicrosomal antibodies are detectable in more than 90% of patients with chronic autoimmune thyroid disease; nearly 100% of individuals with Hashimoto's thyroiditis and more than 80% of patients with Graves' disease have positive titers.[88] Although antithyroglobulin antibodies are more specific than AMA, they are less sensitive and, therefore, they are not as useful in the detection of autoimmune thyroid disease.[14] Elevated levels of AMA are also frequently positive in a variety of other organ-specific autoimmune diseases, such as lupus, rheumatoid arthritis,

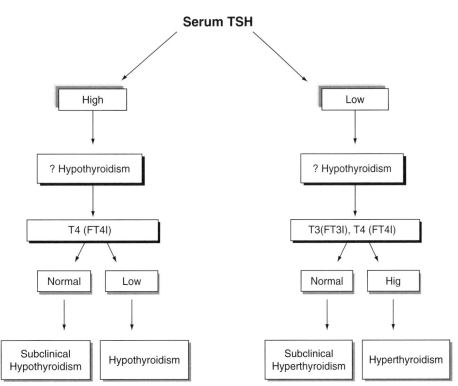

Figure 118-2. Algorithm for using the TSH level in the evaluation of thyroid function.

autoimmune anemia, Sjögren's syndrome, type 1 diabetes mellitus, and Addison's disease.[144]

Approximately 15% of adults (especially women) in the United States have elevated AMA titers.[150] Prevalence of positive AMA titers increases with age, as does the incidence of primary hypothyroidism. The presence of a positive AMA titer should alert one to the possibility of hypothyroidism. Individuals with positive AMA and elevated TSH levels, even with normal serum total T_4 levels (subclinical hypothyroidism), had a 3% to 5% per year likelihood of clinical hypothyroidism developing.[69] In this manner, determination of AMA levels may be useful in both the diagnosis of individuals with suspected autoimmune thyroid disease and in providing prognostic information when used in conjunction with TSH levels.

Thyroid-Stimulating Antibody Measurement

The immune pathogenesis of Graves' disease was first suspected in the mid-1950s, when it was observed that injecting sera of patients with Graves' disease into rats produced a prolonged uptake of radioactive iodine in the rat thyroid glands. Hence, the term *LATS*, or long acting thyroid stimulator, was coined.[1] Later LATS was characterized as a 7S immunoglobulin, and in recent years several assays have been developed for the detection of LATS, or thyroid stimulating antibodies (TSAb). Two methods are commonly used: one dependent on generation of cyclic AMP and the other a radioreceptor method that relies on the TSH binding inhibitory properties of the immunoglobulin. The cyclic AMP–generating assay is termed thyroid-stimulating immunoglobulin (TSI), and it is detectable in 90% to 95% of hyperthyroid patients with Graves' disease. The other assay detects both stimulating and blocking antibodies termed TBII; it is detected in up to 85% of patients with hyperthyroid Graves' disease.[126] Thyroid-stimulating antibody measurements are not indicated for the routine diagnostic evaluation of suspected Graves' disease, but they may be useful when the diagnosis of Graves' disease is not evident.

Radioactive Iodine Uptake Test

The thyroidal radioactive iodine uptake (RAIU) test is performed by administering an isotope of iodine (usually ^{123}I) orally and then measuring the percentage of the ^{123}I trapped by the thyroid gland. The test is usually performed 24 hours after administration of the isotope, although this may be done earlier. Before the development of sensitive and specific assays for thyroid hormones, the RAIU was used as an adjunct to differentiate hyperthyroid from hypothyroid states, with elevated and low RAIU values implying hyperthyroidism and hypothyroidism, respectively. Today, however, its principle usefulness is in differentiating hyperthyroidism into high or low uptake states. RAIU generally provides an accurate estimate of the thyroid gland's functional activity, provided the iodide pool has not been expanded by iodine-containing drugs or radiocontrast materials.

THYROTOXICOSIS

Thyrotoxicosis represents the clinicopathologic and biochemical syndrome that results from exposure to excessive concentrations of thyroid hormones. The syndrome is usually categorized as overt or subclinical. Overt thyrotoxicosis is defined as high serum T_4 and T_3 concentrations and low serum TSH concentrations, whereby most patients have symptoms and signs of this entity. Subclinical thyrotoxicosis is defined as normal serum T_4 and T_3 concentrations and low serum TSH concentrations; most patients in this category have no symptoms or signs of this disorder. Thyrotoxicosis may develop suddenly or gradually, it may be transient or persistent, and it may be of little importance or life threatening. Accordingly, the diagnosis may be obvious and may be confirmed easily by relatively few simple laboratory studies or, conversely, it may be exceedingly difficult, requiring repeated serial investigations or prolonged clinical observation.

Thyrotoxicosis is a rather common disorder. The overall prevalence rates of overt and subclinical thyrotoxicosis resulting from clinical surveys in the United States and Europe demonstrate an incidence of approximately 0.5 to 1 and 10 to 40 per 1000 people, respectively.[34,80,125,176] Within these ranges, the rates are generally higher in older persons, especially women, and seem to be lower in community-based screening programs.

Thyrotoxicosis is about 10 times more common in women than in men, especially with regard to overt thyrotoxicosis. The etiology is Graves' disease in 60% to 85% of patients, toxic nodular goiter in 10% to 30%, and toxic thyroid adenoma in 2% to 20%, with the remainder being represented by some type of thyroiditis.[28,180] The frequency of toxic multinodular goiter and toxic adenoma varies the most, being higher in areas of lower iodine intake.[180] Most individuals identified with Graves' disease are 30 to 60 years old, whereas those with toxic multinodular goiter or toxic thyroid adenoma are in the span of 40 to 70 years old.[136]

Pathophysiology

Thyroid toxicosis results from the unregulated release of T_4 and T_3 from the thyroid gland or the ingestion of excessive amounts of T_4, T_3, or both. It may be caused by increased T_4 and T_3 synthesis and release because of intrinsic thyroid disease, excessive TSH, or, theoretically, excessive TRH secretion, or the production of other thyroid-stimulating hormones, such as TSH receptor stimulating autoantibody and chorionic gonadotropin. It may also be caused by the destruction of thyroid tissue with the subsequent release of stored T_3 and T_4.

Most patients with thyroid toxicosis have increased production of both T_4 and T_3 and increased serum T_4 and T_3 concentrations. The increases in the production rate of T_3 and serum T_3 concentrations are characteristically greater than are those found in T_4. Some patients with thyrotoxicosis have high serum T_3 concentrations but normal serum T_4 concentrations. This is called T_3 thyrotoxicosis; in these patients, T_3 production is increased relative to that of T_4, even more than is the case in the usual patient with thyrotoxicosis. There are, however, no characteristic clinical manifestations of T_3. It is most common in patients whose thyrotoxicosis is due to a toxic thyroid adenoma or recurrent Graves' disease, but it may be due to hyperthyroidism of any cause. It is more common in regions where iodine intake is limited and thus is rare in the United States. The abnormality responsible for it is probably relative intrathyroidal iodide deficiency. The causes of thyrotoxicosis may be found in Table 118-2. The cause of thyrotoxicosis can usually be identified with reasonable certainty by history and physical examination: the most important findings to elicit concern are the duration of symptoms, the degree and pattern of thyroid enlargement, and the presence or absence of thyroid pain and tenderness.

Graves' Disease

Graves' disease is by far the single most common cause of thyrotoxicosis. It most commonly occurs in women 30 to 60 years old but may occur in children and in adult men and women of any age. It is fundamentally an autoimmune disorder consisting of one or more of the following: hyperthyroidism (with thyrotoxicosis), diffuse thyroid enlargement, infiltrative ophthalmopathy (exophthalmos), localized myxedema (dermopathy), and thyroid acropachy. Toxic goiter may appear alone or may be seen before, during, or after the patient has ophthalmopathy develop. Ocular signs range from mild periorbital puffiness to severe extraocular muscle dysfunction with proptosis, corneal ulceration, and optic neuritis and blindness. The extrathyroidal manifestations of Graves' disease can occur in the absence of thyroid disease.

The major gross anatomic abnormality in patients with Graves' thyrotoxicosis is diffuse thyroid enlargement. Microscopic examination reveals hypertrophy and hyperplasia of the thyroid follicular cells.

The natural history of Graves' thyrotoxicosis varies considerably in different patients. Some patients have a single episode of thyrotoxicosis (and Graves' disease) that subsides spontaneously in a few months or years. Other patients have lifelong thyrotoxicosis, and still others have repeated remissions and relapses. In patients who are treated with an antithyroid drug, the occurrence of a remission of Graves' disease means that prolonged therapy is not required. Although the disease potentially undergoes spontaneous remission, prolonged antithyroid medication, ^{131}I ablation, or surgery is usually necessary to control the thyrotoxicosis.

Well-differentiated thyroid cancer is approximately two times more prevalent in patients with Graves' disease than the general population.[110] Well-differentiated thyroid cancers may contain TSH receptors that can be stimulated by the thyroid-stimulating immunoglobulins. These tumors associated with Graves' disease tend to be larger and more aggressive and have more local invasion with more regional lymph node metastases than cancers occurring without Graves' disease.[15] When a palpable, hypofunctional thyroid nodule is found in a patient with Graves' disease, it has about 45% probability of being a thyroid malignancy.[15] Therefore, a palpable hypofunctional nodule in a diffuse toxic goiter of Graves' disease should be regarded with great suspicion and, if proven to be malignant, should be managed aggressively.[110]

An antithyroid drug and radioactive iodine (^{131}I) are the two best treatments for patients with Graves'

TABLE 118-2

ETIOLOGY OF THYROTOXICOSIS

Graves' disease
Thyroiditis
  Subacute thyroiditis
  Painless (silent) thyroiditis
  Postpartum thyroiditis
  Raditation-induced thyroiditis
Exogenous thyrotoxicosis
  Thyroid hormone–induced thyrotoxicosis
  Iodine-induced thyrotoxicosis
  Drug and cytokine-induced thyrotoxicosis
Toxic uninodular goiter (toxic thyroid adenoma)
Toxic multinodular goiter
Autosomal-dominant and sporadic thyrotoxicosis
  McCune-Albright syndrome
Ectopic thyrotoxicosis (struma ovarii)
Thyroid carcinoma
Thyrotropin-dependent thyrotoxicosis
Pregnancy-related thyrotoxicosis
  Gestational thyrotoxicosis
  Trophoblastic tumors

thyrotoxicosis. Both methods are effective, safe, and relatively inexpensive. They represent treatments for hyperthyroidism rather than for the autoimmune process itself, although some antithyroid drugs may also have an immunosuppressive effect. The antithyroid drugs used in the United States are methimazole (MMI) and propylthiouracil (PTU). These drugs inhibit thyroid hormone biosynthesis by inhibiting the oxidation and organification of iodine and the coupling of iodotyrosines, reactions that are catalyzed by thyroid peroxidase.[169] PTU also inhibits the thyroidal and extrathyroidal conversion of T_4 to T_3.[114] Both medications are concentrated in the thyroid, and intrathyroidal concentrations, especially of MMI, remain high for considerably longer than do serum concentrations.[84]

MMI and PTU have immunosuppressive actions that may contribute to the occurrence of remissions of Graves' disease. Both drugs reduce the number of intrathyroidal T cells and inhibit lymphocyte function, including thyroid autoantibody production in vitro, although the latter actions require very high concentrations.[179]

The initial goal of antithyroid drug therapy is to inhibit thyroidal T_4 and T_3 synthesis almost completely. Neither drug has an affect on the release of thyroid hormones stored in the thyroid gland, and their onset of action is thus relatively slow, depending on the severity of disease, size of the goiter, drug dosage, and timing. Release of intrathyroidal hormone stores, which may be substantial, continues until they are depleted.

Adverse reactions to antithyroid drugs are uncommon and probably occur with equal frequency with either MMI or PTU. Pruritus, urticaria or other rashes, arthralgia or myalgia, and fever occur in approximately 5% of patients taking either drug.[44] Both drugs may result in dysgeusia. The most dangerous adverse effect is agranulocytosis, occurring in 0.2% or less of patients taking these medications.[176] Rare adverse affects include aplastic anemia, thrombocytopenia, hepatocellular hepatitis (PTU), or cholestatic hepatitis (MMI), and a lupuslike vasculitis (PTU).[61,103]

Inorganic iodine inhibits thyroid hormone secretion, primarily by inhibiting thyroglobulin proteolysis, and also inhibits thyroidal iodine transport, oxidation, and organification.[169] These actions require only a few milligrams of iodine daily and may be administered in dosages of 5 to 10 drops of a saturated solution of potassium iodide (Lugol's solution) several times daily. This compound is often given in preparation for thyroidectomy, both for its antithyroid action and because it reduces thyroid blood flow, theoretically reducing hemorrhage at the time of surgery. Lithium carbonate demonstrates antithyroid action similar to those of inorganic iodine and has proved effective in doses of 300 mg three or four times daily.[94] Cholestyramine, when added to thioamides and β-blockers, leads to a more rapid decrease in thyroid hormone levels, especially in the first few weeks.[114]

β-blockers are valuable in the management of hyperthyroidism. Independent of alteration of thyroid function, these drugs minimize many of the sympathetic overdrive symptoms found in hyperthyroidism such as tachycardia, excessive sweating, nervousness, tremors, and hyperdynamic cardiac activity. They are contraindicated in patients with severe thyrotoxic cardiomyopathy and heart failure but may benefit patients with atrial fibrillation and heart failure.[92] β-blockers are useful for the reduction of symptoms of thyrotoxicosis before and for several weeks after ^{131}I therapy, before subtotal thyroidectomy, in thyroiditis, and in thyroid storm.

In the United States, radioiodine is the preferred management for most adults and for children who have thionamides fail or who are poorly compliant with these medications. The goal of ^{131}I therapy is to reduce the amount of functioning thyroid tissue and, therefore, its efficacy is independent of whether a remission of Graves' disease occurs. A major advantage of ^{131}I therapy for patients with Graves' thyrotoxicosis are that usually only a single dose is necessary, it reduces thyroid size to normal in most patients, and it is safe.[40] Thionamides should be stopped for about 3 days before and after radioiodine therapy, which is usually effective in 2 to 4 months.

Radioiodine usually causes a transient exacerbation of thyrotoxicosis and rarely precipitates thyroid storm. This occurs within 1 to 2 weeks and is caused by radiation-induced thyroiditis; it is a major problem in seriously thyrotoxic or elderly patients. Thyrotoxicosis may also be exacerbated by stopping thionamides before radioiodine therapy. Hypothyroidism is not so much a complication of ^{131}I treatment as an almost inevitable consequence of it. Early hypothyroidism, defined as occurring within a year after treatment, is caused by the acute destructive effects of [131]I. Its frequency ranges from 40% to as high as 80% in patients treated with higher doses of radioiodine.[13] Lower doses result in early hypothyroidism less often and persistent thyrotoxicosis more often.

Some physicians have been reluctant to treat young adults and especially adolescents and children with [131]I. The reasons are that it might cause thyroidal or other tumors or gonadal damage, or the patient may be pregnant, which is an absolute contraindication to the treatment. [131]I crosses the placenta and can destroy the fetal thyroid, and therefore care must be taken to ensure that any young woman about to be treated with ^{131}I is not pregnant.

Surgical therapy for thyrotoxic Graves' disease is effective and expeditious. The classic operation for surgical treatment of Graves' disease is subtotal thyroidectomy. Implementing this operation either unilaterally or bilaterally, a narrow margin of thyroid tissue in the superolateral aspect of the thyroid where the recurrent laryngeal nerve enters the larynx is preserved by dividing across thyroid tissue at that location.[113] This operation provides the additional benefit of preserving the blood supply to the superior parathyroid gland on one or both sides. The intended goal of the subtotal thyroidectomy is to leave between 3 and 6 g of thyroid tissue providing the benefit that patients become euthyroid without hormone replacement therapy.[163] The amount of thyroid tissue remnant preserved directly impacts the recurrence rate of hyperthyroidism and the development of long-term hypothyroidism.[165] For patients who have larger remnants preserved, an increased incidence of recurrent hyperthyroidism is noted that can often be treated with radioactive iodine ablation efficiently because of the preserved small amount of residual thyroid tissue.[164] Patients in whom more complete thyroid removal is performed are generally guaranteed to have resolution of their hyperthyroidism; however, long-term hypothyroidism will be the outcome of therapy.[134]

Those favoring more complete surgical resection of thyroid tissue in the form of near total thyroidectomy for Graves' disease point out that long-term hypothyroidism may be easily remedied by appropriate hormone replacement therapy, whereas recurrent hyperthyroidism, as a result of leaving behind a larger than intended thyroid remnant, carries with it the need for further treatment.[95] Arguments have been raised in favor of subtotal thyroidectomy as a means by which complications such as permanent hypoparathyroidism and recurrent laryngeal nerve injury may be avoided.[95] However, the rate of permanent recurrent laryngeal nerve injury approaches zero, as does the rate of long-term hypocalcemia, in patients operated by experienced surgeons.[183] The general recommendation for the surgical approach in patients with indications for thyroidectomy is a near total thyroidectomy, thus completely eliminating the potential for recurrent or persistent hyperthyroidism.[117,181]

The absolute indications for surgical treatment for Graves' disease are in those patients who have significant adverse reactions to thionamide drugs and cannot be appropriately blocked before radioactive iodine administration.[129] Patients included in this category are those with very severe skin reactions, hepatic damage, or patients with agranulocytosis. Other indications for surgical therapy in patients with Graves' disease include those with very large thyroid glands in excess of 75 g and those patients in whom neoplasia is either suspected or proven within the setting of diffuse toxic nodular goiter.

Relative indications for surgical therapy are in young women of childbearing age, who wish to attempt achieving pregnancy or who are in the process of lactating and want to continue to do so. An additional relative indication for surgery as opposed to radioactive iodine is in those patients with moderate or severe ocular symptoms related to Graves' ophthalmopathy. Ophthalmopathy may be worsened with radioactive iodine administration secondary to the development of tissue edema and worsening of the ocular symptoms.[182]

Patients undergoing surgery for Graves' thyrotoxicosis require preoperative preparation so as not to induce thyrotoxicosis on induction of general anesthesia and subsequent manipulation of the thyroid intraoperatively. This is accomplished by administering antithyroid drug treatment 4 to 6 weeks and inorganic iodine treatment for 7 to 10 days preoperatively. Treatment with a β-adrenergic antagonist drug for several weeks, with or without concomitant inorganic iodide for 10 to 14 days, also has proved to be safe and effective preoperative therapy.[130]

Postoperative problems after thyroidectomy include wound hematoma, transient or permanent hypocalcemia, vocal paresis or paralysis, recurrent thyrotoxicosis, and transient or permanent hypothyroidism. The frequency of nonthyroid complications is low, especially in experienced surgical hands. Transient hypocalcemia may occur secondary to temporary hypoparathyroidism or the healing of thyrotoxic osteopenia. The incidence of wound hematoma is less than 1% as is the incidence of permanent hypoparathyroidism.[185] In addition, the risk of permanent injury to the recurrent laryngeal nerves in the setting of initial surgery is a fraction of 1%.[4]

Thyroiditis

The thyrotoxicosis that occurs in all forms of thyroiditis is caused by T_4 and T_3 release from thyroglobulin as a result of thyroid inflammation and disruption of thyroid follicles. Because the stores of thyroglobulin are limited and the new T_4 and T_3 synthesis ceases, the thyrotoxicosis is generally transient. Approximately half of patients with subacute or granulomatous thyroiditis have clinical manifestations of thyrotoxicosis, and a significant proportion of the remainder have high serum T_4 and T_3 concentrations.[42] This illness is dominated by nonspecific systemic manifestations of inflammation, including fever, malaise, and myalgias. In addition, localized symptoms of thyroid pain and tenderness are also noted that may be severe. Approximately 50% of the patients have a history of a recent upper respiratory tract infection preceding the illness. Any manifestations of thyrotoxicosis together with thyroid pain and tenderness are usually short-lived, lasting approximately 4 to 6 weeks or less. This inflammatory and thyrotoxic phase may be followed by transient hypothyroidism, but permanent hypothyroidism is rare. The thyroid gland is usually firm in consistency and may be quite hard. Cervical lymphadenopathy is distinctly uncommon. If pursued, thyroid radionuclide uptake scanning is generally low and ultrasonography reveals thyroid hypoechogenicity.[16]

Indirect evidence suggests that subacute thyroiditis may be a viral illness, but conclusive proof is lacking. The disorder has been associated with mumps, influenza, adenovirus, and other viral infections, and small epidemics of subacute thyroiditis have been reported.[171]

Both the inflammatory and the thyrotoxic components of subacute thyroiditis may be so mild and transient that no therapy is required. More often, thyroid pain and tenderness result in sufficient discomfort to warrant antiinflammatory therapy. Salicylates in doses of 2.4 to 3.6 g daily or high doses of other nonsteroidal antiinflammatory medications usually provide effective relief. Patients with severe thyroid pain and tenderness or those who do not improve readily and quickly with one of these medications should be treated with prednisone in a dose of approximately 40 mg daily for 3 to 4 weeks, after which the dose should be gradually reduced and then discontinued to minimize the likelihood of recurrence. Antiinflammatory therapy promptly relieves not only the symptoms of subacute thyroiditis but in addition probably reduces thyroid hormone release, thus accelerating recovery from thyrotoxicosis. The thyrotoxicosis itself usually requires no therapy, but in patients in whom thyrotoxic symptoms may become a problem, a β-adrenergic drug may be administered for approximately 1 to 2 weeks.

Thyrotoxicosis, which is caused by thyroid inflammation in the absence of thyroid pain and tenderness, is known as painless or silent thyroiditis and has also been termed subacute lymphocytic thyroiditis. It is an uncommon cause of thyroid toxicosis. Unlike Graves' disease, it occurs in near equal proportions of men and women. The thyroid gland is not painful or tender and does not appear enlarged, or perhaps only slightly enlarged. In contrast to subacute thyroiditis, there is generally no history of antecedent upper respiratory tract infection. None of the extrathyroidal manifestations of Graves' disease are generally present in this disorder. When present, the thyrotoxicosis associated with painless thyroiditis lasts 2 to 6 weeks and is followed by either recovery or transient hypothyroidism that lasts an additional 2 to 8 weeks. Approximately

half of the patients later had goitrous autoimmune thyroiditis, hypothyroidism, or both. Painless thyroiditis with thyrotoxicosis may likely represent a variant form of chronic autoimmune thyroiditis.

Radiation-induced thyroid follicular necrosis and inflammation occur regularly after ^{131}I therapy and occasionally are sufficiently intense to cause exacerbations of thyrotoxicosis, with or without thyroid pain and tenderness. These complications of ^{131}I therapy are most likely to occur 1 to 2 weeks after treatment, last a week or two, and then subside spontaneously.

Acute suppurative thyroiditis is most commonly caused by *Staphylococcus aureus, Streptococcus hemolyticus,* or *Streptococcus pneumoniae* but occasionally is caused by other organisms such as *Fusobacterium* and *Haemophilus*.[139] This bacterial infection of the thyroid gland may be the result of trauma, hematologic seeding from a distant infected site, or direct extension from a deep cervical infection. The infection is usually localized to a single lobe and most commonly develops an abscess cavity that may rupture through the glans capsule, extending into the mediastinum or the deep neck spaces along fascial planes. This disorder is especially common in children in whom a prodrome of malaise is followed by the acute onset of fever, neck pain and tenderness, severe systemic symptoms, and marked leukocytosis. Referred pain to the homolateral mandible and ear may be present and typically the child will fix the head and neck in a single position similar to torticollis. Localized tenderness over the gland and pain on head movement is commonly noted. This disorder may be difficult to distinguish from subacute nonsuppurative thyroiditis, but the pain is generally more severe, the thyroid hormone levels are generally normal, the erythrocyte sedimentation rate is normal, and the leukocyte count is high. Although the diagnosis is generally made on clinical grounds, needle aspiration of the abscess cavity will establish the bacterial organism causing the infection.

The initial therapy is the administration of high-dose antibiotics, usually penicillinase-resistant penicillin together with a cephalosporin, although antibiotics that cover anaerobic organisms should be considered. Antibiotic therapy that is started before the cavitary phase of the infection may be successful in limiting the progression of infection. However, once an abscess has been demonstrated on needle aspiration, surgical drainage is usually required. Drainage may involve a partial thyroidectomy to remove all evidence of abscess and necrotic tissue and to prevent recrudescence. The neck should be drained externally until purulence ceases, and antibiotics should be continued for at least 2 weeks after the surgical procedure. Both thyrotoxicosis during the course of infection and posttreatment hypothyroidism rarely develop in this entity in contrast to other types of inflammatory thyroiditis.

Exogenous Thyrotoxicosis

Thyrotoxicosis may occur as a result of either intentional or accidental administration of inappropriately high doses of thyroid hormone initiated by caregivers or patients themselves. Important clues to the presence of exogenous thyrotoxicosis are the absence of thyroid enlargement or the failure of thyroid enlargement to regress much if the treatment was given for this purpose. This occurs together with normal or low serum T_4 concentrations if the patient is taking T_3 or preparations containing T_3. These patients also demonstrate low thyroid radioiodine uptake values and low serum thyroglobulin concentrations. Despite the ability of iodine supplementation to decrease the size of goiter and improve thyroid function in patients located in regions of endemic goiter, it has the potential to induce thyrotoxicosis in these same patients. This usually occurs as a result of a preexisting thyroid abnormality that results in autonomous thyroid secretion—for example, Graves' disease or, more commonly, a nodular goiter—but insufficient iodine intake to permit excessive production of T_4 and T_3. Iodine-induced thyrotoxicosis may also occur in nonendemic goiter regions.[162] Most of these patients have autonomously functioning thyroid tissue, such as a multinodular goiter or a thyroid adenoma, that transports iodide poorly.

Amiodarone, because it contains iodine, can cause iodine-induced thyrotoxicosis in patients with nodular goiter.[10] It may also cause painless thyroiditis that is sufficiently severe to cause thyrotoxicosis, apparently because of a direct toxic effect of the drug or one of its metabolites.

Approximately 2% of patients who are treated with interferon-α have thyrotoxicosis develop, caused mostly by painless thyroiditis but sometimes overt Graves' disease.[64] This thyrotoxicosis is generally more subclinical than overt.

Toxic Thyroid Adenoma

Toxic uninodular goiters or toxic thyroid adenoma are autonomously functioning thyroid neoplasms.[31] Among patients with these adenomas, about 20% have overt and 20% subclinical thyrotoxicosis at the time of diagnosis.[77] Although these neoplasms occur in adults of all ages and occasionally in children, most patients demonstrating thyrotoxicosis are in older age groups. Hemorrhagic infarction of a nontoxic thyroid adenoma may result in a transient thyrotoxicosis.[65]

The characteristic finding in patients with toxic thyroid adenoma is a solitary thyroid nodule, which is usually 3 cm or more in diameter. Radionuclide uptake imaging of the thyroid demonstrates intense nuclear uptake in the location of the palpable nodule and nearly complete absence of uptake in the remainder of the thyroid gland.

Management of the toxic adenoma is required unless spontaneous infarction occurs, because the resultant thyrotoxicosis is usually permanent. Definitive treatment may be obtained by either surgical resection of the adenoma through thyroid lobectomy or ^{131}I ablative therapy. Definitive ^{131}I therapy carries a slight to moderate risk of either transient or permanent hypothyroidism after completion of therapy, although with appropriate dosing of ^{131}I, this may be minimized. Surgical resection may be carried out after 4 to 6 weeks of antithyroid drug administration as well as a 7- to 10-day course of inorganic iodine therapy in the form of Lugol's solution. Complications after lobectomy are generally exceedingly rare, and the surgical resection is usually definitive, resulting in no evidence of recrudescent thyrotoxicosis or evidence of hypothyroidism.[60] An alternative approach that is performed more commonly in Europe than in the United States is the percutaneous administration of ethanol directly into the adenoma by use of ultrasound needle guidance. Although there may be some discomfort associated with the injections, long-term complications are rare, and it seems to be a safe procedure done in appropriately experienced hands. The shortcoming of this technique is that it may require multiple treatment sessions. This approach may be desirable in patients who are poor candidates for surgical resection and wish to avoid exposure to radioiodine.

Toxic Multinodular Goiter

Thyrotoxicosis may occur late in the natural history of multinodular goiter, usually in women 50 years old or older. The characteristic patient with this disorder has a long history of thyroid enlargement with insidious development of subclinical and then subsequently overt thyrotoxicosis. These patients generally do not demonstrate ophthalmopathy or localized myxedema and do not undergo spontaneous remissions; thyrotoxicosis generally persists until the autonomous thyroid tissue is destroyed.

^{131}I is generally the treatment of choice for patients with thyrotoxicosis caused by a multinodular goiter, primarily because spontaneous remission does not occur and because surgical resection generally requires removal of most of the thyroid gland.

Patients who are not candidates for radioiodine therapy or who refuse this modality may undergo surgery after preparation with an antithyroid medication and inorganic iodine therapy, similar to patients being treated for Graves' disease surgically. The usual operation is either bilateral subtotal thyroidectomy or near total thyroidectomy with preservation of a 3- to 6-g remnant of thyroid tissue. Surgery is more effective in rapidly reducing the effects of thyrotoxicosis than is ^{131}I and is attractive in terms of volume reduction of goiter size. Surgery may be more likely to result in long-term or permanent hypothyroidism.[12]

Ectopic Thyrotoxicosis

The only recognized etiologies of thyrotoxicosis caused by excessive ectopic thyroid hormone secretion are dermoid tumors and teratomas of the ovary. Most of the uncommon patients with substantial amounts of thyroid tissue in their tumors (struma ovarii) who have thyrotoxicosis also have Graves' disease or a multinodular goiter.[27] Thus, they have one of the common causes of thyrotoxicosis, affecting both the thyroid gland and the ectopic thyroid tissue within the ovarian tumor. In the absence of a functional thyroid gland because of surgical removal or radioiodine ablation, the ovarian tumor may be the only source of excessive thyroid hormone in these patients when it contains a toxic thyroid adenoma.[109]

Special Situations in Thyrotoxicosis
Subclinical Thyrotoxicosis

Subclinical thyrotoxicosis is characterized chemically by the demonstration of a normal serum T_4 and T_3 with low TSH concentrations. Most patients with subclinical thyrotoxicosis are asymptomatic, but a few may demonstrate nonspecific symptoms or physical signs compatible with overt thyrotoxicosis. The course of this disorder is generally variable, with some patients demonstrating resolution within a period of weeks to years, others maintaining a state of subclinical thyrotoxicosis, and a smaller percentage (approximately 10%) demonstrating the development of overt thyrotoxicosis.[107] There seems to be some increased risk of progression to overt thyrotoxicosis in patients who also have thyroid adenomas, multinodular goiters, or history of Graves' disease.[58,147]

If the disorder is due to overt administration of exogenous thyroid hormone, the treatment of choice is to reduce the dosage of thyroid hormone supplementation. If the disorder is secondary to native thyroid disease, treatment is rarely required, primarily because the disorder generally remains asymptomatic. If the disorder is associated with a solitary thyroid adenoma, surgical resection of the adenoma or ^{131}I therapy may be the treatment options. In the setting of multinodular goiter or Graves' disease, patients may be treated with either ^{131}I and/or antithyroid medication.

Thyroid Storm

Severe, life-threatening thyrotoxicosis is referred to as thyroid storm. This disorder usually occurs abruptly in a thyrotoxic patient who has had an acute infection or other medical illness, an injury, or a major operation. It may also occur after ^{131}I therapy, discontinuation of an antithyroid medication, or spontaneously.

The index clinical findings in patients with thyroid storm are fever greater than 38.5°C, tachycardia, and generally some type of central nervous system dysfunction. Central nervous system abnormalities that may be noted include anxiety, agitation and delirium, possibly acute psychosis or seizures, and as a terminal event, coma. Severe cardiovascular effects such as congestive heart failure or atrial fibrillation may also be present.[30]

Determinative laboratory abnormalities in patients with thyroid storm are generally not found. Serum T_4 and T_3 concentrations may be high but no more so than in ordinary thyrotoxicosis. Serum free T_4 and T_3 concentrations may be somewhat more elevated than in less ill patients with thyrotoxicosis.[25]

The treatment of thyroid storm should be directed toward decreasing production of T_4 and T_3, peripheral production of T_3, and the peripheral actions of thyroid hormone, as well as administering supportive treatment to maintain adequate cardiovascular and central nervous system function. Antithyroid medications should be given in large doses, if necessary by nasogastric tube or rectally. Propranolol given orally or intravenously is the most immediately effective treatment for the tachycardia and neuromuscular dysfunction of thyroid storm. Glucocorticoids are usually given in large doses, such as 50 mg of hydrocortisone or 2 mg dexamethasone intravenously every 8 hours. The rationale for glucocorticoid therapy is that adrenocorticotropic hormone (ACTH) and cortisol secretion may not increase sufficiently to meet cortisol requirements in patients who are quite ill and in whom cortisol degradation is increased. Inorganic iodine should be given orally or by nasogastric tube in a dose of 50 to 100 mg four times daily to inhibit the thyroidal release of T_4 and T_3 after administration of the antithyroid medication. Additional supportive systemic therapy should include treatment to reduce hyperpyrexia and appropriate parenteral fluid and electrolyte support.

HYPOTHYROIDISM
Prevalence

Hypothyroidism affects women fourfold to sixfold more often than men and rises with increasing age. The National Health and Nutrition Examination Survey (NHANES III), a sample of 17,353 persons age ≥12 years representing the geographic and ethnic distribution of the US population from 1988 to 1994, reported a prevalence of clinical hypothyroidism at 0.3% and subclinical hypothyroidism at 4.3%.[81] Thyroid peroxidase antibodies were elevated in 11.3%, and thyroglobulin antibodies were elevated in 10.4%. Thyroid peroxidase antibody positivity was associated with hypothyroidism (and hyperthyroidism), but thyroglobulin antibodies were not.

Etiology

Hypothyroidism can be classified (in order of decreasing frequency) as thyroid (primary), pituitary (secondary), or hypothalamic (tertiary) failure and thyroid hormone receptor resistance. Causes of primary hypothyroidism are shown in Box 118-1. Worldwide, the most common cause of hypothyroidism is iodine deficiency. In iodine-sufficient areas, such as the United States, the most common cause is chronic autoimmune (Hashimoto's) thyroiditis. With current administered doses of ^{131}I for patients with

Graves' disease, approximately 90% become hypothyroid by the first year.[47] External neck irradiation in a cohort of 1677 patients with Hodgkin's disease followed for a mean of 9.9 years was associated with a cumulative incidence of hypothyroidism of 30.6%, highlighting the importance of continued clinical and biochemical evaluation.[78]

Clinical Features

The severity of clinical features depends on the severity of thyroid hormone deficiency rather than etiology. Persons with mild hypothyroidism with elevated TSH but normal free T_4 (subclinical hypothyroidism) may have few or no symptoms. At the opposite extreme, persons with severe hypothyroidism may have myxedema coma. Even in persons with overt biochemical hypothyroidism, severity of symptoms is variable. In general, patients are more symptomatic if hypothyroidism develops rapidly. Elderly patients demonstrate fewer symptoms than younger patients.[56] Common symptoms of hypothyroidism such as fatigue, constipation, dry skin, and cold intolerance may be mistakenly misinterpreted as part of the normal aging process.

Hypothyroidism should be suspected in persons with goiter and risk factors (Box 118-2). With the widespread use of the serum TSH assay, hypothyroidism is frequently detected at an earlier stage. The classic symptoms and signs of hypothyroidism are now less frequently found (Box 118-3).

Otolaryngologic Manifestations

Hearing loss. Hearing loss may be conductive, mixed, or sensorineural in origin. It occurs more frequently and with greater severity in congenital than in adult hypothyroidism.[122] Progressive mixed hearing loss is reported in one half to nearly all children with endemic cretinism,[116] but only approximately 30% to 40% of adults with myxedema have bilateral sensorineural hearing loss. Substantial deafness persists

---

BOX 118-1
CAUSES OF PRIMARY (THYROIDAL) HYPOTHYROIDISM

Thyroid agenesis
Destruction of thyroid tissue
  Surgical removal
  Therapeutic irradiation (^{131}I or external radiation)
  Autoimmune (Hashimoto's) thyroiditis
  Replacement by cancer and infiltrative diseases
    (amyloidosis, scleroderma)
  Postthyroiditis (acute or subacute)
  Postlaryngectomy alone or with external irradiation
Inhibition of thyroid hormone synthesis and/or release
  Iodine deficiency
  Iodine administration in persons with underlying
    autoimmune thyroiditis (amiodarone, iodine-
    containing expectorants, kelp, SSKI, Lugol's solution,
    povidone-iodine, iodine-containing radiocontrast
    agents)
  Other medications with antithyroid action
    (methimazole, propylthiouracil, lithium, interferon-α,
    interferon-β, interleukin-2)
  Inherited enzyme defects
Transient
  After surgery or ^{131}I therapy
  Postpartum
  Recovery from thyroiditis
  Autoimmune (Hashimoto's) thyroiditis
  After withdrawal of thyroid hormone in euthyroid
    patients.

Modified from Braverman, Utiger *Introduction to hypothyroidism.* In Braverman LE, Utiger RD editors: *Werner and Ingbar's the thyroid: a fundamental and clinical text*, ed 7, Philadelphia, 1996, Lippincott-Raven, p 736.

BOX 118-2
RISK FACTORS FOR HYPOTHYROIDISM

Older age
Female gender
Graves' disease
Hashimoto's disease
Other autoimmune disease (e.g., type 1 diabetes, adrenal
  insufficiency, vitiligo)
Postthyroidectomy
Goiter
Prior neck irradiation
Laryngectomy alone or with external irradiation
Drugs: lithium, amiodarone, iodine-containing compounds

SYMPTOMS AND SIGNS OF HYPOTHYROIDISM

General: Fatigue, weakness, lethargy
  Weight gain
  Cold intolerance
Ear, nose, throat: Macroglossia
  Hearing loss, vertigo, tinnitus
  Hoarseness of voice
  Middle ear effusion
  Blurred vision
CNS: Slowed speech, movement, and mentation
  Delayed relaxation phase of deep tendon reflexes
Gastrointestinal: Constipation
  Anorexia, nausea, vomiting
  Dysphagia
  Ascites
Cardiovascular: Bradycardia
  Diastolic hypertension
  Pericardial effusion
Integumentary: Dry, rough, thick skin
  Coarse hair
  Nonpitting edema (myxedema)
  Periorbital edema
  Loss of lateral eyebrows
  Decreased perspiration
  Carotenemia
Musculoskeletal: Arthralgia
  Carpel tunnel syndrome
Pulmonary: Pleural effusion
  Dyspnea on exertion
Genitourinary: Menstrual irregularity (oligomenorrhea,
  menorrhagia)

Modified from Watanakunakorn and others: *Arch Intern Med* 16:183, 1965.

after T_4 therapy in 10% of children with congenital hypothyroidism.[49] Although it mainly occurs in primary hypothyroidism, deafness has been reported with panhypopituitarism.[52]

Children with cretinism may have anomalous ossicles involving any bone in the middle ear and also may have atrophy of the organ of Corti.[115] The tectorial membrane is the first structure to change, followed by degeneration of hair cells at the basal turn of the cochlea, with prolongation of wave I; outer hair cells remain intact.[67] Patients with acquired hypothyroidism who have hearing loss may display similar abnormalities. Only a few adults and almost no children with a well-established hearing loss improve with thyroid hormone therapy.

Some adults with severe myxedema have bilaterally symmetric and progressive sensorineural hearing loss that worsens as the severity of hypothyroidism

increases. Conductive losses also may occur as a result of edema of the eustachian tube mucosa.

Vertigo. Vertigo is experienced in as many as two thirds of patients with hypothyroidism. Attacks are usually mild and brief and are not associated with electronystagmography changes or concurrent hearing loss.[17]

Hoarseness. Gradual and progressive hoarseness occurs in hypothyroidism caused by mucopolysaccharide infiltration of the vocal cords and possibly by tissue edema in the ambiguous nucleus or the cricothyroid muscles.[133] Finding bilaterally edematous, mobile vocal cords should raise the suspicion of hypothyroidism. Hoarseness almost invariably dissipates with thyroid hormone replacement alone.

Goitrous Hypothyroidism

The most common cause of goitrous hypothyroidism in adults in the United States is autoimmune thyroiditis (Hashimoto's disease).[111] Other less common causes are drugs (lithium, amiodarone, sulfisoxazole, large doses of iodides, p-aminosalicylic acid, interferon, and antithyroid drugs), infiltration of the gland with tumor or inflammatory processes, and familial defects in thyroid hormonogenesis.

Transient Hypothyroidism

Hypothyroidism resulting from Hashimoto's thyroiditis is transient in approximately 10% of cases. Spontaneous remission is associated with the presence of a larger goiter, a high initial TSH level, and a family history of thyroid disease.[43] Autoimmune thyroid dysfunction may become apparent after surgery for Cushing's disease.[166] Smoking increases the metabolic effects of overt and subclinical hypothyroidism in a dose-dependent way.[119]

Excessive Iodine Intake

In iodine-sufficient areas of the world such as the United States, excess iodine intake can cause hypothyroidism in persons with autoimmune thyroiditis, ^{131}I or surgically treated Graves' disease, and hemithyroidectomy-treated patients for thyroid nodules.[177] Hypothyroidism may develop in persons taking amiodarone, especially among those with an underlying thyroid abnormality. Thyroid autoantibodies are risk factors for the development of hypothyroidism.[108]

Endemic Goiter

Endemic goiter is uncommon in the United States, but TSH levels are elevated in more than 50% of patients with this disorder, many of whom have no clinical features of thyroid failure.[18]

Familial Hypothyroidism

Kindreds with hypothyroidism usually have inherited defects in hormogenesis but rarely may have generalized thyroid hormone resistance.[173]

Nongoitrous Hypothyroidism

Nongoitrous hypothyroidism is most often caused by thyroid disease—most commonly autoimmune diffuse thyroid atrophy and management of Graves' disease with ^{131}I, thionamides, or thyroidectomy—but may be caused by pituitary and hypothalamic disorders.[39,167]

Hypothyroidism After Laryngectomy and Radiotherapy

Hypothyroidism may start within 4 months of surgery but may not become clinically apparent for 1 year.[51] In a multivariate analysis of 221 patients, risk factors for hypothyroidism were high radiation dose, combination of radiotherapy and cervical surgery, time from therapy, and no shielding of the midline neck. Patients receiving irradiation to the neck—particularly those undergoing neck dissections or total laryngectomy—should have routine thyroid function studies performed every 3 to 6 months the first year after management and annually thereafter.

Pituitary and Hypothalamic Hypothyroidism

Pituitary and hypothalamic hypothyroidism is uncommon and includes large pituitary tumors and pituitary apoplexy. Hypothalamic causes include lymphocytic hypophysitis, tumors, infarctions, trauma, and infiltrative diseases.

Subclinical Hypothyroidism
Diagnosis

The diagnosis of subclinical hypothyroidism is made by an elevated TSH with normal free T_4 or a free thyroxine index. Clinically, there are no or a few mild symptoms of hypothyroidism. Some patients may have goiter, especially when antithyroid antibodies are positivity.

Prevalence

In population-based studies, the prevalence of subclinical hypothyroidism is approximately 8% in women and 3% in men, higher in whites (vs blacks), and in persons >75 years (vs 55–64 years).[8,172] The National Health and Examination Survey (NHANES III) reported that in the 16,533 participants who reported no known thyroid disease, goiter, or thyroid hormone use, 4.3% had subclinical hypothyroidism.[81]

Natural History

Progression from subclinical to overt hypothyroidism is not inevitable in all persons. In a large population study in Great Britain followed for more than 20 years, women with both an elevated TSH and elevated antithyroid antibody titers progressed to overt hypothyroidism at a rate of 4.3% per year, greater than those with elevated TSH alone (2.6% per year) or antithyroid antibodies alone (2.1%/year).[177] In this study, there was no increase in all cause or cardiac mortality in those with subclinical hypothyroidism at baseline. In a natural history study of 26 elderly subjects with subclinical hypothyroidism, one third had overt biochemical hypothyroidism develop within 4 years of follow-up. Progression to overt hypothyroidism occurred in those with an initial TSH >20 µIU/mL and in 80% with high titer antimicrosomal antibodies >1:1600.[139] In a more recent prospective study of 82 women with subclinical hypothyroidism, the cumulative incidence of overt hypothyroidism occurred in 43% of women with TSH 6 to 12 and in 77% with TSH >12, and in no woman with a TSH <6 followed for 10 years. Thyroid peroxidase antibody positivity was associated with development to overt hypothyroidism.[82]

Effects on Lipids, Hypothyroid Symptoms, and Mood

Treatment of subclinical hypothyroidism prevents progression to overt hypothyroidism. Other potential benefits of therapy include improvement in hypothyroid symptoms and mood, lipid profile, and decrease in thyroid volume by 20%.

The relationship between subclinical hypothyroidism and effects of lipid profile are inconsistent. Some studies show that persons with subclinical hypothyroidism have an atherogenic lipid profile (higher total cholesterol, low-density lipoprotein [LDL] cholesterol, lipoprotein[a], apolipoprotein B and lower high-density lipoprotein [HDL] cholesterol) than euthyroid persons,[3,35,96] but other studies show no difference.[21,97,128] In the largest cross-sectional study of 25,862 subjects in the United States, those with subclinical hypothyroidism had a higher total cholesterol than the euthyroid group (223 mg/dL vs 216, $P < .003$ and had higher LDL cholesterol than the euthyroid group (144 mg/dL vs 140, $P < .003$).[34] In small studies, thyroxine therapy of patients with subclinical hypothyroidism leads to an increase in HDL cholesterol[36] and decrease in total and LDL cholesterol.[7,21,35] Meta-analysis of thyroxine therapy in subclinical hypothyroidism shows a 10 mg/dL decrease in LDL cholesterol and 7.9 mg/dL decrease in total cholesterol concentration.[48] Greater improvement was seen in those with baseline total cholesterol levels ≥240 vs those with total cholesterol <240.

Thyroxine therapy leads to significant increases in cardiac output, mean arterial pressure, and decreased systemic vascular resistance.[62] In a survey of post-menopausal women, subclinical hypothyroidism is associated with an increased risk of myocardial infarction (odds ratio, 2.3) and aortic atherosclerosis (odds ratio, 1.7) but no subsequent risk of myocardial infarction at 4.6 years of follow-up.[76] Whether thyroid hormone therapy in subclinical hypothyroidism improves cardiac mortality remains unclear.

Subclinical hypothyroidism is associated with depression in some[75] but not in all studies.[132] Similarly, some randomized placebo-controlled trials in persons with subclinical hypothyroidism show improvement in symptoms of hypothyroidism,[45,123] but one reported no difference.[83] Depressed patients with subclinical hypothyroidism have a poorer response to antidepressant therapy than depressed patients who are euthyroid.[85] Persons with subclinical hypothyroidism show impairment in neurobehavioral scores, such as memory, which improve with thyroxine therapy.

Treatment of subclinical hypothyroidism is reasonable in pregnant women to avoid impairment of intellectual potential of the fetus[74] and in women who have ovulatory dysfunction with infertility.[45]

Treatment

Thus, those with subclinical hypothyroidism and positive thyroid peroxidase antibodies, TSH >10, are prone to have overt hypothyroidism develop and should receive thyroid hormone replacement. Risk of overt disease may depend on etiology of subclinical hypothyroidism. Persons receiving radioactive iodine therapy or high-dose external radiation are likely to progress to overt hypothyroidism and should probably be treated with thyroid hormone. Other patients who may benefit include persons with goiter, elevated total or LDL cholesterol, pregnancy, and ovulatory dysfunction with infertility.[45] Small doses are usually needed, such as 50 to 75 μg daily, with monitoring of TSH and dose titration in 4 to 6 weeks until TSH is normalized. Those with coronary artery disease should begin at a lower dose of 25 μg daily.

Nonthyroidal Illness

TSH elevation may occur in conditions other than hypothyroidism. These include recovery from non-thyroidal illness, also known as "sick euthyroid syndrome." Hospitalized and critically ill patients may have a decreased free thyroxine index or free T_4 concentration by radioimmunoassay. However, when measured by equilibrium dialysis, free T_4 is normal or elevated. In one report, serum total T_4 levels <3 μg/dL were associated with mortality in 84% of critically ill patients.[156] In a randomized prospective study, thyroxine treatment in an intensive care unit did not alter mortality.[24]

Laboratory Diagnosis

There is a set point for optimal serum free T_4 concentration in a given individual. Because of the log-linear relationship between serum TSH and T_4 concentrations, small changes in free T_4 from this set point lead to relatively large changes in TSH by negative feedback. Thus, the most sensitive test for hypothyroidism is an elevated serum TSH. In subclinical hypothyroidism, TSH is elevated, whereas free T_4 remains normal. If the disorder progresses to overt hypothyroidism, free T_4 is decreased (see Table 118-3 for thyroid function tests in hypothyroidism and other low thyroxine syndromes). Radioactive iodine uptake is not indicated for the diagnosis of hypothyroidism because low, normal, or high values can occur, depending on the cause.

Central hypothyroidism caused by pituitary or hypothalamic disorder demonstrates a low free T_4 and

---

TABLE 118-3

THYROID FUNCTION TESTS IN HYPOTHYROIDISM AND OTHER LOW THYROXINE SYNDROMES

	Free	T_4T_3	TSH
Hypothyroid hypothyroidism			
Primary hypothyroidism			
Overt	Low	N_1/low	High
Subclinical	N_1	N_1	High
Pituitary (secondary)	Low	Low/N_1	N_1/low/slightly high
Hypothalamic (tertiary)	Low	Low/N_1	N_1/low/slightly high
Euthyroid hypothyroidism			
Low TBG	N_1	Low	N_1
Nonthyroidal illness			
Mild	N_1	Low	N_1
Severe	Low	Low	N_1

TSH that is low, inappropriately normal, or mildly elevated. TRH stimulation testing of TSH has traditionally been used to distinguish between these two entities but is unreliable.[63,157]

Management

Oral synthetic L-thyroxine (T_4) is the therapy of choice to correct hypothyroidism. Gastrointestinal absorption is 81%.[66] Because the plasma half-life of T_4 is long (6.7 days),[73] once-daily administration leads to stable T_4 and T_3 concentrations. There are a number of brand name (Euthyrox, Levothroid, Levoxyl, Synthroid, Unithroid) and generic preparations of T_4, each available in varying doses with different color-coded tablets to allow dose titration at precise increments. In one study, comparison of two brand-name and two generic preparations in the United States demonstrated bioequivalency.[53] Thus, equivalent doses of different formulations of T_4 are generally interchangeable. However, one should repeat the TSH level 4 to 6 weeks after switching.[46,66] In young, otherwise healthy adults, a full replacement dose can be prescribed at 1.6 μg/kg per day for nonmalignant conditions. In persons with known coronary disease, multiple coronary risk factors, and the elderly who may have previously silent coronary disease, conservative therapy with an initial dose of 25 μg/day is advisable. One should repeat TSH measurements with dose adjustment every 4 to 6 weeks (4–6 half-lives of T_4) until serum TSH normalizes or cardiac symptoms arise that may limit therapy to less than a full replacement dose. In persons without residual thyroid tissue, for example, the patient with thyroid cancer who has undergone thyroidectomy, the mean T_4 dose required to achieve euthyroidism is generally higher, 2.1 μg/kg/day.[70]

In persons with primary hypothyroidism, the goal of therapy is to normalize the serum TSH level. After initiation or change in dose of thyroxine, TSH should be repeated in 4 to 6 weeks. Ultimately, TSH measurements annually are needed, or sooner depending on clinical status. In those with central hypothyroidism, free T_4 alone should be normalized, also with repeat measurements free in 4 to 6 weeks. The use of patient's symptoms to judge the adequacy of T_4 dosing is frequently inaccurate. When subjective symptoms were used to determine T_4 dosing, patients chose a dose that produced mild hyperthyroidism.[37]

Potential adverse effects to overtreatment with an excessive dose of T_4 include bone loss in post-menopausal but not premenopausal women[9,174] and in elderly patients, cardiac complications, including cardiac arrhythmias, heart failure, angina, and myocardial infarction.[109] Occasionally, patients have manic behavior develop with T_4 replacement. Severe behav-

ioral manifestations of T_4 therapy for juvenile hypothyroidism are uncommon, but mild behavioral symptoms and poorer school achievement may occur in approximately 25% of patients, who represent the most severe cases at the time of diagnosis.[142]

Poor patient adherence to taking thyroid hormone leads to therapeutic failure. Alternatives to a daily regimen include twice weekly[170] or once weekly regimens.[72] These should probably not be used in persons with coronary artery disease. A number of medications may bind to and interfere with intestinal absorption of thyroxine, including aluminum hydroxide,[106] ferrous sulfate,[33] sucralfate,[32] cholestyramine,[81] and calcium carbonate.[157] Thyroid hormone administration should be separated in time from these medications by a few hours.

Thyroid hormone preparations that contain T_3 alone (e.g., Cytomel), combinations of T_4 and T_3 (e.g., Thyrolar), and desiccated thyroid extract (Armour thyroid) should not be used for the treatment of hypothyroidism. Serum T_3 levels fluctuate widely because of the short half-life of T_3. Temporary T_3 therapy is indicated in persons with thyroid cancer who have undergone thyroidectomy and await thyroid remnant ablation to shorten the period of hypothyroidism. T_3 can be discontinued 2 weeks before [131]I.[68] In addition, temporary switching from T_4 to T_3 therapy in persons undergoing thyroid hormone withdrawal whole-body scanning also reduces the period of hypothyroidism.

Thyroid hormone requirements are increased during pregnancy by an average of 45%[106] because of an estrogen-mediated increase in thyroxine-binding globulin, fetal T_4 transfer, and increased T_4 clearance. Serum TSH should be obtained at each trimester of pregnancy. If the T_4 dose requires adjustment, TSH should be remeasured in 4 weeks with further dose adjustment as necessary. After delivery, the prepregnancy T_4 dose should be resumed.[86] A hypothyroid woman starting oral estrogen therapy such as with hormone replacement therapy may also require a higher thyroid hormone dose,[6] and TSH should be obtained 3 months after initiation of estrogen to determine whether a dose increase is needed. Increases in dose may be necessary in patients who start medications that increase T_4 catabolism (phenytoin, carbamazepine, phenobarbital, rifampin), have gastrointestinal malabsorption, or nephrotic syndrome develop.[2] A decreased thyroid hormone dose requirement may be seen in the elderly[149] and in androgen-treated women treated with breast cancer.[5]

Myxedema Coma

Myxedema coma, a thyroid emergency, is a late manifestation of hypothyroidism and is characterized by coma or precoma with severe clinical manifestations of myxedema. An underlying infection or other precipitating cause of the myxedema coma is usually present. Patients characteristically have extreme hypothermia, bradycardia, pleural and pericardial effusions, hyponatremia, hypoventilation, respiratory acidosis, and hypoxia. Focal or generalized seizures typically precede the coma.

Management is with large doses of intravenous T_4 and hydrocortisone. Although management is usually instituted without laboratory confirmation, the clinical diagnoses should be certain before large doses of intravenous T_4 are given. Supportive care includes intubation and assisted ventilation, cautious warming, support of blood pressure, and management of infection. Mortality rates are approximately 50% and depend on the severity of superimposed illnesses and underlying coronary heart disease.

Surgery

With mild to moderate hypothyroidism, postoperative complications are frequent but are rarely serious or lasting, and necessary surgery should not be postponed simply to replete thyroid hormone.[98] This is not true for patients with severe myxedema, who should be given preoperative thyroid hormone, except in the most urgent surgical emergencies or uncontrolled ischemic heart disease.

In euthyroid patients, total T_4 tends to decrease in the first postoperative day then spontaneously normalizes in 7 days; the same occurs in hypothyroid patients, but T_4 levels do not normalize until thyroid supplementation is given.[89] However, it is usually not necessary to increase the postoperative dose of T_4 and almost never necessary to use parenteral T_4 unless the patient cannot take medication by mouth for several weeks. If parenteral T_4 therapy is necessary, half of the patient's usual daily T_4 dose is ordinarily given while attention is given to the patient's cardiac status, because this therapy may precipitate cardiac arrhythmias, angina, and heart failure.

Cardiac and pulmonary problems are prevalent in the elderly patient with hypothyroidism. The prevalence of coronary artery disease is high, but the diagnosis is easily overlooked, as patients often have few symptoms because of their low metabolic activity or because they fail to communicate their symptoms clearly.[17] Pericardial effusions are often apparent and rarely cause tamponade. Patients with severe hypothyroidism also respond poorly to stress by having hypothermia and hypotension develop, and they do not have tachycardia develop in response to infection or hypotension. Shock responds poorly to vasoconstrictors.

Patients with severe hypothyroidism often display upper airway obstruction caused by oropharyngeal muscle dysfunction and tissue infiltration with mucopolysaccharide.[127] They may have central sleep apnea, insensitivity to hypoxia and hypercarbia,[57] and respiratory muscle weakness,[153] changes that often lead to severe postoperative hypoxia and difficulty in weaning from a ventilator. These defects are reversible with T_4 replacement therapy, but obstructive sleep apnea may be more closely related to obesity and male gender than hypothyroidism.[131]

A von Willebrand disease–like defect is common in hypothyroidism, which may lead to bleeding.[101,120] It resolves promptly with infusion of desmopressin, suggesting that it acts through the β-adrenergic resceptor.[107] This can be helpful in the acute management of bleeding. It resolves permanently with T_4 therapy.[29,59]

REFERENCES

1. Adams DD, Purves HD: Abnormal responses in the assay of thyrotropin, *Proc Univ Otago Med Sch* 34:11, 1956.
2. Afrasiabi MA and others: Throid function studies in the nephritic syndrome, *Ann Intern Med* 90:335, 1979.
3. Althaus BU and others: LDL/HDL-changes in subclinical hypothyroidism: possible risk factors of coronary heart disease, *Clin Endocrinol (Oxf)* 28:157, 1988.
4. Andaker L and others: Surgery for hyperthyroidism: hemithyroidectomy plus contralateral resection or bilateral resection? A prospective randomized study of postoperative complications and long-term results, *World J Surg* 16:765, 1992.
5. Arafah BM: Decreased levothyroxine requirement in women with hypothyroidism during androgen therapy for breast cancer, *Ann Intern Med* 121(4):247, 1994.
6. Arafah BM: Increased need for thyroxine in women with hypothyroidism during estrogen therapy, *N Engl J Med* 344:1743, 2001.
7. Arem R and others: Effect of L-thyroxine therapy on lipoprotein fractions in overt and subclinical hypothyroidism, with special reference to lipoprotein(a), *Metabolism* 44:1559, 1995.
8. Bagchi N and others: Thyroid dysfunction in adults over age 55 years. A study in an urban US community, *Arch Intern Med* 150:785, 1990.
9. Banovac K and others: Evidence of hyperthyroidism in apparently euthyroid patients treated with thyroxine, *Arch Intern Med* 149:809, 1998.
10. Bartalena L and others: Treatment of amiodarone-induced thyrotoxicosis, a difficult challenge: results of a prospective study, *J Clin Endocrinol Metab* 81:2930, 1996.
11. Bates JM, St. Germain DL, Galton VA: Expression profiles of the three iodothyronine deiodinase, D1, D2, and D3, in the developing rat, *Endocrinology* 140:844, 1999.
12. Bayot MR, Chopra IJ: Coexistence of struma ovarii and Graves' disease, *Thyroid* 5:469, 1995.
13. Beckers C: Regulations and policies on radioiodine 131I therapy in Europe, *Thyroid* 7:221, 1997.
14. Beever K and others: Highly sensitive assays of autoantibodies to thyroglobulin and to thyroid peroxidase, *Clin Chem* 35:1949, 1989.
15. Belfiore A and others: Increased aggressiveness of thyroid cancer in patients with Graves' disease, *J Clin Endocrinol Metab* 70:830, 1990.

16. Bennedaek FN, Hegedus L: The value of ultrasonography in the diagnosis and followup of subacute thyroiditis, *Thyroid* 7:45, 1997.

17. Bhatia PF and others: Audiological and vestibular function tests in hypothyroidism, *Laryngoscope* 87:2082, 1997.

18. Biel MA, Maisel RA: Indications for performing hemithyroidectomy for tumors requiring total laryngectomy, *Am J Surg* 150:435, 1985.

19. Biondi B and others: Cardiac effects of long term thyrotropin-suppressive therapy with levothyroxine, *J Clin Endocrinol Metab* 77:334, 1993.

20. Bitton RN, Wexler C: Free triiodothyronine toxicosis: a distinct entity. *Am J Med* 1990; 88:531-533.

21. Bogner U and others: Subclinical hypothyroidism and hyperlipiproteinaemia: indiscriminant L-thyroxine treatment not justified, *Acta Endocrinol (Copenh)* 128:202, 1993.

22. Boyages SC, Halpern JP: Endemic cretinism: toward a unifying hypothesis, *Thyroid* 3:59, 1993.

23. Brent GA: The molecular basis of thyroid hormone action, *N Engl J Med* 331:847, 1994.

24. Brent GA and others: Thyroxine therapy in patients with severe nonthyroidal illnesses and low serum thyroxine concentration, *J Clin Endocrinol Metab* 63:1, 1986.

25. Brooks MH, Waldstein SS: Free thyroxine concentrations in thyroid storm, *Ann Intern Med* 93:694, 1980.

26. Brown J and others: Autoimmune thyroid disease—Graves' and Hashimoto's, *Ann Intern Med* 88:379, 1978.

27. Brown WW, Shetty KR, Rosenfeld PS: Hyperthyroidism due to struma ovarii: demonstration by radioiodine scan, *Acta Endocrinol (Copenh)* 73:266, 1973.

28. Brownlie BEW, Wells JE: The epidemiology of thyrotoxicosis in New Zealand: Incidence and geographical distribution in North Canterbury, 1983-1985, *Clin Endocrinol (Oxf)* 33:249, 1990.

29. Bruggers CS, McElligott K, Rallison ML: Acquired von Willebrand disease in twins with autoimmune hypothyroidism: response to desmopressin and L-thyroxine therapy, *J Pediatr* 125:911, 1994.

30. Burch HB, Wartofsky L: Life-threatening thyrotoxicosis. Thyroid storm, *Endocrinol Metab Clin North Am* 22:263, 1993.

31. Burch HB and others: Diagnosis and management of the autonomously functioning thyroid nodule: the Walter Reed Army Medical Center experience, 1975-1996, *Thyroid* 8:871, 1998.

32. Campbel JA and others: Sucralfate and the absorption of L-thyroxine, *Ann Intern Med* 121:152, 1994.

33. Campbell NR and others: Ferrous sulfate reduces thyroxine efficacy in patients with hypothyroidism, *Ann Intern Med* 117:1010, 1992.

34. Canaris GJ and others: The Colorado thyroid disease prevalence study. *Arch Intern Med* 160:526, 2000.

35. Caraccio N and others: Lipoprotein profile in subclinical hypothyroidism: response to levothyroxine replacement, a randomized placebo-controlled study, *J Clin Endocrinol Metab* 87:1533, 2002.

36. Caron P and others: Decreased HDL cholesterol in subclinical hypothyroidism: the effect of L-thyroxine therapy, *Clin Endocrinol (Oxf)* 33519, 1990.

37. Carr D and others: Fine adjustment of thyroxine replacement dosage: comparison of the thyrotrophin releasing hormone test using a sensitive thyrotrophin assay with measurement of free thyroid hormones and clinical assessment, *Clin Endocrinol (Oxf)* 28:325, 1988.

38. Cavalieri RR and others: Thyroid hormone export in rat FRTL-5 thyroid cells and mouse NIH-3T3 cells is carrier-mediated, verapamil-sensitive, and stereospecific, *Endocrinology* 140:4948, 1999.

39. Cevallos JL and others: Low-dosage ^{131}I therapy of thyrotoxicosis (diffuse goiters): a five-year follow-up study, *N Engl J Med* 290:141, 1974.

40. Chiovato L and others: Outcome of thyroid function in Graves' patients treated with radioiodine: role of thyroid-stimulating and thyrotropin-blocking antibodies and of radioiodine-induced damage, *J Clin Endocrinol Metab* 83:40, 1998.

41. Chopra IJ and others: Thyroid function in nonthyroidal illnesses, *Ann Intern Med* 98:946, 1983.

42. Christiansen NJ and others: Serum thyroxine in the early phase of subacute thyroiditis, *Acta Endocrinol (Copenh)* 64:359, 1970.

43. Comtois R, Faucher L, Lafleche L: Outcome of hypothyroidism caused by Hashimoto's thyroiditis, *Arch Intern Med* 155:1404, 1995.

44. Cooper DS: Antithyroid drugs for the treatment of hyperthyroidism caused by Graves' disease, *Endocrinol Metab Clin North Am* 27:225, 1998.

45. Cooper DS and others: L-thyroxine therapy in subclinical hypothyroidism: a double-blind, placebo-controlled trial, *Ann Intern Med* 101:18, 1984.

46. Copeland PM: Two cases of therapeutic failure associated with levothyroxine brand interchange, *Ann Pharmacother* 29;482, 1995.

47. Cunnien AJ and others: Radioiodine-induced hypothyroidism in Graves' disease: factors associated, *J Nucl Med* 23:978, 1982.

48. Danese MD and others: Clinical review 115:effect of thyroxine therapy on lipoproteins in patients with mild thyroid failure: a quantitative review of the literature, *J Clin Endocrinol Metab* 85:2993, 2000.

49. Debruyne F, Vanderschueren-Lodeweyckx M, Bastinjns P: Hearing in congenital hypothyroidism, *Audiology* 22:404, 1983.

50. DeGroot LJ, Rue PA: Roentgenographic contrast agents inhibit triiodothyronine binding to nuclear receptors in vitro, *J Clin Endocrinol Metab* 49:538, 1979.

51. de Jong JM and others: Primary hypothyroidism as a complication after treatment of tumors of the head and neck, *Acta Radiol* 21:299, 1982.

52. de Luca F and others: Sensorineural deafness in congenital hypopituitarism with severe hypothyroidism, *Acta Paediatr Scand* 74:148, 1985.

53. Dong BJ and others: Bioequivalence of generic and brand-name levothyroxine products in the treatment of hypothyroidism, *JAMA* 277:1205, 1997.

54. Doucet J and others: Does age play a role in the clinical presentation of hypothyroidism? *J Am Geriatr Soc* 42:984, 1994.

55. Dunn JT: *Sources of dietary iodine in industrialized countries.* In Delange F, Dunn JT, Glinoer D, editors: *Iodine deficiency in Europe: a continuing concern,* New York, 1993, Plenum Press, p 17.

56. Dunn JT, Dunn AD: *Thyroglobulin: chemistry, biosynthesis, and proteolysis.* In Braverman LE, Utiger RD, editors: *The thyroid,* ed 8, Philadelphia, 2000, Lippincott Williams & Wilkins, p 91.

57. Duranti R and others: Control of breathing in patients with severe hypothyroidism, *Am J Med* 95:29, 1993.

58. Elte JWF, Bussemaker JK, Haak A: The natural history of euthyroid multinodular goiter, *Postgrad Med J* 66:186, 1990.

59. Erfurth EMT and others: Effect of acute desmopressin and of long-term thyroxine replacement on hemostasis in hypothyroidism, *Clin Endocrinol (Oxf)* 42:373, 1995.

60. Erickson D and others: Treatment of patients with toxic multinodular goiter, *Thyroid* 8:277, 1998.

61. Escobar-Morreale HF and others: Methimazole-induced severe aplastic anemia: unsuccessful treatment with recombinant granulocyte-monocyte colony-stimulating factor, *Thyroid* 7:67, 1997.

62. Faber J and others: Hemodynamic changes after levothyroxine treatment in subclinical hypothyroidism, *Thyroid* 12:319, 2002.

63. Faglia G and others: Plasma thyrotropin response to thyrotropin releasing hormone in patients with pituitary and hypothalamic disorders, *J Clin Endocrinol Metab* 37:5951, 1973.

64. Fernandez-Soto L and others: Increased risk of autoimmune thyroid disease in hepatitis C vs hepatitis B before, during and after discontinuing interferon therapy, *Arch Intern Med* 158:1445, 1998.

65. Ferrari C, Reschini E, Paracchi A: Treatment of autonomous thyroid nodule: a review, *Eur J Endocrinol* 135:383, 1996.

66. Fish LH and others: Replacement dose, metabolism, and bioavailability of levothyroxine in the treatment of hypothyroidism. Role of triiodothyronine in pituitary feedback in humans, *N Engl J Med* 316:764, 1987.

67. Francois M and others: Audiological assessment of eleven congenital hypothyroid infants before and after treatment, *Acta Otolaryngol (Stockh)* 113:39, 1993.

68. Goldman JM and others: Influence of triiodothyronine withdrawal time on 131I uptake post thyroidectomy for thyroid cancer, *J Clin Endocrinol Metab* 50:734, 1980.

69. Gordin A, Lamberg BA: Spontaneous hypothyroidism in symptomless autoimmune thyroiditis: a long term followup study, *Clin Endocrinol* 15:537, 1981.

70. Gordon MB and others: Variations in adequate levothyroxine therapy in patients with different causes of hypothyroidism, *Endocr Pract* 5:233, 1999.

71. Grande C: Hypothyroidism following radiotherapy for head and neck cancer: multivariate analysis of risk factors, *Radiother Oncol* 25:31, 1992.

72. Grebe SK and others: Treatment with hypothyroidism with once weekly thyroxine, *J Clin Endocrinol Metab* 82:870, 1997.

73. Gregerman RI and others: Thyroxine turnover in euthyroid man with special reference to changes with age, *J Clin Invest* 41:2065, 1962.

74. Haddow JE and others: Maternal thyroid deficiency during pregnancy and subsequent neuropsychological development of the child, *N Engl J Med* 341:549, 1999.

75. Haggerty JJ Jr and others: Subclinical hypothyroidism: a modifiable risk factor for depression? *Am J Psychiatry* 150:508, 1993.

76. Hak AE and others: Subclinical hypothyroidism is an independent risk factor for atherosclerosis and myocardial infarction in elderly women: the Rotterdam Study, *Ann Intern Med* 132:270, 2000.

77. Hamburger JI, Taylor CL: Transient thyrotoxicosis associated with acute hemorrhagic infarction of autonomously functioning thyroid nodules, *Ann Intern Med* 91:406, 1979.

78. Hancock SL and others: Thyroid diseases after treatment of Hodgkin's disease, *N Engl J Med* 325:599, 1991.

79. Harmon SM and others: Levothyroxine-cholestyramine interaction reemphasized, *Ann Intern Med* 115:658, 1991.

80. Helfand M, Redfern CC: Screening fro thyroid disease: an update, *Ann Intern Med* 129:144, 1998.

81. Hollowell JG and others: Serum TSH, T4, and thyroid antibodies in the United States population (1988 to 1994): National Health and Nutrition Examination Survey (NHANES III), J Clin Endocrin Metab 87:489, 2002.

82. Huber G and others: Prospective study of the spontaneous course of subclinical hypothyroidism: prognostic value of thyrotropin, thyroid reserve, and thyroid antibodies, *J Clin Endocrinol Metab* 87 3221, 2002.

83. Jaeschke R and others: Does treatment with L-thyroxine influence health status in middle-aged and older adults with subclinical hypothyroidism? *J Gen Intern Med* 11:744, 1996.

84. Jansson R and others: Intrathyroidal concentrations of methimazole in patients with Graves' disease, *J Clin Endocrinol Metab* 57:129, 1983.

85. Joffe RT and others: Major depression and subclinical (grade 2) hypothyroidism, *Psychoneuroendocrinology* 17:215, 1992.

86. Kaplan MM: Management of thyroxine therapy during pregnancy, *Endocr Pract* 2:281, 1996.

87. Kaptein EM: Clinical applications of free thyroxine determinations, *Clin Lab Med* 13:653, 1993.

88. Kaufman KD and others: Recombinant human thyroid peroxidase generated in eukaryotic cells: a source of specific antigen for the immunological assay of antimicrosomal antibodies in the sera of patients with autoimmune thyroid disease, *J Clin Endocrinol Metab* 70:724, 1990.

89. Kawasuji M and others: Coronary artery bypass surgery in patients with angina pectoris and hypothyroidism, *Eur J Cardiothorac Surg* 5:230, 1991.

90. Kim PS, Arvan P: Endocrinopathies in the family of endoplasmic reticulum (ER) storage diseases: disorders of protein trafficking and the role of ER molecular chaperones, *Endocrine Rev* 19:173, 1998.

91. Klee GG, Hay ID: Biochemical thyroid function testing, *Mayo Clin Proc* 69:469, 1994.

92. Klein I and others: Symptom rating scale for assessing hyperthyroidism, *Arch Intern Med* 148:387, 1988.

93. Kohrle J: Local activation and inactivation of thyroid hormones: the deiodinase family, *Mol Cell Endocrinol* 151:103, 1999.

94. Kristensen O, Andersen HH, Pallisgaard G: Lithium carbonate in the treatment of thyrotoxicosis: a controlled trial, *Lancet* 1:603, 1976.

95. Kuma K and others: Natural course of Graves' disease after subtotal thyroidectomy and management of patients with postoperative thyroid dysfunction, *Am J Med Sci* 302:8, 1991.

96. Kung AW and others: Elevated serum lipoprotein(a) in subclinical hypothyroidism, *Clin Endocrinol (Oxf)* 43:445, 1995.

97. Kutty KM and others: Serum lipids in hypothyroidism—a re-evaluation, *J Clin Endocrinol Metab* 46:55, 1978.

98. Ladenson PW and others: Complications of surgery in hypothyroid patients, *Am J Med* 77:261, 1984.

99. Larsen PR and others: Revised nomenclature for tests of thyroid hormones and thyroid related proteins in serum, *J Clin Endocrinol Metab* 64:1089, 1987.

100. Lazarus JH: The effects of lithium therapy on thyroid and thyrotropin-releasing hormone, *Thyroid* 8:909, 1998.

101. Levesque H and others: Acquired von Willebrand's syndrome associated with decrease of plasminogen activator and its inhibitor during hypothyroidism, *Eur J Med* 2:284, 1993.

102. Levy O, De la Vieja A, Carrasco N: The Na+/I− symporter (NIS): recent advances, *J Bioenergetics Biomembranes* 30:195, 1998.

103. Liaw Y-F and others: Hepatic injury during propylthiouracil therapy in patients with hyperthyroidism. A cohort study, *Ann Intern Med* 118:424, 1993.

104. Liel Y and others: Nonspecific intestinal adsorption of levothyroxine by aluminum hydroxide, *Am J Med* 97:363, 199.

105. Liu L and others: Elevated plasma levels of VWF: Ag in hyperthyroidism are medicated through beta-adrenergic receptors, *Endocr Res* 19:123, 1993.

106. Mandel SJ and others: Increased need for thyroxine during pregnancy in women with primary hypothyroidism, *N Engl J Med* 323:91, 1990.

107. Marqusse E, Haden ST, Utiger RD: Subclinical thyrotoxicosis, *Endocrinol Metab Clin North Am* 27:37, 1998.

108. Martino E and others: Amiodarone iodine-induced hypothyroidism: risk factors and follow-up in 28 cases, *Clin Endocrinol (Oxf)* 26:227, 1987.

109. Mazzaferi EL: Adult hypothyroidism, *Postgrad Med* 79:75, 1986.

110. Mazzaferri EL: Thyroid cancer and Graves' disease, *J Clin Endocrinol Metab* 70:826, 1990.

111. McConahey WM: Hashimoto's thyroiditis, *Med Clin North Am* 56:885, 1972.

112. Meier CA, Burger AG: *Effects of drugs and other substances on thyroid hormone synthesis and metabolism.* In Braverman LE, Utiger RD, editors: *The thyroid: a fundamental and clinical text,* ed 8, Philadelphia, 2000, Lippincott Williams and Wilkins, p 265.

113. Menegaux F, Reprecht T, Chigot JP: The surgical treatment of Graves' disease, *Surg Gynecol Obstet* 176:277, 1993.

114. Mercardo M and others: Treatment of hyperthyroidism with a combination of methimazole and cholestyramine, *J Clin Endocrinol Metab* 81:3191, 1996.

115. Meyerhoff WL: The thyroid and audition, *Laryngoscope* 86:483, 1976.

116. Meyerhoff WL: Hypothyroidism and the ear: electrophysical, morphological and chemical considerations, *Laryngoscope* 89:1, 1979.

117. Miccoli P and others: Surgical treatment of Graves' disease. Subtotal or total thyroidectomy? *Surgery* 120:1020, 1996.

118. Michot JL and others: Relationship between thyroid peroxidase, H_2O_2 generating system and NADPH-dependent reductase activities in thyroid particulate fractions, *Mol Cell Endocrinol* 41:211, 1985.

119. Muller B and others: Impaired action of thyroid hormone associated with smoking in women with hypothyroidism, *N Engl J Med* 333:964, 1995.

120. Myrup B, Bregenfrd C, Faber J: Primary haemostasis in thyroid disease, *J Intern Med* 238:59, 1995.

121. Nelson JC, Tomel RT: Direct determination of free thyroxine in undiluted serum by equilibrium dialysis, *Clin Chem* 34:1737, 1988.

122. Nilsson LR and others: Nonendemic goiter and deafness, *Acta Paediatr* 53:117, 1964.

123. Nystrom E and others: A double-blind cross-over 12-month study of L-thyroxine treatment of women with "subclinical" hypothyroidism, *Clin Endocrinol (Oxf)* 29:63, 1988.

124. Ohtaki S and others: Thyroid peroxidase: experimental and clinical integration, *Endocrine J* 43:1-, 1996.

125. Okamura K and others: Thyroid disorders in the general population of Hisayama, Japan, with special reference to prevalence and sex differences, *Int J Epidemiol* 16:545, 1987.

126. Oppenheim DS: TSH and other glycoprotein producing pituitary adenomas: alpha-subunit as a tumor marker, *Thyroid Today* 14:1, 1991.

127. Orr WC, Males JL, Imes NK: Myxedema and obstruction sleep apnea, *Am J Med* 70:1061, 1981.

128. Parle JV and others: Circulating lipids and minor abnormalities of thyroid function, *Clin Endocrinol (Oxf)* 37:411, 1992.

129. Patwardhan NA and others: Surgery still has a role in Graves' hyperthyroidism, *Surgery* 114:1108, 1993.

130. Peek CM and others: Combination of potassium iodide and propranolol in preparation of patients with Graves' disease for thyroid surgery, *N Engl J Med* 302:883, 1980.

131. Pelttari L and others: Upper airway obstruction in hypothyroidism, *J Intern Med* 236:177, 1994.

132. Pop VJ and others: Are autoimmune thyroid dysfunction and depression related? *J Clin Endocrinol Metab* 83:3194, 1998.

133. Rapp MF and others: Laryngeal involvement in scleromyxedema: a case report, *Otolaryngol Head Neck Surg* 104:362, 1991.

134. Razack MS and others: Total thyroidectomy for Graves' disease, *Head Neck* 19:378, 1997.

135. Refetoff S, DeWind T, DeGroot LF: Familial syndrome combining deaf-mutism stippled epiphyses, goiter, and abnormally high PBI: possible target organ refractoriness to thyroid hormone, *J Clin Endocrinol Metab* 27:2779, 1967.

136. Reinwein D and others: The different types of hyperthyroidism in Europe: results of a prospective survey of 924 patients, *J Endocrinol Invest* 11:193, 1988.

137. Rich EJ, Menelman PM: Acute suppurative thyroiditis in pediatric patients, *Pediatr Infect Dis J* 6:936, 1987.

138. Romaldini JH and others: Effect of L-thyroxine administration on antithyroid antibody levels, lipid profile, and thyroid volume in patients with Hashimoto's thyroiditis, *Thyroid* 6:183, 1996

139. Rosenthal MJ and others: Thyroid failure in the elderly. Microsomal antibodies as discriminant for therapy, *JAMA* 258209, 1987.

140. Ross DS: *Subclinical hyperthyroidism.* In: Braverman LE, Utiger RD, editors: *Werner and Ingbar's the thyroid: a fundamental and clinical text,* ed 6, Philadelphia, 1991, JB Lippincott, p 1249.

141. Ross DS: Hyperthyroidism, thyroid hormone therapy and bone, *Thyroid* 4:319, 1994.

142. Rovet JF and others: Psychologic and psychoeducational consequences of thyroxine therapy for juvenile acquired hypothyroidism, *J Pediatr* 122:543, 1993.

143. Royaux IE and others: Pendrin, the protein encoded by the Pendred syndrome gene (PDS), is an apical porter of iodide in the thyroid and is regulated by thyroglobulin in FRTL-5 cells, *Endocrinology* 141:839, 2000.

144. Ruf J and others: Bispecific thyroglobulin and thyroperoxidase autoantibodies in patients with various thyroid and autoimmune diseases, *J Clin Endocrinol Metab* 79:1404, 1994.

145. Sakata S, Nakamura S, Miura K: Auto-antibodies against thyroid hormone or iodothyronines: implications in diagnosis, thyroid function, treatment and pathogenesis, *Ann Intern Med* 103:579, 1985.

146. Salvatore D and others: Type 2 iodothyronine deiodinase is highly expressed in human thyroid, *J Clin Invest* 98:962, 1996.

147. Sandrock D and others: Long-term follow-up in patients with autonomous thyroid adenoma, *Acta Endocrinol (Copenh)* 128:51, 1993.

148. Sawin CT and others: The aging thyroid: increased prevalence of elevated serum thyrotropin in the elderly, *JAMA* 242:247, 1979.

149. Sawin CT and others: Aging and the thyroid. Decreased requirement for thyroid hormone in older hypothyroid patients, *Am J Med* 75:206, 1983.

150. Sawin CT and others: Low serum thyrotropin concentrations as a risk factor for atrial fibrillation in order persons, *N Engl J Med* 331:1249, 1994.

151. Scanlon MF, Toft AD: *Regulation of thyrotropin secretion.* In: Braverman LE, Utiger RD, editors: *The thyroid,* ed 8, Philadelphia, 2000, Lippincott Williams & Wilkins, p 234.

152. Schussler GC: The thyroxine-binding proteins, *Thyroid* 10:141, 2000.

153. Siafakas NM and others: Respiratory muscle strength in hypothyroidism, *Chest* 102:189, 1992.

154. Singer PA and others: Treatment guidelines for patients with hyperthyroidism and hypothyroidism, *JAMA* 273:808, 1995.

155. Singh N and others: Effect of calcium carbonate on the absorption of levothyroxine, *JAMA* 283:2822, 2000.

156. Slag MF and others: Hypothyroxinemia in critically ill patients as a predictor of high mortality, *JAMA* 245:43, 1981.

157. Snyder PJ and others: Diagnostic value of thyrotropin-releasing hormone in pituitary and hypothalamic disorders, *Ann Intern Med* 81:751, 1974.

158. Spencer CA: Clinical evaluation of free T_4 techniques, *J Endocrinol Invest* 9:57, 1986.

159. Spencer CA, Nicoloff JT: Serum TSH measurement: a 1990 status report, *Thyroid Today* 13:1, 1990.

160. Spencer CA, Wang CC: Thyroglobulin measurement: techniques, clinical benefits, and pitfalls, *Endocrinol Metab Clin North Am* 24:841, 1995.

161. Spencer CA and others: Applications of a new chemiluminometric thyrotropin assay to subnormal measurements, *J Clin Endocrinol Metab* 70:453, 1990.

162. Stanbury JB and others: Iodine-induced hyperthyroidism: Occurrence and epidemiology, *Thyroid* 8:83, 1998.

163. Sugino K and others: Follow-up evaluation of patients with Graves' disease treated by subtotal thyroidectomy and risk factor analysis for post-operative thyroid dysfunction, *J Endocrin Invest* 16:195, 1993.

164. Sugino K and others: Early recurrence of hyperthyroidism in patients with Graves' disease treated by subtotal thyroidectomy, *World J Surg* 19:648, 1995.

165. Sugino K and others: Management of recurrent hyperthyroidism in patients with Graves' disease treated by subtotal thyroidectomy, *J Endocrin Invest* 18:415, 1995.

166. Takasu N and others: Simple and reliable method for predicting the remission of Graves' disease: revised triiodothyronine-suppression test, indexed by serum thyroxine, *J Endocrinol Invest* 18:288, 1995.

167. Tamai H and others: Development of spontaneous hypothyroidism in patients with Graves' disease treated with antithyroidal drugs: clinical, immunological, and histological findings in 26 patients, *J Clin Endocrinol Metab* 69:49, 1989.

168. Tamai H and others: Methimazole-induced agranulocytosis in Japanese patients with Graves' disease, *Clin Endocrinol (Oxf)* 30:525, 1989.

169. Taurog A: *Hormone synthesis: thyroid iodine metabolism.* In Braverman LE, Utiger RD, editors: *The thyroid: a fundamental and clinical text,* ed 8, Philadelphia, 2000, Lippincott Williams and Wilkins, p 61.

170. Taylor J and others: Twice-weekly dosing for thyroxine replacement in elderly patients with primary hypothyroidism, *J Int Med Res* 22:273, 1994.

171. Tomer Y, Davies TF: Infection, thyroid disease, and autoimmunity, *Endocr Rev* 14:107, 1993.

172. Tunbridge WM and others: The spectrum of thyroid disease in a community: the Wickham survey, *Clin Endocrinol* 7:481, 1977.

173. Usala SJ, Weintraub BD: *Familial thyroid hormone resistance: clinical and molecular studies.* In Mazzaferri EL, editor: *Advances in endocrinology metabolism,* no 2, St Louis, 1991, Mosby.

174. Uzzan B and others: Effects on bone mass of long term treatment with thyroid hormones: a meta-analysis, *J Clin Endocrinol Metab* 81:4278, 1996.

175. Vagenakis AG and others: Adverse effects of iodides on thyroid function, *Med Clin North Am* 59:1075, 1975.

176. Vanderpump MPJ and others: The incidence of thyroid disorders in the community: a twenty-year follow-up of the Whickham survey, *Clin Endocrinol (Oxf)* 43:55, 1995.

177. Vanderpump MP and others: The incidence of thyroid disorders in the community: a twenty-year follow-up of the Whickam Survey, *Clin Endocrinol (Oxf)* 43:55, 1995.

178. Vassart G, Dumont JE: The thyrotropin receptor and the regulation of thyrocyte function and growth, *Endocr Rev* 13:596, 1992.

179. Weetman AP: The immunomodulatory effects of antithyroid drugs, *Thyroid* 4:145, 1994.

180. Williams I and others: Aetiology of hyperthyroidism in Canada and Wales, *J Epidemiol Comm Health* 37:245, 1983.

181. Winsa B and others: Total thyroidectomy in therapy-resistant Graves' disease, *Surgery* 116:1068, 1994.

182. Winsa B and others: Retrospective evaluation of subtotal and total thyroidectomy in Graves' disease with and without endocrine ophthalmology, *Eur J Endocrinol* 132:406, 1995.

183. Yamashita H and others: Postoperative tetany in patients with Graves' disease: a risk factor, *Clin Endocrinol* 47:71, 1997.

MANAGEMENT OF THYROID NEOPLASMS

Stephen Y. Lai
Susan J. Mandel
Randal S. Weber

INTRODUCTION

Thyroid carcinoma is relatively uncommon, accounting for approximately 2% of all malignancies.[1] Nonetheless, thyroid neoplasms represent more than 90% of all endocrine tumors. In 2002, the estimated annual incidence of thyroid cancer in the United States will be 20,700 cases, and approximately 1300 patients (6%) will die from thyroid cancer.

Although thyroid cancer is relatively rare, the incidence of thyroid nodules is significantly higher, affecting approximately 4% to 7% of the U.S. population.[133] While the overwhelming majority of these nodules are benign, the challenge is to identify the 5% or so of those patients with a malignant lesion. Furthermore, a subset of thyroid cancers is particularly aggressive with a potential for devastating morbidity. No reliable indicators are currently available to determine which patients will develop aggressive or recurrent disease, although risk categories based on clinical and pathologic criteria do yield important prognostic information.

The great majority of thyroid carcinomas are well-differentiated tumors of follicular cell origin.[91,100] These lesions are histologically defined as papillary, follicular, and Hürthle cell carcinoma. A recent survey of 53,856 patients described the overall incidence of thyroid cancer in the United States.[100] In this report, approximately 79% of cases were papillary carcinoma, 13% follicular carcinoma, and approximately 3% Hürthle cell. A small proportion (6%) of patients with these lesions have a family history of thyroid cancer. Medullary thyroid cancer, which arises from parafollicular C cells, accounts for about 4% of thyroid carcinomas. Approximately 30% of patients with these lesions have a strong genetic contribution. Anaplastic carcinomas, lymphoma, and metastatic disease comprise a small portion of thyroid malignancies.

The most common presentation of a thyroid cancer is the development of a thyroid mass or nodule. Assessment of the lesion requires a careful history, physical examination, fine-needle aspiration cytology (FNAC), and perhaps imaging studies. With correct diagnosis and management, most patients with well-differentiated thyroid carcinomas have an excellent prognosis. Indeed, the 10-year disease-specific mortality rate is less than 7% for papillary thyroid cancer and less than 15% for follicular thyroid cancer.[100,134] Controversy regarding the treatment of thyroid carcinomas and the extent of thyroidectomy to be performed arises because of the indolent course of the majority of thyroid cancers. Interventions for thyroid cancer have been difficult to evaluate because of the long follow-up and the large number of patients needed to determine differences in survival. Furthermore, the morbidity that may accompany any aggressive intervention needs to be balanced with the generally good prognosis of thyroid cancer patients.

In this chapter, we begin with a review of the surgical anatomy and embryology of the thyroid gland. After a brief overview of the present understanding of pathogenetic mechanisms leading to thyroid cancer, we review risk factors and staging of thyroid carcinomas. We describe an algorithm for the evaluation of a thyroid nodule and assess available diagnostic tools. A review of the different forms of thyroid cancer, ranging from well-differentiated carcinomas to anaplastic and other less common malignancies, is followed by a discussion of surgical management and postoperative adjuvant treatment.

SURGICAL ANATOMY AND EMBRYOLOGY

The thyroid medial anlage derives from the ventral diverticulum from the endoderm of the first and second pharyngeal pouches at the foramen cecum.[94,191] The diverticulum descends from the base of tongue to its adult pretracheal position through a midline anterior path with the primitive heart and great vessels during weeks 4 to 7 of gestation. The proximal portion of this structure retracts and degenerates into a solid, fibrous stalk; persistence of this tract can lead to the development of a thyroglossal duct cyst with variable amounts of associated thyroid tissue. The lateral thyroid primordia arise from the fourth and fifth pharyngeal pouches and descend to join the central component. Parafollicular C cells arise from the neural crest of the fourth pharyngeal pouch as ultimobranchial bodies and infiltrate the upper portion of the thyroid lobes.[39] Given the predictable fusion of the ultimobranchial bodies to the medial thyroid anlage, C cells are restricted to a zone deep within the middle to upper third of the lateral lobes.[234]

The thyroid gland is composed of two lateral lobes connected by a central isthmus, weighing 15 to 25 g in adults. A thyroid lobe usually measures about 4 cm in height, 1.5 cm in width, and 2 cm in depth. The superior pole lies posterior to the sternothyroid muscle and lateral to the inferior constrictor muscle and the posterior thyroid lamina. The inferior pole can extend to the level of the sixth tracheal ring. Approximately 40% of patients have a pyramidal lobe that arises from either lobe or the midline isthmus and extends superiorly (Figure 119-1).

The thyroid is enclosed between layers of the deep cervical fascia in the anterior neck. The true thyroid capsule is tightly adherent to the thyroid gland and continues into the parenchyma to form fibrous septa separating the parenchyma into lobules. The surgical capsule is a thin, film-like layer of tissue lying on the true thyroid capsule. Posteriorly, the middle layer of the deep cervical fascia condenses to form the posterior suspensory ligament, or Berry's ligament, connecting the lobes of the thyroid to the cricoid cartilage and the first two tracheal rings.

Blood supply to and from the thyroid gland involves two pairs of arteries, three pairs of veins, and a dense system of connecting vessels within the thyroid capsule. The inferior thyroid artery arises as a branch of the thyrocervical trunk (Figure 119-2). This vessel extends along the anterior scalene muscle, crossing beneath the long axis of the common carotid artery to enter the inferior portion of the thyroid lobe. Although variable in its relationship, the inferior thyroid artery lies anterior to the recurrent laryngeal nerve (RLN) in approximately 70% of patients.[99] The inferior thyroid artery is also the primary blood supply for the parathyroid glands.

The superior thyroid artery is a branch of the external carotid artery and courses along the inferior constrictor muscle with the superior thyroid vein to supply the superior pole of the thyroid. This vessel lies posterolateral to the external branch of the superior laryngeal nerve (SLN) as the nerve courses through the fascia overlying the cricothyroid muscle. Care should be taken to ligate this vessel without damaging the SLN. Occasionally, a thyroid ima artery may arise

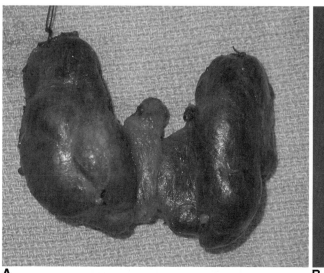 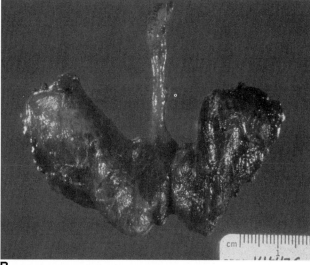

A   **B**

Figure 119-1. A pyramidal lobe of the thyroid gland may occasionally arise from the isthmus. This portion of the thyroid gland can be quite variable in size. This portion of the gland should be carefully identified and removed with the surgical specimen. (**B** Used with permission from Lai SY, Weber RS: *Thyroid cancer.* In Ensley JF and others, editors: *Head and neck cancer: emerging perspectives.* San Diego, 2002, Academic Press, p 419.)

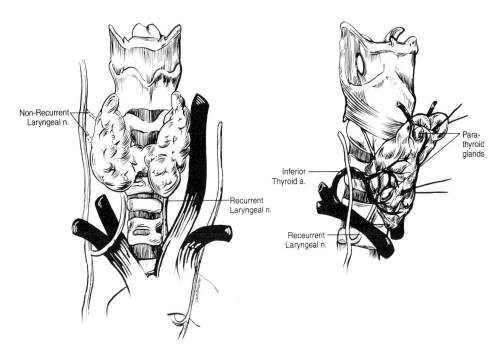

Figure 119-2. The thyroid gland is intimately associated with several important adjacent structures. In the lateral view, the gland has been mobilized medially to demonstrate the recurrent laryngeal nerve and its close relationship to the inferior thyroid artery. This relationship can vary between sides within a patient. Please refer to the text for details. The potential course(s) of the nonrecurrent laryngeal nerve have been indicated *(dashed lines)*. (Used with permission from Lai SY, Weber RS: *Thyroid cancer.* In Ensley JF and others, editors: *Head and neck cancer: emerging perspectives.* San Diego, 2002, Academic Press, p 420.)

from the innominate artery, carotid artery, or aortic arch and supply the thyroid gland near the midline.[99] Many veins within the thyroid capsule drain into the superior, middle, and inferior thyroid veins, leading to the internal jugular or innominate veins. The middle thyroid vein travels without an arterial complement, and division of this vessel permits adequate rotation of the thyroid lobe to identify the RLN and parathyroid glands.

The RLN provides motor supply to the larynx and some sensory function to the upper trachea and subglottic area. Careful management of thyroid carcinomas requires a thorough knowledge of the course of the RLN (see Figure 119-2). During development, the RLN is dragged caudally by the lowest persisting aortic arches. On the right side, the nerve recurs around the fourth arch (subclavian artery); the nerve recurs around the sixth arch (ligamentum arteriosum) on the left side. The right RLN leaves the vagus nerve at the base of the neck, loops around the right subclavian artery, and returns deep to the innominate artery back into the thyroid bed approximately 2 cm lateral to the trachea. The nerve enters the larynx between the arch of the cricoid cartilage and the inferior cornu of the thyroid cartilage. The left RLN leaves the vagus

at the level of the aortic arch and loops around the arch lateral to the obliterated ductus arteriosus. The nerve returns to the neck posterior to the carotid sheath and travels near the tracheoesophageal groove along a more medial course than the right RLN. The nerve will cross deep to the inferior thyroid artery approximately 70% of the time and often branches above the level of the inferior thyroid artery before entry into the larynx.[171] The RLN travels underneath the inferior fibers of the inferior constrictor (i.e., the cricopharyngeus muscle) and behind the cricothyroid articulation to enter the larynx. A "nonrecurrent" laryngeal nerve may rarely occur on the right side and enters from a more lateral course[97] (see Figures 119-2 and 119-4, *C*). Typically, an aberrant retroesophageal subclavian artery (arteria lusoria) or other congenital malformation of the vascular rings is present.

The SLN arises beneath the nodose ganglion of the upper vagus and descends medial to the carotid sheath, dividing into an internal and external branch about 2 cm above the superior pole of the thyroid.[120] The internal branch travels medially and enters through the posterior thyrohyoid membrane to supply sensation to the supraglottis. The external branch extends medially along the inferior constrictor muscle to enter the cricothyroid muscle. Along its course, the nerve travels with the superior thyroid artery and vein. The nerve typically diverges from the superior thyroid vascular pedicle about 1 cm from the thyroid superior pole.

Proper management of the parathyroid glands during thyroid surgery is critical to avoid hypoparathyroidism. The superior parathyroid glands are derived from the fourth pharyngeal pouch, whereas the inferior counterparts originate from the third pharyngeal pouch. The parathyroid glands are caramel-colored glands weighing 30 to 70 mg. The subtle distinction of tan and yellow coloration permits differentiation from adjacent fatty tissue, although with trauma, the glands can become mahogany in color. Eighty percent of patients have four glands and at least 10% have more than four glands.[226] The glands are situated on the undersurface of the thyroid gland in fairly predictable locations. The superior glands are located at the level of the cricoid cartilage, usually medial to the intersection of the RLN and the inferior thyroid artery.[226] The inferior glands are more variable in location than their superior counterparts. These glands may be on the lateral or posterior surface of the lower pole. In many patients, the position of the parathyroid glands on one side is similar to the other side and should be a useful guide.

MOLECULAR BASIS FOR THYROID NEOPLASMS

A number of genetic and molecular abnormalities have been described in thyroid neoplasms. As with other head and neck cancers, an accumulation of genetic alterations appears to be required for progression to a thyroid carcinoma. The specific molecular events and their order continue to be defined.

Alterations noted in the development of thyroid carcinomas include changes in total cellular DNA content. The loss of chromosomes, or aneuploidy, has been noted in 10% of all papillary carcinomas but is present in 25% to 50% of all patients who die from these lesions.[202] Similarly, the development of follicular adenomas is associated with a loss of the short arm of chromosome 11 (11p) and transition to a follicular carcinoma appears to involve a deletions of 3p, 7q, and 22q.[64,113]

Several oncogenes, altered genes that contribute to tumor development, have been identified in early thyroid tumor progression. Mutations in the thyroid-stimulating hormone (TSH)-receptor and G-protein mutations are found in hyperfunctioning thyroid nodules.[231] These changes can lead to the constitutive activation of cell-signaling pathways, such as the adenylate cyclase-protein kinase A system. Point mutations of the G-protein *ras* found in thyroid adenomas and multinodular goiters are believed to be an early mutation in tumor progression.[149] The *ras* mutations are more commonly found in follicular carcinomas than in papillary thyroid carcinomas. The resultant activation of the phosphatidylinositol 3′-kinase (PI3K) signal transduction pathway and AKT, a PI3K-related serine/threonine kinase, also appears to be specific to follicular thyroid carcinoma.[167]

Other genetic changes have also been associated with certain types of thyroid carcinoma. Gene rearrangements involving tropomycin-receptor-kinase A (TRK-A), a receptor for nerve growth factor, are associated with papillary carcinomas. Mutations in *met*/hepatic growth factor have been linked to papillary and poorly differentiated thyroid carcinomas. Different types of galectin, carbohydrate-binding proteins, appear to be differentially expressed in papillary and anaplastic carcinomas and may be useful in distinguishing benign from malignant thyroid lesions.[63,98] In Cowden's disease (familial goiter and skin hamartomas), inactivating mutations of the phosphatase and tensin homolog (PTEN) gene have been identified.[85] PTEN may inhibit phosphorylation and kinase activity of AKT1, leading to the development of follicular adenomas and carcinomas.[167] The PAX8/PPARγγ1 (peroxisome proliferator-activated receptor) rearrangement appears to be unique to follicular thyroid carcinoma.[114] PAX8 is expressed at high levels during thyroid development, and the PAX/PPARγγ1 gene product appears to function as a dominant negative, blocking the activation of wild-type PPARγγ1. Furthermore, mutations in the tumor-suppressor gene *p53*, a transcriptional regulator, appear to be involved in insular thyroid carcinomas and the progression from papillary to anaplastic carcinoma.[65,207]

The role of mutations of the *ret* oncogene in the development of papillary and medullary thyroid carcinomas has been extensively studied.[69] Located on chromosome 10, *ret* codes for a transmembrane tyrosine kinase receptor that binds glial cell line–derived neurotrophic factor (GDNF). During embryogenesis, RET protein is normally expressed in the nervous and excretory systems. Abnormalities in RET expression results in developmental defects, including the disruption of the enteric nervous system (Hirschsprung's disease). Presumably, *ret* gene mutations result in the activation of the *ras*/JNK/ERK1/2 signaling pathways, resulting in further genomic instability and prevention of entry into the apoptotic pathway.[205]

Medullary thyroid cancer and pheochromocytoma arise from neural crest cells containing *ret* point mutations. These point mutations have been well documented in patients with familial medullary thyroid cancer, multiple endocrine neoplasia (MEN) IIA, and MEN IIB.[60,183] Additionally, somatic mutations of *ret* are also found in approximately 25% of sporadic medullary thyroid carcinomas. Many of these are identical to the codon 918 mutation found as a germline mutation in MEN IIB, although other codons are more infrequently involved.[233]

Rearrangements of the *ret* gene by fusion with other genes also create transforming oncogenes. Although more than 10 rearrangements have been described, three oncogene proteins—RET/PTC1, RET/PTC2, and RET/PTC3—account for most of the rearrangements found in papillary thyroid cancers and are more frequently associated with childhood thyroid carcinomas.[223] However, not all patients with papillary carcinomas express a RET/PTC gene.[206] There are marked geographic differences, and the gene rearrangement is strongly associated with radiation exposure. Following the Chernobyl nuclear disaster, 66% of the papillary thyroid cancers removed from affected patients had RET/PTC1 or RET/PTC3 rearrangements.[185] The RET/PTC3 rearrangement is most commonly associated with a "solid" follicular variant of papillary thyroid carcinoma, whereas RET/PTC1 is associated more often with the classic or diffuse sclerosing variants of papillary thyroid cancer.[184,211]

RISK FACTORS AND ETIOLOGY

While the specific molecular events related to the development of thyroid carcinomas remain to be completely defined, several patient and environmental factors have been closely examined. Epidemiologic studies have not demonstrated a clear association between dietary iodine with thyroid carcinomas.[232] Additionally, there does not appear to be a simple relationship between benign goiter and well-differentiated thyroid carcinomas. Although papillary thyroid carcinomas are not associated with goiter, follicular and anaplastic thyroid carcinomas occur more commonly in areas of endemic goiter. Additionally, two particularly important risk factors, exposure to radiation and a family history of thyroid cancer, have been studied extensively.

Exposure to ionizing radiation increases patient risk for the development of thyroid carcinoma.[12,57] Low-dose ionizing radiation treatments (<2000 cGy) were used in the treatment of "enlarged thymus" to prevent "sudden crib death," enlarged tonsils and adenoids, acne vulgaris, hemangioma, ringworm, scrofula, and other conditions. The risk increases linearly from 6.5 to 2000 cGy and typically has a latency period between 10 and 30 years. Although higher doses of ionizing radiation typically lead to the destruction of thyroid tissue, patients with Hodgkin's disease who receive 4000 cGy also have a higher incidence of thyroid cancer. Palpable thyroid nodularity may be present in 17% to 30% of patients exposed to ionizing radiation.[169] A patient with a history of radiation exposure who presents with a thyroid nodule has up to a 50% chance of having a malignancy.[45] Of these patients with thyroid cancer, 60% have cancer within the nodule, while the remaining 40% have cancer located in another area of the thyroid. The thyroid carcinoma tends to be papillary and frequently multifocal. Additionally, there is a higher risk of cervical metastases.

Similarly, patients exposed to radiation from nuclear weapons and accidents have a higher incidence of thyroid cancer. Children near the Chernobyl nuclear power facility had a 60-fold increase in thyroid carcinoma after the nuclear accident in 1986.[126] Most of these children were infants at the time of the accident, and a great number of these cases developed without the typical latency period. The thyroid gland appears to be particularly vulnerable to ionizing radiation in children and yet relatively insensitive in adults. In the life span study of atomic bomb survivors in Hiroshima and Nagasaki, the risk of thyroid cancer was associated with patient age at the time of the bombings.[162] The risk was greatest for those under 10 years of age, and no increased incidence of thyroid cancer was seen in those older than 20 years of age at the time of exposure.

Finally, familial and genetic contributions need to be fully evaluated. The patient with a family history of thyroid carcinoma may require specific diagnostic testing. Approximately 6% of patients with papillary thyroid cancer have familial disease. Papillary thyroid cancer occurs with increased frequency in certain families with breast, ovarian, renal, or central nervous system malignancies.[140] Gardner's syndrome (familial colonic polyposis) and Cowden's disease are associated with well-differentiated thyroid carcinomas. Furthermore, patients with a family history of medullary thyroid cancer, MEN IIA, or MEN IIB warrant evaluation for the RET point mutation.

TUMOR STAGING AND CLASSIFICATION

A number of staging and classification systems have been devised to stratify patients with thyroid carcinomas. These classifications have identified key patient- and tumor-specific characteristics that predict patient outcome. Risk-grouping has been used to focus aggressive treatment for high-risk patients and to avoid excessive treatment and its potential complications in patients with a lower risk for tumor recurrence or tumor-related death.

TNM Classification

The American Joint Commission on Cancer (AJCC) and the Union International Contre le Cancer adopted a tumor-node-metastasis (TNM) classification system

(Table 119-1). In this system, patient age at presentation influences the clinical staging of a thyroid carcinoma. Eighty-two percent of patients with stage I disease had a 20-year survival of nearly 100%, whereas the 5% of patients with stage IV disease experienced a 5-year survival of only 25%.[49]

AMES

In the AMES system, patient *age*, tumor *size*, *extent* of tumor invasion, and the presence of *metastases* were used to stratify patients into low-risk and high-risk groups (Table 119-2). Low-risk patients were young (men, younger than 41 years; women, younger than 51) without distant metastases and all older patients without extrathyroidal papillary carcinoma, without major invasion of the tumor capsule by follicular carcinoma or with a primary tumor less than 5 cm in diameter. In a review of 310 patients from 1961 to 1980, low-risk patients (89%) had a mortality of 1.8%, compared with a mortality rate of 46% in high-risk patients (11%). Recurrence in low-risk patients was 5% and in high-risk patients was 55%.[27] In DAMES, nuclear DNA content was added to the AMES system to improve risk-stratification for papillary thyroid carcinoma.[158]

AGES and MACIS

In the original AGES system, *age* at diagnosis, histologic tumor *grade*, *extent* of disease at presentation, and tumor *size* were used to calculate a prognostic score.[92] Given the infrequent practice of tumor grading, a more recent modification of the system eliminated histologic tumor grade and incorporated metastasis and extent of resection. The MACIS system accounts for *metastasis*, *age* at diagnosis, *completeness* of surgical resection, extrathyroidal *invasion*, and tumor *size*.[93] The MACIS score is calculated as follows:

3.1 (patient age < 40 years) or 0.08 × age (patient age = 40 years) + 0.3 × tumor size (in cm) + 1 (if extrathyroidal extension) + 1 (if incomplete resection) + 3 (if distant metastases)

Patients were stratified by their prognostic scores into four groups with statistically significant differences in 20-year disease-specific mortality.

TABLE 119-1

TNM STAGING FOR THYROID CANCER

Primary Tumor (T)

T_X	Primary tumor cannot be assessed
T_0	No evidence of primary tumor
T_1	Tumor = 2 cm in greatest dimension, limited to thyroid
T_2	Tumor >2 cm and = 4 cm in greatest dimension, limited to thyroid
T_3	Tumor >4 cm in greatest dimension, limited to the thyroid *or*
	Any tumor with minimal extrathyroid extension (e.g., extension to sternothyroid muscle or perithyroid soft tissues)
T_{4a}	Tumor of any size extending beyond the thyroid capsule to invade subcutaneous soft tissues, larynx, trachea, esophagus, or recurrent laryngeal nerve
T_{4b}	Tumor invades prevertebral fascia or encases carotid artery or mediastinal vessels

All anaplastic carcinomas are considered T_4 tumors.

T_{4a}	Intrathyroidal anaplastic carcinoma—surgically resectable
T_{4b}	Extrathyroidal anaplastic carcinoma—surgically unresectable

Regional Lymph Nodes (N)

N_X	Regional lymph nodes cannot be assessed
N_0	No regional lymph node metastasis
N_1	Regional lymph node metastasis
N_{1a}	Metastasis to level VI (pretracheal, paratracheal, and prelaryngeal/Delphian lymph nodes)
N_{1b}	Metastasis to unilateral, bilateral, or contralateral cervical or superior mediastinal lymph nodes

Distant Metastasis (M)

M_X	Distant metastasis cannot be assessed
M_0	No distant metastasis
M_1	Distant metastasis

TABLE 119-1

TNM STAGING FOR THYROID CANCER—cont'd

Stage Grouping

		<45 yr	≥45 yr
Papillary/Follicular			
	Stage I	any T any N M_0	$T_1 N_0 M_0$
	Stage II	any T any N M_1	$T_2 N_0 M_0$
	Stage III		$T_3 N_0 M_0$
			any T $N_{1a} M_0$
Stage IVA			$T_{4a} N_0 M_0$
			$T_{4a} N_{1a} M_0$
			$T_{1-4a} N_{1b} M_0$
Stage IVB			T_{4b} any N M_0
Stage IVC			any T any N M_1
Medullary			
	Stage I	$T_1 N_0 M_0$	
	Stage II	$T_2 N_0 M_0$	
	Stage III	$T_3 N_0 M_0$	
		$T_{1-3} N_{1a} M_0$	
	Stage IVA	$T_{4a} N_0 M_0$	
		$T_{4a} N_{1a} M_0$	
		$T_{1-4a} N_{1b} M_0$	
	Stage IVB	T_{4b} any N M_0	
	Stage IVC	any T any N M_1	
Anaplastic			
	Stage IVA	T_{4a} any N M_0	
	Stage IVB	T_{4b} any N M_0	
	Stage IVC	any T any N M_1	

American Joint Committee on Cancer: *AJCC cancer staging manual,* ed 6, New York, 2002, Springer.

TABLE 119-2

FACTORS USED IN PROGNOSTIC CLASSIFICATION SYSTEMS

	TNM	AMES	AGES	MACIS
Patient factors				
Age	X	X	X	X
Sex	X	X		
Tumor factors				
Size	X	X	X	X
Histologic grade		X		
Histologic type	X	X	*	*
Extrathyroidal spread	X	X	X	X
Lymph node metastasis	X			
Distant metastasis	X	X	X	X
Incomplete resection				X

*AGES/MACIS classifications for papillary carcinomas only.

Other risk-classification systems with similar diagnostic criteria have also been described.[26,193,196] Although a number of multivariable prognostic scoring systems have been developed, none is universally accepted. The application of these classifications to a single population has demonstrated incompatible findings when compared with the original studies.[82] Furthermore, these systems do not necessarily apply to patients with poorly differentiated and more aggressive thyroid carcinomas.

Nevertheless, some general conclusions can be drawn from these studies regarding the prognosis of patients with well-differentiated thyroid carcinomas. Low risk for tumor recurrence and disease-specific mortality is noted in patients who are younger at diagnosis, have smaller primary tumors that lack extrathyroidal extension or regional/distant metastases and have complete gross resection of disease at the initial surgery. Delay in treatment will negatively affect prognosis. However, the single most significant overall indicator of a poor prognosis is distant metastases, especially to bone.[134] While a single risk-classification strategy is not available, these criteria should guide physicians to use therapeutic strategies that are directed towards the particular disease and risk for an individual patient, rather than applying a general treatment strategy for all patients with a particular form of thyroid carcinoma.

EVALUATION OF A THYROID NODULE

The incidence of thyroid nodular disease is quite high, spontaneously occurring at a rate of 0.08% per year starting in early life and extending into the eighth decade.[169] Although thyroid nodules represent a wide spectrum of disease, the great majority are colloid nodules, adenomas, cysts, and focal thyroiditis, with only a minority (5%) being carcinoma. With a lifetime incidence of 4% to 7%, the annual incidence of thyroid nodules in the United States is about 0.1%, which is approximately 300,000 new nodules each year.[71,119] The vast majority of these nodules are benign and do not require removal. However, with approximately 21,000 new thyroid cancers each year, about one in 20 new thyroid nodules will contain carcinoma and approximately one in 200 nodules will be lethal. The challenge in treating patients with thyroid nodule(s) is to identify those with malignant lesions and to balance the potential morbidity of treatment with the aggressiveness of their disease.

Clinical Assessment: History and Physical Examination

A number of findings should raise the physician's suspicion of malignancy in a patient presenting with a thyroid nodule(s). Both younger and older patients are more likely to have a malignant thyroid nodule. Patients younger than 20 years of age have an approximately 20% to 50% incidence of malignancy when presenting with a solitary thyroid nodule.[138] Nodular disease is more common in older patients, usually men older than 40 and women older than 50 years of age. Even though children may present with more advanced disease and even cervical metastases, malignancy in older patients has a considerably worse prognosis. Men often have more aggressive malignancies than women, but both the overall incidence of thyroid nodules and malignancy is higher in women.

A family history of thyroid carcinoma should be carefully evaluated. Similarly, any history of medullary carcinoma, pheochromocytoma, or hyperparathyroidism should raise suspicion for the MEN syndromes. Additionally, Gardner's syndrome (polyposis coli) and Cowden's disease have been associated with well-differentiated thyroid carcinomas. As described previously, a history of previous head and neck radiation exposure significantly increases the risk of malignancy in those patients with a thyroid nodule.

In evaluating the patient, rapid growth of a preexisting or new thyroid nodule is concerning, although the change may represent hemorrhage into a cyst. Throat or neck pain is rarely associated with carcinoma but frequently occurs with hemorrhage into a benign nodule. Patients should be carefully questioned regarding any compressive or invasive symptoms, such as voice change, hoarseness, dysphagia, or dyspnea. However, the clinician should not rely on these findings alone because unilateral vocal cord paralysis can be present without voice change or swallowing difficulties. Although most patients with thyroid cancer are euthyroid at presentation, symptoms of hyperthyroidism and hypothyroidism should be explored. Patients with large carcinomas that have replaced a significant portion of the normal thyroid gland may be hypothyroid and patients with Hashimoto's thyroiditis may develop lymphoma. Although the history alone cannot determine the presence of thyroid cancer, important historical features are associated with thyroid carcinoma and should not be discounted even if diagnostic tests indicated a benign lesion.

The physical examination of a patient with a thyroid nodule begins with careful palpation of the thyroid to assess the lesion. One should determine whether the lesion is solitary or the dominant nodule in a multinodular gland, although the risk of carcinoma in either setting is the same.[45,133] Having the patient swallow will assist in the examination, as nonthyroid pathology does not typically elevate with the thyroid during swallowing. Palpable nodules are typically 1 cm or larger. Smaller nodules can be found incidentally on radiographic studies for other reasons and may be monitored. Lesions greater than 1 cm in size warrant a complete workup. The firmness of the nodule may be associated with an increased risk of carcinoma by twofold to threefold.[178] Nodules greater than 2 cm in diameter and solid lesions have an increased incidence of harboring carcinoma. The evaluation of larger lesions also requires more caution as the rate of false-negative results during FNA also increases.[143]

Potential substernal extension can be estimated by the relationship of the inferior aspect of the mass to the clavicle. Potential thoracic inlet obstruction due to a substernal goiter can be assessed with Pemburton's maneuver. The patient raises his or her arms over the head, and positive findings of obstruction include subjective respiratory discomfort or venous engorgement, resulting in facial suffusion. Radiographic studies are more definitive in determining substernal involvement.

Further assessment of the patient may reveal the extent of involvement of a thyroid lesion. Palpable cervical nodes adjacent to the thyroid nodule certainly increase the suspicion for malignancy and may even be the only presenting sign of a thyroid carcinoma. However, adenopathy may be present in a patient affected by Hashimoto's thyroiditis, Grave's disease, or infection.[3,4] Large lesions can potentially shift the larynx and trachea within the neck. The mobility of the nodule relative to the laryngotracheal complex and adjacent neck structures should be evaluated. Malignant lesions are more likely to be fixed to the trachea, esophagus, or strap muscles.

All patients with a thyroid lesion should have a complete vocal cord examination. Extension into the thyroid cartilage and larynx may result in a complete vocal cord paralysis that is clinically silent. Laryngoscopy should be performed to assess vocal cord motion.

Despite the importance of the initial clinical assessment, the history and physical examination are unreliable in the prediction of carcinoma. Many of the clinical signs of malignancy are manifest late in the course of disease. Additionally, many of these same findings may be caused by events associated with benign disease (e.g., hemorrhage into a benign nodule). Thus, the clinical assessment should provide a justification and a context for the interpretation of diagnostic studies, such as FNA. Of particular note would be any patient and thyroid nodule features that might be concerning for aggressive carcinoma behavior (Table 119-3).

Diagnostic Studies
Laboratory Studies

The majority of patients who present with a thyroid nodule are euthyroid. The finding of hypothyroidism

---

TABLE 119-3

RISK FACTORS FOR AGGRESSIVE BEHAVIOR OF WELL-DIFFERENTIATED THYROID CARCINOMAS

Patient factors
History
Age
Younger	<20 yr
Older	
male	>40 yr
female	>50 yr

Gender
Male > female
History of radiation exposure/therapy
Family history of thyroid carcinoma

Physical examination
Hard, fixed lesion
Rapid growth of mass
Pain
Lymphadenopathy
Vocal cord paralysis
Aerodigestive tract compromise
Dysphagia
Stridor

Histopathologic factors
(at initial presentation)
Size (>4 cm)
Extrathyroidal spread
Vascular invasion
Lymph node metastasis
Distant metastasis
Histologic type
Tall-cell variant of papillary carcinoma
Follicular carcinoma
Hürthle cell carcinoma

---

or hyperthyroidism tends to shift the workup away from thyroid carcinoma to a functional disorder of the thyroid gland, such as Hasimoto's thyroiditis or a toxic nodule.[2] While many thyroid hormone tests are available, few are needed in the initial patient evaluation. TSH measurement serves as an excellent screening test. Full thyroid function tests can be performed if the TSH level is abnormal.

Measurement of thyroglobulin is generally not performed initially because thyroglobulin is secreted by both normal and malignant thyroid tissue. Levels of thyroglobulin cannot differentiate between benign and malignant processes, unless levels are extremely high, as in metastatic thyroid cancer. Furthermore, antithyroglobulin antibodies can also interfere with the assay. Thyroglobulin levels may be useful in studying patients who have undergone total thyroidectomy for well-differentiated thyroid cancer.

Serum calcitonin levels are not a typical initial test for patients with a thyroid nodule unless the patient has a family history of medullary thyroid cancer or MEN II. However, if FNAC demonstrates or is suspicious for medullary thyroid carcinoma, calcitonin levels should be obtained. Additionally, if the patient has RET oncogene mutations, the existence of a coexisting pheochromocytoma should be evaluated with an abdominal magnetic resonance imaging (MRI) scan and a 24-hour urine collection to measure metanephrines and catecholamines (total and fractionated). The serum calcium level should be measured to exclude hyperparathyroidism.

Fine-Needle Aspiration Cytology

FNAC has replaced radionuclide scanning and ultrasonographic imaging as the central diagnostic test in the initial evaluation of thyroid nodules. The findings are highly sensitive and specific, although the accuracy of FNAC is related to the skill of the aspirator and the experience of the cytopathologist.[132] The procedure is minimally invasive and may be performed quickly with little patient discomfort. Unlike large-bore needle biopsies such as the Tru-cut or Vim-Silverman needle, there are fewer complications. With the advent of this technique, the number of patients requiring surgery has decreased by 35% to 75%, and the cost in managing patients with thyroid nodules has been substantially reduced.[7,16,81] Additionally, the yield of malignancies has almost tripled in those patients who have had thyroid surgery after FNAC.[81,159] The accuracy of an FNA diagnosis of papillary carcinoma is 99% with a false-positive rate of less than 1%.[33]

FNAC should be one of the initial steps in the surgical evaluation of a thyroid nodule. Approximately 15% of all aspirates are inadequate or nondiagnostic, largely because of the sampling from cystic, hemorrhagic, hypervascular, or hypocellular colloid nodules. Reaspiration of the nodule is critical, as a nondiagnostic finding should never be interpreted as a negative finding for carcinoma. In fact, surgical diagnoses following repeated nondiagnostic aspirations revealed malignant nodules in 4% of women and 29% of men.[139] Nodules that are difficult to localize and those that have yielded nondiagnostic aspirates on previous attempts may benefit from ultrasound-guided aspiration.

Cytopathologic evaluation of a successful FNA will categorize a nodule into the following groups: benign, malignant, or suspicious. In 60% to 90% of nodules, FNAC will reveal a benign or "negative" diagnosis. The likelihood of malignancy (false-negative rate) is 1% to 6%.[7,72] The diagnosis of malignancy, particularly papillary (including follicular variant), medullary, and anaplastic carcinomas and lymphomas can be deter-

mined in about 5% of nodules. The likelihood of a false-positive finding is less than 5%.[7,72] Frequently, false positives result from difficulties in interpreting cytology in patients with Hashimoto's thyroiditis, Grave's disease, or toxic nodules. A benign cytology is a macrofollicular lesion or a colloid adenomatous nodule. The remaining "suspicious" samples are composed of lesions that contain abnormal follicular epithelium with varying degrees of atypia. This finding needs to be evaluated in the context of patient history and physical findings that may be suggestive of malignancy.

Follicular neoplasms cannot be classified by FNAC alone. The presence of hypercellular, microfollicular arrays with minimal colloid increases the concern for carcinoma. However, the differentiation between follicular adenoma and follicular carcinoma depends on the histologic finding of capsular or vascular invasion that requires evaluation of the entire thyroid nodule. Occasionally, patients with a diagnosis of follicular neoplasm on FNAC will have an iodine-123 (^{123}I) thyroid scan. If the suspicious nodule is "cold," surgery is indicated. However, if the nodule is hyperfunctioning compared with the surrounding thyroid, surgery can be avoided. Overall, 20% of nodules diagnosed as follicular neoplasms by FNAC will contain thyroid carcinomas.[77]

Similarly, Hürthle cell (oxyphilic) neoplasms can be difficult to evaluate. The presence of Hürthle cells in an aspirate may indicate an underlying Hürthle cell adenoma or carcinoma, but can also be present in thyroid disorders, such as multinodular goiter and Hashimoto's thyroiditis. Carcinomas can be found in up to 20% of nodules identified as follicular and oxyphilic neoplasms.[30] Because of the risk of underlying carcinoma in these cases, surgery is recommended.

Imaging

Ultrasonography is tremendously useful and sensitive. These studies detect nonpalpable nodules and differentiate between cystic and solid nodules. In patients with a difficult neck to examine (e.g., a patient with a history of head and neck irradiation), sonography can also clarify findings. Sonography can identify hemiagenesis and contralateral lobe hypertrophy, which may be misdiagnosed as a thyroid nodule.

These studies provide key baseline information regarding nodule size and architecture. Thus, sonography is also a noninvasive and inexpensive method for following changes in the size of benign nodules. However, there is no role for sonography in screening asymptomatic patients for thyroid nodules. Additionally, these studies are not useful in the evaluation of substernal extent or the involvement of adjacent structures.

These studies can also identify cervical nodes that may contain metastatic disease. Characteristics of lymph nodes suspicious for metastatic deposits include loss of the fatty hilum, increased vascularity, rounded node configuration, and the presence of fine calcifications.[163] Ultrasonography is useful in the evaluation of cervical lymph nodes in patients with a history of thyroid cancer who present with adenopathy or rising thyroglobulin levels.

Computed tomography (CT) and MRI scans are usually unnecessary in the evaluation of thyroid tumors, except for large or retrosternal lesions. Although these studies are not as effective as sonography in the evaluation of thyroid nodules, they are more reliable in evaluating the relationship of the thyroid lesion to adjacent neck structures, such as the trachea and esophagus. These studies are useful in determining substernal extension, identifying cervical and mediastinal adenopathy, and evaluating possible tracheal invasion.[38] Caution must be exercised in the use of iodine-containing contrast material in patients with multinodular goiter if a hyperthyroid state is suspected and in patients with well-differentiated thyroid cancer. In the latter group, iodinated contrast media will preclude the use of postoperative radioactive iodine therapy for 2 to 3 months. Finally, the MRI scan is more accurate than a CT scan in distinguishing recurrent or persistent thyroid tumor from postoperative fibrosis.

Thyroid Isotope Scanning

Radionuclide scanning with ^{123}I or technetium-sestamibi–99m (^{99m}Tc) assesses the functional activity of a thyroid nodule and the thyroid gland. Nodules that retain less radioactivity than the surrounding thyroid tissue are termed "cold," nonfunctioning, or hypofunctional. These cold nodules are thought to have lost functions of fully differentiated thyroid tissue and to be at increased risk of containing carcinoma. In a metaanalysis of patients with scanned nodules that were surgically removed, 95% of all nodules were cold.[3,4] The incidence of malignancy in cold nodules was 10% to 15%, but only 4% in hot nodules.

[99m]Tc scanning only tests iodine transport but can be performed in 1 day and involves less radiation exposure than [123]I. Cold nodules identified with this test will also be cold with iodine scanning. However, any "hot" nodules require ^{123}I scanning for confirmation. [123]I scanning tests both transport and organification of iodine. This test is more expensive and requires 2 days to complete. Cold lesions can be more difficult to visualize because of overlying thyroid tissue and glandular asymmetry, although oblique views during scanning can improve detection. Additionally,

[99m]Tc does not penetrate the sternum and is not useful in confirming substernal extension.

With the evolution of FNAC, radionuclide scanning is not routinely performed in the evaluation of a thyroid nodule. More frequently, "cold" nodules are detected in patients during evaluation for hyperthyroid disorders. However, patients who present initially with a thyroid nodule and are found to be hyperthyroid on preliminary thyroid function testing should have radionuclide scanning to differentiate a toxic nodule vs Grave's disease and a nonfunctioning nodule.

A Rational Approach to Management of a Thyroid Nodule

A number of diagnostic algorithms have been proposed for the evaluation of a thyroid nodule[132,219] (Figure 119-3). In general, evaluation begins with a thorough history and physical examination to identify significant risk factors. Surgery may be deemed appropriate based solely on high-risk factors such as age, sex, history of radiation exposure, rapid nodule growth, upper aerodigestive tract symptoms, and/or fixation.

Baseline TSH screening then determines the diagnostic course. Patients with hyperthyroidism (suppressed serum TSH level) should receive radionuclide scanning to determine the presence of a toxic "hot"

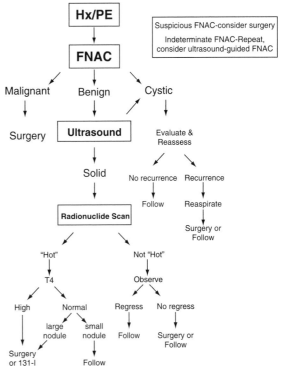

Figure 119-3. An algorithm for the rational approach to the evaluation and management of a thyroid nodule.

nodule or Marine-Lenhart syndrome, or Graves' disease with a concomitant "cold" nodule.[34] A patient with hypothyroidism (elevated serum TSH level) should be appropriately treated by an endocrinologist, and then FNA should be performed. The majority of patients will be euthyroid (normal serum TSH level), and FNA should be performed. Patients with cytologic findings that are diagnostic or strongly suggestive of malignancy should be directed to a surgeon for removal of the lesion.

A diagnosis of follicular neoplasm by FNAC requires surgery to determine the presence of follicular adenoma or follicular carcinoma. An FNAC sample suspicious for medullary carcinoma may be subject to immunohistochemical techniques to detect calcitonin. Before surgical intervention, a patient with an FNAC suggestive of medullary carcinoma will require genetic studies and additional testing that will be discussed later (see section titled "Medullary Carcinoma"). Suspicious findings on FNAC must be assessed in the context of patient risk factors in determining the need for surgery. If a nonsurgical approach is taken, the nodule must be closely monitored, usually with ultrasonography. Benign lesions are usually observed and require surgical removal only in cases of cosmetic or symptomatic concerns. These nodules must be reaspirated to confirm the diagnosis if growth is detected.

REVIEW OF THYROID NEOPLASMS
Thyroid Adenoma
Clinical Presentation

A thyroid adenoma is a true benign neoplasm derived from follicular cells. These follicular lesions are occasionally multiple and may arise in the setting of a normal thyroid, nodular goiter, toxic goiter, or thyroiditis. They occur most commonly in women older than 30 years. Patients usually present with a solitary, mobile thyroid nodule. The thyroid mass is often found incidentally on a routine physical examination and is frequently not associated with any other signs or symptoms. Sudden hemorrhage into the adenoma may cause a sudden increase in size and associated pain.

Pathology

The revised histologic classification of thyroid tumors divides epithelial tumors into the categories of follicular adenoma and other rare tumors (Table 119-4). Follicular adenomas are the most common benign thyroid lesions. Atypical follicular adenomas may demonstrate atypical microscopic features, including excess cellularity, increased mitotic figures, and necrotic foci. Although the great majority of these lesions are benign, they may metastasize even in the absence of microinvasion.[117]

On gross examination, thyroid nodules and adenomas are well circumscribed and demarcated from adjacent normal thyroid tissue. The classic adenoma is fleshy and pale, although areas of necrosis, hemorrhage, and cystic change may be readily apparent. Microscopic findings include large and small follicles with abundant colloid. Cells may be flat, cuboidal, or columnar. The nuclei are small and round with an even chromatin pattern. Mixed populations of macrophages and lymphocytes may be visible, as well as fibrosis, hemosiderin, and calcification. Cystic areas may be present near areas of abundant papillae formation. Adenomas that demonstrate pseudopapillary structures need to be distinguished from papillary carcinoma. The oxyphilic (Hürthle) cell adenoma contains mitochondria-rich eosinophilic cells. Thyroglobulin immunohistochemical staining can distinguish a clear cell adenoma from a parathyroid adenoma and metastasis from a renal carcinoma. This adenoma also needs to be differentiated from the clear cell variant of follicular carcinoma.

Nodules within a nodular goiter may occasionally be hyperfunctional or "hot." These lesions are termed *autonomously hyperfunctioning thyroid adenomas* and may or may not cause thyrotoxicosis. These lesions often occur in women, and those nodules associated with thyrotoxicosis are frequently in patients older than 40 years.

Management and Prognosis

The diagnostic evaluation of a thyroid nodule begins with an FNA that demonstrates follicular neoplasm. Distinguishing follicular or Hürthle cell adenoma from carcinoma depends on histopathologic analysis following surgical excision. Concern for a potential malignancy increases with highly cellular findings or pseudopapillary structures in an FNA sample. The lack of tumor capsule and vascular invasion is characteristic of a follicular adenoma.

Surgical excision involves a thyroid lobectomy. A unilateral partial thyroid lobectomy is no longer an acceptable standard of care. Patients with a history of head-and-neck radiation, other head and neck cancers, potential high-risk factors, and comorbidities may benefit from a total thyroidectomy. Risk of surgical morbidity at the initial surgery must be balanced with the potential risks of reoperation. In most patients, thyroid hormone administration is not necessary when the patient has undergone resection of a single thyroid lobe for a thyroid adenoma.

Autonomously hyperfunctioning thyroid adenomas are usually anatomically and functionally stable. Although most patients do not develop thyrotoxicosis, 20% of patients with lesions greater than 3 cm may develop thyrotoxicosis. Surgery and radioiodine ther-

TABLE 119-4

WORLD HEALTH ORGANIZATION REVISED HISTOLOGIC CLASSIFICATION OF THYROID TUMORS

I. Epithelial tumors
  A. Benign
    1. Follicular adenoma
      a. Architectural patterns
        i. Normofollicular (simple)
        ii. Macrofollicular (colloid)
        iii. Microfollicular (fetal)
        iv. Trabecular and solid (embryonal)
        v. Atypical
      b. Cytologic patterns
        i. Oxyphilic cell type
        ii. Clear cell type
        iii. Mucin-producing cell type
        iv. Signet-ring cell type
        v. Atypical
    2. Others
      a. Salivary gland-type tumors
      b. Adenolipomas
      c. Hyalinizing trabecular tumors
  B. Malignant
    1. Follicular carcinoma
      a. Degree of invasiveness
        i. Minimally invasive (encapsulated)
        ii. Widely invasive
      b. Variants
        i. Oxyphilic (Hürthle) cell type
        ii. Clear cell type
    2. Papillary carcinoma
      a. Variants
        i. Papillary microcarcinoma
        ii. Encapsulated variant
        iii. Follicular variant
        iv. Diffuse sclerosing variant
        v. Oxyphilic (Hürthle) cell type
    3. Medullary thyroid cancer
      a. Variant
        i. Mixed medullary-follicular carcinoma
    4. Undifferentiated (anaplastic) carcinoma
    5. Other carcinomas
      a. Mucinous carcinoma
      b. Squamous cell carcinoma
      c. Mucoepidermoid carcinoma
II. Nonepithelial tumors
III. Malignant tumors
IV. Miscellaneous tumors
  A. Parathyroid tumors
  B. Paragangliomas
  C. Spindle cell tumors with mucous cysts
  D. Teratomas
V. Secondary tumors
VI. Unclassified tumors
VII. Tumor-like lesions
  A. Hyperplastic goiters
  B. Thyroid cysts
  C. Solid cell nests
  D. Ectopic thyroid tissue
  E. Chronic thyroiditis
  F. Riedel's thyroiditis
  G. Amyloid goiter

Hedinger C, editor: *Histological typing of thyroid tumours,* ed 2, Berlin, 1988, Springer-Verlag.

apy can be used to manage these lesions, although many physicians prefer surgery for patients younger than 40 years. These patients may require preoperative medications to control thyrotoxic symptoms. The lesions are typically removed with a unilateral thyroid lobectomy. The remaining thyroid tissue typically returns to normal function after several months. Ethanol injection has become increasingly common, especially in Europe, to manage these lesions.[67]

Thyroid Cyst
Clinical Presentation

Although a thyroid cyst is not a specific diagnosis, this entity is frequently encountered in clinical practice. Approximately 15% to 25% of all thyroid nodules are cystic or have a cystic component.[169] The presence of a cyst does not signify a benign lesion because papillary carcinomas and parathyroid tumors may present with cystic masses. Papillary carcinoma may be present in 14% to 32% of all cystic nodules, although the majority of these lesions are benign adenomas or colloid nodules.[46,173]

Pathology

A thyroid cyst can result from congenital, developmental, or neoplastic causes.[46] Many cysts result from intranodular ischemia causing tissue necrosis and liquefaction. True epithelial-lined cysts are rare. Occasionally, parathyroid or thyroglossal duct cysts can be mistaken for thyroid nodules. However, a parathyroid cyst will contain high parathyroid hormone levels within the clear fluid and a thyroglossal duct cyst will contain columnar epithelium. These lesions may also be differentiated by ultrasound imaging.

Management and Prognosis

When encountered during FNA, a thyroid cyst should be drained completely. This may prove curative in the majority of simple cysts, although one or two additional drainage procedures may be required. However, if a cyst persists after three drainage attempts or reaccumulates quickly, the suspicion for carcinoma should increase. Brown fluid withdrawn from a cyst may represent old hemorrhage into an adenoma, but red fluid is more suspicious for carcinoma.[178] Clear, colorless fluid may be withdrawn from a parathyroid cyst and can be assessed for parathyroid hormone.[88] In suspicious cases, the surgeon and patient should consider an ultrasound-guided FNA to sample a solid component of the lesion or a unilateral thyroid lobectomy to obtain a definitive diagnosis. Given the potential for thyroid carcinoma in cystic lesions, surgical excision for diagnosis is preferable to the injection of sclerosing agents.

Papillary Carcinoma
Clinical Presentation

Papillary carcinoma is the most common form of thyroid malignancy, accounting for 60% to 70% of all thyroid cancer.[105,193] This lesion typically presents in patients 30 to 40 years of age and is more common in women, with a female/male ratio of 2:1. Interestingly, this ratio has decreased steadily over the past 40 years or so as the incidence in men has risen.[28] Papillary carcinomas are the predominant thyroid malignancy in children (75%). Although children more commonly present with advanced disease, including cervical and distant metastases, their prognosis remains quite favorable.

The majority of cases of papillary carcinoma occur spontaneously. Patients with a history of low-dose radiation exposure tend to develop papillary carcinomas (85%–90%).[186] Additionally, these lesions are more common in patients with Cowden's syndrome, Gardner's syndrome, and familial polyposis. Only 6% of papillary carcinomas are associated with familial disease.

Papillary carcinoma can be classified into three categories based on size and extent of the primary lesion.[135,237] Minimal or occult/microcarcinoma tumors are up to 1.5 cm in size and demonstrate no evidence of invasiveness through the thyroid capsule or to cervical lymph nodes. These lesions are typically nonpalpable and are usually incidental findings during operative or autopsy examination. Intrathyroid tumors are greater than 1.5 cm in diameter but are confined to the thyroid gland with no evidence of extrathyroid invasion. Extrathyroid tumors extend through the thyroid capsule to involve the surrounding viscera. This latter form of papillary carcinoma is associated with a substantial morbidity and decreased survival.[70,135]

Most patients present with a slow-growing, painless mass in the neck and are often euthyroid. Often, the primary lesion is confined to the thyroid gland, although up to 30% of patients may have clinically evident cervical nodal disease.[20,137] Histologic studies have demonstrated the strong lymphotropic nature of papillary carcinoma, leading to multifocal disease within the thyroid and regional lymphatics. Microscopic disease has been identified in the cervical nodes of 50% to 80% of patients and in the contralateral lobe in up to 80% of patients with papillary carcinoma at the time of surgery.[153] However, the significance of this microscopic disease is unclear, since clinical recurrence in the neck and in the contralateral lobe occur in fewer than 10% of patients.[213] More likely, the prevalence of microscopic disease suggests that the majority of papillary carcinomas have an indolent course that only occasionally becomes clinically evident. However, definite predictors of the clinical course for papillary carcinoma are not well defined.

Advanced disease may be associated with symptoms of local invasion, including dysphagia, dyspnea, and hoarseness. Occasionally, cervical nodal involvement may be more apparent than the thyroid nodule. Distant metastases, especially to the lungs, are more commonly encountered in children, although up to 10% of all patients may ultimately develop distant disease.[30]

Thyroid cancer is often suspected in these patients after a thorough history and physical examination. The diagnosis is usually established by FNAC. Thyroid function tests are done routinely in the preoperative assessment. Radiographic imaging (CT or MRI) is selectively performed to define extensive local or substernal disease and to evaluate possible lymph node involvement.

Pathology

On gross examination, papillary carcinoma is firm, white, and not encapsulated. The lesion tends to remain flat on sectioning rather than bulging like normal thyroid tissue or benign nodular lesions. Macroscopic calcifications, necrosis, or cystic changes may be readily apparent.[236]

Histologically, these lesions arise from thyroid follicular cells and contain papillary structures that consist of a neoplastic epithelium overlying a true fibrovascular stalk.[171] Cells are cuboidal with a pale, abundant cytoplasm. Large, crowded nuclei with folded and grooved nuclear margins may have intranuclear cytoplasmic inclusions. Prominent nucleoli account for the "Orphan Annie eye" appearance. Laminated calcium densities, psammoma bodies, are likely the remnants of necrotic calcified neoplastic cells and are present in 40% of cases.

Even though a follicular component may predominate, lesions with any papillary features behave clinically as papillary carcinomas. Thus, the designation of "papillary carcinoma" includes mixed papillary follicular carcinoma and the follicular variant of papillary carcinoma. A more unfavorable prognosis is associated with the certain histologic forms of papillary carcinoma, including diffuse sclerosing and tall-cell variants.[121,171] The tall-cell variant is characterized by well-formed papillae covered by cells that are twice as tall as they are wide. The rarer columnar cell variant is characterized by the presence of prominent nuclear stratification.[170]

Papillary carcinomas have a strong tendency for lymphatic spread within the thyroid and to local lymph nodes in the paratracheal and cervical regions. The tendency for intraglandular spread may lead to the multifocal disease often present in patients. However, discrete lesions may be due to de novo formation, especially in patients previously exposed to ionizing radiation.[66]

Local invasion occurs in 10% to 20% of these tumors, leading to involvement of the overlying strap muscles, laryngeal and tracheal framework, RLNs, pharynx, and esophagus. This extension may evolve from the primary lesion or from extracapsular extension of metastatic nodes. Angioinvasion is a clear harbinger of increased risk for recurrence and worse prognosis.[193] Interestingly, a coexisting lymphocytic thyroiditis has been correlated with decreased recurrence and better overall prognosis.

Management and Prognosis

The majority of patients with papillary carcinoma do well regardless of treatment. Prolonged survival, even with recurrent disease, has led to controversy regarding the extent of thyroidectomy for patients with well-differentiated thyroid carcinomas (see section titled "Surgical Management and Technique: Extent of Surgery"). A balance must be achieved between an effective surgical treatment for these malignancies and the potential morbidity of this surgery. A number of studies have attempted to categorize patients by their risk factors and to justify more aggressive surgical intervention for high-risk patients (see section titled "Tumor Staging and Classification").

Minimal papillary thyroid carcinoma is usually identified in a thyroid specimen removed for other reasons. Unilateral thyroid lobectomy and isthmusectomy is usually sufficient surgical treatment unless there is angioinvasion or tumor at the margins of resection. These patients can then be treated with thyroid hormone to suppress TSH and closely followed up with ultrasonography. In patients with a small, encapsulated papillary thyroid carcinoma (<1.5 cm in diameter), a total lobectomy is sufficient.

When patients present with more extensive disease or indications of disease in both lobes, total or near-total thyroidectomy is the procedure of choice.

Additionally, patients stratified into high-risk categories in any of the classification schemes previously described (see section titled "Tumor Staging and Classification") would probably benefit from a more extensive surgical procedure. This would permit possible thyroid hormone suppression therapy and radioiodine ablation of remaining disease.

Multifocal disease is present in as many as 80% of patients in some reports.[121,137] This may represent de novo multicentric tumor formation or intraglandular metastasis. The prevalence of multifocal disease lends credence to the argument for more complete surgical removal of the thyroid gland in patients with papillary thyroid cancer. Patients with partial thyroidectomy had higher local recurrence rates and increased pulmonary and cervical metastases.[31,129] Controversy remains, however, because this increased local recurrence did not compromise disease survival in some studies.[27,40]

Generally, invasive tumors are associated with a compromise in survival. Woolner and others[236] reviewed 1181 thyroid cancer patients and found that no patient died of papillary cancer when the lesion was less than 1.5 cm in size. Only 3% of patients died when the lesion was larger but remained intrathyroid. Mortality rose to 16% of patients when extrathyroid disease was present.

After total thyroidectomy, patients may be monitored by following thyroglobulin levels, which should remain undetectable. Any rise in thyroglobulin levels is suspicious for disease recurrence and will require appropriate screening. Approximately 12% of patients with papillary carcinoma are not cured by initial treatment, leading to a prolonged clinical course.[50] Recurrent disease may occur after many years, involving the thyroid bed (5%–6%), regional lymphatics (8%–9%), or distant sites (4%–11%).[174] Successful treatment of recurrence varies by site of involvement and the patient's initial risk classification.

Local recurrence is a serious complication and is associated with a disease-related mortality of 33% to 50%.[174] Typically, patients with nodal recurrence fare better than those with tumor recurrence in the thyroid bed or distant sites. Studies have been inconsistent regarding the impact of cervical metastases on survival. Patients older than 40 years may have clinically evident nodal disease in 36% to 75% of cases and overall increased mortality.[28,134] Surprisingly, some studies suggest prognosis is better with more cervical node involvement.[93,136] Although the role of cervical metastasis in survival may be controversial, there is an association with an increased recurrence rate, especially in elderly patients.[50,136,189]

Given these findings and the overall prevalence of microscopic cervical disease with uncertain prognostic implications, management of cervical metastasis tends to be conservative. There is no role for elective neck dissection in the clinically disease-free neck, especially given the effectiveness of radioiodine therapy in ablating microscopic disease.[213] In patients with a primary tumor larger than 2 cm in diameter or involving extrathyroidal structures, the central compartment from hyoid bone to mediastinum between the internal jugular veins (levels VI and VII) should be carefully inspected and palpated. In patients with palpable or visible neck disease, a selective neck dissection (levels II–V) should be performed. Although level I is seldom involved, metastatic disease is frequently noted on histologic examination of nodal levels II through V.[160]

The presence of distant metastasis is clearly associated with a worse prognosis. Approximately 10% of patients with papillary thyroid carcinoma develop distant metastasis at some point during their disease course.[30] Most commonly, the lungs are involved, although bone sites and the central nervous system may also be affected.

In nearly every study, patient age at the time of diagnosis is an important prognostic variable.[29,134,136] Older patients (especially older than the age of 40 years) with papillary carcinoma have a worse prognosis. Furthermore, extrathyroidal invasion appears to be more common in older patients. The prognosis for men younger than age 40 is comparable to women of the same age. However, overall survival is worse for men, and the risk of death from papillary thyroid carcinoma may be twice as great.[27,136] Furthermore, in the last 40 years, the increase in incidence of papillary thyroid carcinoma in men has decreased the gender ratio of men to women with the disease from 1:4 to 1:2.[28]

Children clearly fare better with this disease. In patients younger than 15 years of age, 90% demonstrate cervical metastasis at some time during their disease course.[95] Furthermore, up to 20% of children may present with pulmonary metastases.[62] However, neither factor seems to have any impact on survival. Perhaps these differences may be related to biologic differences in the disease process or between age groups.

Finally, the tall-cell variant of papillary thyroid carcinoma is clearly different from other forms of this disease. A review of patients with tall-cell variant papillary carcinoma demonstrates a more aggressive natural history in all age groups and a worse prognosis.[161]

Follicular Carcinoma
Clinical Presentation

Follicular carcinomas represent 10% of thyroid malignancies. The mean age of presentation is 50 years, compared with the younger mean age of patients with papillary carcinoma (35 years). Women more commonly have this lesion, with a female/male ratio of 3:1.[21] These lesions occur more frequently in iodine-deficient areas, especially areas of endemic goiter. Follicular carcinomas have been correlated with pregnancy and with certain HLA subtypes (DR1, DRw, and DR7). Also, a rare form of familial follicular carcinoma is reported in patients with dyshormonogenesis. Interestingly, the overall incidence of follicular carcinoma in decreasing in the United States.

Patients usually present with a solitary thyroid nodule, although some patients may have a history of long-standing goiter and recent rapid size increase. These lesions are typically painless, although hemorrhage into the nodule may cause pain. Cervical lymphadenopathy is uncommon at initial presentation, although distant metastases are more frequently encountered than with papillary carcinomas. In rare cases (1%), the follicular carcinoma may be hyperfunctioning and the patient will present with signs and symptoms of thyrotoxicosis.

Other than characterization of a follicular neoplasm, a definitive preoperative diagnosis is usually not possible by FNAC. Differentiation between follicular adenoma and follicular carcinoma requires an evaluation of the thyroid capsule for invasion or identification of vascular invasion. Typically, about 20% of thyroid nodules demonstrating follicular neoplasm cytology will contain carcinoma.

Unlike papillary carcinoma, follicular thyroid carcinomas are less likely to metastasize via lymphatic pathways (found in fewer than 10% of patients).[38] More commonly, follicular carcinoma spread through local extension and hematogenous spread. Often, the presence of cervical lymph node disease indicates significant local disease and visceral invasion.[28,106] Distant metastasis is also more common in follicular cancers than papillary cancers, especially at presentation.[86,239] A pathologic bone fracture may be the initial presentation of follicular carcinoma. Other common sites include the liver, lung, and brain.

Pathology

Follicular thyroid carcinoma tends to present as solitary, encapsulated lesions. Cytologic analysis of follicular neoplasms reveals small follicular arrays or solid sheets of cells.[171] The follicular structures have lumen that do not contain colloid and the overall architectural pattern depends on the degree of tumor differentiation. Increased cellularity may increase the suspicion for carcinoma, but cytology alone is not sufficient to distinguish between a follicular adenoma and carcinoma.

Histologic findings are necessary to distinguish benign and malignant lesions. Malignant lesions are differentiated by the identification of capsular invasion and potential microvascular invasion of vessels along the tumor capsule.[117,238] Complete capsular evaluation must be performed. Thus, frozen-section analysis is often inadequate, and definitive diagnosis requires complete assessment of permanent sections.

The degree of capsular invasion is important for patient prognosis. Follicular carcinomas can be divided into two broad categories. Minimally invasive tumors demonstrate evidence of invasion into but not through the tumor capsule at one or more sites. These lesions do not exhibit small-vessel invasion. Frankly invasive tumors demonstrate invasion through the tumor and often exhibit vascular invasion.[235] Tumor infiltration and invasion may be apparent at surgery, with tumor present in the middle thyroid or jugular veins.

Many other factors have been investigated as means to differentiate between adenomas and carcinomas. To date, no molecular markers have been clinically useful. DNA ploidy varies in both adenomas and carcinomas with considerable overlap.[104] Aneuploid follicular carcinomas, though, are noted to behave in a more aggressive manner.

Management and Prognosis

Patients diagnosed with an follicular lesion by FNAC should have a thyroid lobectomy with isthmusectomy performed. The pyramidal lobe, if present, should be included in the resection. As described previously, cytologic findings alone cannot determine the presence of adenoma or carcinoma. Intraoperative frozen-section analysis is not helpful given the incomplete assessment of the tumor capsule. However, frozen sections should be analyzed to confirm gross evidence of adjacent cervical lymphadenopathy. A total thyroidectomy is recommended if carcinoma is identified. In patients with a clinical suspicion for follicular carcinoma, the tendency is to perform a more complete resection. Total thyroidectomy is performed in older patients with a nodule greater than 4 cm in size diagnosed by FNAC as follicular neoplasm. In these patients, the risk of carcinoma is approximately 50%.[116]

A diagnosis of follicular carcinoma following a thyroid lobectomy usually necessitates a completion thyroidectomy. Patients with minimally invasive follicular cancer have a very good prognosis, and the initial thyroid lobectomy may be sufficient treatment. However, invasiveness of follicular carcinoma correlates directly with decreased survival. In patients with invasive follicular carcinomas, many surgeons tend toward completion and total thyroidectomy to permit radioiodine scanning for detection and ablation of metastatic disease. More aggressive surgical intervention does not clearly improve survival given that invasiveness already indicates the increased likelihood of distant metastasis. Neck dissection is performed if cervical lymphadenopathy is present. Elective neck dissections are unwarranted because nodal involvement is relatively infrequent.[191]

The recurrence rate after initial management is approximately 30%.[130] Recurrence is related to the degree of invasiveness of the initial lesion, not the extent of initial thyroid surgery. Minimally invasive disease behaves similarly to follicular adenoma and is typically cured with conservative surgical procedures (thyroid lobectomy).[198] Recurrence of minimally invasive follicular carcinoma is approximately 1%. About 15% of those with recurrent or metastatic disease can be cured. The prognosis of these patients relates to the site of recurrence as well as the patient's initial risk stratification. Survival outcomes are significantly poorer in those with capsular invasion and angioinvasion.[220] Those with cervical node recurrence have a 50% cure rate, whereas those with distant metastases have a cure rate of about 9%.[130,174]

Overall, 5-year survival is 70% and decreases to 40% at 10 years for patients with follicular carcinoma. The presence of distant metastasis diminishes 5-year survival to 20%.[41] Factors that worsen the prognosis include age older than 50 years at presentation, tumors greater than 4 cm in size, higher tumor grade, marked vascular invasion, extrathyroidal invasion, and distant metastasis at the time of diagnosis.[191] Extrathyroidal invasion beyond the capsule and into the thyroid parenchyma and local structures is the key factor decreasing patient survival. Clearly, risk stratification demonstrates marked differences in patient survival. In one study, the low-risk group had a 5-year survival rate of 99% and a 20-year survival rate of 86%. In the high-risk group the 5-year survival rate was only 47%, and this decreased to a 20-year survival rate of 8%.[21]

The prognosis of patients with follicular carcinoma has typically been reported to be worse than for those with papillary carcinoma. Some reports that matched age, sex, and stage at time of diagnosis suggest that patients with papillary and follicular carcinomas have similar survival patterns.[55,134] The poor prognosis of those with follicular carcinoma may be related to the increased number of patients who present at an older age and a more advanced disease stage. Additionally, unlike papillary carcinoma, mortality is directly related to recurrence in patients with follicular carcinoma.[28]

Hürthle Cell Tumor
Clinical Presentation

According to World Health Organization classification, Hürthle cell tumor (HCT) is a subtype of follicular cell neoplasm. HCT nodules can be found in patients with Hashimoto's thyroiditis or Graves' disease or within a nodular goiter. These tumors are derived from oxyphilic cells of the thyroid gland. Although the precise function of these cells is unknown, Hürthle cells express TSH receptors and produce thyroglobulin.

Hürthle cell neoplasms are typically diagnosed by FNAC. Approximately 20% of these lesions are malignant. As with follicular lesions, histologic criteria are required to diagnose carcinomas. Hürthle cell carcinomas represent approximately 3% of all thyroid malignancies. The mean age of presentation for patients with Hürthle cell carcinoma may be somewhat older than for follicular carcinoma.[61,77] Hürthle cell carcinomas are more aggressive than follicular carcinomas. They are often multifocal and bilateral at presentation. Additionally, these malignancies are more likely to metastasize to cervical nodes and distant sites.[212]

Pathology

FNAC of HTC typically demonstrates hypercellularity and the presence of eosinophilic cells. These neoplasms are characterized by sheets of eosinophilic cells packed with mitochondria. Cytologic differentiation between adenoma and malignant tumor by FNAC is extremely difficult. Histologic findings of capsular or vascular invasion confirm the presence of Hürthle cell carcinoma.

Management and Prognosis

The clinical approach to an HCT is similar to that for follicular neoplasms. With a Hürthle cell adenoma, resection of the affected lobe and isthmus is sufficient. Invasive findings for a Hürthle neoplasm on formal pathology warrant a total or completion thyroidectomy. Hürthle cell carcinomas tend to be more aggressive than other follicular carcinomas, and they are less amenable to radioiodine therapy given their decreased tendency to uptake radiolabeled iodine. A careful examination for local disease extension or adjacent cervical lymphadenopathy should be performed. The paratracheal region should be carefully palpated and examined. The paratracheal nodes should be removed if disease is obvious during inspection. Also, a comprehensive neck dissection should be undertaken if lateral neck nodes are palpable.

Postoperative management should include TSH suppression and thyroglobulin monitoring. A ^{99m}Tc scan may be useful for detecting persistent local or metastatic disease. A radioiodine scan and ablation can be performed to remove any residual normal thyroid tissue to allow for better surveillance. However, this therapy is unlikely to be effective in tumor ablation, as few (approximately 10%) Hürthle cell carcinomas uptake radioiodine.[59]

Overall, survival rates for HCTüs are significantly worse than for follicular thyroid cancer. The number of patients who die from Hürthle cell carcinoma is greater than those who die from papillary or follicular carcinoma.[208] Additionally, Hürthle cell carcinoma is associated with the highest incidence of distant metastases among the well-differentiated thyroid carcinomas.[176]

Medullary Carcinoma
Clinical Presentation

Medullary thyroid carcinomas (MTCs) are a distinct category of disease and represent approximately 5% of all thyroid carcinomas. These malignancies arise from parafollicular C cells and may secrete calcitonin, carcinoembryonic antigen (CEA), histaminadases, prostaglandins, and serotonin. Measurement of secreted calcitonin is useful for the diagnosis of medullary carcinoma and for postsurgical surveillance for residual and recurrent disease.

MTC demonstrates an intermediate behavior between well-differentiated thyroid cancers and anaplastic carcinomas. Women and men are equally affected by medullary carcinomas.[96] Patients usually present with a neck mass associated with palpable cervical lymphadenopathy (up to 20%).[36] Local pain is more common in these patients, indicating the presence of local invasion, and may be associated with dysphagia, dyspnea, or dysphonia. MTC may present along with papillary thyroid carcinoma because related mutations in *ret* are present in both diseases. Although MTC spreads initially to cervical nodes, distant metastases may be found in the mediastinum, liver, lung, and bone and are present in up to 50% of patients at diagnosis.[58]

The majority (70%) of medullary carcinomas are spontaneous unifocal lesions in patients aged between 50 and 60 years old without an associated endocrinopathy.[36] The remaining 30% of cases affecting younger patients are familial. These hereditary medullary carcinomas are inherited as autosomal-dominant traits with nearly 100% penetrance. Medullary carcinoma in these patients is preceded by multifocal C-cell hyperplasia and leads to disease that is multicentric and bilateral in 90% of cases.[51,166] Familial MTC (FMTC) is not associated with any other endocrine pathology. Two forms of MEN syndrome are associated with MTC. Patients with MEN IIA exhibit MTC, pheochromocytoma, and hyperparathyroidism.[51,145] Patients with MEN

IIB have a marfanoid body habitus and may have MTC, pheochromocytoma, or mucosal neuromas. Although penetrance for MTC approaches 100% in these patients, expression of other features is variable.[75,166]

FNAC diagnosis of MTC is confirmed by elevated serum calcitonin. Additionally, these patients should have testing for mutation of the *ret* protooncogene. Genetic screening has replaced provocative pentagastrin-stimulation testing. Careful screening for hereditary diseases is also necessary when a patient is diagnosed with MTC. Hyperparathyroidism can be assessed by serum calcium levels and appropriate imaging studies. Patients should also be screened for the presence of a pheochromocytoma with 24-hour urinary levels for catecholamines/metanephrines and should undergo an abdominal MRI. An undiagnosed pheochromocytoma could lead to an intraoperative hypertensive crisis and death. Additionally, the detection of any hereditary form of MTC in a patient should lead to family screening. Affected family members can often be identified and treated at earlier stages of disease with improved survival.[15,177]

Pathology

MTC originates from parafollicular C cells of neuroectodermal origin.[190] They descend to join the thyroid gland proper and are concentrated mainly in the lateral portions of the superior poles. Thus, most MTC lesions are located in the middle and upper thyroid poles. In patients with hereditary forms of MTC, the disease is often multifocal. Grossly, the tumor is solid, firm, and has a gray cut surface. The lesion is nonencapsulated but relatively well circumscribed.

These lesions are composed of sheets of infiltrating neoplastic cells that are heterogeneous in shape and size. These cells are separated by collagen, amyloid, and dense irregular calcification. The amyloid deposits are likely polymerized calcitonin and are virtually pathognomonic for MTC, although not all MTC contain amyloid.[203] More aggressive tumors typically have increased mitotic figures, nuclear pleomorphism, and areas of necrosis. Immunohistochemistry for calcitonin and CEA are useful diagnostic studies.

Management and Prognosis

Total thyroidectomy is the treatment of choice in patients with MTC because the lesions have a high incidence of multicentricity and an aggressive disease course. Patients with FMTC or MEN II should have the entire gland removed, even in the absence of a palpable mass.

Given the frequent involvement of cervical nodes, initial surgical management should include bilateral central compartment neck dissection. When central compartment nodes are involved or when palpable lateral cervical nodes are present, treatment including an ipsilateral or bilateral comprehensive neck dissection (levels II–V) should be considered. Additionally, when the primary lesion is greater than 2 cm, the patient should undergo an elective ipsilateral comprehensive neck dissection because nodal metastases may be present in more than 60% of these patients.[17,56] The superior mediastinal lymph nodes (level VII) should be routinely removed as well.

Potentially associated conditions such as hyperparathyroidism and pheochromocytoma must be carefully evaluated and, if necessary, treated before thyroidectomy. A pheochromocytoma may need to be removed before treatment of the thyroid lesion. In the presence of hypercalcemia, the parathyroid glands need to be identified during thyroidectomy. If the parathyroid glands are abnormal, they should be removed. Otherwise, they should be adequately marked to facilitate future identification, especially in patients with MEN IIA.

Children with any of the genetic disorders leading to MTC need to be treated aggressively. Typically a total thyroidectomy should be performed by patient age of 2 to 3 years or before C-cell hyperplasia occurs. Removal of the thyroid gland should prevent development of MTC in these patients and improve survival. However, MTC has been diagnosed in MEN IIB patients as young as 7 months old.[154]

After surgery, patients require close follow-up and monitoring of serum calcitonin and CEA levels. Calcitonin is more sensitive for detecting persistent or recurrent disease, but CEA levels appear to be predictive for survival.[56] Rising or persistent calcitonin levels should increase suspicion for residual or recurrent disease. Localization studies should be performed to identify potential sites of disease involvement. Tumor debulking for metastatic disease or local recurrence can decrease symptoms of flushing and diarrhea and may reduce the risk of death resulting from recurrent central neck disease.[58,230] Unfortunately, though, MTC do not respond to radioiodine therapy or TSH suppression therapy, given their parafollicular C-cell origin.[177] External beam radiation therapy (EBRT) has been controversial for patients with positive tumor margins or unresectable tumor, and there is no effective chemotherapy regimen.

Prognosis for patients with MTC is directly related to disease stage. The overall 10-year survival rate is between 61% and 75% but decreases to 45% if cervical nodes are involved.[107,177] The best outcome is for patients with FMTC, then MEN IIA, sporadic disease, and MEN IIB.

Anaplastic Carcinoma
Clinical Presentation

Anaplastic thyroid carcinomas are one of the most aggressive malignancies, with few patients surviving 6 months beyond initial presentation.[119,122] These lesions represent fewer than 5% of all thyroid carcinomas.[150] These tumors affect patients 60 to 70 years of age and presentation before the age of 50 years is extremely rare. Women are more commonly affected than men, with a ratio of 3:2. Eighty percent of these malignancies may occur with a coexisting carcinoma and may represent transformation of a well-differentiated thyroid cancer.[108,122]

Typically, patients have a long-standing neck mass that enlarges rapidly. This sudden change is often accompanied by pain, dysphonia, dysphagia and dyspnea. Often the mass is quite large and fixed to the tracheolaryngeal framework, resulting in vocal cord paralysis and tracheal compression. More than 80% have jugular lymph node involvement at the time of presentation and greater than 50% have systemic metastases.[52] Most patients will succumb to superior vena cava syndrome, asphyxiation, or exsanguination.

Pathology

In the case of anaplastic thyroid carcinoma, the gross specimen will demonstrate areas of necrosis and macroscopic invasion of surrounding tissues, often with lymph node involvement. Microscopically, sheets of cells with marked heterogeneity are present. Spindle, polygonal, and giant, multinucleated cells are present with occasional foci of differentiated cells. These cells do not produce thyroglobulin, do not transport iodine, and do not express thyroid hormone receptors.[122] These findings can often be established on FNAC, although a formal biopsy is occasional necessary to exclude a diagnosis of lymphoma.

Management and Prognosis

Management of anaplastic carcinoma is extremely difficult, requiring a multidisciplinary approach and close consultation with the patient and family. Surgical debulking may be performed for palliation. Initial therapy should ensure airway protection with a tracheostomy and nutritional support. All treatment forms are disappointing, and median survival is 2 to 6 months.[150,224] One current treatment protocol involves doxorubicin, hyperfractionated radiation therapy, and potentially surgical debulking.[111,210] Although survival beyond 2 years is only 12%, this is the one of the only regimens currently available for these patients.

Retrospective evaluation of various treatment strategies identified a subset of patients who have had long-term survival.[100,209,225] Independent prognostic variables include respectability of local disease, absence of distant metastasis at diagnosis, and adjuvant treatment with radiation therapy. Additionally, many of the long-term survivors had small areas of anaplastic foci within well-differentiated carcinoma.

Other Forms of Thyroid Cancer
Insular Thyroid Carcinoma

Insular carcinoma was named for the clusters of cells that contain small follicles resembling pancreatic islet cells.[32] These tumors are very rare and present as an independent lesion or concomitantly with papillary or follicular thyroid carcinomas. These cells stain with thyroglobulin antibodies, but not for calcitonin. Typically, capsular and vascular invasion is present at the time of diagnosis.

These lesions are very aggressive when compared with follicular and papillary carcinoma and appear to have an increased recurrence and mortality rate when present as an independent process.[24] However, insular carcinoma located within follicular or papillary thyroid cancer does not seem to adversely affect the clinical course. Fortunately, many insular thyroid carcinomas are able to concentrate radioiodine.

Lymphoma

Primary thyroid lymphoma is unusual and represents fewer than 5% of all thyroid malignancies.[201] Women are more commonly affected at a ratio of 3:1, and lymphoma typically presents in those older than 50 years of age. Patients may present with symptoms similar to anaplastic carcinoma, although the rapidly enlarging mass is often painless. Symptoms may also include regional adenopathy, dysphagia, and vocal cord paralysis caused by RLN invasion. Many affected patients are clinically hypothyroid or already receiving thyroid-replacement therapy for conditions such as Hashimoto's disease.[215] Non-Hodgkin's B-cell type lymphoma is most common, although Hodgkin's disease and plasmacytomas do occur.[179] Thyroid lymphoma can arise as part of a generalized lymphomatous condition, as many of these patients have Hashimoto's disease. Current hypotheses as to why this occurs include chronic antigenic lymphocyte stimulation that results in lymphocyte transformation.

A definite diagnosis needs to be made and frequently can be established by FNAC. Occasionally, a needle-core or open cervical lymph node biopsy may be necessary. Given the rare incidence of primary thyroid lymphoma, a comprehensive survey must be performed to exclude the presence of lymphoma at other sites.

Patients typically respond rapidly to chemotherapy, especially CHOP (cyclophosphamide, doxorubicin, vincristine, and prednisone).[53,165] Combined radiation and chemotherapy regimens have also been developed and have been promising. Thyroidectomy and nodal resection may be considered to alleviate symptoms of airway obstruction in patients who do not respond rapidly to treatment, but surgical options are not primary treatment modalities.

The prognosis of patients depends on the histologic grade of the tumor and the presence of extrathyroidal disease. Overall, 5-year survival is about 50%. However, intrathyroid disease survival is 85% and decreases to 40% for patients with extrathyroid disease.

Metastatic Carcinoma

The thyroid is a rare site for metastases from other cancers. However, metastasis can occur from primary lesions in the kidney, breast, lung, and skin (i.e., melanoma). The most common metastatic tumor to the thyroid is from a hypernephroma. Also, approximately 3% of bronchogenic carcinomas metastasize to the thyroid but account for 20% of all metastases to the thyroid.[103]

Typically, the history and physical examination identify the source of the metastasis. FNAC is performed for definitive diagnosis. Thyroidectomy may be considered for palliation, especially when the primary lesion is very slow growing (e.g., renal cell carcinoma).[79]

Squamous Cell Carcinoma

Squamous cell carcinoma of the thyroid is very rare, representing fewer than 1% of thyroid cancers.[142] Older patients are most commonly affected, and the disease can progress rapidly with local invasion and metastasis. During the workup, metastasis from another site within the upper aerodigestive tract needs to be excluded. Early detection and aggressive surgical treatment appears to represent the best option for palliation and cure. As with other squamous cell carcinoma of the head and neck, radiation therapy is probably important, although not well characterized.[216]

SURGICAL MANAGEMENT AND TECHNIQUE
Approach to the Thyroid Gland

Before any thyroid surgery, any voice changes or previous neck surgery should prompt assessment of vocal cord mobility by indirect laryngoscopy. Although many patients with thyroid carcinomas are euthyroid, necessary medical therapy should be instituted for patients demonstrating thyrotoxicosis or hypothyroidism to avoid intraoperative metabolic derangements, such as hypertensive crisis. Details of this management are beyond the scope of the present chapter but should include consultation with an endocrinologist.

The patient should be positioned supine on the operating table with an inflatable pillow or shoulder roll and adequate head support to permit full neck extension for optimal exposure. A symmetrical, transverse incision along a skin crease approximately 1 cm below the cricoid cartilage is made through the platysma. The length of the incision will depend on the size of the thyroid gland. Larger incisions will be necessary for patients with short, thick necks, difficulty with neck extension, or a low-lying thyroid gland. Subplatysmal skin flaps are raised superiorly to the level of the thyroid cartilage notch and inferiorly to the clavicle.

Exposure of the thyroid gland is obtained through a midline, vertical incision through the superficial layer of the deep cervical fascia between the sternohyoid and sternothyroid muscles. The strap muscles are bluntly separated, and dissection proceeds laterally along the thyroid capsule until the ansa cervicalis is noted at the lateral edge of the sternohyoid muscle/medial aspect of the internal jugular vein. Rarely, the strap muscles must be divided to gain access to a large thyroid lobe or tumor. This division should be done high on the muscle to preserve innervation from the ansa hypoglossal nerve. The strap muscles should be reapproximated before skin closure. Any evidence of frank invasion of thyroid carcinoma into the strap muscles should result in the en bloc resection of the section of the affected muscle with the thyroid lobe.

Through blunt dissection, the thyroid lobe is swept anteromedially to the tracheolaryngeal framework (Figure 119-4, A). The middle thyroid vein(s) should be identified, and division of this vessel will improve lateral exposure. The cricoid and trachea should be identified in the midline, and continued mobilization is achieved by sweeping dorsally all tissue along the posterolateral border of the thyroid lobe. Meticulous hemostasis should be maintained to facilitate identification of the SLN, RLN, and parathyroid glands.

The pedicle along the superior thyroid pole is identified early by retracting the thyroid inferiomedially. Dissection should be carried out close to the thyroid capsule to avoid possible injury to the external branch of the SLN. Occasionally, the external branch of the SLN that supplies the cricothyroid muscle can be visualized. The superior pole vessels should be individually identified and isolated for ligation close to the thyroid lobe. At this point, the tissues posterolateral to the superior pole can be swept away from the lobe in a posteromedial direction.

Identification of the RLN is best achieved through an inferior approach in a space defined by Lore and others[124] as the RLN triangle. The triangle is bounded by the trachea medially, the carotid sheath laterally, and the undersurface of the retracted inferior thyroid pole superiorly. Careful dissection in this area parallel to the course of the RLN should safely identify the nerve (Figure 119-4, *B*). A thyroid goiter or unusually large thyroid mass will potentially displace the nerve. The RLN, in these cases, can become fixed to and splay across the undersurface of the enlarged thyroid lobe. Great care needs to be taken in these situations, and identification of the nerve may require a superior approach, identifying the RLN at its entry into the larynx.

Once identified, the RLN should be followed to its laryngeal entry at the level of the cricoid cartilage, passing under or through Berry's ligament and entering the larynx deep to the inferior constrictor muscle. The nerve may divide into multiple branches before entering the larynx.[151] The most difficult portion of the operation is typically in dealing with the dissection where the recurrent nerve passes through Berry's ligament. The RLN is in close proximity to the thyroid, tethered down by the ligament. Bleeding can

occur at this site and should be controlled by gentle pressure before identification of the nerve to avoid injury. Use of electrocautery in this region should be strictly avoided. A small portion of thyroid tissue may be embedded with the ligament, accounting for a remnant of thyroid tissue left following total thyroidectomy.

All vessels are ligated and divided on the capsule to reduce the risk of parathyroid devascularization (Figure 119-5). Ischemic parathyroids and those situated anteriorly on the thyroid gland or removed with the thyroid lobe should be examined. They should be biopsied and confirmed by frozen-section examination. The parathyroid glands can be minced into 1-mm^3 pieces and reimplanted in the ipsilateral sternohyoid muscle or sternocleidomastoid (SCM) muscle with a silk suture/clip to mark the reimplantation site.

Once the lobe is mobilized and key structures are identified, the isthmus can be transected close to the contralateral side. The edge of the isthmus is

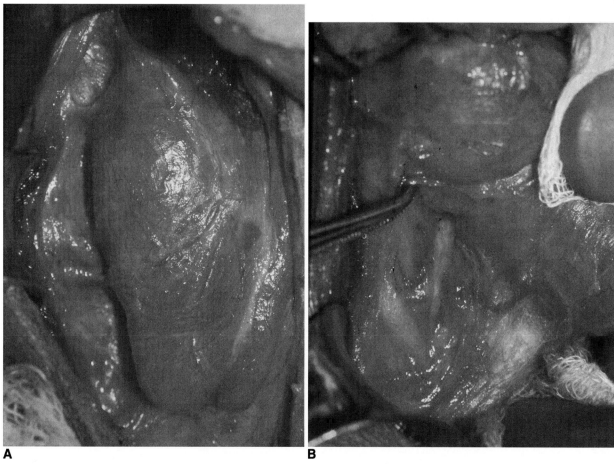

A **B**

Figure 119-4. A, Careful dissection along the lateral portion of the thyroid lobe permits mobilization of the gland medially. The middle thyroid vein(s) should be carefully identified and ligated. **B,** The course of the recurrent laryngeal nerve along the tracheoesophageal groove is demonstrated intraoperatively.

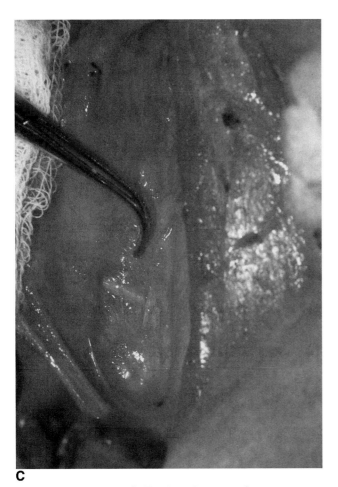

C

Figure 119-4, cont'd C, The lateral course of a nonrecurrent laryngeal nerve has been revealed intraoperatively.

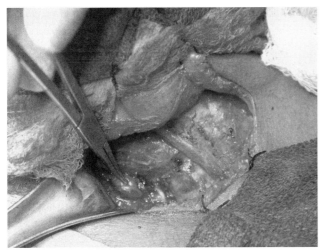

Figure 119-5. A parathyroid gland is demonstrated in close proximity to the recurrent laryngeal nerve. Close dissection and ligation of vessels along the thyroid capsule will ensure that the vascular supply to the parathyroid glands remains intact.

oversewn, and a careful search is made for a pyramidal lobe that should be removed in continuity with the thyroid lobe and isthmus, when present.

For a total thyroidectomy, the same procedure is then repeated on the contralateral side. However, the decision to proceed to excision of the opposite thyroid lobe should depend on the course of the initial thyroid lobectomy. After removal of the thyroid specimen, hemostasis is verified, and a Jackson-Pratt suction drain is placed in the thyroid lobe bed. Divided strap muscles are reapproximated with absorbable sutures and closed along the midline to prevent tracheal adhesion to the skin. The platysma is reapproximated with absorbable sutures, and the skin is closed with a running subcuticular suture.

Special Surgical Situations
Management of Regional Lymphatics

Management of the neck in patients with well-differentiated thyroid carcinomas is typically conservative. Cervical node disease is rare in follicular carcinomas but more common in papillary carcinomas. There is currently no role for elective neck dissection in cases of follicular carcinoma. More controversy exists regarding central compartment (levels VI and VII) dissection in patients with papillary carcinoma.[102,200] If disease is present by palpation or visible inspection, patients with papillary or Hürthle cell thyroid carcinoma will have a concurrent central compartment lymph node dissection with their total thyroidectomy or the completion thyroid lobectomy.

Given the higher frequency of microscopic tumor spread in medullary carcinomas and their lack of radioiodine uptake, elective central compartment lymph node dissection is commonly performed. When these patients present with palpable anterior lymph node disease, bilateral central compartment dissection is performed with the total thyroidectomy and the lateral cervical nodes are carefully inspected. Central compartment dissection should include the Delphian, paratracheal lymphatic, and lymph nodes of the upper mediastinum. The RLN, inferior thyroid artery, and parathyroid glands should be clearly identified, and the lymphatics should be removed en bloc from the level of the cricoid to the innominate artery.

When performing bilateral central compartment dissection, preservation of the parathyroid glands can be difficult. Attempts should be made in the dissection, especially contralateral to the thyroid lesion, to identify and preserve the ascending branch of the inferior thyroid artery that supplies the superior parathyroid gland. If the vascular supply to the parathyroid is compromised, the gland should be biopsied to confirm the presence of parathyroid tissue and placed into a pocket in the sternocleidomastoid muscle. The gland should be minced into 1-mm pieces, and the implantation site should be marked with vascular clips.

When palpable lateral cervical nodes are present and metastatic disease is confirmed by FNAC, a selective neck dissection, including levels II through V should be performed. The submandibular and submental nodes (level I) are rarely involved and should be dissected only when there is clinically positive disease in this region.[128,153] Cervical involvement is frequently ipsilateral to the primary thyroid lesion.[217] Extension of the collar incision superior to the mastoid tip will provide adequate exposure of the lateral neck if palpable disease is present. Careful inspection and dissection should be performed along the spinal accessory nerve because this is a frequent site of metastatic thyroid disease.[191] A more extensive modified radical neck dissection may be necessary to remove gross disease. Radioiodine ablation provides an important adjunctive therapy for the management of cervical disease in these patients.

In patients with medullary thyroid cancer, lymph node metastasis can occur in up to 81% of cases.[144] Retrospective analysis revealed a 10-year survival rate of 67% for those patients with medullary carcinoma treated with neck dissection vs 43% for those who were not.[17] Palpable cervical disease will necessitate central compartment and comprehensive neck dissection. In patients with clinically negative neck disease, surgical treatment should include total thyroidectomy, central compartment dissection, and elective, ipsilateral comprehensive neck dissection. Dissection of the contralateral neck in all patients should be considered, especially when the primary thyroid lesion is 2 cm or greater because bilateral neck dissection may be necessary to maximize regional control.[144]

Intrathoracic Goiter

Fewer than 1% of patients may have a thyroid gland that is partially or completely intrathoracic.[125,192] In the great majority of these patients, the intrathoracic goiter can be removed via a collar incision in the neck without resorting to a sternotomy. The vascular supply, typically originating in the neck, is identified, ligated, and divided. Division of the isthmus may facilitate mobilization of the substernal goiter from beneath the sternum. Large sutures can be placed deeply into the goiter to facilitate traction and blunt dissection to permit delivery of the thyroid through the neck.

Patients with substernal goiters who have had previous thyroid operations, some with invasive malignant tumors, and patients with no thyroid tissue in the neck may require a median sternotomy. Occasionally, the substernal goiter may simply be too large to deliver through a cervical incision. In these cases, the thyroidectomy is usually performed in collaboration with a thoracic surgeon.

Recurrent Laryngeal Nerve Invasion

Surgical situations necessitating the sacrifice of the RLN are quite uncommon. If preoperative vocal cord paralysis is present and carcinoma invasion is seen intraoperatively, the nerve may be sacrificed. More commonly, the RLN should be dissected free of gross disease. In patients with well-differentiated thyroid carcinomas, there is no survival difference between those with RLN sacrifice and those treated postoperatively with radioiodine for gross disease left on the nerve.[165] Given the lack of response by medullary carcinoma to postoperative radioiodine treatment, RLN sacrifice must be considered to achieve complete removal of gross disease.

Sacrifice of the RLN requires the exclusion of nerve infiltration by benign disease processes. Graves' disease, Hashimoto's thyroiditis, and Reidel's thyroiditis can involve the RLN with or without vocal cord paralysis. Benign processes can cause stretch injuries to the RLN that resolve with surgical removal of the mass. Finally, lymphomas can involve the RLN, but treatment is rarely surgical and should not involve excision of the nerve.

Extended Surgical Resection

Surgical treatment of thyroid carcinomas should remove all gross disease, especially in patients with medullary carcinoma. Fixation to the thyroid cartilage or trachea may require partial- to full-thickness removal of those structures (Figure 119-6). A thyroid cartilage lamina can be removed without major morbidity if the internal thyroid perichondrium is left intact. The trachea can be partially resected and repaired to permit en bloc tumor removal. Primary anastomosis can be performed for resections involving up to four tracheal rings.[80] Additionally, tracheal shaving can be performed, leaving the internal mucosa intact. Isolated full-thickness defects can be repaired with composite mucosal-cartilage grafts from the nasal septum. In patients with more extensive skeletal involvement, a partial laryngectomy may be required and has demonstrated improvements in survival.[6,195] Total laryngectomy should be performed in only the most extreme cases of extensive intraluminal invasion. Typically, this would be done after the failure of radioiodine treatment, EBRT, or both. Pharyngeal and esophageal local invasion typically requires resection of the immediate area and primary closure (Figure 119-7).

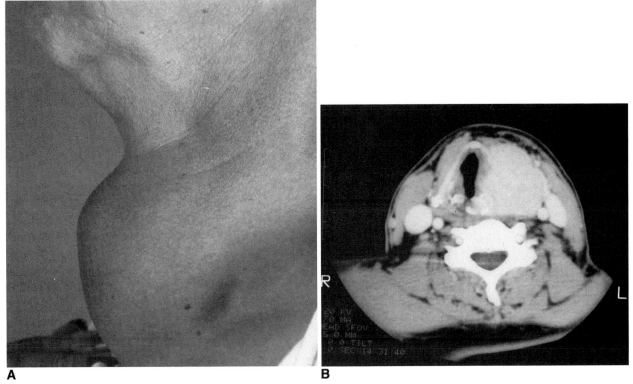

Figure 119-6. A, A lateral neck view demonstrates a large, compressive thyroid mass. **B,** An axial CT scan reveals extensive local invasion by the thyroid lesion involving the thyroid cartilage, larynx, and esophagus.

Reoperative Thyroid Surgery

Reoperative thyroid surgery may be required in a variety of clinical situations. A patient may have had a previous thyroid lobectomy and require a completion thyroidectomy. Recurrence of disease may require reexploration of the thyroid bed or dissection of the cervical lymph nodes, including the central compartment (level VI). Additionally, previous neck surgery, such as a parathyroidectomy, may have involved the thyroid bed.

Reoperative surgery has been associated with a higher incidence of complications than initial thyroid surgery. Scarring and fibrosis from prior surgery may cause difficulty in identifying tissue planes, resulting in an increased risk of injury to the RLN. Potential injury or devascularization of the parathyroid glands on one side of the neck creates increased concern for preservation of the glands on the contralateral side. Older series reported a high incidence of complications in reoperative surgery.[11,213] However, more recent reports indicate that the risk of permanent hypoparathyroidism or RLN injury is less than 2%.[35,115,146,157]

While reoperative thyroid surgery cannot be completely avoided, steps may be taken to minimize the need for reoperation. Before the initial surgery, preoperative preparation should include a thorough evaluation for thyroid mass fixation or RLN palsy/paralysis. In these patients, preoperative imaging and potential coordination with other surgeons will help to prevent unexpected intraoperative findings.

The minimum adequate surgical treatment for a thyroid nodule is a thyroid lobectomy and isthmusectomy. A unilateral subtotal thyroidectomy may encompass a suspected thyroid nodule but leave residual disease behind. En bloc resection of the thyroid lobe can be performed very safely and often eliminates the need to return to the original surgical bed for reexploration.

The effectiveness of FNAC has also directed surgeons to perform the appropriate surgery for a particular disease. The presence of a follicular or Hürthle cell adenoma should direct a surgeon to perform a unilateral thyroid lobectomy, avoiding exploration of the contralateral lobe. In cases of carcinoma, reoperation is safer because the contralateral lobe has been left undisturbed. When a patient has significant

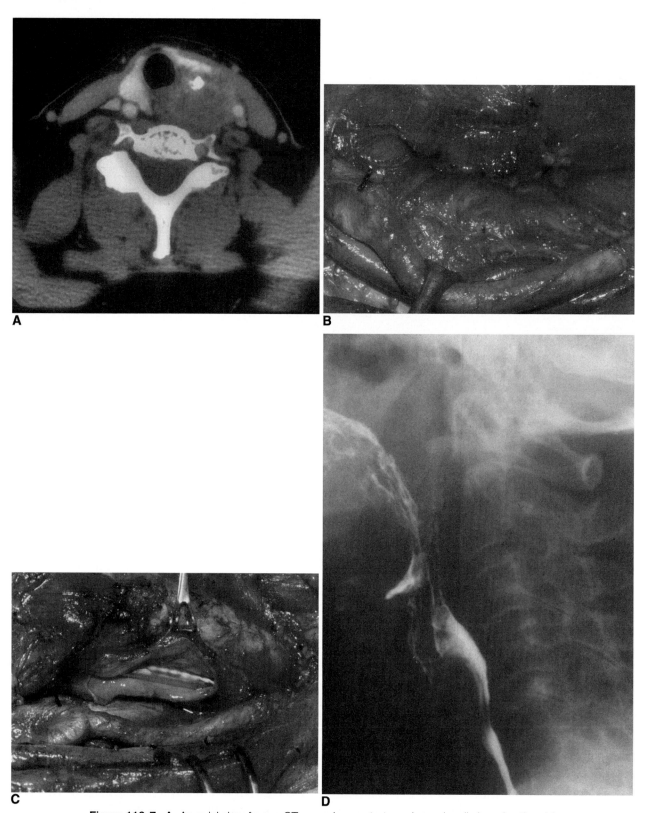

Figure 119-7. A, An axial view from a CT scan demonstrates a large, locally invasive thyroid mass. **B,** The large thyroid mass has been dissected free from adjacent structures but involves the esophagus. **C,** Resection of the thyroid mass required excision of a portion of the esophagus. The esophagus was closed primarily. **D,** A postoperative barium swallow study demonstrated that the esophagus was intact and the patient was able to tolerate a regular diet. (Used with permission from Lai SY, Weber RS: *Thyroid cancer.* In Ensley JF and others, editors: *Head and neck cancer: emerging perspectives,* San Diego, 2002, Academic Press, p 424.)

comorbidities that may preclude reoperation, the contralateral side can be addressed at the initial surgery by performing a total or near-total thyroidectomy. An FNAC that demonstrates papillary carcinoma will prepare a surgeon for total thyroidectomy or more comprehensive surgery for MTC. Furthermore, although intraoperative frozen-section analysis is controversial, frozen-section analysis in conjunction with cytologic examination can be valuable for cases diagnosed on preoperative FNAC as suspicious for papillary thyroid carcinoma.[8,168]

Typically, reoperation should be performed within 3 to 4 days of the initial operation, if definitive pathology is available, or after 3 months. Healing and inflammation during the early and late time points are typically manageable for reoperation. However, no control studies to date have addressed the issue of the degree of inflammation in the neck encountered during repeat surgery.

Before reoperation, the vocal cords should be visualized to identify any potential RLN injury. Imaging studies can be useful in cases of disease recurrence to identify local invasion or cervical disease and potential involvement of the RLN or parathyroid glands. During surgery, the RLN should be followed from a previously undissected area into the surgical bed. The surgeon should be familiar with a number of techniques to identify the RLN. A lateral approach from the medial border of the SCM, a low anterior neck approach, and a medial approach to the superior pole of the thyroid have been described.[146] Intraoperative monitoring of the RLN can be helpful, and an electrophysiologic nerve stimulator can facilitate and confirm nerve identification. Visualization of the RLN remains critical, and the use of loop magnification may be helpful to identify both the RLN and parathyroid glands.

Given the difficulties associated with permanent hypoparathyroidism, preservation of the parathyroid glands is critical in reoperative surgery. As described for initial thyroid surgery, extracapsular thyroid dissection and close vessel ligation will aid in preserving parathyroid gland vascular supply. Prior surgery may have disrupted the normal anatomic locations of the gland or created scarring that makes gland localization difficult. In these cases, all perithyroidal fat should be carefully mobilized and preserved. When reoperation includes central compartment dissection, the parathyroid glands may be removed en bloc with the disease. The surgical specimen needs to be carefully inspected and potential parathyroid tissue should be biopsied. Identified parathyroid tissue should be reimplanted into the sternocleidomastoid muscle. All parathyroid tissue should be preserved when possible. The combination of parathyroid preservation in situ

and autotransplantation of devascularized parathyroid tissue significantly reduces the risk of permanent hypoparathyroidism.[123] Parathyroid tissue that has been reimplanted functions even when other parathyroid glands have been left intact and in the absence of hypocalcemia.[197]

Extent of Surgery

Surgery is the primary modality for treatment of thyroid carcinomas. Although well-differentiated thyroid cancers can be extremely aggressive and lethal, the vast majority of patients have prolonged survival even with residual or recurrent disease. Thus, controversy exists regarding the extent of surgery to be performed in patients with well-differentiated carcinomas. The primary goals of surgical treatment should be to eradicate primary disease, to reduce the incidence of local/distant recurrence, and to facilitate the treatment of metastases. These oncologic goals should be achieved with minimal morbidity.

The large body of literature regarding thyroid carcinoma and its treatment has created a wide variety of terms for describing the extent of thyroid tissue removal. Most surgeons would agree that a subtotal excision of a thyroid nodule is not acceptable and that the minimum amount of thyroid removed should be a lobectomy and isthmusectomy. Some surgeons have advocated in the past a near-total thyroidectomy that preserves the posterior portion of the gland on one side to avoid injury to the RLN and at least one parathyroid gland. A total thyroidectomy involves the complete removal of both thyroid lobes, although radioiodine scans may reveal 2% to 5% residual tissue.[156]

Proponents of a more conservative surgical approach suggest that the thyroid lobectomy and isthmusectomy is sufficient treatment for the great majority of patients (>80%). These patients would be categorized as low-risk in the different classification schemes (see section titled "Tumor Staging and Classification"). The thyroid lobectomy and isthmusectomy are simpler to perform and less time consuming than a total thyroidectomy. The overall risk of morbidity from RLN, superior laryngeal nerve, and parathyroid gland injury is less. Finally, compared with total thyroidectomy, this conservative approach does not adversely affect prognosis and survival.

A large number of studies support the conservative approach. In the AGES classification, low-risk patients with papillary carcinoma had the same 2% 25-year mortality rate regardless of whether they were treated with thyroid lobectomy or total thyroidectomy.[92] A study by Shah and others[193] based risk classifications upon the AJCC staging system. There was no difference in 20-year survival based on surgical treatment for patients with intrathyroidal tumors of less than 4 cm. However, patients treated with total thyroidectomy had an increased risk of complications.

Although survival differences are not found, several studies report an increased incidence of local recurrence in patients treated with only a thyroid lobectomy.[78,188] Some controversy remains regarding the relationship of local recurrence to disease survival, especially with papillary carcinomas.[29,157] Finally, patients categorized as high-risk in these classification systems are treated with near-total or total thyroidectomy and radioiodine-ablation therapy.

A more aggressive surgical approach favors total thyroidectomy in most cases and a lobectomy for small, single lesions. Proponents of this approach favor total thyroidectomy as a better oncologic operation. Removal of the entire thyroid gland encompasses potential extracapsular extension and multicentric lesions. Morbidity of this procedure is relatively low with good technique and an experienced surgeon.[115] Several studies demonstrate improved survival and decreased local/distant recurrence.[50,135,187] Cautionary studies also demonstrate the risk of aggressive disease even in patients determined to be low-risk in the various classification schemes.[5,37]

Postoperative thyroglobulin levels are more valid with removal of all normal thyroid tissue. Total thyroidectomy also facilitates the use of postoperative diagnostic scans to evaluate for metastases and recurrence. Diagnostic radioiodine uptake should ideally be 3% or less after total thyroidectomy. Subsequent radioiodine treatment does not need to be used to ablate excess normal tissue and can be concentrated on the removal of residual carcinoma and distant metastases. Finally, although rare, removal of the entire thyroid reduces the risk of transformation from a well-differentiated thyroid carcinoma to an anaplastic carcinoma.

Clearly, controversy surrounding the extent of surgery will continue to persist since no uniform set of characteristics can be used to classify the aggressiveness of well-differentiated thyroid carcinomas. Results of treatment will also continue to differ among institutions and surgeons. Nevertheless, initial surgery should address gross disease in the thyroid and neck nodes. The extent of the surgery should be guided by the patient's risk factors, operative findings, and intraoperative progress. Ultimately, the primary goal of thyroid surgery should remain the effective eradication of thyroid cancer with minimal morbidity.

Special Treatment Situations
Children

In children, nodular thyroid disease is relatively uncommon, with an incidence between 0.2% and 1.8%.[164] The majority of neck masses occurring in the pediatric population are due to congenital or inflammatory causes. Malignant neck masses may be due to lymphoproliferative disorders, sarcomas, or thyroid carcinomas. Fewer than 6% of pediatric neck tumors are thyroid malignancies.[112] Approximately 10% of all thyroid carcinomas occur in patients younger than 21 years old.[23]

Most children with thyroid neoplasms will present with an asymptomatic mass within either the thyroid or lateral neck. The lesions are often asymptomatic and frequently noted by a parent or pediatrician during a routine physical examination. A complete history should include special attention to family history and radiation exposure. The physical examination should carefully evaluate potential fixation of the thyroid gland to surround neck structures. Vocal cord mobility should be documented by indirect fiberoptic nasolaryngoscopy. Additionally, the central compartment and lateral necks should be carefully palpated. Lymph node metastases are present in more than 50% of children with differentiated thyroid cancer.[87] Local extension was reported in 18%. Additionally, up to 15% of patients have distant metastasis, frequently identified with postoperative radioiodine.[74,199] A chest radiograph may be normal or may demonstrate a fine interstitial reticular pattern, potentially mistaken for miliary tuberculosis. Children with extensive pulmonary involvement may even present with dyspnea on exertion.

The diagnostic workup in children should include both FNAC and ultrasonography. An uncooperative child may require sedation and ultrasound guidance for the FNAC. Given the advanced stage of disease common in children at initial presentation, ultrasound imaging provides valuable information regarding the size and consistency of the thyroid mass. Additionally, ultrasound examination can identify potential regional involvement of the paratracheal or cervical lymphatics.

Although the most common cause of a solitary thyroid nodule in children is a follicular adenoma (68.9%), malignancies are found in 16% to 25% of the nodules.[101,110] The most common malignant histologic type is papillary carcinoma, present in over 80% of these cases. However, unlike thyroid carcinoma in adults, papillary carcinomas are usually follicular in pattern and tall-cell and columnar-cell variants do not occur in the pediatric population.[84,214] Hürthle cell carcinomas may present with multiple lesions and a papillary architecture as a familial syndrome.[109] MTCs constitute about 10% of pediatric thyroid carcinomas, and all family members need to be carefully evaluated for possible familial medullary carcinoma or MEN syndromes.

Management of a child with thyroid carcinoma must balance the potential morbidity associated with treatment against the low probability that the patient will succumb to this disease. The primary goal of surgery is to completely remove gross disease at the primary and regional metastatic sites. A total or near total thyroidectomy is recommended.[23,87,44,221] Multifocal disease is present in 10% to 30% of patients. Additionally, a total or near-total thyroidectomy allows the use of serum thyroglobulin to monitor disease recurrence and facilitates the use of radioiodine to identify and treat distant metastases. Recent studies have demonstrated a low incidence of permanent hypoparathyroidism and RLN injury after total thyroidectomy. Additionally, the recurrence rate is lower for patients undergoing total thyroidectomy than for those with lesser procedures.[229]

Children often present with cervical nodal metastases requiring therapeutic lymphadenectomy. In patients with nodal disease, the paratracheal and pretracheal lymph nodes are involved in 90% of cases.[69] The metastatic deposits are frequently compressive rather than infiltrative with respect to adjacent neck structures. Thus, radical neck dissection is rarely necessary. Patients should have central compartment dissections when cervical disease is present, rather than simple node plucking. Care should be taken to identify and preserve the blood supply to the parathyroid glands. Additionally, lateral neck disease will require a comprehensive lateral neck dissection (levels II–V).

Although children and adolescents commonly present with more advanced disease than adults, their prognosis remains excellent. In several series, young patients have a 10-year survival near 100% and a 2- to 5-year survival rate near 90%.[76] Relapse is most common in the cervical lymphatics and is more common in children than in adults. Recurrence appears to be more common in younger patients and those with papillary histology.[118] Fortunately, cervical disease can be surgically excised, and pulmonary recurrence is responsive to radioiodine therapy.[222]

Pregnancy

Because thyroid neoplasms occur more commonly in women and often during their fertile years, physicians will occasionally need to manage this disease in pregnant women. The incidence of thyroid nodules during pregnancy has been reported as between 2% and 10%.[90,131] Management of these patients must protect the well-being of both mother and fetus and minimize the risks of preterm labor or abortion. A critical difference in thyroid nodule management during pregnancy and breastfeeding is the absolute contraindication for the use of radioactive iodine.[148]

During pregnancy, the thyroid gland physiology is markedly altered. The gland can increase significantly in size due to a relative iodine insufficiency and hormonal changes.[25,73] These physiologic and hormonal changes may increase the incidence of thyroid nodules or cause the enlargement of existing thyroid nodules.

The presence of any discrete thyroid nodule should be evaluated by FNAC.[172] Some authors argue that a pregnant patient beyond 20 weeks of gestation should have the FNAC deferred until after the pregnancy to reduce patient anxiety.[54,131] These authors argue that treatment will likely occur after surgery, and they advocate FNAC only when the nodule demonstrates continued growth or other suspicious features. Others advocate immediate FNAC at any stage of pregnancy.[148]

Ultrasound imaging may be used for initial assessment and continued monitoring. Sonographic evaluation is effective for the evaluation of both thyroid and cervical involvement. CT scans during pregnancy are not recommended, although an MRI, if necessary, may be safely performed.

When the FNAC is benign, the patient should be reassured, and ultrasonography can monitor the nodule for possible growth during pregnancy. A follicular neoplasm may be monitored closely or surgically explored. If the FNAC is suspicious or demonstrates thyroid carcinoma, surgery is recommended at the safest time possible.[90] Thyroid carcinomas identified late in pregnancy should be treated in the immediate postpartum period. Carcinomas diagnosed during the first and early second trimesters may be surgically treated during the 22nd through 26th gestational weeks, when the risk to fetal development and for preterm labor is lowest. The patient can be reassured that thyroidectomy and even cervical lymphadenectomy at midtrimester do not carry significant risks for the fetus. Maternal complications are similar to non-pregnant patients. A recent study, however, suggests no difference in the natural history and prognosis of pregnant patients with a thyroid carcinoma diagnosed early in gestation who defer surgery until after labor.[147] Most patients would likely experience too much stress and anxiety to have an untreated cancer present throughout gestation.

Aggressive thyroid carcinomas that grow rapidly or invade adjacent cervical structures may demand immediate surgical attention. Additionally, a diagnosis of medullary or undifferentiated carcinoma in pregnant patients requires prompt treatment. Fortunately, these tumors are rare and often affect older women. But before commencement of treatment in these cases, the pregnancy should be terminated.

Complications

Among head and neck surgical procedures, thyroid surgery is very safe. Mortality rates are extremely low, and morbidity is relatively low. In general, serious complications occur in fewer than 2% of all thyroid cases.[191] Complications can typically be divided into nonmetabolic and metabolic complications. Of particular concern are injuries to the RLN and the parathyroid glands.

Perioperative complications are fairly unusual in thyroid surgery. Postoperative infections are very unusual, given the abundant blood supply in the thyroid bed. The prevention of scar widening or hypertrophy depends on proper placement of the incision. The incision can often be hidden within existing skin creases. Additionally, the incision should not be placed too low in the neck to avoid the increased skin tension over the sternal notch. Pneumothorax is very rare and often associated with extended procedures that involve subclavicular dissection. Chylous fistula may occur more often on the left side but are usually self-limiting when wound drainage is adequate.

Bleeding Complications

Hemorrhage is uncommon when surgery is performed with meticulous hemostasis. However, bleeding may occur due to an undetected coagulopathy or a technical mishap. Significant hemorrhage in the immediate postoperative period can lead to life-threatening airway compression. A rapidly expanding hematoma requires immediate opening of the surgical incision and evacuation of blood. Airway control can then be established, and the patient can be returned to the operating room for complete exploration to identify bleeding sites. A wound seroma may occur, especially after the removal of a large goiter. Should a fluid collection present, simple needle aspiration should manage the problem and prevent the risk of infection.

Superior Laryngeal Nerve Injury

Injury to the external branch of the SLN is thought to be rare, but the exact frequency is unknown. Often disturbance of SLN function is temporary and unrecognized by the patient and the surgeon.[227] Injury to the SLN will alter function of the cricothyroid muscle. Patients may have difficulty shouting, and singers will find difficulty with pitch variation, especially in the higher frequencies. The external branch of the SLN is not often visualized and lies near the superior pole vessels. Adequate exposure of the superior thyroid pole and close ligation of the individual vessels on the thyroid capsule may prevent SLN injury. Voice therapy may help patients to compensate in cases of SLN injury.

Recurrent Laryngeal Nerve Injury

Injury to the RLN has a much greater impact and is more noticeable than SLN injury. The incidence of permanent RLN paralysis is approximately 1% to 1.5% for total thyroidectomy and less for near-total procedures.[10,68,135] Temporary dysfunction due to nerve traction occurs in 2.5% to 5% of patients.[124] Incidence increases with second and third procedures. RLN injury is also more common in thyroidectomy with neck dissection, although this may reflect more advanced disease states.[152] Disease-specific risk factors for permanent nerve damage include recurrent thyroid carcinoma, substernal goiter, and various thyroiditis conditions. Vocal cord function should be evaluated and documented by indirect laryngoscopy, especially in patients who have had previous surgery.

Unilateral RLN injury leads to a vocal cord in the paramedian position, and the voice may be breathy and lack volume. Concurrent injury of the SLN will result in a more laterally positioned vocal cord and will worsen voice quality and glottic competence.[48] Occasionally, patients may have difficulty with aspiration and pneumonia.[152]

Bilateral RLN injury may present very dramatically. Immediate postoperative stridor and dyspnea may require immediate reintubation and a possible tracheostomy. Occasionally, bilateral RLN injury may not be immediately noticeable, and patients may adapt to the reduced airway. Over time, though, the vocal cords will move to the midline compromising the airway.

Identification and careful dissection along the course of the RLN decreases the incidence of permanent injury. The surgeon should also be aware of the possibility of a nonrecurrent nerve, most commonly on the right side. If the nerve is transected during surgery, microsurgical repair of the nerve is recommended. Although the repair is unlikely to restore normal function, reanastomosis of the RLN may decrease the extent of vocal cord atrophy.[18] Some surgeons advocate anastomosis of the ansa hypoglossal nerve to the distal end of the severed RLN to prevent laryngeal synkinesis and possible vocal cord hyperadduction.[42,218]

Comprehensive management of vocal cord injury is beyond the scope of this chapter. In the majority of cases, RLN injury will be detected postoperatively. Management is supportive, although some surgeons favor reexploration when vocal cord paralysis is noted in the immediate postoperative period. Return of normal vocal cord function occurs as late as 6 to 12 months after temporary RLN injury occurs. Speech therapy can be valuable. Serial examinations should document a potential return of function or compensation by the contralateral vocal cord. In patients with continued vocal incompetence or aspiration, treatment directed toward vocal cord medialization may consist of vocal cord injection, thyroplasty, or arytenoids medialization. In cases of bilateral RLN injury, management is directed at improving the airway while not completely sacrificing airway quality and may involve arytenoidectomy or transverse cordotomy.

Hypocalcemia

Transient symptomatic hypocalcemia after total thyroidectomy occurs in approximately 7% to 25% of cases, but permanent hypocalcemia is less common (0.4%–13.8%).[9,19] The risk of hypoparathyroidism is related to the size and degree of invasion of the tumor, pathology and the extent of procedure and surgeon experience.[83,92] Changes in serum calcium levels are often transient and may not always be related to parathyroid gland trauma or vascular compromise.

Transient hypocalcemia is often related to variations in serum protein binding due to perioperative alterations in acid-base status, hemodilution and albumin concentration. These changes do not produce hypocalcemic symptoms. However, sudden changes in levels of ionized serum calcium can result in perioral and distal extremity paresthesias. As calcium levels continue to decline, patients may experience tetany, bronchospasm, mental status changes, seizures, laryngospasm, and cardiac arrhythmias. Chvostek's sign and Trousseau's sign may develop with increased neuromuscular irritability as serum calcium levels drop below 8.0 mg/dL.

Typically, serum calcium levels are measured in the immediate postoperative period and the next morning for patients with a total or completion thyroidectomy. Patients should demonstrate a stable or rising serum calcium level. Patients undergoing a thyroid lobectomy do not usually require serum calcium monitoring. Findings that should be worrisome for hypoparathyroidism include hypocalcemia, hyperphosphatemia, and metabolic alkalosis.

Treatment for hypocalcemia is typically initiated if the patient is symptomatic or serum calcium levels fall below 7.0 mg/dL. In these patients, cardiac monitoring is warranted. Patients should receive 10 mL of 10% calcium gluconate and 5% dextrose in water intravenously, titrated to symptom resolution and subsequent serum calcium level tests. Oral calcium supplementation should begin with 2 to 3 g of calcium carbonate per day. Additionally, calcitriol (1,25-dihydroxyvitamin D_3) should be initiated. Adjustments in the supplemental calcium and vitamin D should be done in consultation with an endocrinologist.

POSTOPERATIVE MANAGEMENT AND SPECIAL CONSIDERATIONS
Thyroid Hormone Replacement

After total or completion thyroidectomy, exogenous supplementation of thyroid hormone is necessary.[72,134] Long-term supplementation with levothyroxine (T_4) is monitored to suppress TSH to below-normal levels. Patients receiving suppressive therapy have a lower recurrence rate and improved survival.[43,239]

In the immediate postoperative period, patients are frequently given *liothyronine sodium* (Cytomel; T_3). Cytomel has a shorter half-life than thyroxine, decreasing the waiting period before radioiodine body scanning and possible enabling ablative therapy to be performed.

Radiation Treatment

Radiolabeled iodine has been used for more than 40 years to ablate normal thyroid tissue and to treat residual tumor and metastases.[182] The ^{131}I isotope emits β particles that penetrate and destroy tissue within a 2-mm zone. Patients classified as high-risk with papillary carcinoma and most patients with follicular carcinoma are considered for treatment.[86] Despite poor radioiodine uptake in Hürthle cell and medullary carcinomas, these patients will often be treated to provide any possible benefit.

Whole-body scans stage the patient and determine the need and potential benefit of radioiodine therapy. Elevated TSH levels are necessary to enhance uptake of iodine by thyroid cancer cells. Thus, patients are taken off thyroid hormone suppression therapy for 4 to 6 weeks before scanning and placed on a low-iodine diet. Additionally, the administration of exogenous TSH has proved safe and effective for stimulating radioiodine uptake and for detecting serum thyroglobulin in patients undergoing evaluation for thyroid cancer persistence and recurrence.[89,141]

At our institution, ^{123}I has replaced ^{131}I for the initial diagnostic radioiodine scan. The physical properties of ^{123}I permit better image quality and decrease possible stunning of functioning thyroid cells by the β particle emission of [131]I.[127] This permits the maximal benefit of ^{131}I in ablation after the diagnostic procedure.[194]

After the diagnostic scan, therapeutic ablative doses of ^{131}I can be given. Typically, 100 mCi of ^{131}I is given for uncomplicated cases with only thyroid bed uptake. Although a lower dose of 30 mCi has commonly been used, studies have demonstrated this is not as effective. Recent data from our institution have revealed that 60 mCi is as effective as 100 mCi for thyroid bed ablation (A. Alavi/S. Mandel, personal communication.) Patients with uptake in cervical nodes or distant metastases will receive 125 to 200 mCi.[13,14] Doses higher than 200 mCi have not been shown to be more effective in most cases.

Diverse alternatives and protocols exist regarding the use of radioiodine therapy. Surgeons who favor total thyroidectomy for most thyroid carcinomas argue that removal of normal tissue enhances radioiodine ablation therapy. However, proponents of more conservative treatment suggest that radioiodine therapy can be used to remove even a remaining thyroid lobe before whole-body scanning for residual tumor or metastases. Additionally, the use of ^{123}I for diagnostic scanning has only recently gained favor. Continued work in this area should improve patient outcomes and decrease disease recurrence.

External Beam Radiotherapy and Chemotherapy

Given the effectiveness of surgery and radioiodine treatment for the majority of thyroid carcinomas, experience with EBRT and chemotherapy is more limited. EBRT appears to improve local control of well-differentiated carcinomas, especially when used in combination with doxorubicin.[22,199,217] However, the effect of EBRT on survival is uncertain.[22,180] Palliation of patients with distant metastasis of well-differentiated carcinomas, especially to the bone, appears to be improved with EBRT.[217]

Limited success with EBRT in combination with doxorubicin/cisplatin has been noted with anaplastic carcinomas.[47,209] However, this disease remains uniformly fatal, and palliation through local control and airway protection are the only realistic goals. Patients with metastatic medullary carcinoma may benefit from EBRT and chemotherapy to decrease local recurrence.[175,181] Typically, patients with regional nodal metastases recognized during surgery will receive postoperative EBRT. In general, the poorer outcomes for patients with medullary and anaplastic carcinomas have not been significantly altered by EBRT and chemotherapy.

Follow-up Management

Patients treated for thyroid carcinomas will require long-term follow-up and monitoring. In addition to regular physical examination, thyroid hormone and TSH levels are monitored to ensure adequate suppression. Thyroglobulin levels should be closely monitored and diagnostic radioiodine scanning should be performed. These tests should be performed annually for the first 2 years and then every 5 years for 20 years.[204] Typically, thyroglobulin levels should be less than 2 ng/mL after total thyroidectomy and radioiodine ablation therapy (less than 3 ng/mL if the patient is off thyroid replacement therapy). Rising serum thyroglobulin levels are highly sensitive (97%) and specific (100%) for thyroid cancer recurrence.[155] Elevation of thyroglobulin levels warrant repeat radioiodine scanning and therapy. Recent studies have demonstrated the sensitivity of serum thyroglobulin measurements for predicting thyroid cancer recurrence after a patient has received two injections of recombinant human TSH.[228]

Patients with medullary carcinomas require serial measurements of calcitonin and CEA. Suspected recurrences may also be detected with pentagastrin-stimulation test. Please refer to the "Medullary Carcinoma" section for further details.

SUMMARY

A great deal of literature addresses the treatment of thyroid carcinomas. Questions remain unresolved regarding the extent of thyroidectomy to perform in patients with well-differentiated carcinomas and the effect on patient survival. Since the great majority of patients with well-differentiated thyroid carcinomas do well, failure to resolve issues like this are tolerated. Additionally, studies to address these issues require very large cohorts with long-term follow-up that needs to extend 20 to 30 years.

Nevertheless, surgeons need to remain wary of the devastating progression of disease in medullary and anaplastic thyroid carcinomas. Despite clinical classification schemes, even well-differentiated carcinomas can have unpredictably aggressive clinical manifestations. As our understanding of the molecular and genetic mechanisms of thyroid carcinomas improve, better diagnostic tests should improve our ability to treat these cancers.

REFERENCES

1. Ahmedin J and others: Cancer statistics, *CA Cancer J Clin* 52:23, 2002.
2. Ahuja S, Ernst H: Hyperthyroidism and thyroid carcinoma, *Acta Endocrinol* 142:146–151, 1991.
3. Ashcraft M, van Herle A: Management of thyroid nodules I, *Head Neck* 3:216–227, 1981.
4. Ashcraft M, van Herle A: Management of thyroid nodules II, *Head Neck* 3:297–322, 1981.
5. Attie J, Bock G, Moskowitz GW: Postoperative radioactive evaluation of total thyroidectomy for thyroid carcinoma: reappraisal and therapeutic implications, *Head Neck* 14:297–302, 1992.
6. Ballantyne A: Resections of the upper aerodigestive tract for locally invasive thyroid cancer, *Am J Surg* 168:636–639, 1994.
7. Baloch Z and others: Fine-needle aspiration of thyroid: an institutional experience, *Thyroid* 8:565, 1998.
8. Basolo F and others: Usefulness of Ultrafast Papanicolaou–stained scrape preparations in intraoperative management of thyroid lesions, *Mod Pathol* 12:653, 1999.
9. Beahrs O: *Complications in thyroid and parathyroid surgery.* In Conley J, editor: *Complications in head and neck surgery.* Philadelphia, 1979, WB Saunders.

10. Beahrs O: Complications of surgery of the head and neck, *Surg Clin North Am* 57:823–829, 1977.

11. Beahrs OH, Vandertell DJ: Complications of secondary thyroidectomy, *Surg Gynecol Obstet* 117:535, 1963.

12. Becker F and others: Adult thyroid cancer after head and neck irradiation in infancy and childhood, *Ann Intern Med* 83:347–351, 1975.

13. Beirwaltes W: The treatment of thyroid cancer with radioactive I, *Semin Nucl Med* 8:79–94, 1978.

14. Beirwaltes W and others: Survival time and "cure" in papillary and follicular thyroid carcinoma with distant metastases: statistics following University of Michigan therapy, *J Nucl Med* 23:561–568, 1982.

15. Bergholm U, Adami HO, Bergstrom R: Clinical characteristics in sporadic and familial medullary thyroid carcinoma, *Cancer* 63:1196–1204, 1989.

16. Bisi H, Camargo R, Filho A: Role of fine needle aspiration cytology in the management of thyroid nodules: review of experience with 1925 cases, *Diagn Cytopathol* 8:504–510, 1991.

17. Block M: Surgical treatment of medullary carcinoma of the thyroid, *Otol Clin North Am* 23:453–473, 1990.

18. Boles R, Fritzell B:, Injury and repair of the recurrent laryngeal nerves in dogs, *Laryngoscope* 70:1405–1418, 1969.

19. Bourrel C and others: Temporary post thyroidectomy hypocalcemia, *Arch Otolaryngol Head Neck Surg* 102:496–501, 1993.

20. Breaux E, Guillamondegui O: Treatment of locally invasive carcinomas of the thyroid: how radical? *Am J Surg* 140:514–517, 1980.

21. Brennan M and others: Follicular thyroid cancer treated at the Mayo Clinic, 1946–1970: initial manifestations, pathological findings, therapy and outcome, *Mayo Clinic Proc* 66:11–22, 1991.

22. Brunt LM, Wells SH: Advances in the diagnosis and treatment of medullary carcinoma, *Surg Clin North Am* 67:263–279, 1987.

23. Buckwalter J, Gurll NJ, Thomas CG Jr: Cancer of the thyroid in youth, *World J Surg* 5:15, 1981.

24. Burman K, Ringel M, Wartofsky L: Unusual types of thyroid neoplasms, *Endocrinol Metab Clin North Am* 25:49–68, 1996.

25. Burrow G: Thyroid status in normal pregnancy, *J Clin Endocrinol Metab* 71:274–275, 1990.

26. Byar D and others: A prognostic index for thyroid carcinoma: a study of the EORTC Thyroid Cancer Cooperative Group, *Eur J Cancer* 15:1033, 1979.

27. Cady B, Rossi R: An expanded view of risk-group definition in differentiated thyroid carcinoma, *Surgery* 104:947–953, 1988.

28. Cady B and others: Changing clinical, pathologic, therapeutic and survival pattern in differentiated thyroid carcinoma, *Ann Surg* 184:541–553, 1976.

29. Cady B and others: Further evidence of the validity of risk group definition, *Surgery* 98:1171–1178, 1985.

30. Callender D and others: *Cancer of the thyroid.* In Suen E, editor: *Cancer of the head and neck,* ed 3. Philadelphia, 1996, WB Saunders.

31. Carcangiu M, Zampi G, and Pupi A: Papillary carcinoma of the thyroid: a clinicopathologic study of 241 cases treated at the University of Florence, Italy, *Cancer* 55:805–828, 1985.

32. Carcangiu M, Zampi G, Rosai J: Poorly-differentiated ("insular") thyroid carcinoma: a reinterpretation of Langham's "Wuchernde Struma," *Am J Surg Pathol* 8: 655–668, 1984.

33. Caruso D, Mazzaferri E: Fine needle aspiration in the management of thyroid nodules, *Endocrinologist* 1:194–202, 1991.

34. Chandramouly B and others: Marine-Lenhart syndrome: Graves' disease with poorly functioning nodules, *Clin Nucl Med* 17:905–906, 1992.

35. Chao T and others: Completion thyroidectomy for differentiated thyroid carcinoma, *Otolaryngol Head Neck Surg* 118:896, 1998.

36. Chong F and others: Medullary carcinoma of the thyroid gland, *Cancer* 35:695–704, 1975.

37. Chonkich GD, Petti GH: Treatment of thyroid carcinoma, *Laryngoscope* 102:486–491, 1992.

38. Clark O: Thyroid nodules and thyroid cancer: surgical aspects, *West J Med* 133:1–8, 1980.

39. Copp D, Cockcroft D, Kuch Y: Calcitonin from ultimobranchial glands of dogfish and chickens, *Science* 158:924–925, 1967.

40. Crile GJ, Antunez A, Esselstyn C: The advantages of subtotal thyroidectomy and suppression of TSH in the primary treatment of papillary carcinoma of the thyroid, *Cancer* 55:2691–2697, 1985.

41. Crile G, Pontius K, Hawk W: Factors influencing the survival of patients with follicular carcinoma of the thyroid gland, *Surg Gynecol Obstet* 160:409–413, 1985.

42. Crumley R, Izdensk K: Voice quality following laryngeal reinnervation by ansa hypoglossal transfer, *Laryngoscope* 96:611–616, 1986.

43. Cunningham M and others: Survival discriminants for differentiated thyroid cancer, *Am J Surg* 160:344–347, 1990.

44. Danese D and others: Thyroid carcinoma in children and adolescents, *Eur J Pediatr* 156:190, 1997.

45. Daniels G: Thyroid nodules and nodular thyroids: a clinical overview, *Comprehen Ther* 22:239–250, 1996.

46. de los Santos E and others: Cystic thyroid nodules: the dilemma of malignant lesions, *Arch Intern Med* 150:1422, 1990.

47. deBesi P and others: Combined chemotherapy with bleomycin, adriamycin and platinum in advanced thyroid cancer, *J Endocrinol Metab* 14:475–480, 1991.

48. Dedo H: The paralyzed larynx: an electromyographic study in dogs and humans, *Laryngoscope* 80:1455–1517, 1970.

49. DeGroot L and others: Does the method of management of papillary thyroid carcinoma make a difference in outcome? *World J Surg* 18:123–130, 1994.

50. DeGroot L and others: Natural history, treatment and course of papillary thyroid carcinoma, *J Clin Endocrinol Metab* 71:414–424, 1990.

51. DeLellis R: Biology of disease: multiple endocrine neoplasia syndromes revisited, *Lab Invest* 72:494–505, 1995.

52. Demeter J and others: Anaplastic thyroid carcinoma: risk factors and outcome, *Surgery* 110:956–963, 1991.

53. Divine R, Edis A, Banks P: Primary lymphoma of the thyroid: a review of the Mayo Clinic experience through 1978, *World J Surg* 5:33–38, 1981.

54. Doherty C and others: Management of thyroid nodules during pregnancy, *Laryngoscope* 105:251–255, 1995.

55. Donohue J, Goldfien S, Miller T: Do the prognosis of papillary and follicular thyroid cancer differ? *Am J Surg* 148:168–173, 1984.

56. Donovan DT, Gagel RF: *Medullary thyroid carcinoma and the multiple endocrine neoplasia syndromes.* In Falk S, editor: *Thyroid disease: endocrinology, surgery, nuclear medicine and radiotherapy,* ed 2. Philadelphia, 1997, Lippincott-Raven.

57. Duffy BJ, Fitzgerald PJ: Cancer of the thyroid in children: a report of 28 cases, *J Clin Endocrinol* 10:1296–1308, 1950.

58. Ellenhorn J, Shah J, Brennan MF: Impact of therapeutic regional lymph node dissection for medullary carcinoma of thyroid gland, *Surgery* 114:1078–1082, 1993.

59. El-Naggar A, Batsakis J, Luna M: Hürthle cell tumors of the thyroid: a flow cytometric DNA analysis, *Arch Otol Head Neck Surg* 114:520–521, 1988.

60. Eng C and others: The relationship between specific RET proto-oncogene mutations and disease phenotype in multiple endocrine neoplasia type 2: International RET Mutation Consortium Analysis, *JAMA* 276:1575, 1996.

61. Evans H, Vassilopoulou-Sellin R: Follicular and Hurthle cell carcinomas of the thyroid: a comparative study, *Am J Surg Pathol* 22:1512, 1998.

62. Exelby P, Frazell E: Carcinoma of the thyroid in children, *Surg Clin North Am* 49:249–259, 1969.

63. Faggiano A and others: Differential expression of galectin 3 in solid cell nests and C cells of human thyroid, *J Clin Pathol* 56:142–143, 2003.

64. Fagin J: Molecular pathogenesis of human thyroid neoplasms, *Thyroid Today* 18:1–6, 1994.

65. Fagin J and others: High prevalence of mutations of the p53 gene in poorly differentiated human thyroid carcinomas, *J Clin Invest* 91:179, 1993.

66. Favas M, Schneider A, Stachvra M: Thyroid cancer occurring as a consequence of head and neck irradiation, *N Engl J Med* 294:1019, 1976.

67. Ferrari C: Value of ethanol injection in the treatment of the autonomous thyroid nodule, *J Endocrinol Invest* 18:465, 1995.

68. Flynn M, Lyons KJ, Tartar JW: Local complications after surgical resection for thyroid cancer, *Am J Surg* 168:404-407, 1994.

69. Frankenthaler R and others: Lymph node metastasis from papillary-follicular thyroid carcinoma in young patients, *Am J Surg* 160:341, 1990.

70. Frazell E, Foote F:, Papillary cancer of the thyroid, *Cancer* 11:895, 1958.

71. Gharib H: Management of thyroid nodules: another look, *Thyr Today* 20:1, 1997.

72. Gharib H, Goellner JR: Fine needle aspiration biopsy of the thyroid: an appraisal, *Ann Intern Med* 118:282–289, 1993.

73. Glinoer D, Lemone M: Goiter in pregnancy: a new insight into an old problem, *Thyroid* 2:65–70, 1992.

74. Goepfert H, Dichtel W, Samaan N: Thyroid cancer in children and teenagers, *Arch Otolartyngol* 110:72, 1984.

75. Goodfellow P, Wells S: RET gene and its implications for cancer, *J Natl Cancer Inst* 87:1515–1523, 1995.

76. Gordin J, Sallin S: Thyroid cancer in childhood, *Endocrinol Metab Clin North Am* 19:649, 1990.

77. Grant C: Operative and postoperative management of the patient with follicular and Hurthle cell carcinoma: do they differ? *Surg Clin North Am* 75:395–403, 1995.

78. Grant C and others: Local recurrence in papillary thyroid carcinoma: is the extent of surgical resection important? *Surgery* 104:954–962, 1988.

79. Green L and others: Renal cell carcinoma metastatic to the thyroid, *Cancer* 63:1810–1815, 1989.

80. Grillo HC, Zannini P: Resectional management of airway invasion by thyroid carcinoma, *Ann Thorac Surg* 42:287–298, 1986.

81. Hamburger J: Consistency of sequential needle biopsy findings for thyroid nodules: management implications, *Arch Intern Med* 147:97–99, 1982.

82. Hannequin P, Liehn JC, Delisle MJ: Multifactorial analysis of survival in thyroid cancer: pitfalls of applying the results of published studies to another population, *Cancer* 58:1749–1755, 1986.

83. Harach H, Franssila KO, Wasenus VM: Occult papillary carcinoma of the thyroid: a "normal" finding in Finland. A systematic autopsy study, *Cancer* 56:531–538, 1985.

84. Harach HR, Williams ED: Childhood cancer in England and Wales, *Br J Cancer* 72:777, 1995.

85. Harach H and others: Thyroid pathologic findings in patients with Cowden disease, *Ann Diagn Pathol* 3:331, 1999.

86. Harness J and others: Follicular carcinoma of the thyroid gland: trends and treatment, *Surgery* 96:972–980, 1984.

87. Harness J and others: Differentiated thyroid carcinoma in children and adolescents, *World J Surg* 16:547, 1992.

88. Hathaway H: Diagnosis and management of the thyroid nodule, *Otolaryngol Clin North Am* 23:303–337, 1990.

89. Haugen B and others: A comparison of recombinant human thyrotropin and thyroid hormone withdrawal for the detection of thyroid remnant or cancer, *J Clin Endocrinol Metab* 84:3877–3885, 1999.

90. Hay I: Nodular thyroid disease diagnosed during pregnancy: how and when to treat, *Thyroid* 9:667–675, 1999.

91. Hay I, Klee GG: Thyroid cancer diagnosis and management, *Clin Lab Med* 13:725–734, 1993.

92. Hay I and others: Ipsilateral lobectomy versus bilateral lobar resection in papillary thyroid carcinoma: a retrospective analysis of surgical outcome using a novel prognostic scoring system, *Surgery* 102:1088–1095, 1987.

93. Hay I and others: Predicting outcome in papillary thyroid carcinoma: development of a reliable prognostic scoring system in a cohort of 1779 patients surgically treated at one institution during 1940 through 1989, *Surgery* 114:1050–1058, 1993.

94. Hayes B, Anthony A, Kersham R: Anatomy and development of the thyroid gland, *Ear Nose Throat J* 64:10, 1985.

95. Hayles A and others: Management of the child with thyroid cancer, *JAMA* 173:21, 1960.

96. Hazard J: The C-cell of the thyroid gland and medullary thyroid carcinoma: a review, *Am J Pathol* 88:213–250, 1977.

97. Henry J, Audiffret J, Denizot A: The nonrecurrent inferior laryngeal nerve: review of 33 cases, including two on the left side, *Surgery* 104:977, 1988.

98. Herrmann M and others: Immunohistochemical expression of galectin-3 in benign and malignant thyroid lesions, *Arch Pathol Lab Med* 126:710–713, 2002.

99. Hollingshead W: Anatomy of the endocrine glands, *Surg Clin North Am* 39:1115–1140, 1958.

100. Hundhal S and others: A National Cancer Data Base report on 53,856 cases of thyroid carcinoma treated in the U.S., 1985–1995, *Cancer* 83:2638, 1998.

101. Hung W: Solitary thyroid nodules in 93 children and adolescents: a 35-year experience, *Horm Res* 52:15, 1999.

102. Hutter R, Frazell E, Foote F: Elective radical neck dissection: an assessment of its use in the management of papillary thyroid cancer, *Cancer* 20:87–93, 1970.

103. Ivy H: Cancer metastatic to the thyroid: a diagnostic problem, *Mayo Clin Proc* 59:856–859, 1984.

104. Johannessen J and others: The diagnostic value of flow cytometric DNA measurements in selected disorders of the human thyroid, *Am J Clin Pathol* 77:20–25, 1982.

105. Jossart G, Clark OH: Well-differentiated thyroid cancer, *Curr Probl Surg* 21:933–1012, 1994.

106. Kahn N, Perzin K: Follicular carcinoma of the thyroid, *Pathol Annu* 18:221–253, 1983.

107. Kakudo K, Carney JR, Sizemore GW: Medullary carcinoma of the thyroid: biological behavior of the sporadic and familial neoplasm, *Cancer* 55:2818–2821, 1985.

108. Kapp D, LiVolsi V, Sanders M: Anaplastic carcinoma following well-differentiated thyroid cancer: etiological considerations, *Yale J Biol Med* 55:521–528, 1982.

109. Katoh R, Harach HR, Williams ED: Solitary, multiple and familial oxyphil tumors of the thyroid gland, *J Pathol* 186:292, 1998.

110. Khurana K and others: The role of fine-needle aspiration biopsy in the management of thyroid nodules in children, adolescents and young adults: a multi-institutional study, *Thyroid* 9:383, 1999.

111. Kim J, Leeper R: Treatment of locally advanced thyroid carcinoma with combination of doxorubicin and radiation therapy, *Cancer* 60:2372–2375, 1987.

112. Kirkland R and others: Solitary thyroid nodules in 30 children and report of a child with a thyroid abscess, *Pediatrics* 51:85, 1973.

113. Kitamura Y and others: Genetic alterations in thyroid carcinomas, *Nippon Ika Diagaku Zasshi* 66:319, 1999.

114. Kroll T and others: PAX8-PPARgamma1 fusion oncogene in human thyroid carcinoma, *Science* 289:1357, 2000.

115. Kupferman M and others: Safety of completion thyroidectomy following unilateral lobectomy for well-differentiated thyroid cancer, *Laryngoscope* 112:1209–1212, 2002.

116. Lange W, Choritz H, Hundeshagen H: Risk factors in follicular thyroid carcinoma: a retrospective follow-up study covering a fourteen year period with emphasis on morphologic findings, *Am J Surg Pathol* 10:246–255, 1986.

117. Lange W and others: The differentiation of atypical adenomas and encapsulated follicular carcinoma in the thyroid gland, *Virchows Arch A Pathol Anat Histopathol* 385:125–141, 1980.

118. La Quaglia M and others: Recurrence and morbidity in differentiated thyroid carcinoma in children, *Surgery* 104:1149–1156, 1988.

119. Leeper R: Thyroid carcinoma, *Med Clin North Am* 69:1079–1096, 1985.

120. Lennquist S, Kahlin C, Smeds S: The superior laryngeal nerve in thyroid surgery, *Surgery* 102:1000–1008, 1987.

121. LiVolsi V: Papillary neoplasms of the thyroid, pathologic and prognostic features, *Am J Clin Pathol* 3:426–434, 1992.

122. LiVolsi V, Merino M: *Pathology of thyroid tumors.* In Thawley S and others, editors: *Comprehensive management of head and neck tumors.* Philadelphia, 1987, WB Saunders.

123. Lo C, Lam K: Postoperative hypocalcemia in patients who did or did not undergo parathyroid autotransplantation during thyroidectomy: a comparative study, *Surgery* 124:1081, 1998.

124. Lore J, Kim DJ, Elias S: Preservation of the laryngeal nerves during total thyroid lobectomy, *Ann Otol Rhinol Laryngol* 86:777–788, 1977.

125. Mack E: Management of patients with substernal goiters, *Surg Clin North Am* 75:377–394, 1995.

126. Malone J and others: Thyroid consequences of Chernobyl accident in the countries of the European Community, *J Endocrinol Invest* 14:701–717, 1991.

127. Mandel S and others: Superiority of iodine-123 compared with iodine-131 scanning for thyroid remnants in patients with differentiated thyroid cancer, *Clin Nucl Med* 26:6–9, 2001.

128. Marchetta F, Saro K, Matskura H: Modified neck dissection for carcinoma of the thyroid gland, *Am J Surg* 120:452, 1970.

129. Massin J and others: Pulmonary metastases in differentiated thyroid carcinoma: study of 58 cases with implications for the primary tumor treatment, *Cancer* 53:982–992, 1984.

130. Maxon HR, Smith HS: Radioactive 131I in the diagnosis and treatment of metastatic well-differentiated thyroid carcinoma, *Endocrine Metab Clin North Am* 19:695–717, 1990.

131. Mazzaferri E: Evaluation and management of common thyroid disorders in women, *Am J Obstet Gynecol* 176:507–514, 1997.

132. Mazzaferri E: Management of a solitary thyroid nodule, *N Engl J Med* 320:553–559, 1993.

133. Mazzaferri E: Thyroid cancer in thyroid nodules: finding a needle in a haystack, *Am J Med* 93:359–362, 1992.

134. Mazzaferri E, Jhiang SM: Long-term impact of initial surgical and medical therapy on, papillary and follicular thyroid cancer, *Am J Med* 97:418–428, 1994.

135. Mazzaferri E, Young R: Papillary thyroid carcinoma: a 10 year follow-up report of the impact of therapy in 576 patients, *Am J Med* 70:511–518, 1981.

136. Mazzaferri E and others: Papillary thyroid carcinoma: the impact of therapy in 576 patients, *Medicine* 56:171–196, 1977.

137. McConahey W and others: Papillary thyroid carcinoma treatment at Mayo Clinic 1946 through 1970: initial manifestations, pathologic findings, treatment and outcome, *Mayo Clin Proc* 61:978–996, 1986.

138. McHenry C and others: Nodular thyroid disease in children and adolescents, *Ann Surg* 54:444–447, 1988.

139. McHenry C, Walfish PG, Rosen IB: Non-diagnostic fine needle aspiration biopsy: a dilemma in management of nodular thyroid disease, *Am J Surg* 59:415–419, 1993.

140. McTiernan A, Weiss NS, Daling JR: Incidence of thyroid cancer in women in relation to known or suspected risk factors for breast cancer, *Cancer Res* 47:292–295, 1987.

141. Meier C, Braverman LE, Ebner SA: Diagnostic use of recombinant human thyrotropin in patients with thyroid carcinoma (phase I/II study), *J Clin Endocrinol Metab* 78:188–196, 1994.

142. Meissner W, Adler A: Papillary carcinoma of thyroid, *Arch Pathol* 656:518, 1958.

143. Miller J, Kinsi SR, Hamburger JI: Diagnosis of malignant follicular neoplasm of the thyroid by needle biopsy, *Cancer* 55:2812–2817, 1985.

144. Mobley J, DeBenedetti MK: Patterns of nodal metastases in palpable medullary thyroid carcinoma: recommendations for extent of node dissection, *Ann Surg* 229:880–887, 1999.

145. Moley J: Medullary thyroid cancer, *Surg Clin North Am* 75:405–420, 1995.

146. Moley J and others: Preservation of the recurrent laryngeal nerves in thyroid and parathyroid reoperations, *Surgery* 125:673, 1999.

147. Moosa M, Mazzaferri EL: Outcome of differentiated thyroid cancer diagnosed in pregnant women, *J Clin Endocrinol Metab* 82:2862–2866, 1997.

148. Morris P: Thyroid cancer complicating pregnancy, *Obstet Gynecol Clin North Am* 25:401–408, 1998.

149. Namba H, Rubin SA, Fagin JA: Point mutations of ras oncogenes are an early event in thyroid tumorigenesis, *Mol Endocrinol* 4:1474–1479, 1990.

150. Nel C, van Heerden JL, Goellner J: Anaplastic carcinoma of thyroid: a clinicopathologic study of 82 cases, *Mayo Clin Proc* 60:51–58, 1985.

151. Nemiroff PM, Katz AD: Extralaryngeal divisions of the recurrent laryngeal nerve: surgical and clinical significance, *Am J Surg* 144:466–469, 1982.

152. Netterville J, Aly A, Ossoff RH: Evaluation and treatment of complications of thyroid and parathyroid surgery, *Otolaryngol Clin North Am* 23:529–552, 1990.

153. Noguchi S, Murakami N: The value of lymph node dissection in patients with differentiated thyroid cancer, *Surg Clin North Am* 67:251–261, 1987.

154. O'Riordain D and others: Multiple endocrine neoplasia type 2B: more than an endocrine disorder, *Surgery* 118:936–942, 1995.

155. Ozata M, Suzuki S, Miyamoto T: Serum thyroglobulin in the follow-up of patients with treated differentiated thyroid cancer, *J Clin Endocrinol Metab* 79:98, 1994.

156. Park H, Park YH, Zhou XH: Detection of thyroid remnant/metastasis without stunning: an ongoing dilemma, *Thyroid* 7:277–280, 1997.

157. Pasieka J and others: The incidence of bilateral well-differentiated thyroid cancer found at completion thyroidectomy, *World J Surg* 16:711–717, 1992.

158. Pasieka J and others: Addition of nuclear DNA content to the AMES risk-group classification for papillary thyroid cancer, *Surgery* 112:1154–1160, 1992.

159. Pepper G, Zwicker D, Rosen Y: Fine needle aspiration of the thyroid nodule: results of a start-up project in a general teaching hospital setting, *Arch Intern Med* 149:594–596, 1989.

160. Pingpank JJ and others: Tumor above the spinal accessory nerve in papillary thyroid cancer that involves lateral neck nodes: a common occurrence, *Arch Otolaryngol Head Neck Surg* 128:1275–1278, 2002.

161. Prendiville S and others: Prognostic implications of the tall cell variant of papillary thyroid carcinoma, *Otolaryngol Head Neck Surg* 122:352–357, 2000.

162. Prentice R and others: Radiation exposure and thyroid cancer incidence among Hiroshima and Nagasaki residents, *Natl Cancer Inst Monogr* 62:207, 1982.

163. Price D: Radiographic evaluation of the thyroid and the parathyroids, *Radiol Clin North Am* 31:991, 1993.

164. Rallison M and others: Thyroid nodularity in children, *JAMA* 233:1069, 1975.

165. Rasbach D and others: Malignant lymphoma of the thyroid gland: a clinical and pathologic study of 20 cases, *Surgery* 6:1166–1170, 1985.

166. Raue F, Frank-Raue K, Grauer A: Multiple endocrine neoplasia type 2: clinical features and screening, *Endocrinol Metab Clin North Am* 23:137–156, 1994.

167. Ringel M and others: Overexpression and overactivation of AKT in thyroid carcinoma, *Cancer Res* 61:6105, 2001.

168. Rodriguez J and others: Comparison between preoperative etiology and intraoperative frozen-section biopsy in the diagnosis of thyroid nodules, *Br J Surg* 81:1151, 1994.

169. Rojeski M, Gharib H: Nodular thyroid disease, *N Engl J Med* 313:418–436, 1985.

170. Rosai J: Papillary carcinoma, *Monogr Pathol* 35:138, 1993.

171. Rosai J, Carcangui ML, DeLellis RA, editors: *Tumors of the thyroid gland. In Atlas of thyroid pathology.* Washington, DC, 1992, AFIP.

172. Rosen I, Korman M, Walfish PG: Thyroid nodular disease in pregnancy: current diagnosis and management, *Clin Obstet Gynecol* 40:81–89, 1997.

173. Rosen I, Provias JP, Walfish PG: Pathologic nature of cystic thyroid nodules selected for surgery by needle aspiration biopsy, *Surgery* 100:606, 1986.

174. Rossi R and others: Malignancy of the thyroid gland: the Lahey Clinic experience, *Surg Clin North Am* 65:211–230, 1985.

175. Rougier P and others: Medullary thyroid carcinoma: prognostic factors and treatment, *Int J Radiat Oncol Biol Phys* 9:161–169, 1983.

176. Ruegemer J and others: Distant metastases in differentiated thyroid carcinoma: a multivariate analysis of prognostic variables, *J Clin Endocrinol Metab* 67:501, 1988.

177. Saad M and others: Medullary thyroid carcinoma: a study of the clinical features and prognostic factors in 161 patients, *Medicine* 63:319–342, 1984.

178. Sadler G and others: *Thyroid and parathyroid. In Schwartz S, editor: Principles of Surgery, ed 7, vol 2.* New York, 1999, McGraw-Hill, pp 1661–1713.

179. Salhany KE, Pietra GG: Extranodal lymphoid disorders, *Am J Clin Pathol* 99:472–485, 1993.

180. Samaan N, Schultz PN, Hickey RC: Medullary thyroid carcinoma: prognosis of familial versus sporadic disease and the role of radiotherapy, *J Clin Endocrinol Metab* 67:801–805, 1988.

181. Samaan N, Yang K, Schultz P: Diagnosis, management and pathogenetic studies in medullary thyroid carcinoma syndrome, *Henry Ford Hosp Med J* 37:132, 1989.

182. Samaan N and others: The results of various modalities of treatment of well-differentiated thyroid carcinoma: a retrospective review of 1599 patients, *J Clin Endocrinol Metab* 75:714, 1992.

183. Santoro M and others: Activation of RET as a dominant transforming gene by germline mutations of MEN 2A and MEN 2B, *Science* 267:381, 1995.

184. Santoro M and others: Gene rearrangement and Chernobyl related thyroid cancers, *Br J Cancer* 82:315, 2000.

185. Santoro M and others: Molecular defects in thyroid carcinomas: role of the ret oncogene in thyroid neoplastic transformation, *Eur J Endocrinol* 133:513–522, 1995.

186. Scheider A and others: Incidence, prevalence and characteristics of radiation-induced thyroid tumors, *Am J Surg* 64:243–252, 1978.

187. Schlumberger M, Tubiana M, DeVathaire F: Long term results of treatment of 283 patients with lung and bone metastases from differentiated thyroid carcinoma, *J Clin Endocrinol Metab* 63:960–967, 1986.

188. Segal K and others: Papillary carcinoma of the thyroid, *Otolaryngol Head Neck Surg* 113:356–363, 1995.

189. Sellers J: Prognostic significance of cervical lymph node metastasis in differentiated thyroid carcinoma, *Am J Surg* 164:578–581, 1992.

190. Sessions R, Harrison LB, Forastiere AA: *Tumors of the salivary glands and paragangliomas. In DeVita V, Hellman S, Rosenberg SA, editors: Cancer: principles and practice of oncology, ed 5.* Philadelphia, 1996, Lippincott-Raven.

191. Sessions R and others: *Cancer of the thyroid gland. In Harrison LB, Sessions RB, Hong WK, editors: Head and neck cancer: a multidisciplinary approach.* Philadelphia, 1999, Lippincott-Raven.

192. Shah A, Alfonso AE, Jaffe BM: Operative treatment of substernal goiters. *Head Neck* 11:325–330, 1989.

193. Shah J and others: Prognostic factors in differentiated carcinoma of the thyroid gland, *Am J Surg* 164:658–661, 1992.

194. Shankar L and others: Comparison of 123I scintigraphy at 5 and 24 hours in patients with differentiated thyroid cancer, *J Nucl Med* 43:72–76, 2002.

195. Shelton V, Skolnick G, Berlinger FG: Laryngotracheal invasion by thyroid carcinoma, *Ann Otol Rhinol Laryngol* 91:363–369, 1982.

196. Sherman S and others: Prospective multicenter study of treatment of thyroid carcinoma: initial analysis of staging and outcome. The National Thyroid Cancer Treatment Copperative Study Registry Group, *Cancer* 83:1012, 1998.

197. Sierra M and others: Prospective biochemical and scintigraphic evaluation of autografted normal parathyroid glands in patients undergoing thyroid operations, *Surgery* 124:1005–1010, 1998.

198. Silverman M: *Pathology of thyroid and parathyroid glands.* In Cady B, Rossi R: *Surgery of the thyroid and parathyroid glands*, Philadelphia, 1991, WB Saunders.

199. Simpson W and others: Papillary and follicular thyroid cancer: impact of treatment in 1578 patients, *Int J Radiat Oncol Biol Phys* 14:1063–1075, 1988.

200. Siperstein AE, Clark OH: *Surgical therapy.* In Braverman L, Utiger RD, editors: *Wener and Ingbar's the thyroid: a fundamental and clinical text,* ed 7. Philadelphia, 1996, Lippincott-Raven.

201. Sirota DK, Segal RL: Primary lymphomas of the thyroid gland, *JAMA* 242:1743–1746, 1979.

202. Sozzi G and others: Cytogenetic and molecular genetic characterization of papillary thyroid carcinomas, *Genes Chromosomes Cancer* 5:212–218, 1992.

203. Stepanas A and others: Medullary thyroid carcinoma: importance of serial calcitonin measurements, *Cancer* 43:825–837, 1979.

204. Szanto J, Vincze B, Sinkovics I: Postoperative thyroglobulin level determination to follow-up patients with highly differentiated thyroid cancer, *Oncology* 46:99, 1989.

205. Takahashi M and others: Molecular mechanisms of development of multiple endocrine neoplasia 2 by RET mutations, *J Intern Med* 243:509, 1998.

206. Takahashi M and others: Oncogenic activation of the ret proto-oncogene in thyroid cancer, *Crit Rev Oncog* 6:35–46, 1995.

207. Takeuchi Y and others: Mutations of p53 in thyroid carcinoma with an insular component, *Thyroid* 9:377, 1999.

208. Tallini G, Carcangiu ML, Rosai J: Oncocytic neoplasms of the thyroid gland, *Acta Pathologica Japonica* 42:305, 1992.

209. Tan R and others: Anaplastic carcinoma of the thyroid: a 24-year experience, *Head Neck* 17:41–48, 1995.

210. Tennvall J and others: Combined doxorubicin, hyperfractionated radiotherapy and surgery in anaplastic thyroid carcinoma: report on two protocols. The Swedish Anaplastic Thyroid Cancer Group, *Cancer* 74:1348–1354, 1994.

211. Thomas G and others: High prevalence of RET/PTC rearrangements in Ukranian and Belarussian post-Chernobyl thyroid papillary carcinomas: a strong correlation between RET/PTC3 and the solid follicular variant, *J Clin Endocrinol Metab* 84:4232, 1999.

212. Thompson M and others: Hürthle cell lesions of the thyroid gland, *Surg Gynecol Obstet* 139:555–560, 1973.

213. Tollefsen H, Shah JP, Huvos AG: Papillary carcinoma of the thyroid: recurrence in the thyroid gland after initial surgical treatment, *Am J Surg* 124:468–472, 1972.

214. Tronko M and others: Thryoid carcinoma in children and adolescents in Ukraine after the Chernobyl nuclear accident: statistical data and clinicomorphologic characteristics, *Cancer* 86:149, 1999.

215. Tsang R and others: Non-Hodgkin's lymphoma of the thyroid gland: prognostic factors and treatment outcome: the Princess Margaret Hospital Lymphoma Group, *Int J Radiat Oncol Biol Phys* 27:559–604, 1993.

216. Tubiana M, Haddad E, Schlumberger M: External radiotherapy in thyroid cancers, *Cancer* 55:2062–2071, 1985.

217. Tubiana M and others: Long-term results and prognostic factors in patients with differentiated thyroid carcinoma, *Cancer* 55:794–804, 1985.

218. Tucker H: Reinnervation of unilateral paralyzed larynx, *Ann Otol Rhinol Laryngol* 86:789–794, 1977.

219. Tyler D and others: Indeterminate fine-needle aspiration biopsy of the thyroid: identification of subgroups at high risk for invasive carcinoma, *Surgery* 116:1054–1060, 1994.

220. van Heerden J, Hay I, Goellner J: Follicular thyroid carcinoma with capsular invasion alone: a non-threatening malignancy, *Surgery* 112:1136–1138, 1992.

221. Vassiopoulou-Sellin R and others: Differentiated thyroid cancer in children and adolescents: clinical outcome and mortality after long-term follow-up, *Head Neck* 20:549, 1998.

222. Vassiopoulou-Sellin R and others: Pulmonary metastases in children and young adults with differentiated thyroid cancer, *Cancer* 71:1348–1351, 1993.

223. Vecchio G, Santoro M: Oncogenes and thyroid cancer, *Clin Chem Lab Med* 38:113, 2000.

224. Venkatesh Y, Ordonez N, Schultz P: Anaplastic carcinoma of thyroid: a clinicopathologic study of 121 cases, *Cancer* 66:321–330, 1990.

225. Voutilainen P and others: Anaplastic thyroid carcinoma survival, *World J Surg* 23:975, 1999.

226. Wang C: The anatomic basis of parathyroid surgery, *Ann Surg* 183:271-275, 1976.

227. Ward P, Berci G, Calcaterra TC: Superior laryngeal nerve paralysis, an often overlooked entity, *Trans Am Acad Ophthalmol Otolaryngol* 84:78–89, 1977.

228. Wartofsky L, editor: Using baseline and recombinant human TSH-stimulated Tg measurements to manage thyroid cancer without diagnostic 131I scanning, *J Clin Endocrinol Metab* 87:1486–1489, 2002.

229. Welch-Dinauer C and others: Clinical features associated with metastasis and recurrence of differentiated thyroid cancer in children, adolescents and young adults, *Clin Endocrinol* 49:619, 1998.

230. Wells S, Baylin S, Gann P: Medullary thyroid carcinoma: relationship of method of diagnosis to pathologic staging, *Ann Surg* 188:377–383, 1978.

231. Williams E: Mechanisms and pathogenesis of thyroid cancer in animals and man, *Mutat Res* 333:123–129, 1995.

232. Williams E and others: Thyroid cancer in an iodine rich area, *Cancer* 39:215–222, 1977.

233. Wohllk N and others: Relevance of RET proto-oncogene mutations in sporadic medullary thyroid carcinoma, *J Clin Endocrinol Metab* 81:3740, 1996.

234. Wolfe H and others: Distribution of calcitonin containing cells in the normal and neonatal human thyroid gland: a correlation of morphology with peptide content, *J Clin Endocrinol Metab* 41:1076, 1975.

235. Woolner L: Thyroid carcinoma: pathologic classification with data on prognosis, *Semin Nucl Med* 1:481–502, 1971.

236. Woolner L and others: Classification and prognosis of thyroid carcinoma: a study of 885 cases observed in a 30 year period, *Am J Surg* 102:354–387, 1961.

237. Woolner L and others: Occult papillary carcinoma of the thyroid gland: a study of 140 cases observed over a thirty year period, *J Clin Endocrinol* 20:89–105, 1960.

238. Yamashina M: Follicular neoplasms of the thyroid, *Am J Surg Pathol* 16:392–400, 1992.

239. Young R and others: Pure follicular carcinoma: impact of treatment in 214 patients, *J Nucl Med* 21:733–737, 1980.

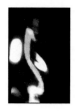

CHAPTER ONE HUNDRED AND TWENTY

SURGICAL MANAGEMENT OF PARATHYROID DISORDERS

Phillip K. Pellitteri
Robert A. Sofferman
Gregory W. Randolph

INTRODUCTION

The recorded history of hyperparathyroidism in modern medicine is relatively short. Sir Richard Owen, a renowned British anatomist and curator, is generally acknowledged as being the first to describe the existence of the parathyroid glands in 1852.[377] The discovery occurred subsequent to the death of the Zoological Society of London's Indian rhinoceros, the postmortem of which was conducted by Owen and subsequently reported to the Zoological Society. In 1877, the Swedish histologist Ivar Sandstrom reported the existence of distinct glandular tissue adjacent to the thyroid in a dog.[342] Over the subsequent 2 years, similar findings in other small mammals led to the search for, and ultimate discovery of, a similar organ in humans (glandulae parathyroideae), which Sandstrom reported on in 1880.

The earliest reports of clinical hyperparathyroidism involved bone disease, or osteitis fibrosa cystica, as termed by von Recklinghausen.[397] However, these reports, did not associate the characteristic changes in bone from hyperparathyroidism with parathyroid gland abnormalities. Askanazy,[15] in 1903, reported on an autopsy performed on a patient with osteomalacia and nonfusing long bone fractures in whom a large (>4 cm) tumor was seen adjacent to the thyroid gland, noting that it might represent a parathyroid tumor. It was not until Jacob Erdheim, a Viennese pathologist, discovered parathyroid gland morphologic and histologic abnormalities in patients with bone disease that an association between osteomalacia and parathyroid gland function was suspected. Erdheim studied the parathyroid glands by autopsy on all patients who died with bone disease and noted that many patients with osteomalacia and osteofibrosis cystica demonstrated enlarged parathyroid glands. He postulated that these glandular enlargements were secondary to compensatory hyper-

plasia and that the bone disease was the primary initiating factor.[109] Following up on initial experiments performed in rats by Eugene Gley, a French physiologist, Erdheim demonstrated that cautery destruction of the parathyroid glands in rats produced not only tetany, as shown by Gley, but also the typical dental changes consistent with calcium not being laid down.

Numerous reports of large parathyroid glands and bone disease followed until Schlagenhaufer suggested, at a meeting in Vienna in 1915, that if only a single parathyroid gland was thought to be enlarged, it should be excised.[341] The event that followed this suggestion years later would usher in the future treatment of parathyroid disease. Anton von Eiselberg, a pupil of Theodore Billroth, is noted as having performed the first parathyroid transplant. After performing total thyroidectomy in cats, von Eiselberg autografted the thyroid gland and a parathyroid gland into the animal's abdominal wall. Postoperatively the animals showed no sign of tetany, and, when subjected to histologic examination, these grafts demonstrated evidence of neovascularization.[396] William Halsted's experience with chronic hypocalcemia in thyroidectomy prompted him to study parathyroid transplantation experimentally in dogs. He demonstrated that even very small portions of parathyroid tissue surviving autograft could be lifesaving in these animals and that their removal would result in tetany and death. In addition, he used intravenous calcium gluconate solution to treat animals after experimental thyroidectomy. These experiments and others sparked his ever-present mandate to perform thyroidectomy carefully and meticulously, avoiding injury to the parathyroid glands and their blood supply.[148]

Halsted worked with Herbert Evans, a medical student at Johns Hopkins, to define the blood supply to the parathyroid glands by use of a vascular casting technique and emphasized that tetany after thyroidectomy was caused more by interruption of the vascular supply to the parathyroid glands than by their inadvertent removal.

From a clinical standpoint the treatment of parathyroid disease was to change significantly with the work of Felix Mandle. Albert Gahne, a tram conductor, lived in Vienna after a bout with tuberculosis, which he acquired while serving in the Army during the years 1914 to 1918. He subsequently had bone pain and muscle fatigue in 1921 from which he became disabled. In 1924, after a fall that resulted in a fractured femur, he came under the treatment of Mandle, who recognized these events as being consistent with parathyroid disease. Believing that this might represent compensatory parathyroid hyperplasia as postulated by Erdheim, Mandle administered fresh parathyroid extract to Albert without improvement. Subsequently, Mandle transplanted fresh parathyroid glands obtained from the victim of a street accident into Albert, which again did not result in any resolution of symptoms. Recalling Schlagenhaufer's suggestion of nearly 10 years earlier, Mandel explored the neck of the now severely crippled tram conductor and removed a parathyroid tumor.[233] Albert experienced a remarkable and immediate improvement in bone pain and nearly 4 years later was walking with a cane free of pain. The disease recurred, and the patient was subsequently reexplored but did not survive after the procedure.[18] This experience illustrated several important issues that would come to influence future work with surgical parathyroid disease, including clinical use of parathyroid transplantation in humans and the treatment of recurrent disease by re-exploration.

That same year (1924), Hanson developed a potent extract of the parathyroid glands, which, when injected into animals, led to increased serum calcium, decreased phosphate, and elevated output of calcium in the urine. When used chronically, this extract would produce osteoporosis in the animals.[77] The association of elevated blood calcium levels and parathyroid dysfunction was well acknowledged when Charles Martell, a sea captain, was evaluated at the Massachusetts General hospital in 1927 and found to have hypercalcemia and generalized demineralization of the skeleton believed to be caused by hyperparathyroidism. The first two of a total of six operations performed on Captain Martell was by Dr. E. Richardson, Chief of Surgery at MGH. These first two neck explorations yielded only a single normal parathyroid gland on each side without identification of abnormal tissue.[319] A third neck exploration was performed in New York in 1929 by Dr. Russell Patterson without success. As renal function began to deteriorate with increasing symptoms of hyperparathyroidism, he returned to MGH under the care of Fuller Albright and Oliver Cope. Cope had experience in several parathyroid explorations under the supervision of Churchill and began cadaver dissection in preparation for re-exploration of Martell, which he did on three occasions in 1932 without success. At the urging of Captain Martell, who had read extensively about his own disease and the potential locations of ectopic parathyroid tissue, a mediastinal exploration, the seventh surgical procedure on Martell, was planned by Churchill. With Cope assisting, Churchill identified and removed most of a 3-cm tumor from the mediastinum, leaving an attached remnant portion with its vascular pedicle intact to avoid profound hypocalcemia. Despite these measures, tetany developed postoperatively that required treatment with calcium supplementation. Several weeks after surgery, Captain Martell experienced renal colic from an impacted ureteral stone, which required surgery. Unfortunately, this remarkable patient died from laryngospasm after an operation to relieve obstruction from the impacted stone. Interestingly, although the series of procedures performed on Captain Martell received more notoriety, the first successful parathyroidectomy performed in the United States took place in 1928 at Barnes Hospital of Washington University by Dr. Isaac Olsch. In this instance, a large adenoma was removed, precipitating a profound fall in serum calcium that required massive doses of parathyroid extract[149,319] and intravenous calcium to save the patient.

The Nobel work of Berson and Yalow in 1963 paved the way for accurate identification of parathyroid hormone levels in serum and heralded a new era in the presentation of patients with parathyroidism. Coupled with this, multichannel autoanalyzing systems rapidly assessed blood chemical components, including calcium, in a routine fashion, thus changing the manner in which patients with hyperparathyroidism present for treatment. Instead of renal stones and bone abnormalities, patients are asymptomatic without significant subjective complaints and very few (if any) clinical signs. In most instances, the only abnormality facing the surgeon is an elevated serum calcium and parathyroid hormone level. It is on these findings and the assessment of risk of end organ damage that the modern-day surgeon treating parathyroid disorders must base his or her management decisions.

ETIOLOGY AND PATHOGENESIS OF HYPERPARATHYROIDISM

Parathyroid adenomas seem to be monoclonal or oligoclonal neoplasms, whereby the mechanism of propagation is thought to be clonal expansion of cells that have an altered sensitivity to calcium.[12] Arnold's work indicates that the molecular events that seem to trigger clonal propagation are heterogeneous. The genetic mutational events that occur in hyperparathyroidism have been characterized in a minority of tumors. Among those events identified are genetic rearrangements of the PRAD1, or parathyroid adenomatosis 1 oncogene, also known as cyclin D1. This protooncogene is located in the vicinity of the regulatory region of the gene for parathyroid hormone (PTH) production[13,118] (Figure 120-1). Subsequent realignment of DNA in this event now combines a growth promoter (PRAD1) with a regulatory region that controls PTH synthesis. This genetic realignment has not been uniformly demonstrated in most parathyroid adenomas, with only a minimal number having been shown to manifest rearrangement.

Another common molecular event, postulated to occur in parathyroid neoplasia, is alteration in tumor suppressor gene expression (Figure 120-2). For this gene to be inactivated and thus product deficient, both alleles on the gene must be affected by the mutational event. Thus, tumorigenesis occurs as a sequential event by inactivation of both copies of the suppressor gene.[11] The most well known of these is the MEN1 tumor suppressor gene that demonstrates somatic mutations in both gene copies in 20% of patients with primary hyperparathyroidism.[164] Not surprisingly, this gene was initially recognized in patients with the MEN1 syndrome.[371] Evidence of loss of suppressor gene function on chromosome 1p has been postulated as being an even more common event in the development of sporadic parathyroid adenomas. It has been suggested that patients with this chromosomal abnormality may be subject to the same constellation of endocrine changes found in MEN1 syndrome.[11] Suspected loss of tumor suppressor gene function has been identified in other chromosomal loci in patients with parathyroid adenomas, including sites 15q, 9p, 6q, and 1q.[11]

Point mutations in the calcium-sensing receptor gene that reduced the activity of this gene have been explained as the basis for familial hypocalciuric hypercalcemia (FHH) and neonatal severe hyperparathyroidism.[306] Thus, it would seem that this gene would represent a likely candidate for molecular rearrangement and altered calcium-sensing function in patients with hyperparathyroidism. To date, however, a calcium-sensing receptor gene mutation or allelic inactivation has not been demonstrated in these patients. It has been postulated that alterations in the calcium-sensing function in primary hyperparathyroidism may represent postgenomic events related to reduced RNA or protein receptor activity in the parathyroid cell clone.[202] Whether this may represent the primary cause for, or secondary effect of, hypercalcemia remains to be determined. Abnormalities in the parathyroid cells' vitamin D receptor similarly may represent changes occurring

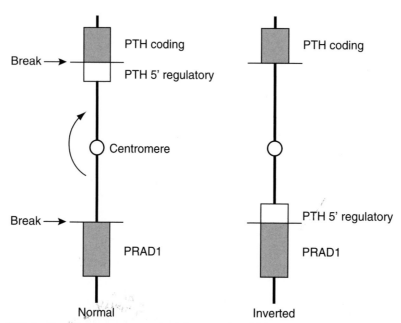

Figure 120-1. Genetic rearrangement of the parathyroid hormone gene in primary hyperparathyroidism. Pericentromeric inversion of chromosome 11 illustrating PRAD 1 and PTH gene rearrangement. (From Arnold A: *J Clin Endocrinol Metab* 77:1108, 1993. The Endocrine Society; reprinted with permission.)

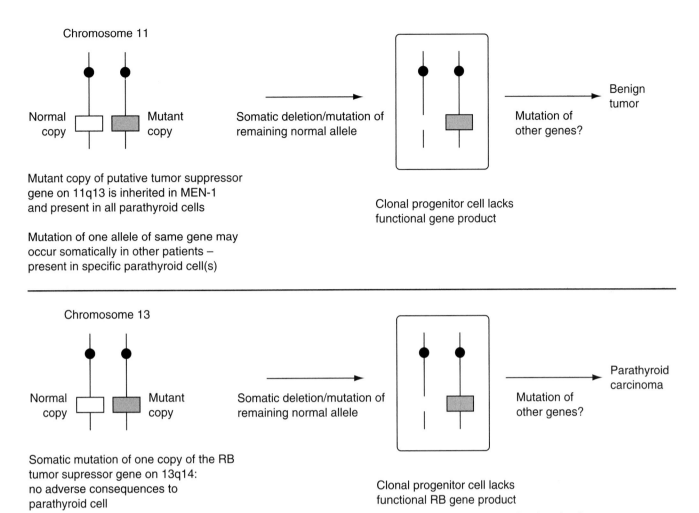

Figure 120-2. Hypothesized roles of inactivated tumor suppressor genes in the development of parathyroid neoplasia. (From Arnold A: *J Clin Endocrinol Metab* 77:1108, 1993. The Endocrine Society; reprinted with permission.)

secondary to hypercalcemia and not a primary genetic event. An inactivating mutation in the gene coding for this receptor has been postulated in primary hyperparathyroidism, but results from these investigations are conflicting.[49]

Firm evidence supports the theory that ionizing radiation can represent the etiologic factor in several human cancers. Tisell[385] observed that there seems to be an association between exposure to ionizing radiation to the head and neck at an early age and the late development of hyperparathyroidism. This finding is supported by other independent observations in which hyperparathyroidism has developed, presumably as a late complication of radiation therapy to the head and neck, similar to the finding noted with differentiated thyroid cancer.

CALCIUM HOMEOSTASIS AND PARATHYROID HORMONE SECRETION AND REGULATION

Calcium homeostasis is maintained by the complex interrelationship of parathyroid hormone, vitamin D and its derivatives, and calcitonin. The polypeptide parathyroid hormone (PTH) contains 84 amino acids. Once secreted by the parathyroid glands, it undergoes degradation into the amino(N) and carboxyl(C)-terminal fragments. The N-terminal fragment is biologically active but is rapidly cleared from the circulation, whereas the C-terminal fragment is biologically inert, is predominately cleared from the circulation by the kidney, and, therefore, persists for a longer time, particularly in patients with renal failure.[142,310] The intact 1-84 molecule is the major circulating form of biologically active parathyroid hormone; therefore, assays that measure the intact hormone more clearly reflect dynamic changes in PTH metabolism compared with the previous polyvalent assays that measured a predominately inactive section of the PTH molecule.[281]

The release of PTH is regulated predominately by serum ionized calcium levels. Parathyroid hormone is secreted in response to a decrease in serum-ionized calcium and is inhibited by an increase of serum-ionized calcium. Ionized calcium is considered to be the physiologically active component of total serum calcium.

The major target end organs for PTH action are the kidneys, skeletal system, and intestine.[274] Parathyroid hormone functions by binding to receptor sites in bone and kidney, which results in stimulation of the production of cyclic adenosine monophosphate (cAMP), which acts to carry out the cellular response of that specific target tissue to PTH.

The primary response to PTH by the kidney is to increase the tubular resorption of calcium and to decrease the tubular resorption of phosphorus.[248,362] The action of PTH on bone to regulate serum calcium is through the remodeling effect of osteoclast and osteoblast activity. The osteoblasts and their precursor cells in bone have a parathyroid hormone receptor site, and binding to this site results in the production of cAMP. The osteoclasts do not have a PTH receptor site but are stimulated indirectly through the cAMP response in the osteoblasts.[245] The last important function of PTH occurs by increasing the rate of conversion in the kidney of 25-hydroxy vitamin D_3 (calcifediol) to 1,25-dihydroxy vitamin D_3 (calcitriol).[240] The coordinated actions of PTH on bone, kidney, and intestine increase the flow of calcium into the extracellular fluid and as a consequence increases the serum calcium levels.

Parathyroid hormone is therefore the primary regulator of rapid changes of extracellular calcium levels. The action of vitamin D affects delayed changes in calcium balance as opposed to the more immediate direct action of PTH.[274] Calcitonin plays a much smaller role in calcium homeostasis. Calcitonin is secreted by the parafollicular cells of the thyroid gland and inhibits bone resorption. Calcitonin tends to be decreased in postmenopausal women and may be increased by estrogen administration in these patients. Extremely high levels of calcitonin found in medullary carcinoma of the thyroid gland do not result in hypocalcemia.[119]

Several endogenous substances, including peptides, steroid hormones, and amines, have been found to influence PTH release.[40,42] However, calcium represents the most potent regulator of PTH secretion. Minor alterations within the physiologic calcium concentration range can induce considerable secretory responses (i.e., reduction of ionized plasma calcium by 0.04 mM/L may elevate serum parathyroid hormone by 100% or more). The rapid effect of extracellular calcium on PTH release suggests that calcium directly interferes with the release process, but the nature of this interference has only been partly clarified. It has been demonstrated that external calcium mainly regulates secretion of newly synthesized hormone, which may bypass the relatively few secretory granules in the parathyroid's chief cells.[143] Intracellular degradation with release of carboxy-terminal PTH fragments occurs especially at high extracellular calcium concentrations. This attenuates the biologic activity of the secretory product, because the calcium-regulating properties of PTH reside predominantly in its amino terminal portion.

Messenger RNA levels for PTH are increased within hours by low extracellular calcium, consistent with the effects of calcium on PTH secretion.[266,420] Furthermore, calcitriol (1,25-dihydroxy vitamin D_3) lowers parathyroid hormone mRNA levels and inhibits parathyroid hormone secretion.[351]

Abnormalities in calcium-controlled PTH release represent a fundamental characteristic of the pathologic parathyroid tissue from hypercalcemic patients with parathyroid adenoma and hyperplasia of varying etiologies.[159,399] The representative disturbance is characterized by variable calcium insensitivity of PTH secretion. The extent of the calcium insensitivity of ionized calcium and PTH release correlates to the degree of hypercalcemia in the patient.[399]

Intact parathyroid hormone 1-84 is rapidly cleared from the human circulation and has a half-life of only a few minutes.[323] Parathyroid hormone clearance mainly depends on high capacity uptake of Kupffer's cells in the liver and on glomerular filtration. A small amount of PTH, however, appears in the urine because of tubular resorption and proteolysis. Circulating PTH is heterogeneous and contains various carboxy terminal peptide sequences arising by cleavage, mainly at residues 33 to 43. Although approximately 15% of intact PTH 1-84 is metabolized to such circulating fragments, they make up at least half, and sometimes substantially more, of the immunoactive PTH in the circulation.[235] The metabolism of such fragments depends virtually only on an intact renal function; consequently, they are accumulated to considerable degrees in renal insufficiency. In contrast, very few amino terminal PTH fragments exist in the circulation of euparathyroid individuals, although these fragments may become appreciable in both primary and secondary hyperparathyroidism.

The diagnosis of primary hyperparathyroidism and evaluation of the extent or severity of secondary hyperparathyroidism have been facilitated by the development of immunometric "sandwich" assays.

These assays use a pair of antibodies that recognize different regions of the PTH protein sequence.[22,31,44] Because of cooperative effort of the antibodies, such a sandwich assay is more sensitive than either of the antibodies alone in displacement radioimmunoassays. With careful selection of antibodies, the immunometric assays are specific and sensitive for intact PTH, which allows identification of insufficient PTH secretion of hypoparathyroidism, as well as a wide range of PTH levels without sample dilution. The immunometric analyzing process is swifter than radioimmunoassays. With a reduction in the incubation times, the analysis may be accomplished in 15 to 30 minutes and, consequently, may be applicable intraoperatively.[183,283]

Clinical analysis with immunometric PTH assays usually discriminates hypercalcemic patients with hyperparathyroidism from patients with other causes of hypercalcemia. This is particularly evident with regard to malignancies of nonparathyroid origin, although some 5% to 10% of these patients demonstrate intact serum PTH in the low normal range. Nonparathyroid tumors that produce intact PTH are exceptionally rare. These include ovarian and small cell carcinomas, as well as thymoma.[280,369,422]

PARATHYROID ANATOMY AND HISTOPATHOLOGY
The Normal Parathyroid Gland

The usual weight, size, and fat content of a normal parathyroid gland remain variable. The weight of a normal gland has been recorded to be as low as 40 mg, and a limit of 50 to 60 mg has been suggested.[102] One study demonstrated that the weights of normal parathyroid glands have a skewed distribution.[102] The mean total weight in the study was 29.5 ± 17.8 mg, with an upper limit of 65 mg. However, the actual value for the 98th percentile was 75 mg, and this correlates with the operative findings typically noted in primary hyperparathyroidism.

The influence of chronic illness, race, and other individual variations may affect the weights of normal parathyroid glands. In patients with chronic illness, total glandular weights are lower; in men and black patients, total glandular weights are higher. Glands that are removed from the patient may show wide variations in weight. One gland may be much smaller than another, and sometimes two glands may be small.

The dimensions of normal glands are rarely mentioned in the literature. Normal dimensions of 3 to 6 mm in length, 2 to 4 mm in width, and 0.5 to 2 mm in thickness, as well as an average of three dimensions of $5 \times 3 \times 1$ mm, have been proposed.[55] Normal glands as large as 12 mm and greater have been reported.[400]

Glandular weight, rather than glandular dimension, is accepted as a better measure of size. For the surgeon, knowing the normal dimensions of parathyroid glands is extremely important. In most operative situations, enlargement of parathyroid glands is determined by the surgeon in the operating room through a judgment of size rather than assessment of weight. The determination of weight or density requires the removal of the glands, which may not be indicated in all circumstances.

The stromal fat content of parathyroid glands is the hallmark in the evaluation of their functional status. Detailed studies of normal glands have demonstrated wide variations in fat content.[87,101] The accepted percentage of normal fat content is approximately 50%. One study indicated that more than 75% of normal parathyroid glands had less than 30% stromal fat, 50% had less than 10%, and only a small number had 40%.[87] The variability of fat content reported by different studies suggests that measurement of stromal fat within parathyroid glands has become nearly useless as a indicator of function.[87,101] In children and adolescents, parathyroid glands contain very sparse amounts of fat. After adolescence, stromal fat progressively increases until 25 to 30 years of age, and then, subsequently, fat content is largely determined by constitutional factors. Women seem to have a tendency to have higher glandular fat content, which may be related to total body fat concentrations.[140]

The characteristic cellular content of the normal gland is dominated by chief cells with rare water-clear cells. The concentration of oxyphilic cells tends to increase with age and is noted to be relatively rare in young individuals. Oxyphilic cell concentrations seem to be more common in adults older than 40 years of age.

The presence of four parathyroid glands is the usual number found in human beings. In dissection studies of 428 human subjects by Gilmore, four parathyroid glands were found in 87% of all patients, and three parathyroids were found in 6.3%.[132] Akerström and others[5] reported comparable rates in an autopsy study of 503 individuals. Four parathyroids were found in 84% and three parathyroid glands in 3% of all patients in this study. The presence of supernumerary parathyroid glands is a rare occurrence, which otherwise may have important clinical consequences, especially with respect to patients with hyperparathyroidism resulting from multiple gland disease. In a series of 2015 patients who were operated on for primary hyperparathyroidism, a hyperfunctioning supernumerary fifth parathyroid was the source of hypercalcemia in 15 patients (0.7%).[329] Nine of these patients required reoperation to remove the supernumerary gland representing the parathyroid tumor. Most of these fifth gland tumors were located in the mediastinum, either in the thymus (n = 7) or related to the aortic arch (n = 3). Edis and Levitt[106] reported a rate of persistent hyperparathyroidism of 10% resulting from an enlarged supernumerary parathyroid gland in patients with secondary hyperparathyroidism. Wang,[406] in a series of 762 patients with primary hyperparathyroidism, documented six patients with persistent hyperparathyroidism caused by hyperfunctional supernumerary glands (0.6%), all of which were located in or in close association with the thymus. In the previously mentioned study by Gilmore, supernumerary parathyroid glands were observed in 29 of 428 specimens (6.7%).[132] Five parathyroids were observed in 25 specimens (5.8%), 6 parathyroids in 2 specimens (0.05%), 8 parathyroids in 1 specimen, and 12 parathyroids in 1 other specimen. From both the Gilmore and Akerström studies, it is evident that supernumerary parathyroids are most commonly found within the thymus or in relation to the thyrothymic tract.[5,132]

Parathyroid Gland Location

The location of parathyroid glands may be quite variable as a consequence of the variation in degree of migratory descent during development. Additional influences on these variable locations involve displacement of enlarged parathyroid glands during the development of hyperparathyroidism. Enlarged parathyroid glands will tend to migrate in a fibroareolar plane that offers little resistance as a result of gravity and the action of swallowing and variations in intrathoracic pressure.[78]

Eighty percent of the superior parathyroid glands are found at the cricothyroid junction approximately 1 cm cranial to the juxtaposition of the recurrent laryngeal nerve and the inferior thyroid artery.[5] The superior parathyroids, which are intimately associated to the posterior capsule of the superior thyroid pole, are usually covered by an extension of the pretracheal fascia that envelopes the thyroid gland and connects it to both the hypopharynx/esophagus and the carotid sheath. The relationship of these superior parathyroid glands with the pretracheal fascia is such that the glands themselves are allowed freedom of movement under this "pseudocapsule." This feature discriminates parathyroid glands from thyroid nodules that cannot move freely because they are enveloped by the true capsule of the thyroid gland.

Normal superior parathyroid glands may be found in the retroesophageal or paraesophageal space in approximately 1% of all instances.[382] These spaces represent sites where enlarged superior parathyroid glands potentially descend to the superior/posterior mediastinum.

The inferior parathyroid glands tend to have a more variable location. More than 50% of the inferior parathyroid glands are situated near the lower pole of the thyroid gland. Twenty-eight percent of the inferior parathyroids are found within the thyrothymic ligament or within the anterior superior mediastinal thymic gland. The migratory pattern of inferior parathyroid glands tends to follow a pathway into the anterior superior mediastinum, where as many as one third of all missed parathyroid tumors may be found.

The incidence of intrathyroidal parathyroid glands is controversial. Akerström noted true superior intrathyroidal parathyroid glands in three instances (0.2%) among 503 autopsy specimens.[341] Wang[402] considered the superior parathyroid gland the most likely to be intrathyroidal, primarily because of the close embryologic relationship of the primordium of the superior parathyroid gland with the lateral complex of the thyroid. However, in a series by Wheeler in which 8 intrathyroidal parathyroid tumors were noted in 7 of 200 patients (3.5%) undergoing neck exploration, 7 of these intrathyroidal glands were considered to originate from the inferior position. The overall incidence of intrathyroidal parathyroid glands ranges from approximately 0.5% to 3% as reported in the literature.[21,74,161,197]

Morphologic Characteristics of Parathyroid Glands

The visible discrimination between normal and abnormal hyperfunctioning parathyroid glands is essential to successful parathyroid surgery. The appearance of both normal and abnormally functioning parathyroid glands is quite variable and dependent on the anatomic position and relationship to the thyroid capsule. Parathyroid glands that are located in loose connective tissue generally have a shape that is more characteristically oval, bean, or teardrop appearance. When parathyroid glands are closely juxtaposed to the thyroid capsule compressed by the pretracheal fascia, their appearance tends to be more conforming, resulting in a flat shape with well-defined edges. The color of normal parathyroid glands ranges from yellowish brown to reddish brown. In general, the color may depend on the amount of stromal fat, oxyphilic cell concentration, and degree of vascularity.[89] Normal glands tend to be more reddish brown or rust colored in younger patients, whereas older individuals demonstrate parathyroid glands of a more yellow brown or tobacco color. Enlarged hyperfunctional parathyroid glands demonstrate a color variation from dark brown to light yellow. Enlarged glands occurring in either secondary or tertiary hyperparathyroidism may have a lighter gray tone to the coloration. Parathyroid carcinoma can also demonstrate a mottled gray to white surface appearance.

Vascular Anatomy of the Parathyroid Glands

Normal parathyroid glands most commonly are supplied by a single dominant artery (80%).[88] The length of the dominant artery supplying the parathyroid gland may vary from 1 to 40 mm. In most instances, both the superior and inferior parathyroid glands derive their dominant arterial blood supply from the inferior thyroid artery. However, ligation of the inferior thyroid artery during thyroid surgery may not always compromise the blood supply to the superior parathyroid gland. Abundant arterial anastomoses exist between the parathyroid glands and include anastomoses with thyroid arteries and dominant arteries of the larynx, pharynx, esophagus, and trachea. Twenty percent or more of the superior parathyroid glands may be vascularized solely by the superior thyroid artery. In an autopsy study by Delattre,[88] 10% of the inferior parathyroid glands derived their dominant arterial supply from a branch of the superior thyroid artery. In most of these instances, the inferior thyroid artery was noted to be absent. Primary mediastinal parathyroid glands have demonstrated an arterial supply that represents a thymic branch of the internal mammary artery.[403]

The venous drainage distribution of the parathyroid glands in general runs parallel to the arterial vessels and drains by way of the neighboring thyroid venous tributaries into the internal jugular system. Similarly, lymphatics from the parathyroid glands drain with those of the thyroid gland into the paratracheal and deep cervical lymphatic basins.

Histopathology of the Parathyroid Glands

The parathyroid glands are enveloped in their own thin collagenous connective tissue capsule. This capsule extends septae into the gland, which separates the parenchyma into elongated chords or clusters of functional secretory cells. Blood vessels, lymphatics, and nerves travel along the septae to reach the interior of the gland.[191]

The major functional parenchymal cells of the parathyroid glands are the chief cells, which are slightly eosinophilic staining and measure 5 to 8 mμm in diameter. The chief cells contain many cytoplasmic granules (200 to 400 nm in diameter) that arise from the Golgi complex and represent the secretory granules.[191] These granules contain parathyroid hormone, which is synthesized from a precursor of pre-proparathyroid hormone. With increasing age, the secretory cells of the parathyroid glands may be replaced by adipose cells, which may comprise 50% to 60% of the gland in older individuals.

The second cell type comprising parathyroid glandular parenchyma is the oxyphilic cell. Although their function is unknown, it is believed that oxyphil cells and a third cell type, sometimes described as intermediate cells, may represent inactive phases of a single cell type.[125] Oxyphil cells are less numerous, somewhat larger (6–10 mμm in diameter), and stain more deeply with eosin than chief cells. Oxyphil cells tends to be more mitochondrial rich, which may explain the increased ability of abnormal parathyroid glands with high oxyphilic cell concentrations to concentrate technetium 99m sestamibi.[300]

By electron microscopy, chief cells show Golgi apparatus among dispersed granular endoplasmic reticulum and few secretory granules. The resting chief cells contain abundant lipid and glycogen, whereas, during active phase, the chief cells are smaller in size and contain decreased amounts of glycogen and lipid.[189] The oxyphilic cells are characterized by their large size and numerous cytoplasmic mitochondria.[189]

Single Glandular Enlargement or Parathyroid Adenoma

Single glandular enlargement, or adenoma, is the single most common cause of hyperparathyroidism. Because of the variation in pathologic interpretation and patient population, however, the reported incidence of parathyroid adenoma varies widely between 30% and 90%.[73,90,129,189] In larger series of patients, where more uniformly accepted pathologic criteria were followed, approximately 80% to 85% of patients with primary hyperparathyroidism were found to have solitary parathyroid adenoma.[73,90,129]

Parathyroid adenoma may occur in any of the four parathyroid glands but may involve inferior glands more commonly than superior glands.[300]

The gross appearance of parathyroid adenomas is variable, but generally they are oval or bean-shaped, red brown in color, and soft in consistency.[114,417] Adenomas may be bilobed or multilobulated in conformation. In up to 70% of adenomas, a rim of normal parathyroid tissue may be found around the hypercellular portion of the replaced normal gland. However, the absence of this characteristic does not exclude the presence of a parathyroid adenoma. The incised surface of an adenoma may appear smooth, nodular, or may show obvious areas of cystic change. Under light microscopy, adenomas appear similar to normal parathyroid glands, exhibiting a thin fibrous capsule with a cellular framework arranged in nests and cords invested by a rich capillary network. Other growth patterns include follicular, pseudopapillary, and acinar patterns. Chief cells are the dominant cell types in most parathyroid adenomas. Oxyphil cells and transitional oxyphil cells are usually seen in varying proportions interspersed between the collections of chief cells.[114,390,417] The chief cells in adenomas may be larger than found in normal glands and may also exhibit a greater degree of nuclear pleomorphism and giant cell formation.[225,328] Nuclear atypia, however, is of limited value in distinguishing between parathyroid adenoma and carcinoma. Mitotic figures are uncommon in adenomas; however, they may be seen in a small percentage of cases.[335]

Variations in single glandular enlargement representative of parathyroid adenoma may occur and include the subtypes oncocytic adenoma, lipoadenoma, large clear cell adenoma, water-clear cell adenoma, and atypical adenoma. *Oncocytic adenoma* is a rare subtype of parathyroid adenoma (4.4%–8.4% of adenomas) that is composed predominantly (>80%–90%) or exclusively of oxyphil cells.[19,307] Previously adenomas of the oncocytic variety were thought to be nonfunctional; however, oxyphil adenomas associated with hyperparathyroidism have been reported.[14,70,418] Similar to typical adenomas, oncocytic tumors occur more frequently in women and are found most often in the sixth or seventh decade.[14,70] Grossly, the tumors tend to be large and have been reported to range in size from 0.2 to 61 g; they are soft, spherical, ellipsoid, lobulated, or nodular and range in color from light tan to dark orange-brown or mahogany.[70,292] Microscopically, the adenomas are composed predominantly of polygonal cells with abundant brightly eosinophilic granular cytoplasm and small round central hyperchromatic nuclei. Fat stain shows reduced cytoplasmic fat as per typical adenomas. Numerous mitochondria are densely packed throughout the cytoplasm on ultrastructural examination.

Lipoadenoma is another rare subtype of adenoma that was first described in 1958 as a parathyroid hamartoma.[288] The initial description was that of a nonfunctioning mass; subsequent reports documented that these lesions can be responsible for hyperparathyroidism.[1,85,150] The tumor is composed of a lobulated yellow-tan mass composed of nests, acini, and cords of chief cells and occasional oxyphil and clear cells, intimately associated with large areas of adipose tissue and/or myxoid stroma. A rim of normal parathyroid tissue may be present at the periphery.

Water-clear cell adenomas have been described, although their existence was initially doubted.[54] In contrast to the *large clear cell adenomas* that accumulate glycogen, true water-clear cell adenomas demonstrate a glycogen-free cytoplasm that is filled with membrane-bound vesicles.[138]

Atypical adenoma is the term that is used to describe parathyroid adenomas that exhibit atypical cytologic features without definite evidence of malignancy; that is, vascular and/or soft tissue invasion or metastases.[217] It is important to distinguish these benign lesions from parathyroid carcinoma. The malignant potential of atypical adenomas in terms of recurrent or metastatic behavior is uncertain. These lesions may exhibit conspicuous mitoses, adherence to surrounding tissues, trabecular cellular arrangements, capsular invasion, or broad fibrous bands.[91] One such lesion described consisted of a multifocal spindle cell proliferation that was mitotically active, averaging 8 mitoses per 10 high-power fields within an otherwise typical parathyroid adenoma.[9]

Multiple Enlarged Glands or Parathyroid Gland Hyperplasia

Primary parathyroid hyperplasia is defined as proliferation of the parenchymal cells leading to an increase in gland weight in multiple parathyroid glands in the absence of a known stimulus for parathyroid hormone secretion. Two types of parathyroid hyperplasia are seen: the common chief cell hyperplasia and the rare water cell or clear cell hyperplasia.[90,129]

Chief Cell Hyperplasia

Oliver Cope, in 1958, first demonstrated chief cell hyperplasia as a cause of primary hyperparathyroidism.[80] It accounts for approximately 15% of hyperparathyroidism in reported series; however, some reports have indicated that about half of primary hyperparathyroidism may be produced by hyperplasia. A variation in this reporting is generally attributable to discrepancies in pathologic interpretation of abnormal parathyroid glands. The stimulus for this disorder is not known; some studies have indicated the role of a possible circulating factor that can induce proliferation of parathyroid cells in culture. Approximately 30% of patients with chief cell hyperplasia have some type of familial hyperparathyroidism or one of the syndromes of multiple endocrine neoplasia (MEN).[4,90,129,405] Molecular studies have demonstrated that hyperplasias are ultimately associated with monoclonal proliferations.[13,118]

Grossly, there is enlargement of all four glands. The glands may be of variable size, or they may be uniformly enlarged. By light microscopy, the dominant cell types are chief cells; however, one may also observe intermixed oxyphil cells and transitional oxyphil cells. The cellular proliferations may also give rise to nodular formation, and this can cause asymmetric gland enlargement.[90,129]

The amount of cytoplasmic fat in the chief cells is either reduced or absent.[90,129] The chief cell in the nodular areas may be totally devoid of any fat, whereas the cells between the nodules may contain fat. Abnormal nuclei or mitoses are distinctly rare.[129]

Water-Clear Cell Hyperplasia

This form of hyperplasia is rare and is characterized by a proliferation of vacuolated water-clear cells in multiple parathyroid glands. It demonstrates a female predilection and leads to pronounced hypercalcemia and severe clinical disease. This represents the only parathyroid disorder in which the superior glands are larger than the inferior parathyroid glands. The glands affected by water-clear cell hyperplasia tend to be larger and more irregular in shape, with lobular extensions to surrounding soft tissue. By light microscopy, the glands demonstrate diffuse proliferations of clear cells characterized by clear cytoplasm and small dense nuclei. On high-power magnification, the cytoplasm is filled with small vacuoles. Cytoplasmic lipid is generally not present; however, moderate amounts of glycogen may be identified. The histologic appearance of water-clear cell hyperplasia bears a resemblance to that of renal cell carcinoma.[222]

Secondary parathyroid hyperplasia as a consequence of renal failure cannot be distinguished from primary hyperplasia, with the exception that early in the disorder there seems to be a greater tendency for the glands to be more uniform in size.[141] As the disease progresses, asymmetry becomes more evident in renal-induced disease. The degree of glandular enlargement tends to reflect the severity of the underlying renal disorder.[349] The largest glands are noted in patients whose renal disease began in childhood.[134]

Parathyroid Carcinoma

Parathyroid carcinoma is a rare malignant neoplasm derived from the parenchymal cells of the parathyroid glands. It has been reported to be responsible for 0.1% to 5.0% of cases of primary hyperparathyroidism.[285,358,391,404,419] It remains uncertain as to whether parathyroid carcinoma actually begins within preexisting benign parathyroid lesions.[209,358] Carcinoma has been postulated to arise in the setting of primary parathyroid hyperplasia, notably familial hyperplasia.[97,146,201] Only rare patients with parathyroid carcinoma have a history of prior neck irradiation.[285,358]

Morphologic features diagnostic of parathyroid malignancy are difficult in terms of definition and practical application during surgery. In one series of 40 patients with metastatic parathyroid cancer, as many as 50% were thought to have benign disease by the operating surgeon and consulting pathologist dur-ing the time of initial exploration.[332] Metastases are the only certain sign of malignancy. However, metastatic behavior at the time of presentation is distinctly rare.[404]

Parathyroid carcinomas are characteristically large tumors, with as many as 30% to 50% being palpable at the time of presentation.[391,404] The tumors may measure up to 6 cm in diameter, with a mean of approximately 3 cm.[404] Although the average weights of carcinomas are reported to be greater than those of adenomas, there seems to be great overlap, indicating that weight alone may not be a major distinguishing characteristic between benign and malignant lesions. Carcinomas generally arise in the usual parathyroid locations, although they have been described in ectopic supernumerary glands within the mediastinum.[196] Most parathyroid carcinomas are firm or hard in consistency and demonstrate a gray to white surface color as opposed to adenomas, which tend to be soft and tan in appearance. Adherence of the lesion to surrounding tissues is common, and these glands may be noted to extend to involve the soft tissues around the thyroid gland or the thyroid parenchyma itself. This may not prove to be a valuable differentiating feature, because previous hemorrhage into a benign adenoma may be associated with fibrosis and adherence to adjacent structures in benign disease.[358]

Metastases at the time of presentation are unusual but may rarely be found in regional lymph node basins.[332] As opposed to regional metastases, parathyroid carcinoma is more often associated with widespread local infiltration, with invasion into contiguous structures such as thyroid gland, strap muscles, trachea and the recurrent laryngeal nerve. Advanced metastases may occur and may be found in the lungs, bone, cervical and mediastinal lymph nodes, liver, and occasionally kidney and adrenal glands.[332,339] Pulmonary metastases are by far the most common distant metastasis noted.[332]

Microscopic diagnosis of parathyroid carcinoma is a difficult task. The entire gland is traversed by broad fibrous bands that seem to originate from the capsule and extend into the substance of tumor leading to a lobulated appearance. The cells may be clear or rarely oxyphilic and are arranged in nests and trabeculae.[285] The cell may be uniformly bland or may demonstrate metaplasia, but the cases with minimal atypical findings may be difficult to distinguish from an adenoma.[111,348,419]

Mitosis can be seen in most instances and has been suggested as a primary factor in diagnosing parathyroid carcinoma.[174] However, mitotic figures may also be seen in parathyroid adenoma and hyperplasia, and their absence does not rule out a diagnosis of carcinoma.[58,359] It is generally acknowledged that mitoses in parathyroid lesions should be of concern, especially because the follow-up in reported benign cases of parathyroid tumor exhibiting mitoses has been limited. Increased mitotic activity in unequivocal parathyroid carcinoma is an indicator of poor prognosis.[26]

The only reliable indicator of malignancy in parathyroid carcinoma is invasion of the surrounding structures and/or metastases.[26] Features such as desmoplastic reaction, mitotic activity, nuclear atypica and necrosis may be more common in carcinoma than in benign lesions but do not constitute criteria sufficient for a diagnosis of malignancy.[26] In the absence of an infiltrative growth pattern, the parathyroid lesion demonstrating some other feature of malignancy including mitoses may be designated as "atypical adenoma."[386] Nonfunctioning parathyroid carcinomas have been rarely described, tending to be large and consisting of clear or oxyphil cells.[246,421]

Parathyroid carcinoma usually grows slowly and can be an indolent tumor. Multiple recurrences after surgical resection are common and may occur over a 15- to 20-year period.[348,419] Patients with parathyroid carcinoma often die as a result of the effects of excessive PTH section and uncontrolled hypercalcemia rather than growth of the tumor mass. Surgical excision of recurrence or metastases may provide excellent palliation by reducing tumor burden and, consequently, hormone production.[350,425]

SURGICAL EMBRYO-ANATOMIC RELATIONSHIPS IN THE CENTRAL NECK

Parathyroid tissue originates from primordial pharyngeal endoderm formed in the third and fourth pharyngeal pouches during the fifth week of embryologic development (Figure 120-3). The epithelial lining of the dorsal wing of the third pharyngeal pouch differentiates into primordial parathyroid glandular tissue, whereas the ventral portion of the pouch differentiates into the thymus. As the thymus migrates medially and inferiorly, it pulls the inferior parathyroid gland (parathymus) with it into the thymic tail. Eventually, the main portion of the thymus migrates to its final position in the upper thoracic region, and its tail involutes, leaving the developing parathyroid gland to come to its position on the dorsal surface of the inferior pole of the thyroid gland. This glandular tissue eventually forms the inferior parathyroid gland. Simultaneously, the epithelium of the dorsal wing of the fourth pharyngeal pouch begins to differentiate into parathyroid glandular tissue. After separation from the regressing pouch, it becomes associated with the lateral portion of the caudally migrating thyroid and is carried a short distance

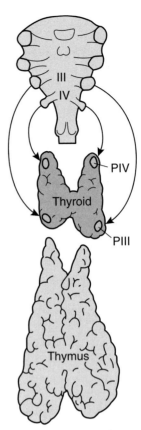

Figure 120-3. Illustration demonstrating embryologic derivation and subsequent descent of the parathyroid glands with associated structures.

medially and inferiorly until it resides posterior to the superior pole of the thyroid gland. This tissue eventually develops into the superior parathyroid gland. This embryologic pattern of development has significant implications for the identification of ectopic or normal glandular variance during the course of parathyroidectomy. The longer embryologic migration results in an extensive area of potential dispersal for the normal inferior parathyroid gland. In 61% of cases, they are situated at the level of the inferior poles of the thyroid lobes on the posterior, lateral, or anterior aspects. In 26% of cases, they are situated in the thyrothymic ligament or on the upper, cervical portion of the thymus. More rarely, in 7% of cases, they are situated higher up, at the level of the middle third of the posterior aspect of the thyroid lobes and may then be confused with the superior parathyroid gland. Because the embryonic descent of the thymus extends from the angle of the mandible to the pericardium, anomalies of migration of the parathymus, whether excessive or insufficient, are responsible for high or low ectopic locations of the inferior parathyroid gland. The incidence of higher ectopia along the carotid sheath, from the angle of the mandible to the lower pole of the thyroid, does not seem to exceed 1% to 2%.[5,117,221] Alternatively, if their separation from the thymus is delayed, the inferior parathyroid gland may be pulled inferiorly into the anterior mediastinum to a varying degree. In this circumstance, they are usually within the thymus, at the posterior aspect of its capsule, or still in contact with the great vessels of the mediastinum. Lower ectopic regions such as these are noted in 3.9% to 5% of instances.[162,221]

The superior parathyroid glands follow the thyroid migration of the ultimo branchial bodies, which travel toward the lateral part of the main medial thyroid rudiment. In contradistinction to the inferior glands, the superior parathyroids have a relatively limited descent within the neck. They remain in contact with the posterior part of the middle third of the thyroid lobes. This relatively limited course of embryonic migration explains why they remain relatively stable in their regional distribution when not pathologic. Thus, in most instances, they are grouped at the posterior aspect of the thyroid lobes, in an area 2 cm in diameter, whose center is situated about 1 cm above the crossing of the inferior thyroid artery and the recurrent laryngeal nerve.[221,381] Because of the more extensive descent of the inferior parathyroid gland, the descent of the parathymus will result in the inferior and superior glands crossing during development. This embryonic crossing of the glands explains why their grouping at the level of the inferior thyroid artery, at the junction of the middle and inferior thirds of thyroid lobe, is in many respects quite close, depending on the degree of migration of the inferior parathyroid gland.

Because of the short migratory descent of the superior parathyroid gland, the area of dispersal of these glands is limited, and thus congenital ectopic positions of the superior gland are unusual. In 13% of instances, the glands are on the posterior aspect of the superior pole of the thyroid lobe in a laterocricoid, lateropharyngeal, or cricothyroid position. In less than 1% of instances, they are above the upper pole of the lobe. In 1% to 4% of instances they are clearly posteriorly behind the pharynx or esophagus. Parathyroid glands that are found in the posterior superior mediastinum are usually neoplastic superior parathyroid glands that have migrated as a consequence of gravity and changes in intrathoracic pressure.[381]

CLINICAL FEATURES OF PRIMARY HYPERPARATHYROIDISM
Incidence

The incidence of hyperparathyroidism has changed dramatically over the past three decades. In the early 1970s, before the widespread use of multichannel autoanalysis of blood chemistry, Heath reported an annual incidence of 7.8 cases per 100,000 persons in Rochester, Minnesota.[154] After the introduction of routine serum calcium assessment later in the 1970s, the incidence rate rose dramatically to 51 cases per 100,000 persons per year. After the most prevalent or clinically significant cases were managed, the incidence declined to 27 cases annually per 100,000, and recent reports indicate that within the population associated with this area of Minnesota, a steady decline in the incidence of hyperparathyroidism since the late 1970s has been noted. This cannot be explained by the more limited routine use of multichannel autoanalyzing of blood, which has become part of cost-saving measures in the late 1990s; nor has this declining incidence been similarly experienced in other populations nationally or internationally. A higher rate of incidence was noted in the "Stockholm Study," which examined more than 15,000 subjects over a 2-year period (1971–1973) with a follow-up at 10 years. The early rate was assessed at 6 cases per 1000 persons that, at the 10-year follow-up, was verified to be 4.4 cases per 1000 persons. This rate has not changed appreciably over a 20-year period, in contrast to the Rochester experience.[69] One may postulate that the Rochester experience is unique in that after securing a very high incidence rate promulgated by routine calcium screening, higher prevalence cases were eliminated to reveal a lower base incidence rate in a population that receives its treatment at a single major center.

There seems to be a distinct predilection for this disease to have higher incidence in women, especially those patients beyond menopause. The highest prevalence rate among women in the Stockholm experience confirmed at the 10-year follow-up was approximately 13 per 1000, which represented a female/male ratio of about 4:1. This experience is similar to that of other published reports.[29,145,154,188,416] Several of these studies based on serum calcium screening have shown that the prevalence of primary hyperparathyroidism in the general population is at 0.1% to 0.3% and in women older than 60 years more than 1%.[69,154,295] The clear female preponderance points to the fact that every woman has a 1% risk of experiencing primary hyperparathyroidism during her lifetime. It has been estimated, however, that approximately 90% of people with primary hyperparathyroidism remain undiagnosed.[223] The screening of serum calcium has been a particularly important factor leading to the detection of patients with mild symptoms or no symptoms, especially among postmenopausal women.

Presentation

The concept of clinical features associated with primary hyperparathyroidism has changed during recent years. So-called classic, specific symptoms (i.e., bone disease, renal stones, and hypercalcemic crisis) represent obvious manifestations of the disease. The relative proportion of patients with osteitis fibrosis cystica, nephrolithiasis, and hypercalcemic crisis has continuously decreased in clinical series because of the increase in the number of patients with nonspecific or inapparent symptoms. Currently, osteitis fibrosis occurs in about 1% of patients and only 10% to 20% of patients have renal stones.[153,212,322] Nonspecific symptoms will include malaise, fatigue, depression and other psychiatric symptoms, sleep disturbance, loss of weight, abdominal pains, constipation, vague musculoskeletal pains in the extremities, and muscular weakness. The term "asymptomatic hyperparathyroidism" has been commonly applied when the disorder is detected during health screenings and population studies or coincidentally during medical examinations. The usual presenting abnormality in these patients is an abnormally elevated serum calcium level detected on routine blood chemistry screening. Despite the lack of obvious abnormalities noted at the time of diagnosis, caution should be exercised before declaring that a patient is asymptomatic. A number of seemingly asymptomatic patients may manifest subtle or even "silent sequelae" of hyperparathyroidism at the time of presentation. In fact, these patients may be more appropriately described as minimally symptomatic in that nonspecific symptoms and unidentified complications of hyperparathyroidism would be eliminated by parathyroidectomy.[375] Some of these nonspecific entities include emotional complaints, muscular fatigue, constipation, bone and joint pain, and silent objective findings such as asymptomatic renal calculi and decreased bone mineral density. In most patients with asymptomatic or minimally symptomatic hyperparathyroidism, these symptoms are subtle and may be so common in the general population that they preclude establishment of a causal relationship to primary hyperparathyroidism.

Among patients in whom symptoms are present or evolving at the time of diagnosis, two populations may be identified. In the first group, the disease progresses insidiously over several years and eventually presents as renal colic. The second group manifest symptoms over a considerably shorter period of time with marked elevations in serum calcium leading to weight loss, acute gastrointestinal symptoms, anorexia, bone pain, and occasionally pathologic fracture. Traditionally, clinical manifestations are described according to the organ system affected.

Kidney/Urinary Tract

Historically, greater than 50% of patients with hyperparathyroidism have renal symptoms manifested by nephrolithiasis and nephrocalcinosis. This percentage decreased significantly to approximately 4% after the widespread use of screening tests for serum calcium levels.[156] Most stones are composed of calcium oxylate; however, calcium phosphate stones may also occur. The symptoms associated with urolithiasis include renal colic, hematuria, and pyuria. Metabolic acidosis may also be a part of the clinical syndrome.

Skeletal System

Abnormalities of the skeletal system in the form of osteitis fibrosis cystica, once a common malady in patients with primary hyperparathyroidism, are now rarely encountered (<10%). These changes include subperiosteal erosion of the distal phalanges, bone wasting and softening, and chondrocalcinosis as a result of bone demineralization. Bone disease may prevent as bone pain, pathologic fracture, cystic bone changes, or focal areas of bone swelling (epulis of the jaw or "brown tumors") representing accumulations of osteoclasts, osteoblasts, and fibrous matrix. Symptoms attributable to joint pathology include gout and pseudogout.

Bone loss in hyperparathyroidism occurs at cortical bone sites generally sparing trabecular bone.[368] Because of this finding, the role of hyperparathyroidism in osteoporosis is not clear, especially for patients in whom symptoms are minimal or absent and in whom the disease is mild.

Postmenopausal women with primary hyperparathyroidism exhibiting early signs of osteoporosis seem to be at significant risk for more severe bone disease and resultant sequelae (i.e., vertebral and hip fractures). It is in this population of patients that the benefit of parathyroidectomy is most apparent.[352]

Neuromuscular

Muscle weakness, particularly in the proximal extremity muscle groups, together with progressive fatigue and malaise, may occur in symptomatic primary hyperparathyroidism. Electromyographic changes may be seen in these patients together with atrophy of the skeletal muscle on biopsy.[119,238,291] Although the severe symptoms are rarely encountered, some signs of muscle fatigue and weakness may be present in as many as 40% of patients with mild primary hyperparathyroidism.[267] Usually, these subtle symptoms are manifested as muscle aches and fatigue on rising from a chair or climbing stairs. Progression of the disease may ultimately result in weakness that limits activity and ambulation over a short period of time (weeks to months). This "neuromuscular syndrome" is noted to improve in 80% to 90% of the patients affected after parathyroidectomy.[142,310]

Neurologic

Neurologic manifestations of primary hyperparathyroidism are represented by a spectrum of symptoms ranging from anxiety and mild emotional disturbance to frank psychosis. Depression, nervousness, and cognitive dysfunction may commonly occur to varying degrees in primary hyperparathyroidism. Cerebral dysfunction characterized by organic brain syndrome is more common in elderly patients with an underlying mild cognitive abnormality exposed to hypercalcemia. Other neurologic changes occasionally seen in patients with hyperparathyroidism include deafness, dysphagia, dysosmia, and dysesthesia.[243] Many of the psychiatric symptoms in patients with primary hyperparathyroidism are improved after parathyroidectomy.[142,219] Fifty percent of patients with depression or anxiety, or both, will improve after surgery. A favorable affect has also been shown in about 50% of patients with organic brain syndrome and dementia. Some older people experience dramatic improvement; however, it is impossible to predict whether any specific patient will improve after surgery.[219]

Gastrointestinal

Gastrointestinal disorders that may occur in hyperparathyroidism include acid peptic disease, pancreatitis, and cholelithiasis. Peptic ulceration occurs with increased frequency in these patients secondary to increased serum gastrin and gastric acid secretion stimulated by hypercalcemia. Hyperparathyroidism may be the heralding manifestation of endocrine disease in patients with MEN 1 syndrome. Those patients exhibiting the Zollinger-Ellison syndrome demonstrate the highest incidence of peptic ulceration. The lower gut may be affected by hyperparathyroidism as well. Frequently patients with "asymptomatic disease" complain of sluggish bowels or constipation that improves after surgery and achievement of normocalcemia.

Cardiovascular

Hypertension may occur in as many as 50% of patients with hyperparathyroidism.[160] Convincing evidence of a pathogenic mechanism does not exist, however, and parathyroidectomy results in a reduction in blood pressure in a minority of these patients.[211] Swedish investigators reported an association with myocardial ischemia and left ventricular dysfunction in patients with hyperparathyroidism of varying symptomology, which exhibited reversibility after parathyroidectomy.[273]

Hypercalcemic Abnormalities

Hypercalcemic syndrome occurring as a result of hyperparathyroidism includes polydipsia and polyuria, anorexia, vomiting, constipation, muscle weakness and fatigue, mental status changes, and skin abnormalities.

Those patients who have markedly elevated serum calcium levels approaching 15 mg/dL may be seen with severe mental status changes or coma, a so-called hypercalcemic crisis. If untreated, this condition may progress to acute renal failure and the onset of dysrhythmias, which may precipitate sudden death.[81] Other abnormalities include metastatic calcifications at the corneal/scleral junction, so-called band keratopathy, shortened Q-T interval on electrocardiogram, ectopic calcium deposits in various organs, and pruritus. In addition, some patients may have a nonspecific debility manifested by anorexia, fatigue, anemia, weight loss, and advancing osteitis, all of which are reversible after parathyroidectomy.

Clinical Course of Untreated Hyperparathyroidism

There have been several 8- to 10-year prospective studies that have demonstrated a relatively benign course of untreated mild hyperparathyroidism in most patients, with no significant progression of symptoms, hypercalcemia, bone marrow density loss, or renal function impairment. No pathologic fractures or kidney stones developed during these observation periods.[86,296] However, there was evidence of disease progression in up to 27% of patients, including marked hypercalcemia, hypercalcuria, or loss of bone mineral density up to 10%.[354]

The clinical manifestations of hyperparathyroidism tend to relate to the level of hypercalcemia, even if this is not always evident because of slowed disease progression, individual susceptibility, and gender- and age-dependent symptoms. Younger men are particularly prone to experience renal stones, sometimes even with only mild hypercalcemia. For renal stones, the individual susceptibility is more than the level of hypercalcemia, and the risk of this particular symptom is probably more efficiently revealed by the patient history. In postmenopausal women, renal stones occur infrequently (generally <5%) and are often clinically silent. Osteitis fibrosis cystica is currently an uncommon finding in patients with primary hyperparathyroidism and is most often seen in patients with severe and longstanding hypercalcemia. Bone density measurements have, however, demonstrated an average reduction in cortical bone of 17% among current patients with primary hyperparathyroidism, and the bone loss tends to be the most pronounced in postmenopausal women.[86,255,354] Total and trabecular bone mass is often reduced, but to a lesser degree than that of cortical bone.[212] No bone loss has been detected in postmenopausal women with borderline hypercalcemia, but losses are significant when the serum calcium level was >2.74 mM/L.[255]

Clinically evident renal failure is currently an unusual complication of primary hyperparathyroidism. Reduction of creatinine clearance and urinary concentrating capacity, however, occur in more than one third of patients with mild hypercalcemia, indicating that impairment of glomerular and tubular function may occur silently.[255] Serum creatinine measurements are crude estimates and will rise only after creatinine clearance is substantially reduced. Serum creatinine levels also decrease with declining muscle mass of aging.[255]

Rare patients with initially mild hypercalcemia but rapidly advancing disease may have parathyroid carcinoma.[309] In addition, stepwise "clinical progression" may occur during observation in patients with primary hyperparathyroidism, possibly representing development of secondary mutations that cause accelerated growth of the tumor. Bleeding in parathyroid tumor may also cause an abrupt rise in serum calcium levels. Thus, a history of mild primary hyperparathyroidism has been reported in up to one third of patients with hypercalcemic crisis. Because it is not yet possible to predict whether progressive disease will occur in any patient, extended follow-up is crucial if surgery is deferred in primary hyperparathyroidism.[25,115,336] Younger patients seem to be at greater risk for progressive disease. Accordingly, medical surveillance is inappropriate in younger patients and in those with more marked hypercalcemia. The indications for surgical intervention and the alternative of medical surveillance will be discussed later in this chapter.

DIAGNOSIS OF HYPERPARATHYROIDISM
Evaluation of Hypercalcemia

Hypercalcemia has been reported as occurring in 1% to 3.9% of the general adult population and 0.2% to 2.9% of hospitalized patients.[120] These patients have widely variable clinical symptoms, depending on the severity of the elevated serum calcium. In most situations, mild hypercalcemia is asymptomatic, but severe hypercalcemia may become life threatening, especially when the serum calcium is elevated above 14.0 mg/dL.

The definition of hypercalcemia depends on the range of normal serum calcium. In general, this is reported as 8.5 to 10.5 mg/dL. Variations in this normal range, as reported by various laboratories, depends largely on differences in assay procedures. Forty-seven percent of circulating serum calcium

binds to proteins, and approximately 10% binds primarily to albumin and/or complexes to circulating anions such as bicarbonate, phosphate, citrate, or sulfate. The remaining 43% is found as the free ionized form. Only the free ionized form of serum calcium exerts physiologic effects. Serum ionized calcium is the major regulator of PTH secretion.

Several factors may influence measured serum total or ionized calcium. Alterations in serum albumin level will increase or decrease serum total calcium without affecting the ionized calcium level. Seventy percent of the circulating calcium that is bound to protein is albumin bound, having 12 calcium-binding regions per molecule. Under normal circumstances, only approximately 20% of these specific calcium-binding sites are actually occupied by serum calcium. Decreases in serum albumin to <4.0 g/dL decrease total calcium by 0.8 mg/dL for each 1.0 g/dL decrease in serum albumin. Correspondingly, increases in serum albumin >4.0 g/dL increase serum total calcium by 0.8 mg/dL for 1.0 g/dL increase in serum albumin. Dehydration may increase total serum calcium because of the resulting hemoconcentration. Acidosis increases serum ionized calcium by decreasing binding of calcium to albumin, and alkalosis decreases ionized calcium by increasing binding of calcium to albumin, without affecting serum total calcium. Under most clinical circumstances, it is adequate and appropriate to measure serum total calcium, but serum ionized calcium should be measured in those clinical situations that may be associated with changes in albumin concentration or serum pH.[346]

Serum calcium reflects the balance between calcium influx into and calcium efflux from extracellular fluid. Calcium influx into extracellular fluid is derived from intestinal absorption, skeletal resorption, and renal reabsorption, and calcium efflux from extracellular fluid is determined by intestinal secretion, skeletal uptake, and renal excretion. Hypercalcemia, accordingly, usually results when the rate of calcium influx into the extracellular fluid exceeds the rate of calcium efflux from the extracellular fluid.

The differential diagnosis of hypercalcemia is varied and extensive. It remains valid that the most common etiology of hypercalcemia in nonhospitalized patients is primary hyperparathyroidism and that the most common source of hypercalcemia in hospitalized patients is malignancy. In most circumstances, the differential diagnosis of hypercalcemia may be categorically divided into that which is mediated by PTH and those causes that are not (see Tables 120-1 to 120-3). Hypercalcemia that is mediated by PTH is most frequently caused by primary hyperparathyroidism (Table 120-1). In addition, physiologic secondary

TABLE 120-1
CAUSES OF PTH-MEDIATED HYPERCALCEMIA
Primary hyperparathyroidism
Parathyroid adenoma
Parathyroid lipoadenoma
Parathyroid hyperplasia
Parathyroid carcinoma
Neck or mediastinal parathyroid cyst
Secondary hyperparathyroidism
Tertiary hyperparathyroidism

hyperparathyroidism, which is defined as hyperparathyroidism caused by a physiologic source without associated renal insufficiency or pathologic secondary hyperparathyroidism with associated renal failure, may result in parathyroid hormone–mediated hypercalcemia.

Secondary hyperparathyroidism from a nonrenal physiologic source may occur in patients with insufficient calcium intake, decreased intestinal calcium absorption, insufficient vitamin D intake or malabsorption, or renal hypercalciuria and represents the homeostatic attempt to maintain a normal serum calcium level by any means necessary. It is important to distinguish physiologic secondary hyperparathyroidism from primary hyperparathyroidism before embarking on surgical correction of presumed primary hyperparathyroid disease.

Pathologic secondary hyperparathyroidism and tertiary hyperparathyroidism occur as a result of renal insufficiency or renal failure. Hyperparathyroidism associated with these conditions results from subtle ionized hypocalcemia persisting over months to years, resulting in chronic stimulation of the parathyroid glands. Parathyroid glands may become autonomous after long-standing renal disease and, as a consequence, no longer respond to regulation by serum-ionized calcium in the course of developing tertiary hyperparathyroidism. An important entity that must be considered in the differential diagnosis of hypercalcemia is familial hypocalciuric hypercalcemia (FHH).[214,237] This disorder has the ability to mimic the serum biochemical appearance of primary hyperparathyroidism but is not treated surgically. Familial hypocalciuric hypercalcemia is an autosomal-dominant disorder that is linked to chromosomes 3q, 19p, and 19q and is largely caused by inactivating mutations in the parathyroid cell calcium-sensing receptor.[43] Patients with FHH have low 24-hour urinary calcium excretion relative to their hypercalcemia. At present, the most useful study to distinguish FHH from primary hyperparathyroidism is the 24-hour urinary calcium/creatinine clearance ratio.[237]

Patients with FHH typically have ratios of <0.01, whereas patients with primary hyperparathyroidism have ratios >0.01.

The second most common etiology of hypercalcemia is malignancy (Table 120-2). The humoral hypercalcemia of malignancy (HHM), which is caused by excessive parathyroid hormone–related protein (PTHrp) secretion by tumors of various types represents the most common source of malignancy-associated hypercalcemia.[139] An extensive list of solid tumors has been reported to secrete excessive PTHrp, including cancers of the lung, esophagus, head and neck, kidney, ovary, bladder, breast, and pancreas. Others that have been variably noted to secrete PTHrp include thymic carcinoma, islet cell carcinoma, malignant carcinoid, and hepatic carcinomas. Patients with adult T-cell leukemia or lymphoma or B-cell lymphoma have also been variably demonstrated to produce excess PTHrp.[176,259,263]

Ectopic PTH secretion has been demonstrated in small cell lung cancer, small cell ovarian carcinoma, squamous cell lung carcinoma, ovarian adenocarcinoma, thymoma, papillary thyroid carcinoma, hepatocellular carcinoma, and undifferentiated neuroendocrine tumor.[175,280] Ectopic 1,25-dihydroxy vitamin D has been found to be secreted by B-cell lymphomas, Hodgkin's disease, and lymphomatoid granulomatosis.[3,38,324,340,343] Excessive cytokine production, which may result in hypercalcemia, has been associated with T-cell lymphomas and leukemias, non-Hodgkin's lymphomas, and other hematologic malignancies.

TABLE 120-2
CAUSES OF HYPERCALCEMIA OF MALIGNANCY
PTHrp secretion by lung, esophagus, head and neck, renal cell, ovary, bladder, and pancreatic cancers, thymic carcinoma, islet cell carcinoma, carcinoid, sclerosing hepatic carcinoma
Ectopic PTH secretion by small cell lung cancer, small cell ovarian carcinoma, squamous cell lung carcinoma, ovarian adenocarcinoma, thymoma, papillary thyroid carcinoma, hepatocellular carcinoma, undifferentiated neuroendocrine tumor
Ectopic 1,25 dihydroxyvitamin D production by B-cell lymphoma, Hodgkin's disease, lymphomatoid granulomatosis
Lytic bone metastases caused by multiple myeloma, lymphomas, breast cancer, invasive sarcoma
Tumor production of other cytokines by T-cell lymphomas/leukemias, non-Hodgkin's lymphoma, and other hematologic malignancies

Another source of hypercalcemia resulting from malignancy is that of calcium released by extensive lytic bone metastasis as a consequence of multiple myeloma, lymphomas, breast cancer, or invasive sarcomas.[260]

A broad list of causes of non-PTH–mediated hypercalcemia is noted in Table 120-3. Nine tumors, including ovarian dermoid cysts or uterine fibroids, may occasionally secrete PTHrp or other bone-resorbing cytokines.[203] Endocrine disorders, including thyrotoxicosis (resulting from increased bone resorption), pheochromocytoma (caused by coexisting primary hyperparathyroidism in multiple endocrine neoplasia syndrome), adrenal insufficiency or crisis (caused by volume depletion or hemoconcentration), and VIPomas (resulting from excess secretion of vasoactive intestinal peptide causing dehydration and metabolic acidosis), may also cause non-PTH–mediated hypercalcemia.[47,261,363,394,395] Granulomatous disease in the absence of malignancy or endocrine disorder may be a source of hypercalcemia, especially in younger and middle-aged patients and may present with elevated serum calcium levels. The source of this hypercalcemia is generally increased production of 1,25-dihydroxy vitamin D and has been demonstrated in patients with sarcoidosis, Wegner's granulomatosis, berylliosis, silicone- or paraffin-induced granulomatosis, eosinophilic granuloma, focal or disseminated tuberculosis, histoplasmosis, coccidioidomycosis, candidiasis, leprosy, and cat scratch disease.*

Medications may serve as the etiology of hypercalcemia through a variety of mechanisms. Excessive vitamin D intake or, hypervitaminosis D, may stimulate intestinal calcium absorption, and thiazide diuretics may directly inhibit renal calcium excretion.[302,308] Lithium compounds may interfere with the ability of calcium to interact with both parathyroid and renal calcium-sensing receptors, thereby increasing PTH secretion by the parathyroid glands.[144] A number of other agents, including estrogens, antiestrogens, or androgens, aminophylline or theophylline, ganciclovir, recombinant growth hormone in AIDS patients, and hypervitaminosis A, may affect other physiologic mechanisms resulting in hypercalcemia.** A spectrum of miscellaneous disorders that can also be associated with hypercalcemia are listed in Table 120-3.

Primary Hyperparathyroidism—Diagnosis

The diagnosis of primary hyperparathyroidism is usually straightforward and is based on minimal criteria

---

*References 2, 8, 30, 104, 133, 168, 192, 201, 206, 297, 320, 365, 398.
**References 32, 127, 215, 244, 330, 338, 389.

TABLE 120-3

CAUSES OF NON-PTH–MEDIATED, NONMALIGNANT HYPERCALCEMIA

Benign tumors: PTH resecreting ovarian dermoid cyst or uterine fibroid
Endocrine disease
  Thyrotoxicosis
  Pheochromocytoma
  Addison's disease
  Islet cell pancreatic tumors
  VIPoma
Granulomatous disorders
  Sarcoidosis
  Wegener's granulomatosis
  Berylliosis
  Silicone- and paraffin-induced granulomatosis
  Eosinophilic granuloma
  Tuberculosis (focal, disseminated, MAC in AIDS)
  Histoplasmosis
  Coccidioidomycosis
  Candidiasis
  Leprosy
  Cat-scratch disease
Drugs
  Vitamin D excess (oral or topical)
  Vitamin A excess
  Thiazide diuretics
  Lithium
  Estrogens and antiestrogens
  Androgens
  Aminophylline, theophylline
  Ganciclovir
  Recombinant growth hormone treatment of AIDS patients
  Foscarnet
  8-chloro-cyclic AMP
Miscellaneous
  Familial hypocalciuric hypercalcemia
  Immobilization with or without Paget's disease of bone
  End-stage liver failure
  Total parenteral nutrition
  Milk-alkali syndrome
  Hypophosphatasia
  Systemic lupus erythematosus
  Juvenile rheumatoid arthritis
  Recent hepatitis B vaccination
  Gaucher's disease with acute pneumonia
  Aluminum intoxication (chronic hemodialysis)
  Manganese intoxication
  Primary oxalosis

---

involving the serum total calcium and measurement of intact PTH levels. In general, patients will usually have increased serum total calcium levels, with overtly increased or inappropriately high normal parathyroid hormone levels. Some patients with surgically proven primary hyperparathyroidism will have a high normal serum total calcium level and inappropriately high normal or increased parathyroid hormone levels. It is important to recognize that patients with primary hyperparathyroidism almost always have documented increased serum total or ionized calcium sometime during their course, recognizing that serum calcium exhibits some variation over time. Patients in whom serum calcium documentations are noted to be in the mid to lower normal range over time may prove difficult with reference to establishing a diagnosis of primary hyperparathyroidism, even if they are found to have increased intact PTH levels. This is due to the possibility that these patients have physiologic secondary hyperparathyroidism as has been discussed earlier in this section. Patients with mid to lower normal serum calcium levels associated with increased intact parathyroid hormone levels should be further evaluated to make sure that they do not have low calcium or vitamin D intake, calcium or vitamin D malabsorption, inability to convert 25-hydroxy vitamin D to biologically active 1,25-dihydroxy vitamin D, or significant hypercalciuria. These entities could explain why parathyroid hormone levels are increased in the setting of mid to low normal serum calcium determinations.

Patients with primary hyperparathyroidism usually have serum phosphate levels in the low-normal to mildly decreased range. Patients with simultaneously high normal or increased serum calcium and high normal or increased serum phosphate should be investigated further for intestinal hyperabsorptive states or hypervitaminosis D.

Intact PTH, determined by the current immunoradiometric (IMRA) or immunochemiluminometric (ICMA) assays, is mildly increased or inappropriately high normal for the level of simultaneously measured serum calcium in patients with primarily hyperparathyroidism. The use of current assays prevents any cross-reactivity between PTH and PTH-related protein, making the distinction between primary hyperparathyroidism and PTH-related protein-mediated hypercalcemia of malignancy certain. Patients with primary hyperparathyroidism almost always have suppressed PTH-related protein levels when checked, and patients with PTH-related protein-mediated hypercalcemia of malignancy almost always have suppressed intact PTH levels. Patients who are receiving thiazide diuretics or lithium compounds may demonstrate mild hypercalcemia and increased intact PTH levels without coexisting primary hyperparathyroidism, and so it is important to remove these medications for at least 1 month before assessing levels of serum total calcium and intake parathyroid hormone to make the correct diagnosis. Those hypercalcemic

patients who are being treated with thiazides or lithium therapy and who have coexisting primary hyperparathyroidism will have persistent hypercalcemia and increased intact parathyroid hormone levels after discontinuation of the medication.

Accurate diagnosis of primary hyperparathyroidism is essential before surgical exploration and attempted parathyroidectomy. Careful attention to the biochemical parameters as described, with special notice of the serum total calcium, phosphate, and intact parathyroid hormone levels, is essential in making the correct diagnosis. A 24-hour total urinary calcium level is also important in eliminating the possibility of FHH from the differential diagnosis.

LOCALIZATION STUDIES AND THEIR APPLICATION

Although a comprehensive bilateral exploration of all appropriate cardinal parathyroid locations in the surgical management of hyperparathyroidism remains the "gold standard" and must be fundamental to the armamentarium of all parathyroid surgeons, the development of more effective imaging methods or parathyroid localization have permitted surgeons to use more limited procedures in neck exploration, while achieving the same, or improved, surgical outcomes as those achieved by four-gland exploration.[300,387] Aside from the application of these imaging techniques for parathyroid localization in more limited, focused explorations of the neck for primary hyperparathyroidism, the use of localization studies before re-exploration for persistent or recurrent hyperparathyroidism has been universally accepted.[99,278,410] Localization methods may be operationally classified as *preoperative* (invasive or noninvasive) and *intraoperative* (Table 120-4).

Noninvasive Preoperative Localization
Pertechnetate (Tc 99m) Thallous Chloride (Tl 201) Imaging

Thallium uptake by parathyroid adenomas was initially reported by Fukunaga and others.* Subsequently, Ferlin and Young performed the clinical application using technetium-99m together with thallium 201.[113,424] Subtraction of the resulting two images helped to locate the abnormal parathyroid gland or glands. This technique required prolonged patient immobilization for obtaining images, because the patient remained in the same position for both radionuclide administrations. Results of this localization technology have been variable, with sensitivity rates as low as 27% and as high as 82% reported.[152,311] Improved sensitivity

*References 32, 99, 121, 127, 144, 215, 244, 278, 308, 330, 338, 387, 389, 410.

TABLE 120-4

LOCALIZATION STUDIES IN HYPERPARATHYROIDISM

Noninvasive preoperative methods
  Ultrasonography
  Radioiodine or technetium thyroid scan
  Thallium-technetium scintigraphy
  Technetium-99m sestamibi scintigraphy
  Computed tomography scan
  Magnetic resonance imaging
Invasive preoperative methods
  Fine-needle aspiration
  Selective arteriography or digital subtraction
    angiography
  Selective venous sampling for parathyroid
    hormone assay
  Arterial injection of selenium-ethionine
Intraoperative methods
  Intraoperative ultrasonography
  Toluidine blue or methylene blue
  Urinary adenosine monophosphate
  Quick parathyroid hormone intraoperative

has been reported by the application of single-photon emission computed tomography (SPECT) techniques with 3D images.[269] The previously noted advantages of this imaging technique are widespread availability, minimum irradiation, and low risk. However, false-positive results attributable to patient motion during the examination or as a result of concurrent thyroid abnormalities have resulted in poor acceptance of this technique as a reliable preoperative localization method for limited parathyroid exploration.

Sestamibi-Technetium 99m Scintography

In 1988, Coakly and others[72] reported the use of technetium Tc 99m sestamibi for cardiac function studies. Chiu[64] demonstrated the incorporation of technetium 99 (Tc 99m) into the cytoplasm and mitochondria of mouse fibroblasts in response to certain stimuli. Parathyroid cells have large numbers of mitochondria that enable sestamibi to enter parathyroid tissue more intensely than into the neighboring thyroid parenchyma.[334] O'Doherty[290] compared radionuclide uptake in parathyroid tissue and noted a greater uptake per gram for sestamibi than for thallium-201.

In 1992, Taillefer[372] proposed a dual-phase scan with technetium-99m sestamibi and cervicothoracic planar parathyroid scintigraphy. In this method, the patient is intravenously injected with 20 to 25 millicuries of technetium-99m sestamibi. Subsequent images are obtained at 10 to 15 minutes and then at 2 to 3 hours after the injection. Late phase is usually preferable for detecting parathyroid adenomas,

because the thyroid and thyroid nodules clear of uptake faster than do parathyroid neoplasms. Geoffrey has demonstrated that 70% of delayed images are best seen at 2 hours and only 15% at 4 hours.[187] In certain circumstances, oblique or lateral images can be obtained to attempt to add a third dimension to the study. The advantages of the technique include the ability to use this imaging method without patient immobilization between images.

The sensitivity reported for solitary adenomas is as high as 100%, with a specificity of approximately 90%.[2,53,383] Few false-positive results have been reported with this imaging technique and are predominantly caused by solid thyroid nodules, predominantly adenomas.[301] Hurthle cell carcinoma and malignant thyroid lymph node metastases have also been noted to result in false-positive sestamibi imaging results; however, cystic lesions of the thyroid gland have not.[17,300]

False-negative results may be attributable to smaller parathyroid adenoma size or suboptimal dosing of technetium-99m sestamibi.[300] Intrathyroid, mediastinal, and deep cervical parathyroid glands have been located with technetium-99m sestamibi, and thus location seems to be independent of its efficiency (representing an advantage over technetium/thallium subtraction scanning). The presence of multiple-gland disease in the form of double parathyroid adenomas has been demonstrated by this technique (Figure 120-4).[300] However, sestamibi, like thallium-201, also is inaccurate in patients with diffuse four-gland parathyroid hyperplasia.

Technetium-99m sestamibi has been combined with ^{123}I and recorded simultaneously in nonoverlapping windows and subtraction. In a series by Hindie, 25 of 27 solitary adenomas were identified with a sensitivity of 94%.[167] In the same population, examination with technetium-99m sestamibi as the sole radionuclide identified 22 of these 27 patients correctly for a sensitivity of 79%. Neumann has used technetium-99m sestamibi/^{123}I subtraction and SPECT in patients with secondary hyperparathyroidism for a sensitivity of 77%.[268] In this series of 13 patients with recurrent secondary hyperparathyroidism, all hyperplastic parathyroids were predicted and then subsequently correctly identified at surgery.

Technetium-99m Sestamibi with SPECT

The application of SPECT uses a camera collimator that rotates 360 degrees around the patient in the axial plane and in essence portrays a 3D image as the sequence progresses from mandible through the thorax. Some investigators have demonstrated a superior sensitivity/localization in the early phase compared with cervicothoracic planar images, whereas the

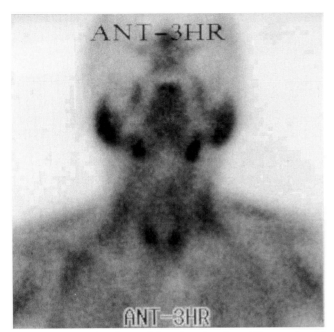

Figure 120-4. Two-hour delayed technetium-99m sestamibi nuclear scan in a patient with hyperparathyroidism secondary to double parathyroid adenomata. Nuclear uptake is clearly demonstrated bilaterally on the image, indicating the location of both adenomas confirmed at surgery.

delayed images are approximately equivalent.[50] The images do appear to have a higher resolution and have two definite recognized advantages over planar sestamibi images: (1) anatomic localization in ectopic adenomas within the carotid sheath, and (2) localization of mediastinal lesions to the anterior or posterior compartment, allowing planning of surgery by lateral thoracotomy vs median sternotomy.[289]

Ultrasonography

High-resolution ultrasonography (10 or 12 MHz) was introduced by Edis and Evans in 1979.[105] It provides for sonographic exploration of the thyroid, carotid, and jugular areas and the cervical area between the thyroid cartilage and the sternal margin. The advantages of this technique is that it is easy to perform, is well tolerated by the patient, does not require the injection of a radiotracer, and can be performed rapidly and at low cost. Disadvantages include localization of enlarged parathyroid glands in the retroesophageal, retrotracheal, retrosternal, and deep cervicothoracic inlet regions. Intrathyroid parathyroid adenomas have reportedly been localized more efficiently with ultrasound than with other techniques, although they may be confused with cystic thyroid lesions.[216] The sensitivity of ultrasonography in identifying abnormal parathyroid glands varies according to the ultrasonographer's experience, the

frequency of the transducer, the resolution of the image, and parathyroid gland size.[135]

Gray-scale ultrasound with high-resolution linear array transducers represent the ideal modality for parathyroid study. Both transverse and longitudinal scans are required. Transverse scans are useful in identifying the adenoma, whereas longitudinal scans better demonstrate its relationship to the thyroid and its internal architecture and vascularity. A parathyroid adenoma typically appears as a hypoechoic mass posterior or inferior to the thyroid gland in its usual extracapsular location. Retrothyroid lesions tend to oval or flat, whereas intrathyroid lesions are usually spherical. Some parathyroid adenomas may demonstrate cystic portions within, but calcification is rare. Given that the most common false-positive image with a technetium-99m sestamibi image is that caused by a thyroid adenoma (Figure 120-5), this particular entity may be reconciled with adjunctive ultrasonography. A discrete blood supply to the mass within the thyroid parenchyma identified by color Doppler suggests a diagnosis of intrathyroidal parathyroid adenoma rather than a lesion of the thyroid itself (Figure 120-6).

False-positive ultrasonographic studies have resulted from thyroid nodules, adenopathy, and even esophageal lesions.[135] The presence of surgical clips can also make interpretation more difficult. The overall false-positive rare has been reported to be approximately 15% to 20%.[216,252,321]

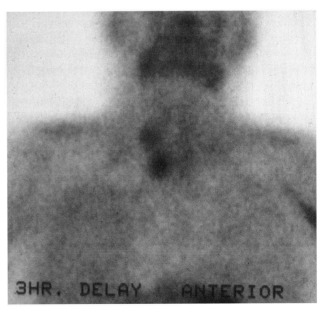

Figure 120-5. Technetium-99m sestamibi nuclear scan in a patient with hyperparathyroidism and nodular thyroid disease. Nuclear uptake in right lower cervical region on delayed image represents uptake by a thyroid adenoma.

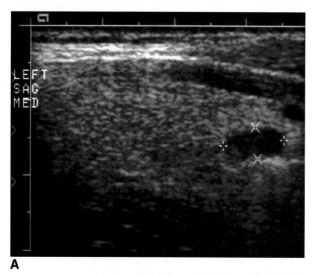

A

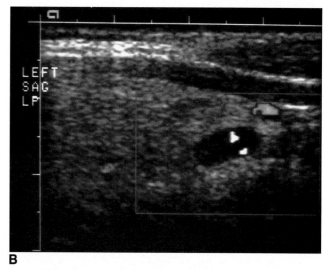

B

Figure 120-6. A small but hyperfunctioning parathyroid adenoma is demonstrated on sagittal ultrasonography **(A)** to be completely within the thyroid gland. Color Doppler ultrasonography **(B)** shows a discrete blood supply *(black arrows)* that differs from the more diffuse perinodular vascular support for a thyroid adenoma from its surrounding parent gland.

Computed Tomography

Computed tomography (CT) is a less-sensitive method than magnetic resonance imaging (MRI). It is relatively expensive, exposes the patient to radiation, and requires the administration of contrast to obtain optimum imaging. It may be useful for ectopic parathyroid glands (retrotracheal, retroesophageal, and mediastinal) but is less effective for those parathyroid adenomas that reside in a normal anatomic location. Metal clips distort the image of CT. Furthermore, perithyroidal lymph nodes and ectopic vasculature may make identification of adenoma difficult.[204] This technique does not selectively image endocrine tissue and thus is not physiologically based, supplying only anatomic information. False-positive results are usually more frequent than with other techniques and may reach as high as 50%, making this technique impractical for most clinical situations.[110,200]

Magnetic Resonance Imaging

Magnetic resonance imaging is generally thought to be superior to CT imaging, because it does not require the administration of radioiodinated contrast and there is no interference from surgical clips left in the neck after initial exploration. A parathyroid neoplasm usually has a low signal intensity in T1-weighted imaging (similar to muscle or thyroid) and a high signal intensity (more than or the same as fat) in T2-weighted imaging (Figure 120-7).[16]

Magnetic resonance imaging may be more useful for identifying ectopic parathyroid tissue. In an investigation evaluating patients undergoing reoperation

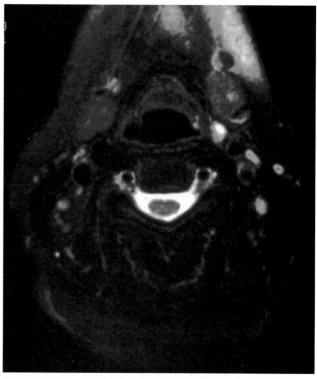

Figure 120-7. Magnetic resonance imaging demonstrating a mass in the left submandibular triangle consistent with an undescended superior parathyroid adenoma.

for recalcitrant hyperparathyroidism, Rodriguez noted that MRI localized 79% of ectopic glands and only 59% of those enlarged glands situated in a normal position.[186] Parathyroid adenomas located in a superior position have been noted to be difficult to locate posterior to the thyroid at the level of the cricoid cartilage.[165]

The sensitivity for MRI has been reported to be superior to that for CT imaging, ranging from 50% to 80%.[110,186] MRI, like that of thallium-201 scanning, demonstrates false-positive findings as a consequence of enlarged lymph nodes.[166] Thyroid adenomata may also lead to false-positive results with MRI.

Both MRI and CT imaging offer limited application in preoperative localization, although the relative cost of these procedures and their inconsistent results generally preclude their universal use before initial exploration. However, they are important modalities to be used in patients who have recalcitrant hyperparathyroidism and require re-exploration.

Invasive Preoperative Localization

Invasive localization studies are indicated when the combined results of noninvasive tests are negative, equivocal, or conflicting, generally in the setting of recalcitrant hyperparathyroidism before re-exploration.

Parathyroid Arteriography

Appropriate parathyroid arteriography includes examination of both thyrocervical trunks (search for glands in the superior mediastinum, tracheoesophageal sulcus or intrathyroid or juxtathyroid glands), the internal mammary arteries (glands in the thymus and the anterior mediastinum) and carotids (juxtathyroid or undescended glands), and sometimes the selected catheterization of the superior thyroid artery. Parathyroid adenomas appear highly vascularized and oval or round in shape. The sensitivity reported for conventional arteriography is approximately 60%, although the results obtained with digital subtraction arteriography are slightly better.[250,253,254]

Selective Venous Sampling For PTH

Angiography is performed primarily to outline the venous drainage, facilitating sampling for PTH assay. This investigation is expensive and technically difficult. Sampling must be obtained as selectively as possible from the smallest venous branch to document the exact location of the parathyroid tumor.[251] However, published reports suggest that sampling from large veins such as the internal jugular vein, innominate vein and superior vena cava may yield optimal results.[271] A twofold gradient between the PTH concentration in peripheral blood and that in the selectively sampled venous tributary establishes the site of the venous drainage from the tumor.

This technique is generally thought to be the most sensitive, lateralizing about 80% of the parathyroid

tumors.[137,186,253,370] It seems to be just as effective in localizing mediastinal glands as it is for cervical glands and is dependent on physiologic properties of the parathyroid gland rather than size. It may be helpful in multiple gland disease and has the ability to reconcile an equivocal noninvasive study such that localization may be achieved.

Ultrasound-Guided Fine-Needle Aspiration

Fine-needle aspiration (FNA) of a parathyroid tumor performed under sonographic guidance may offer an improvement over the results obtained with ultrasound. Fine-needle aspiration may provide for direct cytologic examination, or it may facilitate the use of a bioassay of the aspirate to determine PTH level. When the aspirate is positive for PTH, it confirms the presence of parathyroid tissue within the enlarged gland.[100] Parathyroid hormone determination is generally more helpful than cytology examination for diagnosing parathyroid lesions because of the difficulty in differentiating between parathyroid and thyroid tissue in such a limited sample.[195] In one study, reported by Tikkakoski, 100% of patients with abnormal parathyroid glands were diagnosed by bioassay but only 60% by cytologic examination.[384]

Intraoperative Localization Methods

High-resolution intraoperative ultrasound may be useful in a number of operative settings, primarily that of re-exploration for hyperparathyroidism in a neck that demonstrates significant surgical fibrosis.

The injection of methylene blue or toluidine blue is of little value, because the pathologic gland has to be identified.[37] Methylene blue has been used in the setting of reoperation within 1 to 2 days after initial parathyroidectomy for persistent hyperparathyroidism. Postoperative edema and seroma fluid makes re-exploration difficult in this circumstance and the blue color may be helpful in identifying parathyroid tissue.

Radio-guided parathyroid gland identification and removal has been advocated by Norman and colleagues.[275,276] Hand-held gamma probes developed for operating room use are used to detect the gland concentrating technetium 99m sestamibi, which is injected on the day of operation, usually within approximately 2 hours of the operation. The initial scan provides information regarding localization of putative adenomas and the presence of delayed uptake of nuclear material within the thyroid gland. Should excessive delayed activity be present in the thyroid, the patient is subjected to thyroid suppression for 6 to 8 weeks before operation to reduce background radiation in the thyroid bed and increase the accuracy of the probe. This is the usual circumstance in reoperative settings. After identification and removal of the abnormal gland or glands, the final abnormal gland removed is checked for the degree of radioactivity ex vivo against background tissues in the surgical bed. On the basis of previous reported data, excised glandular tissue emitting radiation >20% of that found in tissues in the surgical bed was confirmed as the hyperfunctional parathyroid tissue implicated in disease.[275]

SURGICAL MANAGEMENT
Indications For Exploration

The decision to perform surgical exploration in the medically stable patient with primary hyperparathyroidism is predicated on the potential for development of complications from prolonged exposure to hypercalcemia and the long-term benefit of surgery. In general, patients should be assessed for the risk of complications developing on the basis of disease severity at the time of diagnosis, and those previously diagnosed in whom complications have arisen over a short interval since diagnosis and are at significant risk of further problems.

Patient age should not represent an exclusive determinate of candidacy for surgery; rather, general medical condition and the potential for pursuing an active lifestyle should play a more prominent role in determining the recommendation for treatment. In general, younger patients who potentially will have longer exposure to hypercalcemia are at a substantially greater risk for complications developing.

The severity of hypercalcemia represents a consideration in the decision to perform surgery. Although no absolute level of serum calcium provides stringent criteria for surgery, most endocrine surgeons consider a serum calcium level of 11.5 mg/dL or greater as an absolute indication for surgery. Surgery in postmenopausal women should be given special consideration independent of the severity of hypercalcemia and/or absence of symptoms. Women in this population are at greater risk for development of long-term skeletal complications from generalized demineralization and osteopenia (i.e., hip and vertebral fractures).[199]

A major factor to be considered in determining the need for surgery is the potential for long-term benefits and prospects for cure. In 85% to 90% of patients, hyperparathyroidism occurs as a result of a single adenoma. Exploration and removal of the adenoma is curative in >95% of patients, and the long-term benefit and potential for cure is high. Primary hyperplasia occurs in approximately 10% to 12% of patients with hyperparathyroidism. Surgery in these patients involves subtotal parathyroidectomy, with the amount of tissue left ultimately determining the long-term

benefit of the surgery. Because of the variable amount of parathyroid tissue left in the neck and thus potential for variable activity, the prospect for cure is less reliable than for patients with adenoma. These patients have cure rates significantly reduced from those in whom an adenoma is removed.[45]

Given the considerations mentioned previously, the decision to perform surgery on patients who seem asymptomatic and who have no obvious metabolic complications is somewhat problematic. Although early surgical intervention seems to be favored, stringent criteria as to whether these patients should undergo surgery have not been clearly defined. About 50% of asymptomatic patients will go on to have metabolic complications from hyperparathyroidism within 5 to 7 years of the onset of hypercalcemia.[82] As a result of some of the uncertainties about the indications for surgery in asymptomatic patients, a consensus conference held by the National Institutes of Health in 1990 addressed the question of management in this clinical situation.[265] Recommendations for surgical management and/or surveillance for patients with primary hyperparathyroidism derived from that conference predated much of what has evolved over the course of the past decade with respect to clinical experience with asymptomatic primary hyperparathyroidism, the evolution of contemporary surgical technique, and development of newer technologies in preoperative localization. Accordingly, this conference was reconvened in early 2002 in an effort to reevaluate the original recommendations from the 1990 symposium and contemporize recommendations on the management of asymptomatic primary hyperparathyroidism.[264] The following is a review of the indications for surgery as suggested by the conference:

1. Serum calcium is >1.0 mg/dL above the upper limit of normal.
2. Creatinine clearance is reduced >30% for age in the absence of another cause.
3. Twenty-four hour urinary calcium is >400 mg/dL.
4. Patients are younger than 50 years of age.
5. Bone mineral density measurement at the lumbar spine, hip, or distal radius is reduced >2.5 standard deviations (by T score).
6. Patients request surgery, or patients are unsuitable for long-term surveillance.

These recommended indications are conservative; they provide a framework for surgical decision making but are not absolute or universal. The decision to perform surgery on a patient with primary hyperparathyroidism and metabolic complications is straightforward.

The decision is less clear in asymptomatic patients and must be guided by the potential benefits of surgery, the patient's risk of complications developing from disease, the wishes of the patient, and, importantly, the experience of the surgeon. The success rate of surgery and the incidence of complications after parathyroidectomy have been documented to vary greatly, depending on the surgeon's experience. In one study, experienced Swedish surgeons achieved normal calcium in >90% of patients, with recurrent laryngeal nerve complications realized in less than 1%. However, surgeons who perform fewer than 10 parathyroidectomies per year had a success rate of 70%, with 15% of patients remaining hypercalcemic and 14% becoming permanently hypocalcemic.[230] Therefore, in weighing potential benefits of surgery again risks for patients with asymptomatic hyperparathyroidism, the experience of the surgeon should be a primary consideration.

Although patients with mild to moderate hypercalcemia seldom experience rapid elevation in serum calcium level, the risk of symptoms developing and risks for potential end-organ damage increase with time. As a result, patients with untreated primary hyperparathyroidism are at risk for major morbidity and mortality from cardiovascular disease.[272,304] The benefits derived from parathyroidectomy in patients with occult or minimally symptomatic disease have been discussed previously in this chapter under "Clinical Manifestations of Hyperparathyroidism." In addition, parathyroidectomy seems to offer a distinct and measurable advantage in patients with mild asymptomatic primary hyperparathyroidism as indicated by the results of a randomized trial in which patients were subjectively surveyed by use of a standardized health survey instrument.[375] In this investigation, patients with mild symptomatic hyperparathyroidism were randomly assigned to surgery or observation and then assessed every 6 months after randomization for 2 years with the SF-36 Health Survey, an instrument that measures wellness.[407] Function was significantly improved in patients after parathyroidectomy compared with patients who were observed.

Technique of Parathyroidectomy
Anesthesia and Preparation

Exploration of the neck in patients with hyperparathyroidism is generally performed under general anesthesia with endotracheal intubation. In patients who are medically unfit for general anesthesia, parathyroid exploration for removal of solitary adenoma localized preoperatively may be performed under local anesthesia supplemented by intravenous sedation.[63,179]

Positioning of the patient on the operating table is very important. The patient's neck should be hyperextended dorsally to provide optimal access to the neck, particularly in those patients with a short wide neck, to provide access to the cervicothoracic junction. The arms of the patient should lie along aside the body to allow the surgeon and the assistant to stand on both sides of the neck comfortably. Long ventilation tubes are helpful in facilitating placement of the ventilator at some distance from the operating table, which allows for rotation of the operating table away from the anesthesia personnel. Patients in whom exploration is being performed in a directed or minimally invasive fashion should have an accessible intravascular site, intravenous or intraarterial, from which a peripheral sample of blood may be drawn to assess PTH levels intraoperatively. After the complete positioning and preparation of the patient on the operating table, the table may be adjusted in the reverse Trendelenburg position to decrease venous congestion around the thyroid bed and central are of the neck.

Exploration of the Neck

A low transverse cervical incision (Kocher) is designed two fingerbreadths above the suprasternal notch, usually over a natural skin crease, and is carried down through the platysma. The incision may be tailored according to the surgeon's preference with respect to the type of exploration being carried out. More directed, focused procedures require a shorter incision than a traditional bilateral four-gland exploration. In any event, the incision should not extend beyond the sternocleidomastoid muscles. After incising the platysma, the cranial skin–platysma flap is dissected upward to the notch of the thyroid cartilage and the caudal–platysma flap is dissected inferiorly to the suprasternal notch. A self-retaining retractor is useful in spreading the cranial and caudal flaps to expose the midline strap muscles in the region of the thyroid bed and central neck structures. The midline raphe of the strap muscles is identified and separated from the thyroid notch to the suprasternal notch, thus allowing the sternohyoid muscles to be retracted laterally. It is usually unnecessary to divide the sternohyoid muscles. The sternothyroid muscle is then separated over the thyroid lobe on the side of the neck to be explored first, carefully elevating the muscle away from the thyroid capsule. Unlike the plane between the strap muscles, which is predominantly avascular, the plane separating the sternothyroid muscle from the true thyroid capsule may be quite vascular, and particular attention to hemostasis is important in carrying out this maneuver. Hemostasis during parathyroid exploration cannot be overemphasized, because blood-stained tissues will hinder the ability of the surgeon to identify both abnormal and normal parathyroid glands within the fatty tissue of the central neck. The thyroid lobe on the side being explored is then retracted anteromedially to access the potential space posterior to the thyroid lobe. This is facilitated by exposing the dominant middle thyroid venous tributaries and dividing and ligating them to access this region. Ligation of the superior and/or inferior thyroid artery is not necessary for adequate rotation of the thyroid anteromedially during this maneuver.

Once this region has been accessed, blunt dissection of fibroareolar tissue facilitates evaluation of the area where both normal and abnormal parathyroid glands generally reside. This will permit visualization and/or palpation of enlarged parathyroid tissue with minimal dissection so as to prevent staining the tissues with blood. It is essential to maintain anteromedial retraction of the thyroid gland to expose the angle of visualization and subsequent exploration (Figure 120-8). This is further facilitated by opening the fascial sheath (pretracheal fascia) connecting the carotid sheath and the thyroid gland. This maneuver provides access to the paraesophageal and retroesophageal spaces. Although identification of the recurrent laryngeal nerve is not generally mandatory, dissection in either the retroesophageal or paraesophageal space will require visualization of the nerve to prevent injury.

A systematic approach to the surgical identification of the parathyroid glands is essential to ensure a high success rate and to avoid missing abnormal glands. It is important to develop a methodical and disciplined sequence of exploration so as to minimize the potential for missing either normal or abnormal glands. The ability to palpate abnormal glands cannot be overemphasized. Often glands within the paraesophageal

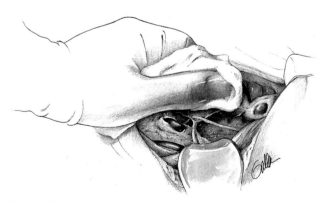

Figure 120-8. Exposure achieved through anteromedial rotation of the thyroid gland with demonstration of superior and inferior parathyroid gland positions.

space just dorsal to the juxtaposition of the recurrent laryngeal nerve and the inferior thyroid artery may be quite readily palpated before they are seen. Palpation in this area will generally direct the surgeon to this region, so that focal areas of meticulous dissection may be carried out, thus minimizing the potential for significant tissue staining by blood and inadvertent devascularization of normal parathyroid glands. Initial palpation along the posterior aspect of the thyroid capsule, especially adjacent to the superior pole above the inferior thyroid artery entrance to the gland, will, at times, demonstrate the presence of an enlarged superior parathyroid gland closely situated against the true thyroid capsule underneath a covering of pretracheal fascia.

Depending on surgical preference, the usual trend is to identify the inferior glands initially. They tend to be larger and more anterior; however, their location may also be less predictable and constant. Typically, they are found adjacent to the inferior pole of the thyroid gland or within a tongue of thymic tissue inferior to the thyroid, the so-called thyrothymic ligament. Commonly, they may be located anterior and slightly medial to the juxtaposition of the inferior thyroid artery and recurrent laryngeal nerve. The superior parathyroid glands are most commonly found along the posterior capsule of the thyroid gland at a point slightly lateral and posterior to the juxtaposition between the recurrent nerve and inferior thyroid artery. Blunt dissection along the posterior capsule will often reveal the superior gland to be suspended in a teardrop fashion within a centimeter of the entrance of the recurrent laryngeal nerve under the cricothyroid muscle. A helpful maneuver in exposing this superior location is to divide the sternothyroid muscle close to the superior thyroid pole to provide maximal medial mobilization without devascularizing the superior pole of the thyroid gland.

Parathyroid glands are often (partially) surrounded by fat. Accordingly, any lobule of fat that is noted at sites that may harbor parathyroid glands should be carefully inspected. This is facilitated by opening the thin fascia that covers the fat lobule and applying pressure, allowing the parathyroid gland to extrude or "blossom" out of the fat. Most normal parathyroid glands will have a light brown or tobacco color. This color is important in differentiating parathyroid glands from fat, which is generally more yellow, than from thyroid nodules, which are more rust red in color. Parathyroid glands also enjoy a degree of freedom of mobility along the true thyroid capsule in relationship to the thyroid gland. It is quite helpful to bluntly dissect along the thyroid capsule with a Kitner (peanut) dissector to visualize moving structures within fat and adjacent to the true thyroid capsule.

The close relationship of the pretracheal fascia over-lying these pseudo-subcapsular parathyroid glands will allow this freedom of movement on blunt dissection. In contradistinction, a thyroid nodule mimicking a parathyroid gland does not enjoy this freedom of movement and is more firmly attached to the central thyroid lobe without a plane of cleavage between it and the thyroid gland and without a vascular pedicle. Perithyroidal lymph nodes, particularly those within the thyrothymic ligament, may be confused with parathyroid glands. However, the consistency of lymph nodes is more firm than that of parathyroid glands, and lymph nodes are also noted to be more of a translucent white-gray than parathyroid glands.

During the exploration for both normal and abnormal parathyroid glands, the vascular anatomy of these glands should be observed. Dissection of the superior parathyroid glands should be initiated at the outermost tip of this gland to prevent injury to the parathyroid vessels, which usually ascend from arterial anastomoses originating from the inferior thyroid artery. The dissection of the inferior parathyroid gland should begin at the caudal end of the parathyroid, because the vascular pedicle generally enters on the upper or cranial side of the inferior parathyroid gland. Suspected devitalization of a normal parathyroid gland during dissection generally requires that it be autotransplanted within cervical muscle. Accordingly, this involves sharply fragmenting the gland into cubic millimeter pieces and implanting them in a hemostatic fashion within the sternocleidomastoid muscle of the same side.

Once identified, the abnormal gland is removed and sent for pathologic analysis. A thorough search is conducted to locate the second gland on the same side; if found, it, too, is biopsied and sent for pathologic determination. If the enlarged gland is reported as hypercellular and the second gland normal or suppressed, the operation proceeds by accessing the viscerovertebral angle of the opposite side. Surgical preference and the type of procedure advocated (directed unilateral vs traditional bilateral) determine the extent of exploration at this point. In the event that the second gland biopsied on the side explored first is found to be abnormal, or if it appears enlarged, all four glands should be identified and histologically examined. In this instance, the presumptive diagnosis is hyperplasia that will require subtotal (3½ gland) parathyroidectomy. The distinction between adenoma and hyperplastic parathyroid tissue is difficult or impossible on frozen section analysis; therefore, the surgeon cannot rely on single-gland histologic analysis for definitive therapy.

The appearance of parathyroid tissue, both normal and diseased, is generally readily recognizable, pro-vided the fibroareolar tissues remain free of excessive blood staining. In contrast to normal parathyroid tissue, parathyroid adenomata appear rust or beefy red in situ. They may be mottled or variegated in their coloring and will usually lighten on resection. In contrast, hyperplastic glands will generally appear darker than adenoma, usually a dark rust, brown, or chocolate color resembling more the color of thyroid tissue.

Failure to identify a missing gland suspected of being an adenoma, or in the case of hyperplasia, failure to locate all glands mandates a thorough dissection in an effort to locate abnormally located or ectopic parathyroid tissue. A systematic approach is undertaken to examine all areas potentially harboring an ectopic gland. It is imperative that the surgeon know which gland is missing, with the understanding that a search is predicated on the likely variable or ectopic sites. Surgical dissection should address all areas accessible through a cervical approach, including the removal of thymic tissue within the superior mediastinum, examination of the retroesophageal space and carotid sheath to the hyoid, and thyroid lobectomy (lobotomy), if necessary. Approximately 90% of all parathyroid adenomas are resectable through a transcervical approach, and thus a missing gland is usually harbored in an ectopic location accessible to the surgeon at initial operation.

Closure of the Incision

After completion of the surgical exploration, the operative field is irrigated with warm saline solution and inspected for adequate hemostasis. Particular attention to any normal parathyroid glands that were isolated and dissected is important to document apparent viability. Parathyroid glands judged to be poorly vascularized or of compromised viability should be autotransplanted as discussed previously. Depending on the extent of exploration, the body habitus of the patient with respect to depth of dissection within the cervicothoracic junction, and the degree of bleeding encountered, a drain may or may not be used. In most cases, drainage of the wound is not required, because most dissections are limited and hemostatic. Depending on surgical preference, the skin may be closed in either a cuticular or subcuticular fashion after reapproximation of the strap muscles in the midline and closure of the platysma. An occlusive dressing is placed to prevent fluid collection under the incision.

Postoperative Care

Successful parathyroid exploration with removal of a solitary adenoma results in a decrease in total serum calcium level that usually reaches a nadir approximately 48 hours after the operation. Postoperative hypocalcemia may be seen in patients with severe skeletal depletion of calcium, resulting in "bone hunger." In some patients, symptoms of hypocalcemia or tetany may develop while the serum calcium level is normal. This may be due to a rapid decrease in serum calcium after removal of the parathyroid tumor, causing an increased neural excitability, but may also persist after calcium replacement resulting from accompanying hypomagnesemia.[136]

Depending on surgeon preference, postoperative total serum calcium levels should be measured at least once within the first 24 hours after operation either in the hospital or in an outpatient facility. Normocalcemia at 6 months postoperatively is the usual standard assessment for surgical success, and thus both total serum calcium level and intact PTH level should be assessed at both 1 month and 6 months postoperatively.

Surgical Strategy and Approach to Exploration

The optimal surgical approach in managing primary hyperparathyroidism is one in which normocalcemia is achieved while minimizing potential surgical morbidity, including recurrent laryngeal nerve injury, postexploration hypocalcemia, and persistent/recurrent hyperparathyroidism requiring reoperation. In addition, the approach selected should be individualized to the patient and disease entity (suspected single vs multiple gland disease) and should be time and cost efficient. The development of a surgical strategy in managing patients with primary hyperparathyroidism has in recent years evolved from the routine performance of bilateral cervical exploration to a more directed unilateral approach. In theory, because most patients with primary hyperparathyroidism have a single hyperfunctioning adenoma as the offending lesion, it follows that the ideal surgical approach would involve directed removal of the solitary abnormal gland in the least–invasive and atraumatic manner. Incorporating this theoretic ideal into a practical and reliable surgical approach had previously been limited by two constraints. The first of these was accurate preoperative localization of the abnormal gland, and the second was an inability to intraoperatively confirm removal of all hyperfunctioning parathyroid tissue without performing a bilateral cervical exploration and examining all four parathyroid glands.

Traditionally, the argument for a bilateral cervical exploration in patients with suspected adenoma has been the demonstrated high success rate in achieving normocalcemia with a conventional bilateral approach in experienced hands (>95% cure), the inability to accurately predict which side to selectively explore, and the potential risk of missing unsuspected multiple gland disease such as double adenoma or unsuspected hyperplasia.* Recent technologic advances have helped address these areas of concern, and there is now growing consensus for a less-extensive, directed exploration in the approach to primary hyperparathyroidism. The first impetus to this shift in surgical philosophy was provided by improvements in preoperative imaging for the accurate localization of hyperfunctioning solitary adenomas through the use of technetium-99m sestamibi imaging (see "Noninvasive Preoperative Localization"). The second major advance involved the quest for a more precise and timely means of judging surgical success, which led to the development of assays to measure the intact parathyroid hormone (iPTH) molecule. With the ability to biochemically confirm removal of all hyperfunctioning parathyroid tissue intraoperatively, the theoretic advantages of a directed unilateral cervical approach have increasingly become reality.[182,184,298]

Single-Gland Disease

Directed unilateral cervical exploration. This surgical approach uses both preoperative localization with technetium-99m sestamibi and the implementation of intraoperative assay for parathyroid hormone determination (IOPTH) for the surgical management of primary hyperparathyroidism secondary to anticipated parathyroid adenoma. In the initial preoperative evaluation, all patients with disease entities exhibiting multiple-gland hyperplasia, such as those with familial hyperparathyroidism and MEN types 1 or 2A, are determined to be candidates for standard bilateral cervical exploration and do not have localizing studies performed before initial operation. A preoperative technetium 99m sestamibi scan is obtained on all other patients with primary hyperparathyroidism, and, depending on surgical preference, may be combined with high-resolution ultrasound evaluation of the thyroid bed and central neck. If the scan is inconclusive or equivocal, as judged by both the surgeon and nuclear medicine specialist, a standard bilateral cervical exploration is planned and carried out, whether an enlarged gland is found on the side explored first or not. Failure to localize with an optimally performed technetium-99m sestamibi scan, in the absence of significant thyroid disease, is strongly suggestive of sporadic diffuse hyperplasia.[51,193] If the nuclear scan identifies a discrete nuclear focus on delayed imaging, suggestive of adenoma, a directed exploration to the side localized is performed, and biochemical confirmation of removal of all hyperfunctioning parathyroid tissue is obtained through the use of IOPTH. It has been previously demonstrated that the most precipitous

---

*References 27, 170, 194, 314, 344, 409.

decrease in PTH levels occurs 5 minutes after removal of all hyperfunctioning parathyroid tissue.[193] The short half-life of PTH (roughly 2–5 minutes) allows peripheral blood samples to be obtained intraoperatively for rapid PTH testing anywhere from 7 to 10 minutes after excision of all suspected hyperfunctioning parathyroid tissue.[282] Accordingly, a peripheral blood sample for rapid PTH assays is drawn at the time of abnormal gland identification (baseline) and subsequently 10 minutes after removal of all suspected hyperfunctioning parathyroid tissue. Degradation in the serum PTH level exceeding 50%, noted in the postexcision PTH level compared with the preexcision level, provides biochemical confirmation of removal of all hyperfunctioning parathyroid tissue, allowing the procedure to be concluded without identification or biopsy of any other parathyroid glands. If the postexcision PTH level is degrades less than 50% of the baseline preexcision level, suggesting the presence of residual hyperfunctioning parathyroid tissue, a standard bilateral cervical exploration is performed.

Intraoperative PTH determination may be carried out by a number of methods, one of which uses a radioimmunoassay developed through a simple, previously described modification of an intact PTH overnight assay method.[116] The iPTH assay is a two-antibody sandwich system. One antibody (the capture antibody) is fixed to a plastic bead; the second is conjugated with a measurable marker. The amount of iPTH present in a plasma sample can be determined by measuring the amount of the marker material remaining after all unbound solutions have been removed. Results of this rapid PTH assay are generally available within 8 to 10 minutes after submission to the radioimmunoassay laboratory. To overcome problems associated with sensitivity of the rapid immunoradiometric assay, researchers began conjugating the labeling antibody with chemiluminescent tracers to avoid the handling issues of their radioactive predecessors.[182,184,193] Since the introduction of the immunochemiluminometric assay (ICMA) in 1993, researchers have experimented with several different variations on this theme, and some manufacturers now offer so-called quick kits. Experience with this assay is consistent among the investigators in that a decrease of 50% or greater between the postexcision and baseline preexcision PTH values is indicative of removal of all hyperfunctioning parathyroid tissue.* The major drawback of these kits is their high cost. However, because the assay negates the need for frozen section analysis in most cases, the overall cost is only slightly more expensive than the traditional

unilateral approach.[182] These modifications can provide a cost-effective alternative to preformed kits, especially when weighed against the potential costs of a missed ectopic adenoma.[300]

The kinetics of postadenoma resection are important to understand if logical management strategies are based on this objective data. Libutti and others[218] demonstrate the half-life of PTH varies within a short brief window, 0.42 to 3.81 minutes. Randolph and others[315] have demonstrated that the lowest values occur within 1 to 3 days. In up to 38% of patients with successful resection of a single parathyroid adenoma and return to normocalcemia, intact PTH levels may remain elevated at 1 month. Suggested mechanisms are cortical bone remineralization, increase in calcium receptor set point, and a relative secondary hyperparathyroidism.

In situations in which localization studies are inconclusive or equivocal (lacking mutual agreement by both surgeon and radiologist) or clinical circumstances suggest multiple gland disease (MEN, familial hyperparathyroidism), a traditional bilateral cervical exploration is advocated. Specifically, both sides of the neck are explored in an attempt to identify at least four parathyroid glands, independent of whether the first side explored yields an enlarged gland or not. Routine biopsy of all normal-appearing glands is not recommended. Instead, incisional biopsy of glands is performed selectively. Intraoperative PTH determination remains an important adjunct in the bilateral approach in that this modality serves to biochemically confirm removal of all hyperfunctioning parathyroid tissue and thus reduces the chance of missing ectopic multiglandular disease, whether as a result of "double adenoma" or ectopic supernumerary glands.

Minimally invasive techniques. Surgical techniques that derive from the basic cervical exploration described previously have been termed "minimally invasive" techniques primarily as a result of modifications resulting from advancements in technology. Scan directed surgery under local or regional anesthesia has been advocated by a number of investigators reporting excellent surgical results.[218,315] These techniques capitalize on the ability to administer effective regional anesthesia to the awake, sedated patient to perform directed unilateral focused exploration with removal of a localized solitary parathyroid adenoma. The technique uses preoperative utilization with technetium-99m sestamibi by use of both planar and SPECT imaging and intraoperative PTH assay for biochemical confirmation of removal of all hyperfunctioning parathyroid tissue. Advantages of this technique have been reported as improved patient comfort postoperatively, the performance of ambulatory procedures, and reduced cost.[218] Disadvantages

---

*References 51, 116, 180, 181, 193, 256, 282, 360, 388.

of the technique include the potential for conversion to a comprehensive bilateral dissection in the event that the adenoma is not found in the area indicated by the scan (thus necessitating general anesthesia) and the potential for patient anxiety and/or discomfort requiring conversion to general anesthesia.

The ability to accurately localize solitary parathyroid adenomata with technetium 99m sestamibi has allowed a number of investigators to pursue intraoperative nuclear mapping to isolate and recover the enlarged parathyroid gland representing the adenoma. This has been termed radio-guided parathyroidectomy and uses preoperative administration of technetium 99m sestamibi immediately before the operation combined with intraoperative use of the hand-held gamma detection device (gamma probe).[28,178,275] In this technique, the patient is administered approximately 18 to 20 millicuries of technetium-99m sestamibi approximately 2 hours before surgery. The timing of the preoperative injection may be modified by the visualized washout sequence demonstrated by the solitary parathyroid gland on review of delayed images. After appropriate positioning of the patient on the operating table, intravenous sedation is administered. The gamma probe is applied to the anterior surface of the neck to measure the radioactivity of the thyroid isthmus, which is used to determine the background radioactive count. The threshold of the gamma probe is then set to filter out background radioactivity. Radioactive counts are then measured in each quadrant of the neck, and a marking pen is used to mark the area of maximal radioactivity, the location of which should correspond to the location of the adenoma on the sestamibi scan. The size of the incision, accordingly, may be considerably smaller than that used for conventional four-gland bilateral parathyroid exploration. The area to be incised is anesthetized with a local anesthetic, and a small 2- to 3-cm incision is made directly over the area of maximal radioactivity. A gamma probe is then used to guide the surgical dissection by repeatedly placing it into the operative field allowing a precise surgical dissection. Once the adenoma is found, it is carefully dissected close to its capsule, its pedicle is identified, clipped, and divided, ensuring first that the recurrent laryngeal nerve is not within the dissected field. Radioactivity of the removed parathyroid adenoma (ex vivo) and the operative basin is measured, the sum of which should roughly equal the radioactivity in the corresponding quadrant of the neck before making the incision. In most cases, frozen section analysis is not necessary, but a permanent histopathologic assessment on the specimen is performed. As experience with this procedure has increased, the technique has been applied more selectively to exclude the following clinical situations: deep retroesophageal lesions, ectopic glands, superior adenomas in men, and persistent or recurrent hyperparathyroidism.[178]

Endoscopic parathyroid exploration. Parathyroid exploration performed in humans was first described by Gagner in 1996.[306] With the advent of improved technology and video-assisted endoscopic technology, several pioneering investigators have evaluated this technique in the management of hyperparathyroidism.[124,163,177,247] This procedure is generally carried out under general anesthesia on patients who have demonstrated focal areas of nuclear uptake on delayed imaging with technetium 99m sestamibi scanning for parathyroid localization. The instrumentation allows for minimal access surgery through several very small incisions placed either in the cervical region, the upper chest wall, or the axilla.[163,177,247] In a larger series, of video-assisted parathyroidectomy with limited use of insufflation has been recorded by Miccoli in 137 patients.[247] Potential advantages of the endoscopic approach to parathyroid removal include excellent cosmesis, negligible discomfort, and minimal problems with cervical motion. Investigators advocating this technique have indicated that the selection process in determining which patients are candidates for the procedure is a crucial aspect with regard to surgical success. In general, the criteria for consideration of the procedure include initial explorations, single-gland disease, and the absence of significant thyroid enlargement or multinodularity. All patients must have a preoperative localization study performed with unequivocal focus of nuclear uptake on delayed imaging. In addition, all patients should have PTH levels assessed intraoperatively with the intraoperative PTH assay to biochemically confirm removal of the suspected hyperfunctional parathyroid gland. Although endoscopic cervical exploration for parathyroid disease represents the least invasive and most focused of the minimally invasive surgical techniques, the time required to perform this procedure may be extensive and thus in some ways counterproductive to limiting anesthesia time and cost.[123] At this point, although this procedure shows promise, the role of endoscopic parathyroid exploration remains undefined.

Multiple-Gland Disease

True double adenoma. The incidence of double parathyroid adenomas seems to increase with age. Synchronous double adenomas have been variably reported at rates ranging from 1% to 2% to as high as 10% in patients older than 60 years of age.[151,379] Approximately 50% of true double adenomas will image accurately to each of the two locations (see Figure 120-4). Bilateral exploration is required despite high suspicion on localization because of the possibility of asymmetric hyperplasia. Intraoperative PTH assay provides biochemical confirmation that all hyperfunctional parathyroid tissue has been removed, in that a sequential drop in PTH levels will be noted after successive excision of the first and then second enlarged gland (Figure 120-9). At least one other normal gland should be identified, but surgical biopsy and histologic analysis of additional glands are not necessary, provided the final postexcision PTH level ultimately decreases beyond 50% of the preexcision level intraoperatively to within a normal range.

Sporadic hyperplasia. Multiglandular disease secondary to diffuse hyperplasia of the parathyroid glands may occur in as many as 10% to 15% of patients with sporadic primary hyperparathyroidism. The approach to these patients includes performance of a nuclear imaging study using technetium 99m sestamibi preoperatively unless the patient is known to have one of the MEN disorders.

A scan that does not indicate an unequivocal area of nuclear uptake on delayed images raises the surgeon's suspicion of diffuse hyperplasia. Forty percent of equivocal scans were associated with the ultimate finding of multiglandular hyperplasia at exploration in a series performed by one of the authors (PKP) (Figure 120-10). The presence of an equivocal scan demonstrating the absence of a distinct focus of delayed uptake of nuclear material mandates the performance of a bilateral exploration with histologic identification of at least one abnormal and one normal gland and the assurance that no additional grossly enlarged glands exist on either side. After removal of all enlarged

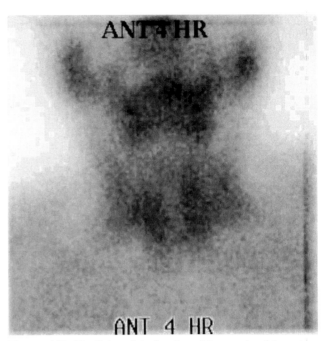

Figure 120-10. Delayed technetium-99m sestamibi nuclear scan performed on a patient with hyperparathyroidism secondary to diffuse four-gland hyperplasia. Note the absence of any focus of nuclear uptake on the image.

glands (either single or multiple) and the demonstration of a histologically normal gland (in the event of less than four-gland disease), rapid PTH assessment (Figure 120-11) is performed to confirm the removal of all hyperfunctional parathyroid tissue, per the same protocol used in the directed exploration strategy. Failure to achieve this degree of parathyroid hormone degradation mandates further exploration, either for

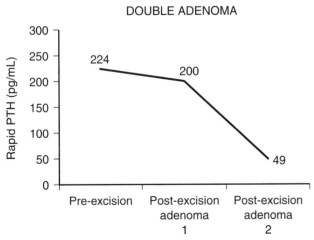

Figure 120-9. Sequential serum parathyroid hormone levels assessed by intraoperative rapid PTH immunoassay (IOPTH) after removal of the first and then second parathyroid adenoma in a patient with hyperparathyroidism and double adenomata.

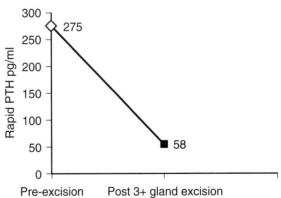

Figure 120-11. Sequential serum parathyroid hormone levels as assessed by intraoperative rapid PTH immunoassay comparing hormone level obtained before and then 10 minutes after a 3½-gland subtotal parathyroidectomy in a patient with diffuse 4-gland hyperplasia.

an ectopically located gland or, uncommonly, a supernumerary gland.

Once all hyperplastic glands have been located in situ, the three largest glands are removed and histologically confirmed. Subtotal excision of the remaining gland follows, leaving at least one third to one half of the gland as a viable vascularized remnant. Titration of PTH levels is helpful by use of rapid parathyroid hormone assay. Should the postexcision level fall below 10 pg/mL, consideration should be given to cryopreservation of parathyroid tissue excised from the fourth gland. Although this is rarely necessary, this approach is favored over routine forearm autotransplantation of parathyroid tissue in that additional surgery is avoided and because a measurable PTH level detected intraoperatively is generally predictive of euparathyroid function and normocalcemia.[300,367]

Familial hyperparathyroidism. Familial hyperparathyroidism accounts for <5% of all cases of hyperparathyroidism.[390] It is composed of a spectrum of autosomal-dominant inherited diseases that include MEN 1, MEN 2A, non-MEN, and familial neonatal hyperparathyroidism. In contrast to sporadic hyperparathyroidism, patients with familial hyperparathyroidism are younger and more likely to have multiglandular disease and persistent or recurrent hyperparathyroidism after parathyroidectomy. Subtotal or total parathyroidectomy in combination with bilateral transcervical thymectomy is more frequently necessary for definitive treatment rather than simple excision of an adenoma, which is all that is required for approximately 80% of patients with sporadic primary hyperparathyroidism. It is imperative that long-term follow-up of patients with familial hyperparathyroidism be performed for early detection and treatment of other endocrine neoplasms associated with these disorders and for the diagnosis of recurrent hyperparathyroidism. In addition, screening of family members represents an important aspect of the overall management of familial hyperparathyroidism. As a result of the identification of causative genetic components in these disorders, the ability for genetic screening of family members and allowing for a global treatment plan for those individuals identified as gene carriers is now possible.

MEN 1. MEN 1 is an autosomal-dominant inherited syndrome characterized by the presence of neoplastic lesions involving the parathyroid glands, the anterior pituitary, the pancreas, and the duodenum. In addition, patients may have carcinoid tumors of the bronchus or thymus, tumors of the ovaries, thyroid gland, adrenal glands, and multiple lipomas. This is an uncommon disorder, occurring in 2 to 20 of every 100,000 persons.[24] Not all patients with MEN 1 have the complete syndrome, indicating a variable degree of penetrance. Primary hyperparathyroidism is the most common manifestation of MEN 1, occurring in >95% of patients, usually before the age of 30, and as the initial manifestation of the syndrome.[35,94,208] Pancreatic endocrine tumors are most often multiple and are distributed throughout the pancreas. Nonfunctioning tumors, gastroma, and insulinoma are the islet cell tumors that are most often associated with MEN 1. A pituitary tumor is diagnosed in 30% to 40% of patients and is most commonly a prolactinoma. The syndrome of hyperparathyroidism may occur up to 10 years before the onset of other endocrine disorders, and, as such, MEN 1 should be considered in any patient diagnosed with primary hyperparathyroidism at an early age or with multiglandular disease.[208] The hyperparathyroidism in MEN 1 is due to diffuse four-gland parathyroid hyperplasia.*

In general, the clinical manifestations of primary hyperparathyroidism in patients with MEN 1 are similar to those found in patients with sporadic primary hyperparathyroidism. Some of the symptoms in primary hyperparathyroidism associated with MEN 1 may be masked by the Zollinger-Ellison syndrome or insulinoma.[208] Alternatively, the symptoms associated with hyperparathyroidism may also aggravate the clinical manifestations of the Zollinger-Ellison syndrome as a result of calcium stimulation of gastrin secretion.[208]

Biochemical findings (serum calcium and PTH levels) in patients with MEN 1 are similar to those found in patients with sporadic primary hyperparathyroidism, and, as such, the diagnosis is made by documenting hypercalcemia associated with an elevated or inappropriately highly PTH level.[207] If a patient with hyperparathyroidism has a family history of the same disorder and/or other endocrinopathies, further screening for tumors of the pituitary gland and pancreas is warranted.[94] This should consistent of serum prolactin levels, glucose, basal serum gastrin, and pancreatic polypeptide levels.

Wermer,[415] in 1954, noted that 50% of the offspring of individuals affected with the MEN 1 syndrome inherited the disorder (without gender differentiation) and that this inheritance did not skip generations. This pattern of inheritance is characteristic of an autosomal-dominant trait with a high degree of penetrance.[94,190]

The MEN 1 locus has been mapped to a section of chromosome 11.[213] This was further shown to involve a mutation at the 11q13 locus.[213] After this, the MEN 1 gene has been identified as a tumor suppressor gene that encodes the protein menin.[59] Greater than 90%

---

*References 94, 158, 208, 232, 293, 392.

of patients with MEN 1 have known germ line menin gene mutations, and most MEN 1 families have their own unique mutation.[337] The predisposition to MEN 1 is a heterozygotic mutation.[207]

The finding of multiple abnormal parathyroid glands and, commonly, supernumerary glands in patients with MEN 1 represents a formidable management dilemma in these patients. The inability to recognize a supernumerary gland at the time of initial exploration for this disorder is a well-documented cause of persistent disease.[79,107,208,312]

The surgical approach should consist of a routine bilateral neck exploration with identification of all four parathyroid glands. The extensiveness of surgical resection of the parathyroid glands, once identified, is controversial, with advocates of both subtotal and total parathyroidectomy. A number of authors have reported their experience with subtotal parathyroidectomy in patients with MEN 1 and hyperparathyroidism with differing degrees of surgical success.[208,293,312,392] Edis[107] reported that 82% of patients with chief cell hyperplasia had normal parathyroid function at least 1 year after subtotal parathyroidectomy. Of these, however, only 6 of 55 actually had hyperparathyroidism secondary to the MEN 1 syndrome. In 12 patients undergoing subtotal parathyroidectomy for the hyperparathyroidism of MEN 1 as reported by Prinz,[312] only 5 ultimately achieved normocalcemia. It has been postulated that the difference in success rates between the hyperparathyroidism attributable to sporadic four-gland hyperplasia and that associated with the MEN 1 syndrome may be due to persistent exposure of a trophic factor. A potential parathyroid mitogenic humoral factor was identified by Brande[34] in 1986 from the serum of patients with familial MEN 1 syndrome. The mitogenic activity of this humoral factor persisted in the patient's plasma for up to 4 years after total parathyroidectomy.[34] As a consequence, any parathyroid remnant remaining after subtotal parathyroidectomy will be exposed to this humoral factor, thus potentially increasing the chance of recurrence. This theory was supported by a finding by Prinz, who reported a patient with persistent hypoparathyroidism who required calcium supplementation for 10 years after subtotal parathyroidectomy before recurrent disease developed. The re-exploration of this patient demonstrated that remnant parathyroid hyperplasia was the etiology of recurrence.[34]

Total parathyroidectomy with autotransplantation of fragmented parathyroid tissue has been advocated by other investigators as the procedure of choice for the initial operation for patients with primary parathyroid hyperplasia because of the MEN 1 syndrome.[412,413] In this procedure, four glands are identified and removed with sectioning of the most morphologically normal-appearing gland into cubic centimeter fragments. These are then implanted into the brachioradialis muscle of the nondominant forearm. Sections from this gland may be also be cryopreserved and successfully autotransplanted if the primary autograft does not function. Wells has pioneered this approach, and has reported that 30% of the patients developed recurrent, graft-dependent hyperparathyroidism.[413] It should be noted that autotransplantation of cryopreserved parathyroid autografts have been successful in only 50% of patients, resulting in permanent hypoparathyroidism.[241] The concept that a humoral factor may be initiating growth in the remnant parathyroid tissue is further supported by the finding of Malette, who reported a higher incidence of graft-dependent recurrence in patients with MEN 1 treated with total parathyroidectomy with autotransplantation than in patients with sporadic hyperplasia undergoing the same operation.[232] MEN 1–associated hyperparathyroidism is associated with the finding of supernumerary parathyroid glands. This factor contributes to the potential for missed glands at the time of initial operation, thus increasing the risk of recurrence. The implementation of intraoperative PTH determination (IOPTH) has been helpful in reconciling this problem in patients with hyperparathyroidism associated with the MEN 1 syndrome.[300]

Primary surgical explorations in patients with MEN 1 and hyperparathyroidism may result in cure rates >90%. The requisite for identifying all four parathyroid glands in these patients is emphasized in a report by O'Riordan.[293] In this series, immediate cure was noted in 94% of patients; however, hypercalcemia was noted to be persistent in 19% of patients in whom fewer than four glands were visualized at initial operation compared with 3% of patients in whom four glands or more were noted at initial surgery. In general, both persistent and recurrent disease rates are higher in patients who have less than total parathyroidectomy performed and in whom fewer than four glands are found at the time of initial operation.[94,293]

MEN type 2A (MEN 2A). Multiple endocrine neoplasia type 2A (MEN 2A) is a syndrome characterized by medullary thyroid carcinoma, pheochromocytoma, hyperparathyroidism, lichen planus amyloidosis, and Hirschsprung's disease. This disorder first came to clinical light in 1932, when Eisenberg and Wallerstein first reported a pheochromocytoma and concurrent thyroid carcinoma in a patient at autopsy.[108] Sipple in 1961 estimated that the incidence of thyroid cancer in patients with pheochromocytoma was 14 times higher than that of the normal population, and Cushman subsequently reported a family with hereditary thyroid carcinoma and pheochromocytoma in which one affected member had a parathyroid tumor.[83,356] Thus came the description and characterization of the syndrome, formerly known as Sipple's syndrome, now known as multiple endocrine neoplasia type 2A.[364]

The penetrance of the independent entities for patients with MEN 2A syndrome is variable with the exception of medullary thyroid carcinoma that is seen in essentially all affected individuals. Pheochromocytoma and hyperparathyroidism, however, both demonstrate variable penetrance, with pheochromocytoma occurring in 70% of individuals affected and hyperparathyroidism reported least commonly in approximately 20% to 35% of affected patients.[48,65,171,316,317]

Hyperparathyroidism is usually diagnosed as a result of screening patients or family members with MEN 2A or incidentally during thyroidectomy for C cell hyperplasia or medullary thyroid carcinoma.[23] A review of 67 patients with hyperparathyroidism associated with the MEN 2A syndrome by Raue noted that 75% were diagnosed at the time of thyroidectomy for either C cell hyperplasia or medullary thyroid carcinoma. These patients demonstrated normal serum calcium and PTH levels preoperatively, and thus the diagnosis was made on the basis of intraoperative morphology or histology.[316] Uncommonly, a diagnosis of hyperparathyroidism is made as a result of the development of clinical symptoms that are similar to those encountered in sporadic primary hyperparathyroidism.[317]

MEN 2A–associated hyperparathyroidism usually develops after the third decade of life in the form of mild hypercalcemia with rarely demonstrated hypercalcemic crises.[171,316] It is generally acknowledged that the hyperparathyroidism associated with the MEN 2A syndrome is less aggressive than its counterpart noted for MEN 1 or non-MEN syndromes.[293,317] Patients with MEN 2A generally have lower serum calcium levels, fewer symptoms or complications of hypercalcemia, less frequent multiple gland involvement, and a lower incidence of persistent or recurrent disease after surgical treatment than patients with the MEN 1 or non-MEN variety of hyperparathyroidism. A circulating humoral factor that stimulates parathyroid cell proliferation has not been postulated to exist in association with the hyperparathyroidism associated with MEN 2A syndromes.

Similar to MEN 1, MEN 2A is a genetic disease that is transmitted in an autosomal-dominant fashion and with a high degree of penetrance but with variable expression. In the late 1980s, the inherited defect of the MEN 2 syndrome was mapped to the pericentromeric region of chromosome 10.[239,355] Subsequent work identified the ret protooncogene as a segment on chromosome 10 that encodes for a specific cell surface receptor complex, the exact function of which is poorly characterized. Mutations in the segment of the ret protooncogene coding for the extracellular domain of the tyrosine kinase receptor protein are responsible for producing the MEN 2A phenotype.[258] Although the mutation has been well characterized for its association with medullary thyroid carcinoma, the exact relationship to parathyroid disease is unknown.

In the event that parathyroid exploration for hyperparathyroidism associated with MEN 2A syndrome is required, the presence of a pheochromocytoma must be excluded in patients before surgery. Surgery on a patient with an unrecognized pheochromocytoma may result in a hypertensive crisis intraoperatively with potential catastrophic sequelae. Accordingly, these patients should be screened for the presence of a catecholamine-producing neoplasm of the adrenal, and thus a plasma collection for catecholamines, metanephrine, and nonmetanephrine levels should be performed before parathyroid exploration. Once this is assured, the surgical approach in these patients is generally more conservative than in patients with MEN 1–associated hyperparathyroidism. A bilateral neck exploration is performed with identification of all four parathyroid glands. Although the hyperparathyroidism associated with patients affected with MEN 2A demonstrates a higher incidence of multiglandular disease than patients with sporadic primary hyperparathyroidism, it is not as high as found in patients with MEN 1 syndrome. Subtotal parathyroidectomy with removal of only the obviously morphologically enlarged parathyroid glands is the approach of choice in patients with MEN 2–associated hyperparathyroidism. Transcervical thymectomy is generally not necessary, because supernumerary gland involvement is uncommon in these patients. In the event that all four glands are involved, transcervical thymectomy may be performed concurrent with subtotal parathyroidectomy. In surgery for medullary thyroid carcinoma, normal parathyroid glands in the superior position are generally preserved with resection of the inferior parathyroid and subsequent autotransplantation, so that lymph nodes in the central neck compartment and the anterior mediastinum are not missed.

Surgical exploration for patients with MEN 2A–associated hyperparathyroidism is generally quite effective. Cance and Wells[48] reported a 100% surgical success rate and 3% recurrence rate in treating patients with primary hyperparathyroidism associated with MEN 2A. Unlike MEN 1, where the extensiveness of parathyroid gland resection is important in defining operative success, the degree of parathyroid gland resection does not seem to significantly influence the success rate in patients operated for hyperparathyroidism associated with MEN 2A syndrome. O'Riordan has reported a 100% cure rate with no recurrences whether total parathyroidectomy, subtotal parathyroidectomy, or excision of enlarged glands independently was performed.[293]

Non-MEN familial hyperparathyroidism (NMFH).

Non-MEN familial hyperparathyroidism (NMFH), also known as familial isolated hyperparathyroidism, refers to hyperparathyroidism occurring in the absence of other endocrinopathies in patients with at least one first-degree relative with surgically proven hyperparathyroidism and no personal or family history of MEN.

Familial hyperparathyroidism occurs in young patients with a mean age at diagnosis of approximately 36 years. Some of these patients experience this disorder as children, although it is rare before 10 years of age.[172] In contradistinction, patients with sporadic primary hyperparathyroidism typically are seen during their fifth or sixth decades of life.[390] Familial hyperparathyroidism seems to be more aggressive than sporadic or MEN 2A-related hyperparathyroidism; frequently patients with this disorder will manifest profound hypercalcemia and more frequently be seen with hypercalcemic crisis.[172,173] Renal lithiasis occurs in one third to half of patients reported with familial hyperparathyroidism and will commonly also manifest other nonspecific signs and symptoms such as fatigue, weakness, hypertension, and peptic ulcer disease.[172] It has been postulated that familial hyperparathyroidism may be associated with an increased risk for the development of parathyroid cancer.[172,242,408] A high incidence of persistent or recurrent disease after treatment seems to be a characteristic feature of the clinical profile of non–MEN-related familial hyperparathyroidism. Of the 97 patients reported in the literature, persistent or recurrent disease has been noted to occur at a rate of 33%. This degree of recalcitrant disease contrasts markedly with the very low rate of recurrent disease after treatment in patients with sporadic hyperparathyroidism undergoing parathyroidectomy. This characteristic bears strong consideration in planning the appropriate operative strategy in patients with non–MEN-related familial hyperparathyroidism.

Before initiating treatment for this disorder, it is important to exclude all other familial sources for hyperparathyroidism, as well as the entity known as benign FHH. Once these other entities have been excluded, patients with non-MEN–related familial hyperparathyroidism should be considered for parathyroid exploration because of the aggressive biologic behavior of this disorder. There is a high incidence of both multiglandular and supernumerary gland disease accounting for the high rate of recalcitrance after initial surgery. Similar to the other familial hyperparathyroidism disorders, a bilateral neck exploration with identification of all four parathyroid glands is performed. Either subtotal or total parathyroidectomy together with bilateral cervical thymectomy is generally performed with autotransplantation of parathyroid tissue as necessary, depending on the extent of parathyroid gland resection. If only one or two parathyroid glands are morphologically abnormal and enlarged, the goal of therapy is to resect all abnormal parathyroid tissue from one side of the neck and leave existing remnant parathyroid tissue in only one side.[172] Intraoperative PTH determination is helpful in determining the degree of hyperfunctional parathyroid tissue remaining after subtotal parathyroidectomy in these patients and may serve as an indicator of remnant parathyroid function once abnormally enlarged glands have been removed. Both the visualization and subsequent removal of abnormally enlarged glands and the intraoperative PTH findings serve to guide the extensiveness of surgery in patients who manifest this disorder and have less than four glands appearing abnormal. It is important that these patients be followed long term to recognize if and when recalcitrant disease occurs.

Familial neonatal hyperparathyroidism.

Neonatal hyperparathyroidism is a rare condition characterized by severe hypercalcemia occurring in association with severe hypotonia, poor feeding, constipation, failure to thrive and respiratory distress. The clinical manifestations of this disorder become evident during the first week of life; however, it may not become manifest until the age of 3 months or older.[172] Most patients with familial neonatal hyperparathyroidism have occurred in families with a known history of benign FHH. The disease locus for FHH has been identified on the long arm of chromosome 3, and patients with FHH are heterozygous for the mutation, with one affected allel.[155,157] The occurrence of two defective alleles is believed to cause severe neonatal hyperparathyroidism.[305] Most patients with this disorder will require urgent parathyroid exploration and resection of all four glands. Total parathyroidectomy is advocated together with parathyroid autotransplantation, bilateral transcervical thymectomy, and cryopreservation of parathyroid tissue because of the high recalcitrance rate for this disorder.

Renal failure–induced hyperparathyroidism.

The indications for parathyroid exploration in patients

with renal failure–induced hyperparathyroidism may be characterized as those manifested before and after renal transplantation. Surgery is generally indicated when medical therapy fails to control progressive secondary hyperparathyroidism.[96,169,228] The clinical manifestations occurring in this disorder include persistent or worsening skeletal symptoms, intractable pruritus, and soft tissue calcifications.[93] The presence of biopsy-proven high turnover bone disease and/or calciphylaxis in a patient with chronic renal failure with secondary hyperparathyroidism are additional indications for a parathyroidectomy.[95,103,224] Parathyroidectomy may be indicated in some patients after successful renal transplantation because of the development of clinical manifestations similar to those of primary hyperparathyroidism, including hypercalcemia with nephrolithiasis, pancreatitis, central nervous system manifestation, and overt bone demineralization.[84] The presence of mild hypercalcemia in and of itself does not seem to be a serious threat to the patient after renal transplantation, but impaired kidney function in the presence of high parathyroid hormone levels and hypercalcemia represents an indication for parathyroidectomy, as is the association of kidney stones and long-standing hypercalcemia.[61,61,68,303]

In general, preoperative localization studies are not recommended before initial exploration or renal failure–induced hyperparathyroidism. This is principally because of the need to perform bilateral exploration with visualization of all four parathyroid glands and the finding that nuclear imaging with technetium-99 sestamibi is not as effective for localization as it is for single-gland disease. In contrast to the directed exploration protocols for minimally invasive operations performed for solitary adenoma, the operation of choice for patients with renal-induced hyperparathyroidism at initial surgery is traditional four-gland bilateral exploration. The surgical principle of "not removing anything before seeing everything" is aptly applied in this situation.

The two most widely used initial surgical procedures for the management of renal failure–induced hyperparathyroidism are subtotal parathyroidectomy and total parathyroidectomy with parathyroid autotransplantation with or without cryopreservation of parathyroid tissue. If subtotal parathyroidectomy is the procedure of choice, the smallest most normal-appearing parathyroid gland is selected to represent the remnant gland left in situ. The pole opposite the vascular pedicle is excised, leaving approximately one third to one half of the entire gland as a vascularized remnant. It is important that all parathyroid glands be in situ when this is accomplished, so that should the remnant prove to be nonviable after its section-

ing, the next most normal-appearing gland be selected for the remnant and the initial remnant completely removed. It is generally easier to leave a superior remnant with a viable pedicle than an inferior because of the proximity of the vascular pedicle to the normal position of the gland. The remnant is marked with a nonreabsorbable suture or metal surgical clip. In the event that only three parathyroid glands are found after a comprehensive exploration, all three are removed. This circumstance has been noted to result in approximately 30% of patients with persistent hyperparathyroidism.[357] In the event total parathyroidectomy and autotransplantation with or without cryopreservation is planned, all four glands are removed after discovery, with the most normal-appearing gland selected as the autograft.[411] Ten to 15 mm^3 fragments of the selected autotransplant gland are placed into several intramuscular pockets in the brachioradialis muscle of the nondominant forearm in a hemostatic fashion, because hemorrhage into the implant beds may result in poor "take" of the grafts.[413] Cryopreservation of the remaining portion of this autotransplant gland should be performed in the event that sufficient parathyroid function does not develop after revascularization of the implants.

A number of reports supporting one procedure vs the other are noted in the literature, but objective controlled trials dealing specifically with renal-induced hyperparathyroidism are rare. Of the few trials conducted, the only prospective randomized series was reported by Rothmund, who found that parathyroidectomy with autotransplantation was superior to subtotal thyroidectomy in controlling symptoms in a group of 40 patients with renal-induced hyperparathyroidism.[326] In this series, in which follow-up was noted over a mean of 4 years, four patients who were randomly assigned to the subtotal parathyroidectomy cohort experienced recurrent disease. The elimination of bone pain was significantly improved proportionally in patients who underwent total parathyroidectomy with autotransplantation. Three independent reports compared both techniques in a retrospective analysis and found that both procedures resulted in similar outcomes.[229,373,414] In assessing the merit of each technique, one should keep in mind that most surgeons will find the procedure they routinely use and have more experience with to be the most applicable and appropriate in dealing with patients with this disorder.

The success of subtotal parathyroidectomy depends mainly on the size and viability of the remnant parathyroid gland left in situ. Remnants that are nodular are more likely to grow and result in recurrent hyperparathyroidism. This procedure has a theoretical advantage of producing less postoperative hypocalcemia, because the remnant continues to function. The main disadvantage is that in the event that these remnants become hyperfunctional, the reoperations on many occasions are tedious, difficult technically, and carry increased risk of complications such as injury to the recurrent laryngeal nerve. In general, successful subtotal parathyroidectomy alleviated bone pain to a lesser degree than those total parathyroidectomies with autotransplantation but carried less risk of postoperative low turnover bone disease.[92]

The success of total parathyroidectomy with autotransplantation mainly depends on the nodularity of the gland from which the graft is obtained and number and weight of the fragments that are implanted. As in recurrent disease within a nodular remnant after subtotal parathyroidectomy, graft-dependent recurrence is three times greater when implanting a nodular gland instead of a diffusely hyperplastic one.[376] The advantage of autotransplantation is represented by the fact that should hyperparathyroidism recur in the graft remnant, this may be partially resected under local anesthesia and with minimal potential complications. Several studies published theories that show a 5% to 38% rate of postoperative hypercalcemia attributable to a hyperfunctional graft with a 2% to 6% chance of recurrence requiring graft resection and a 5% to 30% chance of hypocalcemia lasting more than 12 months secondary to poor graft viability and function.*

Re-Exploration for Recalcitrant Hyperparathyroidism

The distinction between *persistent* (hypercalcemia persisting or recurring within 6 months after initial operation) and *recurrent* (hypercalcemia recurring after 6 months of normocalcemia after the initial surgery) hyperparathyroidism after a prior cervical or mediastinal exploration for hypercalcemia has been applied loosely but poses an equitable management dilemma and technical challenge to the surgeon.

It has been estimated that 2% to 10% of surgical failures may be attributed to an incorrect diagnosis.[71,236] Accordingly, the first requirement for success in reoperative parathyroid surgery is proper diagnosis. By definition, hyperparathyroidism (primary or secondary) must be proven by elevation of serum calcium levels associated with high or inappropriately elevated PTH levels. Elevated serum chloride and decreased serum phosphate levels are frequently noted. In addition, urinary calcium should be appropriately elevated to exclude a diagnosis of FHH. If all these parameters are not present, other causes of hypercal-

cemia must be considered, because a repeat surgical exercise is almost guaranteed to be unsuccessful.[380] The diagnosis of hyperparathyroidism is currently more straightforward with immunoradiometric and immunochemiluminescent assays of PTH levels. Diagnostic errors in hyperparathyroidism can result from medications (calcium, vitamin D, furosemide, thiazide diuretics, calcitonin, lithium), FHH, malignancy (bone metastasis or humoral hypercalcemia), granulomatous disease, acute renal failure, bone disease (Paget's, immobilization), hyperthyroidism, or adrenal insufficiency.

The indications for surgical intervention in secondary cases must be solid, because the morbidity and technical difficulty is increased. In general, the guidelines for surgery in primary hyperparathyroidism, as outlined in the National Institutes of Health 2002 Consensus Conference, serve as a framework for surgical decision making in patients requiring further treatment after initial failed exploration.

Causes of failed exploration. The most common finding on parathyroid re-exploration by the experienced parathyroid surgeon is a missed single adenoma. Akerström reported on 84 parathyroid re-explorations in 69 patients with primary hyperparathyroidism. Thirty-seven of these patients had missed adenomas, four of these patients had double "adenomas," and only one adenoma was resected on the initial exploration.[6] Most of the remaining patients had persistent hyperparathyroidism secondary to inadequate resection of parathyroid hyperplasia, with only four patients demonstrating recurrent "single" adenomas. Rotstein and colleagues analyzed their series of 28 reoperations for primary hyperparathyroidism. They identified solitary adenomas in 24 patients, with 2 patients each having hyperplasia and carcinoma.[327] Norman and Denham have used the technique of minimally invasive radio-guided parathyroidectomy for reoperative disease and resected 23 solitary adenomas from 24 patients.[277] Jaskowiak and others[185] reviewed their experience at the National Institutes of Health with 288 patients with persistent/recurrent hyperparathyroidism. Two hundred twenty-two (77%) of these patients were ultimately demonstrated to have solitary adenomas.

In patients with secondary hyperparathyroidism, hyperplasia is the expected histopathology. Cattan and others[56] explored 89 patients for persistent or recurrent secondary hyperparathyroidism; 53 of these patients had undergone subtotal parathyroidectomy, whereas 36 had prior total parathyroidectomy with autotransplantation. They identified hypertrophy of the remnant as the principal cause of recurrence in the subtotal group. In the group receiving total

---

*References 7, 126, 130, 131, 257, 294, 325, 361.

parathyroidectomy, recurrence was located in the autotransplant in half; hyperplastic disease was identified in the neck or mediastinum in the other half.

Equally as important as the finding that the cause of recalcitrant hyperparathyroidism is a solitary adenoma in most patients, through the observation that, in most of these cases, the adenoma is in a "standard" location. In the Akerström report, only 8 patients required sternotomy for ectopic adenomas identified in the mediastinum despite 17 sternotomies being performed. In 5 of the 17 patients who had sternotomy, the offending lesion was ultimately identified in a normal location in the neck.[6] Of the more unusual ectopic locations, one was ventral to the left atrium, one was ventral to aortic root, and one was in the aortopulmonary window. Furthermore, only one gland was truly intrathyroid, despite 19 thyroid lobectomies performed as part of the re-exploration. In the series by Norman and Denham,[277] only one gland was in the mediastinum (just anterior to the right atrium), whereas two were intrathyroid. Jaskowiak and others identified adenomas in the posterior superior mediastinum, specifically in the tracheoesophageal groove in 27% of their patients (59 of 215). This was the most common location of the adenoma in the failed first exploration. This site is easily explored transcervically and should be considered as an inferior extension of the normal superior gland position. Furthermore, the authors point out that these adenomas were almost always in direct apposition to the recurrent laryngeal nerve, perhaps suggesting that inadequate dissection around the nerve initially contributed to the failure. Another 24.3% of patients had their adenomas in the normal positions adjacent to the thyroid gland.[234]

In the NIH series, the most common ectopic site was within the thymus or mediastinum, accounting for 16.7%.[234] This value is lower than other reports of 22% intrathymic tumors at the initial operation and 38% for reoperation.[393] An intrathyroidal lesion was noted in 10% (22 patients) of their study population. A similar percentage of patients had undescended parathyroid glands. These so-called parathymus lesions are located at the bifurcation of the carotid artery, high in the neck, and represent an inferior gland that is arrested in the descent from the third brachial pouch. Other "typical" ectopic locations included lesions within the carotid sheath and the retroesophageal space. Unusual ectopic locations include the aortopulmonary window in two patients, the hypopharynx at the base of the tongue in one patient, the wall of the nasopharynx near the nasal septum in one patient, and within the vagus nerve high in the neck at the level of C1 to C2 vertebrae. Furthermore, three patients had lesions "seeded" within the strap muscles, most likely because of the first exploration.[234]

Preoperative assessment. Because a missed single adenoma located in a "standard" position accounts for most patients whose initial procedures fail, accessing the records from the original exploration, including the operative note and the pathology report, is essential. Notes from the original operation may describe in detail the thoroughness of the exploration: which parathyroid glands remain in situ, whether the recurrent laryngeal nerve was identified and thoroughly skeletonized, and whether any "atypical" but regional areas were explored. Pathology reports should document what histologic items were identified (i.e., whether all normal parathyroid glands were biopsy proven). Ideally, all four glands should be identified before calling an initial exploration negative.

No matter what the original surgical and pathologic reports state, endocrine surgeons universally agree that preoperative imaging studies are an essential component of reoperative parathyroid surgery. A variety of invasive and noninvasive techniques are available to image or localize abnormal parathyroid glands, and these have been discussed previously.

Operative risk: re-exploration. Once a decision has been made to pursue re-exploration for persistent or recurrent hyperparathyroidism, the patient and surgeon must review and mutually understand the inherent risks of such surgery. The risk of injury to the recurrent laryngeal nerve, a potentially very problematic complication, is greater in reexplored necks than that for initial exploration. In two large studies, the incidence of vocal paralysis exceeded 6% after parathyroid re-exploration, in sharp contrast to the exceedingly low rate (less than 1%) realized after initial bilateral exploration.[299] Although more limited approaches to parathyroid re-exploration (targeted exploration; minimally invasive radio-guided surgery) are likely to result in a reduced incidence of nerve injury after reoperation, it remains that surgical treatment of the operated neck will always be associated with increased risk. In addition to an incidence of recurrent nerve injury, re-exploration carries with it a greater likelihood for postoperative hypocalcemia, both temporary and permanent.[36] Finally, although the success rate for reoperative parathyroid surgery may exceed 90% in experienced hands, this remains substantially less than the near perfect rate of success for initial surgery. Thus, it is important that, together with reconfirmation of the diagnosis and careful patient preparation, a candid discussion of the risks associated with reoperation be held with the patient.

Operative strategy. After the decision to proceed with re-exploration and having performed a review of the initial operative procedure and localization studies, the surgeon then considers the operative approach. Ideally, the objective is to remove a single gland without extensive dissection, which may result in injury to the surrounding structures (i.e., recurrent laryngeal nerve or devascularization of remaining parathyroid tissue). The likelihood of accomplishing this objective depends on two factors: the experience of the initial operating surgeon and the demonstration of an enlarged parathyroid gland on correlative localization studies. In most cases, reoperation after initial surgery by an experienced surgeon will be difficult and tedious, because the initial dissection will have been comprehensive, and the surgical bed will have significant fibrosis. In contradistinction, the extensiveness of initial exploration, and resulting degree of fibrosis, may be significantly less in patients having had the original surgery performed by a relatively inexperienced surgeon. In both of these circumstances, the localizing studies will be of prime importance in targeting the putative hyperfunctional gland and limiting the reoperative dissection.

The best of all scenarios, and the most common, is unequivocal localization to a cervical site that may also include the anterior superior mediastinum. The previous neck incision is generally used for access, in some cases by excising the old scar completely. The usual superior/inferior flaps are raised, and access is gained to the side of the neck indicated by the localization studies. A lateral to medial approach to dissection is undertaken to avoid the dense scarification and fibrosis in the region of the tracheoesophageal groove where the recurrent laryngeal nerve resides. In this manner, dissection proceeds medially from the sternomastoid muscle superficial to the great vessels and then directly to the region overlying the cervical spine. This approach exploits the concept of the viscerovertebral angle as described by Tenta.[378] This potential anatomic space is defined as that area bordered laterally by the carotid sheath structures, medially by the trachea and esophagus, anteriorly by the thyroid, and posteriorly by the cervical spine (Figure 120-12). In accessing this region, the surgeon may take advantage of a tissue plane with relatively little vascularity and fibrosis. This area will allow the surgeon to examine the superior mediastinum inferiorly, the retroesophageal compartment medially and as far superiorly as the hyoid bone, all within planes of dissection that separate with relative freedom. Although not necessary in most cases, the recurrent laryngeal nerve may be identified and isolated for protection by following this approach, because dense fibrosis is infrequently encountered over the prevertebral space,

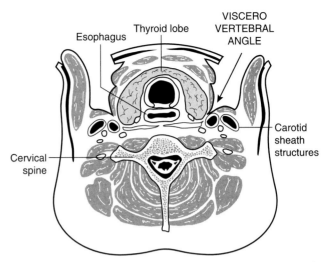

Figure 120-12. The viscerovertebral angle (VVA) approach relative to parathyroid exploration.

even after a thorough initial exploration. In the event a gland is suspected in the superior retrothyroidal area, the nerve should be identified, because it may be lateral to a medially displaced superior gland. Most missed adenomas, which are accessible through a cervical incision, may be approached by use of this technique, which also allows for thyroid lobectomy should an intrathyroidal gland be suspected. A situation wherein localization studies indicate a mediastinal location usually mandates a thoracic approach, either by median sternotomy or lateral thoracotomy, depending on the involved area within the mediastinum. An enlarged gland identified within the anterior mediastinum is usually associated with the thymus and may be accessed by median sternotomy. These glands are usually found at the level of the innominate vein within thymic tissue but may also be found adjacent to the aortic arch or between the thymus and pleura. Should the localizing studies demonstrate a posterior-based mediastinal gland, a lateral or posterolateral thoracotomy should be strongly considered to avoid attempts at dissection through critical structures in the anterior mediastinum. These posterior glands may reside in the aortopulmonary window or the retroesophageal region. One should be aware that the recurrent laryngeal nerve might be injured when approaching the posterior mediastinum through a left lateral thoracotomy. Despite what may be interpreted as compelling localization results, the surgeon should be prepared to perform concurrent cervical exploration in the event that initial intraoperative PTH levels do not confirm removal of all hyperfunctional parathyroid tissue.

The most problematic preoperative scenario to confront is that in which localization fails to identify any suspicious site. It is in this situation that reoperative surgery for hyperparathyroidism is potentially the least successful and the most morbid. Failure to localize usually mandates a bilateral cervical exploration that comprehensively and methodically addresses all potential sites that may harbor a missing gland or glands. A properly constructed initial operative note that accurately documents remaining histologically identified parathyroid glands and regions explored is of utmost importance and potential value for the reoperating surgeon. An orderly systematic approach to re-exploration is required in these circumstances to locate the missing gland(s) and limit morbidity. The order in which regions are approached may vary according to the surgeon; however, it is important that all potential areas be accessed to increase the chance of success and avoid a failed re-exploration. The preferred approach is to explore each side through the viscerovertebral angle by a lateral to medial orientation (see Figure 120-12). Regions of dissection are then addressed in the following manner: the anterior superior mediastinum is dissected first, with careful attention to the thyrothymic ligament and tracheoesophageal groove region adjacent to the recurrent nerve (Figure 120-13). Cervical thymectomy, if not performed during initial surgery, is completed at this time (Figure 120-14). Dissection then turns to the retropharyngeal, retroesophageal region, where blunt dissection within the prevertebral space will allow for digital exploration superiorly above the cricoid larynx and inferiorly into the posterior mediastinum. Enlarged glands in this anatomic plane may often be felt before they are seen by use of these techniques. Next, the thyroid lobe is mobilized, possibly truncating the superior vascular pedicle to rotate the gland anteromedially so that the posterior thyroid

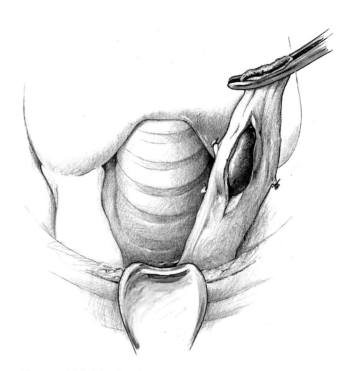

Figure 120-14. Cervical thymectomy demonstrating an intrathymic inferior parathyroid adenoma.

capsule may be closely examined for a folded, lobulated parathyroid gland under the capsular fascia (Figure 120-15). With this maneuver, the thyroid lobe is palpated for any nodular densities that may be suspicious for an intrathyroidal parathyroid gland. The

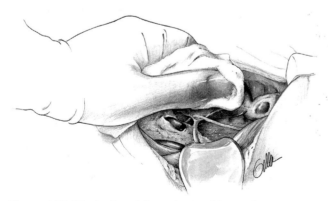

Figure 120-13. A gloved finger inserted beneath the pretracheal fascia overlying the cervical spine demonstrates the "pseudo" ectopic location of a descended superior parathyroid adenoma in the tracheoesophageal groove.

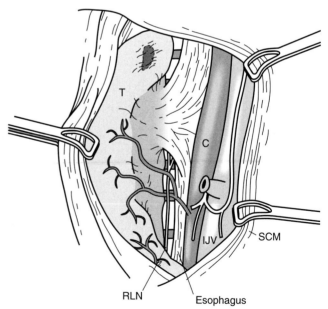

Figure 120-15. Superior parathyroid adenoma located under the pretracheal fascia over the posterior aspect of the thyroid gland, a "pseudo" subcapsular parathyroid gland. T, Thyroid gland; C, carotid sheath; RLN, recurrent laryngeal nerve; SCM, sternomastoid muscle; IJV, internal jugular vein.

carotid sheath is then opened from the superior medi-astinum to the hyoid bone, inspecting and palpating for nodular structures within the sheath (Figure 120-16). Failing identification on the side explored first, the dissection proceeds contralaterally in the same manner with orderly inspection of all regions noted previously. In the event that a bilateral exploration fails to identify the offending gland, thyroid lobectomy or lobotomy is usually performed on the side suspected of harboring the missing gland. During these exercises, it is important to document carefully all normal parathyroid tissue found, or in the instance that glands are not identified, the putative missing parathyroid gland by position.

If all maneuvers previously described are unsuccessful in identifying the missing gland, the procedure is terminated, and further measures are undertaken to identify the gland's position by imaging and possibly angioinvasive studies. Mediastinal exploration should not be performed in this setting, predominantly because of the lack of localization and element of time involved with the unsuccessful bilateral cervical exploration just completed.

Special Circumstances
Unsuccessful Localization

In most situations, failure to localize to a discrete area of the neck after sestamibi imaging occurs as a result of unrecognized multinodular thyroid disease (Figure 120-17). In the absence of a nodular thyroid gland,

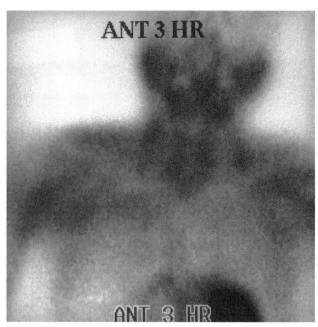

Figure 120-17. Technnectium-99m sestamibi nuclear scan in a patient with hyperparathyroidism and nodular thyroid disease.

one must suspect diffuse hyperplasia or less likely, an ectopically located gland, either cervical or mediastinal. One must be careful that an appropriately dosed (minimum 23 to 26 millicuries) and correctly conducted nuclear scan has been carried out in all studies. Single-positron emission computed tomography technetium-99m sestamibi imaging might be helpful in reconciling equivocal planar images.[62,270] A failure to localize on delayed nuclear imaging mandates the performance of a standard bilateral exploration.

The false-positive sestamibi scan; that is, discrete areas of delayed nuclear uptake representing false-positive localizations demonstrated at surgery, may occur. Almost without exception, this occurs as a result of unsuspected nodular thyroid disease. Nodular thyroid abnormalities accounting for false-positive scans are usually solid in consistency. In contrast, cystic thyroid lesions were not associated with a false-positive localization study. This suggests the importance of performing high-resolution ultrasound evaluation in patients with nodular thyroid disease, in that the finding of a cystic nodule would decrease suspicion that the localization result represents a false-positive study. Even in the presence of solid nodular thyroid disease, both subcapsular and intrathyroidal abnormal parathyroid glands have been encountered that have imaged correctly. This emphasizes the importance of evaluating all nodularity within or associated with the thyroid gland in the event that these abnormal parathyroid glands are located in a "hidden" region either between thyroid

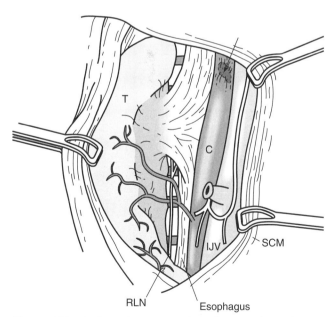

Figure 120-16. Ectopic parathyroid adenoma *(arrow)* illustrated within the carotid sheath. T, Thyroid gland; C, carotid sheath; RLN, recurrent laryngeal nerve; SCM, sternomastoid muscle; IJV, internal jugular vein.

nodules or tightly held under the pretracheal fascia representing the "pseudocapsule" over the thyroid gland (Figure 120-18). More likely, however, is that solid thyroid nodularity with a false-positive sestamibi image is consistent with an adenomatous thyroid nodule, thus mandating bilateral cervical exploration.

Mediastinal Exploration

Initial or re-exploration for parathyroid disease may require exploration of the mediastinum. Ectopic parathyroid glands located within the mediastinum and below the level of the thymus account for a small percentage (0.2%) of all abnormally located glands.[132] In contrast, in the re-operative setting, both Wang and Norton have shown that a more substantial proportion, 18% and 20%, respectively, of ectopically located adenomas reside in the mediastinum accessible only through a mediastinal approach.[278,401] These inferior parathyroid glands are associated in almost all circumstances with the thymus with which they descend during embryonic development, having arisen with the thymus as a third pharyngeal pouch derivative.

Several approaches to the mediastinum are available for exploration. The choice of approach used depends on the location of the putative adenoma. Localization studies that, in combination, corroborate and specify the mediastinal location are required before undertaking exploration. It has been the experience of most investigators that technetium-99 sestamibi imaging together with MRI represent the optimal combination of physiologic- and anatomic-based imaging for localization (Figure 120-19). The techniques available for approaching the mediastinum include transcervical substernal with thymectomy with anterior retraction of the sternum for superior mediastinal glands; median sternotomy with direct approach to the anterior middle and caudal mediastinal compartments; posterolateral thoracotomy for selective posteriorly based glands in the lower mediastinal compartment; and endoscopic, minimally invasive mediastinal dissection for selectively focused exploration.[313] Most glands will be approached through a median sternotomy, owing to this technique's capability to safely address a number of areas within the mediastinum and the lower cervical region immediately posterior to the clavicular heads and manubrium. This technique also allows uninterrupted visualization of both recurrent laryngeal nerves, thus preventing inadvertent injury to these structures within the mediastinum.

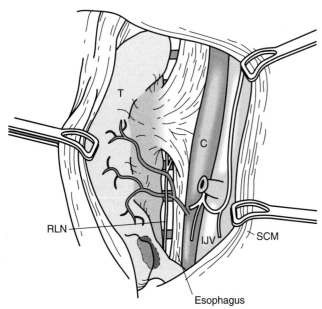

Figure 120-18. Inferior parathyroid adenoma demonstrated deep to the true thyroid capsule between nodular thyroid projections. T, Thyroid gland; C, carotid sheath; RLN, recurrent laryngeal nerve; SCM, sternomastoid muscle; IJV, internal jugular vein.

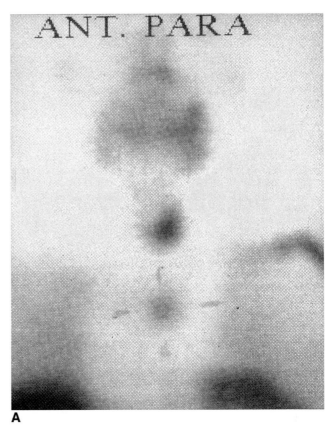

Figure 120-19. Technetium-99m sestamibi scan **(A)** and magnetic resonance imaging scan **(B)** in a patient with a mediastinal parathyroid adenoma. The area of nuclear uptake noted on the sestamibi scan correlates anatomically with the nodule demonstrated in the aortopulmonary window on MRI. Adenoma was removed via left lateral thoracotomy.

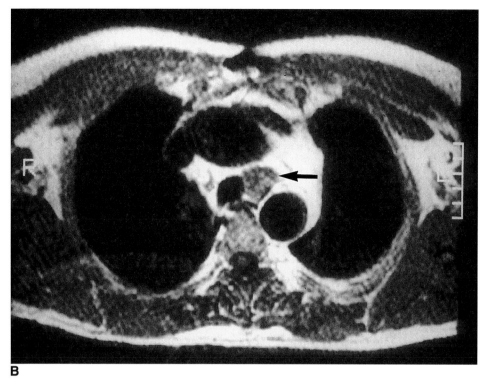

B

Figure 120-19, cont'd Technetium-99m sestamibi scan **(A)** and magnetic resonance imaging scan **(B)** in a patient with a mediastinal parathyroid adenoma. The area of nuclear uptake noted on the sestamibi scan correlates anatomically with the nodule demonstrated in the aortopulmonary window on MRI. Adenoma was removed via left lateral thoracotomy.

Surgical adjuncts that may aid in the intraoperative localization of adenomas and may be used after median sternotomy include intraoperative ultrasound and gamma probe after preoperative sestamibi injection.

Gamma Radiation Detection Device

Minimally invasive surgical exploration with a gamma radiation detection device (gamma probe) has been developed and advocated by Norman[275] and associates to actively facilitate and expedite initial surgery for parathyroid adenoma (See "Intraoperative Localization Methods").[75] This method exploits both the nuclear uptake characteristics of parathyroid adenoma with respect to technetium-99 sestamibi and the ability of the gamma probe to intraoperatively localize these glands in the neck after preoperative sestamibi injection.

This technique has been applied by one of the authors (PKP) in mediastinal exploration after sternotomy with satisfactory results (Figure 120-20). Despite uptake of sestamibi by myocardial tissue, background radioactivity within the mediastinum seems to be less than that of thyroid tissue, thus facilitating a focused dissection with minimal disturbance of surrounding mediastinal structures. Reoperation

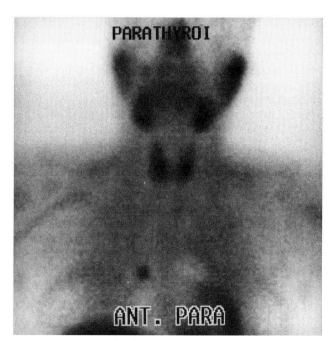

Figure 120-20. Technetium-99m sestamibi imaging showing mediastinal parathyroid that represented a fifth hyperplastic gland missed at initial surgery, at which time four hyperplastic glands were removed.

for multiple-gland disease in secondary and tertiary hyperparathyroidism has been aided with the use of the gamma probe when supernumerary glands are present. In one notable instance in this series, three additional parathyroid glands (two cervical, one mediastinal) were recovered in a patient with tertiary hyperparathyroidism who previously underwent documented four-gland parathyroidectomy during preparation for cadaveric renal transplantation. The gamma probe was instrumental in identifying one of the cervical glands and one mediastinal gland that was the only parathyroid gland that localized accurately on initial sestamibi imaging. The gamma probe may also be applied for removal of hyperfunctional parathyroid tissue autotransplanted to the forearm in the setting of secondary/tertiary hyperparathyroidism.

Parathyroid Carcinoma

Parathyroid carcinoma is reported to be the cause of primary hyperparathyroidism in only 0.1% to 4% of persons affected.[75,147,393,404] Parathyroid carcinoma occurs with equal frequency in male and female patients; in contrast, parathyroid adenomas occur more frequently in women.[174] The epidemiology of parathyroid carcinoma offers few clues about its etiology and pathogenesis. The development of cancer of the parathyroid glands has been linked to chronic renal failure and dialysis[33,249,374] and with familial hyperparathyroidism syndromes including MEN 1 and 2A and the hereditary hyperparathyroidism-jaw tumor syndrome.[423] The hyperparathyroidism-jaw tumor syndrome is characterized by recurrent parathyroid adenomas, fibroosseous tumors of the mandible, and Wilms' tumors.[423]

In general, patients with parathyroid cancer have higher serum calcium levels, higher levels of intact parathyroid hormone, and more profound metabolic abnormalities than do patients with parathyroid adenoma or hyperplasia. Approximately 70% of patients with parathyroid carcinoma have serum calcium levels >14 mg/dL and intact parathyroid hormone levels of at least five times the upper limit of normal.[10,284,287,348,419] Approximately 80% of patients with parathyroid cancer are either symptomatic or have some metabolic abnormality associated with their disease, and 40% were found to have a palpable neck mass.[284,419] This contrasts with the presentation in patients with benign causes of hyperparathyroidism in that up to 50% of that cohort are asymptomatic in diagnosis, and the presence of a neck mass is rare.

A definitive preoperative diagnosis of parathyroid carcinoma is impossible to make; metabolic manifestations of parathyroid cancer overlap with those of patients with parathyroid adenoma. A high index of suspicion of parathyroid carcinoma should be maintained especially in patients with serum calcium levels >14 mg/dL and a palpable neck mass.[284,348,419] Recurrent laryngeal nerve palsy seen in a patient with hyperparathyroidism is also highly suggestive of parathyroid cancer.[345]

The definitive treatment of parathyroid cancer is en bloc resection of the tumor and areas of potential local invasion and/or regional metastasis. Parathyroid cancer will frequently recur in the central neck compartment and typically exhibits a natural history marked by recurrent hypercalcemia. Therefore, performance of the appropriate surgical procedure during the initial operation is critical and is one of the most important prognostic factors in parathyroid cancer.[333] The integrity of the parathyroid capsule should be maintained during dissection by use of an en bloc resection of the ipsilateral central neck contents including the thyroid lobe and tracheoesophageal soft tissues and lymphatics.[347] Structures such as the recurrent laryngeal nerve, esophageal wall, or strap muscles may require sacrifice if the tumor adheres to them; this will reduce the risk of tumor spillage and local recurrence. The increased local control achieved with resection of the recurrent laryngeal nerve outweighs the complication of vocal cord paralysis, which may be managed by phonosurgical rehabilitative procedures.

A central compartment neck dissection together with resection of soft tissues within the superior anterior mediastinum is important to appropriately stage any lymph node involvement that is not directly palpable during the initial surgery. Lymph node metastasis lateral to the jugular vein is rare in parathyroid cancer during the initial presentation.[284] Accordingly, prophylactic modified radical or selective dissection of levels 1 through 5 is not generally recommended. Neck dissection is reserved for patients with lymph node metastasis detected radiographically or by clinical examination in the jugular distribution or for patients with massive soft tissue invasion of lateral neck structures.

Although cure after resection of recurrent parathyroid carcinoma is rare, aggressive resection of local recurrence is recommended to control severe hypercalcemia. Selected patients will achieve prolonged disease-free intervals after one or more surgical procedures for recurrence in the neck or anterior superior mediastinum.[112]

In addition to the approach for both initial surgery of parathyroid carcinoma and local recurrence, an aggressive surgical approach to metastatic parathyroid cancer has been advocated to control marked hypercalcemia. Ovara has reported on lung resection for metastasis from parathyroid cancer in which 32% of patients resected achieved a significant reduction in total serum calcium levels and 14% achieved long-term survival ranging anywhere from 9 to 30 years.[286] Surgery for locally recurrent parathyroid cancer may be guided by preoperative localization studies to better define the extent and location of recurrent parathyroid cancer (Figure 120-21). Localization studies should be interpreted with caution, however, because not all tumor foci may be detected, and in patients with very high intact parathyroid hormone levels, benign lesions of bone (brown tumors) may mimic metastases.[198,227,331,336]

The low incidence of parathyroid cancer has made it difficult to study the roles of radiation and chemotherapy. A report issued by the National Cancer Database described the use of radiation therapy in combination with surgery in <7% of the 286 cases included.[174] Other reports have advocated the importance of complete en bloc resection followed by radiation therapy to increase local control.[67,220] However, the results of these reports must be tempered by the finding that patients in these series may not have had advanced resectable disease, a finding that characterized investigations where radiation therapy was thought to be a factor that worsened prognosis for parathyroid cancer.

Chemotherapy has a very limited role in the management of parathyroid cancer. Some response to therapy has been noted with a combination of 5-fluorouracil, cyclophosphamide and dacarbazine, as well as the combination of methotrexate, doxorubicin, cyclophosphamide, and lomustine. However, it must be emphasized, that these agents were not administered in a controlled study environment, and patient numbers were exceedingly few.[46,57]

Hyperparathyroidism During Pregnancy

Hyperparathyroidism during pregnancy is rare, and pregnant women usually represent a very small fraction of the total number of patients treated for this disease.[205] As in nonpregnant patients, a single parathyroid adenoma is the most likely to be found as the cause of hyperparathyroidism, although hyperplasia and carcinoma have been reported.[128,210,262]

During pregnancy, there is a degree of protection in the mother against hypercalcemia provided by calcium transport across the placenta.[262] Large amounts of calcium depress the fetal parathyroid function and result in fetal hypoparathyroidism. After delivery, when maternal calcium is no longer available, neonatal tetany develops as a consequence of hypercalcemia and this, in fact, is the most common presenting sign for maternal hyperparathyroidism in pregnancy.[128] Additional fetal complications described in mothers with hyperparathyroidism include abortion, prematurity, intrauterine growth restriction, and stillbirth.[205] Although many pregnant women are asymptomatic, presenting symptoms of hyperparathyroidism during pregnancy may include muscle weakness, abdominal symptoms, disorientation, and even coma and death.[210] The risk of obstetric complications has been shown to be significantly greater in women who do not undergo surgery for hyperparathyroidism while pregnant.[210] Some investigators believe that neonatal hypocalcemia is transient and treatable, whereas maternal disease can be successfully controlled medically when the diagnosis is already known.[128,226] The opposing opinion is that regardless of symptom complex severity, all pregnant patients with hyperparathyroidism should undergo neck exploration to prevent the array of potential maternal and fetal complications.[279]

There seems to be uniform agreement that in severely symptomatic patients, surgery should not be postponed until after delivery. The ideal safe period for parathyroidectomy is the second trimester, when chances of pregnancy loss or premature labor as a consequence of surgical intervention are minimal.[279] If the diagnosis is made during the third trimester, parathyroid exploration can usually be postponed until after labor and delivery. Preoperative hypercalcemia may be successfully controlled with fluids, diuretics, and orally administered phosphate. However, mithramycin, an antineoplastic agent, should be

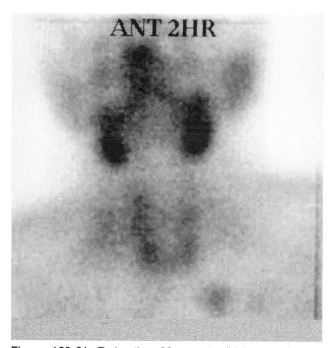

Figure 120-21. Technetium-99m sestamibi image demonstrating delayed uptake in the left superior mediastinum in a patient with recurrent parathyroid carcinoma.

avoided during pregnancy, because it is highly toxic to the fetal bone marrow, liver, and kidney. The most severe cases of hypercalcemia may require hemodialysis for appropriate control and stabilization.[262]

MEDICAL MANAGEMENT OF HYPERPARATHYROIDISM

It may be necessary in selected patients with hyperparathyroidism to consider medical therapy, including those in whom significant comorbidity may render patients at risk for significant complications as a consequence of surgical exploration or those patients with unresectable parathyroid carcinoma and uncontrolled hypercalcemia. Consideration for medical therapy should be weighed in relation to the patient's symptom complex, age, and overall medical condition/health status.

A limited number of general management schemes may be used to treat hypercalcemia. Expansion of intravascular volume by hydration together with the administration of loop diuretics should enhance urinary calcium excretion. Pharmaceuticals that reduce osteoclastic bone resorption, such as bisphosphonates, calcitonin, and plicamycin, may be used for various clinical settings.

The type of treatment used generally depends on the severity of the hypercalcemia and resultant clinical setting. In patients not fulfilling any criteria for surgery and in the absence of any circumstances that would make the patient no longer suitable for medical monitoring as currently accepted, no treatment is recommended except adequate hydration and avoidance of thiazide diuretics and immobilization. Estrogens have a theoretical advantage of potentially lowering serum calcium while providing known beneficial effects on bone in the prevention of osteoporosis in the postmenopausal women. The potential for the development of malignancies of the uterus and breast with estrogen use limits the practicality of this approach to reduce calcium levels. In addition, estrogen may raise levels of parathyroid hormone. Considering these variables, estrogen should be used cautiously in these patients, and, if needed to control calcium levels, surgical exploration should be more strongly considered.

For patients in whom calcium levels are 12 mg/dL or less, enhancement of urinary calcium excretion should be the initial approach. Most patients in this category are volume depleted as a result of the loss of water resulting from hypercalciuria. Volume correction with appropriate oral intake of salt and fluids will most often correct the serum calcium level. Diuresis should be implemented carefully in these patients, because the use of diuretics may worsen volume depletion and exacerbate hypercalcemia. If diuresis is

warranted to enhance calciuria, loop diuretics such as furosemide may be used. Thiazide compounds, which may worsen hypercalcemia, are to be avoided.

The use of oral phosphate salts has been advocated in the treatment of mild hypercalcemia in controlled situations.[39] This approach may lower the serum calcium by up to 1 mg/dL through a series of complex mechanisms involving decreased calcium absorption from the gut, decrease in circulating 1,25 dihydroxy vitamin D, and the reciprocal lowering of serum calcium by increasing serum levels of phosphorus. Bisphosphonates, among the most effective inhibitors of bone resorption, conceptually offered an alternative in treatment for mild hypercalcemia caused by primary hyperparathyroidism but thus far have not provided for a substantial reduction in serum calcium levels.[318] However, recent clinical evidence has suggested that the postmenopausal osteoporosis dose of alendronate (10 mg/day) effectively reversed bone loss in hyperparathyroidism.[66] Alendronate increased bone density within 1 year by >5% in the spine, similar to its effect in postmenopausal osteoporosis. Accordingly, it may be inferred that bone loss associated with hyperparathyroidism may be controlled by bisphosphonates treatment and could protect the bone in cases in which surgery is contraindicated.

Long-term medical management of hypercalcemia in patients with mild hyperparathyroidism or those in whom surgery may carry unacceptable risks remains problematic. Direct reduction of parathyroid hormone levels by manipulating the calcium-sensing receptors on parathyroid cells has ushered in a new class of pharmaceuticals called calcimimetic agents.[76,353] These agents act at the level of the parathyroid cell calcium receptor as a G-protein, such that when coupled with the receptor, the receptor G-protein complex recognizes calcium as its ligand.[41] In the presence of increased extracellular calcium, the receptor complex is activated, which results in a signal to the cell by way of a G-protein transducing pathway to raise intracellular calcium, thus inhibiting parathyroid hormone secretion. One such calcimimetic agent under investigation is R-568, which was found to increase cytoplasmic calcium and reduce parathyroid hormone secretion in vitro.[76] Further investigational experience was noted in postmenopausal women with primary hyperparathyroidism in which administration of R-568 resulted in decreased parathyroid hormone secretion and reduced serum calcium concentrations.[440] Larger clinical trials will further clarify the therapeutic potential of these calcimimetic compounds, but it seems that they may offer a therapeutic alternative to parathyroidectomy in the long-term management of hypercalcemia, selected in patients with mild hyperparathyroidism or those in whom surgery is contraindicated or not possible (i.e., parathyroid carcinoma).

SUMMARY

The management of hyperparathyroidism mandates a thorough, methodologic approach to diagnosis, patient evaluation and preparation, and the development of a comprehensive therapeutic strategy. Advances in nuclear imaging and the ability to rapidly assess the serum level of parathyroid hormone have allowed the fundamental surgical approach to become accurately directed, more refined, and less extensive, leading to improvements in outcome and reductions in treatment time, morbidity, and cost.

Although these changes have revolutionized the manner in which surgeons approach disorders of the parathyroid glands, they may not be universally applicable and thus should not serve as a substitute for a well-founded and traditional knowledge base in surgical embryology, anatomy, and technique. Most patients with hyperparathyroidism who undergo surgical therapy benefit symptomatically and metabolically.

REFERENCES

1. Abul-Haj SK, Conklin H, Hewitt WC: Functioning lipoadenoma of the parathyroid gland: report of a unique case, *N Engl J Med* 266:121, 1962.
2. Adams JS and others: Isolation and structural identification of 1,25-dihydroxyvitamin D3 produced by cultured alveolar macrophages in sarcoidosis, *J Clin Endocrinol Meta.* 60:960, 1985.
3. Adams JS and others: Vitamin D metabolite mediated hypercalcemia and hypercalciuria in patients with AIDS and non-AIDS-associated lymphoma, *Blood* 73:235, 1989.
4. Adams PH and others: Primary chief cell hyperplasia of the parathyroid glands, *Ann Intern Med* 63:454, 1965.
5. Akerström G, Malmaeus J, Bergström R: Surgical anatomy of human parathyroid glands, *Surgery* 95:14, 1984.
6. Akerström G and others: Causes of failed primary exploration and technical aspects of re-operation in primary hyperparathyroidism, *World J Surg* 16:562, 1992.
7. Albertucci M and others: Surgical treatment of the parathyroid gland in patients with end-stage renal disease, *Surg Gynecol Obstet* 167:49, 1988.
8. Albitar S and others: Multisystem granulomatous injuries 28 years after paraffin injections, *Nephrol Dial Transplant* 12:1974, 1997.
9. Alpers CE, Clark OH: Atypical spindle cell pattern (carcinoma?) arising in a parathyroid adenoma, *Surg Pathol* 2:15, 1989.
10. Anderson BJ and others: Parathyroid carcinoma: features and difficulties in diagnosis and management, *Surgery* 94:906, 1983.
11. Arnold A: Genetic basis of endocrine disease 5: molecular genetics of parathyroid gland neoplasia, *J Clin Endocrinol Metab* 77:1108, 1993.
12. Arnold A and others: Monoclonality and abnormal parathyroid hormone genes in parathyroid adenomas, *N Engl J Med* 318:658, 1988.
13. Arnold A and others: Molecular cloning and chromosomal mapping of DNA rearranged with the parathyroidal hormone

14. given in parathyroidal adenoma, *J Clin Invest* 83:2034, 1989.
14. Arnold BM and others: Functioning oxyphil cell adenoma of the parathyroid gland: evidence for parathyroid secretory activity of oxyphil cells, *J Clin Endocrinol Metab* 38:458, 1974.
15. Askanazy M: Uber ostitis deformans ohne osteideo Genebe, *Arb Pathol Inst Tübingen* 4:398, 1904.
16. Auffermann W and others: Diagnosis of recurrent hyperparathyroidism: Comparison of MR imaging and the other techniques, *AJR Am J Roentgenol* 150:1027, 1988.
17. Balon HR, Fink Bennet D, Stoffer SS: Technetium 99m sestamibi uptake by recurrent cell carcinoma of the thyroid, *J Nucl Med* 33:1393, 1992.
18. Bauer W, Albright F, Aub J: A case of osteitis fibrosa cystica (osteomalacia) with evidence of hyperactivity of the parathyroid bodies: metabolic study, *J Clin Invest* 8:229, 1930.
19. Bedetti CD, Dekker A, Watson CG: Functioning oxyphil cell adenoma of the parathyroid gland: a clinicopathologic study of ten patients with hyperparathyroidism, *Hum Pathol* 15:1121, 1984.
20. Benz RL and others: Successful treatment of postparathyroidectomy hypocalcemia using continuous ambulatory intraperitoneal calcium (CACI) therapy, *Perit Dial Int* 9:285, 1989.
21. Black EM, Zimmer JF: Hyperparathyroidism, with particular reference to treatment, *Arch Surg* 72:830, 1956.
22. Blind E and others: Measurement of intact human parathyrin by an extracting two-site immunoradiometric assay, *Clin Chem* 33:1376, 1987.
23. Block MA, Jackson CE, Tashjian AHJ: Management of parathyroid glands in surgery for medullary thyroid carcinoma, *Arch Surg* 110:617, 1975.
24. Boey JA and others: Occurrence of other endocrine tumors in primary hyperparathyroidism, *Lancet* 2:781, 1975.
25. Bondeson A-G, Bondeson L, Thompson NW: Clinicopathological peculiarities in parathyroid disease with hypercalcemic crisis, *Eur J Surg* 159:613, 1993.
26. Bondeson L, Sandelin K, Grimelius L: Histopathological variable and DNA cytometry in parathyroid carcinoma, *Am J Surg Pathol* 17:820, 1993.
27. Bonjer HJ and others: Single and multigland disease in primary hyperparathyroidism: clinical followup, histopathology, and flow cytometric DNA analysis, *World J Surg* 16:737, 1992.
28. Bonjer HJ and others: Intraoperative nuclear guidance in benign hyperparathyroidism and parathyroid cancer, *Eur J Nucl Med* 24:246, 1997.
29. Boonstra C, Jackson C: Serum calcium survey for hyperparathyroidism: results in 50,000 clinic patients, *Am J Clin Pathol* 55:523, 1971.
30. Bosch X: Hypercalcemia due to endogenous overproduction of active vitamin D in identical twins with cat-scratch disease, *JAMA* 279:532, 1998.
31. Bouillon R and others: Immunoradiometric assay of parathyrin with polyclonal and monoclonal region-specific antibodies, *Clin Chem* 36:271, 1990.
32. Bourke JF, Berth-Jones J, Hutchinson PE: Hypercalcemia with topical calcipotriol, *BMJ* 306:1334, 1993.
33. Boyle NH and others: Parathyroid carcinoma secondary to prolonged hyperplasia in chronic renal failure and in coeliac disease, *Eur J Surg Oncol* 25:100, 1999.
34. Brandi ML and others: Parathyroid mitogenic activity in plasma from patients with familial multiple endocrine neoplasia type 1, *N Engl J Med* 314:1287, 1986.

35. Brandi ML and others: Familial multiple endocrine neoplasia type I: a new look at pathophysiology, *Endocrine Rev* 8:391, 1987.

36. Brennan M and others: Results of re-operation for persistent and recurrent hyperparathyroidism, *Ann Surg* 194:671, 1981.

37. Brennan MF, Norton JA: Reoperation for persistent and recurrent hyperparathyroidism, *Ann Surg* 120:40, 1985.

38. Breslau NA and others: Hypercalcemia associated with increased serum calcitriol levels in three patients with lymphoma, *Ann Intern Med* 100:1, 1984.

39. Broadus AE and others: A detailed evaluation of oral phosphate therapy in selected patients with primary hyperparathyroidism, *J Clin Endcrinol Metab* 56:953, 1983.

40. Brown EM: PTH secretion in vivo and in vitro: regulation by calcium and other secretagogues, *Miner Electrolyte Metab* 8:130, 1982.

41. Brown EM, Pollak M, Seidman CE: Calcium ion sensing cell surface receptors, *N Engl J Med* 333:234, 1995.

42. Brown EM and others: Secretory control in normal and abnormal parathyroid tissue, *Recent Progr Horm Res* 43:337, 1987.

43. Brown EM and others: Calcium-ion-sensing cell-surface receptors, *N Engl J Med* 333:234, 1995.

44. Brown RC and others: Circulating intact parathyroid hormone measured by a two-site immunochemiluminometric assay, *J Clin Endocrinol Metab* 65:407, 1987.

45. Bruining H and others: Causes of failure in operation for hyperparathyroidism, *Surgery* 101:562, 1987.

46. Bukowski RM and others: Successful combination chemotherapy for metastatic parathyroid carcinoma, *Arch Intern Med* 144:339, 1984.

47. Burman KD and others: Ionized and total serum calcium and parathyroid hormone in hyperthyroidism, *Ann Intern Med* 84:668, 1976.

48. Cance WG, Wells SA Jr: Multiple endocrine neoplasia type IIa, *Curr Probl Surg* 22:1, 1985.

49. Carling T and others: Vitamin D receptor polymorphisms correlate to parathyroid cell function in primary hyperparathyroidism, *J Clin Endocrinol Metab* 82:1772, 1997.

50. Carty S and others: Concise parathyroidectomy and the impact of preoperative SPECT 99m Tc-sestamibi scanning and intraoperative quick parathormone assay, *Surgery* 122:1107, 1997.

51. Carty SE and others: Concise parathyroidectomy: the impact of preoperative SPECT 99mTC sestamibi scanning and intraoperative quick parathormone assay, *Surgery* 122:1107, 1997.

52. Casas AT and others: Prospective comparison of technetium 99 m sestamibi/iodine 123 scan versus high resolution ultrasonography for the preoperative localization of abnormal parathyroid glands in patients with previously unoperated primary hyperparathyroidism, *Am J Surg* 166:369, 1993.

53. Casas AT and others: Impact of technetium 99m sestamibi localization on operative time and success of operations for primary hyperparathyroidism, *Am Surgeon* 60:1217, 1994.

54. Castleman B, Mallory TB: Pathology of the parathyroid gland in hyperparathyroidism: study of 25 cases, *Am J Pathol* 11:1, 1935.

55. Castleman B, Roth SI: *Tumors of the parathyroid glands: atlas of tumor pathology*, Second Series, Fasicle 14, Washington, DC: Armed Forces Institute of Pathology, 1978.

56. Cattan P and others: Re-operation for secondary uremic hyperparathyroidism: are technical difficulties influenced by initial surgical procedure? *Surgery* 127:562, 2000.

57. Chahinian AP and others: Metastatic nonfunctioning parathyroid carcinoma: ultrastructural evidence of secretory granules and response to chemotherapy, *Am J Med Sci* 282:80, 1981.

58. Chaitin BA, Goldman RL: Miotic activity in benign parathyroid disease [letter], *Am J Clin Pathol* 76:363, 1981.

59. Chandrasekharappa SC and others: Positional cloning of the gene for multiple endocrine neoplasia–type 1, *Science* 276:404, 1997.

60. Chatterjee SN and others: Persistent hypercalcemia after successful renal transplantation, *Nephron* 17:1, 1976.

61. Chatterjee SN and others: The high incidence of persistent secondary hyperparathyroidism after renal homotransplantation, *Surg Gynecol Obstet* 143:440, 1976.

62. Chen CC and others: Comparison of parathyroid imaging with technetium 99m-pertechnetate/sestamibi subtraction double phase technetium-99m-sestamibi oral technetium 99m sestamibi SPECT, *J Nucl Med* 38:834, 1997.

63. Chen H, Sokoll L, Udelsman R: Outpatient minimally invasive parathyroidectomy: a combination of sestamibi–SPECT localization, cervical block anesthesia and intraoperative parathyroid hormone assay, *Surgery* 126:1016, 1999.

64. Chiu ML and others: Effect of mitochondrial and plasmamembrane potentials on accumulation of hexakis (2 methoxyisobutylisonitrile) technetium in cultured mouse fibroblasts, *J Nucl Med* 31:1646, 1990.

65. Chong GC and others: Medullary carcinoma of the thyroid gland, *Cancer* 35:695, 1975.

66. Chow C and others: Oral alendronate increases bone mineral density in postmenopausal women with primary hyperparathyroidism, *J Clin Endocrinol Metab* 88:581, 2003.

67. Chow E and others: Parathyroid carcinoma—the Princess Margaret Hospital experience, *Int J Radiat Oncol Biol Phys* 41:569, 1998.

68. Christensen MS, Nielsen HE: The clinical significance of hyperparathyroidism after renal transplantation, *Scand J Urol Nephrol (suppl 42)*:130, 1977.

69. Christensson T and others: Prevalence of hypercalcemia in a health screening in Stockholm, *ALDA Med Scand* 200:131, 1976.

70. Christie AC: The parathyroid oxyphil cells, *J Clin Pathol* 20:591, 1967.

71. Clark OH, Way LW, Hunt TK: Recurrent hyperparathyroidism, *Ann Surg* 184:391, 1976.

72. Coakley AJ and others: 99m-technetium sestamibi: A new agent for parathyroid imaging, *Nucl Med Commun* 10:791, 1989.

73. Coffey RJ, Lee TC, Canary JJ: The surgical treatment of primary hyperparathyroidism: a 20 year experience, *Ann Surg* 185:518, 1977.

74. Coffey RJ, Potter JF, Canary JJ: Diagnosis and surgical control of hyperparathyroidism, *Ann Surg* 161:732, 1965.

75. Cohn K and others: Parathyroid carcinoma: the Lahey Clinic experience, *Surgery* 98:1095, 1985.

76. Collins MT and others: Treatment of hypercalcemia secondary to parathyroid carcinoma with a novel calcimimetric agent, *J Clin Endocrinol Metab* 93:1083, 1998.

77. Collip J: Extraction of a parathyroid hormone which will prevent or control parathyroid tetany and which regulates the levels of blood calcium, *J Biol Chem* 63:395, 1925.

78. Cope O: Surgery of hyperparathyroidism: the occurrence of parathyroids in the anterior mediastinum and the division of the operation into two stages, *Ann Surg* 114:706, 1941.

79. Cope O: Hyperparathyroidism—too little, too much surgery [editorial]? *N Engl J Med* 295:100, 1976.

80. Cope O and others: Primary chief-cell hyperplasia of the parathyroid glands: a new entity in the surgery of hyperparathyroidism, *Ann Surg* 28:163, 1958.

81. Corsello SM and others: Acute compliance in the course of "mild" hyperparathyroidism, *J Endocrinol Invest* 14:971, 1991.

82. Cristesson T: Primary hyperparathyroidism—pathogenesis, incidence and natural history. In M Rothmund, SA Wells Jr (eds): *Progress in surgery*, vol 18. Basel, 1986, Karger.

83. Cushman PJ: Familial endocrine tumors: report of two unrelated kindreds affected with pheochromocytomas, one also with multiple thyroid carcinomas, *Am J Med* 32:352, 1962.

84. D'Alessandro AM and others: Tertiary hyperparathyroidism after renal transplantation: operative indications, *Surgery* 106:1049, 1989.

85. Daroca PJ Jr and others: Functioning lipoadenoma of the parathyroid gland, *Arch Pathol Lab Med* 101:28, 1977.

86. Davies M: Current therapy. Primary hyperparathyroidism: aggressive or conservative treatment? *Clin Endocrinol* 36:325, 1992.

87. Dekker A, Dunsford HA, Geyer SJ: The normal parathyroid gland at autopsy: the significance of stromal fat in adult patients, *J Pathol* 128:127, 1979.

88. Delattre JF and others: Les variations des parathyroïdes. Nombre 2, situation et vascularization artérielle. Étude anatomique et applications chirurgicales, *J Chir* (Paris) 199:633, 1982.

89. DeLellis RA: *Tumors of the parathyroid gland*, Third Series, Fascicle 6, Armed Forces Institute of Pathology, Washington, DC, 1993, p 1.

90. DeLellis RA: *Tumors of the parathyroid glands,* Third Series, Fascicle 6, Armed Forces Institute of Pathology; Washington, DC, 1993, p 25.

91. DeLellis RA: *Tumors of the parathyroid gland*, Series 3, Fascicle 6, Armed Forces Institute of Pathology, Washington, DC: 1993, p 85.

92. Delmonico FL and others: Parathyroid surgery in patients with renal failure, *Ann Surg* 200:644, 1984.

93. Demeure MJ and others: Results of surgical treatment for hyperparathyroidism associated with renal disease, *Am J Surg* 160:337, 1990.

94. Deveney CW: *Multiple endocrine neoplasia type 1*. In Clark OH, Duh QY, editors: *Textbook of endocrine surgery*, Philadelphia, 1997, WB Saunders, p 556.

95. DeVita MV and others: Assessment of renal osteodystrophy in hemodialysis patients, *Medicine* 71:284, 1992.

96. Diethelm AG, Edwards RP, Whelchel JD: The natural history and surgical treatment of hypercalcemia before and after renal transplantation, *Surg Gynecol Obstet* 154:481, 1982.

97. Dinnen JS and others: Parathyroid carcinoma in familial hyperparathyroidism, *J Clin Pathol* 30:966, 1977.

98. Dolgin C and others: Twenty-five year experience with primary hyperparathyroidism at Columbia Presbyterian Medical Center, *Head Neck Surg* 2:92, 1979.

99. Doppman J and others: Parathyroid adenomas in the aortopulmonary window [see comments], *Radiology* 201:456, 1996.

100. Doppman JL, Krudy AG, Marx SJ: Aspiration of enlarged parathyroid glands for parathyroid hormone assay, *Radiology* 148:31, 1983.

101. Dufour DR, Wilkerson SY: The normal parathyroid revisited: percentage of stromal fat, *Hum Pathol* 13:717, 1982.

102. Dufour DR, Wilkerson SY: Factors related to parathyroid weight in normal persons, *Arch Pathol Lab Med* 107:167, 1983.

103. Duh QY, Lim RC, Clark OH: Calciphylaxis in secondary hyperparathyroidism: diagnosis and parathyroidectomy, *Arch Surg* 126:12, 1991.

104. Edelson GW, Talpos GB, Bone HG III: Hypercalcemia associated with Wegener's granulomatosis and hyperparathyroidism: etiology and management, *Am J Nephrol* 13:275, 1993.

105. Edis AJ, Evans PC: High-resolution real-time ultrasonography and preoperative localization of parathyroid tumors, *N Engl J Med* 301:532, 1979.

106. Edis AJ, Levitt MD: Supernumerary parathyroid glands: Implications for the surgical treatment of secondary hyperparathyroidism, *World J Surg* 11:398, 1987.

107. Edis AJ, van Heerden JA, Scholz DA: Results of subtotal parathyroidectomy for primary chief cell hyperplasia, *Surgery* 86:462, 1979.

108. Eisenberg AA, Wallerstein HW: Pheochromocytoma of the suprarenal medulla (paraganglioma): a clinicopathology study, *Arch Pathol* 14:818, 1932.

109. Erdheim J: Tetania parathyreopriva, *Mih Grenzes Mes Chir* 16:632, 1906.

110. Erdman WA and others: Noninvasive localization of parathyroid adenomas: a comparison of x-ray, computerized tomography, ultrasound, scintigraphy and MRI, *Magn Reson Imaging* 102:917, 1989.

111. Evans HL: Criteria for diagnosis of parathyroid carcinoma [abstract], *Lab Invest* 66:35A, 1992.

112. Favia G and others: Parathyroid carcinoma: sixteen new cases and suggestions for correction management, *World J Surg* 22:1225, 1998.

113. Ferlin G and others: New perspectives localizing enlarged parathyroids by technetium thallium substraction scan, *J Nucl Med* 24:438, 1983.

114. Fialkow PJ and others: Multicellular origin of parathyroid "adenomas," *N Engl J Med* 297:695, 1977.

115. Fitzpatrick LA, Bilezikian JP: Acute primary hyperparathyroidism, *Am J Med* 82:275, 1987.

116. Fleetwood MK and others: Rapid PTH assay by simple modification of Nichols intact PTH-parathyroid hormone assay kit, *Clin Chem* 42:1498, 1996.

117. Fraker DL and others: Undescended parathyroid adenoma: an important etiology for failed operations for primary hyperparathyroidism, *World J Surg* 14:342, 1990.

118. Friedman E and others: Genetic abnormalities in sporadic parathyroid adenoma, *J Clin Endocrinol Metab* 71:293, 1990.

119. Friedman J, Raisz LG: Thyrocalcitonin inhibitor of bone resorption in tissue culture, *Science* 150:1465, 1965.

120. Frolich A: Prevalence of hypercalcemia in normal and hospitalized populations, *Danish Med Bull* 45:436, 1998.

121. Fukunaga M, Morita R, Yokenuga Y: Accumulation of 201 Tc chloride in a parathyroid adenoma, *Clin Nucl Med* 4:229, 1979.

122. Gagner M: Endoscopic subtotal parathyroidectomy in patients with primary hyperparathyroidism, *Br J Surg* 83:875, 1996.

123. Gagner M: *Endoscopic parathyroidectomy*. In Inabnet W, Gagner M, editors: *Minimally invasive endocrine surgery,* Philadelphia, Lippincott William & Wilkins, 2002.

124. Gagner M, Breton G: Endoscopic parathyroidectomy, thyroidectomy, esophageal myotomy and cervical lymph node dissection, *Surg Endosc* 10:232, 1996.

125. Gartner LP, Haitt JL: *Histology*, Philadelphia, WB Saunders, 1997.

126. Garvin PJ and others: Management hypercalcemic hyperparathyroidism after renal transplantation, *Ann Surg* 120:578, 1985.

127. Gayet S and others: Foscarnet-induced hypercalcemia in AIDS [letter], *AIDS* 11:1068, 1997.

128. Gelister JSK and others: Management of hyperparathyroidism in pregnancy, *Br J Surg* 76:1207, 1989.

129. Ghandur-Mnaymneh L, Kimura N: The parathyroid adenoma. A histopathologic clarification with a study of 172 cases of primary hyperparathyroidism, *Am J Pathol* 115:70, 1984.

130. Giangrande A, and others: Ultrasound-guided percutaneous fine-needle ethanol injection into parathyroid glands in secondary hyperparathyroidism, *Nephrol Dial Transplant* 7:412, 1992.

131. Giangrande A and others: Chemical parathyroidectomy for recurrence of secondary hyperparathyroidism, *Am J Kidney Dis* 24:421, 1994.

132. Gilmour JR: The gross anatomy of the parathyroid glands, *J Pathol* 46:133, 1938.

133. Gkonos PJ, London R, Hendler ED: Hypercalcemia and elevated 1,25-dihydroxyvitamin D levels in a patient with end stage renal disease and active tuberculosis, *N Engl J Med* 311:1683, 1984.

134. Golden A, Kerwin DM: *The parathyroid glands.* In Bloodworth JMB Jr., editor: *Endocrine pathology general and surgical,* ed 2, Baltimore/London, 1982, Williams & Wilkins.

135. Gooding GAW: Sonographic imaging of the thyroid and parathyroid, *Radiol Clin North Am* 31:967, 1993.

136. Granberg PO and others: Parathyroid tumors, *Curr Probl Cancer* 9:32, 1985.

137. Granberg PO and others: Selective venous sampling for localization of hyperfunctioning parathyroid glands, *Br J Surg* 73:118, 1988.

138. Grenko RT and others: Water-clear cell adenoma of the parathyroid: a case report with immunohistochemistry and electron microscopy, *Arch Pathol Lab Med* 119:1072, 1995.

139. Grill V and others: Parathyroid hormone-related protein: elevated levels in both humoral hypercalcemia of malignancy and hypercalcemia complicating metastatic breast cancer, *J Clin Endocrinol Metab* 73:1309, 1991.

140. Grimelius L and others: Anatomy and histopathology of human parathyroid gland, *Pathol Annu* 16:1, 1981.

141. Grimelius L and others: *The parathyroid glands.* In Kovacs K, Asa SL, editors: *Functional endocrine pathology,* Boston, Blackwell Scientific Publications, 1991.

142. Habener JF and others: Immunoreactive parathyroid hormone in circulation of man, *Nature* 238:152, 1972.

143. Habener JT, Rosenblatt M, Potts JT: Parathyroid hormone: biochemical aspects of biosynthesis, secretion, action, and metabolism, *Physiol Rev* 64:985, 1984.

144. Haden ST and others: Alterations in parathyroid dynamics in lithium-treated subjects, *J Clin Endocrinol Metab* 82:2844, 1979.

145. Haff R, Black W, Ballinger W: Primary hyperparathyroidism: changing clinical, surgical and pathologic aspects, *Ann Surg* 171:85, 1970.

146. Haghighi P and others: Concurrent primary parathyroid hyperplasia and parathyroid carcinoma, *Arch Pathol Lab Med* 107:349, 1983.

147. Hakaim AG, Esselstyn CB Jr: Parathyroid carcinoma: 50-year experience at The Cleveland Clinic Foundation, *Cleve Clin J Med* 60:331, 1993.

148. Halsted W, Evans H: The parathyroid glandules: their blood supply and their preservation in operation upon the thyroid gland, *Ann Surg* 46;489, 1907.

149. Hanson A: An elementary chemical study of the parathyroid glands of cattle, *Milit Surgeon* 52:280, 1923.

150. Hargreaves HK, Wright TC Jr: A large functioning parathyroid lipoadenoma found in the posterior mediastinum, *Am J Clin Pathol* 76:89, 1981.

151. Harness JK and others: Multiple adenomas of the parathyroids: do they exist? *Arch Surg* 114:468, 1979.

152. Hauty M and others: Technetium thallium scintiscanning for localizing of parathyroid adenomas and hyperplasia: a reappraisal, *Am J Surg* 153:479, 1987.

153. Heath DA: Primary hyperparathyroidism: clinical presentation and factors influencing clinical management, *Endocrinol Metab Clin North Am* 17:631, 1989.

154. Heath H, Hodgson S, Kennedy M: Primary hyperparathyroidism. Incidence, morbidity, and potential economic impact in a community, *N Engl J Med* 302:189, 1980.

155. Heath H III: Familial benign hypercalcemia—from clinical description to molecular genetics, *World J Med* 160:554, 1994.

156. Heath H III, Hodgson S, Kennedy N: Primary hyperparathyroidism incidence, mortality and potential economic impact in a community, *N Engl J Med* 302:189, 1980.

157. Heath H III and others: Genetic linkage analysis in familial benign (hypocalciuric) hypercalcemia: evidence for locus heterogeneity, *Am J Hum Genet* 53:193, 1993.

158. Hellman P and others: Findings and long term results of parathyroid surgery in multiple endocrine neoplasia type 1, *World J Surg* 16:718, 1992.

159. Hellman P and others: *Pathophysiology of hyperparathyroidism.* In Åkerström G, Rastad J, Juhlin C, editors: *Current controversy in parathyroid operation and reoperation,* Austin, TX, 1994, RG Landes Co, p 9.

160. Hellström J, Birke G, Edvall CA: Hypertension in hyperparathyroidism, *Br J Urol* 30:13, 1958.

161. Hellström J, Ivemark BI: Primary hyperparathyroidism: clinical and structural findings in 138 cases, *Acta Chir Scand* 294S:1, 1962.

162. Henry JF, Denizot A: *Anatomic and embryologic aspects of primary hyperparathyroidism.* In Barbier J, Henry JF, editors: *Primary hyperparathyroidism,* Paris, 1992, Springer-Verlag, p 5.

163. Henry JF and others: Minimally invasive videoscopic parathyroidectomy by lateral approach, *Langenbecks Arch Surg* 384:298, 1999.

164. Heppner C and others: Somatic mutation of the men 1 gene in parathyroid tumors, *Nat Genet* 16:375, 1997.

165. Higgins CB: Role of magnetic resonance imaging in hyperparathyroidism, *Radiol Clin North Am* 31:1017, 1993.

166. Higgins CB, Aufferman W: MRI imaging of thyroid and parathyroid glands: a review of current status, *AJR Am J Roentgenol* 151:1095, 1988.

167. Hindie E and others: Parathyroid imaging using simultaneous double window recording of technetium-99m-sesstamibi and iodine-123, *J Nucl Med* 39:1100, 1998.

168. Hoffman VH, Korzeniowski OM: Leprosy, hypercalcemia, and elevated serum calcitriol levels, *Ann Intern Med* 105:890, 1986.

169. Hognestad J, Flatmark A: Hyperparathyroidism in uremia and after kidney transplantation, *Scand J Urol Nephrol (suppl 42)*:137, 1977.

170. Howe JR: Minimally invasive parathyroid surgery, *Surg Clin North Am* 80:1399, 2000.

171. Howe JR, Norton JA, Wells SA Jr: Prevalence of pheochromocytoma and hyperparathyroidism in multiple endocrine neoplasia type 2a: results of long-term follow-up, *Surgery* 114:1070, 1993.

172. Huang SM: *Familial hyperparathyroidism.* In Clark OH, Duh QY, editors: *Textbook of endocrine surgery,* Philadelphia, WB Saunders, 1997, p 385.

173. Huang SM and others: Familial hyperparathyroidism without multiple endocrine neoplasia, *World J Surg* 21:22, 1997.

174. Hundahl SA and others: Two hundred eighty-six cases of parathyroid carcinoma treated in the U.S. between 1985-1995: a national cancer data base report, *Cancer* 86:538, 1999.

175. Iguchi H and others: Hypercalcemia caused by ectopic production of parathyroid hormone in a patient with papillary adenocarcinoma of the thyroid gland, *J Clin Endocrinol Metab* 83:2653, 1998.

176. Ikeda K and others: Development of a sensitive two-site immunoradiometric assay for parathyroid hormone-related peptide: evidence for elevated levels in plasma from patients with adult T-cell leukemia/lymphoma and B-cell lymphoma, *J Clin Endocrinol Metab* 79:1322, 1994.

177. Ikeda Y and others: Endoscopic neck surgery by the axillary approach, *J Am Coll Surg* 191:336, 2000.

178. Inabnet WB: *Radioguided parathyroidectomy under local anesthesia.* In Inabnet WB, Gagner M, editors: *Minimally invasive endocrine surgery,* Philadelphia, 2002, Lippincott William & Wilkins.

179. Inabnet WB and others: Unilateral neck exploration under local anesthesia: the approach of choice for asymptomatic primary hyperparathyroidism, *Surgery* 126:1004, 1999.

180. Inabnet W and others: Radio guidance is not necessary during parathyroidectomy, *Arch Surg* 137:967, 2002.

181. Irvin GL, Dembrow VD, Prudhomme DL: Clinical usefulness of an intraoperative "quick parathyroid hormone" assay, *Surgery* 114:1019, 1993.

182. Irvin GL, Deriso GT: A new, practical intraoperative parathyroid hormone assay, *Am J Surg* 168:466, 1994.

183. Irvin GL and others: Clinical usefulness of an intraoperative "quick parathyroid hormone" assay, *Surgery* 114:1019, 1993.

184. Irvin GL and others: A new approach to parathyroidectomy, *Ann Surg* 219:574, 1994.

185. Jaskowiak N and others: A prospective trial evaluating a standard approach to re-operation for missed parathyroid adenoma, *Ann Surg* 224:308, 1996.

186. Jeelos KC and others: Persistent and recurrent hyperparathyroidism assessment with gache pentate dimeglumine enhanced MR imaging, *Radiology* 177:373, 1990.

187. Jofre J and others: Optimal imaging for delayed images in the diagnosis of abnormal parathyroid tissue with Tc-99m-sestamibi, *Clin Nucl Med* 24:594, 1999.

188. Johasson H, Thoren L, Werner I: Hyperparathyroidism. Clinical experiences from 208 cases, *Upsal J Med Sci* 77:41, 1972.

189. Johannessen JV: *Parathyroid glands.* In Johannessen JV, editor: *Electron microscopy in human medicine,* vol 10. New York, 1981, McGraw-Hill, p 111.

190. Johnson GJ and others: Clinical and genetic investigation of a large kindred with MEA, *N Engl J Med* 277:1379, 1967.

191. Junqueira LC, Carneiro J, Kelly RO: *Basic histology,* ed 9, Stamford, CT, Appleton & Lange, 1998.

192. Jurney TH: Hypercalcemia in a patient with eosinophilic granuloma, *Am J Med* 76:527, 1984.

193. Kao PC, van Heerden JA, Taylor RL: Intraoperative monitoring of parathyroid procedures by a 15-minute parathyroid hormone immunochemiluminometric assay, *Mayo Clin Proc* 69:532, 1994.

194. Kaplan EL, Yashiro T, Salti G: Primary hyperparathyroidism in the 1990s. Choice of surgical procedures for this disease, *Ann Surg* 215:300, 1992.

195. Karstrupp S and others: Ultrasound guided, histological, fine needle biopsy from suspect parathyroid tumours: success rate and reliability of histological diagnosis, *Br J Radiol* 62:981, 1989.

196. Kastan DJ and others: Carcinoma in a mediastinal fifth parathyroid gland, *JAMA* 257:1218, 1987.

197. Katz AD, Hopp D: Parathyroidectomy: review of 338 consecutive cases for histology, location and reoperation, *Am J Surg* 144:411, 1982.

198. Kebebew E and others: Localization and reoperation results for persistent and recurrent parathyroid carcinoma, *Arch Surg* 136:878, 2001.

199. Kenny A and others: Fracture incidence in postmenopausal women with primary hyperparathyroidism, *Surgery* 118:109, 1995.

200. Kern KA, Shawker TH, Jones BL: Intraoperative ultrasound on reoperative parathyroid surgery: an initial evaluation, *World J Surg* 10:631, 1986.

201. Khantarijian HM and others: Hypercalcemia in disseminated candidiasis, *Am J Med* 74:721, 1983.

202. Kifor O and others: Reduced immunostaining for the extracellular calcium sensing receptor in primary and uremic secondary hyperparathyroidism, *J Clin Endocrinol Metab* 81:1598, 1996.

203. Knecht TP and others: The humoral hypercalcemia of benignancy. A newly appreciated syndrome, *Am J Clin Pathol* 105:487, 1996.

204. Kohri K and others: Comparison of imaging methods for localization of parathyroids tumors, *Am J Surg* 164:140, 1992.

205. Kort KC, Shiller HJ, Numann PJ: Hyperparathyroidism and pregnancy, *Am J Surg* 177:66, 1999.

206. Kozeny GA and others: Hypercalcemia associated with silicone-induced granulomas, *N Engl J Med* 311:1103, 1984.

207. Kraimps JL, Barbier J: *Familial hyperparathyroidism in multiple endocrine neoplasia syndromes.* In Clark OH, Duh QY, editors: *Textbook of endocrine surgery,* Philadelphia, WB Saunders, 1997, p 381.

208. Kraimps JL and others: Hyperparathyroidism in multiple endocrine neoplasia syndrome, *Surgery* 112:1080, 1992.

209. Kramer WM: Association of parathyroid hyperplasia with neoplasia, *Am J Clin Pathol* 53:275, 1970.

210. Kristofferson A and others: Primary hyperparathyroidism and pregnancy, *Surgery* 97:326, 1985.

211. Lafferty FW: Primary hyperparathyroidism: changing clinical spectrum, prevalence of hypertension, and discriminant analysis of laboratory tests, *Arch Intern Med* 41:1761, 1981.

212. Lafferty FW, Hubay CA: Primary hyperparathyroidism: a review of the long-term surgical and nonsurgical morbidities as a basis for a rational approach to treatment, *Arch Intern Med* 149:789, 1989.

213. Larsson C and others: Multiple endocrine neoplasia type 1 gene maps to chromosome 11 and is lost in insulinoma, *Nature* 332:85, 1988.

214. Law WM Jr, Heath H III: Familial benign hypercalcemia (hypocalciuric hypercalcemia): clinical and pathogenetic studies in 21 families, *Ann Intern Med* 102:511, 1985.

215. Legha SS and others: Tamoxifen-induced hypercalcemia in breast cancer, *Cancer* 47:2803, 1981.

216. Levin K, Clark OH: The reasons of failure in parathyroid surgery, *Arch Surg* 124:911, 1989.

217. Levin KE, Galanet M, Clark OH: Parathyroid carcinoma versus parathyroid adenoma in patients with profound hypercalcemia, *Surgery* 101:649, 1987.

218. Libuttis S: Kinetic analysis of the rapid intraoperative parathyroid hormone assay in patients during operation for hyperparathyroidism, *Surgery* 126:1145, 1999.

219. Lieberman VA and others: Metabolic and calcium kinetic studies in idiopathic hypercalciuria, *J Clin Invest* 47:2580, 1968.

220. Lillemoe KD, Dudley NE: Parathyroid carcinoma: pointers to successful management, *Ann R Coll Surg Engl* 67:222, 1985.

221. Linch D, Watson L, Cowie A: Ectopic parathyroid adenomas, *J R Soc Med* 73:638, 1980.

222. LiVolsi VA, Asa SL: The parathyroid glands in endocrine pathology, Philadelphia, Churchill-Livingstone, 2002.

223. Ljunghall S and others: Primary hyperparathyroidism: epidemiology, diagnosis and clinical picture, *World J Surg* 15:681, 1991.

224. Llach F: Parathyroidectomy in chronic renal failure: indications, surgical approach and the use of calcitriol, *Kidney Int* 29(suppl):S63, 1990.

225. Lloyd HM, Jacobi JM, Cooke RA: Nucleare diameter in parathyroid adenomas, *J Clin Pathol* 32:1278, 1979.

226. Lowe DK and others: Hyperparathyroidism and pregnancy, *Am J Surg* 145:611, 1983.

227. Lu G, Shih WJ, Xiu JY: Technetium-99m MIBI uptake in recurrent parathyroid carcinoma and brown tumors, *J Nucl Med* 36:811, 1995.

228. Lundgren G and others: The role of parathyroidectomy in the treatment of secondary hyperparathyroidism before and after renal transplantation, *Scand J Urol Nephrol* 31(suppl 42):149, 1997.

229. Malmaeus J and others: Parathyroid surgery in chronic renal insufficiency, *Acta Chir Scand* 148:229, 1982.

230. Malmaeus J and others: Parathyroid surgery in Scandinavia, *Acta Chir Scand* 54:409, 1988.

231. Mallette LE and others: Parathyroid carcinoma in familial hyperparathyroidism, *Am J Med* 57:642, 1974.

232. Mallete LE and others: Autogenous parathyroid grafts for generalized primary hyperplasia: contrasting outcome in sporadic hyperplasia versus multiple endocrine neoplasia type 1, *Surgery* 101:738, 1987.

233. Mandle F. Attempt to treat generalized fibrous osteitis by extirpation of parathyroid tumor [Orgara C, transl, 1984], *Zentrabl Chir* 53:260, 1926.

234. Martin JK and others: Persistent postoperative hyperparathyroidism, *Surg Gynecol Obstet* 151:764, 1980.

235. Martin KJ and others: The peripheral metabolism of parathyroid hormone, *N Engl J Med* 302:1092, 1979.

236. Marx SJ and others: Familial hypocalciuric hypercalcemia: recognition among patients referred after unsuccessful parathyroid exploration, *Ann Intern Med* 92:351, 1980.

237. Marx SJ and others: The hypocalciuric or benign variant of familial hypercalcemia: clinical and biochemical features in fifteen kindreds, *Medicine* 60:397, 1981.

238. Massry SG, Coburn JW: The hormonal and non-hormonal control of renal excretion of calcium and magnesium, *Nephron* 10:66, 1973.

239. Matthew CGP and others: A linked genetic marker for multiple endocrine neoplasia type 2A on chromosome 10, *Nature* 328:527, 1987.

240. Mawer EB and others: Vitamin D metabolism and parathyroid function in man, *Clin Sci Met Med* 48:349, 1975.

241. McHenry CR, Senger DB, Calandro NK: The effect of cryopreservation on parathyroid cell viability and function, *Am J Surg* 174:481, 1997.

242. McHenry CR and others: Parathyroid crisis of unusual features in a child, *Cancer* 71:1923, 1993.

243. McLeod MK, Monchik JM, Martin HF: The role of ionized calcium in the diagnosis of subtle hypercalcemia in symptomatic primary hyperparathyroidism, *Surgery* 95:667, 1984.

244. McPherson ML and others: Theophylline-induced hypercalcemia, *Ann Intern Med* 105:52, 1986.

245. McSheehy PMJ, Chambers TJ: Osteoblastic cells mediate osteoclastic responsiveness to parathyroid hormone, *Endocrinology* 118:824, 1986.

246. Merlano M and others: Nonfunctioning parathyroid carcinoma. A case report, *Tumori* 71:193, 1985.

247. Miccoli P and others: Minimally invasive video-assisted parathyroidectomy: lesson learned from 137 cases, *J Am Coll Surg* 191:613, 2000.

248. Michelangoli VP, Hunt NH, Martin TJ: States of activation of chick kidney adenylate-cyclase induced by parathyroid hormone and guanylyl nucleotides, *J Endocrinol* 72:69, 1977.

249. Miki H and other: Parathyroid carcinoma in patients with chronic renal failure on maintenance hemodialysis, *Surgery* 120:897, 1996.

250. Miller DL: Preoperative localization and interventional treatment of parathyroid tumours. When and how? *World J Surg* 15:706, 1991.

251. Miller DL: Endocrine angiography and venous sampling, *Radiol Clin North Am* 31:1051, 1993.

252. Miller DL, Doppman JL, Shawker TH: Localization of parathyroid adenomas in patients who have undergone surgery: noninvasive methods, *Radiology* 162:133, 1987.

253. Miller DL and others: Localization of parathyroid adenomas in patients who have undergone surgery: Part II. Invasive procedures, *Radiology* 162:138, 1987.

254. Miller DL and others: Superselective DSA versus superselective conventional arteriography, *Radiology* 170:1003, 1989.

255. Mitlak BH and others: Asymptomatic primary hyperparathyroidism, *J Bone Miner Res* 6:S103, 1991.

256. Moncitik JM and others: Minimally invasive parathyroid surgery in 103 patients with local/regional anesthesia without exclusion criteria, *Surgery* 131:502, 2002.

257. Mozes MF and others: Total parathyroidectomy and autotransplantation in secondary hyperparathyroidism, *Arch Surg* 115:378, 1980.

258. Mulligan LM and others: Germline mutation of the RET protooncogene in multiple endocrine neoplasia type 2A, *Nature* 363:458, 1993.

259. Mundy GR, Guise TA: Hormonal control of calcium homeostasis, *Clin Chem* 45:1347, 1999.

260. Mundy GR, Yoneda T, Guise TA: *Hypercalcemia in hematologic malignancies and in solid tumors associated with extensive localized bone destruction.* In: Favus MJ, editor: *Primer on the metabolic bone diseases and disorders of mineral metabolism*, ed 4 Philadelphia, 1999, Lippincott Williams & Wilkins, p 183.

261. Mune T and others: Production and secretion of parathyroid hormone-related protein in pheochromocytoma: participation of an α-adrenergic mechanism, *J Clin Endocrinol Metab* 76:757, 1993.

262. Nader S: *Other endocrine disorders*. In Creasy RB, Resnik R, editors: *Maternal fetal medicine—principals and practice*, ed 3, Philadelphia, 1994, Saunders, p 1004.

263. Nagai Y and others: Role of interleukin 6 in uncoupling of bone *in vivo* in a human squamous carcinoma co-producing PTHrp and interleukin 6, *J Bone Miner Res* 13:664, 1998.

264. National Institutes of Health Conference: *Asymptomatic primary hyperparathyroidism*, Washington DC, NIH, 2002.

265. National Institutes of Health Conference: Diagnosis and management of asymptomatic primary hyperparathyroidism: consensus development conference statement, *Ann Intern Med* 114:593, 1991.

266. Naveh-Many T and others: Calcium regulates parathyroid hormone messenger ribonucleic acid (mRNA), but not calcitonin mRNA in vivo in the rat: Dominant role of 1,25-dihydroxy-vitamin D, *Endocrinology* 83:1053, 1989.

267. Neer R and others: Multicompartmental analysis of calcium kinetics in normal adult males, *J Clin Invest* 46:1364, 1967.

268. Neumann D, Esselstyn C, Madera A: Sestamibi/iodine subtraction single photon emission computed tomography in reoperative secondary hyperparathyroidism, *Surgery* 128:22, 2000.

269. Neumann DR: Simultaneous dual isotope SPECT imaging for the detection and characterization of parathyroid pathology, *J Nucl Med* 33:131, 1992.

270. Newmann DR and others: Comparison of double phase 99m Tc-sestamibi with 123I-99m Tc-sestamibi subtraction SPECT in hyperparathyroidism, AJR *AM J Roentgenol* 169:1671, 1997.

271. Nilsson BE and others: Parathyroid localization by catheterization of large cervical and mediastinal veins to determine serum concentrations of intact parathyroid hormone, *World J Surg* 18:605, 1994.

272. Nilsson I and others: Endothelial vasodilatory dysfunction in primary hyperparathyroidism is reversed after parathyroidectomy, *Surgery* 126:1049, 1999.

273. Nilsson I and others: Left ventricular systolic and diastolic function and exercise testing in primary hyperparathyroidism—effects of parathyroidectomy, *Surgery* 128:895, 2000.

274. Nordin BEC and others: *Plasma calcium homeostasis*. In Talmage RV, Owen M, Parsons JA, editors: *Calcium-regulating hormones*, New York, 1975, Excerpta Medica, p 239.

275. Norman J, Chheda H: Minimally invasive parathyroidectomy facilitated by intraoperative nuclear mapping, *Surgery* 122:998, 1997.

276. Norman J, Chheda H, Farrell C: Minimally invasive parathyroidectomy for primary hyperparathyroidism: decreasing operative time and potential complications while improving cosmetic results, *Ann Surg* 64:391, 1998.

277. Norman J, Denham D: Minimally invasive radio-guided parathyroidectomy in the re-operative neck, *Surgery* 124:1088, 1998.

278. Norton J: Re-operation for missed parathyroid adenoma. *Ann Surg* 31:273, 1997.

279. Nudelman J and others: The treatment of hyperparathyroidism during pregnancy, *Br J Surg* 71:217, 1984.

280. Nussbaum S, Gaz R, Arnold A: Hypercalcemia and ectopic secretion of parathyroid hormone by an ovarian carcinoma with rearrangement of the gene for parathyroid hormone, *N Engl J Med* 323:1324, 1990.

281. Nussbaum SR and others: Highly sensitive two-site immunoradiometric assay of parathyrin and its clinical utility in evaluating patients with hypercalcemia, *Clin Chem* 33:1364, 1987.

282. Nussbaum SR and others: Intraoperative measurement of parathyroid hormone in the surgical management of hyperparathyroidism, *Surgery* 104:1221, 1988.

283. Nussbaum SR and others: Intraoperative measurement of PTH 1-84: A potential use of the clearance of PTH to assess surgical cure of hyperparathyroidism, *Surgery* 104:1121, 1988.

284. Obara T, Fujimoto Y: Diagnosis and treatment of patients with parathyroid carcinoma: an update and review, *World J Surg* 15:738, 1991.

285. Obara T, Fujimoto Y: Diagnosis and treatment of patients with parathyroid carcinoma: an update and review, *World J Surg* 15:738, 1991.

286. Obara T and others: Surgical and medical management of patients with pulmonary metastasis from parathyroid carcinoma, *Surgery* 114:1040; discussion 1048, 1993.

287. Obara T and others: Functioning parathyroid carcinoma: clinicopathologic features and rational treatment, *Semin Surg Oncol* 13:134, 1997.

288. Ober WB, Kaiser GA: Hamartoma of the parathyroid, *Cancer* 11:601, 1958.

289. O'Doherty M: Radionuclide parathyroid imaging, *J Nucl Med* 38:840, 1997.

290. O'Doherty MJ and others: Parathyroid imaging with technetium 99m sestamibi: preoperative localization and tissue uptake studies, *J Nucl Med* 33:313, 1992.

291. Omdahl J, DeLuca HF: Regulation of vitamin D metabolism and function, *Physiol Rev* 53:327, 1973.

292. Ordoñez NG and others: Functioning oxyphil cell adenomas of parathyroid gland: Immunoperoxidase evidence of hormonal activity in oxyphil cells, *Am J Clin Pathol* 78:681, 1982.

293. O'Riordan DS and others: Surgical management of primary hyperparathyroidism in multiple endocrine neoplasia types 1 and 2, *Surgery* 114:1031, 1993.

294. Page B and others: Correction of severe secondary hyperparathyroidism in two dialysis patients: Surgical removal versus percutaneous ethanol injection, *Am J Kidney Dis* 19:378, 1992.

295. Palmer M and others: Prevalence of hypercalcemia in a health survey: A 14-year follow-up study of serum calcium values, *Eur J Clin Invest* 18:39, 1988.

296. Parfitt AM Rao DS, Kleerekoper M: Asymptomatic primary hyperparathyroidism discovered by multichannel biochemical screening: clinical course and considerations bearing on the need for surgical intervention, *J Bone Miner Res* 6(suppl 2):S97, 1991.

297. Parker MS and others: Hypercalcemia in coccidioidomycosis, *Am J Med* 76: 341, 1984.

298. Patel PC and others: Use of a rapid intraoperative parathyroid hormone assay in the surgical management of parathyroid disease, *Arch Otolaryngol Head Neck Surg* 124:559, 1998.

299. Patow C, Norton J, Brennan M: Vocal cord paralysis and re-operative parathyroidectomy: a prospective study, *Ann Surg* 203:282, 1986.

300. Pellitteri PK: Directed parathyroid exploration: evolution and evaluation of this approach in a single-institution review of 346 patients, *Laryngoscope* 113:1857, 2003.

301. Pellitteri PK, Patel P: *Surgical management of primary hyperparathyroidism*. In Pellitteri PK, McCaffery TV, editors: *Endocrine surgery of the head and neck*, Canada, 2003, Delmar-Thomson, p 359.

302. Pettifor JM and others: Serum levels of free 1,25-dihydroxyvitamin D in vitamin D toxicity, *Ann Intern Med* 122:511, 1995.

303. Pieper R and others: Secondary hyperparathyroidism and its sequelae in renal transplant recipients, *Scand J Urol Nephrol* 11(suppl 42):144, 1977.

304. Piovesan A, Molineri N, Casosso F, et al: Left ventricular hypertrophy in primary hyperparathyroidism: Effects of successful parathyroidectomy. *Clin Endocrinol* 50:321-328, 1999.

305. Pollack MR and others: Mutations in the human Ca^{2+} sensing receptor gene cause familial hypocalciuric hypercalcemia and neonatal severe hyperparathyroidism, *Cell* 75:1297, 1993.

306. Pollak M and others: Mutations in the human Ca^{2+}-sensing receptor gene cause familial hypocalciuric hypocalcemia and neonatal severe hyperparathyroidism, *Cell* 75:1297, 1993.

307. Poole GV Jr and others: Oxyphil cell adenoma and hyperparathyroidism, *Surgery* 92:799, 1982.

308. Porter and others: Treatment of hypoparathyroid patients with chlorthalidone, *N Engl J Med* 298:577, 1978.

309. Posen S and others: Is parathyroidectomy of benefit in primary hyperparathyroidism? *Q J Med* 15:241, 1985.

310. Potts JT Jr, Deftos LJ: *Parathyroid hormone, calcitonin, vitamin D, bone and bone mineral metabolism*. In Bondy PK, Rosenberg LE, editors: *Duncan's diseases of metabolism*, Philadelphia, 1974, WB Saunders, p 1225.

311. Price DC: Radioisotopic evaluation of the thyroid and the parathyroids, *Radiol Clin North Am* 31:991, 1993.

312. Prinz RA and others: Subtotal parathyroidectomy for primary chief cell hyperplasia of the multiple endocrine neoplasia type 1 syndrome, *Ann Surg* 193:26, 1981.

313. Prinz RA and others: Thoracoscopic excision of enlarged mediastinal parathyroid glands, *Surgery* 116:999, 1994.

314. Proye CAG and others: Single and multigland disease in seemingly sporadic primary hyperparathyroidism revisited: where are we in the 1990s? A plea against unilateral parathyroid exploration, *Surgery* 112:1118, 1992.

315. Randolph GW: *Surgery of the thyroid and parathyroid glands*, Philadelphia, Saunders, 2003.

316. Raue F, Frank-Raue K, Grauer A: Multiple endocrine neoplasia type 2, clinical features and screening, *Endocrinol Metab Clin North Am* 23:137, 1994.

317. Raue F and others: Primary hyperparathyroidism in multiple endocrine neoplasia type 2A, *J Int Med* 238:369, 1995.

318. Reasner CA and others: Acute changes in calcium homeostasis during treatment of primary hyperparathyroidism with risedronate, *J Clin Endocrinol Metab* 77:1067, 1993.

319. Richardson E, Aub J, Bauer W: Parathyroidectomy in osteomalacia, *Ann Surg* 90:730, 1929.

320. Rizzato G: Clinical impact of bone and calcium metabolism changes in sarcoidosis, *Thorax* 53:425, 1998.

321. Rodríguez JM and others: Localization procedures in patients with persistent or recurrent hyperparathyroidism, *Arch Surg* 129:870, 1994.

322. Ronni-Sivula H, Sivula A: Long-term effect of surgical treatment on the symptoms of primary hyperparathyroidism, *Ann Clin Res* 17:141, 1985.

323. Rosenblatt M, Kronenberg HM, Potts JT: *Parathyroid hormone: physiology, chemistry, biosynthesis, secretion, metabolism and mode of action*. In DeGroot LJ, editor: *Endocrinology*, vol 2. Philadelphia, 1989, WB Saunders, p 848.

324. Rosenthal NR and others: Elevations in circulating 1,25(OH)$_2$D in three patients with lymphoma-associated hypercalcemia, *J Clin Endocrinol Metab* 60:29, 1985.

325. Rothmund M, Wagner PK: Total parathyroidectomy and autotransplantation of parathyroid tissue for renal hyperparathyroidism, *Ann Surg* 197:7, 1983.

326. Rothmund M, Wagner PK, Schark C: Subtotal parathyroidectomy versus total parathyroidectomy and autotransplantation in secondary hyperparathyroidism: a randomized trial, *World J Surg* 15:745, 1991.

327. Rotstein L and others: Re-operative parathyroidectomy in the era of localization technology, *Head Neck* 20:535, 1998.

328. Rudberg C and others: Alterations in density, morphology, and parathyroid hormone release of dispersed parathyroid cells from patients with hyperparathyroidism, *Acta Pathol Microbiol Immunol Scand (A)* 94:253, 1986.

329. Russell CF, Grant CS, van Heerden JA: Hyperfunctioning supernumerary parathyroid glands, *Mayo Clin Proc* 57:121, 1982.

330. Sakoulas G and others: Hypercalcemia in an AIDS patient treated with growth hormone, *AIDS* 11:1353, 1997.

331. Sandelin K, Thomas NW, Bondeson L: Metastatic parathyroid carcinoma: dilemmas in management, *Surgery* 110:978; discussion 986, 1991.

332. Sandelin K, Tullgren O, Farnebo LO: Clinical course of metastatic parathyroid cancer, *World J Surg* 18:594, 1994.

333. Sandelin K and others: Prognostic factors in parathyroid cancer: a review of 95 cases, *World J Surg* 16:724, 1992.

334. Sandrock D and others: Light and electromicroscopic analyses of parathyroid tumors explain results of T120 Tc99m parathyroid scintigraphy, *Eur J Med* 15:410, 1989.

335. San-Juan J and others: Significance of mitotic activity and other morphologic parameters in parathyroid adenomas and their correlation with clinical behavior [abstract], *Am J Clin Pathol* 92:523, 1989.

336. Sarfati E and others: Acute primary hyperparathyroidism, *Br J Surg* 76:979, 1989.

337. Sato F, Duh QY: *Multiple endocrine neoplasia syndrome*. In Prinz RA, Staren ED, editors. *Endocrine surgery*, Georgetown, TX, Landes Bioscience, 2000, p 263.

338. Saunders M and others: A novel cyclic adenosine monophosphate analog induces hypercalcemia via production of 1,25-dihydroxyvitamin D in patients with solid tumors, *J Clin Endocrinol Metab* 83:4044, 1997.

339. Schantz A, Castleman B: Parathyroid carcinoma: a study of 70 cases, *Cancer* 31:600, 1973.

340. Schienman SJ and others: Hypercalcemia with excess serum 1,25-dihydroxyvitamin D in lymphomatoid granulomatosis/angiocentric lymphoma, *Am J Med Sci* 301:178, 1991.

341. Schlagenaufer F: Zwei Fälle von Parathyreoideatumoren, *Wien Klin Wochenschr* 28:1362, 1915.

342. Seiple C: *On a new gland in man and several mammals (Glandulae Parathyroideae)* [Sandström I, (transl], Baltimore, Johns Hopkins Press, 1938.

343. Seymour JF, Gagel RF: Calcitriol: the major humoral mediator of hypercalcemia in Hodgkin's disease and non-Hodgkin's lymphomas, *Blood* 82:1383, 1993.

344. Shaha AR, Jaffe BM: Cervical exploration for primary hyperparathyroidism, *J Surg Oncol* 52:14, 1993.

345. Shane E: Parathyroid carcinoma, *Curr Ther Endocrinol Metab* 6:565, 1997.

346. Shane E: *Hypercalcemia*. In Favus MJ, editor: *Primer on the metabolic bone diseases and disorders of mineral metabolism*, ed 4, Philadelphia, 1999, Lippincott Williams & Wilkins, p 183.

347. Shane E: Clinica review 122: parathyroid carcinoma, *J Clin Endocrinol Metab* 86:485, 2001.

348. Shane E, Bilezikian JP: Parathyroid carcinoma: a review of 62 patients, *Endocrinol Rev* 3:218, 1982.

349. Shelling DH: *The parathyroids in health and disease*, St. Louis: C.V. Mosby, 1935.

350. Shortell CK and others: Carcinoma of the parathyroid gland: a 30-year experience, *Surgery* 110:704, 1991.

351. Shvil Y and others: Regulation of parathyroid cell gene expression in experimental uremia, *J Am Soc Nephrol* 1:99, 1990.

352. Silverberg S, Shane E, de la Cruz L: Skeletal disease in primary hyperparathyroidism, *J Bone Miner Res* 4:283, 1989.

353. Silverberg SJ and others: Short-term inhibition of parathyroid hormone secretion by a calcium-receptor agonist in patients with primary hyperparathyroidism, *N Engl J Med* 337:1506, 1997.

354. Silverberg SJ and others: A 10-year prospective study of primary hyperparathyroidism with or without parathyroid surgery, *N Engl J Med* 341:1249, 1999.

355. Simpson NE and others: Assignment of multiple endocrine neoplasia type 2A on chromosome 10 by linkage, *Nature* 328:528, 1987.

356. Sipple JH: The association of pheochromocytoma with carcinoma of the thyroid gland, *Am J Med* 31:163, 1961.

357. Sitges-Serra A, Caralps-Riera A: Hyperparathyroidism associated with renal disease: pathogenesis, natural history, and surgical treatment, *Surg Clin North Am* 67:359, 1987.

358. Smith JF, Coombs RRH: Histologic diagnosis of carcinoma of the parathyroid gland, *J Clin Pathol* 37:1370, 1984.

359. Snover DC, Foucar K: Mitotic activity in benign parathyroid disease, *Am J Clin Pathol* 75:345, 1981.

360. Sofferman RA, Sandage J, Tang ME: Minimal access parathyroid surgery using intraoperative parathyroid hormone assay, *Laryngoscope* 108:1497, 1998.

361. Solbiati L and others: Percutaneous ethanol injection of parathyroid tumors under US guidance: treatment for secondary hyperparathyroidism, *Radiology* 155:607, 1985.

362. Spiegel AM and others: Clinical implications of guanine nucleotide-binding proteins as receptor-effector couplers, *N Engl J Med* 312:26, 1985.

363. Stewart AF and others: Hypercalcemia in pheochromocytoma: evidence for a novel mechanism, *Ann Intern Med* 102:776, 1985.

364. Steiner AL, Goodman AD, Powers SR: Study of a kindred with pheochromocytoma, medullary thyroid carcinoma, hyperparathyroidism and Cushing's disease: multiple endocrine neoplasia type 2, *Medicine* 47:371, 1968.

365. Stoeckle JD, Hard HL, Weber AL: Chronic beryllium disease: long-term follow-up of sixty cases and selective review of the literature, *Am J Med* 46:545, 1969.

366. Stokkel MP, van Eck-Smit BL: Tc-99m MIBI in a patient with parathyroid carcinoma. What to expect from it, *Clin Nucl Med* 21:142, 1996.

367. Stratmann SL and others: Comparison of quick parathyroid assay for uniglandular and multiglandular parathyroid disease, *Am J Surg* 184:518, 2002.

368. Strewer G: Indications for surgery in patients with minimally symptomatic primary hyperparathyroidism, *Surg Clin North Am* 75:439, 1995.

369. Strewler GJ and others: Production of parathyroid hormone by a malignant nonparathyroid tumor in a hypercalcemia patient, *J Clin Endocrinol Metab* 76:1373, 1993.

370. Sugg SL and others: Prospective evaluation of selective venous sampling for parathyroid hormone concentrations in patients undergoing reoperations for primary hyperparathyroidism, *Surgery* 114:1004, 1993.

371. Tahara H and others: Genetic localization of novel candidate tumor suppression gene loci in human parathyroid adenomas, *Cancer Res* 56:599, 1996.

372. Taillefor R and others: Detection and localization of parathyroid adenomas in patients with hyperparathyroidism using a single radionuclide imaging procedure with technetium 99m sestamibi (double phase), *J Nucl Med* 33:1801, 1992.

373. Takagi H and others: Subtotal versus total parathyroidectomy with forearm autograft for secondary hyperparathyroidism in chronic renal failure, *Ann Surg* 200:18, 1984.

374. Takami H, Kameyama K, Nagakubo I: Parathyroid carcinoma in a patient receiving long-term hemodialysis, *Surgery* 125:239, 1984.

375. Talpos G and others: Randomized trial of parathyroidectomy in mild asymptomatic primary hyperparathyroidism: patient description and effects on the SF-36 health survey, *Surgery* 128:1013, 2000.

376. Tanaka Y and others: Factors related to the recurrent hyperfunction of autografts after total parathyroidectomy in patients with severe secondary hyperparathyroidism, *Surg Today* 23:220, 1993.

377. Taylor S: Hyperparathyroidism: retrospect and prospect, *Ann R Coll Surg* 58:255, 1976.

378. Tenta LT, Keyes GR: Transcervical parathyroidectomy microsurgical autotransplantation and visceroverterbral arm, *Otolaryngol Clin North Am* 13:169, 1980.

379. Tetelman S and others: Double parathyroid adenomas: clinical and biochemical characteristics before and after parathyroidectomy, *Am Surg* 218:300, 1993.

380. Thompson GB and others: Re-operative parathyroid surgery in the era of sestamibi scanning and intraoperative parathyroid hormone monitoring, *Arch Surg* 134:699, 1999.

381. Thompson NW: *Surgical anatomy of hyperparathyroidism*. In Rothmund M, Wells SA Jr, editors: *Parathyroid surgery*, Basel, 1986, Karger, p 59.

382. Thompson NW, Eckhauser FE, Harness JK: The anatomy of primary hyperparathyroidism, *Surgery* 92; 814, 1982.

383. Thulé P and others: Preoperative localization of parathyroid tissue with technetium 99m sestamibi Y 123 subtraction scanning, *J Clin Endocrinol Metab* 78:77, 1994.

384. Tikkakosky T and others: Parathyroid adenomas: Preoperative localization with ultrasound combined with fine needle biopsy, *J Laryngol Otol* 62:981, 1989.

385. Tisell L and others: Kan Strålterapi iducera hyperparathyroidism, *Svensk Kirurgi* 32:83, 1975.

386. Trigonio C and others: Parathyroid carcinoma—problems in diagnosis and treatment, *Clin Oncol* 10:11, 1984.

387. Udelsman R: Six hundred fifty-six consecutive explorations for primary hyperparathyroidism, *Ann Surg* 235:665, 2002.

388. Udelsman R, Donovan PI, Sokoll LJ: One hundred consecutive minimally invasive parathyroid explorations, *Ann Surg* 232:331, 2000.

389. Valentin-Opran A and others: Estrogens and antiestrogens stimulate release of bone-resorbing activity in cultured human breast cancer cells, *J Clin Invest* 75:726, 1985.

390. van Heerden JA, Grant CS: Surgical treatment of primary hyperparathyroidism: an institutional perspective, *World J Surg* 15:688, 1991.

391. van Heerden JA and others: Cancer of the parathyroid glands, *Arch Surg* 114:475, 1979.

392. Van Heerden JA and others: Primary hyperparathyroidism in patients with multiple endocrine neoplasia syndromes, *Arch Surg* 118:533, 1983.

393. van Heerden JA and others: Cancer of the parathyroid glands, *Arch Surg* 114:475, 1997.

394. Vasikaran SD, Tallis GA, Braund WJ: Secondary hypoadrenalism presenting with hypercalcemia, *Clin Endocrinol* 41:261, 1994.

395. Verner JV, Morrison AB: Endocrine pancreatic islet disease with diarrhea, *Arch Intern Med* 133:492, 1974.

396. Von Eiselsberg A: Über Erfolgreiche Einbeilung der Katzenshilddrüse in die Bauchdecke und Autreten von Tetanie nach deren extirpation, *Wien Klin Wochenschr* 5:81, 1892.

397. Von Recklinghausen F: Die fibrose oder deformierende ostitis, die osteomalacie und die osteoplastiche Karzinosk in ihren gegenseitigen Beziehumgen. Excerpted from Taylor S: *History of hyperparathyroidism*. In *Progr Surg* 18:1, 1968.

398. Walker JV and others: Histoplasmosis with hypercalcemia, renal failure, and papillary necrosis: confusion with sarcoidosis, *JAMA* 237:1350, 1977.

399. Wallfelt C and others: Relationship between external and cytoplasmic calcium concentrations, parathyroid hormone release and weight of parathyroid glands in human hyperparathyroidism, *J Endocrinol* 16:457, 1988.

400. Wang C: The anatomic basis of parathyroid surgery, *Ann Surg* 183:271, 1976.

401. Wang CA: Parathyroid re-exploration: a clinical and pathological study of 112 cases, *Ann Surg* 186:140, 1977.

402. Wang CA: Hyperfunctioning intrathyroid parathyroid gland: a potential cause failure in parathyroid surgery, *J R Soc Med* 74:49, 1981.

403. Wang CA: Surgical management of primary hyperparathyroidism, *Curr Probl Surg* 12:1, 1985.

404. Wang CA, Caz RD: Natural history of parathyroid carcinoma: Diagnosis, treatment, and results, *Am J Surg* 149:522, 1985.

405. Wang CA, Cassstleman B, Cope O: Surgical management of hyperparathyroidism due to primary hyperplasia: a clinical and pathologic study of 104 cases, *Ann Surg* 195:384, 1982.

406. Wang CA and others: Hyperfunctioning supernumerary parathyroid glands, *Surg Gynecol Obstet* 148:711, 1979.

407. Ware J, Sherbourne C: The MOS 36-item, short-term health survey (SF-36): I, conceptual framework and item selection, *Med Care* 30:473, 1992.

408. Wassif WS and others: Familial isolated hyperparathyroidism: a distinct genetic entity and increased risk of parathyroid cancer, *J Clin Endocrinol Metab* 77:1485, 1993.

409. Weber CJ, Sewell CW, McGarity WC: Persistent and recurrent sporadic primary hyperparathyroidism: histopathology, complications, and results of reoperation, *Surgery* 116:991, 1994.

410. Weber CJ and others: Value of technetium 99m sestamibi iodine 123 imaging in reoperation parathyroid surgery, *Surgery* 114:1011, 1993.

411. Wells SA Jr and others: Transplantation of the parathyroid glands in man: clinical indications and results, *Surgery* 78:34, 1975.

412. Wells SA Jr and others: Parathyroid autotransplantation in primary parathyroid hyperplasia, *N Engl J Med* 295:57, 1976.

413. Wells SA Jr and others: Long-term evaluation of patients with primary parathyroid hyperplasia managed by total parathyroidectomy and heterotopic autotransplantation, *Ann Surg* 192:451, 1980.

414. Welsh CL and others: Parathyroid surgery in chronic renal failure: Subtotal parathyroidectomy or autotransplantation? *Br J Surg* 71:591, 1984.

415. Werner P: Genetic aspects of adenomatosis of endocrine glands, *Am J Med* 16:363, 1954.

416. Williamson E, Van Peevan H: Patient benefits in discovering occur hyperparathyroidism, *Arcot Intern Med* 133:430, 1974.

417. Williams ED: Pathology of the parathyroid glands, *J Clin Endocrinol Metab* 3:285, 1974.

418. Wolpert HR, Vickery AL Jr, Wang CA: Functioning oxyphil cell adenomas of the parathyroid gland: a study of 15 cases, *Am J Surg Pathol* 13:500, 1989.

419. Wynne AG and others: Parathyroid carcinoma: clinical and pathologic features in 43 patients, *Medicine* 71:197, 1992.

420. Yamamoto M and others: Hypocalcemia increases and hypercalcemia decreases the steady state level of parathyroid hormone messenger ribonucleic acid in the rat, *J Clin Invest* 83:1053, 1989.

421. Yamashita H and others: Light and electron microscopic study of nonfunctioning parathyroid carcinoma, *Acta Pathol Jpn* 34:123, 1984.

422. Yoshimoto K and others: Ectopic production of parathyroid hormone by small cell lung cancer in a patient with hypercalcemia, *J Clin Endocrinol Metab* 68:976, 1989.

423. Yoshimoto K and others: Familial isolated primary hyperparathyroidism with parathyroid carcinomas: clinical and molecular features, *Clin Endocrinol (Oxf)* 48:67, 1998.

424. Young AE and others: Localization of parathyroid adenomas by thallium 201 and technetium 99m, *BMJ* 286:1384, 1983.

425. Zisman E and others: Production of parathyroid hormone by metastatic parathyroid carcinoma, *Am J Med* 45:619, 1968.

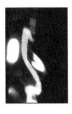

PARANASAL SINUSES: MANAGEMENT OF THYROID EYE DISEASE (GRAVES' OPHTHALMOPATHY)

‖ Douglas A. Girod

INTRODUCTION

In 1835, Robert Graves described a clinical syndrome that included such symptoms as hypermetabolism, diffuse enlargement of the thyroid gland, and exophthalmos. Although others also had recognized this entity, it was Graves who defined the thyroid as playing a central role in the disease. Graves' disease is now recognized as a multisystem disorder characterized by one or more of the following: (1) hyperthyroidism associated with diffuse hyperplasia of the thyroid gland; (2) infiltrative ophthalmopathy (leading to exophthalmos); and (3) infiltrative dermopathy (localized pretibial myxedema). Recent work has helped to establish Graves' disease as an autoimmune process targeted at the thyroid-stimulating hormone (TSH) receptor in the thyroid.[49,61,65] In addition, retroocular fibroblasts have been found to play a key role in the development and progression of the ophthalmopathy seen in some patients with Graves' disease.[2,3]

Despite these advances in the understanding of Graves' disease pathogenesis, only limited progress has been made in the management of the disease. Therapy is still primarily directed at the manifestations of the disease in a palliative fashion rather than at preventing the underlying destructive autoimmune process. This chapter will focus on the evaluation and management of the ophthalmic manifestations of Graves' disease.

PATHOPHYSIOLOGY

Extensive research in recent years has led to important insights into the pathologic mechanisms involved in Graves' disease and Graves' ophthalmopathy. As the understanding progresses, so should the ability to deal with this challenging disorder.

Graves' Disease

Current theory describing the development of Graves' disease involves autoreactive T cells, which arise either through an escape from clonal deletion, through failure of suppressor T-cell activity, or through molecular mimicry to become reactive to TSH receptors.[7,27] The majority of the T cells responsible for the reaction are located in the thyroid gland itself. Subsequent thyroid damage from any etiology (e.g., chronic thyroiditis, radiotherapy, smoking, drugs) results in the release of the thyroid autoantigen (TSH receptors). As the autoimmune process amplifies, T lymphocytes are activated, and humoral immunity produces antibodies to the TSH receptor that are stimulatory, resulting in hyperthyroidism. In some patients, underlying chronic thyroiditis may dramatically reduce thyroid reserve or TSH receptor–blocking antibodies may be present, resulting in the "euthyroid" patient with Graves' disease.

Graves' Ophthalmopathy

The extraocular muscles are the site of the most clinically evident changes in patients with Graves' ophthalmopathy. Although the muscles are enlarged on computed tomography (CT) scan, the myocytes themselves appear fairly normal histopathologically.[40] There is an associated intense proliferation of perimysial fibroblasts and dense lymphocytic infiltration. Early reports of circulating autoantibodies against eye muscle antigen in sera from patients with Graves' ophthalmopathy led to the theory that the disease was a result of an autoimmune response directed against the extraocular eye muscle fibers.[47] This theory began to lose favor as study of these autoantibodies proved them to be neither tissue or disease specific. The lack of histologic evidence of cytotoxicity against eye muscle in vivo also argues against this theory.

Attention has now focused on the retrobulbar fibroblast as playing a key role in the pathogenesis of Graves' ophthalmopathy. These fibroblasts have several capabilities that place them at the center of the changes seen in the eye. They secrete a range of glycosaminoglycans (predominately hyaluronate), the deposition of which is a hallmark of Graves' ophthalmopathy and causes interstitial edema as a result of its intensely hydrophilic nature. These cells can also produce major histocompatibility complex class II molecules, heat shock proteins, and lymphocyte adhesion molecules, which allow them to act as target and effector cells in the ongoing immune process in those with Graves' ophthalmopathy.[36] In addition, autoantibodies against fibroblast antigens have been found in a majority of patients with Graves' ophthalmopathy. These antibodies share some characteristics with TSH receptor antibodies (TRAbs).[3] More recently, probes to TSH receptor messenger ribonucleic acid (mRNA) have labeled mRNA within the retrobulbar fibroblasts of patients with Graves' ophthalmopathy.[7] Thus, the "fibroblast antigen" may be similar to all or part of the TSH receptor, and therefore it represents a shared thyroid–eye antigen. Such an antigenic similarity would explain the immune cross-reactivity between these two seemingly unrelated tissue sites.

Lymphocytes also are active in the ongoing immune process of Graves' ophthalmopathy. Orbital lymphocyte infiltrates have been found to be primarily T cells, including CD4+ (T helper cells) and CD8+ (T suppressor and cytotoxic cells). Cytokines released by T cells have been shown to induce fibroblast proliferation and collagen and glycosaminoglycan deposition. Recently, Grubeck-Loebenstein and others[32] cultured retrobulbar suppressor and cytotoxic T cells out of tissues removed at the time of orbital decompression and found them capable of targeting the retrobulbar fibroblasts. Interactions with fibroblasts resulted in pronounced T-cell cytokine production and fibroblast proliferation without evidence of fibroblast cytotoxicity. Thus, the T-cell–retrobulbar fibroblast interaction may be responsible for the clinical manifestations of Graves' ophthalmopathy.

Burch and Wortofsky[7] have proposed a hypothetical sequence of events that led to the initiation and progression of Graves' ophthalmopathy based on an extensive review of the recent literature (Figure 121-1).

EPIDEMIOLOGY/ETIOLOGY

An accurate estimate of the prevalence of Graves' ophthalmopathy is difficult to determine and depends in part on the diagnostic criteria used to define the presence of ophthalmopathy. For example, "lid lag" and "stare" are nonspecific signs and can be seen with thyrotoxicosis stemming from etiologies other than Graves' disease. In an exhaustive review of the literature, Burch and Wartofsky[7] found an incidence of ophthalmopathy in patients with Graves' disease of 10% to 25% if these nonspecific signs were excluded and 30% to 45% if lid findings were included as diag-

nostic criteria. When intraocular pressure on upgaze or CT findings also were included, the incidence increased to nearly 70%. Fortunately, the most severe form of Graves' ophthalmopathy with optic nerve involvement and visual impairment occurs in only 2% to 5% of patients with Graves' disease.[53,80]

EFFECTS OF GENETICS AND SEX

The role of genetic predisposition and major histocompatibility complex (MHC) antigen patterns in those with Graves' ophthalmopathy has been extensively studied but remains poorly characterized.[7] Ethnicity appears to play some role, as Tellez and others[76] found that Europeans with Graves' disease were six times more likely to develop ophthalmopathy than Asian patients with Graves' disease. More important are the influences of sex on the development of Graves' disease and the associated ophthalmopathy. A strong 3:1 female-to-male preponderance exists for Graves' disease,[55,77] which decreases to about 2:1 for those with Graves' ophthalmopathy. Overall, male patients with Graves' disease have a higher incidence of ophthalmopathy that is more severe and tends to develop later in life.[7]

EFFECTS OF TOBACCO

Several studies have reported an increased incidence of goiter in tobacco smokers compared with nonsmokers, attributing this to thiocyanate, a known goitrogen that is present in inhaled tobacco smoke.[10,16] Studies have also reported an association between smoking and the incidence and severity of Graves' ophthalmopathy.[4,76] This relationship was not found in patients with other forms of thyroid disease and suggests the tobacco effects are specific to Graves' disease. It is possible that the decrease in female preponderance in Graves' ophthalmopathy, especially in the more severe forms, may be a reflection of the higher incidence of smoking among male patients rather than a true sex difference.[7]

EFFECTS OF THYROID STATUS

The role of thyroid hormonal status in the development and severity of Graves' ophthalmopathy has been particularly difficult to ascertain because of the overlap of thyrotoxicosis with antithyroid therapy in this patient population. Thyrotoxicosis alone is thought to have little direct effect on the autoimmune process. It serves as a fairly poor marker for disease severity because the prevalence and course of hyperthyroidism correlate poorly with that of Graves' ophthalmopathy.[7] An improvement in eye status with maintenance of euthyroidism during antithyroid therapy may be more a reflection of improving immune function than a decreased circulating thyroid hormone.

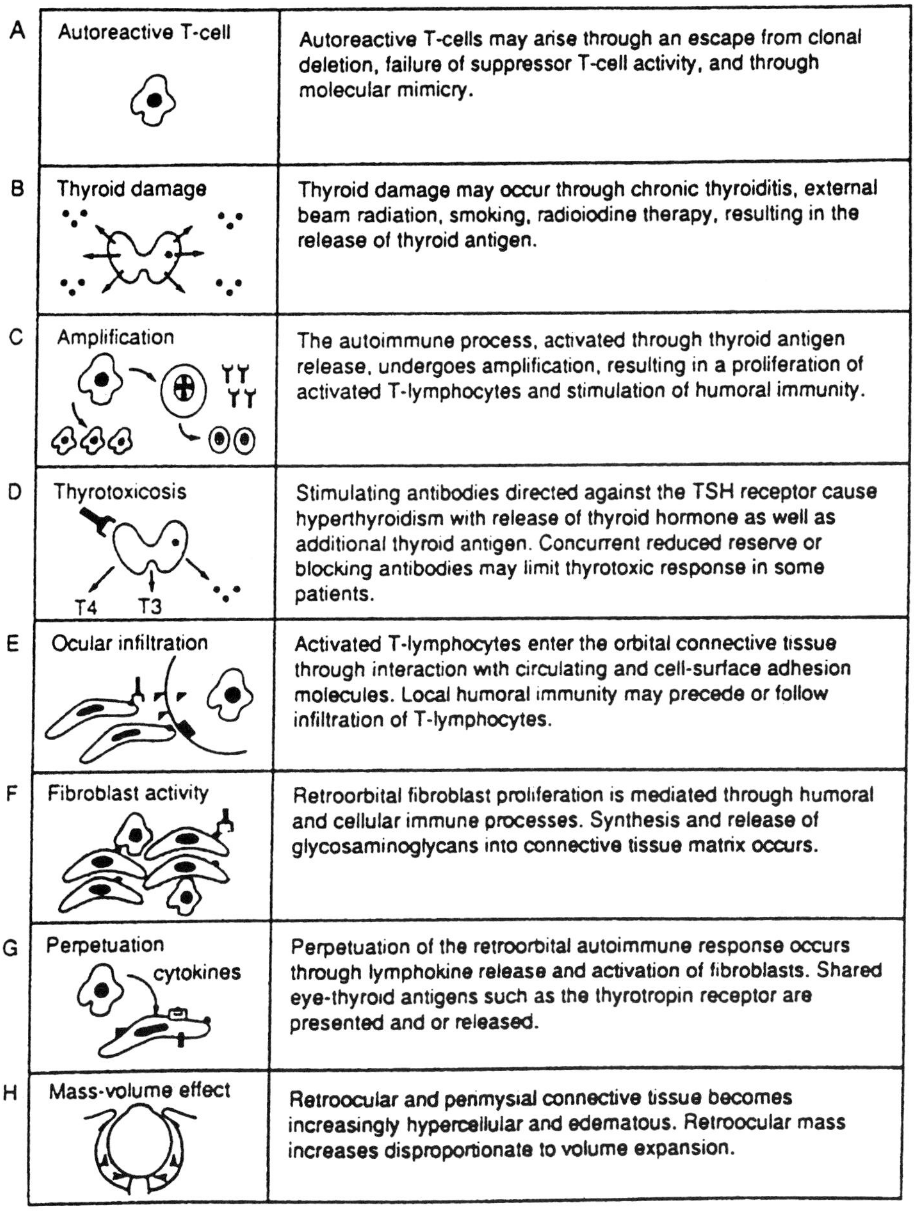

A	Autoreactive T-cell	Autoreactive T-cells may arise through an escape from clonal deletion, failure of suppressor T-cell activity, and through molecular mimicry.
B	Thyroid damage	Thyroid damage may occur through chronic thyroiditis, external beam radiation, smoking, radioiodine therapy, resulting in the release of thyroid antigen.
C	Amplification	The autoimmune process, activated through thyroid antigen release, undergoes amplification, resulting in a proliferation of activated T-lymphocytes and stimulation of humoral immunity.
D	Thyrotoxicosis T4 T3	Stimulating antibodies directed against the TSH receptor cause hyperthyroidism with release of thyroid hormone as well as additional thyroid antigen. Concurrent reduced reserve or blocking antibodies may limit thyrotoxic response in some patients.
E	Ocular infiltration	Activated T-lymphocytes enter the orbital connective tissue through interaction with circulating and cell-surface adhesion molecules. Local humoral immunity may precede or follow infiltration of T-lymphocytes.
F	Fibroblast activity	Retroorbital fibroblast proliferation is mediated through humoral and cellular immune processes. Synthesis and release of glycosaminoglycans into connective tissue matrix occurs.
G	Perpetuation cytokines	Perpetuation of the retroorbital autoimmune response occurs through lymphokine release and activation of fibroblasts. Shared eye-thyroid antigens such as the thyrotropin receptor are presented and or released.
H	Mass-volume effect	Retroocular and perimysial connective tissue becomes increasingly hypercellular and edematous. Retroocular mass increases disproportionate to volume expansion.

Figure 121-1. Proposed sequence of events leading to the initiation and progression of Graves' ophthalmopathy based on the current literature. (From Burch HB, Wartofsky L: *Endocr Rev* 14:747, 1993.)

Elevated circulating TSH levels appear to promote eye disease in patients with Graves' disease. Hamilton and others[35] have reported an increased incidence of progressive ophthalmopathy with the hypothyroidsm, which followed antithyroid therapy. Tamaki and others[75] described a marked improvement in eye status and a reduction of circulating TRAb in two patients receiving thyroid hormone replacement during antithyroid therapy. The mechanism by which elevated TSH achieves its influence is not clear, but it may serve to upregulate TSH receptors (apparent autoantigens, to be discussed) in thyrocytes[39] and possibly lymphocytes.[23]

NATURAL HISTORY

On summarizing the available literature on the natural history of Graves' ophthalmopathy, Burch and Wartofsky[7] noted the disease tended to progress through a phase of rapid progression (6–24 months), followed by a prolonged plateau phase with subsequent slow but incomplete regression of eye changes. Lid retraction and soft tissue changes, such as chemosis and eyelid edema, tended to be short-lived with improvement or resolution over 1 to 5 years (60%–90%). Ophthalmoplegia resolved incompletely and less rapidly, although 30% to 40% of patients showed some improvement in ocular motility without specific therapy. Proptosis is the eye finding least likely to improve or resolve spontaneously (10%). Trobe[79] reviewed 32 patients with untreated Graves' optic neuropathy and found that vision improved spontaneously in most, but 21% had a final visual acuity of 20/100 or worse, with five patients progressing to near blindness. Facing potential loss of sight, it is not surprising that attempts at medical and surgical intervention, some of them heroic, have occurred for the past 80 years.

CLINICAL FEATURES
Thyroid Disease

A patient with Graves' ophthalmopathy will most commonly visit an endocrinologist for management of thyroid disease or an ophthalmologist for evaluation of eye complaints. A thorough history, examination, and high level of suspicion are required to make the diagnosis. Classically, the patient is experiencing hyperthyroidism, and the expected hypermetabolic findings are present at the time of presentation with eye disease. However, in a review of more than 800 cases from the literature, Burch and Wortofsky[7] found that 20% of patients presented with eye disease before any manifestation of hyperthyroidism, 39% presented concurrently with thyroid and eye disease, and 41% presented with eye disease after clinical hyperthyroidism already was evident. In 80% of the patients in whom both diseases eventually manifested, both became clinically evident within 18 months of each other, although some patients either may never demonstrate thyroid and eye disease or many years may separate the two.

Pretibial Myxedema

Pretibial myxedema, or thyroid dermopathy, is the localized thickening of the skin, usually in the pretibial area. It occurs in up to 4.3% of patients with Graves' disease but at a higher rate (12%–15%) in patients with Graves' ophthalmopathy[20,50] and usually is a late manifestation. Conversely, almost all patients with pretibial myxedema have Graves' ophthalmopathy, although the dermopathy may precede the ophthalmopathy. Symptomatic lesions consist of shiny, erythematous to brown plaques, nodules, or areas of nonpitting edema, which most commonly occur in the anterior or lateral aspects of the leg or at sites of old or recent trauma. Involvement of other body sites is rare. Almost all patients have high circulating levels of TRAbs, although the true pathogenesis of the dermopathy is not understood. Pretibial myxedema usually is of cosmetic importance only, but if the feet or hands become massively swollen, it can cause functional difficulties.

GRAVES' OPHTHALMOPATHY

As described previously, Graves' disease occurs more commonly in women and over a broad age range (16 to 81 years), with a mean age in the fifth and sixth decade.[11,28,87] Eye involvement in those with Graves' disease is bilateral in the majority of patients, although 5% to 14% of patients will have unilateral disease depending on the method of detection.[7] With careful testing (i.e., CT scan) 50% to 90% of these patients will have changes in both eyes. In contrast, major asymmetry in the extent of eye involvement is common. Thus, Graves' ophthalmopathy remains the most common etiology of "unilateral" proptosis in adults.[8]

Ophthalmopathy Classification

The spectrum of eye changes ranges from eyelid retraction (resulting in the appearance of a "stare"), to proptosis, corneal exposure and ulceration, diplopia, and loss of vision. A clinical classification system for eye involvement by Graves' disease was proposed by Werner,[91] approved by the American Thyroid Association (ATA), and subsequently modified[92] in 1977. The ATA's detailed classification is shown in Table 121-1. This classification is strictly clinical and has been helpful for reporting purposes. Unfortunately, the disease does not necessarily progress systematically through the classes and may skip one or more classes entirely. In addition, the classification system has been criticized for not considering disease activity (stable or rapidly progressing), which is critical for making patient treatment decisions.[84]

In response to these deficiencies and several other proposed classification schemes, an international ad hoc committee representing the American, European, Asia-Oceanic, and Latin America Thyroid Associations recommended in 1992 a new characterization of Graves' ophthalmopathy, which is shown in Table 121-2. This system is recommended for use in attempting objective clinical assessment and documenting disease activity, as in clinical studies. The older ATA classification system is still used for educational purposes and clinical evaluation.

Eye Findings

Lid lag and the appearance of a "stare" are seen in the mildest form (ATA class I disease) of eye involvement by Graves' disease. This is thought to occur initially as the result of an increased sympathetic sensitivity to catecholamines as seen with those with hyperthyroidism.[9] As the disease progresses and the lymphocytic inflammatory reaction infiltrates the extraocular muscles and orbital fat, the fibroblasts proliferate and deposit glycosaminoglycans, predominantly hyaluronic acid.[66,69] The resulting muscle and fat enlargement

TABLE 121-1

DETAILED CLASSIFICATION OF THE EYE CHANGES OF GRAVES' DISEASE

Classes	Grades	Ocular Symptoms and Signs
0		No signs or symptoms
1		Only signs, no symptoms (signs limited to upper lid retraction and stare, with or without lid lag and proptosis)
2		Soft tissue involvement with symptoms and signs
	o	Absent
	a	Minimal
	b	Moderate
	c	Marked
3		Proptosis 3 mm or more in excess of upper normal limit, with or without symptoms
	o	Absent
	a	3- to 4-mm increase over upper normal
	b	5- to 7-mm increase
	c	8 or more mm increase
4		Extraocular muscle involvement (usually with diplopia, other symptoms or signs)
	o	Absent
	a	Limitation of motion at extremes of gaze
	b	Evident restriction of motion
	c	Fixation of a globe or globes
5		Corneal involvement (primarily a result of lagophthalmos)
	o	Absent
	a	Stippling of cornea
	b	Ulceration
	c	Clouding, necrosis, perforation
6		Sight loss (caused by optic nerve involvement)
	o	Absent
	a	Disc pallor or choking, or visual field defect: vision 20/20 to 20/60
	b	Same, but vision 20/70 to 20/200
	c	Blindness (i.e., failure to perceive light, vision less than 20/200)

combines with interstitial edema to cause an increase in intraocular pressure.

Intraocular pressure is increased in primary gaze (straight ahead) and even more so in upward gaze (supraduction). This increase in intraocular pressure can lead to a misdiagnosis of glaucoma, with a subsequent delay in appropriate therapy.[28] Over time, increases in intraocular pressure also produce conjunctival chemosis, excessive lacrimation, periorbital edema, and photophobia (ATA class II disease).

As enlargement of orbital muscle and fat progresses, the volume of the orbital contents increases. The orbital cavity has four fixed bony walls with an average volume of 26 mL.[29] In healthy people, the globe takes up 30% of this volume, with retrobulbar and peribulbar structures taking up the remaining 70% of the volume. With nowhere else to expand, an increase of only 4 mL in the volume of the orbital contents will result in 6 mm of proptosis (ATA class III disease).

As the extraocular muscles become increasingly enlarged by edema and infiltration, they also become dysfunctional, resulting in reduced ocular mobility and diplopia (ATA class IV disease). Over time, the inflammatory response provokes the deposition of collagen by the fibroblasts, replacing the normally elastic muscles of the eye and ultimately causing a permanent fibrotic, restrictive ophthalmoplegia.

Progressive proptosis also dramatically interferes with the protective mechanisms of the cornea, causing exposure, desiccation, irritation, and ultimately, ulceration (ATA class V disease). Corneal ulceration becomes a vision-threatening problem, with a risk of permanent corneal scarring, and requires immediate attention.

In its most severe form, Graves' ophthalmopathy involves the optic nerve to impair vision (ATA class VI disease). Optic nerve involvement typically presents as a painless gradual loss of visual acuity or visual field,[53] although it can occur precipitously over days to weeks. Although originally thought to be caused by ischemia or venous congestion of the nerve as a result of increased intraocular pressure, there now is convincing evidence to support crowding and compression

TABLE 121-2

CHARACTERIZATION OF GRAVES' OPHTHALMOPATHY: RECOMMENDATIONS OF AN INTERNATIONAL AD HOC COMMITTEE*

Category of Disease	Objective Criteria Monitored
Eyelid	Maximal lid fissure width
	Upper lid to limbus distance
	Lower lid to limbus distance
Cornea	Exposure keratitis assessed by rose bengal or fluorescein staining (indicate presence or absence)
Extraocular muscles	Single binocular vision in central 30° of vision (indicate presence or absence, with or without prisms)
	One or more of the following measurement techniques:
	Maddox rod test
	Alternate cover test
	Hess chart measurements
	Lancaster red-green test
	Optional
	Intraocular pressure in downward gaze
	CT or MRI
Proptosis	Exophthalmometer reading (CT or MRI measurement may also be used for measurement)
Optic nerve	Visual acuity
	Visual fields
	Color vision
Activity score	Sum of one point each for any of the following:
	Spontaneous retrobulbar pain
	Pain with eye movement
	Eyelid erythema
	Eyelid edema or swelling
	Conjunctival injection
	Chemosis
	Caruncle swelling
Patient self-assessment	Satisfaction with the following (indicate change with therapy in each using a scale such as: greatly improved, improved, unchanged, worse, much worse):
	Appearance
	Visual acuity
	Eye discomfort
	Diplopia

*Consensus of an 18-member ad hoc committee comprised of representatives from the American, European, Asia-Oceanic, and Latin America Thyroid Associations. (From 1992 Classification of eye changes of Graves' disease, *Thyroid* 2:235.)
CT, Computed tomography; MRI, magnetic resonance imaging.

of the optic nerve at the orbital apex by the enlarged extraocular muscles as the etiology of nerve dysfunction.[62]

Optic nerve function is measured in several ways, one or all of which may be impaired. In one study of 31 patients with optic nerve involvement,[28] visual acuity was 20/25 or worse in 100% of eyes; color vision was decreased in 64%; and visual fields were decreased in 70%, with inferior scotomata and cecocentral scotomata defects most common. Impaired visual fields or color vision also may be found in patients with normal visual acuity.[11]

Clinical Evaluation
Differential Diagnosis

Graves' ophthalmopathy presents a spectrum of clinical manifestations that are reminiscent of other clinical entities. Eye changes range from minimal—requiring a detailed eye examination or CT scan for identification—to dramatic, disfiguring, and vision-threatening changes that eclipse the manifestations of the underlying thyroid disease. The high prevalence of asymmetric eye involvement may also lead the clinician to suspect a unilateral disease process rather than a systemic one. Although the differential diagnosis for proptosis is extensive (Table 121-3), most other disease entities have only superficial similarities to Graves' ophthalmopathy and can be quickly ruled out. Most importantly, the clinician should maintain a high degree of suspicion if the diagnosis of Graves' ophthalmopathy is to be made in a timely fashion.

TABLE 121-3

DIFFERENTIAL DIAGNOSIS OF PROPTOSIS

Endocrine

    Graves' ophthalmopathy
    Cushing's syndrome

Orbital neoplasms

    Primary neoplasms
    Hemangioma
    Lymphoma (may be systemic)
    Optic nerve glioma
    Choroidal melanoma
    Lacrimal gland tumors
    Meningioma
    Rhabdomyosarcoma

Extension of
   paranasal sinus
   tumors

Metastatic disease

    Malignant melanoma
    Breast carcinoma
    Lung carcinoma
    Kidney
    Prostate

Inflammatory

    Orbital pseudotumor
    Orbital myositis

Granulomatous

    Sarcoidosis
    Wegener's granulomatosis

Infectious

    Orbital cellulitis
    Syphilis
    Mucormycosis
    Parasitic (trypanosomiasis,
      schistosomiasis,
      cystocercosis, echinococcal
      disease)

Vascular
Miscellaneous

    Carotid-cavernous fistula
    Lithium therapy
    Cirrhosis
    Obesity
    Amyloidosis
    Dermoid and epidermoid cysts
    Foreign body

Thyroid Function

A full endocrinology workup is essential in the diagnosis and management of Graves' disease. Laboratory testing should include thyroid function tests and a TSH level. In some apparently euthyroid patients, more detailed dynamic testing of thyroid function may be required to uncover thyroid dysfunction. These studies include the suppression of radioiodine uptake with T_3 to assess for non–TSH-mediated thyroid stimulation, the thyrotropin-releasing hormone (TRH) stimulation test to determine the presence of low-grade suppression of the hypothalamic–pituitary axis, and TSH stimulation tests of thyroid reserve. Serologic evaluation for evidence of thyroid autoimmunity can also be performed, including microsomal antibody, thyroglobulin antibody, and TRAb assays. Overall, with sufficient scrutiny, most if not all patients with euthyroid ophthalmopathy can be shown to have some degree of thyroid dysfunction.[7]

Eye Evaluation

A thorough examination by a skilled ophthalmologist is critical for the diagnosis and management of Graves' ophthalmopathy. Serial eye examinations are required to monitor disease activity, progression, and response to therapy. The eye examination should include attention to soft tissue changes, including lid edema and retraction, chemosis, scleral injection, limitation of ocular motility, documentation of proptosis (Hertel exophthalmometer) and intraocular pressure in primary and upward gaze (Schiotz tonometer), strabismus and visual function in the form of acuity (Snellen's wall chart), color vision (Ishihara's color plates), and visual fields (Goldmann perimetry).

Imaging Studies

CT scans of the orbit can be helpful in the diagnosis of Graves' ophthalmopathy in the euthyroid patient and are essential if surgical intervention is being considered. Typical findings include a twofold to eightfold enlargement of the extraocular muscle bodies, sparing the tendinous portions (Figure 121-2). The changes will be bilateral in 90% of patients, although asymmetry in the extent of involvement is the rule. The medial and inferior rectus muscles are involved most commonly, although any or all of the muscles may be enlarged.[41] The orbital and extraocular muscle volume can be estimated using CT images.[21,22,33] Although estimates of extraocular muscle volume have correlated with the presence of optic neuropathy, subsequent studies have not found a correlation between muscle volume estimates and the severity of optic neuropathy or the effectiveness of decompression,[28,34] thus limiting the usefulness of these estimates.

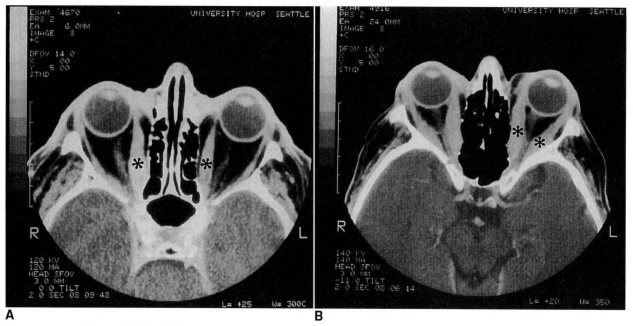

Figure 121-2. Axial computed tomography scans through the orbits in two patients with Graves' ophthalmopathy, demonstrating **(A)** medial rectus muscle enlargement (asterisks) with normal lateral rectus muscle size and **(B)** medial and lateral rectus muscle enlargement (asterisks) with orbital apex crowding, causing optic neuropathy.

Ultrasound (orbital echography) has been reported to be reliable and effective in evaluating extraocular muscle size.[15] Although not as beneficial in the initial diagnosis and surgical planning as the CT scan in those with Graves' disease, it is proposed as an inexpensive, noninvasive method for monitoring response to therapy (steroids or radiation).

Magnetic resonance imaging (MRI) of the orbits has proved excellent for the evaluation of the soft tissues of the orbit. Extraocular muscle volume can be readily estimated from a single coronal MRI section.[73] Studies have suggested that T2-weighted MRI images may provide a sensitive measure of active inflammation in the orbit, giving much needed information on disease activity.[38,42] Unfortunately, MRI provides little detail of the bony anatomy of the orbit, which is required if the possibility of surgical intervention is being entertained.

Nuclear medicine studies such as single photon emission computed tomography (SPECT) imaging using 99mTc-DTPA and gallium-67 have also been used to image the orbit and give reliable information as to the level of disease activity with in the extraocular muscles.[24,48]

Management of Graves' Ophthalmopathy

A multispecialty team approach for the treatment of patients with Graves' disease and Graves' ophthal-mopathy is recommended because of the multiple organ systems involved and the variety of diagnostic and therapeutic modalities needed to provide optimal care of this complex entity. Team members representing endocrinology, radiology, nuclear medicine, radiotherapy, ophthalmology, otolaryngology–head and neck surgery, and neurosurgery will be involved to varying degrees. A coordinating member of the team (usually the endocrinologist for Graves' disease and the ophthalmologist for Graves' ophthalmopathy) is critical for maintaining records, tracking disease progression, and providing continuity of care for long periods.[78]

Medical Therapy

Thyroid therapy. The management of the thyroid in those with Graves' disease remains somewhat controversial, and a complete discussion is beyond the scope of this chapter. The impact of thyroid management on Graves' ophthalmopathy is only now becoming clear. As previously discussed, the correlation between the severity of hyperthyroidism and the prevalence or course of Graves' ophthalmopathy is poor at best. For patients with thyrotoxicosis, the thyroid may be managed with antithyroid drugs (i.e., propylthiouracil and methimazole), radioiodine ablation (iodine-131), or thyroidectomy (usually subtotal). Reports on the effect of each of these modalities on the development or progression of ophthalmopathy are conflicting in the literature, although in a recent prospective study, Tallstedt and others[74] randomly assigned 168 patients into groups receiving either antithyroid drugs, radioiodine ablation, or surgery. There was no difference in the rate of new onset or progression of existing ophthalmopathy between the antithyroid drug and surgery groups (10%–16%), but the radioiodine ablation group showed a higher incidence (33%) of these problems.

One possible mechanism for the increase in those with ophthalmopathy receiving radioiodine ablation includes transient hypothyroidism and the release of thyroid antigens, promoting an acceleration of the autoimmune process. In support of this hypothesis, investigators have found that TRAb levels briefly decrease and then show a sustained increase after iodine-131 ablation for Graves' disease.[6] However, after thyroidectomy, TRAb levels showed a transient increase followed by a gradual decrease.[5] Potentially least concerning were TRAb levels, which gradually declined after antithyroid therapy alone. Thus, it would seem that radioiodine ablation of the thyroid may not be the best option for the management of thyrotoxicosis in patients with Graves' disease. As mentioned previously, thyroid hormone replacement and suppression during antithyroid drug therapy or after radioiodine or surgical ablation (before the onset of measurable hypothyroidism) appear to result in a decrease in the prevalence or progression of ophthalmopathy in those with Graves' disease and therefore should be considered.[75]

Local therapy. The majority of patients with Graves' ophthalmopathy will experience a self-limited disease course requiring only local measures for symptomatic relief. Corneal exposure and drying respond well to eyedrops and nocturnal taping of the eyelid. Some have found the use of diuretics useful in decreasing swelling. Sunglasses help with photophobia, and prisms may help with mild strabismus. Topical guanethidine eyedrops have been found to reduce lid retraction and lid lag, reportedly by sympathetic blockade of Muller's muscle in the upper lid, but they are poorly tolerated and rarely used.

Steroid therapy. High-dose corticosteroids (prednisone, 80–100 mg/day) are commonly used as the first-line management of more severe Graves' ophthalmopathy. The administration of high doses is maintained for 2 to 4 weeks, followed by a slow taper over several months. Patients experience rapid relief of pain, erythema, and conjunctival edema and improved vision. Trobe, Glaser, and Laflamme[80] reported a 48% success rate after 2 months of therapy.

Unfortunately, steroids may only be temporizing, with recurrence of visual loss on taper. Improvement in proptosis and ophthalmoplegia may also be seen with corticosteroid therapy but generally less so, and these conditions are more likely to recur on steroid withdrawal. The multiple adverse effects of steroid therapy are well known and include glucose intolerance, weight gain, psychosis, peptic ulcer disease, and osteoporosis with vertebral fracture. Thus, corticosteroid therapy should be considered temporizing, while either regression and stabilization of disease or definitive therapy are awaited.

Immunosuppression with cyclosporine also has been evaluated for those with Graves' ophthalmopathy and has been found to be less effective than prednisone in single-agent therapy.[7] The beneficial effects of both drugs appear to be additive, and maintenance cyclosporine therapy may be corticosteroid-sparing. Careful drug level monitoring is necessary to avoid nephrotoxicity. Other common adverse effects include hypertension, liver enzyme elevation, gum hypertrophy, and paresthesias. Plasmapheresis to remove circulating antibodies and other immunomodulatory drugs have also been used, but the results suggest further evaluation before widespread use.

Radiotherapy

Radiotherapy to the orbit has been used for more than 85 years for patients with Graves' ophthalmopathy. Traditionally this is accomplished by delivering 20 Gy in 10 fractions over 2 weeks. The fractions are delivered to a field just behind the lateral canthus to spare the cornea and lens. In a 1989 review of the literature, Sautter-Bihl and Heinze[67] found a good to excellent response overall in 35% to 92% of patients and improvement of impaired visual acuity in 33% to 85% of patients treated with orbital radiation. The mechanism of action of radiation to the orbit is thought to be, in large part, an effect on the lymphocytes infiltrating the orbital muscles and fat during the inciting stages of the disease. Thus, patients treated early in the course of the disease with pronounced soft tissue involvement are most likely to benefit. Proptosis, ophthalmoplegia, and optic neuropathy are less responsive, and patients with long-standing stable disease are not likely to benefit. The portion of the radiation dose delivered to the lens is less than 5% and has not been reported to be harmful.

However, more recent studies have cast considerable doubt on the efficacy of radiotherapy for Grave's ophthalmopathy. In 2003, Gerling and colleagues[26] found no difference in the documented improvement when patients were treated with very low dose radiotherapy (2.4 Gy) and more standard doses (16 Gy). In another study, improvement in symptoms and clinical findings was not different between patients treated with steroids alone compared with those treated with steroids plus 24 Gy of radiotherapy.[63] In a prospective randomized trial treating one orbit of each patient with 20 Gy of radiotherapy, Gorman and others[31] were unable to show any significant benefit over the nontreated orbit at 1 year. Long-term follow-up in an uncontrolled fashion also found no benefit from the radiotherapy.[30] Because radiotherapy has potential long-term adverse effects, its usefulness in Grave's ophthalmopathy should be questioned.

Surgical Therapy

Indications for surgical decompression of the orbit have evolved over the years and have included cosmetic management of proptosis, lid lag, and stare as well as the management of optic neuropathy.[9,11,17,25] New-onset strabismus after orbital decompression has been reported in as many as 30% to 64% of the patients, suggesting that patient selection should be done with caution.[25,61] As a result, many centers perform orbital decompression primarily in the setting of optic nerve involvement combined with failure to respond or inability to tolerate steroid therapy or for the relapse of symptoms with the taper of steroid therapy.[28,53] Radiotherapy is generally reserved for those who refuse, cannot tolerate, or fail surgical decompression, although some still advocate primary radiotherapy.[64,81]

The goal of surgical decompression of the orbit is simply to expand the bony orbital confines to make room for the increased volume of the orbital contents. Surgical decompression was first described by Dollinger,[12] who advocated removal of the lateral orbital wall for decompression into the temporal fossa (Krönlein's procedure). Twenty years later, Naffziger[60] reported removal of the orbital roof with decompression into the anterior cranial fossa via a transcranial approach. Decompression into the paranasal sinuses was first advocated by Sewell,[70] who described decompression into the ethmoid air cells, and Hirsch,[37] who later reported inferior decompression into the maxillary sinus by removal of the orbital floor. Walsh and Ogura[86] combined the inferior and medial approaches into a single transantral decompression of two orbital walls using the Caldwell-Luc approach (Figure 121-3). This approach is extracranial, decompresses two walls of the orbit into the largest empty space, and allows gravity to aid in the expansion of orbital contents into the paranasal sinuses. For these reasons, it has become the most widely used technique.

Predicting the results of transantral decompression in patients with severe Graves' ophthalmopathy remains a challenge. In a retrospective analysis of 428 patients, Fatourechi and others[19] reported that young

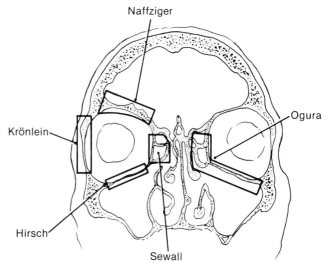

Figure 121-3. Diagram of a coronal section through the skull and paranasal sinuses showing portions of the orbit removed for various methods of orbital decompression.

men with long-standing eye symptoms were likely to have more severe initial proptosis. Only the severity of the initial proptosis and the longer postoperative follow-up period correlated with greater recession of proptosis after decompression. Failure of corticosteroid or orbital radiotherapy did not affect the degree of recession of proptosis or improvement in visual acuity. A greater degree of recession of proptosis postoperatively was associated with better visual acuity but also with a greater likelihood of persistent strabismus. Patient satisfaction with postoperative eye appearance was associated only with procedures performed for cosmetic indications.

Transantral orbital decompression.

Surgical technique. The transantral decompression (Walsh-Ogura method) of the orbital floor and medial wall is performed during general anesthesia with an oral Ray endotracheal tube secured in place. The eyes are protected with topical ointment and are not taped to allow examination of the pupil during the procedure. Intravenous broad-spectrum antibiotics and high-dose corticosteroids (dexamethasone, 8 to 10 mg) are given before the surgery. A curved sublabial incision with a standard Caldwell-Luc antrostomy and ethmoidectomy is performed (Figure 121-4). Care is taken to identify and preserve the inferior orbital nerve in its bony canal. An extensive ethmoidectomy should be performed while preserving the lamina papyracea, middle turbinate insertion, and fovea ethmoidalis (Figure 121-5). The remaining mucosa is then carefully stripped from the maxillary sinus roof, keeping in mind that the inferior orbital nerve will be partially or completely dehiscent in 29% of patients.[45]

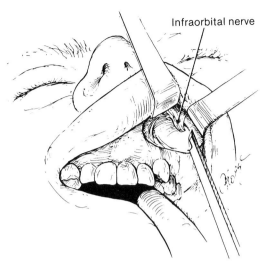

Figure 121-4. Sublabial buccogingival incision that exposes the anterior wall of the maxillary sinus. An osteotome is used to create the antrostomy.

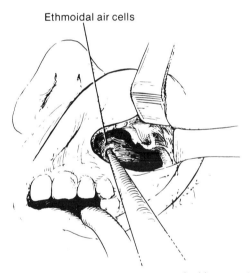

Figure 121-5. Ethmoidal cells are entered with a curette and subsequently removed by curettage and bone-biting forceps.

The bone of the maxillary sinus roof (orbital floor) medial to the infraorbital nerve is then carefully removed (Figure 121-6). This maneuver can be performed using a drill with cutting or diamond burrs or with small osteotomes, as long as the underlying periorbita is not violated. Some surgeons find the operating microscope useful at this stage of the procedure. The lamina papyracea (medial orbital wall) is then gently fractured medially and removed up to the posterior ethmoid neurovascular bundle, preserving the periorbita. A No. 12 scalpel blade is used to make incisions in the posterior-to-anterior direction through the periorbital fascia, which allows the immediate

herniation of orbital fat through the incision and into the sinuses (Figure 121-7). This process is begun medial and superior to avoid the loss of visualization as the fat herniates from the orbit. The number of incisions required is determined intraoperatively by assessing the degree of residual proptosis after each incision. Calcaterra and Thompson[9] recommend operating on the more severe eye first with planned incomplete recession because an additional 1 to 2 mm of recession develops during the first 3 months after surgery. The less severe eye then is decompressed to match the position of the first eye. Four to six incisions in the periorbita usually will be adequate.[90] Finally, a large nasoantral window is created, and the sinus is packed with a large Penrose drain coated in antibiotic ointment, which is brought out through the nose for removal the next day. The sublabial incision then is closed with absorbable suture. The patient is given antibiotics and corticosteroids intravenously overnight and then orally after discharge from the hospital.

Immediately after surgery, all patients (unless it is medically contraindicated) are given high-dose corticosteroids with a slow taper. The rate of steroid taper is determined by the clinical response to the surgery. In one study, steroid use was discontinued in 80% of patients within 2 months of surgery.[28]

Surgical outcome. The results of transantral orbital decompression surgery depend on the indications for the operation. For those with optic neuropathy, Walsh-Ogura decompression was effective in improving vision in 92% of patients (Figure 121-8). Equally important, these patients had stabilization of their disease with successful taper of steroid therapy. Major improvement in proptosis in the range of 1 to 12 mm can be achieved (Figure 121-9, *A*), with an average improvement of 3.4 to 5.3 mm.[25,28,73,74] This decrease in proptosis is of functional and cosmetic benefit and is not seen with either medical or radiotherapy. Major reduction in intraocular pressure (100% of patients; Figure 121-9, *B*), improvement of extraocular motility (36%), and improvement of strabismus (47%) are other benefits of decompression.

Transantral decompression failed to stabilize the disease in 3% to 8% of patients who underwent surgery for severe ophthalmopathy.[25,28] In this setting, repeat CT scanning with coronal cuts can be helpful to assess the adequacy of the decompression and to decide between further surgery using the same approach or via a lateral or superior approach[18] or proceeding with radiotherapy.

The earlier the diagnosis of Graves' optic neuropathy is made and intervention initiated, the better the outcome will be. When preoperative visual acuity was limited to detecting hand motion or worse, decompression

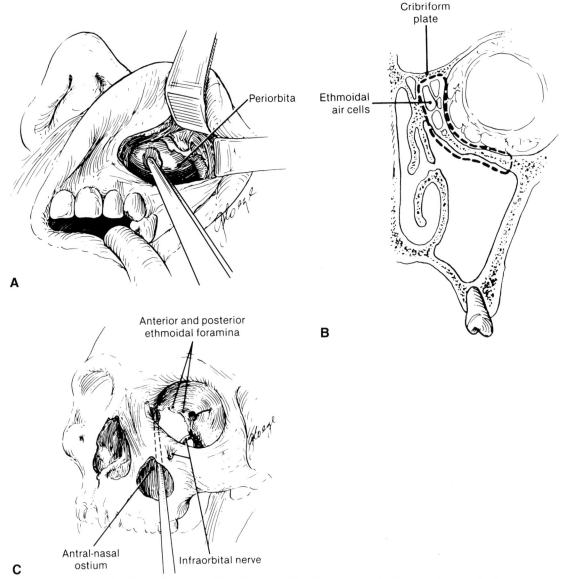

Figure 121-6. A, Removal of the floor of orbit after eggshell fracturing of bone. **B,** Coronal section of paranasal sinuses showing the extent of bone removal. **C,** View of the skull showing completion of ethmoidectomy and removal of the lamina papyracea.

provided little improvement in vision (see Figure 121-8).[28] When visual acuity allowed counting fingers or better, all patients experienced a favorable outcome.

Ocular dysmotility and strabismus remain a major problem in surgical patients despite decompression. Extraocular motility was impaired (primarily in supraduction) in 92% of patients undergoing decompression; only one third showed improvement, and 9% experienced a worsening of motility postoperatively.[28] Strabismus (diplopia) was present preoperatively in 67% to 85% of patients and in 71% to 80% of patients postoperatively.[25,28] Once the eye disease was stable, 70% of patients underwent extraocular muscle surgery

to correct diplopia, and some were able to be corrected with prisms alone. One long-term follow-up evaluation (average, 8.8 years) of 355 patients with decompression reported only 17% having double vision most or all of the time.[25]

Transantral decompression for cosmetic indications should be evaluated carefully because it carries the risk of lower patient acceptance of adverse effects than when vision is threatened. Fatourechi and others[17] reviewed the outcomes of 34 patients who underwent transantral decompression for cosmesis and noted a dramatic improvement in proptosis (average, 5.2 mm), but no major change in asymmetry between the eyes. Postoperative diplopia developed in 73% of patients

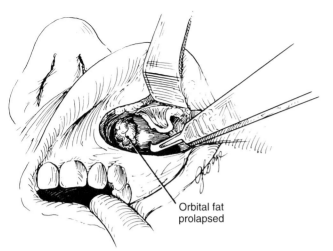

Figure 121-7. Radial incisions in the intact periorbita with a scalpel, permitting prolapse of orbital fat into the sinuses.

who did not suffer from diplopia preoperatively. Half of the patients underwent subsequent extraocular muscle surgery and eyelid surgery. On long-term follow-up evaluation (average, 12 years after surgery) of 29 patients, 82% reported they were satisfied with their current eye status. Thus, decompression surgery for cosmetic indications may be appropriate in a select group of patients who are willing to undergo subsequent eye muscle surgery for diplopia.

Surgical complications. Patients uniformly complain of hypoesthesia in the distribution of the inferior orbital nerve immediately after decompression as a result of intraoperative stretching of the nerve with retraction. This resolves spontaneously over several months in more than 95% of patients. In one large series, Garrity and others[25] reported other infrequent complications, including sinusitis (4%), lower eyelid entropion (9%), cerebrospinal fluid leaks (3%), and

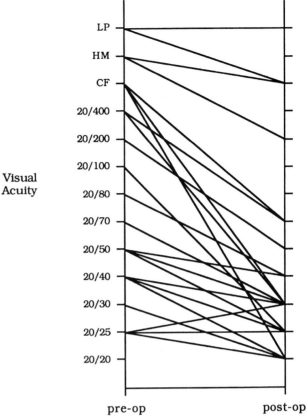

Figure 121-8. Preoperative (left) and postoperative (right) best corrected visual acuity for 36 eyes in 20 patients undergoing transantral orbital decompression for Graves' optic neuropathy. CF, Counts fingers; HM, hand motion; LP, light perception. (From Girod and others: *Arch Otolaryngol Head Neck Surg* 119:229, 1993.)

frontal lobe hematoma (0.2%). Blindness from nerve injury or orbital hemorrhage is rare but does occur.[24,51] Although theoretically possible, orbital infection has not been reported.

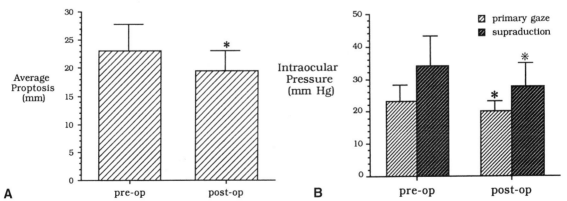

Figure 121-9. A, Preoperative *(left)* and postoperative *(right)* average proptosis for the 36 eyes undergoing decompression in Figure 121-8. **B,** Intraocular pressure in the same eyes in primary gaze and upward gaze before and after decompression surgery. *P < .05.

Modifications of transantral orbital decompression. The transantral orbital decompression has held up well to the test of time since its description in 1957. Only in the past several years have advances in surgical technique and instrumentation led to the description of major modifications to the Walsh-Ogura operation. A transorbital approach using a modified blepharoplasty (subciliary) incision provides excellent exposure to the anterior orbital floor and decreases the risk to the infraorbital nerve.[53] This approach also provides access for a lateral orbital wall decompression without disrupting the orbital rim or canthal tendon, thus providing a three-wall decompression.[1] This method is reported to have a lower incidence of postoperative strabismus, although the reason for this is unclear. Others have reported using the transconjuctival approach for the antral-ethmoidal decompres-

sion.[51,89] The major criticism of these anterior approaches is limited exposure to the medial orbit, which can restrict the degree of decompression around the orbital apex as is required in patients with optic neuropathy.

Endoscopic orbital decompression. With the rapid development and dissemination of endoscopic instrumentation and techniques for transnasal paranasal sinus surgery, it is not surprising that this technology has been applied to include antral-ethmoidal decompression of the orbit. Despite concerns about adequate anterior orbital floor access, Kennedy and others[44] reported equivalent results with transantral decompression and endoscopic decompression. Reports of an average of 3.2- to 5.1-mm reduction of proptosis with an endoscopic decompression of the medial and inferior orbital walls compare well to the traditional

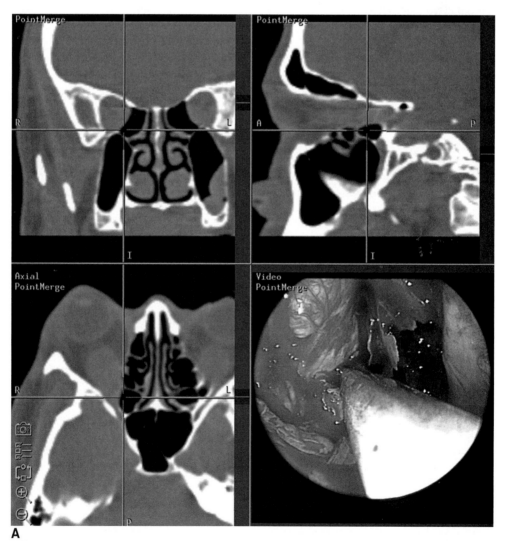

A

Figure 121-10. View from a CT image–guided system during orbital decompression surgery. **A,** Images showing initial periorbita incision at the orbital apex with herniation of orbital fat seen on the video image.

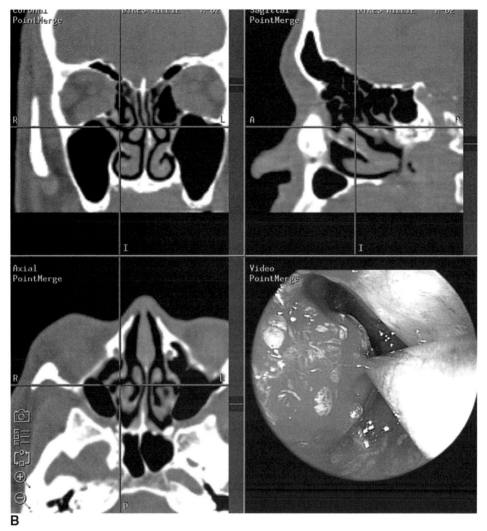

Figure 121-10, cont'd. B, Images showing inferomedial periorbita incision with extensive orbital fat decompression into the sinus cavity. The degree of decompression can be readily assessed on the CT images. To view this image in color, please go to *www.ototext.com* or the Electronic Image Collection CD, bound into your copy of Cummings Otolaryngology—Head and Neck Surgery, 4th edition.

approach.[57,58,88] Metson and Samaha[58] reported a modification to the standard endoscopic decompression that preserves a horizontal sling of periorbita to support the globe position without limiting the degree of decompression. This has resulted in a significant decrease in the incidence of new onset or worsening diplopia after surgery.

Recent advances in image-guided surgery have resulted in improved intraoperative localization during endoscopic sinus surgery. This technology has found a role in endoscopic orbital decompression surgery as well. The use of the CT-guided technology allows a safer and more aggressive decompression of the orbital apex, orbital nerve (if indicated), and superior medial orbital wall. The inferior orbital nerve can also be easily identified and preserved. Equally helpful is the ability to assess and measure the degree of orbital content decompression into the sinuses intraoperatively using measurements on the CT scans (Figure 121-10).

Combined endoscopic and open approach to orbital decompression. For a more thorough optic nerve decompression, Khan and others[46] have described a combined transconjunctival-endoscopic decompression of the orbit. The addition of a small medial external skin incision also aided the retraction of the orbital contents to allow the dissection of the medial wall beyond the posterior ethmoidal neurovascular bundle up to the optic canal. Experience with 72 orbital decompressions in 41 patients resulted in an average reduction of proptosis of 3.65 mm, an 89% improvement in vision and minimal complications.[68] Others have combined the endoscopic orbital decompression with a percutaneous lateral orbital wall decompression via the upper lid crease resulting in additional decompression (up to 6.9 mm).[57,82] In addition, Metson and others[56] have successfully performed combined endoscopic and lateral wall decompressions during local anesthesia, which has the advantage of avoiding general anesthesia and permitting intraoperative monitoring of visual function, critical for surgery on an only-seeing eye. In this setting, if both eyes are to be decompressed, they are done so in stages.

Balanced orbital decompression. In an attempt to reduce the incidence of new-onset diplopia after orbital decompression surgery, several authors have advocated removing the medial and lateral walls of the orbit without decompressing the orbital floor. This "balanced" approach decompresses equally medially and laterally and is thus less likely to affect the position of the globe.[43,82,85] Postoperative new-onset diplopia is reported in 0% to 15% of patients with this technique. The degree of decompression with this two-wall approach can be comparable to the three-wall medial-inferior-lateral decompression if orbital fat is resected at the time of the decompression.[82]

Other approaches for orbital decompression.

A modification of the Walsh-Ogura method called the *three-wall orbital decompression* refers to the addition of the lateral wall decompression to the standard antral-ethmoidal decompression. This addition can be achieved by any combination of approaches, including a modified blepharoplasty incision, a sublabial or transconjunctival incision plus an anterior orbitotomy, or through a bicoronal forehead flap. The advantage of the three-wall decompression is that it allows the further enlargement of the orbital volume by expansion into the temporal fossa and the paranasal sinuses. Metson, Dallow, and Shore[57] were able to increase the recession of proptosis from an average of 3.2 to 5.6 mm with the addition of the lateral decompression to the endoscopic antral-ethmoid decompression. Other authors[52,83] prefer the bicoronal approach to the three-wall decompression, even for unilateral decompressions. Although dramatic decompression is reported (average, 7.5 mm), a high complication rate can be expected, including infraorbital hypesthesia (70%), supraorbital hypesthesia (60%), and frontalis palsy (30%).[52]

A two-wall decompression of the superior-lateral orbit can be achieved through a bicoronal incision with subsequent frontal craniotomy[54,60] or a lateral rim approach.[14] This allows decompression of the orbital contents into the anterior cranial fossa and temporal fossa. Expansion of orbital contents into the empty paranasal sinuses with the help of gravity would be predicted to provide a more adequate decompression, although in a cadaveric study, Stanley and others[72] found the superior-lateral decompression to be as effective as the antral-ethmoidal decompression in withstanding intraocular pressure increases and in allowing orbital recession. The craniotomy approach has the advantages of direct access to the optic canal for superior decompression and of potential additional medial orbital wall decompression via the ethmoid sinuses. The orbital rim approach has the advantage of less dural exposure and the ability to advance the superior orbital rim with plates, screws, and bone grafts to further increase orbital volume.[14] Because the superior-lateral decompression is a more involved procedure with the violation of the cranial cavity, irrespective of the approach, most centers reserve it for recalcitrant patients in whom antral-ethmoidal decompression has failed.

Classical descriptions of orbital decompression have always referred to the removal of one or more orbital bony walls. Trokel, Kazim, and Moore[81] have reported successful decompression of the orbit strictly by the removal of orbital fat via superior and inferior orbitotomies without any bone removal. This procedure was reserved primarily for cosmetic indications in patients with inactive disease. An average reduction in proptosis of 1.8 mm was achieved, although patients with large amounts of fat seen by CT scan and with greater preoperative proptosis had more dramatic reductions. Importantly, there were no new long-term motility problems commonly reported with bony orbital decompression for cosmesis, which may be an important decompression option for cosmetic indications in an attempt to reduce postoperative strabismus and the need for subsequent eye muscle surgery.

Ancillary procedures

Extraocular muscle surgery.

Extraocular motility problems resulting from Graves' ophthalmopathy are not likely to resolve spontaneously with disease regression and are mostly refractory to medical management. It is also the manifestation of eye involvement most likely to develop or worsen after orbital decompression.[71] Although disturbing, this is not surprising because irreversible extraocular muscle fibrosis is seen late in the disease. In one study, up to 70% of patients with decompression ultimately underwent eye muscle surgery for strabismus once the eye disease was stable.[25]

The indications for eye muscle surgery are diplopia in the primary and reading positions, with the goal being to restore single vision in these positions. It is unlikely that eye muscle surgery will achieve single vision in all positions because of the baseline restrictive ophthalmoplegia induced by the disease. Dyer[13] reviewed 290 patients with Graves' ophthalmopathy requiring eye muscle surgery and found 59% required a single surgery, 30% required two procedures, and

12% required three or more procedures to achieve single vision in the primary and reading positions.

The timing of eye muscle surgery is critical for predictable results. Patients not requiring orbital decompression for Graves' ophthalmopathy should manifest stable disease with corticosteroid administration for 6 months to avoid subtle changes in the muscles over time. If these patients have serious proptosis, orbital decompression should be considered before eye muscle surgery, which may exacerbate the proptosis and corneal problems.[13] In addition, a decompression is likely to alter the position of the globes and thus disturb the gaze, and it should therefore be completed before eye muscle surgery. Because recession of the globe is progressive for several months after an orbital decompression, it is advisable to delay eye muscle surgery for 2 to 3 months.

Eyelid surgery. Surgery on the eyelids may be required early or late in the management of Graves' ophthalmopathy. Early in the disease, a lateral tarsorrhaphy may be needed to urgently provide corneal coverage and protection as a temporizing measure while medical therapy is instituted. Late in the course of the disease, eyelid surgery may be indicated for cosmesis and corneal protection in patients with permanent lid retraction. Multiple upper eyelid procedures have been described, including excision or recession of Müller's muscle, levator aponeurosis transection or recession with or without scleral grafts, and levator myotomy.[7] Similar procedures have been described for the lower lid. In the overall rehabilitation of the eye, eyelid surgery should be delayed for 1 year after control of the hyperthyroidism and at least 6 months after the eye disease stabilizes.

SUMMARY

Although recent studies on the etiology of Graves' disease suggest a common thyroid–eye antigen (TSH receptor), this difficult and debilitating disease is still not preventable. Further advances in the identification of the specific autoantigenic site in the eye and the thyroid and in antigen-specific immunotherapy are necessary before a major shift in management can occur. Until that time, therapy for Graves' disease and the associated Graves' ophthalmopathy will remain palliative. A team approach to these patients is warranted given multiple organ system involvement and the complexity of manifestations encountered. Only through close collaboration between team members can optimal therapy be provided.

REFERENCES

1. Antoszyk JH, Tucker N, Codere F: Orbital decompression for Graves' disease: exposure through a modified blepharoplasty incision, *Ophthalmic Surg* 23:516, 1992.

2. Bahn RS and others: Human retroocular fibroblasts in vitro: a model for the study of Graves' ophthalmopathy, *J Clin Endocrinol Metab* 65:665, 1987.

3. Bahn RS, Heufelder AE: Retroocular fibroblasts: important effector cells in Graves' ophthalmopathy, *Thyroid* 2:89, 1992.

4. Bartalena L and others: More on smoking habits and Graves' ophthalmopathy, *J Endocrinol Invest* 12:733, 1989.

5. Bech K and others: The acute changes in thyroid stimulating immunoglobulins, thyroglobulin, and thyroglobulin antibodies following subtotal thyroidectomy, *Clin Endocrinol (Oxf)* 16:235, 1982.

6. Bech K, Madsen N: Influence of treatment with radioiodine and propylthiouracil on thyroid stimulating immunoglobulins in Graves' disease, *Clin Endocrinol (Oxf)* 13:417, 1980.

7. Burch HB, Wartofsky L: Graves' ophthalmopathy: current concepts regarding pathogenesis and management, *Encocr Rev* 14:747, 1993.

8. Calcaterra TC, Hepler RS, Hanafee WN: The diagnostic evaluation of unilateral exophthalmos, *Laryngoscope* 2:231, 1974.

9. Calcaterra TC, Thompson JW: Antral-ethmoidal decompression of the orbit in Graves' disease: 10-year experience, *Laryngoscope* 90:1941, 1980.

10. Christensen SB and others: Influence of cigarette smoking on goiter formation, thyroglobulin, and thyroid hormone levels in women, *J Clin Endocrinol Metab* 58:615, 1984.

11. DeSanto LW: The total rehabilitation of Graves' ophthalmopathy, *Laryngoscope* 90:1652, 1980.

12. Dollinger J: Die drickentlastung der augenhokle durch entfernung der ausseren obitalwand bei hochgradien exophthalmus und koneskutwer hornhauter kronkung, *Dtsch Med Wochenschr* 37:1888, 1911.

13. Dyer, JA: *Ocular muscle surgery.* In Gorman CA, Campbell RJ, Dyer JA, editors: *The eye and orbit in thyroid disease,* New York, 1984, Raven Press.

14. Elisevich K and others: Decompression for dysthyroid ophthalmopathy via the orbital rim approach, technical note, *J Neurosurg* 80:580, 1994.

15. Erickson BA and others: Echographic monitoring of response of extraocular muscles to irradiation in Graves' ophthalmopathy, *Int J Radiat Oncol Biol Phys* 31:651, 1995.

16. Ericsson UB, Lindgarde F: Effects of cigarette smoking on thyroid function, the prevalence of goitre, thyrotoxicosis and autoimmune thyroiditis, *J Clin Endocrinol Metab* 229:67, 1991.

17. Fatourechi V and others: Graves' ophthalmopathy: results of transantral orbital decompression performed primarily for cosmetic indications, *Ophthalmology* 101:938, 1994.

18. Fatourechi V and others: Orbital decompression in Graves' ophthalmopathy associated with pretibial myxedema, *J Endocrinol Invest* 16:433, 1993.

19. Fatourechi V and others: Predictors of response to transantral orbital decompression in severe Graves' ophthalmopathy, *Mayo Clin Proc* 69:841, 1994.

20. Fatourechi V, Pajouhi M, Fransway AF: Dermopathy of Graves' disease (pretibial myxedema), *Medicine (Baltimore)*, 107:257, 1994.

21. Feldon SE, Weiner JM: Clinical significance of extraocular muscle volumes in Graves' ophthalmopathy: a quantitative computed tomography study, *Arch Ophthalmol* 100:1266, 1982.

22. Forbes G and others: Ophthalmopathy of Graves' disease: computerized volume measurements of the orbital fat and muscle, *Am J Neuroradiol* 7:651, 1986.

23. Francis T and others: Lymphocytes express thyrotropin receptor specific mRNA as detected by the PCR technique, *Thyroid* 1:223, 1991.

24. Galuska L and others: SPECT using 99m Tc-DTPA for the assessment of disease activity in Graves' ophthamopathy: a comparison with the results from MRI, *Nucl Med Commun* 23(12):1211, 2002.

25. Garrity JA and others: Results of transantral orbital decompression in 428 patients with severe Graves' ophthalmopathy, *Am J Ophthalmol* 116:533, 1993.

26. Gerling J and others: Retrobulbar irradiation for thyroid-associated orbitopathy: double-blind comparison between 2.46y and 16 Gy, *Int J Radiat Oncol Biol Phys* 55(1):182, 2003.

27. Ginsberg J: Diagnosis and management of Graves' disease, *CMAJ-JAMC* 165(5):575, 2003.

28. Girod DA, Orcutt JC, Cummings CW: Orbital decompression for the preservation of vision in Graves' ophthalmopathy, *Arch Otolaryngol Head Neck Surg* 119:229, 1993.

29. Gorman CA: The presentation and management of endocrine ophthalmopathy, *Clin Endocrinol Metab* 7:67, 1978.

30. Gorman CA and others: The aftermath of orbital radiotherapy for grave ophthalmopathy, *Ophthalmology* 109(11):2100, 2002.

31. Gorman CA and others: A prospective, randomized, double-blind, placebo controlled study of orbital radiotherapy for Graophthalmopathy, *Ophthalmology* 108(9):1523, 2001.

32. Grubeck-Loebenstein B and others: Retrobulbar cells from patients with Graves' ophthalmopathy are CD8+ and specifically recognized autologous fibroblasts, *J Clin Invest* 93:2738, 1994.

33. Hallin ES, Feldon SE: Graves' ophthalmopathy: I. Simple CT estimates of extraocular muscle volume, *Br J Ophthalmol* 72:674, 1988.

34. Hallin ES, Feldon SE, Luttrell J: Graves' ophthalmopathy: III. Effect of transantral orbital decompression on optic neuropathy, *Br J Ophthalmol* 72:683, 1988.

35. Hamilton RD and others: Ophthalmopathy of Graves' disease: a comparison between patients treated surgically and patients treated with radioiodine, *Mayo Clin Proc* 42:812, 1967.

36. Heufelder AE, Bahn RS: Modulation of Graves' orbital fibroblast proliferation by cytokines and glucocorticoid receptor agonists, *Invest Ophthalmol Vis Sci* 35:120, 1994.

37. Hirsch O: Surgical decompression for malignant exophthalmosis, *Arch Otolaryngol Head Neck Surg* 51:325, 1950.

38. Hosten N and others: Graves' ophthalmopathy: MR imaging of the orbit, *Radiology* 172:759, 1989.

39. Huber GK and others: Positive regulation of human thyrotropin receptor mRNA by thyrotropin, *J Clin Endocrinol Metab* 72:1394, 1991.

40. Hufnagel TJ and others: Immunohistochemical, ultrastructural studies of the exenterated orbital tissues of a patient with Graves' disease, *Ophthalmology* 91:1411, 1984.

41. Jelks GW, Jelks EB, Ruff, G: Clinical and radiographic evaluation of the orbit, *Otolaryngol Clin North Am* 21:13, 1988.

42. Just M and others: Graves' ophthalmopathy: role of MR imaging in radiotherapy, *Radiology* 179:187, 1991.

43. Kacker A and others: "Balanced" orbital decompression for severe Graves' orbitopathy: technique with treatment algorithm, *Otolaryngol Head Neck Surg* 128(2):228, 2003.

44. Kennedy DW and others: Endoscopic transnasal orbital decompression, *Arch Otolaryngol Head Neck Surg* 116:275, 1990.

45. Kent KJ, Merwin GE, Rarey KE: Margins of safety with transantral orbital decompression, *Laryngoscope* 98:815, 1988.

46. Khan JA and others: Combined transconjunctival and external approach for endoscopic orbital apex decompression in Graves' disease, *Laryngoscope* 105:203, 1995.

47. Kodama K and others: Demonstration of a circulating autoantibody against soluble eye-muscle antigen in Graves' ophthalmopathy, *Lancet* 2:1353, 1982.

48. Konuk and others: Orbital gallium-67 scintigraphy in Graves' ophthalmopathy, *Thyroid* 12(7):603, 2002.

49. Kosugi S and others: The extracellular domain of the TSH receptor has an immunogenic epitope reactive with Graves' sera but unrelated to receptor function as well as epitopes having different roles for high affinity TSH binding, the activity of thyroid stimulating antibodies, *Thyroid* 1:321, 1991.

50. Kriss JP: Pathogenesis and treatment of pretibial myxedema, *Endocrinol Metab Clin North Am* 16:409, 1987.

51. Kulwin DR, Cotton RT, Kersten RC: Combined approach to orbital decompression, *Otolaryngol Clin North Am* 23:381, 1990.

52. Leatherbarrow B, Lendrum J, Mahaffey PJ: Three wall orbital decompression for Graves' ophthalmopathy, *Eye* 5:456, 1991.

53. Lindberg JV, Anderson RL: Transorbital decompression: indications and results, *Arch Ophthalmol* 99:113, 1981.

54. MacCarty CS and others: Ophthalmopathy of Graves' disease treated by removal of roof, lateral walls, and lateral sphenoid ridge: review of 46 cases, *Mayo Clin Proc* 45:488, 1970.

55. Marcocci D and others: Studies on the occurrence of ophthalmopathy in Graves' disease, *Acta Endocr (Copenh)* 120:473, 1989.

56. Metson R and others: Endoscopic orbital decompression under local anesthesia, *Otolaryngol Head Neck Surg* 113:661, 1995.

57. Metson R, Dallow RL, Shore JW: Endoscopic orbital decompression, *Laryngoscope* 104:950, 1994.

58. Metson R, Samaha M: Reduction of diplopia following endoscopic orbital decompression: the orbital sling technique, *Laryngoscope* 112(10):1753, 2002.

59. Mourits MP and others: Orbital decompression for Graves' ophthalmopathy by inferomedial, by inferomedial plus lateral, and by coronal approach, *Ophthalmology* 97:636, 1990.

60. Naffziger H: Progressive exophthalmos following thyroidectomy: its pathology and treatment, *Ann Surg* 94:582, 1931.

61. Nagy E and others: Graves' IgG recognizes linear epitopes in the human thyrotropin receptor, *Biochem Biophys Res Commun* 188:28, 1992.

62. Neigel JM and others: Dysthyroid optic neuropathy: the crowded orbital apex syndrome, *Ophthalmology* 95:1515, 1988.

63. Ohtsuka K and others: Effect of steroid pulse therapy with and without orbital radiotherapy on Graves' ophthalmopath, *Am J Ophthalmol* 135(3):285, 2003.

64. Pigeon P and others: High voltage radiotherapy and surgical orbital decompression in the management of Graves' ophthalmopathy, *Horm Res* 26:172, 1987.

65. Rees Smith B, McLachlan SM, Furmaniak J: Autoantibodies to the thyrotropin receptor, *Endocrinology* 9:106, 1988.

66. Riley FD: Orbital pathology in Graves' disease, *Mayo Clin Proc* 47:974, 1972.

67. Sautter-Bihl ML, Heinze HG: Radiotherapy of Graves' ophthalmopathy, *Dev Ophthalmol* 20:139, 1989.

68. Schaefer SD and others: Endoscopic and transconjunctival orbital decompression for thyroid-related orbital apex compression, *Laryngoscope* 113(3):508, 2003.

69. Sergott RC, Glaser JS: Graves' ophthalmopathy: a clinical and immunologic review, *Surv Ophthalmol* 26:1-21, 1981.

70. Sewell EC: Operative control of progressive exophthalmosis, *Arch Otolaryngol Head Neck Surg* 24:621, 1936.

71. Shorr N, Neuhaus RW, Baylis HA: Ocular motility problems after orbital decompression for dysthyroid ophthalmopathy, *Ophthalmology* 89:323, 1982.

72. Stanley RJ and others: Superior and transantral orbital decompression procedures: effects on increased intraorbital pressure and orbital dynamics, *Arch Otolaryngol Head Neck Surg* 115:369, 1989.

73. Szues-Farkas A and others: Using morphologic parameters of extraocular muscles for diagnosis and follow-up of Graves' ophthalmopathy: diameters, areas, or volumes? *Am J Roentgenol*, 179(4):1005, 2002.

74. Tallstedt L and others: Occurrence of ophthalmopathy after treatment for Graves' hyperthyroidism, *N Engl J Med* 326:1733, 1992.

75. Tamaki H and others: Improvement of infiltrative ophthalmopathy in parallel with a decrease of thyroid-stimulating antibody activity in two patients with hypothyroid Graves' disease, *J Endocr Invest* 12:47, 1989.

76. Tellez M, Cooper J, Edmonds C: Graves' ophthalmopathy in relation to cigarette smoking and ethnic origin, *Clin Endocr (Oxf)* 36:291, 1992.

77. Teng CS and others: Thyroid-stimulating immunoglobulins in ophthalmic Graves' disease, *Clin Endocr (Oxf)* 6:207, 1977.

78. Terwee C and others: Long-terms effects of Graves' ophthalmopathy on health-related quality of life, *Eur J Endocrinol* 146(6):751, 2002.

79. Trobe JD: Optic nerve involvement in dysthyroidism, *Ophthalmology* 88:488, 1981.

80. Trobe JD, Glaser JS, Laflamme P: Dysthyroid optic neuropathy: clinical profile, rationale for management, *Arch Ophthalmology* 96:1199, 1978.

81. Trokel S, Kazim M, Moore S: Orbital fat removal. Decompression for Graves' orbitopathy, *Ophthalmology* 100:674, 1993.

82. Unal M and others: Balanced orbital decompression combined with removal in Graves ophthalmopathy: do we really need to remove the third wall? *Ophthal Plast Reconstr Surg* 19(2):112, 2003.

83. van der Wal KG and others: Surgical treatment of proptosis bulbi by three-wall orbital decompression, *J Oral Maxillofac Surg* 53:140, 1995.

84. Van Dyk HJL: Orbital Graves' disease: a modification of the "NO SPECS" classification, *Ophthalmology* 88:479, 1981.

85. Vaseghi M and others: Minimally invasive orbital decompression for Graves' ophthalmopathy, *Ann Otol Rhinol Laryngol* 112(1):57, 2003.

86. Walsh TE, Ogura JH: Transantral orbital decompression for malignant exophthalmos, *Laryngoscope* 67:544, 1957.

87. Warren JD, Spector JG, Burde R: Long-term follow-up and recent observations on 305 cases of orbital decompression for dysthyroid orbitopathy, *Laryngoscope* 99:35, 1989.

88. Wee and others: Endoscopic orbital decompression for Graves' ophthalmopathy, *J Laryngol Otol* 116(2):6, 2002.

89. Weisman RA, Osguthorpe JD: Orbital decompression in Graves' disease, *Arch Otolaryngol Head Neck Surg* 120:831, 1994.

90. Weisman RA, Savino PJ: Management of endocrine orbitopathy, *Otolaryngol Clin North Am* 21:93, 1988.

91. Werner SC: Classification of the eye changes of Graves' disease, *J Clin Endocrinol Metab* 29:982, 1969.

92. Werner SC: Modification of the classification of the eye changes of Graves' disease: recommendations of the ad hoc committee of the American Thyroid Association, *J Clin Endocrinol Metab* 44:203, 1977.

Index